BORON  BOULPAEP

CONCISE
Medical Physiology

BORON ⬛ BOULPAEP

CONCISE
Medical
Physiology

Walter F. Boron, MD, PhD
Distinguished University Professor
David N. and Inez Myers/Antonio Scarpa Chairman
Department of Physiology and Biophysics
Case Western Reserve University School of Medicine
Cleveland, Ohio

Emile L. Boulpaep, MD
Professor
Department of Cellular and Molecular Physiology
Yale University School of Medicine
New Haven, Connecticut

ELSEVIER

Elsevier
1600 John F. Kennedy Blvd.
Ste 1600
Philadelphia, PA 19103-2899

BORON & BOULPAEP CONCISE MEDICAL PHYSIOLOGY   ISBN: 978-0-323-65530-9

Copyright © 2021 by Elsevier, Inc. All rights reserved.

ISBN: 978-0-323-65530-9

Publisher: Elyse O'Grady
Senior Content Development Specialist: Mary Hegeler
Publishing Services Manager: Catherine Jackson
Senior Project Manager: Kate Mannix
Design Direction: Amy Buxton

Printed in India

Last digit is the print number: 9   8   7   6   5   4   3   2

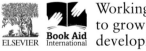

EDITORS

Walter F. Boron, MD, PhD
Distinguished University Professor
David N. and Inez Myers/Antonio Scarpa Chairman
Department of Physiology and Biophysics
Case Western Reserve University School of Medicine
Cleveland, Ohio

Emile L. Boulpaep, MD
Professor
Department of Cellular and Molecular Physiology
Yale University School of Medicine
New Haven, Connecticut

CONTRIBUTORS

Peter S. Aronson, MD
C.N.H. Long Professor of Internal Medicine
Professor of Cellular and Molecular Physiology
Section of Nephrology
Department of Internal Medicine
Yale University School of Medicine
New Haven, Connecticut

Eugene J. Barrett, MD, PhD
Professor
Departments of Medicine and Pharmacology
University of Virginia School of Medicine
Charlottesville, Virginia

Paula Q. Barrett, PhD
Professor
Department of Pharmacology
University of Virginia School of Medicine
Charlottesville, Virginia

Henry J. Binder, MD
Professor Emeritus of Medicine
Department of Internal Medicine—Digestive Diseases
Yale University School of Medicine
New Haven, Connecticut

Walter F. Boron, MD, PhD
Distinguished University Professor
David N. and Inez Myers/Antonio Scarpa Chairman
Department of Physiology and Biophysics
Case Western Reserve University School of Medicine
Cleveland, Ohio

Emile L. Boulpaep, MD
Professor
Department of Cellular and Molecular Physiology
Yale University School of Medicine
New Haven, Connecticut

Lloyd Cantley, MD, FASN
Professor
Department of Internal Medicine
Department of Cellular and Molecular Physiology
Yale University School of Medicine
New Haven, Connecticut

Michael J. Caplan, MD, PhD
C.N.H. Long Professor and Chair
Department of Cellular and Molecular Physiology
Yale University School of Medicine
New Haven, Connecticut

Barry W. Connors, PhD
Professor and Chair
Department of Neuroscience
Alpert Medical School
Brown University
Providence, Rhode Island

Arthur DuBois, MD[†]
Professor Emeritus of Epidemiology and Public Health and
    Cellular and Molecular Physiology
John B. Pierce Laboratory
New Haven, Connecticut

Gerhard Giebisch, MD[†]
Professor Emeritus of Cellular and Molecular Physiology
Department of Cellular and Molecular Physiology
Yale University School of Medicine
New Haven, Connecticut

Fred S. Gorelick, MD
Professor
Departments of Internal Medicine and Cell Biology
Yale University School of Medicine
New Haven, Connecticut

Peter Igarashi, MD
Nesbitt Chair and Head
Department of Medicine
University of Minnesota
Minneapolis, Minnesota

W. Jonathan Lederer, MD, PhD
Director and Professor, Center for Biomedical Engineering
    and Technology and Department of Physiology
University of Maryland School of Medicine
Baltimore, Maryland

George Lister, MD
Jean McLean Wallace Professor of Pediatrics
Professor of Cellular and Molecular Physiology
Yale School of Medicine
New Haven, Connecticut

[†]Deceased

v

Charles M. Mansbach II, MD†
Professor of Medicine and Physiology
University of Tennessee Health Science Center
Memphis, Tennessee

Christopher R. Marino, MD
Professor of Medicine
University of Tennessee Health Science Center
VA Medical Center
Memphis, Tennessee

Edward J. Masoro, PhD†
Professor Emeritus of Physiology
University of Texas Health Science Center at San Antonio
San Antonio, Texas

Sam Mesiano, PhD
William H. Weir Professor of Reproductive Biology
Department of Reproductive Biology
Case Western Reserve University School of Medicine
and
Department of Obstetrics and Gynecology
University Hospitals of Cleveland
Cleveland, Ohio

Edward G. Moczydlowski, PhD
Professor Emeritus of Physiology
California Northstate University
Elk Grove, California

Shaun F. Morrison, PhD
Professor
Department of Neurological Surgery
Oregon Health & Science University
Portland, Oregon

Kitt Falk Petersen, MD
Professor
Section of Endocrinology
Department of Internal Medicine
Yale University School of Medicine
New Haven, Connecticut

Bruce R. Ransom, MD, PhD
Professor and Chair
Department of Neuroscience
City University of Hong Kong
Kowloon Tong, Hong Kong

George B. Richerson, MD, PhD
Professor & Chairman
Department of Neurology
University of Iowa Carver College of Medicine
Iowa City, Iowa

Steven S. Segal, PhD
Professor
Department of Medical Pharmacology and Physiology
University of Missouri School of Medicine
Columbia, Missouri

Gerald I. Shulman, MD, PhD, FACP, MACE
Investigator, Howard Hughes Medical Institute
George R. Cowgill Professor of Physiological Chemistry
Professor of Medicine (Endocrinology/Metabolism) and
    Cellular & Molecular Physiology
Co-Director, Yale Diabetes Research Center
Yale University School of Medicine
New Haven, Connecticut

Frederick J. Suchy, MD
Chief Research Officer
Director, Children's Hospital Colorado Research Institute
Professor of Pediatrics
Associate Dean for Child Health Research
University of Colorado School of Medicine
Aurora, Colorado

EDITORIAL CONSULTANTS

Stephen W. Jones, PhD
Professor
Department of Physiology and Biophysics
Case Western Reserve University School of Medicine
Cleveland, Ohio

Joseph C. LaManna, PhD
The Jeannette M. and Joseph S. Silber Professor for the
    Study of Brain Sciences
Department of Physiology and Biophysics
Case Western Reserve University School of Medicine
Cleveland, Ohio

Sam A. Mesiano, PhD
William H. Weir Professor of Reproductive Biology
Department of Reproductive Biology
Case Western Reserve University School of Medicine
and
Department of Obstetrics and Gynecology
University Hospitals of Cleveland
Cleveland, Ohio

Andrea M.P. Romani, MD, PhD
Associate Professor
Department of Physiology and Biophysics
Case Western Reserve University School of Medicine
Cleveland, Ohio

William P. Schilling, PhD
Professor
Rammelkamp Center for Education and Research
MetroHealth Medical Center and Department of
    Physiology and Biophysics
Case Western Reserve University School of Medicine
Cleveland, Ohio

---

†Deceased

PREFACE

We thank the physiological community for making our full-length text *Medical Physiology* such a success. However, we understand that some curricula are too abbreviated for students to make full use of our classical text. Therefore, with the encouragement of Elsevier, we have developed this Concise Edition. The three-fold philosophy that has guided us in the full-length editions has endured as we prepared the Concise Edition.

First, we combine the expertise of several authors with the consistency of a single pen. We achieve this singleness of pen by editing the Concise Edition jointly and in real time—monitor to monitor—using desktop-sharing software. After more than three decades, we have become so accustomed to each other's writing styles that we can literally finish each other's sentences.

Second, we still integrate physiological concepts from the level of DNA and epigenetics to the human body, and everything in between.

Third, we complete the presentation of important physiological principles by putting them in a clinical context.

Aside from Part I, which is a brief introduction to the discipline of physiology (Chapter 1), the book consists of nine major parts. Part II (Physiology of Cells and Molecules) reflects that, increasingly, the underpinnings of modern physiology have become cellular and molecular. Chapter 2 (Functional Organization of the Cell), Chapter 3 (Signal Transduction), and Chapter 4 (Regulation of Gene Expression) provide the essentials of cell biology and molecular biology necessary for understanding cell and organ function. The other chapters in Part II cover the *cellular* physiology of transport, excitability, and muscle—all of which are classic topics for traditional physiology texts. In this book we have extended each of these subjects to the *molecular* level. The remainder of the book will frequently send the reader back to the principles introduced in Part II.

Parts III to IX address individual organ systems. In each case, the first chapter provides a general introduction to the system. Part III (The Nervous System) is untraditional in that it deliberately omits those aspects of the physiology of the central nervous system that neuroscience courses generally treat and that require extensive knowledge of neuroanatomical pathways. Rather, Part III focuses on cellular neurophysiology, including synaptic transmission in the nervous system, sensory transduction, and neural circuits. In addition, Part III also treats two subjects—the autonomic nervous system and the neuronal microenvironment—that are important for understanding other physiological systems.

Finally, Part X (Physiology of Cells and Molecules) is an integrated, multisystem approach to metabolism, temperature regulation, exercise, adaptations to special environments, and aging.

THE EBOOK

Although you can still enjoy our book while reading the print version, you can also access the content on a computer, tablet, or smart phone. Regardless of the platform for accessing the eBook, the student may access crosslinks within the text.

ACKNOWLEDGMENTS

A textbook is the culmination of successful collaborations among many individuals. First, we thank our chapter authors and others who contributed to the Third Edition of the full-length text. We list the chapter authors under Contributors on pages *v* and *vi*. We are especially grateful to the faculty of the Department of Physiology and Biophysics who taught students in the Physician Assistant (PA) Program at Case Western Reserve University. Besides Walter Boron, this group includes Stephen W. Jones, Joseph C. LaManna, Sam Mesiano, Andrea Romani, and William P. Schilling. With extensive experience using this book to teach medical and graduate students, these faculty members undertook the arduous task of carefully extracting selected material from the full-length Third Edition of our text. The challenge was to be concise while still remaining as comprehensive as possible. We thank our PA students who beta-tested this redacted version of the text. In the meantime, we meticulously edited the beta version of the Concise Edition to ensure that it flows properly—and still reads as though it comes from a single pen.

At Elsevier, we are most grateful to Elyse O'Grady, Executive Content Strategist, for her trust and endurance. Mary Hegeler, Senior Content Development Specialist, was the project's communications hub, responsible for coordinating all parties working on the textbook and for assembling the many elements that comprise the final product. Her meticulous care was indispensable. We thank Kate Mannix, Senior Project Manager, for overseeing production of the textbook. Striving for consistency, Elsevier did us the favor of assigning a single copy editor—Jenny Korte—to the entire project. We were especially impressed with her meticulous copyediting. Moreover, because she read the manuscript as a dedicated student, she identified several logical or scientific errors, including inconsistencies between chapters.

As we do for the full-length editions, we again invite the reader to enjoy learning physiology. We hope that this Concise Edition piques your interest in physiology enough that you decide to consult the full-length edition! If you are pleased with our effort, tell others. If not, tell us.

Walter F. Boron, MD, PhD
Emile L. Boulpaep, MD

CONTENTS*

*Throughout this text, you will see numbered red targets ◉. These highlight locations referred to elsewhere in the book. Callouts to these locations are gray ◉. Together, these icons help cross-link important related concepts and information.

†Deceased

VIDEO CONTENTS

INTRODUCTION

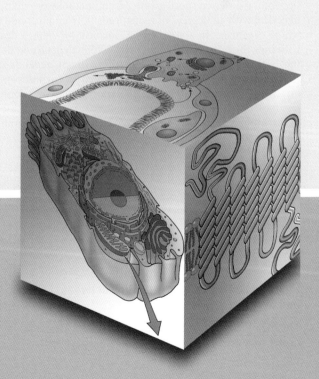

CHAPTER 1

FOUNDATIONS OF PHYSIOLOGY

Emile L. Boulpaep and Walter F. Boron

What is physiology?

Physiology is the dynamic study of life. Physiology describes the "vital" functions of living organisms and their organs, cells, and molecules. For centuries, the discipline of physiology has been closely intertwined with medicine. Although physiology is not primarily concerned with structure—as is the case for anatomy, histology, and structural biology—structure and function are inextricably linked because the living structures perform the functions.

For some, physiology is the function of the whole person (e.g., exercise physiology). For many practicing clinicians, physiology may be the function of an individual organ system, such as the cardiovascular, respiratory, or gastrointestinal system. For still others, physiology may focus on the cellular principles that are common to the function of all organs and tissues. This last field has traditionally been called *general physiology*, a term that is now supplanted by *cellular and molecular physiology*. Although one can divide physiology according to varying degrees of reductionism, it is also possible to define a branch of physiology—for example, *comparative physiology*—that focuses on differences and similarities among different species. Indeed, comparative physiology may deal with all degrees of reductionism, from molecule to whole organism. In a similar way, *medical physiology* deals with how the human body functions, which depends on how the individual organ systems function, which depends on how the component cells function, which in turn depends on the interactions among subcellular organelles and countless molecules. Thus, medical physiology takes a global view of the human body, but in doing so, it requires an integrated understanding of events at the level of molecules, cells, and organs.

It should come as no surprise that the boundaries of physiology are not sharply delineated. Conversely, physiology has its unique attributes. For example, physiology has evolved over the centuries from a more qualitative to a more quantitative science. Indeed, many of the leading physiologists were—and still are—trained as chemists, physicists, mathematicians, or engineers.

Physiological genomics is the link between the organ and the gene

The life of the human body requires not only that individual organ systems do their jobs but also that these organ systems work "hand in hand" with each other. They must share information. Their actions must be interdependent. The cells within an organ or a tissue often share information, and certainly the individual cells must act in concert to perform the proper function of the organ or tissue. In fact, cells in one organ must often share information with cells in another organ and make decisions that are appropriate for the health of the individual cell as well as for the health of the whole person.

In most cases, the sharing of information between organs and between cells takes place at the level of atoms or molecules. Cell-to-cell messengers or intracellular messengers may be as simple as H^+ or K^+ or Ca^{2+}. The messengers may also be more complex chemicals. A cell may release a molecule that acts on a neighboring cell or that enters the bloodstream and acts on other cells a great distance away. In other cases, a neuron may send an axon a centimeter or even a meter away and rapidly modulate, through a neurotransmitter molecule, the activity of another cell or another organ. Cells and organs must interact with one another, and the method of communication is almost always molecular.

The grand organizer—the master that controls the molecules, the cells, and the organs and the way they interact—is the genome, together with its epigenetic modifications. Traditionally, the discipline of physiology has, in its reductionistic journey, always stopped at about the level of cells and certain subcellular organelles as well as their component and controlling molecules. The discipline of physiology left to molecular biology and molecular genetics the business of how the cell controls itself through its DNA. The modern discipline of physiology has become closely intertwined with molecular biology, however, because DNA encodes the proteins in which physiologists are most interested.

Physiological genomics (or functional genomics) is a new branch of physiology devoted to the understanding of the roles that genes play in physiology. Traditionally, physiologists have moved in a reductionistic direction from organ to cell to molecule to gene. One of the most fascinating aspects of physiological genomics is that it has closed the circle and linked organ physiology directly with molecular biology. Perhaps one of the most striking examples is the knockout mouse. Knocking out the gene encoding a protein—that, according to conventional wisdom, is very important—will sometimes have no obvious effect or sometimes unexpected effects. It is up to the physiologist, at least in part, to figure out why. It is perhaps rather sobering to consider that, to truly understand the impact of a transgene or a knockout on the physiology of a mouse, one would have to carefully re-evaluate the totality of mouse physiology. To grasp the function of a gene product, the physiologist must retrace the steps up the reductionistic road and achieve an integrated understanding of that gene's function at the level of the cells, organs, and whole body. Physiology is unique among the basic medical sciences in that it is both broad in its scope (i.e., it deals with multiple systems) and integrative in its outlook.

Not uncommonly, important physiological parameters, such as blood pressure, may be under the control of many genes. Certain polymorphisms in several of these many genes could have a cumulative effect that produces high blood pressure. How would one identify which polymorphisms of which genes may underlie high blood pressure? This sort of complex problem does not easily lend itself to a physiologist's controlled studies. One approach would be to study a population of people, or strains of experimental animals, and use statistical tools to determine which polymorphisms correlate with high blood pressure in a population. Indeed, epidemiologists use "data science" to study group effects in populations. However, even after the identification of variants in various genes, each of which may make a small contribution to high blood pressure, the physiologist has an important role. First, the physiologist, performing controlled experiments, must determine whether a particular genetic variant does indeed have at least the potential to modulate blood pressure. Second, the physiologist must determine the mechanism of the effect.

⊙ 1-1 Cells live in a highly protected milieu intérieur

In his lectures on the phenomena of life, Claude Bernard noted in 1878 on the conditions of the constancy of life, which he considered a property of higher forms of life. According to Bernard, animals have two environments: the "milieu extérieur," which physically surrounds the whole organism, and the "milieu intérieur," in which the tissues and cells of the organism live. This internal environment is neither the air nor the water in which an organism lives but rather—in the case of the human body—the well-controlled liquid environment that Bernard called "the organic liquid that circulates and bathes all the anatomic elements of the tissues, the lymph or the plasma." In short, this internal environment is what we today call the extracellular fluid. He argued that physiological functions continue in a manner indifferent to the changing environment because the milieu intérieur isolates the organs and tissues of the body from the vagaries of the physical conditions of the environment. Indeed, Bernard described the milieu intérieur as if an organism had placed itself in a greenhouse.

According to Bernard's concept of milieu intérieur, some fluids contained within the body are not really inside the body at all. For example, the *contents* of the gastrointestinal tract, sweat ducts, and renal tubules are all outside the body. They are all continuous with the milieu extérieur.

Bernard compares a complex organism to an ensemble of anatomical elements that live together inside the milieu intérieur. Therefore, in Section II of this textbook, we examine the physiology of these cells and molecules. In Section III,

we examine how the nervous system exploits excitability to process information.

Another theme developed by Bernard was that the "fixité du milieu intérieur" (the constancy of the extracellular fluid) is the condition of "free, independent life." He explains that organ differentiation is the exclusive property of higher organisms and that each organ contributes to "compensate and equilibrate" against changes in the external environment. In that sense, several organ systems permit the body to live within an adverse external environment. Indeed, the cardiovascular system (Section IV), the respiratory system (Section V), the urinary system (Section VI), the gastrointestinal system (Section VII), and the endocrine system (Section VIII) create and maintain a constant internal environment. Individual cell types in various organ systems act in concert to support the constancy of the internal milieu, and the internal milieu in turn provides these cells with a culture medium in which they can thrive.

The discipline of physiology also deals with those characteristics that are the property of a living organism as opposed to a nonliving organism. Four fundamental properties distinguish the living body. First, only living organisms exchange matter and energy with the environment to continue their existence. Several organ systems of the body participate in these exchanges. Second, only living organisms can receive signals from their environment and react accordingly. The principles of sensory perception, processing by the nervous system, and reaction are discussed in the chapters on excitable membranes (Section II) and the nervous system (Section III). Third, what distinguishes a living organism is the life cycle of growth and reproduction, as discussed in the chapters on reproduction (Section IX). Finally, the living organism is able to adapt to changing circumstances. This is a theme that is developed throughout this textbook but especially in the chapters on everyday life (Section X).

Homeostatic mechanisms—operating through sophisticated feedback control mechanisms—are responsible for maintaining the constancy of the milieu intérieur

Homeostasis is the control of a vital parameter. The body carefully controls a seemingly endless list of vital parameters. Examples of tightly controlled parameters that affect nearly the whole body are arterial pressure and blood volume. At the level of the milieu intérieur, tightly regulated parameters include body core temperature and plasma levels of a wide range of solutes. Homeostasis also occurs at the level of the single cell. Thus, cells regulate many of the same parameters that the body as a whole regulates: volume, the concentrations of many small inorganic ions, and energy levels.

One of the most common themes in physiology is the **negative-feedback mechanism** responsible for homeostasis. Negative feedback requires at least four elements. First, the system must be able to sense the vital parameter (e.g., glucose level) or something related to it. Second, the system must be able to compare the input signal with some internal reference value called a *setpoint*, thereby forming a difference signal. Third, the system must multiply the error signal by some proportionality factor (i.e., the gain) to produce some sort of output signal (e.g., release of insulin). Fourth, the output signal must be able to activate an effector mechanism (e.g., glucose uptake and metabolism) that opposes the source of the input signal and thereby brings the vital parameter closer to the setpoint (e.g., decrease of blood glucose levels back to normal).

A single feedback loop often does not operate in isolation but rather as part of a larger network of controls. Thus, a complex interplay may exist among feedback loops within single cells, within a tissue, within an organ or organ system, or at the level of the whole body. After studying these individual feedback loops in isolation, the physiologist may find that two feedback loops act either synergistically or antagonistically. For example, insulin lowers blood glucose levels, whereas epinephrine and cortisol have the opposite effect. Thus, the physiologist must determine the relative weights of feedback loops in **competition** with one another. Finally, the physiologist must also establish **hierarchy** among various feedback loops. For example, the hypothalamus controls the anterior pituitary, which controls the adrenal cortex, which releases cortisol, which helps control blood glucose levels.

Another theme of homeostasis is **redundancy.** The more vital a parameter is, the more systems the body mobilizes to regulate it. If one system should fail, others are there to help maintain homeostasis. It is probably for this reason that genetic knockouts sometimes fail to have their expected deleterious effects. The result of many homeostatic systems controlling many vital parameters is a milieu intérieur with a stable composition.

Whether at the level of the milieu intérieur or the cytoplasm of a single cell, homeostasis occurs at a price: energy. When a vital parameter (e.g., the blood glucose level) is well regulated, that parameter is not in equilibrium. **Equilibrium** is a state that does not involve energy consumption. Instead, a well-regulated parameter is generally in a **steady state.** That is, its value is constant because the body or the cell carefully matches actions that lower the parameter value with other actions that raise it. The net effect is that the vital parameter is held at a constant value.

An important principle in physiology, to which we have already alluded, is that each cell plays a specialized role in the overall function of the body. In return, the body—which is the sum of all these cells—provides the milieu intérieur appropriate for the life of each cell. As part of the bargain, each cell or organ must respect the needs of the body as a whole and not run amok for its own greedy interests. For example, during exercise, the system that controls body core temperature sheds heat by elaborating sweat for evaporation. However, the production of sweat ultimately reduces blood volume. Because the body as a whole places a higher **priority** on the control of blood volume than on the control of body core temperature, at some point the system that controls blood volume will instruct the system that controls body core temperature to reduce the production of sweat. Unfortunately, this juggling of priorities works only if the individual stops exercising; if not, the result may be heat stroke.

The **adaptability** of an organism depends on its ability to alter its response. Indeed, flexible feedback loops are at the root of many forms of physiological adaptation. For instance, at sea level, experimentally lowering the level of oxygen (the sensory stimulus) in the inspired air causes an increase in breathing (the response). However, after **acclimatization** at high altitude to low oxygen levels, the same low level of oxygen (the same sensory stimulus) causes one to breathe much faster (a greater response). Thus, the response may depend on the previous history and therefore the "state" of the system. In addition to acclimatization, genetic factors can also contribute to the ability to respond to an environmental stress. For example, certain populations of humans who have lived for generations at high altitude withstand hypoxia better than lowlanders do, even after the lowlanders have acclimatized as fully as they can.

Medicine is the study of "physiology gone awry"

Medicine borrows its physicochemical principles from physiology. Medicine also uses physiology as a reference state (e.g., the "physiological value" of a parameter such as blood glucose). It is essential to know how organs and systems function in the healthy person to grasp which components may be malfunctioning in a patient. A large part of clinical medicine is simply dealing with the abnormal physiology brought about by a disease process. One malfunction (e.g., heart failure) can lead to a *primary* pathological effect (e.g., a decrease in cardiac output) that—in chain-reaction style—leads to a series of *secondary* effects (e.g., fluid overload) that are the appropriate responses of physiological feedback loops. Indeed, as clinician-physiologists have explored the basis of disease, they have discovered a great deal about physiology.

Physiologists have developed many tools and tests to examine normal function. A large number of **functional tests**—used in diagnosis of a disease, monitoring of the evolution of an illness, and evaluation of the progress of therapy—are direct transfers of technology developed in the physiology laboratory. Typical examples are cardiac monitoring, pulmonary and renal function tests, as well as the assays used to measure plasma levels of various ions, gases, and hormones. The understanding of physiology summarized in this book comes from some experiments on humans but mostly from research on other mammals and even on squids and slime molds. However, our ultimate focus is on the human body.

REFERENCES

Bernard C. Leçons sur les phénomènes de la vie communs aux animaux et aux végétaux. *Cours de physiologie générale du Museum d'Histoire Naturelle.* Paris: Baillière et Fils; 1878.

Cannon WB. *The Wisdom of the Body.* New York: WW Norton; 1932.

Smith HW. *From Fish to Philosopher.* New York: Doubleday; 1961.

PHYSIOLOGY OF CELLS AND MOLECULES

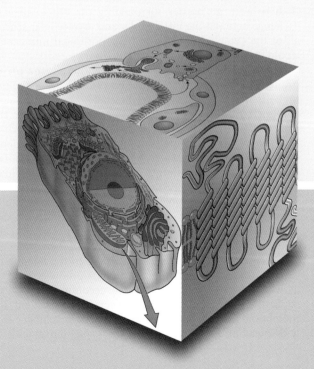

CHAPTER 2

FUNCTIONAL ORGANIZATION OF THE CELL

Michael J. Caplan

The modern treatment of physiology that is presented in this textbook is as much about the interactions of molecules in cells as it is about the interactions of organs in organisms. It is necessary, therefore, at the outset to discuss the structure and characteristics of the cell. Our discussion focuses first on the architectural and dynamic features of a generic cell. We then examine how this generic cell can be adapted to serve in diverse physiological capacities. Through adaptations at the cellular level, organs acquire the machinery necessary to perform their individual metabolic tasks.

STRUCTURE OF BIOLOGICAL MEMBRANES

The surface of the cell is defined by a membrane

The chemical composition of the cell interior is very different from that of its surroundings. The biochemical processes involved in cell function require the maintenance of a precisely regulated intracellular environment. The cytoplasm is an extraordinarily complex solution, the constituents of which include myriad proteins, nucleic acids, nucleotides, and sugars that the cell synthesizes or accumulates at great metabolic cost. The cell also expends tremendous energy to regulate the intracellular concentrations of numerous ions. If there were no barrier surrounding the cell to prevent exchange between the intracellular and extracellular spaces, all of the cytoplasm's hard-won compositional uniqueness would be lost by diffusion in a few seconds.

The requisite barrier is provided by the **plasma membrane,** which forms the cell's outer skin. The plasma membrane is *impermeable* to large molecules such as proteins and nucleic acids, thus ensuring their retention within the cytosol. It is *selectively permeable* to small molecules such as ions and metabolites. However, the metabolic requirements of the cell demand a plasma membrane that is much more sophisticated than a simple, passive barrier that allows various substances to leak through at different rates. Frequently, the concentration of a nutrient in the extracellular fluid (ECF) is several orders of magnitude lower than that required inside the cell. If the cell wishes to use such a substance, therefore, it must be able to *accumulate* it against a concentration gradient. A simple pore in the membrane cannot concentrate anything; it can only modulate the rate at which a gradient dissipates. To accomplish the more sophisticated feat of creating a concentration gradient, the membrane must be endowed with special machinery that uses metabolic energy to drive the *uphill* movements of

substances—**active transport**—into or out of the cell. In addition, it would be useful to rapidly modulate the permeability properties of the plasma membrane in response to various metabolic stimuli. Active transport and the ability to control passive permeabilities underlie a wide range of physiological processes, from the electrical excitability of neurons to the resorptive and secretory functions of the kidney.

The cell membrane is composed primarily of phospholipids

Biochemical analysis reveals that the plasma membrane is composed of two principal constituents: lipid and protein.

Most of the lipid associated with the plasma membrane belongs to the molecular family of **phospholipids.** In general, phospholipids share a **glycerol** backbone, two hydroxyl groups of which are esterified to various **fatty-acid** or **acyl groups** (Fig. 2.1A). These acyl groups may have different numbers of carbon atoms and also may have double bonds between carbons. For glycerol-based phospholipids, the third glycerolic hydroxyl group is esterified to a **phosphate** group, which in turn is esterified to a small molecule referred to as a **head group.** The identity of the head group determines the name as well as many of the properties of the individual phospholipids. For instance, glycerol-based phospholipids that bear an ethanolamine molecule in the head group position are categorized as **phosphatidylethanolamines** (see Fig. 2.1A).

Phospholipids form complex structures in aqueous solution

The unique structure and physical chemistry of each phospholipid (see Fig. 2.1B) underlie the formation of biological membranes and explain many of their most important properties. Fatty acids are nonpolar molecules. Their long carbon chains lack the charged groups that would facilitate interactions with water, which is polar. Consequently, fatty acids dissolve poorly in water but readily in organic solvents; thus, fatty acids are **hydrophobic.** On the other hand, the head groups of most phospholipids are charged or polar. These head groups interact well with water and consequently are very water soluble. Thus, the head groups are **hydrophilic.** Because phospholipids combine hydrophilic heads with hydrophobic tails, their interaction with water is referred to as **amphipathic.**

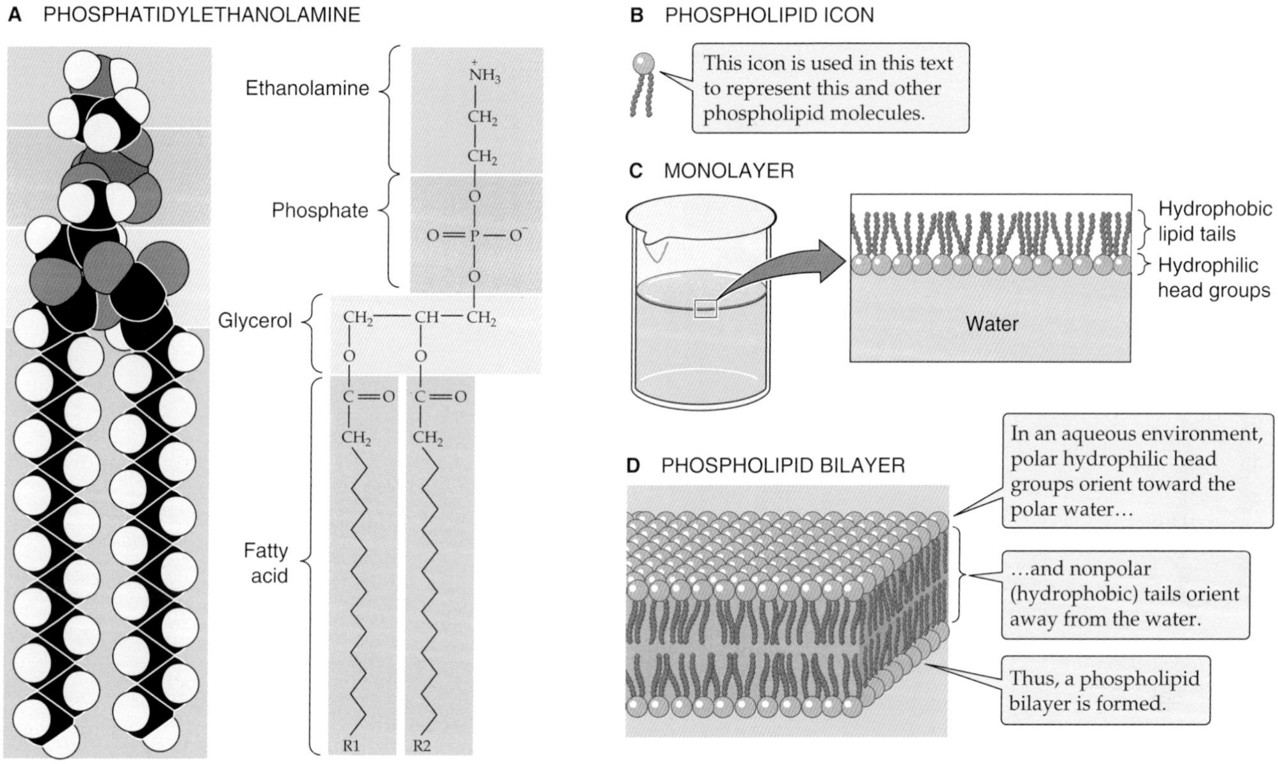

A PHOSPHATIDYLETHANOLAMINE

B PHOSPHOLIPID ICON

This icon is used in this text to represent this and other phospholipid molecules.

C MONOLAYER

Hydrophobic lipid tails

Hydrophilic head groups

Water

D PHOSPHOLIPID BILAYER

In an aqueous environment, polar hydrophilic head groups orient toward the polar water…

…and nonpolar (hydrophobic) tails orient away from the water.

Thus, a phospholipid bilayer is formed.

Ethanolamine

Phosphate

Glycerol

Fatty acid

Figure 2.1 Phospholipids.

When mixed with water, phospholipids organize themselves into structures that prevent their hydrophobic tails from making contact with water while simultaneously permitting their hydrophilic head groups to be fully dissolved. When added to water at fairly low concentrations, phospholipids form a **monolayer** (see Fig. 2.1C) on the water's surface at the air-water interface. It is energetically less costly to the system for the hydrophobic tails to stick up in the air than to interact with the solvent.

At still higher concentrations, phospholipids spontaneously form **bilayers** (see Fig. 2.1D). In these structures, the phospholipid molecules arrange themselves into two parallel sheets or **leaflets** that face each other tail to tail. The hydrophilic head groups form the surfaces of the bilayer; the hydrophobic tails form the center of the sandwich. The hydrophilic surfaces insulate the hydrophobic tails from contact with the solvent, leaving the tails free to associate exclusively with one another.

The *glycerol-based* phospholipids, the most common membrane lipids, include the phosphatidylethanolamines described above (see Fig. 2.1A), as well as the **phosphatidylinositols** (Fig. 2.2A), **phosphatidylserines** (see Fig. 2.2B), and **phosphatidylcholines** (see Fig. 2.2C). The second major class of membrane lipids, the **sphingolipids** (derivatives of *sphingosine*), is made up of three subgroups: **sphingomyelins** (see Fig. 2.2D), **glycosphingolipids** such as the galactocerebrosides (see Fig. 2.2E), and **gangliosides** (not shown in figure). Cholesterol (see Fig. 2.2F) is another important membrane lipid.

⊙ **2-1** Although phospholipids can diffuse in the plane of a lipid bilayer membrane, they do not diffuse between adjacent leaflets (Fig. 2.3). The rate at which phospholipids spontaneously "flip-flop" from one leaflet of a bilayer to the other is extremely low. As mentioned above, the center of a bilayer membrane consists of the fatty-acid tails of the phospholipid molecules and is an extremely hydrophobic environment. For a phospholipid molecule to jump from one leaflet to the other, its highly hydrophilic head group would have to transit this central hydrophobic core, which would have an extremely high energy cost. This caveat does not apply to cholesterol (see Fig. 2.3), whose polar head is a single hydroxyl group. The energy cost of dragging this small polar hydroxyl group through the bilayer is relatively low, which permits relatively rapid cholesterol flip-flop.

Phospholipid bilayer membranes are impermeable to charged molecules

The lipid bilayer is ideally suited to separate two aqueous compartments. Its hydrophilic head groups interact well with water at both membrane surfaces, whereas the hydrophobic center ensures that the energetic cost of crossing the membrane is prohibitive for charged atoms or molecules. Pure phospholipid bilayer membranes are extremely impermeable to almost any charged water-soluble substance. Ions such as Na^+, K^+, Cl^-, and Ca^{2+} are insoluble in the hydrophobic membrane core and consequently cannot travel from the aqueous environment on one side of the membrane to the aqueous environment on the opposite side. The same is true of large water-soluble molecules, such as proteins, nucleic acids, sugars, and nucleotides.

Whereas phospholipid membranes are impermeable to water-soluble molecules, small *uncharged* polar molecules can cross fairly freely. This is often true for O_2,

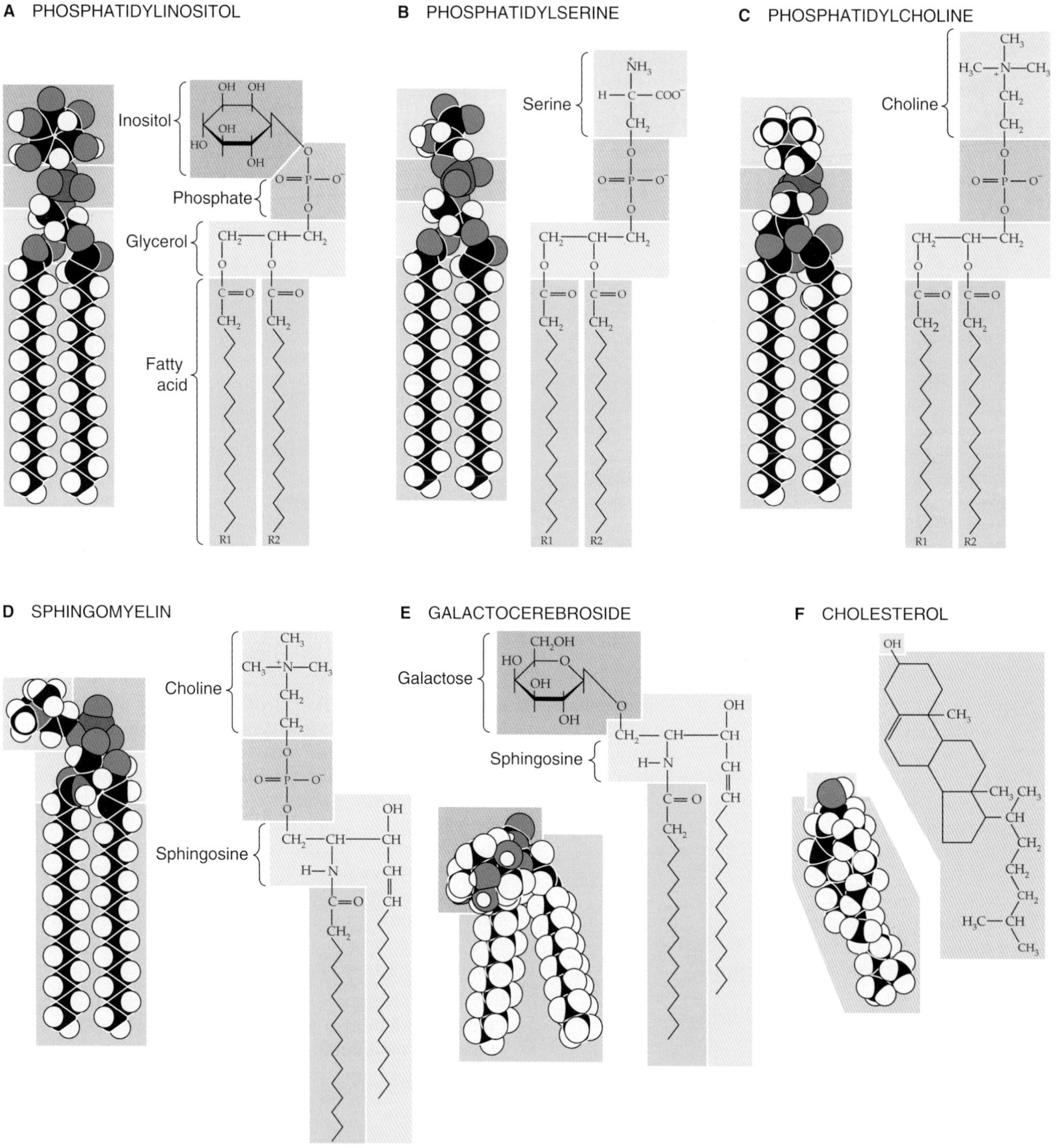
A PHOSPHATIDYLINOSITOL
Inositol
Phosphate
Glycerol
Fatty acid
B PHOSPHATIDYLSERINE
Serine
C PHOSPHATIDYLCHOLINE
Choline
D SPHINGOMYELIN
Choline
Sphingosine
E GALACTOCEREBROSIDE
Galactose
Sphingosine
F CHOLESTEROL

Figure 2.2 Structures of some common membrane lipids.

CO_2, NH_3, and, remarkably, water itself. Water molecules may, at least in part, traverse the membrane through transient cracks between the hydrophobic tails of the phospholipids without having to surmount an enormous energetic barrier. The degree of permeability of water (and perhaps that of CO_2 and NH_3 as well) varies extensively with lipid composition; some phospholipids (especially those with short or kinked fatty-acid chains) permit a much greater rate of transbilayer water diffusion than others do.

The plasma membrane is a bilayer

As may be inferred from the preceding discussion, the membrane at the cell surface is, in fact, a phospholipid bilayer. The membrane's bilayer structure can be visualized directly in the high-magnification electron micrograph depicted in Fig. 2.4. The osmium tetroxide molecule (OsO_4) with which the membrane is stained binds to the head groups of phospholipids. Thus, both surfaces of a phospholipid bilayer appear black in electron micrographs, whereas the membrane's unstained central core appears white.

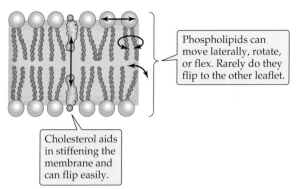

Phospholipids can move laterally, rotate, or flex. Rarely do they flip to the other leaflet.

Cholesterol aids in stiffening the membrane and can flip easily.

Figure 2.3 Mobility of lipids within a bilayer.

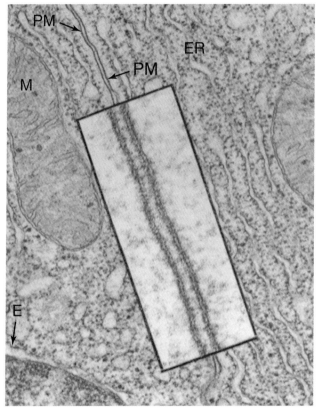

Figure 2.4 Transmission electron micrograph of a cell membrane. The *inset* is a high-magnification view of the plasma membranes *(PM)* of two adjacent cells. Each membrane includes two dense layers with an intermediate layer of lower density. *E*, nuclear envelope; *ER*, endoplasmic reticulum; *M*, mitochondrion. (From Porter KR, Bonneville MR. *Fine Structure of Cells and Tissues.* 4th ed. Philadelphia: Lea & Febiger; 1973.)

The phospholipid compositions of the two leaflets of the plasma membrane are not identical. Labeling studies performed on erythrocyte plasma membranes reveal that the surface that faces the cytoplasm contains phosphatidylethanolamine and phosphatidylserine, whereas the outward-facing leaflet is composed almost exclusively of phosphatidylcholine. It is not entirely clear what advantage this distribution provides to the cell. The lipid asymmetry may be especially important for those phospholipids that are involved in second-messenger cascades. Phosphatidylinositols, for example, give rise to phosphoinositides, which play critical roles in signaling pathways. In addition, the

phosphatidylinositol composition of the cytoplasmic face of an organelle helps to define the identity of the organelle and to govern its trafficking and targeting properties. Finally, the phospholipids that are characteristic of animal cell plasma membranes generally have one saturated and one unsaturated fatty-acid residue.

Membrane proteins can be integrally or peripherally associated with the plasma membrane

◉ **2-2** Membrane proteins can belong to either of two broad classes, peripheral or integral. **Peripherally associated membrane proteins** are neither embedded within the membrane nor attached to it by covalent bonds; instead, they adhere tightly to the cytoplasmic or extracellular surfaces of the plasma membrane (Fig. 2.5A). They can be removed from the membrane, however, by mild treatments that disrupt ionic bonds (very high salt concentrations) or hydrogen bonds (very low salt concentrations).

In contrast, **integral membrane proteins** are intimately associated with the lipid bilayer. They cannot be eluted from the membrane by these high- or low-salt washes. For integral membrane proteins to be dislodged, the membrane itself must be dissolved by adding detergents. Integral membrane proteins can be associated with the lipid bilayer in any of three ways. First, some proteins actually span the lipid bilayer once or several times (see Fig. 2.5B and C) and hence are referred to as **transmembrane proteins.**

◉ **2-3** The second group of integral membrane proteins is embedded in the bilayer without actually crossing it (see Fig. 2.5D). A third group of membrane-associated proteins is not actually embedded in the bilayer at all. Instead, these lipid-anchored proteins are attached to the membrane by a covalent bond that links them either to a lipid component of the membrane or to a fatty-acid derivative that intercalates into the membrane. For example, proteins can be linked to a special type of glycosylated phospholipid molecule (see Fig. 2.5E), which is most often **glycosylphosphatidylinositol (GPI),** on the outer leaflet of the membrane. This family is referred to collectively as the **glycophospholipid-linked proteins.** Another example is a direct linkage to a fatty acid (e.g., a myristyl group) or a prenyl (e.g., farnesyl) group that intercalates into the inner leaflet of the membrane (see Fig. 2.5F).

The membrane-spanning portions of transmembrane proteins are usually hydrophobic α helices

◉ **2-4** How can membrane-spanning proteins remain stably associated with the bilayer in a conformation that requires at least some portion of their amino-acid sequence to be in continuous contact with the membrane's hydrophobic central core? The answer to this question can be found in the special structures of those protein domains that actually span the membrane.

The side chains of the eight amino acids listed in the upper portion of Table 2.1 are hydrophobic. These aromatic or uncharged aliphatic groups are almost as difficult to solvate in water as are the fatty-acid side chains of the membrane phospholipids themselves. Not surprisingly, therefore, these hydrophobic side chains are quite comfortable in

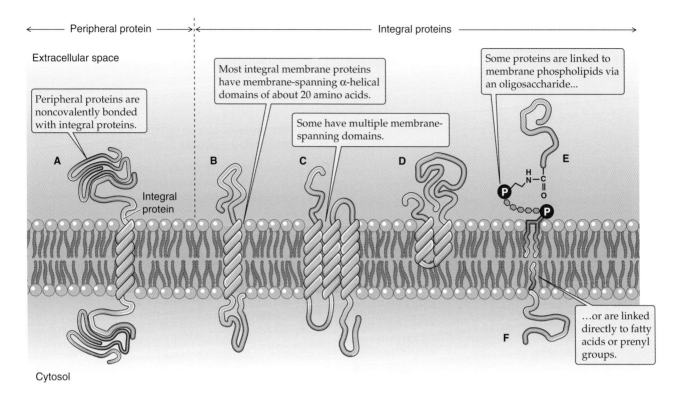

Figure 2.5 Classes of membrane proteins. In (E), protein is coupled via a GPI linkage.

the hydrophobic environment of the bilayer core. Most **membrane-spanning segments**—that is, the short stretches of amino acids that pass through the membrane once—are composed mainly of these nonpolar amino acids, in concert with polar, uncharged amino acids.

The hydrophobic, membrane-spanning segments of transmembrane proteins are specially adapted to the hydrophobic milieu in which they reside. The phospholipid molecules of the membrane bilayer actually protect these portions of transmembrane proteins from energetically unfavorable interactions with the aqueous environment.

Transmembrane proteins can have a single membrane-spanning segment (see Fig. 2.5B) or several (see Fig. 2.5C). Those with a single transmembrane segment can be oriented with either their amino (N) or their carboxyl (C) terminus facing the extracellular space. Multispanning membrane proteins weave through the membrane, and the N and C termini can be exposed to either the cytoplasmic or extracellular compartments. The pattern with which the transmembrane protein weaves across the lipid bilayer defines its membrane **topology.**

The amino-acid sequences of membrane-spanning segments tend to form α helices, with ~3.6 amino acids per turn of the helix (see Fig. 2.5B). In the case of multispanning membrane proteins, their transmembrane helices probably pack together tightly (see Fig. 2.5C).

Many membrane proteins form tight, noncovalent associations with other membrane proteins in the plane of the bilayer. These **multimeric proteins** can be composed of a single type of polypeptide or of mixtures of two or more different proteins. The side-to-side interactions that hold these complexes together can involve the membrane-spanning segments or regions of the proteins that protrude at either surface of the bilayer. By assembling into multimeric complexes, membrane proteins can increase their stability. They can also increase the variety and complexity of the functions that they are capable of performing.

Some membrane proteins are mobile in the plane of the bilayer

As is true for phospholipid molecules (see Fig. 2.3), some transmembrane proteins can diffuse within the surface of the membrane. In the absence of any protein-protein attachments, transmembrane proteins are free to diffuse over the entire surface of a membrane.

Because transmembrane proteins are large molecules, their diffusion in the plane of the membrane is much slower than that of lipids. Even the fastest proteins diffuse ~1000 times more slowly than the average phospholipid. The diffusion of many transmembrane proteins appears to be further impeded by their attachments to the cytoskeleton, just below the surface of the membrane. Tight binding to this meshwork can render proteins essentially immobile. Like phospholipids, proteins can diffuse only in the plane of the bilayer. They cannot flip-flop across it. Thus, a membrane protein's topology does not change over its life span.

FUNCTION OF MEMBRANE PROTEINS

Integral membrane proteins can serve as receptors

⊙ **2-5** All communication between a cell and its environment must involve or at least pass through the plasma

TABLE 2.1   Classification of the Amino Acids Based on the Chemistry of Their Side Chains

	NAME	THREE-LETTER CODE	SINGLE-LETTER CODE	STRUCTURE OF THE SIDE CHAIN
Nonpolar	Alanine	Ala	A	$-CH_3$
	Valine	Val	V	$-CH(CH_3)_2$
	Leucine	Leu	L	$-CH_2CH(CH_3)_2$
	Isoleucine	Ile	I	$-CH-CH_2-CH_3$ with CH_3
	Proline	Pro	P	
	Phenylalanine	Phe	F	$-CH_2-$⬡
	Tryptophan	Trp	W	
	Methionine	Met	M	$-CH_2-CH_2-S-CH_3$
Polar uncharged	Glycine	Gly	G	$-H$
	Serine	Ser	S	$-CH_2-OH$
	Threonine	Thr	T	$-CH-CH_3$ with OH
	Cysteine	Cys	C	$-CH_2-SH$
	Tyrosine	Tyr	Y	$-CH_2-$⬡$-OH$
	Asparagine	Asn	N	$-CH_2-C=O$ with NH_2
	Glutamine	Gln	Q	$-CH_2-CH_2-C=O$ with NH_2
Polar, charged, acidic	Aspartate	Asp	D	$-CH_2-C=O$ with O^-
	Glutamate	Glu	E	$-CH_2-CH_2-C=O$ with O^-
Polar, charged, basic	Lysine	Lys	K	$-CH_2-CH_2-CH_2-CH_2-NH_3^+$
	Arginine	Arg	R	$-CH_2-CH_2-CH_2-NH-C-NH_2$ with NH_2^+
	Histidine	His	H	

membrane. For the purposes of this discussion, we define communication rather broadly as the exchange of any signal between the cell and its surroundings. Except for lipid-soluble signaling molecules such as steroid hormones, essentially all communication functions served by the plasma membrane occur via membrane proteins.

Ligand-binding receptors comprise the group of transmembrane proteins that perhaps most clearly illustrate the concept of transmembrane signaling (Fig. 2.6A). For water-soluble hormones such as epinephrine to influence cellular behavior, their presence in the ECF compartment must be made known to the various intracellular mechanisms whose

A LIGAND-BINDING RECEPTOR

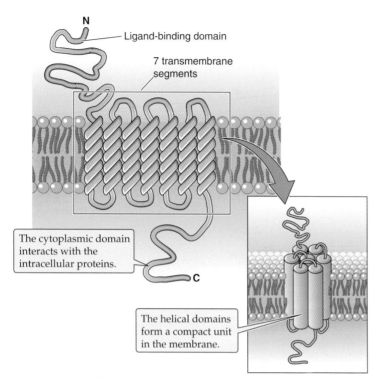

B CELL-MATRIX ADHESION MOLECULE (INTEGRIN)

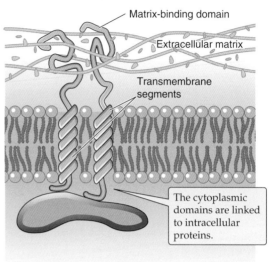

Figure 2.6 Integral membrane proteins that transmit signals from the outside to the inside of a cell. (A) The ligand may be a hormone, a growth factor, a neurotransmitter, an odorant, or another local mediator. (B) An integrin is an adhesion molecule that attaches the cell to the extracellular matrix.

behaviors they modulate. The interaction of a hormone with the extracellular portion of the hormone receptor, which forms a high-affinity binding site, produces conformational changes within the receptor protein that extend through the membrane-spanning domain to the intracellular domain of the receptor. As a consequence, the intracellular domain either becomes enzymatically active or can interact with cytoplasmic proteins that are involved in the generation of so-called second messengers. Either mechanism completes the transmission of the hormone signal across the membrane. The transmembrane disposition of a hormone receptor thus creates a single, continuous communication medium that is capable of conveying, through its own structural modifications, information from the environment to the cellular interior.

Integral membrane proteins can serve as adhesion molecules

◉ **2-6** Cells can also exploit integral membrane proteins as **adhesion molecules** that form physical contacts with the surrounding extracellular matrix (i.e., cell-matrix adhesion molecules) or with their cellular neighbors (i.e., cell-cell adhesion molecules). These attachments can be extremely important in regulating the shape, growth, and differentiation of cells. The **integrins** are examples of matrix receptors or **cell-matrix adhesion molecules.** They comprise a large family of transmembrane proteins that link cells to components of the extracellular matrix (e.g., fibronectin, laminin) at adhesion plaques (see Fig. 2.6B). These linkages produce conformational changes in the integrin molecules that are

transmitted to their cytoplasmic tails. These tails, in turn, communicate the linkage events to various structural and signaling molecules that participate in formulating a cell's response to its physical environment.

◉ **2-7** In contrast to matrix receptors, which attach cells to the extracellular matrix, several enormous superfamilies of **cell-cell adhesion molecules** attach cells to each other. These cell-cell adhesion molecules include the Ca^{2+}-dependent cell adhesion molecules called **cadherins** and Ca^{2+}-independent neural cell adhesion molecules called **N-CAMs.** The two classes of cell-cell adhesion molecules mediate similar sorts of transmembrane signals that help organize the cytoplasm and control gene expression in response to intercellular contacts.

◉ 2-8 Integral membrane proteins can carry out the transmembrane movement of water-soluble substances

Ions and other membrane-impermeable substances can cross the bilayer with the assistance of transmembrane proteins that serve as pores, channels, carriers, and pumps. **Pores** and **channels** serve as conduits that allow water, specific ions, or even very large proteins to flow passively through the bilayer. **Carriers** can either facilitate the transport of a specific molecule across the membrane or couple the transport of a molecule to that of other solutes. **Pumps** use the energy that is released through the hydrolysis of ATP to drive the transport of substances into or out of cells against energy gradients.

Fig. 2.7 shows an example of a type of K^+ channel that is formed by the apposition of four identical subunits, each of which has six membrane-spanning segments. The pore of

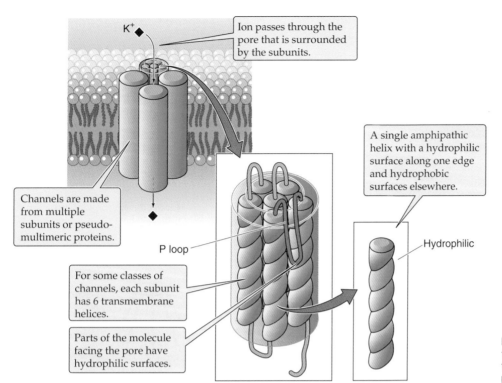

Ion passes through the pore that is surrounded by the subunits.

A single amphipathic helix with a hydrophilic surface along one edge and hydrophobic surfaces elsewhere.

K^+

Channels are made from multiple subunits or pseudo-multimeric proteins.

P loop

Hydrophilic

For some classes of channels, each subunit has 6 transmembrane helices.

Parts of the molecule facing the pore have hydrophilic surfaces.

Figure 2.7 Amphipathic α helices interacting to form a channel through the cell membrane. This is an example of a K^+ channel.

this channel is created by the amphipathic helices as well as by short, hydrophilic loops (P loops) contributed by each of the four subunits.

Integral membrane proteins can also be enzymes

Ion pumps are actually enzymes. They catalyze the hydrolysis of ATP and use the energy released by that reaction to drive ion transport. Many other classes of proteins that are embedded in cell membranes function as enzymes as well. Membrane-bound enzymes are especially prevalent in the cells of the intestine, which participate in the final stages of nutrient digestion and absorption.

Integral membrane proteins can participate in intracellular signaling

Some integral proteins associate with the cytoplasmic surface of the plasma membrane by covalently attaching to fatty acids or prenyl groups that in turn intercalate into the lipid bilayer (see Fig. 2.5F). The fatty acids or prenyl groups act as hydrophobic tails that anchor an otherwise soluble protein to the bilayer. These proteins are all located at the *intra*cellular leaflet of the membrane bilayer and often participate in intracellular signaling pathways. Many of these proteins are involved in relaying the signals that are received at the cell surface to the effector machinery within the cell interior. Their association with the membrane, therefore, brings these proteins close to the cytoplasmic sides of receptors that transmit signals from the cell exterior across the bilayer. The medical relevance of this type of membrane association is beginning to be appreciated. For example, denying certain oncogene products their lipid modifications—and hence their membrane attachment—eliminates their ability to induce tumorigenic transformation.

CELLULAR ORGANELLES AND THE CYTOSKELETON

The cell is composed of discrete organelles that subserve distinct functions

When a eukaryotic cell is viewed through a light microscope, a handful of recognizable intracellular structures can be discerned. Even the simplest nucleated animal cell possesses a wide variety of intricate structures with specific shapes and sizes. These structures are the **membrane-enclosed organelles,** the functional building blocks of cells.

Fig. 2.8 illustrates the interior of a typical cell. The largest organelle in this picture is the **nucleus,** which houses the cell's complement of genetic information. This structure, which is visible in the light microscope, is usually round or oblong, although in some cells it displays a complex, lobulated shape. Depending on the cell type, the nucleus can range in diameter from 2 to 20 μm. With some exceptions, including skeletal muscle and certain specialized cells of the immune system, each animal cell has a single nucleus.

◉ 2-9 Surrounding the nucleus is a web of tubules or saccules known as the **endoplasmic reticulum (ER).** This organelle can exist in either of two forms, rough or smooth. The surfaces of the rough ER tubules are studded with **ribosomes,** the major sites of protein synthesis. Ribosomes can also exist free in the cytosol. The surfaces of the smooth ER, which participates in lipid synthesis, are not similarly endowed. The ER also serves as a major reservoir for calcium ions. The ER membrane is equipped with a Ca pump that uses the energy released through ATP hydrolysis to drive the transport of Ca^{2+} from the cytoplasm into the ER lumen. This Ca^{2+} can be rapidly released in response to messenger molecules and plays a major role in intracellular signaling.

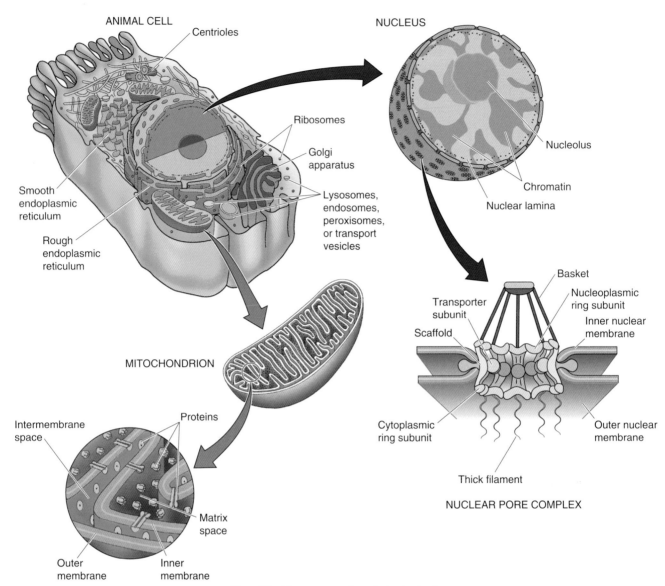

ANIMAL CELL
— Centrioles
Ribosomes
Golgi apparatus
Lysosomes, endosomes, peroxisomes, or transport vesicles
Smooth endoplasmic reticulum
Rough endoplasmic reticulum

NUCLEUS
Nucleolus
Chromatin
Nuclear lamina

MITOCHONDRION

Intermembrane space
Proteins
Matrix space
Outer membrane
Inner membrane

NUCLEAR PORE COMPLEX
Basket
Nucleoplasmic ring subunit
Inner nuclear membrane
Transporter subunit
Scaffold
Cytoplasmic ring subunit
Outer nuclear membrane
Thick filament

Figure 2.8   Ultrastructure of a typical animal cell.

⊙ **2-10** The **Golgi complex** resembles a stack of pancakes. Each pancake in the stack represents a discrete, flat saccule. The number and size of the saccules in the Golgi stack vary among cell types. The Golgi complex is a processing station that participates in protein maturation and targets newly synthesized proteins to their appropriate subcellular destinations.

Perhaps the most intriguing morphological appearance belongs to the **mitochondrion,** which is essentially a balloon within a balloon. The outer membrane and inner membrane define two distinct internal compartments: the intermembrane space and the matrix space. The surface of the inner membrane is thrown into dramatic folds called *cristae.* This organelle is ~0.2 μm in diameter, which is at the limit of resolution of the light microscope. The mitochondrion is the power plant of the cell, a critical manufacturer of ATP. Many cellular reactions are also catalyzed within the mitochondrion.

The cell's digestive organelle is the **lysosome.** This large structure frequently contains several smaller, round vesicles called **exosomes** within its internal space.

The cytoplasm contains numerous other organelles whose shapes are not quite as distinguishing, including **endosomes, peroxisomes,** and **transport vesicles.**

Despite their diversity, all cellular organelles are constructed from the same building blocks. Each is composed of a membrane that forms the entire extent of its surface. The biochemical and physical properties of an organelle's limiting membrane dictate many of its functional properties.

The nucleus stores, replicates, and reads the cell's genetic information

The nucleus serves as a cell's repository for its complement of chromosomal DNA. To conceive of the nucleus as simply a hermetically sealed vault for genetic information, however, is a gross oversimplification. All of the machinery necessary to maintain, to copy, and to transcribe DNA is in the nucleus, which is the focus of all of the cellular pathways that regulate gene expression and cell division.

◉ **2-11** The nucleus is surrounded by a double membrane (see Fig. 2.8). The **outer membrane** is studded with ribosomes and is continuous with the membranes of the rough ER. The **inner membrane** is smooth and faces the intranuclear space, or nucleoplasm. The space between these concentric membranes is continuous with the lumen of the rough ER. The inner and outer nuclear membranes meet at specialized structures known as **nuclear pores,** which penetrate the nuclear envelope and provide a transport pathway between the cytoplasm and the nuclear interior. All RNA transcripts that are produced in the nucleus must pass through nuclear pores to be translated in the cytoplasm. Similarly, all the signaling molecules that influence nuclear function as well as all proteins of the nuclear interior (which are synthesized in the cytoplasm) enter the nucleus through nuclear pores.

Nuclear pores are selective in choosing the molecules that they allow to pass. Cytoplasmic proteins destined for the nuclear interior must be endowed with a **nuclear-localization sequence** to gain entry.

◉ **2-12** The nuclear pore's specificity is provided by the **nuclear pore complex (NPC),** an intricate matrix of several hundred proteins of at least 30 different types that form a pore of variable internal diameter.

Lysosomes digest material derived from the interior and exterior of the cell

In the course of normal daily living, cells accumulate waste. Organelles become damaged and dysfunctional. Proteins denature and aggregate. New materials are constantly being brought into the cells from the extracellular environment through the process of endocytosis. If this material were allowed to accumulate indefinitely, it would ultimately fill the cell and essentially choke it to death. Clearly, cells must have mechanisms for disposing of this waste material.

The lysosome is the cell's trash incinerator. It is filled with a broad assortment of degradative enzymes that can break down most forms of cellular debris. **Proton pumps** embedded within the lysosome's limiting membrane ensure that this space is an extremely acidic environment, which aids in protein hydrolysis.

Material that has been internalized from the cell exterior by endocytosis is surrounded by the membrane of an **endocytic vesicle.** To deliver this material to the lysosome, the membranes of the endocytic vesicles fuse with the lysosomal membrane and discharge their cargo into the lysosomal milieu.

Intracellular structures that are destined for degradation, such as fragments of organelles, are engulfed by the lysosome in a process called **autophagy.** Autophagy results in the formation of membrane-enclosed structures within the lysosomal lumen; hence, the lysosome is often referred to as a multivesicular body. Autophagy allows the cell to degrade old or damaged components. Increased metabolic needs also can stimulate autophagy, allowing the cell to recycle and "burn" its own structural components to generate energy.

The mitochondrion is the site of oxidative energy production

Oxygen-dependent ATP production—or oxidative phosphorylation—occurs in the mitochondrion. Like the nucleus, the mitochondrion (see Fig. 2.8) is a double-membrane structure. The inner mitochondrial membrane contains the proteins that constitute the electron transport chain, which generates pH and voltage gradients across this membrane. The inner membrane uses the energy in these gradients to generate ATP from ADP and inorganic phosphate.

◉ **2-13** The mitochondrion also plays a central role in the process called **apoptosis,** or programmed cell death. Certain external or internal signals can induce the cell to initiate a signaling cascade that leads ultimately to the activation of enzymes that bring about the cell's demise. One of the pathways that initiates this highly ordered form of cellular suicide depends on the participation of the mitochondrion. Apoptosis plays an extremely important role during tissue development and is also involved in the body's mechanisms for identifying and destroying cancer cells.

The cytoplasm is not amorphous but is organized by the cytoskeleton

The cytoplasmic **cytoskeleton** is composed of protein filaments that radiate throughout the cell, serving as the beams, struts, and stays that determine cell shape and resilience. On the basis of their appearance in the electron microscope, these filaments were initially divided into several classes (Table 2.2): thick, thin, and intermediate filaments, as well as microtubules. Subsequent biochemical analysis has revealed that each of these varieties is composed of distinct polypeptides and differs with respect to its formation, stability, and biological function.

◉ 2-14 SPECIALIZED CELL TYPES

All cells are constructed of the same basic elements and share the same basic metabolic and biosynthetic machinery. What distinguishes one cell type from another? Certainly, cells have different shapes and molecular structures. In addition, out of an extensive repertoire of molecules that cells are capable of making, each cell type chooses which molecules to express, how to organize these molecules, and how to regulate them. It is this combination of choices that endows them with specific physiological functions. These specializations are the product of cell differentiation. Each of these cell types arises from a **stem cell.** Stem cells are mitotically active and can give rise to a spectrum of cellular lineages that can range from multiple to limited. Thus, they may be *pluri*potent, *multi*potent, *oligo*potent, or *uni*potent. Clearly, the zygote is the ultimate stem cell because it gives rise to every cell lineage present in the complete organism and is thus *toti*potent. Specific cell types arise from stem cells by activating a differentiation-specific program of gene expression. The interplay of environmental signals, temporal cues, and transcription factors that control the processes of cellular differentiation constitutes one of the great unraveling mysteries of modern biology.

TABLE 2.2　**Components of the Cytoskeleton**

	SUBUNITS	DIAMETER (nm)
Intermediate filaments	Tetramer of two coiled dimers	8–10
Microtubules	Heterodimers of α and β tubulin form long protofilaments, 5 nm in diameter	25
Thin filaments	Globular or G-actin, 5 nm in diameter, arranged in a double helix to form fibrous or F-actin	5–8
Thick filaments	Assembly of myosin molecules	10

Epithelial cells form a barrier between the internal and external milieu

How can an organism tightly regulate its internal fluid environment (i.e., internal milieu) without allowing this environment to come into direct and disastrous contact with the external world (i.e., external milieu)? The body has solved these problems by arranging a sheet of cells—an **epithelium**—between these two disparate environments. Because of their unique subcellular designs and intercellular relationships, epithelial cells form a dynamic barrier that can import or expel substances, sometimes against steep concentration gradients.

Two structural features of epithelia permit them to function as useful barriers (Fig. 2.9). First, epithelial cells connect to one another via tight junctions, which constrain the free diffusion of solutes and fluids around the epithelial cells, between the internal and external compartments. Second, the tight junctions define a boundary between an apical and a basolateral domain of the plasma membrane. Each of these two domains is endowed with distinct protein and lipid components, and each subserves a distinct function. Thus, the surface membranes of epithelial cells are polarized. It is worth touching on a few of the cellular specializations that characterize polarized epithelia and permit them to perform their critical roles.

⊙ **2-15** The **apical membranes** of the epithelial cells (see Fig. 2.9) face the lumen of a compartment that is often topologically continuous with the outside world. For example, in the stomach and intestine, apical membranes form the inner surface of the organs that come into contact with ingested matter.

The **basolateral membranes** of epithelial cells face the ECF compartment—which indirectly makes contact with the blood—and rest on a basement membrane. The **basement membrane** is composed of extracellular matrix proteins that the epithelial cells themselves secrete and include collagens, laminin, and proteoglycans. The basement membrane provides the epithelium with structural support and, most importantly, serves as an organizing foundation that helps the epithelial cells to establish their remarkable architecture.

⊙ **2-16** Each epithelial cell is interconnected to its neighbors by a variety of **junctional complexes** (see Fig. 2.9). The lateral surfaces of epithelial cells participate in numerous types of cell-cell contacts, including tight junctions, adhering junctions, gap junctions, and desmosomes.

Tight Junctions ⊙ **2-17** A **tight junction** (or *zonula occludens*) is a complex structure that impedes the passage of molecules and ions *between* the cells of the epithelial monolayer. This pathway between the cells is termed the **paracellular pathway.** The functional properties of tight junctions are related to their intriguing architecture (see Fig. 2.9). The **claudins,** a large family of proteins, are the principal structural elements of the tight junction. Interactions between the claudins present in the apposing membranes of neighboring cells form the permeability barrier.

Tight junctions play several roles. First, they are **barriers** in that they separate one compartment from another. Second, tight junctions can act as selective **gates** in that they permit certain solutes to flow more easily than others. Third, tight junctions act as **fences** that separate the polarized surfaces of the epithelial plasma membrane into apical and basolateral domains. The presence of distinct populations of proteins and lipids in each plasma-membrane domain is absolutely essential for an epithelium to mediate transepithelial fluid and solute transport.

Adhering Junctions ⊙ **2-18** An adhering junction (or *zonula adherens*) is a belt that encircles an entire epithelial cell just below the level of the tight junction. These cell-cell contacts are mediated by the extracellular domains of members of the **cadherin** family. Formation of these junctions initiates the assembly of a subcortical cytoskeleton, in which **anchor proteins** (e.g., vinculin, catenins, α actinin) link the cytosolic domains of cadherins to a network of **actin filaments** that is associated with the cytosolic surfaces of the lateral membranes. In epithelial tumors, for example, loss of expression of the adhering-junction cadherins tends to correlate with the tumor cell's loss of controlled growth and with its ability to **metastasize**—that is, to leave the epithelial monolayer and form a new tumor at a distant site in the body.

Gap Junctions ⊙ **2-19** The channels that interconnect the cytosols of neighboring cells are called gap junctions. They allow small molecules (less than ~1 kDa) to diffuse freely between cells. In some organs, epithelial cells are interconnected by an enormous number of gap junctions, which organize into paracrystalline hexagonal arrays. Because ions can flow through gap junctions, cells that communicate through gap junctions are electrically coupled.

Desmosomes ⊙ **2-20** A desmosome (or *macula adherens*) holds adjacent cells together tightly at a single, round spot. Desmosomes are easily recognized in thin-section electron micrographs by the characteristic dense plaques of intermediate filaments. **Anchor proteins** link the cytosolic domains of the cadherins to **intermediate filaments** that radiate into the cytoplasm from the point of intercellular contact (see Fig. 2.9). These filaments interact with and organize the cytoplasmic intermediate filaments, thus coupling neighboring cells to one another. Epithelial cells are often coupled to adjacent cells by numerous desmosomes, especially in regions where the epithelium is subject to physical stress.

Epithelial cells are polarized

In many epithelia, the apical surface area is amplified by the presence of a **brush border** that is composed of hundreds of finger-like microvillar projections (see Fig. 2.9). In the case of the small intestine and the renal proximal tubule,

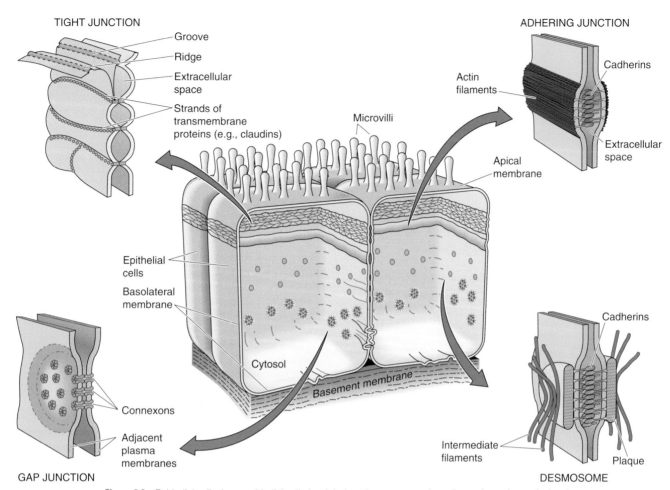

TIGHT JUNCTION
- Groove
- Ridge
- Extracellular space
- Strands of transmembrane proteins (e.g., claudins)

ADHERING JUNCTION
- Actin filaments
- Cadherins
- Extracellular space

Microvilli
Apical membrane

Epithelial cells
Basolateral membrane
Cytosol
Basement membrane

GAP JUNCTION
- Connexons
- Adjacent plasma membranes

DESMOSOME
- Cadherins
- Intermediate filaments
- Plaque

Figure 2.9 Epithelial cells. In an epithelial cell, the tight junction separates the cell membrane into apical and basolateral domains that have very different functional properties.

the membrane covering each microvillus is richly endowed with enzymes that digest sugars and proteins as well as with transporters that carry the products of these digestions into the cells. The presence of a microvillar brush border can amplify the apical surface area of a polarized epithelial cell by as much as 20-fold, thus greatly enhancing its capacity to interact with, to modify, and to transport substances present in the luminal fluid.

The basolateral surface area of certain epithelial cells is amplified by the presence of **lateral interdigitations** and **basal infoldings** (see Fig. 2.9). Although they are not as elegantly constructed as microvilli, these structures can greatly increase the basolateral surface area. In epithelial cells that are involved in large volumes of transport—or in transport against steep gradients—amplifying the basolateral membrane can greatly increase the number of Na-K pumps that a single cell can place at its basolateral membrane.

Although the morphological differences between apical and basolateral membranes can be dramatic, the most important distinction between these surfaces is their protein composition. As noted above, the "fence" function of the tight junction separates completely different rosters of membrane proteins between the apical and basolateral membranes. For example, the Na-K pump is restricted to the basolateral membrane in almost all epithelial cells, and the membrane-bound enzymes that hydrolyze complex sugars and peptides are restricted to apical membranes in intestinal epithelial cells. The polarized distribution of transport proteins is absolutely necessary for the directed movement of solutes and water across epithelia. Furthermore, the restriction of certain enzymes to the apical domain limits their actions to the lumen of the epithelium and therefore offers the advantage of not wasting energy putting enzymes where they are not needed.

CHAPTER 3

SIGNAL TRANSDUCTION

Lloyd Cantley

The evolution of multicellular organisms required the evolution of **cell-to-cell communication** within the organism to coordinate various cells activities, including receiving and processing biological information.

External **signals** such as odorants, metabolites, ions, hormones, growth factors, and neurotransmitters can all serve as **chemical messengers** to link neighboring or distant cells. These messengers interact with specific **cell-surface receptors** and trigger a cascade of secondary events, including the activation of intracellular **second-messenger systems** that mediate the cell's response to that stimulus. However, hydrophobic messengers, such as steroid hormones and some vitamins, can diffuse across the plasma membrane and interact with **cytosolic or nuclear receptors.**

MECHANISMS OF CELLULAR COMMUNICATION

Cells can communicate with one another via chemical signals

◉ 3-1 Cells secrete chemical signals that can induce a physiological response in any (or all) of three ways (Fig. 3.1): by entering the circulation and acting on distant tissues **(endocrine),** by acting on a neighboring cell in the same tissue **(paracrine),** or by stimulating the same cell that released the chemical **(autocrine).** Secreted factors that are produced by cells of one organ and enter the circulation to induce a response in a separate organ are called **hormones,** and the organs that secrete them—such as the pituitary, adrenal, and thyroid glands—are parts of the endocrine system. However, many other cells and tissues not classically thought of as endocrine also produce hormones. For example, the kidney produces 1,25-dihydroxyvitamin D_3, and the salivary gland synthesizes nerve growth factor. Finally, physical contact between one cell and another, or between a cell and the matrix secreted by another cell, can transmit a signal **(juxtacrine).**

For paracrine and autocrine signals to be delivered to their proper targets, their diffusion must be limited. This restriction can be accomplished by rapid endocytosis of the chemical signal by neighboring cells, its destruction by extracellular enzymes, or its immobilization by the extracellular matrix. The events that take place at the neuromuscular junction are excellent examples of paracrine signaling.

Soluble chemical signals interact with target cells via binding to surface or intracellular receptors

Four types of chemicals can serve as extracellular signaling molecules:
1. **Amines,** such as epinephrine
2. **Peptides and proteins,** such as angiotensin II and insulin
3. **Steroids,** including aldosterone, estrogens, and retinoic acid
4. **Other small molecules,** such as amino acids, nucleotides, ions (e.g., Ca^{2+}), and gases (e.g., nitric oxide)

For a molecule to act as a signal, it must bind to a **receptor.** Most receptors are proteins on the cell surface or within the cell that specifically bind a signaling molecule (the ligand) and induce a cellular response by interacting with an effector. In some cases, the receptor is itself the effector, as in ligand-gated ion channels. In most cases, however, interaction of the ligand with its receptor results in association of the receptor with one or more intracellular effector molecules that in turn initiate the cellular response. Effectors include enzymes, channels, transport proteins, contractile elements, and transcription factors. Receptors can be divided into five categories on the basis of their mechanisms of signal transduction.
1. **Ligand-gated ion channels.** Integral membrane proteins, these hybrid receptors/channels are involved in signaling between electrically excitable cells. The binding of a neurotransmitter such as ACh to its receptor results in transient opening of the channel and thus alters the ion permeability of the cell.
2. **G protein–coupled receptors.** These integral plasma-membrane proteins work through multiple intermediaries to activate or inactivate downstream effectors, such as membrane-associated enzymes or channels. This group of receptors is named for the initial intermediary, which is a heterotrimeric GTP-binding complex called a G protein.
3. **Catalytic receptors.** When activated by a ligand, these integral plasma-membrane proteins either add phosphate groups to their substrates—**kinases**—or remove substrate phosphate groups—**phosphatases.**
4. **Nuclear receptors.** These proteins, located in the cytosol or nucleus, are ligand-activated transcription factors. These receptors link extracellular signals to gene transcription.
5. **Receptors that undergo cleavage.** In response to ligand binding, some transmembrane proteins undergo **regulated intramembranous proteolysis (RIP),** creating fragments that signal a cellular response.

A ENDOCRINE

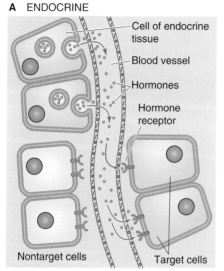

Cell of endocrine tissue

Blood vessel

Hormones

Hormone receptor

Nontarget cells

Target cells

B PARACRINE

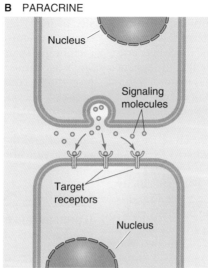

Nucleus

Signaling molecules

Target receptors

Nucleus

C AUTOCRINE

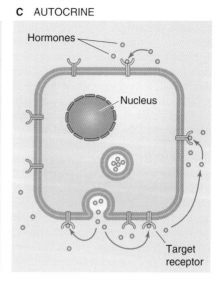

Hormones

Nucleus

Target receptor

Figure 3.1   Modes of intercellular communication.

Signaling events initiated by membrane-associated receptors can generally be divided into six steps:

Step 1: **Recognition** of the signal by its receptor. The same signaling molecule can sometimes bind to more than one kind of receptor via *ionic bonds, van der Waals* interactions, or *hydrophobic interactions.*

Step 2: **Transduction** of the extracellular message into an intracellular signal or **second messenger.**

Step 3: **Transmission** of the second messenger's signal to the appropriate effector, resulting in an amplification of the message or in its transmission to a distant region within the cell.

Step 4: **Modulation** of the expression or activity of effectors such as enzymes, ion channels, cytoskeletal components, and transcription factors.

Step 5: **Response** of the cell to the initial stimulus via summation and integration of input from multiple signaling pathways.

Step 6: **Termination** of the response by feedback mechanisms at any or all levels of the signaling pathway.

Cells can also communicate by direct interactions—juxtacrine signaling

Gap Junctions Neighboring cells can be electrically and metabolically coupled by means of gap junctions formed by the interaction of connexins in two closely apposed cell membranes. These water-filled channels facilitate the passage of inorganic ions and small molecules, such as Ca^{2+} and cyclic 3′,5′-adenosine monophosphate (cAMP), from the cytoplasm of one cell into the cytoplasm of an adjacent cell. Gap junctions are also excellent pathways for the flow of electrical current between adjacent cells, playing a critical role in cardiac and smooth muscle.

The permeability of gap junctions can be rapidly regulated by changes in cytosolic concentrations of Ca^{2+}, cAMP, and H^+ as well as by the voltage across the cell membrane or V_m.

Adhering and Tight Junctions ⊙ **3-2 Adhering junctions** form as the result of the Ca^{2+}-dependent interactions of the extracellular domains of transmembrane proteins called **cadherins** (see ⊙ 2-7). The clustering of cadherins at the site of interaction with an adjacent cell causes secondary clustering of intracellular proteins known as **catenins,** which in turn serve as sites of attachment for the intracellular **actin cytoskeleton.** In addition to playing a homeostatic role, adhering junctions can serve a signaling role during organ development and remodeling.

Similar to adhering junctions, **tight junctions** (see ⊙ 2-17) comprise transmembrane proteins that link with their counterparts on adjacent cells and with intracellular proteins to stabilize the complex and have a signaling role.

Membrane-Associated Ligands Another mechanism by which cells can directly communicate is the interaction of a receptor in the plasma membrane with a ligand that is itself a membrane protein on an adjacent cell. Such membrane-associated ligands can provide spatial clues in migrating cells. For example, an **ephrin** ligand (Eph) expressed on the surface of one cell can interact with an Eph receptor on a nearby cell to regulate such developmental events as axonal guidance in the nervous system and endothelial-cell guidance in the vasculature.

Ligands in the Extracellular Matrix Cells also receive input from their extracellular environment via cell-surface receptors that interact with the extracellular matrix. These receptors, called **integrins** (see ⊙ 2-6), have an extracellular domain that interacts with specific amino-acid sequences in collagen, fibronectin, and laminin proteins. The resulting conformational change in the integrin promotes the accumulation of a cluster of signaling molecules—called a **focal adhesion**—on the cytosolic side of the membrane. Focal adhesions regulate actin cytoskeletal anchoring and turnover, as well as intracellular kinases such as focal-adhesion kinase (FAK) and Src, which control such diverse processes as cell proliferation, cell migration, and cell differentiation.

Second-messenger systems amplify signals and integrate responses among cell types

Once a signal has been received at the cell surface, it is typically amplified and transmitted to specific sites within the cells via second messengers. For a molecule to function as a second messenger, its concentration, activation, and location must be finely regulated. The cell achieves this control by rapidly producing or activating the second messenger and then inactivating or degrading it. To ensure that the system returns to a resting state when the stimulus is removed, counterbalancing activities function at each step of the cascade.

An example of *creating* an active species would be G proteins that elicit the formation of the second messenger **cAMP** (see ◉ 3-8), whereas an example of *degrading* an active species would be G proteins that elicit the breakdown of a related second messenger, cGMP (see ◉ 3-5).

Second-messenger systems also allow both **specificity** and **diversity.** A single signaling molecule can produce distinct responses in different cells, depending on the complement of receptors and signal-transduction pathways that are available in the cell as well as the specialized function that the cell carries out in the organism. For example, ACh stimulates contraction of skeletal muscle cells, inhibits contraction of heart muscle cells, and facilitates the exocytosis of secretory granules by pancreatic acinar cells. These different end points are achieved by interacting with distinct receptors on each cell.

The diversity and specialization of second-messenger systems are important to a multicellular organism, as can be seen in the coordinated response of an organism to a stressful situation. Under these conditions, the adrenal gland releases epinephrine. Different organ systems respond to epinephrine in a distinct manner, such as activation of glycogen breakdown in the liver, constriction of the blood vessels of the skin, dilation of the blood vessels in skeletal muscle, dilation of airways in the lung, and increased rate and force of heart contraction. The overall effect is an **integrated response** that readies the organism for attack, defense, or escape. Integration of these stimuli requires **crosstalk** among the various signaling cascades.

Signal-transduction systems that project to the cell membrane or to the cytoplasm produce **nongenomic** effects, the focus of this chapter.

We will now discuss four of the five major classes of receptors.

RECEPTORS THAT ARE ION CHANNELS

The property that defines the ligand-gated ion channel class of multisubunit membrane-spanning receptors is that the signaling molecule itself controls the opening and closing of an ion channel by binding to a site on the receptor. Thus, these receptors are also called **ionotropic receptors** to distinguish them from the metabotropic receptors, which act via "metabolic" pathways. We will discuss this class of receptors in Chapter 6.

RECEPTORS COUPLED TO G PROTEINS

◉ **3-3 G protein–coupled receptors (GPCRs)** constitute the largest family of receptors on the cell surface, with >1000 members either known or predicted from genome sequences. GPCRs mediate cellular responses to a diverse array of signaling molecules. Despite the chemical diversity of their ligands, most receptors of this class have a similar structure: a single polypeptide chain with seven membrane-spanning α-helical segments, an extracellular N terminus that is glycosylated, a large cytoplasmic loop that is composed mainly of hydrophilic amino acids between helices 5 and 6, and a hydrophilic domain at the cytoplasmic C terminus. Binding of the GPCR to its extracellular ligand regulates this interaction between the receptor and the G proteins, thus transmitting a signal to downstream effectors.

GENERAL PROPERTIES OF G PROTEINS

G proteins are heterotrimers that exist in many combinations of different α, β, and γ subunits

G proteins are members of a superfamily of **GTP-binding proteins.** This superfamily includes the classic heterotrimeric G proteins that bind to GPCRs as well as the so-called small GTP-binding proteins, such as Ras. Both the heterotrimeric and small G proteins can hydrolyze GTP and switch between an active GTP-bound state and an inactive GDP-bound state.

Heterotrimeric G proteins are composed of three subunits, α, β, and γ. At least 18 different α subunits (~42 to 50 kDa), 5 β subunits (~33 to 35 kDa), and 12 γ subunits (~8 to 10 kDa) are present in mammalian tissue. The α subunit binds and hydrolyzes GTP and also interacts with "downstream" effector proteins such as adenylyl cyclase. The βγ complex also functions in signal transduction by interacting with effector molecules distinct from those regulated by the α subunits.

The multiple α, β, and γ subunits demonstrate distinct tissue distributions and interact with different receptors and effectors (Table 3.1). Because of the potential for several hundred combinations of the known α, β, and γ subunits, G proteins are ideally suited to link a diversity of receptors to a diversity of effectors. For example, when epinephrine binds $β_1$ adrenergic receptors in the heart, it *stimulates* adenylyl cyclase, which increases heart rate and the force of contraction. However, in the periphery, epinephrine acts on $α_2$ adrenergic receptors coupled to a G protein that *inhibits* adenylyl cyclase, thereby increasing peripheral vascular resistance and consequently increasing venous return and blood pressure.

Among the first effectors found to be sensitive to G proteins was the enzyme adenylyl cyclase. The heterotrimeric G protein known as G_s was so named because it stimulates adenylyl cyclase. A separate class of G proteins was given the name G_i because it is responsible for the ligand-dependent inhibition of adenylyl cyclase. The toxin from *Vibrio cholerae* activates G_s, whereas the toxin from *Bordetella pertussis* inactivates the cyclase-inhibiting G_i.

G protein activation follows a cycle

In their inactive state, heterotrimeric G proteins are a complex of α, β, and γ subunits, in which GDP occupies the guanine nucleotide–binding site of the α subunit. After ligand binding to the GPCR (Fig. 3.2, step 1), a

TABLE 3.1 Families of G Proteins

FAMILY/SUBUNIT	% IDENTITY	TOXIN	DISTRIBUTION	RECEPTOR	EFFECTOR/ROLE
G_s (α_s)					
$\alpha_{s(s)}$	100	CTX	Ubiquitous	β adrenergic, TSH, glucagon, others	↑ Adenylyl cyclase
$\alpha_{s(l)}$					↑ Ca^{2+} channel
α_{olf}	88	CTX	Olfactory epithelium	Odorant	↑ Adenylyl cyclase Open K^+ channel
G_i (α_i)					
α_{i1}	100	PTX	~Ubiquitous	M_2, α_2 adrenergic, others	↑ IP_3, DAG, Ca^{2+}, and AA, ↓ adenylyl cyclase
α_{i2}	88	PTX	Ubiquitous		
α_{i3}		PTX	~Ubiquitous		
α_{O1A}	73	PTX	Brain, others	Met-enkephalin, α_2 adrenergic, others	
α_{O1B}	73	PTX	Brain, others		
α_{t1}	68	PTX, CTX	Retinal rods	Rhodopsin	↑ cGMP-phosphodiesterase
α_{t2}	68	PTX, CTX	Retinal cones	Cone opsin	
α_g	67	PTX, CTX	Taste buds	Taste	
α_z	60		Brain, adrenal, platelet	?	↓ Adenylyl cyclase
G_q					
α_q	100		~Ubiquitous	M_1, α_1 adrenergic, others	↑ PLC β1, PLC β2, PLC β3
α_{11}	88		~Ubiquitous		
α_{14}	79		Lung, kidney, liver		
α_{15}	57		B cell, myeloid		
α_{16}	58		T cell, myeloid	Several receptors	↑ PLC β1, PLC β2, PLC β3
G_{12}					
α_{12}	100		Ubiquitous		
α_{13}	67		Ubiquitous		

CTX, Cholera toxin; *PTX,* pertussis toxin

conformational change in the receptor–G protein complex facilitates the release of bound GDP and simultaneous binding of GTP to the α subunit (see Fig. 3.2, step 2). This GDP-GTP exchange stimulates dissociation of the complex from the receptor (see Fig. 3.2, step 3) and causes disassembly of the trimer into a free GTP-bound α subunit and separate βγ complex (see Fig. 3.2, step 4). The GTP-bound α subunit interacts in the plane of the membrane with downstream effectors such as adenylyl cyclase and phospholipases (see Fig. 3.2, step 5), or cleavage of its myristoyl or palmitoyl group can release the α subunit from the membrane. Similarly, the βγ subunit can activate ion channels or other effectors.

The α subunit is itself an enzyme that catalyzes the hydrolysis of GTP to GDP and inorganic phosphate (P_i). The result is an *inactive* α-GDP complex that dissociates from its downstream effector and reassociates with a βγ subunit (see Fig. 3.2, step 6); this reassociation terminates signaling and brings the system back to resting state (see Fig. 3.2, step 1). The βγ subunit stabilizes α-GDP and thereby substantially slows the rate of GDP-GTP exchange (see Fig. 3.2, step 2) and dampens signal transmission in the resting state.

⊙ 3-4 Activated α subunits couple to a variety of downstream effectors, including enzymes and ion channels

Activated α subunits can couple to a variety of enzymes. A major enzyme that acts as an effector downstream of activated α subunits is **adenylyl cyclase** (Fig. 3.3A), which catalyzes the conversion of ATP to cAMP. This enzyme can be either activated or inhibited by G-protein signaling, depending on whether it associates with the GTP-bound form of $G\alpha_s$ (stimulatory) or $G\alpha_i$ (inhibitory).

⊙ 3-5 G proteins can also activate enzymes that break down cyclic nucleotides. For example, the G protein called **transducin** contains an α_t subunit that activates the **cGMP phosphodiesterase,** which in turn catalyzes the breakdown of cGMP to GMP (see Fig. 3.3B). This pathway plays a key role in phototransduction in the retina (see ⊙ 15-6).

⊙ 3-6 G proteins can also couple to **phospholipases**, which catabolize phospholipids. This superfamily of phospholipases can be grouped into phospholipases A_2, C, or D on the basis of the site at which the enzyme cleaves the phospholipid. G proteins that include the α_q subunit activate **phospholipase C,** which breaks phosphatidylinositol

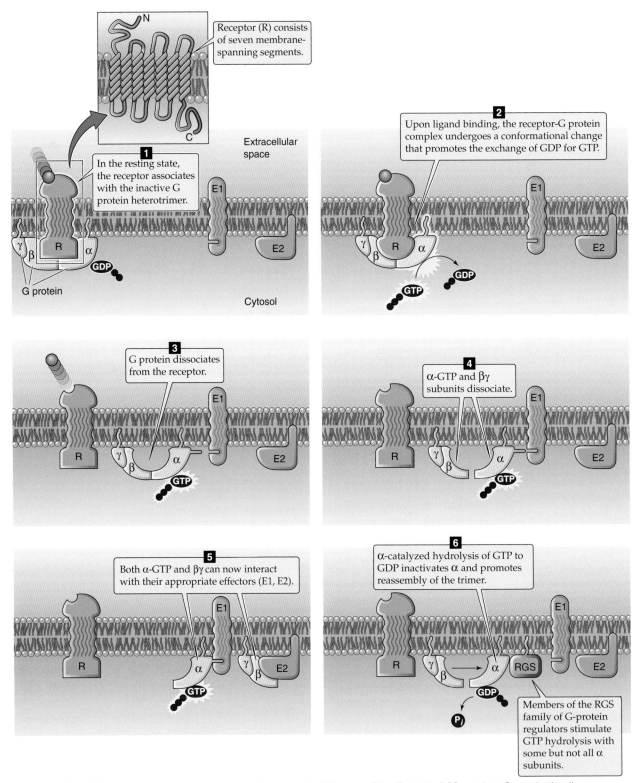

Figure 3.2 Enzymatic cycle of heterotrimeric G proteins. *E1,* Effector 1; *E2,* effector 2; *RGS,* regulator G protein signaling.

4,5-bisphosphate into two intracellular messengers, membrane-associated diacylglycerol and cytosolic IP$_3$ (see Fig. 3.3C). Diacylglycerol stimulates protein kinase C, whereas IP$_3$ binds to a receptor on the endoplasmic reticulum (ER) membrane and triggers the release of Ca^{2+} from intracellular stores.

Some G proteins interact with **ion channels.** Agonists that bind to the β adrenergic receptor activate the L-type Ca^{2+} channel (see ⊙ 7-5) in the heart and skeletal muscle. The α subunit of the G protein G$_s$ stimulates L-type Ca^{2+} channels both directly by binding to the channel, as well as indirectly by a signal-transduction cascade

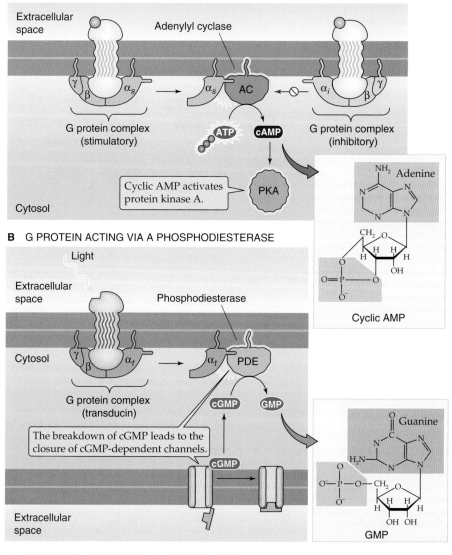

A G PROTEINS ACTING VIA ADENYLYL CYCLASE

Extracellular space

Adenylyl cyclase

γ β α_s

G protein complex (stimulatory)

α_s AC

α_i β γ

G protein complex (inhibitory)

ATP cAMP

Cyclic AMP activates protein kinase A.

PKA

Cytosol

NH₂ Adenine

Cyclic AMP

B G PROTEIN ACTING VIA A PHOSPHODIESTERASE

Light

Extracellular space

Phosphodiesterase

Cytosol

γ β α_t

G protein complex (transducin)

α_t PDE

cGMP GMP

The breakdown of cGMP leads to the closure of cGMP-dependent channels.

cGMP

Extracellular space

Guanine

GMP

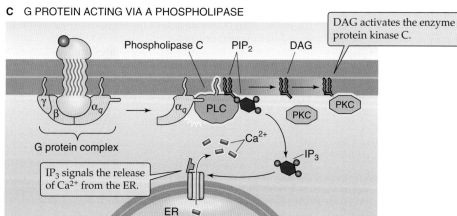

C G PROTEIN ACTING VIA A PHOSPHOLIPASE

Phospholipase C   PIP₂   DAG

DAG activates the enzyme protein kinase C.

γ β α_q

α_q PLC

PKC

PKC

G protein complex

Ca²⁺

IP₃

IP₃ signals the release of Ca²⁺ from the ER.

ER

Figure 3.3 Downstream effects of activated G-protein α subunits. *DAG*, diacylglycerol; *PIP*, 2, phosphatidylinositol 4, 5-bisphosphate; *PLC*, phospholipase C.

that involves cAMP-dependent phosphorylation of the channel.

⊙ 3-7 βγ subunits can activate downstream effectors

Following activation and disassociation of the heterotrimeric G protein, βγ subunits can also interact with downstream effectors. The neurotransmitter ACh

released from the vagus nerve reduces the rate and strength of heart contraction. This action in the atria of the heart is mediated by *muscarinic* M_2 AChRs, members of the GPCR family (see ⊙ **14-5**). Binding of ACh to the muscarinic M_2 receptor in the atria activates a heterotrimeric G protein, which results in the generation of both activated $G\alpha_i$ as well as a free βγ subunit complex. The βγ complex then interacts with a particular class of K^+

channels, increasing their permeability. This increase in K+ permeability keeps the membrane potential relatively negative and thus renders the cell more resistant to excitation. The βγ subunit complex also modulates the activity of adenylyl cyclase and phospholipase C and stimulates phospholipase A₂.

Some βγ complexes can bind to a special protein kinase called the β **adrenergic receptor kinase (βARK).** As a result of this interaction, βARK translocates to the plasma membrane, where it phosphorylates the ligand-receptor complex. This phosphorylation results in the recruitment of β-**arrestin** to the GPCR, which in turn mediates disassociation of the receptor-ligand complex and thus attenuates the activity of the same β adrenergic receptors that gave rise to the βγ complex in the first place. This action is an example of **receptor desensitization.** These phosphorylated receptors eventually undergo endocytosis, which transiently reduces the number of receptors that are available on the cell surface. This endocytosis is an important step in **resensitization** of the receptor system.

Small GTP-binding proteins are involved in a vast number of cellular processes

A distinct group of proteins that are structurally related to the α subunit of the heterotrimeric G proteins are the **small GTP-binding proteins.** More than 100 of these have been identified, and they have been divided into five groups: Ras, Rho, Rab, Arf, and Ran families. These 21-kDa proteins can be membrane associated (e.g., Ras) or may translocate between the membrane and the cytosol (e.g., Rho).

G-PROTEIN SECOND MESSENGERS: CYCLIC NUCLEOTIDES

⊙ 3-8 cAMP usually exerts its effect by increasing the activity of protein kinase A

Activation of Gs-coupled receptors results in the stimulation of **adenylyl cyclase,** which can cause [cAMP]ᵢ to rise 5-fold in ~5 seconds (see Fig. 3.3B). This sudden rise is counteracted by cAMP breakdown to AMP by **cAMP phosphodiesterase.** The downstream effects of this increase in [cAMP]ᵢ depend on the cellular microdomains in which [cAMP]ᵢ rises as well as the specialized functions that the responding cell carries out in the organism. For example, in the adrenal cortex, ACTH stimulation of cAMP production results in the secretion of aldosterone and cortisol (see ⊙ 50-6); in the kidney, a vasopressin-induced rise in cAMP levels facilitates water reabsorption (see ⊙ 38-4). Excess cAMP is also responsible for certain pathological conditions, such as **cholera.**

⊙ 3-9 cAMP exerts many of its effects through **cAMP-dependent protein kinaseA(PKA).** This enzyme catalyzes transfer of the terminal phosphate of ATP to specific **serine or threonine residues** on substrate proteins. PKA phosphorylation sites are present in a multitude of intracellular proteins, including ion channels, receptors, metabolic enzymes, and signaling pathway proteins. Phosphorylation of these sites can influence either the localization or the activity of the substrate.

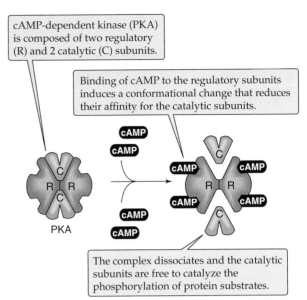

Figure 3.4   Activation of protein kinase A (PKA) by cyclic 3′,5′-adenosine monophosphate (cAMP).

To enhance regulation of phosphorylation events, the cell tightly controls the activity of PKA so that the enzyme can respond to subtle—and local—variations in cAMP levels. One important control mechanism is the use of **regulatory subunits** that constitutively inhibit PKA. In the absence of cAMP, two catalytic subunits of PKA associate with two of these regulatory subunits; the result is a heterotetrameric protein complex that has a low level of catalytic activity (Fig. 3.4). Binding of cAMP to the regulatory subunits induces a conformational change that diminishes their affinity for the catalytic subunits, and the subsequent dissociation of the complex results in activation of kinase activity. Not only can PKA activation have the short-term effects noted above but also the free catalytic subunit of PKA can enter the nucleus, where substrate phosphorylation can activate the transcription of specific PKA-dependent genes (see ⊙ 4-3). Although most cells use the same catalytic subunit, different regulatory subunits are found in different cell types.

Another mechanism that contributes to regulation of PKA is the targeting of the enzyme to specific subcellular locations. PKA targeting is achieved by the association of a PKA regulatory subunit with an **A-kinase anchoring protein (AKAP),** which in turn binds to cytoskeletal elements or to components of cellular subcompartments.

⊙ 3-10 Protein phosphatases reverse the action of kinases

As discussed previously, one way that the cell can terminate a cAMP signal is to use a phosphodiesterase to degrade cAMP. However, because the downstream effects of cAMP often involve phosphorylation of effector proteins at serine and threonine residues by kinases such as PKA, another powerful way to terminate the action of cAMP is to dephosphorylate these effector proteins. Such dephosphorylation events are mediated by enzymes called serine/threonine phosphoprotein phosphatases.

Four groups of **serine/threonine phosphoprotein phosphatases (PPs)** are known: 1, 2a, 2b, and 2c. These enzymes themselves are regulated by phosphorylation at their serine, threonine,

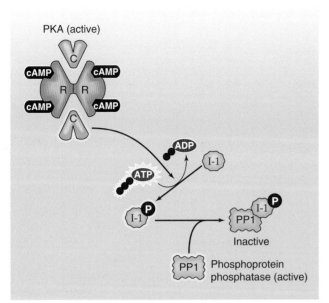

Figure 3.5   Inactivation of phosphoprotein phosphatase 1 (PP1) by protein kinase A (PKA).

and tyrosine residues. The balance between kinase and phosphatase activity plays a major role in the control of signaling events.

PP1 dephosphorylates many proteins phosphorylated by PKA, including those phosphorylated in response to epinephrine (see Fig. 58.3). Another protein, **phosphoprotein-phosphatase inhibitor1(I-1),** can bind to and inhibit PP1. Interestingly, PKA phosphorylates and induces I-1 binding to PP1 (Fig. 3.5), thereby inhibiting PP1 and preserving the phosphate groups added by PKA in the first place.

PP2a, which is less specific than PP1, appears to be the main phosphatase responsible for reversing the action of other protein serine/threonine kinases. The Ca^{2+}-dependent **PP2b,** also known as **calcineurin,** is prevalent in the brain, muscle, and immune cells and is also the pharmacological target of the immunosuppressive reagents FK-506 (tacrolimus) and cyclosporine.

 3-11 In addition to serine/threonine kinases such as PKA, a second group of kinases involved in regulating signaling pathways (see 3-24) are **tyrosine kinases** that phosphorylate their substrate proteins on tyrosine residues. The enzymes that remove phosphates from these tyrosine residues—**phosphotyrosine phosphatases (PTPs)**—are much more variable than the serine and threonine phosphatases. A number of intracellular PTPs contain **Src homology 2 (SH2) domains,** a peptide sequence or motif that interacts with phosphorylated tyrosine groups and thus acts to recruit the phosphatase to its target substrate. Many of the PTPs are themselves regulated by phosphorylation.

G-PROTEIN SECOND MESSENGERS: PRODUCTS OF PHOSPHOINOSITIDE BREAKDOWN

Many messengers bind to receptors that activate phosphoinositide breakdown

 3-12 Although the **phosphatidylinositols (PIs)** are minor constituents of cell membranes, they are largely distributed in the internal leaflet of the membrane and play an important

role in signal transduction. The two major phosphoinositides involved in signal transduction are: **phosphatidylinositol 4,5-bisphosphate (PI(4,5)P2 or PIP2)** and phosphatidylinositol 3,4,5-trisphosphate (PI(3,4,5)P3 or PIP3; see 3-26).

 3-13 Certain membrane-associated receptors act through G proteins (e.g., G_q) that stimulate phospholipase C (PLC) to cleave PIP$_2$ into **inositol 1,4,5-trisphosphate (or IP$_3$)** and **diacylglycerol (DAG),** as shown in Fig. 3.6A. PLCs are classified into three families (β, γ, δ) that differ in their catalytic properties, cell-type–specific expression, and modes of activation. PLCβ is typically activated downstream of certain G proteins (e.g., G_q), whereas PLCγ contains an SH2 domain and is activated downstream of certain tyrosine kinases. Stimulation of PLCβ results in a rapid increase in cytosolic IP$_3$ levels as well as an *early* peak in DAG levels (see Fig. 3.6B). Both products are second messengers. The water-soluble IP$_3$ travels through the cytosol to stimulate Ca^{2+} release from intracellular stores (see next section). DAG remains in the plane of the membrane to activate protein kinase C, which migrates from the cytosol and binds to DAG in the membrane (see 3-17).

Phosphatidylcholines (PCs), which—unlike PI—are an abundant phospholipid in the cell membrane, are also a source of DAG. The cell can produce DAG from PC by either of two mechanisms (see Fig. 3.6C). First, PLC can directly convert PC to phosphocholine and DAG. Second, **phospholipase D (PLD),** by cleaving the phosphoester bond on the other side of the phosphate, can convert PC to choline and phosphatidic acid (PA; also phospho-DAG). This PA can then be converted to DAG via PA-phosphohydrolase.

IP$_3$ liberates Ca^{2+} from intracellular stores

 3-14 As discussed in Chapter 5 (see Fig. 5.9), three major transport mechanisms keep free intracellular Ca^{2+} ($[Ca^{2+}]_i$) below ~100 nM. Increases in $[Ca^{2+}]_i$ from this extremely low baseline allow Ca^{2+} to function as an important second messenger. IP$_3$ generated by the metabolism of membrane phospholipids travels through the cytosol and binds to the IP$_3$ receptor, a ligand-gated Ca^{2+} channel located in the membrane of the *endoplasmic* reticulum (see Fig. 3.6A). The result is a release of Ca^{2+} from intracellular stores and a rise in $[Ca^{2+}]_i$. The **IP3 receptor (ITPR)** is a tetramer composed of subunits of ~260 kDa. The receptor is a substrate for phosphorylation by protein kinases A and C as well as calcium-calmodulin (Ca^{2+}-CaM)–dependent protein kinases.

Structurally related to ITPRs are the Ca^{2+}-release channels known as **ryanodine receptors (RYRs;** see 9-3). Because cytosolic Ca^{2+} activates RYRs, these channels play an important role in elevating $[Ca^{2+}]_i$ in certain cells by a process known as **calcium-induced Ca^{2+} release (CICR;** see 9-11). RYRs are responsible for releasing Ca^{2+} from the *sarcoplasmic* reticulum of muscle and thereby switching on muscle contraction (see 9-2).

$[Ca^{2+}]_i$ can increase as the result not only of Ca^{2+} release from intracellular stores but also of enhanced influx through Ca^{2+} channels in the plasma membrane.

The same mechanisms that normally keep $[Ca^{2+}]_i$ at extremely low levels (see Fig. 5.9) are also responsible for reversing the increases in $[Ca^{2+}]_i$ that occur during signaling events. Increases in $[Ca^{2+}]_i$ activate a Ca pump, the sarcoplasmic and endoplasmic reticulum Ca-ATPase (SERCA; see 5-11) that begins pumping Ca^{2+} back into the ER. In

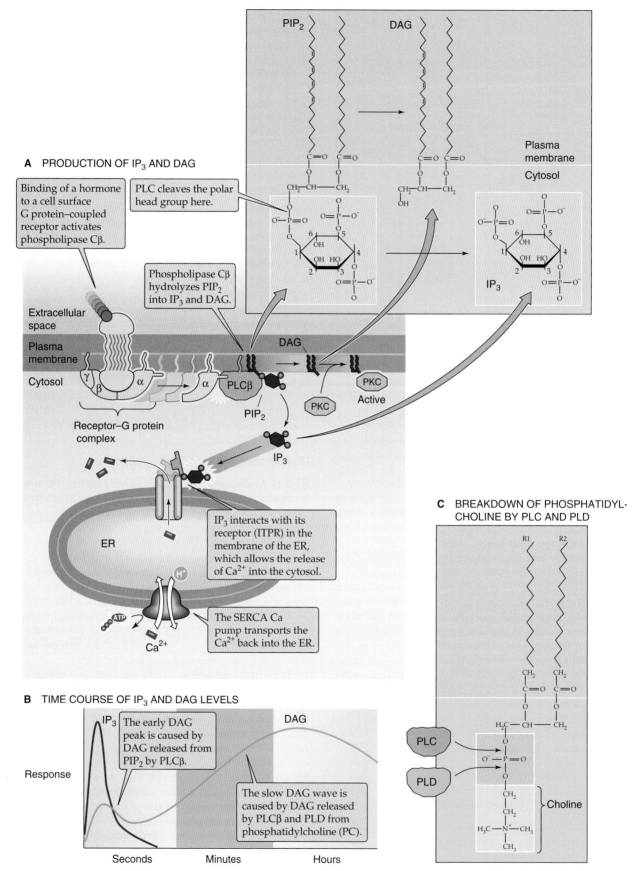

A PRODUCTION OF IP₃ AND DAG

Binding of a hormone to a cell surface G protein–coupled receptor activates phospholipase Cβ.

PLC cleaves the polar head group here.

Phospholipase Cβ hydrolyzes PIP₂ into IP₃ and DAG.

IP₃ interacts with its receptor (ITPR) in the membrane of the ER, which allows the release of Ca²⁺ into the cytosol.

The SERCA Ca pump transports the Ca²⁺ back into the ER.

B TIME COURSE OF IP₃ AND DAG LEVELS

The early DAG peak is caused by DAG released from PIP₂ by PLCβ.

The slow DAG wave is caused by DAG released by PLCβ and PLD from phosphatidylcholine (PC).

C BREAKDOWN OF PHOSPHATIDYL-CHOLINE BY PLC AND PLD

Figure 3.6 Second messengers in the diacylglycerol/ (DAG/IP₃) pathway. *ER*, Endoplasmic reticulum; *SERCA*, sarcoplasmic and endoplasmic reticulum Ca-ATPase.

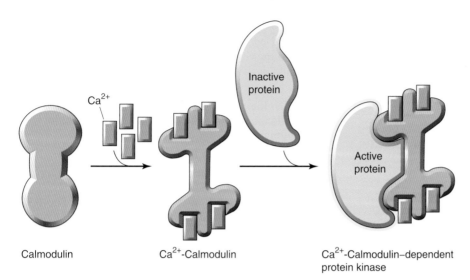

Figure 3.7 Calmodulin (CaM). After four intracellular Ca^{2+} ions bind to CaM, the Ca^{2+}-CaM complex can bind to and activate another protein. In this example, the activated protein is a Ca^{2+}-CaM–dependent kinase.

Calmodulin Ca^{2+}-Calmodulin Ca^{2+}-Calmodulin–dependent protein kinase

Inactive protein

Active protein

Ca^{2+}

addition, a Ca pump (see ◉ 5-10) and Na-Ca exchanger (see Fig. 5.8A) at the plasma membrane extrude excess Ca^{2+} from the cell. These processes are much slower than Ca^{2+} release, so $[Ca^{2+}]_i$ remains high until IP_3 is dephosphorylated, terminating Ca^{2+} release via ITPR and thereby allowing the transporters to restore $[Ca^{2+}]_i$ to basal levels.

Calcium activates calmodulin-dependent protein kinases

◉ **3-15** The effects of changes in $[Ca^{2+}]_i$ are mediated by Ca^{2+}-binding proteins, the most important of which is **calmodulin (CaM).** CaM is a high-affinity cytoplasmic Ca^{2+}-binding protein of 148 amino acids. Each molecule of CaM cooperatively binds four calcium ions. Ca^{2+} binding induces a major conformational change in CaM that allows it to bind to other proteins (Fig. 3.7).

◉ **3-16** Many of the effects of CaM occur as the Ca^{2+}-CaM complex binds to and activates a family of Ca^{2+}-CaM–dependent kinases known as **CaM kinases (CaMKs).** These kinases phosphorylate specific serine and threonine residues of a variety of proteins. An important CaMK in smooth-muscle cells is myosin light-chain kinase (MLCK) (see ◉ 9-14). Another CaMK is glycogen phosphorylase kinase (PK), which plays a role in glycogen degradation (see ◉ 58-10).

DAGs and Ca^{2+} activate protein kinase C

◉ **3-17** As noted above, hydrolysis of PIP_2 by PLC yields not only the IP_3 that leads to Ca^{2+} release from internal stores but also DAG (see Fig. 3.6A). The most important function of DAG is to activate **protein kinase C (PKC),** an intracellular serine/threonine kinase. In mammals, the PKC family comprises at least 15 members that differ in their tissue and cellular localization. This family is further subdivided into three groups that all require membrane-associated phosphatidylserine but have different requirements for Ca^{2+} and DAG. The *classical* PKC family members PKCα, PKCβ, and PKCγ require both DAG and Ca^{2+} for activation, whereas the *novel* PKCs (such as PKCδ, PKCε, and PKCη) require DAG but are independent of Ca^{2+}, and the *atypical* PKCs (PKCζ and PKCλ) appear to be independent of both DAG and Ca^{2+}.

As a consequence, the signals generated by the PKC pathway depend on the isoforms of the enzyme that a cell expresses as well as on the levels of Ca^{2+} and DAG at specific locations at the cell membrane.

In its basal state, PKCα is an inactive, soluble cytosolic protein. When a GPCR activates PLC, both DAG (generated in the inner leaflet of the plasma membrane) and Ca^{2+} (released in response to IP_3) bind to the PKC regulatory domain; this results in translocation of PKCα to the membrane and activation of the PKC kinase domain. Even though the initial Ca^{2+} signal is transient, PKCα activation can be sustained, resulting in activation of physiological responses, such as proliferation and differentiation. Elevated levels of active PKCα are maintained by a slow wave of elevated DAG (see Fig. 3.6B), which is due to the hydrolysis of PC by PLC and PLD.

PKC can also directly or indirectly modulate transcription factors and thereby enhance the transcription of specific genes (see ◉ 4-1). Such genomic actions of PKC explain why phorbol esters are tumor promoters.

G PROTEIN SECOND MESSENGERS: ARACHIDONIC ACID METABOLITES

In addition to DAG, other hydrolysis products of membrane phospholipids can act as signaling molecules. The best characterized of these hydrolysis products is **arachidonic acid (AA).** Phospholipase A_2 initiates the cellular actions of AA by releasing this fatty acid from glycerol-based phospholipids. A series of enzymes subsequently convert AA into a family of biologically active metabolites that are collectively called **eicosanoids** because, like AA, they all have 20 carbon atoms. Three major pathways can convert AA into these eicosanoids (Figs. 3.8 and 3.9). In the first pathway, cyclooxygenase (COX) enzymes produce *thromboxanes (TXs), prostaglandins (PGs),* and *prostacyclins.* In the second pathway, 5-lipoxygenase enzymes produce *leukotrienes (LTs)* and some *hydroxyeicosatetraenoic acid (HETE)* compounds. In the third pathway, the epoxygenase enzymes, which are members of the cytochrome P-450 class, produce other *HETE* compounds as well as *cis-epoxyeicosatrienoic*

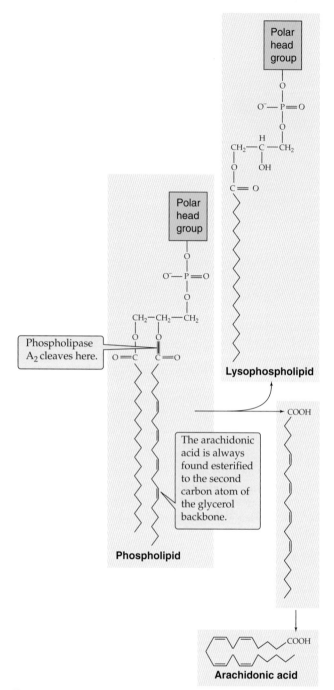

Figure 3.8 Release of arachidonic acid (AA) from membrane phospholipids by phospholipase A_2 (PLA$_2$). AA is esterified to membrane phospholipids at the second carbon of the glycerol backbone. PLA$_2$ cleaves the phospholipid at the indicated position and releases AA as well as a lysophospholipid.

acid (EET) compounds. Eicosanoids have powerful biological activities, including effects on allergic and inflammatory processes, platelet aggregation, vascular smooth muscle, and gastric acid secretion.

Phospholipase A_2 is the primary enzyme responsible for releasing AA

The first step in the **phospholipase A2 (PLA2)** signal-transduction cascade is binding of an extracellular agonist

to a membrane receptor (see Fig. 3.9). Once the receptor is occupied by its agonist, it can activate a G protein that belongs to the G_i/G_o family. The result is rapid hydrolysis of phospholipids that contain AA.

⊙ 3-18 Cyclooxygenases, lipoxygenases, and epoxygenases mediate the formation of biologically active eicosanoids

Once it is released from the membrane, AA can diffuse out of the cell, be reincorporated into membrane phospholipids, or be metabolized (see Fig. 3.9).

In the first pathway of AA metabolism (see Fig. 3.9), **cyclooxygenases** catalyze the stepwise conversion of AA into the intermediates prostaglandin G_2 (PGG$_2$) and prostaglandin H_2 (PGH$_2$). PGH$_2$ is the precursor of the other **prostaglandins,** the **prostacyclins** and the **thromboxanes.**

In the second pathway of AA metabolism, **5-lipoxygenase** initiates the conversion of AA into biologically active **leukotrienes.** For example, in myeloid cells, 5-lipoxygenase converts AA to 5-hydroperoxyeicosatetraenoic acid (5-HPETE), which is short lived and rapidly degraded by a peroxidase to the corresponding alcohol 5-HETE. Alternatively, a dehydrase can convert 5-HPETE to an unstable epoxide, leukotriene A_4 (LTA$_4$), which can be either further metabolized by LTA$_4$ hydrolase to LTB$_4$ or coupled ("conjugated") by LTC$_4$ synthase to the tripeptide glutathione (see ⊙ 46-5). This conjugation—via the cysteine residue of glutathione—yields LTC$_4$.

The third pathway of AA metabolism begins with the transformation of AA by **epoxygenase** (a cytochrome P-450 oxidase). Molecular O_2 is a substrate in this reaction. The epoxygenase pathway converts AA into two major products, **HETEs** and **EETs.**

Prostaglandins, prostacyclins, and thromboxanes (cyclooxygenase products) are vasoactive, regulate platelet action, and modulate ion transport

⊙ **3-19** The metabolism of PGH$_2$ to generate selected prostanoid derivatives is cell specific. For example, platelets convert PGH$_2$ to **thromboxane A2 (TXA2),** a short-lived compound that can aggregate platelets, bring about the platelet release reaction, and constrict small blood vessels. In contrast, endothelial cells convert PGH$_2$ to **prostacyclin I2 (PGI2),** which *inhibits* platelet aggregation and *dilates* blood vessels. Many cell types convert PGH$_2$ to prostaglandins. Acting locally in a paracrine or autocrine fashion, **prostaglandins** are involved in such processes as platelet aggregation, airway constriction, renin release, and inflammation. **Nonsteroidal anti-inflammatory drugs (NSAIDs)** such as aspirin, acetaminophen, ibuprofen, indomethacin, and naproxen directly target cyclooxygenase. NSAID inhibition of cyclooxygenase is a useful tool in the treatment of inflammation and fever and, at least in the case of aspirin, in the prevention of heart disease.

The leukotrienes (5-lipoxygenase products) play a major role in inflammatory responses

Many lipoxygenase metabolites of AA have a role in allergic and inflammatory diseases (Table 3.2). LTB$_4$ is produced by inflammatory cells such as neutrophils and

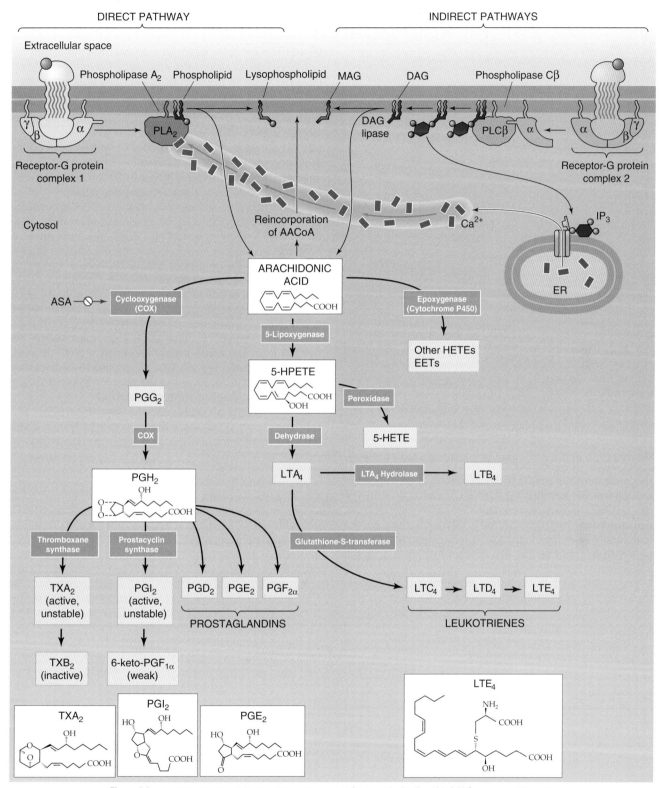

Figure 3.9 Arachidonic acid (AA) signaling pathways. *ASA*, acetylsalicylic acid; *MAG*, monoacylglycerol.

macrophages. The cysteinyl leukotrienes, including **LTC4** and **LTE4**, are synthesized by mast cells, basophils, and eosinophils, cells that are commonly associated with allergic inflammatory responses such as **asthma** and **urticaria.**

The HETEs and EETs (epoxygenase product) tend to enhance Ca²⁺ release from intracellular stores and to enhance cell proliferation The epoxygenase pathway leads to the production of HETEs other than 5-HETE as well as EETs. HETEs and EETs have been implicated in a wide variety of processes. For

TABLE 3.2 Involvement of Leukotrienes in Human Disease

DISEASE	EVIDENCE
Asthma	Bronchoconstriction from inhaled LTE_4; identification of LTC_4, LTD_4, and LTE_4 in serum or urine or both
Psoriasis	Detection of LTB_4 and LTE_2 in fluids from psoriatic lesions
Adult respiratory distress syndrome (ARDS)	Elevated levels of LTB_4 in plasma
Allergic rhinitis	Elevated levels of LTB_4 in nasal fluids
Gout	Detection of LTB_4 in joint fluid
Rheumatoid arthritis	Elevated levels of LTB_4 in joint fluids and serum
Inflammatory bowel disease (ulcerative colitis and Crohn disease)	Identification of LTB_4 in gastrointestinal fluids and LTE_4 in urine

example, in smooth-muscle cells, **HETEs** increase proliferation and migration; these AA metabolites may be one of the primary factors involved in the formation of atherosclerotic plaque. In blood vessels, HETEs can be potent vasoconstrictors. In blood vessels, **EETs** primarily induce vasodilation and angiogenesis, although they have vasoconstrictive properties in the smaller pulmonary blood vessels.

Degradation of the eicosanoids terminates their activity

Inactivation of the products of eicosanoids is an important mechanism for terminating their biological action. In the case of COX products, the enzyme 15-hydroxyprostaglandin dehydrogenase catalyzes the initial reactions that convert biologically active prostaglandins into their inactive 15-keto metabolites. This enzyme also appears to be active in the catabolism of thromboxanes.

As far as the 5-lipoxygenase products are concerned, the specificity and cellular distribution of the enzymes that metabolize leukotrienes parallel the diversity of the enzymes involved in their synthesis.

The metabolic breakdown of the HETE and EET products of epoxygenase is rapid but complex.

RECEPTORS THAT ARE CATALYTIC

A number of hormones and growth factors bind to cell-surface proteins that have—or are associated with—enzymatic activity on the cytoplasmic side of the membrane. Here we discuss five classes of such catalytic receptors (Fig. 3.10):

1. **Receptor guanylyl cyclases** catalyze the generation of cGMP from GTP.
2. **Receptor serine/threonine kinases** phosphorylate serine or threonine residues on cellular proteins
3. **Receptor tyrosine kinases(RTKs)** phosphorylate tyrosine residues on themselves and other proteins.
4. ◉ **3-20 Tyrosine kinase–associated receptors** interact with cytosolic (i.e., not membrane-bound) tyrosine kinases.

5. **Receptor tyrosine phosphatases** cleave phosphate groups from tyrosine groups of cellular proteins.

◉ 3-21 The receptor guanylyl cyclase transduces the activity of atrial natriuretic peptide, whereas a soluble guanylyl cyclase transduces the activity of nitric oxide

Receptor (Membrane-Bound) Guanylyl Cyclase Some of the best-characterized examples of a transmembrane protein with guanylyl cyclase activity (see Fig. 3.10A) are the receptors for the natriuretic peptides. These ligands are a family of related small proteins (~28 amino acids) including **atrial natriuretic peptide (ANP),** B-type or brain natriuretic peptide (BNP), and C-type natriuretic peptide (CNP).

Natriuretic peptide receptors NPRA and NPRB are proteins with an extracellular ligand-binding domain and a single membrane-spanning segment (see Fig. 3.10A). The intracellular domain has two consensus catalytic domains for guanylyl cyclase activity. Binding of ANP to its receptor causes the conversion of GTP to cGMP and raises intracellular levels of cGMP. In turn, cGMP activates a **cGMP-dependent kinase** (PKG or cGK) that phosphorylates proteins at certain serine and threonine residues.

Soluble Guanylyl Cyclase ◉ **3-22** In contrast to the receptor guanylyl cyclase, which is activated by ANP, the cytosolic soluble guanylyl cyclase (sGC) is activated by **nitric oxide (NO).** This sGC is unrelated to the receptor guanylyl cyclase and contains a heme moiety that binds NO.

◉ **3-23** NO is a highly reactive, short-lived free radical. This dissolved gas arises from a family of **NO synthase (NOS)** enzymes that catalyze the reaction

$$L\text{-arginine} + 1.5\ NADPH + H^+ + 2O_2 \qquad (3\text{-}1)$$
$$\rightarrow NO + citrulline + 1.5\ NADP^+$$

The NOS family includes neuronal or nNOS (NOS1), inducible or iNOS (NOS2), and endothelial or eNOS (NOS3). nNOS and iNOS are soluble enzymes, whereas eNOS is linked to the plasma membrane. The activation of NOS begins as an extracellular agonist (e.g., ACh) binds to a plasma-membrane receptor, triggering the entry of Ca^{2+}, which binds to cytosolic CaM and then stimulates NOS. In smooth muscle, NO stimulates the sGC, which then converts GTP to cGMP, activating PKG, which leads to smooth-muscle relaxation.

The importance of NO in the control of blood flow had long been exploited unwittingly to treat **angina pectoris.** Angina is the classic chest pain that accompanies inadequate blood flow to the heart muscle, usually as a result of coronary artery atherosclerosis. Nitroglycerin relieves this pain by spontaneously breaking down and releasing NO, which relaxes the smooth muscles of peripheral arterioles, thereby reducing the work of the heart and relieving the associated pain.

Some catalytic receptors are serine/threonine kinases

We have already discussed how activation of various G protein–linked receptors can initiate a cascade that eventually activates kinases (e.g., PKA, PKC) that phosphorylate proteins at serine and threonine residues. In addition, some receptors are *themselves* serine/threonine kinases—such as the one for transforming growth factor-β (TGF-β)—and are thus catalytic receptors.

The receptors for TGF-β and related factors are glycoproteins with a single membrane-spanning segment and intrinsic

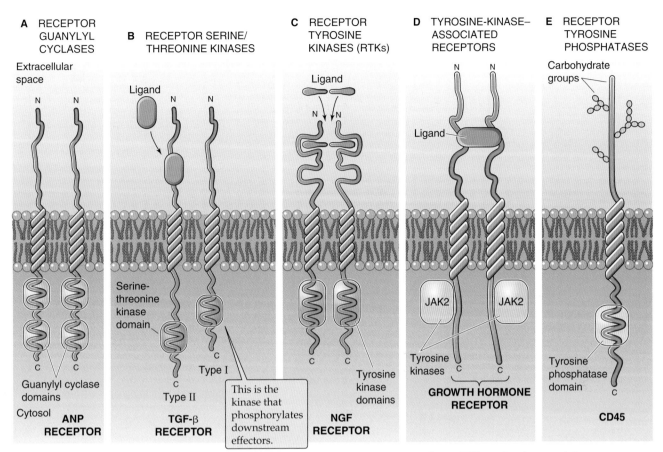

A RECEPTOR GUANYLYL CYCLASES

Extracellular space

N N

Guanylyl cyclase domains

Cytosol **ANP RECEPTOR**

B RECEPTOR SERINE/ THREONINE KINASES

Ligand

N N

Serine-threonine kinase domain

C

Type I

C

Type II

TGF-β RECEPTOR

This is the kinase that phosphorylates downstream effectors.

C RECEPTOR TYROSINE KINASES (RTKs)

Ligand

N N

C C

Tyrosine kinase domains

NGF RECEPTOR

D TYROSINE-KINASE– ASSOCIATED RECEPTORS

N N

Ligand

JAK2 JAK2

Tyrosine kinases

C C

GROWTH HORMONE RECEPTOR

E RECEPTOR TYROSINE PHOSPHATASES

Carbohydrate groups

Tyrosine phosphatase domain

C

CD45

Figure 3.10 Catalytic receptors. *ANP,* Atrial natriuretic peptide; *NGF,* nerve growth factor; *TGF,* transforming growth factor.

serine/threonine-kinase activity. Receptor types I and II (see Fig. 3.10B) are required for ligand binding and catalytic activity. The **type II receptor** first binds the ligand, and this binding is followed by the formation of a stable ternary complex of ligand, type II receptor, and type I receptor. After recruitment of the **type I receptor** into the complex, the type II receptor phosphorylates the type I receptor, thereby activating the serine/threonine kinase activity of the type I receptor.

⊙ 3-24 RTKs produce phosphotyrosine motifs recognized by SH2 and phosphotyrosine-binding domains of downstream effectors

In addition to the class of receptors with intrinsic *serine/threonine* kinase activity, other plasma-membrane receptors have intrinsic *tyrosine* kinase activity. All RTKs phosphorylate themselves in addition to other cellular proteins. Epidermal growth factor (EGF), platelet-derived growth factor (PDGF), vascular endothelial growth factor (VEGF), insulin and insulin-like growth factor type 1 (IGF-1), fibroblast growth factor (FGF), and nerve growth factor (NGF) can all bind to receptors that possess intrinsic tyrosine kinase activity.

Creation of Phosphotyrosine Motifs Most RTKs are single-pass transmembrane proteins that have an extracellular ligand-binding domain and a single intracellular kinase domain (see Fig. 3.10C). Binding of a ligand, such as NGF, facilitates the formation of receptor dimers that in turn promote the direct association and transphosphorylation of the adjacent kinase domains; the result is activation of the receptor complex. The activated receptors then catalyze the addition of phosphate

to tyrosine (Y) residues on the receptor itself as well as specific membrane-associated and cytoplasmic proteins. The resulting **phosphotyrosine (pY) motifs** serve as high-affinity binding sites for the recruitment of a number of intracellular signaling molecules, discussed in the next paragraph. These interactions lead to the formation of a signaling complex and the activation of downstream effectors.

Recognition of pY Motifs by SH2 and Phosphotyrosine-Binding Domains The pY motifs created by tyrosine kinases serve as high-affinity binding sites for the recruitment of cytoplasmic or membrane-associated proteins that contain either an **SH2 domain** or **PTB (phosphotyrosine-binding) domain.**

In contrast to SH2 and PTB domains, which interact with highly regulated pY motifs, **Src homology 3 (SH3)** domains interact constitutively with proline-rich regions in other proteins in a manner that does not require phosphorylation of the motif.

The MAPK Pathway ⊙ 3-25 A common pathway by which activated RTKs transduce their signal to cytosol and even to the nucleus is a cascade of events that includes the increased activity of the small GTP-binding protein Ras and culminate in mitogen-activated protein-kinases (MAPKs). This signaling pathway involves the steps shown in Fig. 3.11.

The Phosphatidylinositol-3-Kinase Pathway ⊙ 3-26 The **phosphatidylinositol-3-kinase (PI3K)** is an SH2 domain–containing protein that commonly signals downstream of RTKs. PI3K is a heterodimer consisting of a p85 regulatory subunit and p110 catalytic subunit. p110 is a lipid kinase that phosphorylates PIP_2 (see ⊙ 3-12) on the 3 position of the inositol ring to form PIP_3.

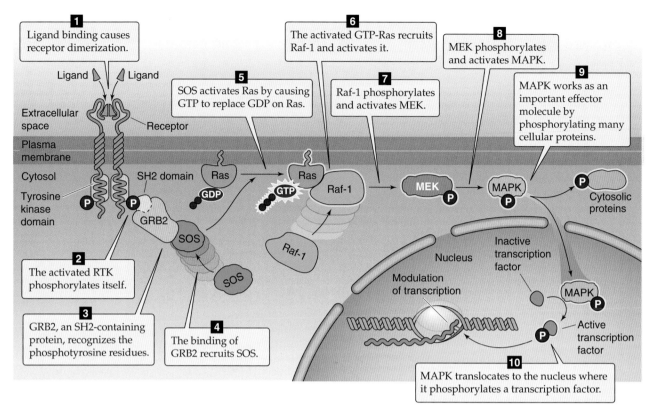

Figure 3.11 Regulation of transcription by the Ras pathway.

Following RTK activation, the newly recruited PI3K produces PIP$_3$ locally in the membrane, where it serves as a binding site for proteins such as 3-phosphoinositide–dependent kinase 1 (PDK1) and PKC (see ⊙ **3-17**). The events downstream of the insulin receptor are a good examples of PDK1 signaling (see Fig. 51.3).

Tyrosine kinase–associated receptors activate cytosolic tyrosine kinases such as Src and JAK

⊙ **3-27** Some of the receptors for cytokines and growth factors that regulate cell proliferation and differentiation do not themselves have *intrinsic* tyrosine kinase activity but can associate with nonreceptor tyrosine kinases (see Fig. 3.10D). Receptors in this class include those for several cytokines, including IL-2, IL-3, IL-4, IL-5, IL-6, leukemia inhibitory factor (LIF), granulocyte-macrophage colony-stimulating factor (GM-CSF), and erythropoietin (EPO). The family also includes receptors for growth hormone (GH), prolactin (PRL), leptin, ciliary neurotrophin factor (CNTF), oncostatin M, and interferon-α (IFN-α), IFN-β, and IFN-γ.

The **tyrosine kinase–associated receptors** typically comprise multiple subunits that form homodimers (αα), heterodimers (αβ), or heterotrimers (αβγ). None of the cytoplasmic portions of the receptor subunits contain kinase domains or other sequences with recognized catalytic function. Instead, tyrosine kinases of the **Src family** and **Janus family** (JAK or Janus kinases) associate noncovalently with the cytoplasmic domains of these receptors. Thus, these are **receptor-associated tyrosine kinases.** Ligand binding to these receptors results in receptor dimerization and activation of the associated tyrosine kinase. The activated kinase then phosphorylates tyrosines on both itself and the receptor.

Thus, tyrosine kinase–associated receptors, together with their tyrosine kinases, function much like the RTKs discussed previously.

Receptor tyrosine phosphatases are required for lymphocyte activation

Tyrosine residues that are phosphorylated by the tyrosine kinases described in the preceding two sections are *de*phosphorylated by PTPs, which can be either cytosolic or membrane spanning (i.e., the receptor tyrosine phosphatases). Both classes of *tyrosine* phosphatases have structures very different from the ones that dephosphorylate *serine* and *threonine* residues. Because the tyrosine phosphatases are highly active, pY groups tend to have a short half-life and are relatively few in number in unstimulated cells.

⊙ 3-28 NUCLEAR RECEPTORS

Steroid and thyroid hormones enter the cell and bind to members of the nuclear receptor superfamily in the cytoplasm or nucleus

A number of important signaling molecules produce their effects not by binding to receptors on the cell membrane but by binding to **nuclear receptors (NRs)**—also called intracellular receptors—that can act as transcription regulators, a concept that we will discuss in more depth in Chapter 4. This family includes receptors for steroid hormones, vitamin D, thyroid hormones, and retinoic acid (Table 3.3). In addition, this family includes related receptors, known as orphan receptors, whose ligands have yet to be identified. Steroid hormones,

TABLE 3.3 Nuclear Receptors

RECEPTOR	FULL NAME	DIMERIC ARRANGEMENT
GR	Glucocorticoid receptor	GR/GR
MR	Mineralocorticoid receptor	MR/MR
PR	Progesterone receptor	PR/PR
ERα, ERβ	Estrogen receptors	ER/ER
AR	Androgen receptor	AR/AR
VDR	Vitamin D receptor	VDR/RXR
TR	Thyroid hormone receptor	TR/RXR
RAR	Retinoic acid receptor	RAR/RXR
PPARα, PPARγ, PPARδ	Peroxisome proliferation–activated receptors α, γ, δ	PPAR/RXR
FXR	Bile acid receptor	FXR/RXR
LXR	Liver X receptor	LXR/RXR
SXR (or PXR)	Steroid and xenobiotic receptor (pregnane X receptor)	SXR/RXR
CAR	Constitutive androstane receptor	CAR/RXR

RXR, Retinoid X receptor.

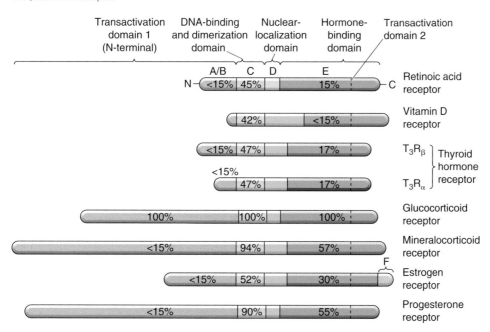

Figure 3.12 Modular construction of intracellular (or nuclear) receptors. The percentages listed inside the A/B, C, and E domains refer to the degrees of amino-acid identity, referenced to the glucocorticoid receptor.

vitamin D, and retinoic acid appear to enter the cell by diffusing through the lipid phase of the cell membrane. Thyroid hormones, which are charged amino-acid derivatives, may cross the cell membrane either by diffusion or by carrier-mediated transport. Once inside the cell, these substances bind to intracellular receptors. The ligand-bound receptors are activated **transcription factors** that regulate the expression of target genes by binding to specific DNA sequences. In addition, steroid hormones can have nongenomic effects (see ⊚ 47-6).

The family of nuclear receptors contains at least 48 genes and has been classically divided into two subfamilies based on structural homology. One subfamily consists of receptors for **steroid hormones,** including the glucocorticoids, mineralocorticoids, and androgens, as well as estrogens and progesterone. These receptors function primarily as *homodimers* (see Table 3.3). The other group includes receptors for **retinoic**

acid, thyroid hormone, and **vitamin D.** These receptors appear to act as *heterodimers.* Yet other nuclear receptors recognize a wide range of **xenobiotics** and metabolites and thereby modulate the expression of genes that encode transporters and enzymes involved in drug metabolism.

The intracellular localization of the different unoccupied receptors varies. The glucocorticoid (GR) and mineralocorticoid (MR) receptors are mainly cytoplasmic, the estrogen (ER) and progesterone (PR) receptors are primarily nuclear, and the thyroid hormone (TR) and retinoic acid (RAR) receptors are bound to DNA in the nucleus. Cytoplasmic receptors are frequently complexed to chaperone (or "heat-shock") proteins. Hormone binding induces a conformational change in these receptors that causes dissociation from the cytoplasmic chaperone and unmasks a nuclear transport signal that allows the hormone-receptor complex to translocate into the nucleus.

Nuclear receptors contain five to six functionally distinct domains (Fig. 3.12) that are differentially conserved among the various members of the family. The N-terminal A/B region differs most widely among receptors and contains the first of two transactivation domains. **Transactivation** is the process by which a ligand-induced conformational change of the receptor results in a change in conformation of the DNA and thus initiates transcription. The C region, the most highly conserved among receptor types, contains the DNA-binding domain and is also involved in **dimerization** (see Table 3.3). It is composed of two "zinc finger" structures. The D, or hinge, region contains the "nuclear localization signal" and may also contain transactivation sequences. The E domain is responsible for hormone binding. Like the C region, it is involved in dimerization via its "basic zipper" region. Finally, like the A/B region, the E region contains a transactivation domain. The small C-terminal F domain is present in only some nuclear receptors and is of unknown function.

Activated nuclear receptors bind to sequence elements in the regulatory region of responsive genes and either activate or repress DNA transcription

One of the remarkable features of nuclear receptors is that they bind very specifically to short DNA sequences—called **hormone response elements**—in the regulatory region of responsive genes. The various nuclear receptors display specific cell and tissue distributions. Thus, the battery of genes affected by a particular ligand depends on the complement of receptors in the cell, the ability of these receptors to form homodimers or heterodimers, and the affinity of these receptor-ligand complexes for a particular response element on the DNA.

In addition to affecting transcription by directly binding to specific regulatory elements, several nuclear receptors modulate gene expression by acting as transcriptional repressors (see ⊙ 4-5). For example, the glucocorticoids, acting via their receptor, can attenuate components of the inflammatory response by suppressing the transcriptional activity of other transcription factors such as activator protein 1 (AP-1) and nuclear factor κB (NF-κB).

CHAPTER 4

REGULATION OF GENE EXPRESSION

Peter Igarashi

FROM GENES TO PROTEINS

Gene expression differs among tissues and—in any tissue—may vary in response to external stimuli

The haploid human genome contains 20,000 to 30,000 distinct genes, but only about one third of these genes are actively translated into proteins in any individual cell. Cells from different tissues have distinct morphological appearances and functions and respond differently to external stimuli, even though their DNA content is identical. For example, although all cells of the body contain an albumin gene, only liver cells (hepatocytes) can synthesize and secrete albumin into the bloodstream. Conversely, hepatocytes cannot synthesize insulin, which pancreatic β cells produce. The explanation for these observations is that expression of genes is regulated so that some genes are active in hepatocytes and others are silent. In pancreatic β cells, a different set of genes is active; others, such as those expressed only in the liver, are silent. How does the organism program one cell type to express liver-specific genes, and another to express a set of genes appropriate for the pancreas? This phenomenon is called **tissue-specific gene expression.**

A second issue is that genes in individual cells are generally not expressed at constant, unchanging levels (constitutive expression). Rather, their expression levels often vary widely in response to environmental stimuli. For example, when blood glucose levels decrease, α cells in the pancreas secrete the hormone glucagon (see ◉ 51-11). Glucagon circulates in the blood until it reaches the liver, where it causes a 15-fold increase in expression of the gene that encodes phosphoenolpyruvate carboxykinase (PEPCK), an enzyme that catalyzes the rate-limiting step in gluconeogenesis (see Fig. 51.7). Increased gluconeogenesis then contributes to restoration of blood glucose levels toward normal. This simple regulatory loop, which necessitates that the liver cells perceive the presence of glucagon and stimulate PEPCK gene expression, illustrates the phenomenon of **inducible gene expression.**

Genetic information flows from DNA to proteins

The "central dogma of molecular biology" states that genetic information flows unidirectionally from DNA to proteins. DNA is a polymer of nucleotides, each containing a nitrogenous base (adenine, A; guanine, G; cytosine, C; or thymine, T) attached to deoxyribose 5′-phosphate. The polymerized nucleotides form a polynucleotide strand in which the sequence of the nitrogenous bases constitutes the genetic

information. With few exceptions, all cells in the body share the same genetic information. Hydrogen-bond formation between bases (A and T, or G and C) on the two complementary strands of DNA produces a double-helical structure.

DNA has two functions. The first is to serve as a self-renewing data repository that maintains a constant source of genetic information for the cell. This role is achieved by DNA replication, which ensures that when cells divide, the progeny cells receive exact copies of the DNA. The second purpose of DNA is to serve as a template for the translation of genetic information into proteins, which are the functional units of the cell. This second purpose is broadly defined as **gene expression.**

Gene expression involves two major processes (Fig. 4.1). The first process—**transcription**—is the synthesis of RNA from a DNA template, mediated by an enzyme called RNA polymerase II. The resultant RNA molecule is identical in sequence to one of the strands of the DNA template except that the base uracil (U) replaces thymine (T). The second process—**translation**—is the synthesis of protein from RNA. During translation, the genetic code in the sequence of RNA is "read" by **transfer RNA (tRNA),** and then amino acids carried by the tRNA are covalently linked together to form a polypeptide chain. In eukaryotic cells, transcription occurs in the nucleus, whereas translation occurs on ribosomes located in the cytoplasm. Therefore, an intermediary RNA, called **messenger RNA (mRNA),** is required to transport the genetic information from the nucleus to the cytoplasm. The complete process, proceeding from DNA in the nucleus to protein in the cytoplasm, constitutes gene expression.

Although the **central dogma of molecular biology** applies to most protein-coding genes, exceptions exist. For example, RNA viruses (such as the human immunodeficiency virus [HIV] that causes acquired immunodeficiency syndrome) contain their genetic information in the sequence of an RNA genome. Upon infection with HIV, the cell "reverse transcribes" the RNA genome into double-stranded DNA that then integrates into the host DNA genome. Transcription of the virally encoded DNA by the host transcriptional machinery produces RNA molecules that become part of new HIV particles. Cells transcribe some genes into RNAs that do not encode proteins. So-called noncoding RNAs include ribosomal RNAs (rRNAs) and tRNA that participate in protein translation, small nuclear RNAs (snRNAs) that are involved in RNA splicing, and microRNAs (miRNAs) that regulate mRNA abundance and translation (see ◉ 4-6).

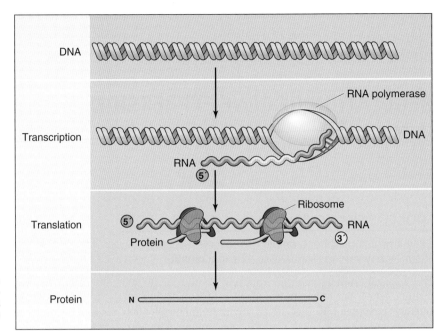

Figure 4.1 Pathway from genes to proteins. Gene expression involves two major processes. First, the DNA is transcribed into RNA by RNA polymerase. Second, the RNA is translated into protein on the ribosomes.

The gene consists of a transcription unit

Fig. 4.2 depicts the structure of a typical eukaryotic protein-coding gene. The **gene** consists of a segment of DNA that is transcribed into RNA. It extends from the site of transcription initiation to the site of transcription termination. The region of DNA that is immediately adjacent to and upstream (i.e., in the 5′ direction) from the transcription initiation site is called the **5′ flanking region.** The corresponding domain that is downstream (3′) to the transcription termination site is called the **3′ flanking region.** (Recall that DNA strands have directionality because of the 5′ to 3′ orientation of the phosphodiester bonds in the sugar-phosphate backbone of DNA. By convention, the DNA strand that has the same sequence as the RNA is called the coding strand, and the complementary strand is called the noncoding strand. The 5′ to 3′ orientation refers to the coding strand.) Although the 5′ and 3′ flanking regions are not transcribed into RNA, they frequently contain DNA sequences, called **regulatory elements,** that control gene transcription. The site where transcription of the gene begins, sometimes called the cap site, may have a variant of the nucleotide sequence 5′-ACTT(T/C)TG-3′ (called the cap sequence), where T/C means T *or* C. The A is the **transcription initiation site.** Transcription proceeds to the **transcription termination site,** which has a less-defined sequence and location in eukaryotic genes. Slightly upstream from the termination site is another sequence called the **polyadenylation signal,** which often has the sequence 5′-AATAAA-3′.

The RNA that is initially transcribed from a gene is called the **primary transcript** (Fig. 4.2) or precursor mRNA (pre-mRNA). Before it can be translated into protein, the primary transcript must be processed into a mature mRNA in the nucleus. Most eukaryotic genes contain **exons,** DNA sequences that are present in the mature mRNA, alternating with **introns,** which are not present in the mRNA. The primary transcript is colinear with the coding strand of the gene and contains the sequences of both the exons and the introns. To produce a mature mRNA that can be translated into protein, the cell must process the primary transcript in four steps.

First, the cell adds an unusual guanosine base, which is methylated at the 7 position, via a 5′-5′ phosphodiester bond to the 5′ end of the transcript. The result is a 5′ methyl **cap.** The presence of the 5′ methyl cap is required for export of the mRNA from the nucleus to the cytoplasm as well as for translation of the mRNA.

Second, the cell removes the sequences of the introns from the primary transcript via a process called **pre-mRNA splicing.** Splicing involves the joining of the sequences of the exons in the RNA transcript and the removal of the intervening introns. As a result, **mature mRNA** (Fig. 4.2) is shorter and not colinear with the coding strand of the DNA template.

The third processing step is cleavage of the RNA transcript about 20 nucleotides downstream from the polyadenylation signal, near the 3′ end of the transcript.

The fourth step is the addition of a string of 100 to 200 adenine bases at the site of the cleavage to form a **poly(A) tail.** This tail contributes to mRNA stability.

The mature mRNA produced by RNA processing not only contains a coding region—the open-reading frame—that encodes protein but also sequences at the 5′ and 3′ ends that are not translated into protein—the 5′ and 3′ untranslated regions (UTRs), respectively. Translation of the mRNA on ribosomes always begins at the codon AUG, which encodes methionine, and proceeds until the ribosome encounters one of the three stop codons (UAG, UAA, or UGA). Thus, the 5′ end of the mRNA is the first to be translated and provides the N terminus of the protein; the 3′ end is the last to be translated and contributes the C terminus.

DNA is packaged into chromatin

Although DNA is commonly depicted as linear, chromosomal DNA in the nucleus is actually organized into a

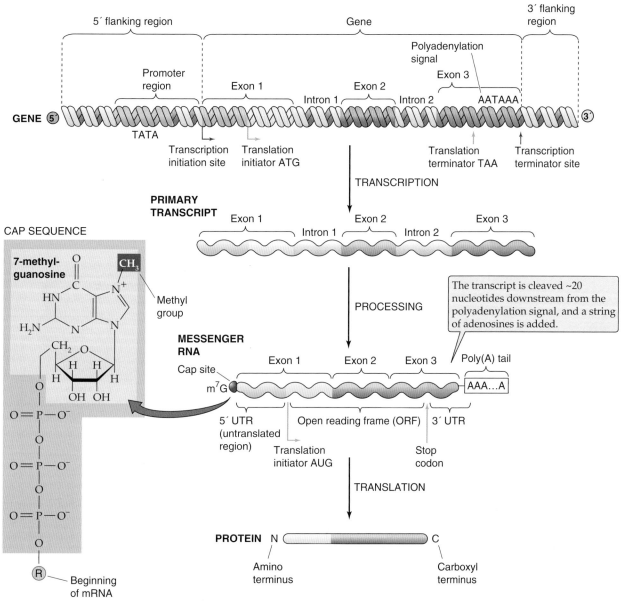

Figure 4.2 Structure of a eukaryotic gene and its products. The figure depicts a gene, a primary RNA transcript, the mature mRNA, and the resulting protein. The 5′ and 3′ numbering of the gene refers to the coding strand. ATG, AATAAA, and the like, are nucleotide sequences. m^7G, 7-methyl guanosine.

higher-order structure called chromatin. This packaging is required to fit DNA with a total length of ~1 m into a nucleus with a diameter of 10^{-5} m. **Chromatin** consists of DNA associated with **histones** and other nuclear proteins. The basic building block of chromatin is the **nucleosome** (Fig. 4.3), each of which consists of a protein core and 147 base pairs (bp) of associated DNA. The protein core is an octamer of the histones H2A, H2B, H3, and H4. DNA wraps twice around the core histones to form a solenoid-like structure. A linker histone, H1, associates with segments of DNA between nucleosomes. Regular arrays of nucleosomes have a beads-on-a-string appearance and constitute the so-called 11-nm fiber of chromatin, which can condense to form the 30-nm fiber.

Chromatin exists in two general forms that can be distinguished cytologically by their different degrees of condensation. **Heterochromatin** is a highly condensed form of chromatin that is transcriptionally inactive. In general, highly organized chromatin structure is associated with *repression* of gene transcription. Heterochromatin contains mostly repetitive DNA sequences and relatively few genes. **Euchromatin** has a more open structure and contains genes that are actively transcribed. Even in the transcriptionally active "open" euchromatin, local chromatin structure may influence the activity of individual genes.

Gene expression may be regulated at multiple steps

Gene expression involves eight steps (Fig. 4.4):

Step 1: **Chromatin remodeling.** Before a gene can be transcribed, some local alteration in chromatin structure

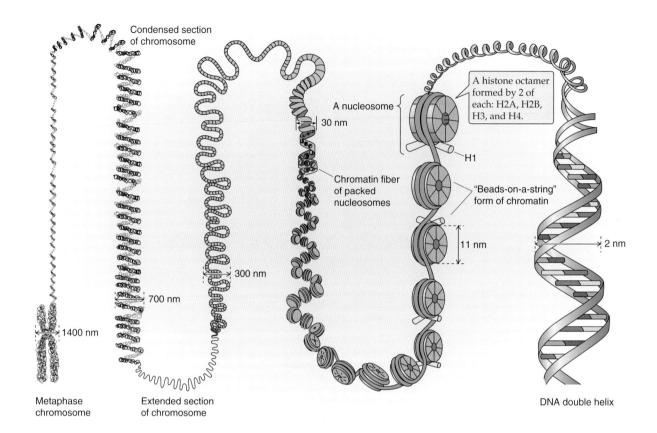

Condensed section of chromosome

A nucleosome

30 nm

A histone octamer formed by 2 of each: H2A, H2B, H3, and H4.

H1

Chromatin fiber of packed nucleosomes

"Beads-on-a-string" form of chromatin

11 nm

2 nm

300 nm

700 nm

1400 nm

Metaphase chromosome

Extended section of chromosome

DNA double helix

Figure 4.3 Chromatin structure.

must occur so that the enzymes that mediate transcription can gain access to the genomic DNA. The alteration in chromatin structure is called chromatin remodeling, which may involve loosening of the interaction between histones and DNA, repositioning of nucleosomes, or local depletion of histones.

Step 2: **Initiation of transcription.** In this step, RNA polymerase is recruited to the gene promoter and begins to synthesize RNA that is complementary in sequence to one of the strands of the template DNA. For most eukaryotic genes, initiation of transcription is the critical, rate-limiting step in gene expression.

Step 3: **Transcript elongation.** During transcript elongation, RNA polymerase proceeds down the DNA strand and sequentially adds ribonucleotides to the elongating strand of RNA.

Step 4: **Termination of transcription.** After producing a full-length RNA, the enzyme halts elongation.

Step 5: **RNA processing.** As noted before, RNA processing involves (a) addition of a 5′ methylguanosine cap, (b) pre-mRNA splicing, (c) cleavage of the RNA strand, and (d) polyadenylation.

Step 6: **Nucleocytoplasmic transport.** The next step in gene expression is the export of the mature mRNA through pores in the nuclear envelope (see ◉ **2-11**) into the cytoplasm. Nucleocytoplasmic transport is a regulated process that is important for mRNA quality control.

Step 7: **Translation.** The mRNA is translated into proteins on ribosomes. During translation, the genetic code on the mRNA is read by tRNA, and then amino acids carried by the tRNA are added to the nascent polypeptide chain.

Step 8: **mRNA degradation.** Finally, the mRNA is degraded in the cytoplasm by a combination of endonucleases and exonucleases.

Each of these steps is potentially a target for regulation (Fig. 4.4, right panel):

1. Gene expression may be regulated by global as well as by local alterations in chromatin structure.
2. An important related alteration in chromatin structure is the state of methylation of the DNA.
3. Initiation of transcription can be regulated by transcriptional activators and transcriptional repressors.
4. Transcript elongation may be regulated by premature termination, in which the polymerase falls off (or is displaced from) the template DNA strand; such termination results in the synthesis of truncated transcripts.
5. Pre-mRNA splicing may be regulated by alternative splicing, which generates different mRNA species from the same primary transcript.
6. At the step of nucleocytoplasmic transport, the cell prevents expression of aberrant transcripts, such as those with defects in mRNA processing. In addition, mutant transcripts containing premature stop codons may be de-

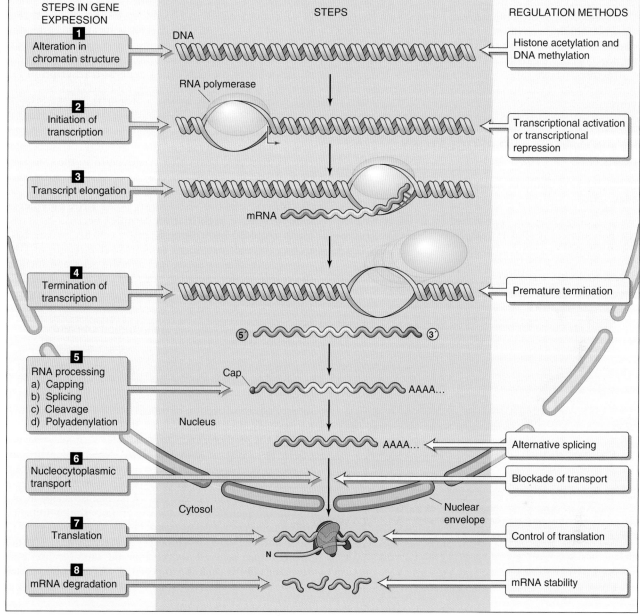

Figure 4.4 Steps in gene expression. Nearly all of the eight steps in gene expression are potential targets for regulation.

graded in the nucleus through a process called nonsense-mediated decay.

7. Control of translation of mRNA is a regulated step in the expression of certain genes, such as the transferrin receptor gene.

8. Control of mRNA stability contributes to steady-state levels of mRNA in the cytoplasm and is important for the overall expression of many genes.

Transcription factors are proteins that regulate gene transcription

⊙ **4-1** A general principle is that gene transcription is regulated by interactions of specific proteins with specific DNA sequences. The proteins that regulate gene transcription are

called **transcription factors.** Many transcription factors recognize and bind to specific sequences in DNA. The binding sites for these transcription factors are called **regulatory elements.** Because they are located on the same piece of DNA as the genes that they regulate, these regulatory elements are sometimes referred to as *cis-acting* factors.

Fig. 4.5 illustrates the overall scheme for the regulation of gene expression. Transcription requires proteins (transcription factors) that bind to specific DNA sequences (regulatory elements) located near the genes they regulate (target genes). Once the proteins bind to DNA, they stimulate (or inhibit) transcription of the target gene. A particular transcription factor can regulate the transcription of multiple target genes. In general, regulation of gene expression can occur at the level of either transcription factors or regulatory elements.

Examples of regulation at the level of transcription factors include variations in the abundance of transcription factors, their DNA-binding activities, and their ability to stimulate (or to inhibit) transcription. Examples of regulation at the level of regulatory elements include alterations in chromatin structure (which influences accessibility to transcription factors) and covalent modifications of DNA, especially methylation.

THE PROMOTER AND REGULATORY ELEMENTS

The basal transcriptional machinery mediates gene transcription

Protein-coding genes are transcribed by an enzyme called **RNA polymerase II (Pol II),** which catalyzes the synthesis of RNA that is complementary in sequence to a DNA

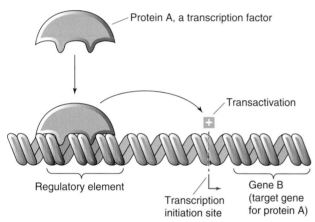

Figure 4.5 Regulation of transcription. Protein A, a transcription factor that is encoded by gene A (not shown), regulates another gene, gene B. Protein A binds to a DNA sequence (a regulatory element) that is upstream from gene B; this DNA sequence is a *cis*-acting element because it is located on the same DNA as gene B. In this example, protein A stimulates (transactivates) the transcription of gene B. Transcription factors also can inhibit transcription.

template. Pol II is a large protein (molecular mass of 600 kDa), comprising 10 to 12 subunits. Although Pol II catalyzes mRNA synthesis, by itself it is incapable of binding to DNA and initiating transcription at specific sites. The recruitment of Pol II and initiation of transcription requires an assembly of proteins called **general transcription factors.** Six general transcription factors are known—TFIIA, TFIIB, TFIID, TFIIE, TFIIF, and TFIIH—each of which contains multiple subunits. These general transcription factors are essential for the transcription of all protein-coding genes, which distinguishes them from the transcription factors discussed below that are involved in the transcription of specific genes. Together with Pol II, the general transcription factors constitute the **basal transcriptional machinery,** which is also known as the **RNA polymerase holoenzyme** or **preinitiation complex** because its assembly is required before transcription can begin. The basal transcriptional machinery assembles at a region of DNA that is immediately upstream from the gene and includes the transcription initiation site. This region is called the **gene promoter** (Fig. 4.6).

The promoter determines the initiation site and direction of transcription

The promoter is a *cis*-acting regulatory element that is required for expression of the gene. In addition to locating the site for initiation of transcription, the promoter also determines the direction of transcription. Perhaps somewhat surprisingly, no unique sequence defines the gene promoter. Instead, the promoter consists of modules of simple sequences (DNA elements). A common DNA element in many promoters is the Goldberg-Hogness **TATA box.** The TATA box has the consensus sequence 5′-GNGTATA(A/T)A(A/T)-3′, where N is any nucleotide. The TATA box is usually located ~30 bp upstream (5′) from the site of transcription initiation. The general transcription factor TFIID—a component of the basal transcriptional machinery—recognizes the TATA box, which is thus believed to determine the site of transcription initiation. TFIID itself is composed of TATA-binding protein

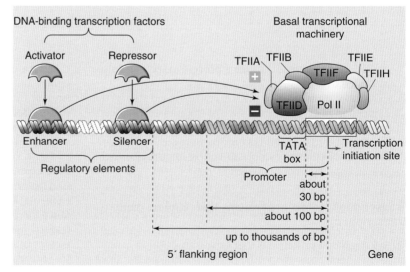

Figure 4.6 Promoter and DNA regulatory elements. The basal transcriptional machinery assembles on the promoter. Transcriptional activators bind to enhancers, and repressors bind to negative regulatory elements.

(TBP) and at least 10 TBP-associated factors (TAFs). The TBP subunit is a sequence-specific DNA-binding protein that binds to the TATA box. TAFs are involved in the activation of gene transcription.

⊙ 4-2 REGULATION OF INDUCIBLE GENE EXPRESSION BY SIGNAL-TRANSDUCTION PATHWAYS

How do cells activate previously quiescent genes in response to environmental cues? How are such external signals transduced to the cell nucleus to stimulate the transcription of specific genes? Transcription factors may be thought of as effector molecules in signal-transduction pathways (see Chapter 3) that modulate gene expression. Several such signaling pathways have been defined. Lipid-soluble steroid and thyroid hormones can enter the cell and interact with specific receptors that are themselves transcription factors. However, most cytokines, hormones, and mitogens cannot diffuse into the cell interior and instead bind to specific receptors that are located on the cell surface. First, we consider three pathways for transducing signals from cell-surface receptors into the nucleus: a cAMP-dependent pathway, a Ras-dependent pathway, and the JAK-STAT pathway. Next, we examine the mechanisms by which steroid or thyroid hormones act via nuclear receptors. Finally, we discuss how transcription factors coordinate gene expression in response to physiological stimuli.

⊙ 4-3 cAMP regulates transcription via the transcription factors CREB and CBP

cAMP is an important second messenger (see ⊙ 3-9) in the response to agonists binding to specific cell-surface receptors. Increases in $[cAMP]_i$ stimulate the transcription of certain genes, including those that encode a variety of hormones, such as somatostatin, the enkephalins, glucagon, and vasoactive intestinal peptide. Many genes that are activated in response to cAMP contain within their regulatory regions a common DNA element called **CRE (cAMP response element)** that has the consensus sequence 5'-TGACGTCA-3'. Several different transcription factors bind to CRE, among them **CREB (CAMP response element–binding protein),** a 43-kDa member of the bZIP family. As shown in Fig. 4.7, increases in $[cAMP]_i$ stimulate protein kinase A (PKA) by causing dissociation of the PKA regulatory subunit. The catalytic subunit of PKA then translocates into the nucleus, where it phosphorylates CREB and other proteins. Activation of CREB is rapid (30 minutes) and declines gradually during a 24-hour period. This phosphorylation greatly increases the affinity of CREB for the coactivator **CBP,** which is a 245-kDa protein containing two domains, one that binds to phosphorylated CREB and another that activates components of the basal transcriptional machinery. Thus, CBP serves as a "bridge" protein that communicates the transcriptional activation signal from CREB to the basal transcriptional machinery. The result of phosphorylation of CREB is a 10- to 20-fold stimulation of CREB's ability to induce the transcription of genes containing a CRE.

How is the transcriptional signal terminated? When $[cAMP]_i$ is high, PKA phosphorylates and activates

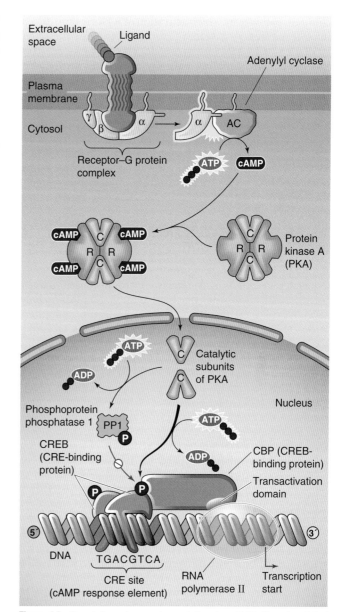

Figure 4.7 Regulation of gene transcription by cAMP. Phosphorylated CREB binds CBP, which has a transactivation domain that stimulates the basal transcriptional machinery. In parallel, phosphorylation activates phosphoprotein phosphatase 1 (PP1), which dephosphorylates CREB, terminating the activation of transcription. *R,* Regulatory subunit of protein kinase A.

phosphoprotein phosphatase 1 in the nucleus. When cAMP levels fall, the still-active phosphatase dephosphorylates CREB.

Receptor tyrosine kinases regulate transcription via a Ras-dependent cascade of protein kinases

⊙ Many growth factors bind to cell-surface receptors that, when activated by the ligand, have tyrosine kinase activity (see Fig. 3.10C). Examples of growth factors that act through such receptor tyrosine kinases (RTKs) are epidermal growth factor (EGF), platelet-derived growth factor (PDGF), insulin, insulin-like growth factor type 1 (IGF-1), fibroblast growth factor (FGF), and nerve growth factor (NGF). The common pathway by which activation of RTKs is transduced into the nucleus is a cascade of events that increase the activity of the small GTP-binding protein Ras (see Fig. 3.11). This **Ras-dependent signaling pathway** culminates in the activation of mitogen-activated protein kinase (MAPK), which translocates to the nucleus, where it phosphorylates a number of nuclear proteins that are transcription factors. Phosphorylation of a transcription factor by MAPK can enhance or inhibit binding to DNA and can stimulate either transactivation or transrepression. Transcription factors that are regulated by the Ras-dependent pathway include c-Myc, c-Jun, c-Fos, and Elk-1. Many of these transcription factors regulate the expression of genes that promote cell proliferation.

Tyrosine kinase–associated receptors can regulate transcription via JAK-STAT

A group of cell-surface receptors termed tyrosine kinase–associated receptors lack *intrinsic* tyrosine kinase activity (see ◉ 3-20). The ligands that bind to these receptors include several cytokines, growth hormone, prolactin, and interferons (IFN-α, IFN-β, and IFN-γ). Although the receptors themselves lack catalytic activity, their cytoplasmic domains are associated with the **Janus kinase (JAK) family** of protein tyrosine kinases.

Binding of ligand to certain tyrosine kinase–associated receptors activates a member of the JAK family, which results in phosphorylation of cytoplasmic proteins, among which are believed to be latent cytoplasmic transcription factors called signal transducers and activators of transcription (STATs). When phosphorylated on tyrosine residues, the STAT proteins dimerize and thereby become competent to enter the nucleus and induce transcription.

A well-characterized example of the JAK-STAT pathway is the activation of **interferon-responsive genes** by IFN-α and IFN-γ. IFN-α activates the JAK1 and Tyk2 kinases that are associated with its receptor (Fig. 4.8A). Subsequent phosphorylation of two different STAT monomers causes the monomers to dimerize. This STAT heterodimer enters the nucleus, where it combines with a third 48-kDa protein to form a transcription factor that binds to a DNA sequence called the IFN-stimulated response element (ISRE). In the case of IFN-γ (Fig. 4.8B), the receptor associates with the JAK1 and JAK2 (rather than Tyk2) kinases, and subsequent phosphorylation of a *single* kind of STAT monomer causes these monomers to dimerize. These STAT homodimers also enter the nucleus, where they bind to the DNA at IFN-γ response elements called IFN-γ activation sites (GASs), without requiring the 48-kDa protein.

Nuclear receptors are transcription factors

◉ 4-4 Steroid and thyroid hormones are examples of ligands that activate gene expression by binding to cellular receptors that are themselves transcription factors. Members of the steroid and thyroid hormone receptor superfamily, also called the nuclear receptor superfamily, are grouped together because they are structurally similar and have similar mechanisms of action. After these hormones enter the cell, they bind to receptors in the cytoplasm or nucleus. Ligand binding converts the receptors into active transcription factors. The

transcription factors bind to specific regulatory elements on the DNA, called **hormone response elements,** and activate the transcription of *cis*-linked genes. The family of nuclear receptors includes receptors that bind glucocorticoids (GR), mineralocorticoids (MR), estrogens (ER), progesterone (PR), androgens (AR), thyroid hormone (TR), vitamin D (VDR), retinoic acid (RAR), lipids (peroxisome proliferator–activated receptor, PPAR), and 9-*cis*-retinoic acid (retinoid X receptor, RXR) as well as bile acids (bile acid receptor, FXR) and xenobiotics (steroid and xenobiotic receptor, SXR; constitutive androstane receptor, CAR) (see Table 3.3).

With the exception of the thyroid hormones, the hormones that bind to these receptors are lipophilic molecules that enter cells by diffusion and do not require interaction with cell-surface receptors. The thyroid hormones differ in that they are electrically charged and may cross the cell membrane via transporters.

Activation of Transcription. Ligand binding activates nuclear receptors through two main mechanisms: regulation of subcellular localization and interactions with coactivators. Some nuclear receptors, such as GR, are normally located in the cytoplasm and are maintained in an inactive state by association with a cytoplasmic anchoring protein (Fig. 4.9A). The protein that retains GR in the cytoplasm is a **molecular chaperone,** the 90-kDa heat shock protein **hsp90.** GR must bind to hsp90 to have a high affinity for a glucocorticoid hormone. When glucocorticoids bind to the GR, hsp90 dissociates from the GR and exposes a nuclear localization signal that permits the transport of GR into the nucleus. The receptor must remain hormone bound for receptor dimerization, which is a prerequisite for binding to the **glucocorticoid response element (GRE)** on the DNA. Other receptors, such as TR, are normally already present in the nucleus before binding the hormone (Fig. 9.4B). For these receptors, binding of hormone is evidently not essential for dimerization or binding to DNA. However, ligand binding is necessary at a subsequent step for transactivation.

Repression of Transcription. ◉ 4-5 Nuclear receptors sometimes function as active repressors, perhaps acting by alternative mechanisms. First, a receptor may form inactive heterodimers with other members of the nuclear receptor family. Second, a receptor may compete with other transcription factors for DNA-binding sites. For example, when the TR—without bound thyroid hormone—interacts with its own DNA response element, the TR acts as a repressor. Finally, nuclear receptors can also inhibit gene transcription by interacting with corepressors, which can recruit histone deacetylases that enhance nucleosome assembly, resulting in transcriptional repression.

POST-TRANSCRIPTIONAL REGULATION OF GENE EXPRESSION

Although initiation of transcription (Fig. 4.4, step 2) is the most frequently regulated step in gene expression, for certain genes subsequent steps are more important for determining the overall level of expression. These processes are generally classified as **post-transcriptional regulation.** The mechanisms for regulating these steps are less well understood than are those for regulating transcription initiation, but some information comes from the study of model genes.

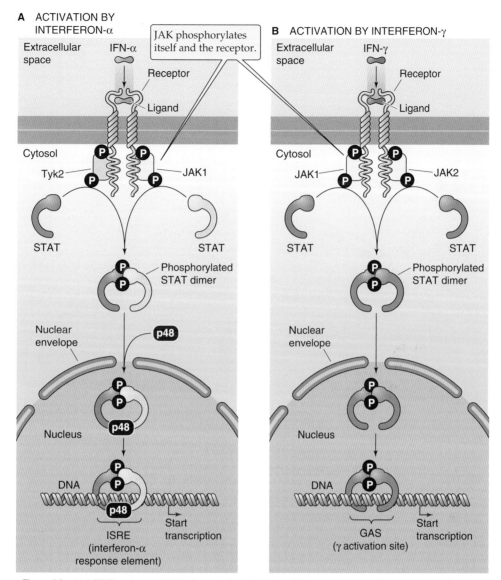

A ACTIVATION BY INTERFERON-α

Extracellular space

IFN-α

JAK phosphorylates itself and the receptor.

Receptor

Ligand

Cytosol

Tyk2   JAK1

STAT   STAT

Phosphorylated STAT dimer

Nuclear envelope

p48

Nucleus

p48

DNA

p48

ISRE (interferon-α response element)

Start transcription

B ACTIVATION BY INTERFERON-γ

Extracellular space

IFN-γ

Receptor

Ligand

Cytosol

JAK1   JAK2

STAT   STAT

Phosphorylated STAT dimer

Nuclear envelope

Nucleus

DNA

GAS (γ activation site)

Start transcription

Figure 4.8 JAK-STAT pathway. (A) Binding of a ligand such as IFN-α to a tyrosine kinase–associated receptor causes JAK1 and Tyk2 to phosphorylate themselves, the receptor, and two different STAT monomers. The phosphorylation of the STAT monomers leads to the formation of a *hetero*dimer, which translocates to the nucleus and combines with a third protein (p48). The complex binds to ISRE and activates gene transcription. (B) Binding of a ligand such as IFN-γ to a tyrosine kinase–associated receptor causes JAK1 and JAK2 to phosphorylate themselves, the receptor, and two identical STAT monomers. The phosphorylation of the STAT monomers leads to the formation of a *homo*dimer, which translocates to the nucleus. The complex binds to the GAS response element and activates gene transcription.

Post-transcriptional processes that we review here are pre-mRNA splicing (step 5) and transcript degradation (step 8).

Alternative splicing generates diversity from single genes

Eukaryotic genes contain introns (Fig. 4.2) that must be removed from the primary transcript to create mature mRNA; this process is called **pre-mRNA splicing.** Splicing involves the joining of two sites on the RNA transcript, the **5′ splice-donor site** and the **3′ splice-acceptor site,** and removal of the intervening intron.

Many genes also undergo **alternative splicing,** which refers to differential splicing of the same primary transcript

to produce mature transcripts that contain different combinations of exons. If the coding region is affected, the resulting splicing variants will encode proteins with distinct primary structures that may have different physiological functions. Thus, alternative splicing is a mechanism for increasing the diversity of proteins that a single gene can produce. Fig. 4.10 summarizes seven patterns of alternative splicing.

Retained Intron In some cases, the cell may choose whether to splice out a segment of RNA. For example, the γA isoform of rat γ-fibrinogen lacks the seventh intron, whereas the γB isoform retains the intron, which encodes a unique C terminus of 12 amino acids (Fig. 4.10A).

**A   TRANSCRIPTIONAL ACTIVATION
BY GLUCOCORTICOID HORMONE**

**B   TRANSCRIPTIONAL ACTIVATION
BY THYROID HORMONE**

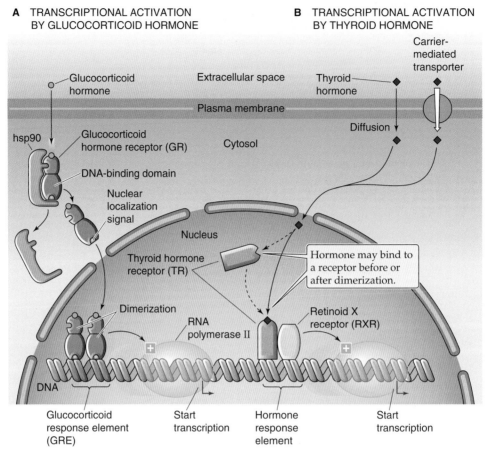

Figure 4.9   Transcriptional activation by glucocorticoid and thyroid hormones. (A) The binding of a glucocorticoid hormone to a cytoplasmic receptor causes the receptor to dissociate from the chaperone hsp90 (90-kDa heat shock protein). The free hormone-receptor complex can then translocate to the nucleus, where dimerization leads to transactivation. (B) The binding of thyroid hormone to a receptor in the nucleus leads to transactivation. The active transcription factor is a heterodimer of the TR and the RXR.

Alternative 3′ Splice Sites   In this case, the length of an intron is variable because the *downstream* boundary of the intron can be at either of two or more different 3′ splice-acceptor sites (Fig. 4.10B). For example, in rat fibronectin, a single donor site may be spliced to any of three acceptor sites. The presence or absence of the amino acids encoded by the sequence between the different splice-acceptor sites results in fibronectin isoforms with different cell adhesion properties.

Alternative 5′ Splice Sites   Here also, the length of the intron is variable. However, in this case, it is the *upstream* boundary of the intron that can be at either of two or more different 5′ splice-donor sites (Fig. 4.10C). For example, cells can generate mRNA encoding 3-hydroxy-3-methylglutaryl–coenzyme A (HMG-CoA) reductase (see ⊙ **46-9**) with different 5′ UTRs by splicing from multiple donor sites for the first intron to a single acceptor site.

Cassette Exons   In some cases, the cell may choose either to splice in an exon or group of exons (**cassette exons**) or not to splice them in (Fig. 4.10D). An example is the α-tropomyosin gene, which contains 12 exons. All α-tropomyosin transcripts contain the invariant exons 1, 4 to 6, 8, and 9. All muscle-like cells splice in exon 7, but hepatoma (i.e., liver tumor) cells do not splice in exon 7; they directly link exon 6 to exon 8.

Mutually Exclusive Exons   In yet other cases, the cell may splice in **mutually exclusive exons** (Fig. 4.10E). One of the Na/K/Cl cotransporter genes *(NKCC2)* is an example. Isoforms containing distinct 96-bp exons are differentially expressed in the kidney cortex and medulla. Because the encoded amino-acid sequence is predicted to reside in the membrane, the isoforms may have different kinetic properties. The α-tropomyosin gene again is another example. Smooth-muscle cells splice in exon 2 but not exon 3. Striated-muscle cells and myoblasts splice in exon 3 but not exon 2. Fibroblasts and hepatoma cells do not splice in either of these two exons.

Alternative 5′ Ends   Cells may select among different alternative promoters, creating alternative 5′ ends, and then splice the selected end to a downstream portion of the pre-mRNA (Fig. 4.10F). For example, the gene that encodes the electrogenic Na/HCO$_3$ cotransporter 1 has 26 exons. The transcript that encodes the NBCe1-A variant expressed heavily in the renal proximal tubule initiates from a promoter located upstream from exon 4 and then continues with exons 5 through 26. The transcript that encodes the NBCe1-B variant expressed heavily in pancreatic ducts initiates from a promoter located upstream from exon 1 and then continues with exons 2 through 26. This use of alternative promoters permits differential regulation of gene expression in kidney versus pancreas.

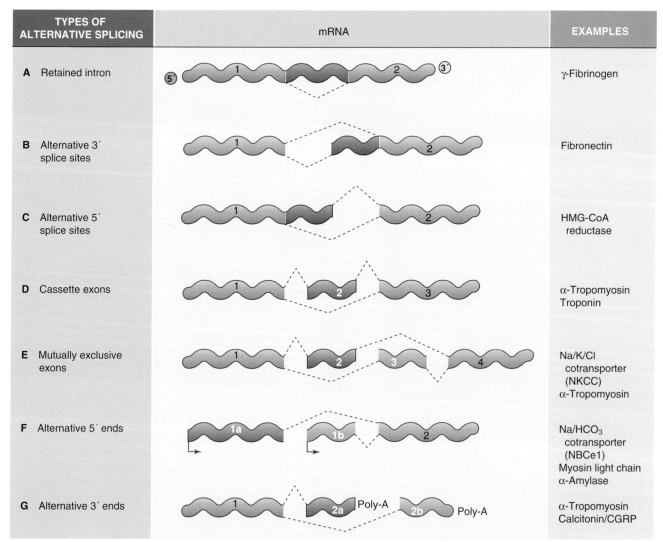

TYPES OF ALTERNATIVE SPLICING	mRNA	EXAMPLES
A Retained intron		γ-Fibrinogen
B Alternative 3′ splice sites		Fibronectin
C Alternative 5′ splice sites		HMG-CoA reductase
D Cassette exons		α-Tropomyosin Troponin
E Mutually exclusive exons		Na/K/Cl cotransporter (NKCC) α-Tropomyosin
F Alternative 5′ ends		Na/HCO₃ cotransporter (NBCe1) Myosin light chain α-Amylase
G Alternative 3′ ends		α-Tropomyosin Calcitonin/CGRP

Figure 4.10 Types of alternative splicing. In (F), the two *red arrows* represent alternative transcription initiation sites. *Poly-A,* Polyadenylic acid.

Alternative 3′ Ends Finally, cells may differentially splice the transcript near the 3′ end of the gene (Fig. 4.10G) and thereby alter the site of cleavage and polyadenylation. Such splicing may also affect the coding region. Again, α-tropomyosin is an example. Striated-muscle cells splice in exon 11, which contains one alternative 3′ UTR. Smooth-muscle cells splice in exon 12 instead of exon 11. Another example is the calcitonin gene, which encodes both the hormone calcitonin and calcitonin gene–related peptide-α (CGRPα). Thyroid C cells produce one splice variant that includes exons 1 to 4 and encodes calcitonin. Sensory neurons, on the other hand, produce another splice variant that excludes exon 4 but includes exons 5 and 6. It encodes a different protein, CGRPα.

These examples illustrate that some splicing variants are expressed only in certain cell types and not in others. Clearly, control of alternative splicing must involve steps other than initiation of transcription because many splice variants have identical 5′ ends. In some genes, the control elements that are required for alternative splicing have been identified, largely on the basis of deletion mutations that result in aberrant splicing. These control elements can reside in either introns or exons and are located within or near the splice sites. The proteins that interact with such elements remain largely unknown, although some RNA-binding proteins that may be involved in regulation of splicing have been identified.

⊙ 4-6 MicroRNAs regulate mRNA abundance and translation

A major form of post-transcriptional gene regulation occurs via small RNA molecules called **microRNAs (miRNAs)**, which mediate a type of post-transcriptional gene regulation. miRNAs are typically ~22 nucleotides in length, too short to encode proteins. Instead, miRNAs play regulatory functions in many physiological and pathophysiological processes. They bind to specific mRNA targets and regulate mRNA abundance and translation. Because this regulation occurs after the transcription of mRNA, it is *post-transcriptional* in nature.

Fig. 4.11 shows the biogenesis and function of miRNAs. Transcription of genomic DNA initially gives rise to a longer primary miRNA (pri-miRNA) transcript, which the

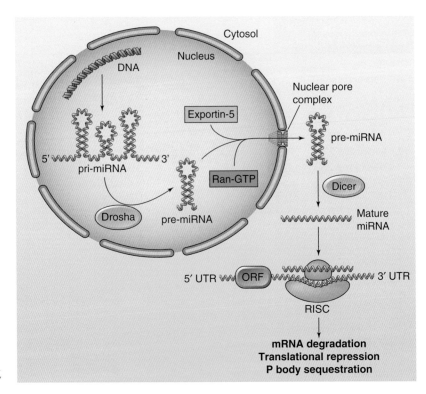

Figure 4.11 miRNA biogenesis and function. *ORF,* Open reading frame.

endonuclease **Drosha** then cleaves to produce a precursor miRNA (pre-miRNA), typically 50 to 70 nucleotides in length. The pre-miRNA forms a hairpin structure because of intramolecular base pairing. The pre-miRNA, complexed with exportin-5 and Ran-GTP, then exits the nucleus via nuclear pores. In the cytoplasm, a second endonuclease called **Dicer** cleaves the pre-miRNA to produce the mature, single-stranded miRNA.

In the cytoplasm, the newly synthesized miRNA associates with a protein complex called the **RNA-induced silencing complex (RISC).** Once complexed with RISC, the miRNA binds via base pairing to an mRNA target. Usually, miRNAs bind to sites located in the 3′ UTR of mRNA, although occasionally it binds to sites in the 5′ UTR (Fig. 4.2). Recall that the 5′ and 3′ UTRs flank the coding region of the mRNA. Binding of the miRNA and the associated RISC complex results in degradation of the mRNA target or inhibits translation of the mRNA. In some cases, the targeted mRNA may be sequestered in subcellular organelles, called **processing bodies (P bodies),** where it is no longer available for translation. Regardless of the exact

mechanism, the net result is that the expression of the protein encoded by the mRNA is inhibited.

The inhibition of gene expression by miRNAs represents a form of **RNA interference.** RNA interference refers to a process, found in most animal and plant species, in which short RNA molecules silence the expression of specific genes.

Since the discovery of the first mammalian miRNA in 2000, hundreds of miRNAs have been identified in humans and other species. The sequences of miRNAs are often evolutionarily conserved, consistent with their important functions.

miRNAs play important roles in embryonic development, stem-cell differentiation, cell proliferation, and cell death. Other physiological processes under the control of miRNAs include insulin secretion, the stress response, renin secretion, and lipid metabolism. By fine-tuning mRNA abundance and translation, miRNAs work in concert with gene transcription to maintain the levels of proteins in cells within an optimal range. Dysregulation of miRNAs commonly plays a role in pathological conditions such as cancer, viral infection, diabetes, and Alzheimer disease.

CHAPTER 5

TRANSPORT OF SOLUTES AND WATER

Peter S. Aronson, Walter F. Boron, and Emile L. Boulpaep

The cells of the human body live in a carefully regulated fluid environment. The fluid inside the cells, the **intracellular fluid (ICF),** occupies what is called the intracellular compartment, and the fluid outside the cells, the **extracellular fluid (ECF),** occupies the extracellular compartment. The barriers that separate these two compartments are the **cell membranes.** For life to be sustained, the body must rigorously maintain the volume and composition of the intracellular and extracellular compartments. To a large extent, such regulation is the result of transport across the cell membrane. In this chapter, we discuss how cell membranes regulate the distribution of ions and water in the intracellular and extracellular compartments.

THE INTRACELLULAR AND EXTRACELLULAR FLUIDS

Total-body water is the sum of the ICF and ECF volumes

Total-body water (TBW) is ~60% of total-body weight in a young adult human male, ~50% of total-body weight in a young adult human female (Table 5.1), and 65% to 75% of total-body weight in an infant. TBW accounts for a lower percentage of weight in females because they typically have a higher ratio of adipose tissue to muscle, and fat cells have a lower water content than does muscle. Because water represents such a large fraction of body weight, acute changes in TBW can be detected simply by monitoring body weight.

The anatomy of the body fluid compartments is illustrated in Fig. 5.1. The prototypical 70-kg male has ~42 L of TBW (60% of 70 kg). Of these 42 L, ~60% (25 L) is intracellular and ~40% (17 L) is extracellular. ECF is composed of blood plasma, interstitial fluid, and transcellular fluid.

Plasma Volume ◉ 5-1 Of the ~17 L of ECF, only ~20% (~3 L) is contained within the cardiac chambers and blood vessels, that is, within the intravascular compartment. The *total* volume of this intravascular compartment is the **blood volume,** ~6 L. The extracellular 3 L of the blood volume is the plasma volume. The balance, ~3 L, consists of the cellular elements of blood: erythrocytes, leukocytes, and platelets. The fraction of blood volume that is occupied by these cells is called the **hematocrit.** The hematocrit is determined by centrifuging blood that is treated with an anticoagulant and measuring **the fraction of the total volume that is occupied by the packed cells.**

Interstitial Fluid About 75% (~13 L) of the ECF is outside the intravascular compartment, where it bathes the non-blood cells of the body. Within this interstitial fluid are two smaller compartments that communicate only slowly with the bulk of the interstitial fluid: dense connective tissue, such as cartilage and tendons, and bone matrix.

The barriers that separate the intravascular and interstitial compartments are the walls of **capillaries.** Water and solutes can move between the interstitium and blood plasma by crossing capillary walls and between the interstitium and cytoplasm by crossing cell membranes.

Transcellular Fluid Finally, ~5% (~1 L) of ECF is trapped within spaces that are completely surrounded by epithelial cells. This transcellular fluid includes the synovial fluid within joints and the cerebrospinal fluid surrounding the brain and spinal cord. Transcellular fluid does *not* include fluids that are, strictly speaking, outside the body, such as the contents of the gastrointestinal tract or urinary bladder.

ICF is rich in K⁺, whereas ECF is rich in Na⁺ and Cl⁻

Not only do the various body fluid compartments have very different volumes, they also have radically different compositions, as summarized in Fig. 5.1. Table 5.2 is a more comprehensive listing of these values. ICF is high in K^+ and low in Na^+ and Cl^-; ECF (interstitial and plasma) is high in Na^+ and Cl^- and low in K^+. The cell maintains a relatively high K^+ concentration ($[K^+]_i$) and low Na^+ concentration ($[Na^+]_i$) by using the Na-K pump to extrude Na^+ actively from the cell and to transport K^+ actively into the cell.

Transcellular fluids differ greatly in composition, both from each other and from plasma, because they are secreted by different epithelia. The two major constituents of ECF, the plasma and the interstitial fluid, have similar composition as far as small solutes are concerned. For most cells, it is the composition of the interstitial fluid enveloping the cells that is the relevant parameter. The major difference between plasma and interstitial fluid is the absence of plasma proteins from the interstitium. These plasma proteins, which cannot equilibrate across the walls of most capillaries, are responsible for the usually slight difference in small-solute concentrations between plasma and interstitial fluid.

TABLE 5.1 Approximate Water Distribution in Adult Humans[a]

	MEN	TYPICAL VOLUME(L)	WOMEN	TYPICAL VOLUME(L)
Total-body water (TBW)	60% of BW	42	50% of BW	35
Intracellular fluid (ICF)	60% of TBW	25	60% of TBW	21
Extracellular fluid (ECF)	40% of TBW	17	40% of TBW	14
Interstitial fluid	75% of ECF	13	75% of ECF	10
Plasma (PV)	20% of ECF	3	20% of ECF	3
Transcellular fluid	5% of ECF	1	5% of ECF	1
Blood (BV)	PV/(1 − Hct)	6	PV/(1 − Hct)	5

BW, Body weight; *Hct*, hematocrit.
[a]All of the above values are approximate and for illustration only. The volumes are rounded to the nearest liter, assuming a BW of 70 kg for both sexes, an Hct for men of 45%, and an Hct for women of 40%.

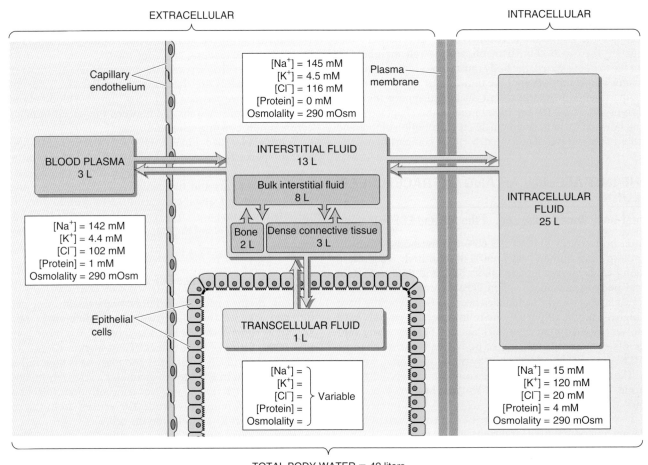

Figure 5.1 Fluid compartments of a prototypical adult human male weighing 70 kg. TBW is divided into four major compartments: ICF *(green)*, interstitial fluid *(blue)*, blood plasma *(red)*, and transcellular water such as synovial fluid *(tan)*. Color codes for each of these compartments are maintained throughout this book.

All body fluids have approximately the same osmolality, and each fluid has equal numbers of positive and negative charges

Osmolality Despite the differences in solute composition among the intracellular, interstitial, and plasma compartments, they all have approximately the same osmolality. Osmolality describes the total concentration of all particles that are free in a solution. Thus, glucose contributes one particle, whereas fully dissociated NaCl contributes two. Particles bound to macromolecules do not contribute at all to osmolality. In all body fluid compartments, humans have an osmolality—expressed as the number of osmotically active particles per kilogram of water—of ~290 milliosmoles/kg H_2O (290 mOsm).

TABLE 5.2 **Approximate Solute Composition of Key Fluid Compartments**

SOLUTE	PLASMA	PROTEIN-FREE PLASMA	INTERSTITIUM	CELL
Na^+ (mM)	142	153	145	15
K^+ (mM)	4.4	4.7	4.5	120
Ca^{2+} (mM)	1.2 (ionized) 2.4 (total)[a]	1.3 (ionized)	1.2 (ionized)	0.0001 (ionized)
Mg^{2+} (mM)	0.6 (ionized) 0.9 (total)[a]	0.6 (ionized)	0.55 (ionized)	1 (ionized) 18 (total)
Cl^- (mM)	102	110	116	20
HCO_3^- (mM)	22[b]	24	25	16
$H_2PO_4^-$ and HPO_4^{2-} (mM)	0.7 (ionized) 1.4 (total)[c]	0.75 (ionized)	0.8 (ionized)	0.7 (free)
Proteins	7 g/dL 1 mmole/L 14 meq/L	—	1 g/dL	30 g/dL
Glucose (mM)	5.5	5.9	5.9	Very low
pH	7.4	7.4	7.4	~7.2
Osmolality (milliosmoles/kg H_2O)	291	290	290	290

[a]Total includes amounts ionized, complexed to small solutes, and protein bound.
[b]Arterial value. The value in mixed-venous blood would be ~24 mM.
[c]Total plasma inorganic phosphate levels are not tightly regulated and vary between 0.8 and 1.5 mM.

Electroneutrality All solutions must respect the principle of bulk electroneutrality: the number of positive charges in the overall solution must be the same as the number of negative charges. If we add up the major cations and anions in the cytosol (Table 5.2), we see that the sum of $[Na^+]_i$ and $[K^+]_i$ greatly exceeds the sum of $[Cl^-]_i$ and $[HCO_3^-]_i$. The excess positive charge reflected by this difference is balanced by the negative charge on intracellular macromolecules (e.g., proteins) as well as smaller anions such as organic phosphates.

There is a similar difference between major cations and anions in blood plasma, where it is often referred to as the **anion gap.** The clinical definition of anion gap is

$$\text{Anion gap}_{\text{plasma}} = [Na^+]_{\text{plasma}} - \left([Cl^-]_{\text{plasma}} + [HCO_3^-]_{\text{plasma}}\right) \quad \textbf{(5.1)}$$

Note that plasma $[K^+]$ is ignored. The anion gap is usually 9 to 14 meq/L.

The differences in ionic composition between the ICF and ECF compartments are extremely important for normal functioning of the body. For example, because the K^+ gradient across cell membranes is a major determinant of electrical excitability, clinical disorders of extracellular $[K^+]$ can cause life-threatening disturbances in the heart rhythm. Disorders of extracellular $[Na^+]$ cause abnormal extracellular osmolality, with water being shifted into or out of essentially all cells, but most importantly brain cells; if uncorrected, such disorders lead to seizures, coma, or death.

SOLUTE TRANSPORT ACROSS CELL MEMBRANES

In passive, noncoupled transport across a permeable membrane, a solute moves down its electrochemical gradient

A substance can passively move across a membrane that separates two compartments when there is both a favorable driving force and an open pathway through which the driving force can exert its effect.

When a pathway exists for transfer of a substance across a membrane, the membrane is said to be **permeable** to that substance. The **driving force** that determines the passive transport of solutes across a membrane is the **electrochemical gradient** or electrochemical potential energy difference acting on the solute between the two compartments. This **electrochemical potential energy difference** includes a contribution from the concentration gradient of the solute—the chemical potential energy difference—and, for charged solutes (e.g., Na^+, Cl^-), a contribution from any difference in voltage that exists between the two compartments—the electrical potential energy difference.

This concept of how force and pathway determine passive movement of solutes is most easily illustrated by the example of passive, noncoupled transport. **Noncoupled transport** of a substance X means that movement of X across the membrane is not directly coupled to the movement of any other solute or to any chemical reaction (e.g., the hydrolysis of ATP). What, then, are the driving forces for the net movement of X? Clearly, if the concentration of X is higher in the outside compartment ($[X]_o$) than in the inside compartment

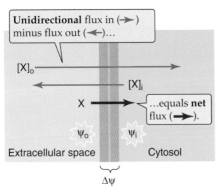

Figure 5.2 Uncoupled transport of a solute across a cell membrane.

([X]$_i$), and assuming no voltage difference, the concentration gradient will act as the driving force to bring about the net movement of X across the membrane from outside to inside (Fig. 5.2). If [X] is the same on both sides but there is a voltage difference across the membrane—that is, the electrical potential energy on the outside (ψ_o) is not the same as on the inside (ψ_i)—this voltage difference will also drive the net movement of X, provided X is charged. The concentration gradient for X and the voltage difference across the membrane are the two determinants of the electrochemical potential energy difference for X between the two compartments. Because the movement of X by such a noncoupled mechanism is not directly coupled to the movement of other solutes or to any chemical reactions, the electrochemical gradient for X is the only driving force that contributes to the transport of X. Thus, the transport of X by a noncoupled, passive mechanism must always proceed "downhill," in the direction down the electrochemical potential energy difference for X.

Regardless of *how* X moves passively through the membrane—whether X moves through lipid or through a membrane protein—the direction of the overall driving force acting on X determines the direction of net transport. In the example in Fig. 5.2, the overall driving force favors net transport from outside to inside (influx). However, X may still move from inside to outside (efflux). Movement of X across the membrane in one direction or the other is known as **unidirectional flux.** The algebraic sum of the two unidirectional fluxes is the **net flux,** or the net transport rate. Net transport occurs only when the unidirectional fluxes are unequal. In Fig. 5.2, the overall driving force makes unidirectional influx greater than unidirectional efflux, which results in net influx.

When no net driving force is acting on X, we say that X is at **equilibrium** across the membrane and there is no net transport of X across the membrane. However, even when X is in equilibrium, there may be and usually are equal and opposite movements of X across the membrane. Net transport takes place only when the net driving force acting on X is displaced from the equilibrium point, and transport proceeds in the direction that would bring X back to equilibrium.

Equilibrium is actually a special case of a **steady state.** In a steady state, by definition, the conditions related to X do not change with time. Thus, a transport system is in a steady state when both the driving forces acting on it and the rate of transport are constant with time. Equilibrium is the

particular steady state in which there is no net driving force and thus no net transport.

A cell can maintain a nonequilibrium steady state for X only when some device, such as a mechanism for actively transporting X, can compensate for the passive movement of X and prevent the intracellular and extracellular concentrations of X from changing with time. This combination of a pump and a leak maintains both the concentrations of X and the passive flux of X.

At equilibrium, the chemical and electrical potential energy differences across the membrane are equal but opposite

As noted in the preceding section, the driving force for the passive, uncoupled transport of a solute is the electrochemical potential energy difference for that solute across the membrane that separates the inside (i) from the outside (o). The electrochemical potential energy difference is:

$$\underbrace{\Delta\tilde{\mu}_X}_{\substack{\text{Electrochemical} \\ \text{potential energy} \\ \text{difference}}} = \underbrace{RT\ln\frac{[X]_i}{[X]_o}}_{\substack{\text{Chemical} \\ \text{potential energy} \\ \text{difference}}} + \underbrace{z_X F(\psi_i - \psi_o)}_{\substack{\text{Electrical} \\ \text{potential energy} \\ \text{difference}}} \tag{5.2}$$

where z_X is the valence of X, T is absolute temperature, R is the gas constant, and F is the Faraday constant. The first term on the right-hand side of Equation 5.2, the difference in chemical potential energy, describes the energy change (joules per mole) as X moves across the membrane if we disregard the charge—if any—on X. The second term, the difference in electrical potential energy, describes the energy change as a mole of charged particles (each with a valence of z_X) moves across the membrane. The difference ($\psi_i - \psi_o$) is the **voltage difference across the membrane (V_m)**, also known as the **membrane potential.**

By definition, X is at equilibrium when the electrochemical potential energy difference for X across the membrane is zero:

$$\Delta\tilde{\mu}_X = 0 \tag{5.3}$$

If we set $\Delta\bar{u}_X$ in Equation 5.2 to zero, as necessary for a state of equilibrium,

$$0 = RT\ln\frac{[X]_i}{[X]_o} + z_X F V_m$$

$$-\frac{RT}{z_X F}\ln\frac{[X]_i}{[X]_o} = V_m \tag{5.4}$$

$$V_m = E_X = -\frac{RT}{z_X F}\ln\frac{[X]_i}{[X]_o}$$

This is the **Nernst equation,** which describes the conditions when an ion is in equilibrium across a membrane. Given values for [X]$_i$ and [X]$_o$, X can be in equilibrium only when the voltage difference across the membrane equals the **equilibrium potential (E_X)**, also known as the Nernst potential. Stated somewhat differently, E_X is the value that the membrane voltage *would have to have* for X to be in equilibrium. If we express the logarithm to the base 10, then for the special case in which the temperature is 29.5°C,

TABLE 5.3 Net Electrochemical Driving Forces Acting on Ions in a Typical Cell[a]

EXTRACELLULAR CONCENTRATION $[X]_0$	INTRACELLULAR CONCENTRATION $[X]_i$	MEMBRANE VOLTAGE V_m	EQUILIBRIUM POTENTIAL (mV) $E_X = -(RT/z_X F)$ ln $([X]_i/[X]_0)$	ELECTROCHEMICAL DRIVING FORCE($V_m - E_X$)
Na$^+$ 145 mM	15 mM	−60 mV	+61 mV	−121 mV
K$^+$ 4.5 mM	120 mM	−60 mV	−88 mV	+28 mV
Ca^{2+} 1.2 mM	10^{-7} M	−60 mV	+125 mV	−185 mV
Cl$^-$ 116 mM	20 mM	−60 mV	−47 mV	−13 mV
HCO$_3^-$ 25 mM	16 mM	−60 mV	−12 mV	−48 mV
H$^+$ 40 nM pH 7.4	63 nM 7.2	−60 mV	−12 mV	−48 mV

[a]Calculated at 37°C using $-RT/z_X F = -26.71$ mV.

$$V_m = E_X = -\frac{(60\ mV)}{z_X} \log_{10} \frac{[X]_i}{[X]_o} \quad \textbf{(5.5)}$$

At normal body temperature (37°C), the coefficient is ~61.5 mV instead of 60 mV. At 20°C, it is ~58.1 mV.

To illustrate the use of Equation 5.5, we compute E_X for a monovalent cation, such as K$^+$. If $[K^+]_i$ is 100 mM and $[K^+]_o$ is 10 mM, a 10-fold concentration gradient, then

$$E_K = -\frac{(60\ mV)}{1} \log_{10} \frac{100}{10} = -60\ mV \quad \textbf{(5.6)}$$

Thus, a 10-fold gradient of a monovalent ion such as K$^+$ is equivalent, as a driving force, to a voltage difference of 60 mV. For a divalent ion such as Ca^{2+}, a 10-fold concentration gradient can be balanced as a driving force by a voltage difference of 60 mV/2, or only 30 mV.

($V_m - E_X$) is the net electrochemical driving force acting on an ion

When dealing with an ion (X), think about the net driving force in voltage (*units:* millivolts) rather than electrochemical potential energy difference (*units:* joules per mole).

A convenient equation expressing the net driving force is

$$\text{Net driving force in volts} = (V_m - E_X) \quad \textbf{(5.7)}$$

In Table 5.3, we use this equation—along with the values in Table 5.2 for extracellular (i.e., interstitial) and intracellular concentrations and a typical V_m of −60 mV—to compute the net driving force of Na$^+$, K$^+$, Ca^{2+}, Cl$^-$, HCO$_3^-$, and H$^+$. When the net driving force is negative, cations will enter the cell and anions will exit. Stated differently, when V_m is more negative than E_X (i.e., the cell is *too negative* for X to be in equilibrium), a cation will tend to enter the cell and an anion will tend to exit.

In simple diffusion, the flux of an uncharged substance through membrane lipid is directly proportional to its concentration difference

So far, we have discussed only the *direction* of net transport, not the *rate*. How will the rate of X transport vary if we vary

the driving force $\Delta \tilde{u}_X$? Unlike determining the direction, determining the rate—that is, the **kinetics**—of transport requires knowing the peculiarities of the actual mechanism that mediates passive X transport.

⊙ **5-2** Here we examine the simplest case, which is **simple diffusion.** How fast does an uncharged, hydrophobic solute move through a lipid bilayer? Gases (e.g., CO$_2$), a few endogenous compounds (e.g., steroid hormones), and many drugs (e.g., anesthetics) are both uncharged and hydrophobic. Imagine that such a solute is present on both sides of the membrane but at a higher concentration on the outside (Fig. 5.2). Because X has no electrical charge and because $[X]_o$ is greater than $[X]_i$, the net movement of X will be *into* the cell. How *fast* X moves is described by its **flux** (J_X); namely, the number of moles of X crossing a unit area of membrane (typically 1 cm^2) per unit time (typically 1 second). Thus, J_X has the units of moles/(square centimeter · second). The better that X can dissolve in the membrane lipid (i.e., the higher the lipid-water **partition coefficient** of X), the more easily X will be able to traverse the membrane-lipid barrier. The flux of X will also be greater if X moves more readily once it is in the membrane (i.e., a higher **diffusion coefficient**) and if the distance that it must traverse is short (i.e., a smaller **membrane thickness**). We can combine these three factors into a single parameter called the **permeability coefficient of X** (P_X). Finally, the flux of X will be greater as the difference in [X] between the two sides of the membrane increases (a large **gradient**).

⊙ **5-3** These concepts governing the simple diffusion are embodied in this simplified version of **Fick's law:**

$$J_X = P_X \left([X]_o - [X]_i \right) \quad \textbf{(5.8)}$$

Thus, net flux is proportional to the concentration *difference* ($[X]_o - [X]_i$). In all cases, the proportionality constant is P_X.

Some substances cross the membrane passively through intrinsic membrane proteins that can form pores, channels, or carriers

Because most ions and hydrophilic solutes of biological interest partition poorly into the lipid bilayer, simple passive diffusion of these solutes through the lipid portion of the membrane is negligible. Noncoupled transport across the

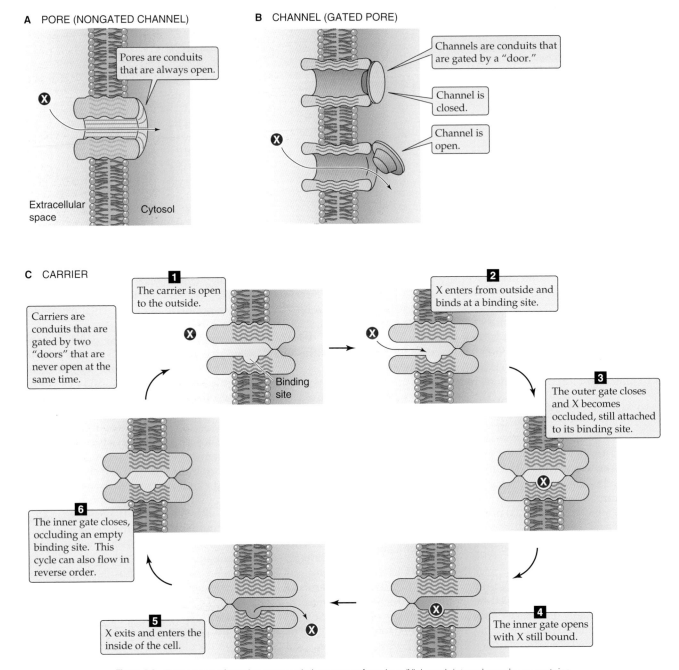

A PORE (NONGATED CHANNEL)

Pores are conduits that are always open.

Extracellular space   Cytosol

B CHANNEL (GATED PORE)

Channels are conduits that are gated by a "door."

Channel is closed.

Channel is open.

C CARRIER

Carriers are conduits that are gated by two "doors" that are never open at the same time.

1 The carrier is open to the outside.

Binding site

2 X enters from outside and binds at a binding site.

3 The outer gate closes and X becomes occluded, still attached to its binding site.

4 The inner gate opens with X still bound.

5 X exits and enters the inside of the cell.

6 The inner gate closes, occluding an empty binding site. This cycle can also flow in reverse order.

Figure 5.3 Three types of passive, noncoupled transport of a solute *(X)* through integral membrane proteins.

plasma membrane generally requires specialized pathways that allow particular substances to cross the lipid bilayer. In all known cases, such pathways are formed from **integral membrane proteins.** Three types of protein pathways through the membrane are recognized:

1. The membrane protein forms a **pore** that is always open (Fig. 5.3A).
2. The membrane protein forms a **channel** that is alternately open and closed because it is equipped with a movable barrier or gate (Fig. 5.3B).
3. The membrane protein forms a **carrier** surrounding a conduit that never offers a continuous transmembrane path because it is equipped with at least two gates that are never open at the same time (Fig. 5.3C).

⊙ 5-4 Gated channels, which alternately open and close, allow ions to cross the membrane passively

Gated **ion channels** consist of one or more polypeptide subunits with α-helical membrane-spanning segments. These channels have several functional components (Fig. 5.3B). The first is a **gate** that determines whether the channel is open or closed, with each state reflecting a different conformation of the membrane protein. Second, the channel generally has one or more **sensors** that can respond to one of several different types of signals: (1) changes in membrane voltage, (2) second-messenger systems that act at the cytoplasmic face of the membrane protein, or (3) ligands, such as neurohumoral agonists, that bind to the extracellular face of the membrane protein. These signals regulate transitions between the open and closed states. A third functional component is a **selectivity filter,** which determines the *classes* of ions (e.g., anions or cations) or the *particular* ions (e.g., Na⁺, K⁺, Ca²⁺) that have access to the channel pore. The fourth component is the actual **open channel pore** (Fig. 5.3B). Each time that a channel assumes the open conformation, it provides a continuous pathway between the two sides of the membrane so that ions can flow through it passively by diffusion until the channel closes again. During each channel opening, many ions flow through the channel pore, usually a sufficient number to be detected as a small current by sensitive recording techniques (see ◉ 6-3).

Na⁺ Channels Because the **electrochemical driving force for Na⁺** ($V_m - E_{Na}$) is always strongly *negative* (Table 5.3), a large, inwardly directed net driving force or gradient favors the passive movement of Na⁺ into virtually every cell of the body. Therefore, an open Na⁺ channel will act as a conduit for the passive entry of Na⁺. One physiological use for channel-mediated Na⁺ entry is the transmission of information. Thus, voltage-gated Na⁺ channels are responsible for generating the action potential (e.g., "nerve impulse") in many excitable cells.

K⁺ Channels The **electrochemical driving force for K⁺** ($V_m - E_K$) is usually fairly close to zero or somewhat *positive* (Table 5.3), so K⁺ is either at equilibrium or tends to move *out* of the cell. In virtually all cells, K⁺ channels play a major role in generating a resting membrane voltage that is inside negative. Other kinds of K⁺ channels play a key role in excitable cells, where these channels help terminate action potentials.

Ca²⁺ Channels The **electrochemical driving force for Ca²⁺** ($V_m - E_{Ca}$) is always strongly *negative* (Table 5.3), so Ca²⁺ tends to move *into* the cell. When Ca²⁺ channels are open, Ca²⁺ rapidly enters the cell down a steep electrochemical gradient. This inward movement of Ca²⁺ plays a vital role in transmembrane signaling for both excitable and nonexcitable cells as well as in generating action potentials in some excitable cells.

Anion Channels Most cells contain one or more types of anion-selective channels through which the passive, noncoupled transport of Cl⁻—and, to a lesser extent, HCO₃⁻—can take place. The **electrochemical driving force for Cl⁻** ($V_m - E_{Cl}$) in most cells is modestly *negative* (Table 5.3), so Cl⁻ tends to move *out of* these cells. In certain epithelial cells with Cl⁻ channels on their basolateral membranes, the passive movement of Cl⁻ through these channels plays a role in the transepithelial movement of Cl⁻ from lumen to blood.

Some carriers facilitate the passive diffusion of small solutes such as glucose

Carrier-mediated transport systems transfer a broad range of ions and organic solutes across the plasma membrane. Each carrier protein has a specific affinity for binding one or a small number of solutes and transporting them across the bilayer. The simplest passive carrier-mediated transporter is one that mediates *facilitated diffusion*. Below, we will introduce *cotransporters* (which carry two or more solutes in the same direction) and *exchangers* (which move them in opposite directions).

All carriers that do not either hydrolyze ATP or couple to an electron transport chain are members of the **solute carrier (SLC) superfamily.** The superfamily includes 54 families (i.e., SLC1 through SLC54). Members of a particular SLC family (e.g., SLC4A1 vs. SLC4A4) may differ in molecular mechanism (i.e., facilitated diffusion, cotransport, exchange), kinetic properties (e.g., solute specificity and affinity), regulation (e.g., phosphorylation), sites of membrane targeting (e.g., plasma membrane versus intracellular organelles), tissues in which they are expressed (e.g., kidney versus brain), or developmental stage at which they are expressed.

Carrier-mediated transport systems behave according to a general kinetic scheme for facilitated diffusion that is outlined in Fig. 5.3C. This model illustrates how, in a cycle of six steps, a carrier can passively move a solute X into the cell.

This mechanism can mediate only the downhill, or passive, transport of X. Therefore, it mediates a type of diffusion, called **facilitated diffusion.** When [X] is equal on the two sides of the membrane, no *net* transport will take place, although equal and opposite *unidirectional* fluxes of X may still occur.

In a cell membrane, a fixed number of carriers is available to transport X. Furthermore, each carrier has a limited speed with which it can cycle through the steps illustrated in Fig. 5.3C. Thus, if the extracellular X concentration is gradually increased, for example, the influx of X will eventually reach a maximal value once all the carriers have become loaded with X. This situation is very different from the one that exists with simple diffusion—that is, the movement of a solute through the lipid phase of the membrane. Influx by simple diffusion increases linearly with increases in $[X]_o$, with no maximal rate of transport (Fig. 5.4A). Thus, the relationship describing carrier-mediated transport follows the same Michaelis-Menten kinetics as do enzymes (Fig. 5.4B):

$$V = \frac{[S]\,V_{max}}{K_m + [S]} \qquad \textbf{(5.9)}$$

This equation describes how the velocity of an enzymatic reaction *(V)* depends on the substrate concentration ([S]), the Michaelis constant (K_m), and the maximal velocity (V_{max}). The comparable equation for carrier-mediated transport is identical, except that fluxes replace reaction velocities:

$$J_X = \frac{[X]\,J_{max}}{K_m + [X]} \qquad \textbf{(5.10)}$$

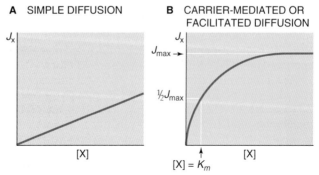

A   SIMPLE DIFFUSION   **B**   CARRIER-MEDIATED OR FACILITATED DIFFUSION

Figure 5.4   Dependence of transport rates on solute concentration.

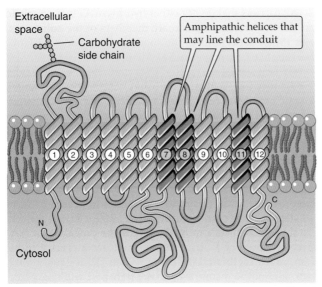

Extracellular space

Carbohydrate side chain

Amphipathic helices that may line the conduit

Cytosol

N

C

Figure 5.5 Structure of the GLUT family of glucose transporters. The 12 membrane-spanning segments are connected to each other by intracellular and extracellular loops.

Thus, K_m is the solute concentration at which J_X is half of the maximal flux (J_{max}). The lower the K_m, the higher the apparent **affinity** of the transporter for the solute.

⊙ **5-5** Examples of membrane proteins that mediate facilitated diffusion are the **GLUT glucose transporters** (Fig. 5.5), members of the SLC2 family. The GLUTs have 12 membrane-spanning segments as well as multiple hydrophilic polypeptide loops facing either the ECF or the ICF. The membrane-spanning segments, as well as other portions of the protein, probably act as the gates and solute-binding sites that allow transport to proceed in the manner outlined in Fig. 5.3C.

The Na-K pump, the most important primary active transporter in animal cells, uses the energy of ATP to extrude Na⁺ and take up K⁺

⊙ **5-6 Active transport** is a process that can transfer a solute uphill across a membrane—that is, against its electrochemical potential energy difference. In **primary active transport,** the energy needed to cause net transfer of a solute against its electrochemical gradient comes from ATP hydrolysis. In **secondary active transport,** the driving force is provided by coupling the *uphill* movement of that solute to the *downhill* movement of one or more other solutes for which a favorable electrochemical potential energy difference exists. For transporters, it is commonly the favorable inwardly directed Na⁺ electrochemical gradient that drives the *secondary* active transport of another solute. Primary active transporters are also referred to as **pumps.** The pumps discussed here are all energized by ATP hydrolysis and hence are **ATPases.**

As a prototypic example of a primary active transporter, consider the nearly ubiquitous **Na-K pump** (or **Na,K-ATPase, NKA**). The Na-K pump is located in the plasma membrane and has both α and β subunits (Fig. 5.6A). The α subunit, which has 10 transmembrane segments, is the catalytic subunit that mediates active transport. The β subunit, which has one transmembrane segment, is essential for proper assembly and membrane targeting of the Na-K pump.

With each forward cycle, the pump couples the extrusion of three Na⁺ ions and the uptake of two K⁺ ions to the intracellular hydrolysis of one ATP molecule.

Although animal cells may have other pumps in their plasma membranes, the Na-K pump is the only primary active transport process for Na⁺. The Na-K pump is also the most important primary active transport mechanism for K⁺. In cells throughout the body, the Na-K pump is responsible for maintaining a low [Na⁺]ᵢ and a high [K⁺]ᵢ relative to ECF.

The Na-K pump exists in two major conformational states: E_1, in which the binding sites for the ions face the inside of the cell; and E_2, in which the binding sites face the outside. The Na-K pump is a member of a large superfamily of pumps known as **E_1-E_2 ATPases** or **P-type ATPases.** It is the ordered cycling between these two states that underlies the action of the pump. Fig. 5.6B is a simplified model showing the eight stages of this catalytic cycle of the α subunit.

Because each cycle of hydrolysis of one ATP molecule is coupled to the extrusion of three Na⁺ ions from the cell and the uptake of two K⁺ ions, the *stoichiometry* of the pump is three Na⁺ to two K⁺, and each cycle of the pump is associated with the net extrusion of one positive charge from the cell. Thus, the Na-K pump is *electrogenic*.

The rate of active transport by the Na-K pump is a saturable function of [Na⁺]ᵢ and [K⁺]ₒ. The transport rate is also a saturable function of [ATP]ᵢ and therefore depends on the metabolic state of the cell. In cells with high Na-K pump rates, such as renal proximal tubules, a third or more of cellular energy metabolism is devoted to supplying ATP to the Na-K pump.

⊙ **5-7** A hallmark of the Na-K pump is that it is blocked by a class of compounds known as **cardiac glycosides,** examples of which are ouabain and digoxin; digoxin is widely used for a variety of cardiac conditions. These compounds have a high affinity for the extracellular side of the E_2-P state of the pump, which also has a high affinity for extracellular K⁺. Thus, the binding of extracellular K⁺ competitively antagonizes the binding of cardiac glycosides. An important clinical correlate is that hypokalemia (a low [K⁺] in blood plasma) potentiates digitalis toxicity in patients.

⊙ 5-8 Besides the Na-K pump, other P-type ATPases include the H-K and Ca pumps

The family of P-type ATPases—all of which share significant sequence similarity with the α subunit of the Na-K pump—includes several subfamilies.

H-K Pump ⊙ **5-9** In the parietal cells of the gastric gland, an H-K pump (HKA) extrudes H⁺ across the apical membrane into the gland lumen. Similar pumps are present in the kidney and intestines. The H-K pump mediates the active extrusion of H⁺ and the uptake of K⁺, all fueled by ATP hydrolysis, probably in the ratio of two H⁺ ions, two K⁺ ions, and one ATP molecule.

Ca Pumps ⊙ **5-10** Most, if not all, cells have a primary active transporter at the plasma membrane that extrudes Ca²⁺ from the cell. These pumps, which are abbreviated **PMCA** (for plasma-membrane Ca-ATPase), exchange one H⁺ for one Ca²⁺ for each molecule of ATP that is hydrolyzed.

⊙ **5-11** Ca pumps (or Ca-ATPases) also exist on the membrane surrounding such intracellular organelles as the sarcoplasmic reticulum (SR) in muscle cells and the endoplasmic

A Na-K PUMP

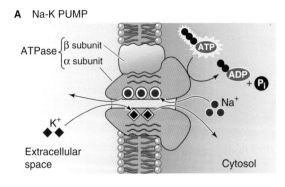

B ENZYMATIC CYCLE OF THE Na-K PUMP

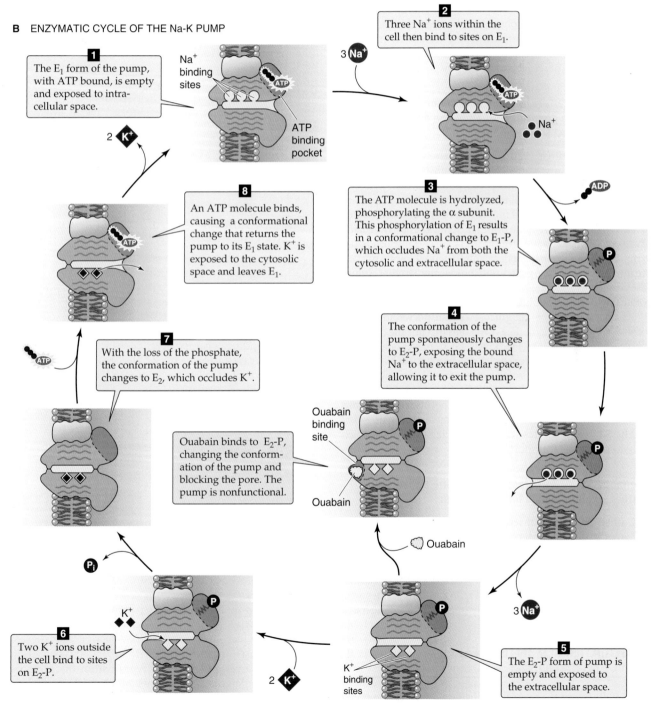

1 The E_1 form of the pump, with ATP bound, is empty and exposed to intracellular space.

2 Three Na^+ ions within the cell then bind to sites on E_1.

3 The ATP molecule is hydrolyzed, phosphorylating the α subunit. This phosphorylation of E_1 results in a conformational change to E_1-P, which occludes Na^+ from both the cytosolic and extracellular space.

4 The conformation of the pump spontaneously changes to E_2-P, exposing the bound Na^+ to the extracellular space, allowing it to exit the pump.

5 The E_2-P form of pump is empty and exposed to the extracellular space.

6 Two K^+ ions outside the cell bind to sites on E_2-P.

7 With the loss of the phosphate, the conformation of the pump changes to E_2, which occludes K^+.

8 An ATP molecule binds, causing a conformational change that returns the pump to its E_1 state. K^+ is exposed to the cytosolic space and leaves E_1.

Ouabain binds to E_2-P, changing the conformation of the pump and blocking the pore. The pump is nonfunctional.

Figure 5.6 Model of the sodium pump.

reticulum (ER) in other cells, where they play a role in the active sequestration of Ca^{2+} into intracellular stores. The **SERCAs** (for sarcoplasmic and endoplasmic reticulum calcium ATPases) appear to transport two H^+ and two Ca^{2+} ions for each molecule of ATP hydrolyzed.

ATP-binding cassette transporters can act as pumps, channels, or regulators

The so-called ABC proteins all have a motif in their amino-acid sequence that is an ATP-binding cassette (ABC). In humans, this family includes at least 49 members in seven subfamilies named ABCA through ABCG. Some are pumps that presumably hydrolyze ATP to provide energy for solute transport. Some may hydrolyze ATP, but they do not couple the liberated energy to perform active transport. In other cases, ATP regulates ABC proteins that function as ion channels or regulators of ion channels or transporters.

⊙ 5-12 Cotransporters, one class of secondary active transporters, are generally driven by the energy of the inwardly directed Na⁺ gradient

Like pumps or primary active transporters, secondary active transporters can move a solute uphill (against its electrochemical gradient). However, unlike the pumps, which fuel the process by hydrolyzing ATP, the secondary active transporters fuel it by coupling the uphill movement of one or more solutes to the downhill movement of other solutes. The two major classes of secondary active transporters are cotransporters (or symporters) and exchangers (or antiporters). Cotransporters are intrinsic membrane proteins that move the "driving" solute (the one whose gradient provides the energy) and the "driven" solutes (which move uphill) in the *same* direction.

As an example, the **Na/glucose cotransporter (SGLT)** is located at the apical membrane of the cells that line the proximal tubule and small intestine (Fig. 5.7A). SGLT2 moves one Na^+ ion with each glucose molecule (i.e., 1:1 stoichiometry of Na^+ to glucose), whereas the SGLT1 isoform moves two Na^+ ions with each glucose molecule. Drugs that inhibit SGLT2 are useful in treating type 2 diabetes in adults because these agents reduce glucose reabsorption in the kidney, thereby lowering plasma [glucose].

Fig. 5.7B–L illustrates several other classes of physiologically important cotransporters.

Exchangers, another class of secondary active transporters, exchange ions for one another

The other major class of secondary active transporters is the exchangers, or antiporters. Exchangers are intrinsic membrane proteins that move one or more "driving" solutes in one direction and one or more "driven" solutes in the *opposite* direction. In general, these transporters exchange cations for cations or anions for anions. Fig. 5.8A–F illustrates several other classes of physiologically important exchangers.

REGULATION OF INTRACELLULAR ION CONCENTRATIONS

Fig. 5.9 illustrates the tools at the disposal of a prototypic cell for managing its intracellular composition. Cells in different

A Na/GLUCOSE COTRANSPORTER (SGLT1-2)

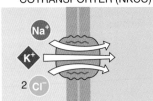

B Na/AMINO ACID COTRANSPORTER

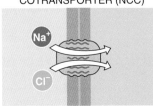

C Na/PHOSPHATE COTRANSPORTER (NaPi)

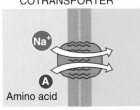

D Na/HCO₃ COTRANSPORTER (NBCe1, e2)

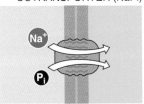

E Na/HCO₃ COTRANSPORTER (NBCe1, e2)

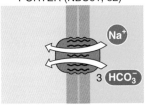

F Na/HCO₃ COTRANSPORTER (NBCn1, n2)

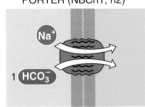

G Na/K/Cl COTRANSPORTER (NKCC)

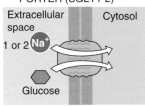

H Na/Cl COTRANSPORTER (NCC)

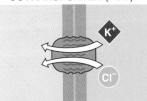

I K/Cl COTRANSPORTER (KCC)

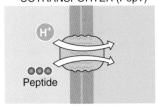

J H/OLIGOPEPTIDE COTRANSPORTER (PepT)

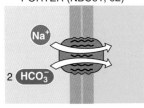

K H/MONOCARBOXYLATE COTRANSPORTER (MCT)

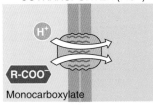

L H/DIVALENT METAL ION COTRANSPORTER (DMT)

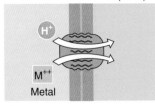

Figure 5.7 Representative cotransporters.

tissues—and even different cell types within the same tissue—have different complements of channels and transporters. Epithelial cells and neurons may segregate specific channels and transporters to different parts of the cell (e.g.,

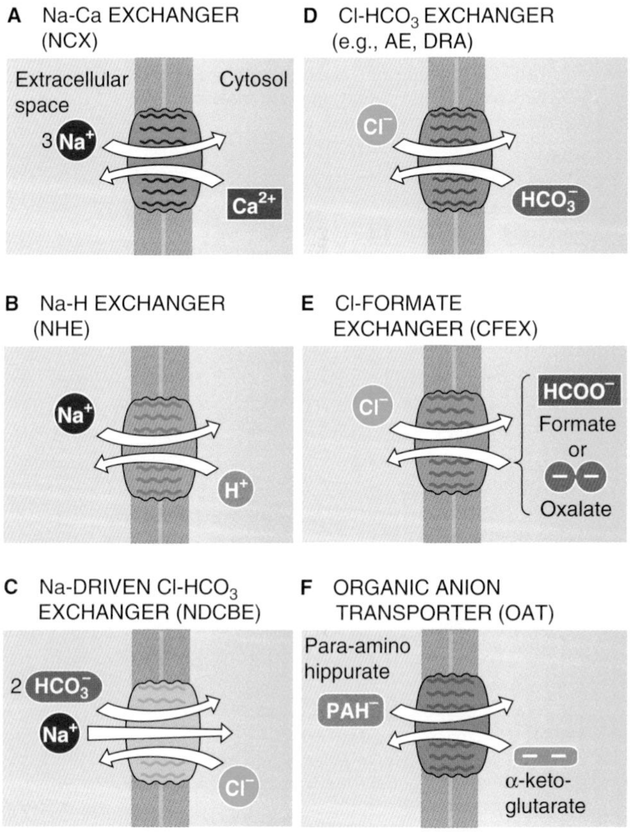

A Na-Ca EXCHANGER (NCX)

D Cl-HCO₃ EXCHANGER (e.g., AE, DRA)

B Na-H EXCHANGER (NHE)

E Cl-FORMATE EXCHANGER (CFEX)

Formate or Oxalate

C Na-DRIVEN Cl-HCO₃ EXCHANGER (NDCBE)

F ORGANIC ANION TRANSPORTER (OAT)

Para-amino hippurate

α-keto-glutarate

Figure 5.8 Representative exchangers.

apical versus basolateral membrane or axon versus soma/dendrite). Thus, different cells may have somewhat different intracellular ionic compositions.

WATER TRANSPORT AND THE REGULATION OF CELL VOLUME

Water transport is driven by osmotic and hydrostatic pressure differences across membranes

⊙ 5-13 Transport of water across biological membranes is always passive. To a certain extent, single H_2O molecules can dissolve in lipid bilayers and thus move across cell membranes at a low but finite rate by simple diffusion. However, the plasma membranes of many types of cells have specialized H_2O channels—the **AQPs**—that serve as passive conduits for H_2O transport. The presence of AQPs greatly increases membrane H_2O permeability.

Water transport across a membrane is always a linear, nonsaturable function of its net driving force. The direction of net passive transport of an uncharged solute is always down its chemical potential energy difference. For H_2O, we must consider two passive driving forces. The first is the familiar chemical potential energy difference, which depends on the difference in **water concentration** on the two sides of the membrane. The second is the energy difference, per mole of H_2O that results from the difference in **hydrostatic pressure** across the membrane.

Dealing with H_2O concentrations is cumbersome and imprecise because $[H_2O]$ is very high (i.e., ~56 M) and does not change substantially in the dilute solutions in which

physiologists are interested. Therefore, it is more practical to work with the inverse of $[H_2O]$, namely, the concentration of osmotically active solutes, or **osmolality.** The units of osmolality are osmoles per kilogram of H_2O, or Osm.

Osm is the total concentration of all osmotically active solutes in the indicated compartment (e.g., Na^+ + Cl^- + K^+ + …).

The *driving force* for H_2O movement from the inside to the outside of the cell includes both an osmotic-pressure difference RT $(Osm_o – Osm_i)$ or $(\pi_o – \pi_i)$ and a hydrostatic-pressure difference $(P_i – P_o)$. The **flux of H_2O** across the membrane (J_V) is:

$$J_V = L_p \left[RT \left(Osm_o - Osm_i \right) + \left(P_i - P_o \right) \right] \tag{5.11}$$

J_V is positive when H_2O flows out of the cell and has the units of $L/(cm^2 \cdot s)$. The proportionality constant L_p is the **hydraulic conductivity.**

Movement of H_2O in and out of cells is driven by osmotic gradients only, that is, by differences in osmolality across the membrane. For example, if the osmolality is greater outside the cell than inside, H_2O will flow out of the cell and the cell will shrink. Such a movement of H_2O driven by osmotic gradients is called **osmosis.** H_2O is at equilibrium across *cell membranes* only when the osmolality inside and outside the cell is the same.

⊙ 5-14 Hydrostatic pressure differences are an important force for driving fluid out across the *walls of capillaries.* Small solutes permeate freely across most capillaries. Thus, any difference in *osmotic* pressure as a result of these small solutes does not exert a driving force for H_2O flow across that capillary. The situation is quite different for plasma proteins, which are too large to penetrate the capillary wall freely. As a result, the presence of a greater concentration of plasma proteins in the intravascular compartment than in interstitial fluid sets up a difference in osmotic pressure that tends to pull fluid back into the capillary. This difference is called the **colloid osmotic pressure** or **oncotic pressure.** H_2O is at equilibrium across the wall of a *capillary* when the colloid osmotic and hydrostatic pressure differences are equal. When the hydrostatic pressure difference exceeds the colloid osmotic pressure difference, the result is movement of H_2O out of the capillary, called **ultrafiltration.**

The gradient in tonicity—or effective osmolality—determines the osmotic flow of water across a cell membrane

TBW is distributed among blood plasma and the interstitial, intracellular, and transcellular fluids. The mechanisms by which H_2O exchanges between interstitial fluid and ICF, and between interstitial fluid and plasma, rely on the principles that we have just discussed.

Water Exchange Across Cell Membranes Because cell membranes are not rigid, hydrostatic pressure differences never arise between cell H_2O and interstitial fluid. Increasing the *hydrostatic* pressure in the interstitial space will cause the cell to compress so that the intracellular hydrostatic pressure increases to a similar extent. Thus, H_2O does not enter the cell under these conditions. However, increasing the interstitial *osmotic* pressure (π_o), and thus generating a $\Delta\pi$, is quite a different matter. If we suddenly increase ECF osmolality by adding an *impermeant* solute such as mannitol, the resulting osmotic gradient across the cell membrane causes H_2O to move out of the cell.

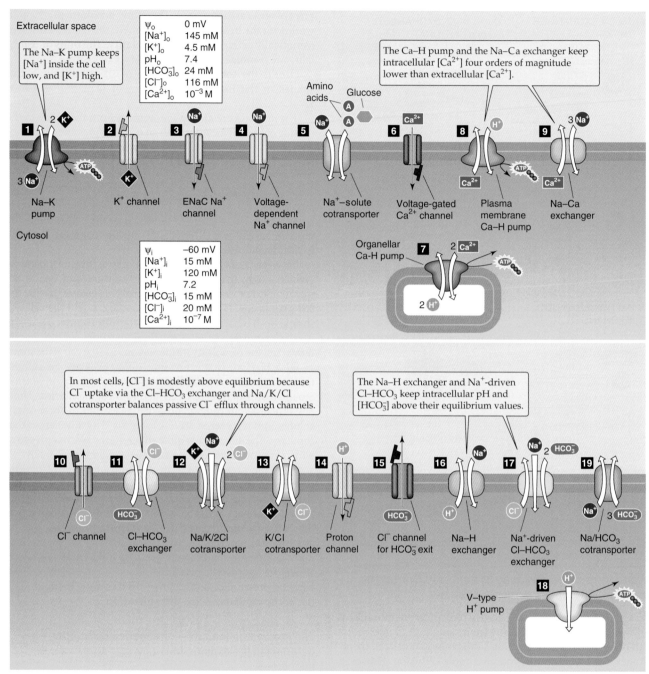

Figure 5.9 Ion gradients, channels, and transporters in a typical cell.

On the other hand, consider what would happen if we suddenly increase ECF osmolality by adding a *permeant* solute such as urea. Urea can rapidly penetrate cell membranes by facilitated diffusion through members of the UT family of transporters; however, cells have no mechanism for extruding urea. Because urea penetrates the membrane more slowly than H_2O does, the initial effect of applying urea is to shrink the cell (Fig. 5.10). However, as urea gradually equilibrates across the cell membrane and abolishes the initially imposed osmotic gradient, the cell swells back to its initial volume. Thus, sustained changes in cell volume do not occur with a change in the extracellular concentration of a permeant solute.

⊙ **5-15** The difference between the effects of mannitol and urea on the final cell volume illustrates the need to distinguish between total osmolality and **effective osmolality** (also known as **tonicity**). In terms of clinically measured solutes, total and effective osmolality of the ECF can be approximated as in Equation 5.12. BUN stands for **blood urea nitrogen**, that is, the concentration of the nitrogen that is contained in the plasma as urea. The clinical laboratory reports the value of $[Na^+]$ in Equation 5.12 in milliequivalents per liter. Because laboratories in the United States report the glucose and BUN concentrations in terms of milligrams per deciliter, we divide glucose by one tenth of the molecular weight of glucose and BUN by one tenth of the summed atomic

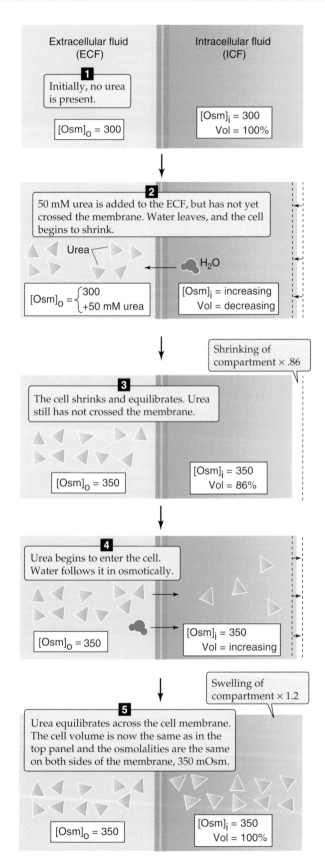

Figure 5.10 Effect of urea on the volume of a single cell bathed in an infinite volume of ECF. We assume that the cell membrane is permeable only to water during the initial moments in steps 2 and 3. Later, during steps 4 and 5, we assume that the membrane is permeable to both water and urea.

weights of the two nitrogen atoms in urea. The computed tonicity does not include BUN because—as we saw above—urea easily equilibrates across most cell membranes. On the other hand, the computed tonicity includes both Na^+ and glucose. It includes Na^+ because Na^+ is *functionally* impermeant owing to its extrusion by the Na-K pump. Tonicity includes glucose because this solute does not appreciably accumulate in most cells as a result of metabolism.

$$\text{Total osmolality (mOsm)} \cong 2 \cdot [Na^+] + \frac{\overset{\text{Glucose}}{(mg/dL)}}{18} + \frac{\overset{\text{BUN}}{(mg/dL)}}{2.8} \quad \textbf{(5.12)}$$

$$\text{Tonicity or effective osmolality (mOsm)} \cong 2 \cdot [Na^+] + \frac{\text{Glucose }(mg/dL)}{18}$$

Osmolality describes the number of osmotically active solutes in a single solution. If we regard a plasma osmolality of 290 mOsm as being normal, solutions having an osmolality of 290 mOsm are **isosmolal,** solutions with osmolalities >290 mOsm are **hyperosmolal,** and those with osmolalities <290 mOsm are hypo-osmolal. On the other hand, when we use the terms *isotonic, hypertonic,* and *hypotonic,* we are comparing one solution with another solution (e.g., ICF) across a well-defined membrane (e.g., a cell membrane). A solution is **isotonic** when its *effective* osmolality is the same as that of the reference solution, which for our purposes is the ICF. A **hypertonic** solution is one that has a higher effective osmolality than the reference solution, and a **hypotonic** solution has a lower effective osmolality.

Shifts of H_2O between the intracellular and interstitial compartments result from alterations in *effective* ECF osmolality, or *tonicity.* Clinically, such changes in tonicity are usually caused by decreases in $[Na^+]$ in the plasma and ECF (hyponatremia), increases in $[Na^+]$ (hypernatremia), or increases in glucose concentration (hyperglycemia). Changes in the concentration of a highly permeant solute such as urea, which accumulates in patients with kidney failure, have no effect on tonicity.

Water Exchange Across the Capillary Wall The barrier separating the blood plasma and interstitial compartments—the capillary wall—is, to a first approximation, freely permeable to solutes that are smaller than plasma proteins. Thus, the only *net* osmotic force that acts across the capillary wall is that caused by the asymmetric distribution of proteins in plasma versus interstitial fluid. Several terms may be used for the osmotic force that is generated by these impermeant plasma proteins, such as protein osmotic pressure, colloid osmotic pressure, and oncotic pressure. These terms are synonymous and can be represented by the symbol $\pi_{oncotic}$. The **oncotic pressure difference ($\Delta\pi_{oncotic}$),** which tends to pull H_2O from the interstitium to the plasma, is opposed by the hydrostatic pressure difference across the capillary wall (ΔP), which drives fluid from plasma into the interstitium. All net movements of H_2O across the capillary wall are accompanied by the small solutes dissolved in this H_2O, at their ECF concentrations; that is, the pathways taken by the H_2O across the capillary wall are so large that small solutes are not *sieved* out.

To summarize, fluid shifts between plasma and the interstitium respond only to changes in the balance between ΔP and $\Delta\pi_{oncotic}$. Small solutes such as Na^+, which freely cross the capillary wall, do not contribute significantly to osmotic driving forces across this barrier and move along with the H_2O in which they are dissolved.

Adding isotonic saline, pure water, or pure NaCl to the ECF will increase ECF volume but will have divergent effects on ICF volume and ECF osmolality

Adding various combinations of NaCl and **solute-free water** to the ECF will alter the volume and composition of the body fluid compartments. Three examples illustrate the effects seen with intravenous therapy. In Fig. 5.11A, we start with a TBW of 42 L (60% of a 70-kg person), subdivided into an ICF volume of 25 L (60% of TBW) and an ECF volume of 17 L (40% of TBW). These numerical values are the same as those in Fig. 5.1 and Table 5.1.

Infusion of Isotonic Saline Consider the case in which we infuse or ingest 1.5 L of isotonic saline, which is a 0.9% solution of NaCl in H_2O (Fig. 5.11B). This solution has an effective osmolality of 290 mOsm in the ECF. This 1.5 L is initially distributed throughout the ECF and raises ECF volume by 1.5 L. Because the effective osmolality of the ECF is unaltered, no change occurs in the effective osmotic gradient across the cell membranes, and the added H_2O moves neither into nor out of the ICF. This outcome is, of course, in accord with the definition of an *isotonic* solution. Thus, we see that adding isotonic saline to the body is an efficient way to expand the ECF without affecting the ICF. Similarly, if it were possible to remove isotonic saline from the body, we would see that this measure would efficiently contract the ECF and again have no effect on the ICF.

Infusion of "Solute-Free" Water Now consider a case in which we either ingest 1.5 L of pure H_2O or infuse 1.5 L of an isotonic (5%) glucose solution (Fig. 5.11C). Infusing the glucose solution intravenously is equivalent, in the long run, to infusing pure H_2O because the glucose is metabolized to CO_2 and H_2O, with no solutes left behind in the ECF. Infusing pure H_2O would be unwise inasmuch as it would cause the cells near the point of infusion to burst.

How do the effects of adding 1.5 L of pure H_2O compare with those in the previous example? At first, the 1.5 L of pure H_2O will be rapidly distributed throughout the ECF and increase its volume from 17 to 18.5 L (Fig. 5.11C, *left side*, "Early"). This added H_2O will also dilute the pre-existing solutes in the ECF, thereby lowering ECF osmolality to 290 mOsm × 17/18.5 = 266 mOsm. Because intracellular osmolality remains at 290 mOsm at this imaginary, intermediate stage, a large osmotic gradient is created that favors the entry of H_2O from the ECF into the ICF. Water will move into the ICF and consequently lower the osmolality of the ICF and simultaneously raise the osmolality of the ECF until osmotic equilibrium is restored (Fig. 5.11C, *right side*, "Final"). Because the added H_2O is distributed between the ICF and ECF according to the initial ICF/ECF ratio of 60%/40%, the final ECF volume is 17.6 L (i.e., 17 L expanded by 40% of 1.5 L). Thus, infusion of solute-free H_2O is a relatively *ineffective* means of expanding the ECF. More of the added H_2O has ended up intracellularly (60% of 1.5 L = 0.9 L of expansion). The major effect of the H_2O has been to dilute the osmolality of body fluids. The initial total-body solute content was 290 mOsm × 42 L = 12,180 milliosmoles.

This same solute has now been diluted in 42 + 1.5 or 43.5 L, so the final osmolality is 12,180/43.5 = 280 mOsm.

Ingestion of Pure NaCl Salt The preceding two "experiments" illustrate two extremely important principles that govern fluid and electrolyte homeostasis; namely, that adding or removing Na^+ will mainly affect ECF volume (Fig. 5.11B), whereas adding or removing solute-free H_2O will mainly affect the *osmolality* of body fluids (Fig. 5.11C). The first point can be further appreciated by considering a third case, one in which we add the same amount of NaCl that is contained in 1.5 L of isotonic (i.e., 0.9%) saline: 1.5 L × 290 mOsm = 435 milliosmoles. However, we will not add any H_2O. At first, these 435 milliosmoles of NaCl will rapidly distribute throughout the 17 L of ECF and increase the osmolality of the ECF (Fig. 5.11D, *left side*, "Early"). The initial total osmolal content of the ECF was 290 mOsm × 17 L = 4930 milliosmoles. Because we added 435 milliosmoles, we now have 5365 milliosmoles in the ECF. Thus, the ECF osmolality is 5365/17 = 316 mOsm. The resulting hyperosmolality draws H_2O out of the ICF into the ECF until osmotic equilibrium is re-established. What is the final osmolality? The total number of milliosmoles dissolved in TBW is the original 12,180 milliosmoles plus the added 435 milliosmoles, for a total of 12,615 milliosmoles. Because these milliosmoles are dissolved in 42 L of TBW, the final osmolality of the ICF and ECF is 12,615/42 = 300 mOsm.

In the new equilibrium state, the ECF volume has increased by 0.9 L, even though no H_2O at all was added to the body. Because the added ECF volume has come from the ICF, the ICF shrinks by 0.9 L. This example further illustrates the principle that the total-body content of Na^+ is the major determinant of ECF volume.

⊙ 5-16 Whole-body Na^+ content determines ECF volume, whereas whole-body water content determines osmolality

Changes in ECF volume are important because they are accompanied by proportional changes in the volume of blood plasma, which in turn affects the adequacy with which the circulatory system can perfuse vital organs with blood (see ⊙ **23-26**). The blood volume that is necessary to achieve adequate perfusion of key organs is sometimes referred to as the **effective circulating volume.** Because the body generally stabilizes osmolality, an increase in extracellular Na^+ content will increase ECF volume:

$$\underbrace{\text{Extracellular } Na^+ \text{ content}}_{\text{millimoles}} = \underbrace{[Na^+]_o}_{\text{millimoles/liter}} \times \underbrace{\text{ECF volume}}_{\text{liters}}$$

$$\cong \left(\frac{\text{Osmolality}}{2}\right) \times \underbrace{\text{ECF volume}}_{\text{liters}} \qquad \textbf{(5.13)}$$

Because cells contain very little Na^+, extracellular Na^+ content is nearly the same as **total-body Na^+** content.

We will see in Chapter 40 how the body regulates effective circulating volume. Increases in effective circulating volume, which reflect increases in ECF volume or total-body Na^+ *content*, stimulate the renal excretion of Na^+. In contrast, the plasma Na^+ *concentration* does *not* regulate renal excretion of Na^+. It makes sense that regulation of Na^+ excretion is not sensitive to the plasma Na^+ concentration because the concentration is not an indicator of ECF volume.

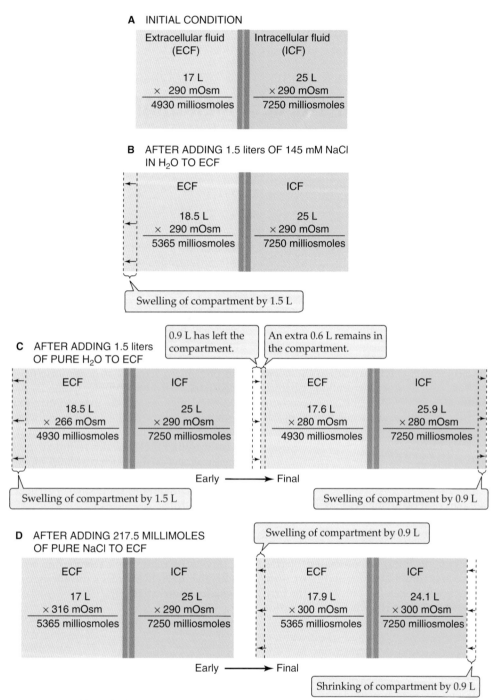

A INITIAL CONDITION

Extracellular fluid (ECF)	Intracellular fluid (ICF)
17 L × 290 mOsm ——— 4930 milliosmoles	25 L × 290 mOsm ——— 7250 milliosmoles

B AFTER ADDING 1.5 liters OF 145 mM NaCl IN H₂O TO ECF

ECF	ICF
18.5 L × 290 mOsm ——— 5365 milliosmoles	25 L × 290 mOsm ——— 7250 milliosmoles

Swelling of compartment by 1.5 L

C AFTER ADDING 1.5 liters OF PURE H₂O TO ECF

0.9 L has left the compartment.   An extra 0.6 L remains in the compartment.

ECF	ICF		ECF	ICF
18.5 L × 266 mOsm ——— 4930 milliosmoles	25 L × 290 mOsm ——— 7250 milliosmoles		17.6 L × 280 mOsm ——— 4930 milliosmoles	25.9 L × 280 mOsm ——— 7250 milliosmoles

Early ——→ Final

Swelling of compartment by 1.5 L   Swelling of compartment by 0.9 L

D AFTER ADDING 217.5 MILLIMOLES OF PURE NaCl TO ECF

Swelling of compartment by 0.9 L

ECF	ICF		ECF	ICF
17 L × 316 mOsm ——— 5365 milliosmoles	25 L × 290 mOsm ——— 7250 milliosmoles		17.9 L × 300 mOsm ——— 5365 milliosmoles	24.1 L × 300 mOsm ——— 7250 milliosmoles

Early ——→ Final

Shrinking of compartment by 0.9 L

Figure 5.11   Effect on body fluid compartments of infusing different solutions.

As discussed, when we hold osmolality constant, Na⁺ content determines ECF volume. What would happen if we held constant the Na⁺ content, which is a major part of **total-body osmoles**? An increase in **TBW** would decrease **osmolality.**

$$\underbrace{\text{Total body osmoles}}_{\text{milliosmoles}} = \underbrace{[\text{Osmolality}]}_{\text{milliosmoles/liter}} \times \underbrace{\text{Total body water}}_{\text{liters}} \quad \textbf{(5.14)}$$

Thus, a net gain or loss of solute-free H₂O has a major impact on the *osmolality* and [Na⁺] of the ECF. Moreover, because a large part (~60%) of the added solute-free water distributes into the ICF, a gain or loss of solute-free H₂O affects ICF more than ECF.

CHAPTER 6

ELECTROPHYSIOLOGY OF THE CELL MEMBRANE

Edward G. Moczydlowski

Electrical currents in a metal wire are conducted by the flow of electrons, but electrical currents across cell membranes are carried by inorganic ions. Many concepts and terms used in cellular electrophysiology are the same as those used to describe electrical circuits. At the molecular level, electrical current across cell membranes flows primarily via ion channels. The flow of ions via channels is the basis of electrical signals that underlie neuronal activity and animal behavior. Opening and closing of such channels is the fundamental process behind electrical phenomena such as the nerve impulse, the heartbeat, and sensory perception. Channel proteins are also intimately involved in hormone secretion, ionic homeostasis, osmoregulation, and regulation of muscle contractility.

IONIC BASIS OF MEMBRANE POTENTIALS

The plasma membranes of most living cells are electrically polarized, with a transmembrane voltage—or a **membrane potential**—in the range of 0.1 V. In Chapter 5, we discussed how the energy stored in this miniature battery can drive a variety of transmembrane transport processes. Electrically excitable cells such as brain neurons and heart myocytes also use this energy for signaling purposes. The brief electrical impulses produced by such cells are called **action potentials.**

Atoms consist of negatively (−) and positively (+) charged elementary particles, such as electrons (e⁻) and protons (H⁺), as well as electrically neutral particles (neutrons). Charges of the same sign repel each other, and those of opposite sign attract. Charge is measured in units of **coulombs (C)**. The **unitary charge** of one electron or proton is denoted by e_0 and is equal to 1.6022×10^{-19} C. Ions in solution have a charge valence (z) that is an integral number of elementary charges. For example, $z = +2$ for Ca^{2+}, $z = +1$ for K^+, and $z = -1$ for Cl^-. The charge of a single ion (q_0), measured in coulombs, is the product of its valence and the elementary charge:

$$q_0 = ze_0 \qquad (6.1)$$

In an aqueous solution or a bulk volume of matter, the number of positive and negative charges is always equal. Charge is also conserved in any chemical reaction.

Membrane potentials can be measured with microelectrodes as well as dyes or fluorescent proteins that are voltage sensitive

The voltage difference across the cell membrane, or the **membrane potential (V_m)**, is the difference between the electrical potential in the cytoplasm (ψ_i) and the electrical potential in the extracellular space (ψ_o). Fig. 6.1A shows how to measure V_m with an intracellular electrode. The sharp tip of a microelectrode is gently inserted into the cell and measures the transmembrane potential with respect to the electrical potential of the extracellular solution, defined as ground (i.e., $\psi_o = 0$). If the cell membrane is not damaged by electrode impalement and the impaled membrane seals tightly around the glass, this technique provides an accurate measurement of V_m. Such a voltage measurement is called an **intracellular recording.** Voltages can be measured with optical techniques in some smaller structures, such as neuronal dendrites.

For an amphibian or mammalian skeletal muscle cell, resting V_m is typically about −90 mV, which means that the interior of the resting cell is ~90 mV more negative than the exterior. There is a simple relationship between the electrical potential difference across a membrane and another parameter, the **electric field (E)**:

$$E = \frac{V_m\} \text{ Electrical potential difference across the membrane}}{a\} \text{ Distance across the membrane}} \qquad (6.2)$$

Accordingly, for a V_m of −0.1 V and a membrane thickness of $a = 4$ nm (i.e., 40×10^{-8} cm), the magnitude of the electric field is ~250,000 V/cm. Thus, despite the small transmembrane *voltage*, cell membranes actually sustain a very large electric *field*. Below, we discuss how this electric field influences the activity of a particular class of membrane signaling proteins called voltage-gated ion channels (see ◉ 7-3).

Skeletal muscle cells, cardiac cells, and neurons typically have resting membrane potentials of approximately −60 to −90 mV; smooth-muscle cells have membrane potentials in the range of −55 mV; and the V_m of the human erythrocyte is only about −9 mV.

Measurements of V_m have shown that many types of cells are electrically excitable. Examples of excitable cells are neurons, muscle fibers, heart cells, and secretory cells

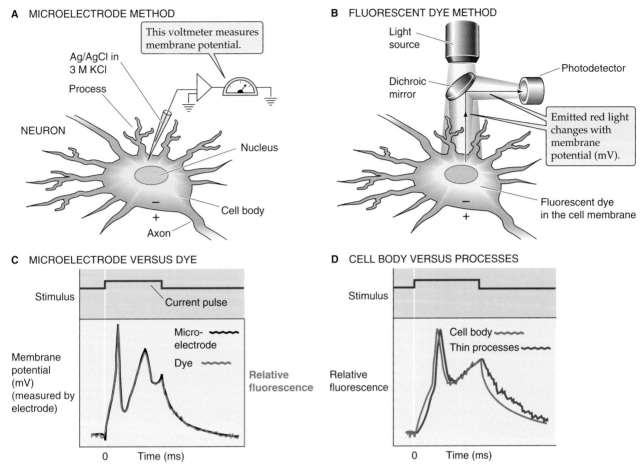

A MICROELECTRODE METHOD

This voltmeter measures membrane potential.

Ag/AgCl in 3 M KCl

Process

NEURON

Nucleus

Cell body

Axon

B FLUORESCENT DYE METHOD

Light source

Dichroic mirror

Photodetector

Emitted red light changes with membrane potential (mV).

Fluorescent dye in the cell membrane

C MICROELECTRODE VERSUS DYE

Stimulus

Current pulse

Membrane potential (mV) (measured by electrode)

Micro-electrode

Dye

Relative fluorescence

Time (ms)

D CELL BODY VERSUS PROCESSES

Stimulus

Cell body

Thin processes

Relative fluorescence

Time (ms)

Figure 6.1 Recording of membrane potential. (C and D, Data modified from Grinvald A. Real-time optical mapping of neuronal activity: From single growth cones to the intact mammalian brain. *Annu Rev Neurosci.* 1985;8:263–305. © Annual Reviews www.annualreviews.org.)

of the pancreas. In such cells, V_m exhibits characteristic time-dependent changes in response to electrical or chemical stimulation. When the cell body, or soma, of a neuron is electrically stimulated, electrical and optical methods for measuring V_m detect an almost identical response at the cell body (Fig. 6.1C). The optical method provides the additional insight that V_m changes are similar but delayed in the more distant neuronal processes inaccessible to a microelectrode (Fig. 6.1D). When the cell is not undergoing such active responses, V_m usually remains at a steady value that is called the **resting potential.** In the next section, we discuss the origin of the membrane potential and lay the groundwork for understanding its active responses.

Membrane potential is generated by ion gradients

An ATP-dependent pump is not the *immediate* energy source underlying the membrane potential. Indeed, the squid giant axon normally has a resting potential of −60 mV. When the electrogenic Na-K pump in the giant axon membrane is specifically inhibited with a cardiac glycoside (see ⊚ 5-7), the immediate positive shift in V_m is only 1.4 mV. Thus, in most cases, the direct contribution of the Na-K pump to the resting V_m is very small.

In contrast, many experiments have shown that cell membrane potentials depend on ionic **concentration gradients.** For a frog muscle fiber, V_m is approximately a linear function of the *logarithm* of $[K^+]_o$ at $[K^+]_o$ values >10 mM (Fig. 6.2). Numerous experiments of this kind have demonstrated that the *immediate* energy source of the membrane potential is not the active pumping of ions but rather the potential energy stored in the ion concentration gradients themselves. Of course, it is the ion pumps—and the secondary active transporters that derive their energy from these pumps—that are responsible for generating and maintaining these ion gradients.

For mammalian cells, Nernst potentials for ions typically range from −100 mV for K⁺ to +100 mV for Ca²⁺

The dependence of V_m on $[K^+]_o$ can be understood in terms of a K⁺-selective membrane, with diffusion of K⁺ down its concentration gradient. Membrane potentials that arise by this mechanism are called **diffusion potentials.** At equilibrium, the diffusion potential of an ion is the same as the equilibrium potential (E_X) given by the **Nernst equation** previously introduced as Equation 5.4.

$$E_X = -\frac{RT}{z_X F} \ln \frac{[X]_i}{[X]_o}$$

(6.3)

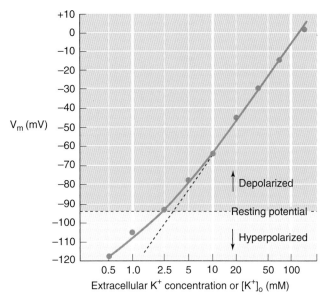

Figure 6.2 Dependence of resting potential on extracellular K⁺ concentration in a frog muscle fiber. The slope of the linear part of the curve is 58 mV for a 10-fold increase in $[K^+]_o$. Note that the horizontal axis for $[K^+]_o$ is plotted using a logarithmic scale. (Data from Hodgkin AL, Horowicz P. The influence of potassium and chloride ions on the membrane potential of single muscle fibers. *J Physiol.* 1959;148:127–160.)

TABLE 6.1 Ion Concentration Gradients in Mammalian Cells

ION	OUT (mM)	IN (mM)	OUT/IN	E_X^* (mV)
Skeletal Muscle				
K⁺	4.5	155	0.026	−95
Na⁺	145	12	12	+67
Ca²⁺	1.0	10⁻⁴	10,000	+123
Cl⁻	116	4.2	28	−89
HCO₃⁻	24	12	2	−19
Most Other Cells				
K⁺	4.5	120	0.038	−88
Na⁺	145.4	15	9.67	+61
Ca²⁺	1.0	10⁻⁴	10,000	+123
Cl⁻	116	20	5.8	−47
HCO₃⁻	24	15	1.6	−13

*Nernst equilibrium potential at 37°C.

The Nernst equation predicts the equilibrium membrane potential for any concentration gradient of a particular ion across a membrane. E_X is often simply referred to as the **Nernst potential.** The Nernst potentials for K⁺, Na⁺, Ca²⁺, and Cl⁻ are written as E_K, E_{Na}, E_{Ca}, and E_{Cl}, respectively.

The linear portion of the plot of V_m versus the logarithm of $[K^+]_o$ for a frog muscle cell (see Fig. 6.2) has a **slope** that is ~58.1 mV for a 10-fold change in $[K^+]_o$, as predicted by the Nernst equation. Indeed, if we insert the appropriate values for R and F into Equation 6.3, select a temperature of 20°C, and convert the logarithm base e (ln) to the logarithm base 10 ($\log_{10}$), we obtain a coefficient of −58.1 mV, and the Nernst equation becomes

$$E_K = (-58.1 \text{ mV}) \log_{10} \frac{[K^+]_i}{[K^+]_o} \tag{6.4}$$

For a negative ion such as Cl⁻, where $z = -1$, the sign of the slope is positive:

$$E_{Cl} = (+58.1 \text{ mV}) \log_{10} \frac{[Cl^-]_i}{[Cl^-]_o} \tag{6.5}$$

For Ca²⁺ ($z = +2$), the slope is half of −58.1 mV, or approximately −30 mV. Note that a Nernst slope of 58.1 mV is the value for a univalent ion at 20°C. For mammalian cells at 37°C, this value is 61.5 mV.

At $[K^+]_o$ values above ~10 mM, the magnitude of V_m and the slope of the plot in Fig. 6.2 are virtually the same as those predicted by the Nernst equation (see Equation 6.4), which suggests that the resting V_m of the muscle cell is almost equal to the K⁺ diffusion potential. When V_m follows the Nernst equation for K⁺, the membrane is said to behave like a

potassium electrode because ion-specific electrodes monitor ion concentrations according to the Nernst equation.

Table 6.1 lists the expected Nernst potentials for K⁺, Na⁺, Ca²⁺, Cl⁻, and HCO₃⁻ as calculated from the known concentration gradients of these physiologically important inorganic ions for mammalian skeletal muscle and typical nonmuscle cells. For a mammalian muscle cell with a V_m of −80 mV, E_K is ~15 mV more negative than V_m, whereas E_{Na} and E_{Ca} are about +67 and +123 mV, respectively, far more positive than V_m. E_{Cl} is ~9 mV more negative than V_m in muscle cells but slightly more positive than the typical V_m of −60 mV in most other cells.

What determines whether the cell membrane potential follows the Nernst equation for K⁺ or Cl⁻ rather than that for Na⁺ or Ca²⁺? As we shall see in the next two sections, V_m depends on the relative permeabilities of the cell membrane to the various ions and the concentrations of ions on both sides of the membrane. Thus, the stability of V_m depends on the constancy of plasma ion concentrations—an important aspect of the homeostasis of the *milieu intérieur* (see ⊙ 1-1). Changes in the ionic composition of blood plasma can therefore profoundly affect physiological function.

Membrane potential depends on ionic concentration gradients and permeabilities

If the membrane is permeable to the monovalent ions K⁺, Na⁺, and Cl⁻—and only to these ions—the **total ionic current** carried by these ions across the membrane is the sum of the individual ionic currents:

$$I_{total} = I_K + I_{Na} + I_{Cl} \tag{6.6}$$

⊙ **6-1** At the resting membrane potential the sum of all ion currents is zero (i.e., $I_{total} = 0$). With some additional assumptions, we get an expression known as the **GHK *voltage* equation** or the **constant-field equation:**

$$V_{rev} = \frac{RT}{F} \ln \left(\frac{P_K[K^+]_o + P_{Na}[Na^+]_o + P_{Cl}[Cl^-]_i}{P_K[K^+]_i + P_{Na}[Na^+]_i + P_{Cl}[Cl^-]_o} \right) \qquad (6.7)$$

Because we derived Equation 6.7 for the case of $I_{total} = 0$, it is valid only when zero net current is flowing across the membrane. Note that the resting V_m depends primarily on the concentrations of the most permeant ion.

Equation 6.7 can explain why the plot of V_m versus $[K^+]_o$ in Fig. 6.2 bends away from the idealized Nernst slope at very low values of $[K^+]_o$ given a small permeability to Na^+ (~1% that of K^+).

The resting potential of most vertebrate cells is dominated by high permeability to K^+, so the resting V_m is typically close to E_K. The resting permeability to Na^+ and Ca^{2+} is normally very low. Skeletal muscle cells, cardiac cells, and neurons typically have resting membrane potentials ranging from –60 to –90 mV.

ELECTRICAL MODEL OF A CELL MEMBRANE

The cell membrane model includes various ionic conductances and electromotive forces in parallel with a capacitor

The current carried by a particular ion varies with membrane voltage. This observation suggests that the contribution of each ion to the electrical properties of the cell membrane may be represented by elements of an electrical circuit. The various ionic gradients across the membrane provide a form of stored electrical energy, much like that of a battery. In physics, the voltage source of a battery is known as an **emf** (electromotive force). The equilibrium potential of a given ion can be considered an emf for that ion. Each of these batteries produces its own ionic **current** across the membrane, and the sum of these individual ionic currents is the total ionic current (see Equation 6.6). According to **Ohm's law,** the emf or voltage *(V)* and current *(I)* are related directly to each other by the **resistance (R)**—or inversely to the reciprocal of resistance, **conductance (G)**:

$$V = IR \text{ Ohm's law}$$
$$= I/G \qquad (6.8)$$

Currents of Na^+, K^+, Ca^{2+}, and Cl^- generally flow across the cell membrane via distinct pathways. At the molecular level, these pathways correspond to specific types of ion channel proteins (Fig. 6.3A). It is helpful to model the electrical behavior of cell membranes by a circuit diagram (Fig. 6.3B). The electrical current carried by each ion flows via a separate parallel branch of the circuit that is under the control of a **variable resistor** and an emf. For instance, the variable resistor for K^+ represents the conductance provided by K^+ channels in the membrane (G_K). The emf for K^+ corresponds to E_K. Similar parallel branches of the

circuit in Fig. 6.3B represent the other physiologically important ions. Each ion provides a component of the total conductance of the membrane, so $G_K + G_{Na} + G_{Ca} + G_{Cl}$ sum to G_m.

The GHK voltage equation (see Equation 6.7) predicts steady-state V_m, provided the underlying assumptions are valid. We can also predict steady-state V_m (i.e., when the net current across the membrane is zero) with another, more general equation that assumes channels behave like separate ohmic conductances:

$$V_m = \frac{G_K}{G_m}E_K + \frac{G_{Na}}{G_m}E_{Na} + \frac{G_{Ca}}{G_m}E_{Ca} + \frac{G_{Cl}}{G_m}E_{Cl} \dots \qquad (6.9)$$

Thus, V_m is the sum of equilibrium potentials (E_X), each weighted by the ion's fractional conductance (e.g., G_X/G_m). Formally, permeability and conductance are different, but qualitatively, if more channels are open, the permeability and conductance are both higher.

One more parallel element, a **capacitor,** is needed to complete our model of the cell membrane as an electrical circuit. A capacitor is a device that is capable of storing separated charge. Because the lipid bilayer can maintain a separation of charge (i.e., a voltage) across its ~4-nm width, it effectively functions as a capacitor. In physics, a capacitor that is formed by two parallel plates separated by a distance *a* can be represented by the diagram in Fig. 6.3C. When the capacitor is charged, one of the plates bears a charge of $+Q$ and the other plate has a charge of $-Q$. Such a capacitor maintains a potential difference *(V)* between the plates. **Capacitance** (C) is the magnitude of the charge stored per unit potential difference:

$$C = \frac{Q}{V} \qquad (6.10)$$

Capacitance is measured in units of farads (F); 1 farad = 1 coulomb/volt. For the particular geometry of the parallel-plate capacitor in Fig. 6.3C, capacitance is directly proportional to the surface area *(A)* of one side of a plate, to the relative permittivity (dielectric constant) of the medium between the two plates (ε_r), and to the vacuum permittivity constant (ε_0), and it is inversely proportional to the distance *(a)* separating the plates.

$$C = \frac{A\varepsilon_r\varepsilon_0}{a} \qquad (6.11)$$

Most membranes have a specific capacitance of 1 $\mu F/cm^2$. We can use Equation 6.11 to estimate the thickness of the membrane. If we assume that the average dielectric constant of a biological membrane is $\varepsilon_r = 5$ (slightly greater than the value of 2 for pure hydrocarbon), Equation 6.11 gives a value of 4.4 nm for *a*—that is, the thickness of the membrane. This value is quite close to estimates of membrane thickness that have been obtained by other physical techniques.

A MODEL OF A CELL MEMBRANE

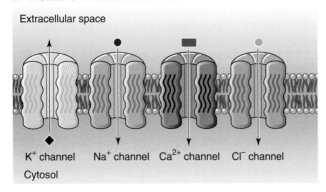

Extracellular space

K⁺ channel   Na⁺ channel   Ca²⁺ channel   Cl⁻ channel

Cytosol

B EQUIVALENT CIRCUIT MODEL

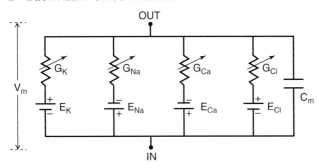

OUT

G_K G_{Na} G_{Ca} G_{Cl} C_m

V_m

E_K E_{Na} E_{Ca} E_{Cl}

IN

C PARALLEL–PLATE CAPACITOR   LIPID MEMBRANE

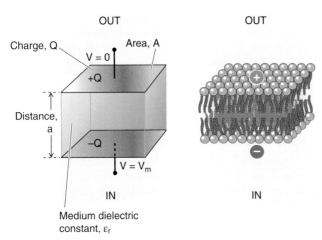

OUT   OUT

Charge, Q   Area, A

V = 0

+Q

Distance,
a

−Q

V = V_m

IN   IN

Medium dielectric
constant, ε_r

Figure 6.3 Electrical properties of model cell membranes.

The separation of relatively few charges across the bilayer capacitance maintains the membrane potential

We can also use the capacitance of the cell membrane to estimate the amount of charge that the membrane actually separates in generating a typical membrane potential. For example, consider a spherical cell with a diameter of 10 μm and a $[K^+]_i$ of 100 mM. This cell needs to lose only 0.004% of its K^+ to charge the capacitance of the membrane to a voltage of −61.5 mV. This small loss of K^+ is clearly insignificant in comparison with a cell's total ionic composition and does not significantly perturb concentration gradients. In general, cell membrane potentials are sustained by a very small separation

of charge. Similarly, changes in membrane potential (e.g., action potentials) require only small ion movements, and thus small changes in bulk ion concentration.

Because of the existence of membrane capacitance, total membrane current has two components (Fig. 6.3), one carried by ions through channels, and the other carried by ions as they charge the membrane capacitance.

Ionic current is directly proportional to the electrochemical driving force (Ohm's law)

Fig. 6.3 compares the equilibrium potentials for Na^+, K^+, Ca^{2+}, and Cl^- with a resting V_m of −80 mV. I_K or I_{Na} becomes zero when V_m equals the reversal potential, which is the same as the E_X or emf for that ion. When V_m is more negative than E_X, the current is negative or inward, whereas when V_m is more positive than E_X, the current is positive or outward. Thus, the ionic current depends on the difference between the actual V_m and E_X. In fact, the ionic current through a given conductance pathway is proportional to the difference $(V_m - E_X)$, and the proportionality constant is the ionic conductance (G_X):

$$I_X = G_X (V_m - E_X) \qquad \textbf{(6.12)}$$

This equation simply restates Ohm's law (see Equation 6.8). The term $(V_m - E_X)$ is often referred to as the **driving force** in electrophysiology. In our electrical model of the cell membrane (Fig. 6.3), this driving force is represented by the difference between V_m and the emf of the battery. The larger the driving force, the larger the observed current. When V_m is more positive than E_K, the driving force is positive, producing an outward (i.e., positive) current. Conversely, at V_m values more negative than E_K, the negative driving force produces an inward current.

In Fig. 6.4, the arrows represent the magnitudes and directions of the driving forces for the various ions. For a typical value of the resting potential (−80 mV), the driving force on Ca^{2+} is the largest of the four ions, followed by the driving force on Na^+. In both cases, V_m is more negative than the equilibrium potential and thus draws the positive ion *into* the cell. The driving force on K^+ is small. V_m is more positive than E_K and thus pushes K^+ out of the cell. In muscle, V_m is slightly more positive than E_{Cl} and thus draws the anion inward. In most other cells, however, V_m is more negative than E_{Cl} and pushes the Cl^- out.

Capacitative current is proportional to the rate of voltage change

The idea that ionic channels can be thought of as conductance elements (G_X) and that ionic current (I_X) is proportional to driving force $(V_m - E_X)$ provides a framework for understanding the electrical behavior of cell membranes. Current carried by inorganic ions flows through open channels according to the principles of electrodiffusion and Ohm's law, as explained above. However, when V_m is changing—as it does during an action potential—another current due to the membrane capacitance

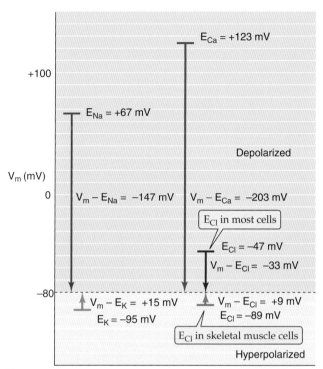

Figure 6.4 Electrochemical driving forces acting on various ions. For each ion, we represent the equilibrium potential (e.g., $E_{Na} = +67$ mV) as a horizontal bar and the net driving force for the ion (e.g., $V_m - E_{Na} = -147$ mV) as an arrow, assuming a resting potential (V_m) of −80 mV. The values for the equilibrium potentials are those for mammalian skeletal muscle given in Table 6.1, as well as a typical value for E_{Cl} in a nonmuscle cell.

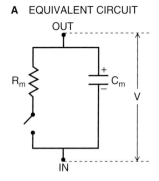

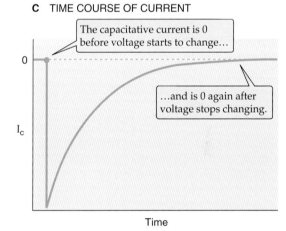

Figure 6.5 Capacitative current through a resistance-capacitance (RC) circuit.

also shapes the electrical responses of cells. This current, which flows only while V_m is changing, is called the capacitative current. How does a capacitor produce a current? When voltage across a capacitor changes, the capacitor either gains or loses charge. This movement of charge onto or off the capacitor is an electrical (i.e., the capacitative) current.

The simple membrane circuit of Fig. 6.5A, which is composed of a capacitor (C_m) in parallel with a resistor (R_m) and a switch, can help illustrate how capacitative currents arise. Assume that the switch is open and that the capacitor is initially charged to a voltage of V_0, which causes a separation of charge (Q) across the capacitor. According to the definition of capacitance (see Equation 6.5), the charge stored by the capacitor is a product of capacitance and voltage.

$$Q = C_m V_0 \tag{6.13}$$

⊙ **6-2** As long as the switch in the circuit remains open, the capacitor maintains this charge. However, when the switch is closed, the charge on the capacitor discharges through the resistor, and the voltage difference between the circuit points labeled "In" and "Out" in Fig. 6.5A decays from V_0 to a final value of zero (see Fig. 6.5B). This voltage decay follows an exponential time course. The time required for the voltage to fall to 37% of its initial value is a characteristic parameter called the **time constant (τ)**, which has units of time:

$$\tau = R_m \cdot C_m \tag{6.14}$$

Thus, the time course of the decay in voltage is

$$V = V_0 e^{-t/RC} \tag{6.15}$$

Fig. 6.5C shows that the **capacitative current** (I_C) is zero before the switch is closed, when the voltage is stable at V_0. When we close the switch, charge begins to flow rapidly off the capacitor, and the magnitude of I_C is maximal. As the charge on the capacitor gradually falls, the rate at which charge flows off the capacitor gradually falls as well until I_C

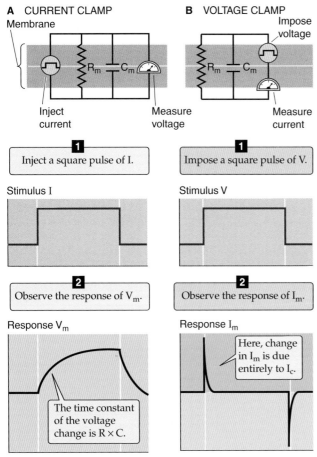

Figure 6.6 Voltage and current responses caused by the presence of a membrane capacitance. For a typical voltage clamp, the time constant for decay of the capacitive current is much faster than the membrane (R × C) time constant.

is zero at "infinite" time. Note, however, that V and I_C relax with the same time constant.

In Fig. 6.5, current and voltage change freely. Fig. 6.6 shows two related examples in which either current or voltage is abruptly changed to a fixed value, held constant for a certain time, and returned to the original value. This pattern is called a square pulse. In Fig. 6.6A, we control, or "clamp," the current and allow the voltage to follow. When we inject a square pulse of current across the membrane, the voltage changes to a new value with a rounded time course determined by the RC value of the membrane. In Fig. 6.6B, we clamp voltage and allow the current to follow. When we suddenly change voltage to a new value, a transient capacitive current flows as charge flows onto the capacitor. The capacitive current is maximal at the beginning of the square pulse, when charge flows most rapidly onto the capacitor, and then falls off exponentially. When we suddenly decrease the voltage to its original value, I_C flows in the direction opposite that observed at the beginning of the pulse. Thus, I_C appears as brief spikes at the beginning and end of the voltage pulse.

A voltage clamp measures currents across cell membranes

Electrophysiologists use a technique called **voltage clamping** to deduce the properties of ion channels. In this method,

specialized electronics are used to inject current into the cell to set the membrane voltage to a value that is different from the resting potential. The device then measures the total current required to clamp V_m to this value. A typical method of voltage clamping involves impaling a cell with two sharp electrodes, one for monitoring V_m and one for injecting the current. Fig. 6.7A illustrates how the technique can be used with a *Xenopus* (i.e., frog) oocyte. When the voltage-sensing electrode detects a difference from the intended voltage, called the command voltage, a feedback amplifier rapidly injects opposing current to maintain a constant V_m. The magnitude of the injected current needed to keep V_m constant is equal, but opposite in sign, to the membrane current and is thus an accurate measurement of the **total membrane current** (I_m).

I_m is the sum of the individual currents through each of the parallel branches of the circuit in Fig. 6.3B. For a simple case in which only one type of ionic current (I_X) flows through the membrane, I_m is simply the sum of the capacitive current and the ionic current:

$$I_m = \underbrace{I_C}_{\substack{\text{Capacitive} \\ \text{current}}} + \underbrace{I_X}_{\substack{\text{Ionic} \\ \text{current}}}$$

$$= I_C + G_X (V_m - E_X)$$

(6.16)

Equation 6.16 suggests a powerful way to analyze how ionic conductance (G_X) changes with time. For instance, if we abruptly change V_m to another value and then hold V_m constant (i.e., we *clamp* the voltage), the capacitive current flows for only a brief time at the voltage transition and disappears by the time that V_m reaches its new steady value (Fig. 6.6B). Therefore, after I_C has decayed to zero, any additional changes in I_m must be due to changes in I_X. Because V_m is clamped and the ion concentrations do not change (i.e., E_X is constant), only one parameter on the right side of Equation 6.16 is left free to vary, G_X. In other words, we can directly monitor changes in G_X because this conductance parameter is directly proportional to I_m when V_m is constant (i.e., clamped).

Fig. 6.7B shows examples of records from a typical voltage-clamp experiment on an oocyte expressing voltage-gated Na⁺ channels. In the experiment, a cell membrane is initially clamped at a resting potential of −80 mV. V_m is then stepped to −120 mV for 10 ms (a step of −40 mV) and finally returned to −80 mV. Such a negative-going V_m change is called a **hyperpolarization.** With this protocol, only brief spikes of current are observed at the beginning and end of the voltage step and are due to the charging of membrane capacitance. No current flows in between these two spikes.

What happens if we rapidly change V_m in the opposite direction by shifting the voltage from −80 to −40 mV (a step of +40 mV)? Such a positive-going change in V_m from a reference voltage is called a **depolarization.** In addition to the expected transient *capacitive* current, a large, inward, time-dependent current flows. This current is an *ionic* current and is due to the opening and closing kinetics of a particular class of channels called voltage-gated Na⁺ channels, which open only when V_m is made sufficiently positive. We can remove the contribution of the capacitive current to

A OOCYTE TWO-ELECTRODE VOLTAGE CLAMP

B VOLTAGE CLAMP METHOD OF MEASURING IONIC CURRENT

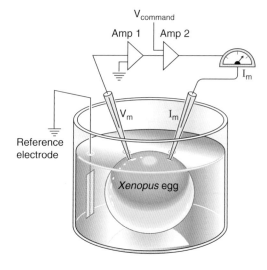

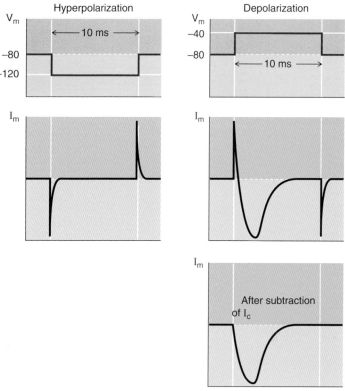

Figure 6.7 Two-electrode voltage clamp.

the total current by subtracting the inverse of the rapid transient current recorded during the hyperpolarizing pulse of the same magnitude. The remaining slower current is inward (i.e., downward or negative going) and represents I_{Na}, which is directly proportional to G_{Na} (see Equation 6.16).

The ionic current in Fig. 6.7B (lower right panel) is called a **macroscopic current** because it is due to the activity of a large population of channels sampled from a whole cell. Why did we observe Na⁺ current only when we shifted V_m in a positive direction from the resting potential? As described below, such Na⁺ channels are actually members of a large family of voltage-sensitive ion channels that are activated by *depolarization*. A current activated by depolarization is commonly observed when an electrically excitable cell, such as a neuron, is voltage clamped under conditions in which Na⁺ is the sole extracellular cation.

A modern electrophysiological method called **whole-cell voltage clamping** involves the use of a single microelectrode both to monitor V_m and to pass current into the cell. In this method, one presses onto the cell surface a glass micropipette electrode with a smooth, fire-polished tip that is ~1 μm in diameter (Fig. 6.8A). Applying slight suction to the inside of the pipette causes a high-resistance seal to form between the circular rim of the pipette tip and the cell membrane. The piece of sealed membrane is called a **patch**, and the pipette is called a **patch pipette**. Subsequent application of stronger suction causes the patch to rupture, creating a continuous, low-resistance pathway between the inside of the cell and the pipette. In this configuration, **whole-cell currents** can be recorded (Fig. 6.8B). Because single cells can be dissociated from many

different tissues and studied in culture, this method has proved very powerful for analyzing the physiological roles of various types of ion channels and their regulation at the cellular level.

⊙ 6-3 The patch-clamp technique resolves unitary currents through single channel molecules

Voltage-clamp studies of ionic currents at the whole-cell (i.e., macroscopic) level led to the question of how many channels are involved in the production of a macroscopic current. Electrophysiologists realized that if the area of a voltage-clamped membrane was reduced to a very small fraction of the cell surface area, it might be possible to observe the activity of a single channel.

This goal was realized when Neher and Sakmann developed the **patch-clamp technique.** Applying suction to a patch pipette creates a high-resistance seal between the glass and the cell membrane, as described in the preceding section for whole-cell voltage clamping. However, rather than rupturing the enclosed membrane patch as in the whole-cell approach, one keeps the tiny membrane area within the patch intact and records current from channels within the patch. A current recording made with the patch pipette attached to a cell is called a **cell-attached recording** (Fig. 6.8A). After a cell-attached patch is established, it is also possible to withdraw the pipette from the cell membrane to produce an **inside-out patch configuration** by either of two methods (Fig. 6.8E and Fig. 6.8F–H). In this configuration, the *intracellular* surface of the patch membrane faces the bath solution. One can also

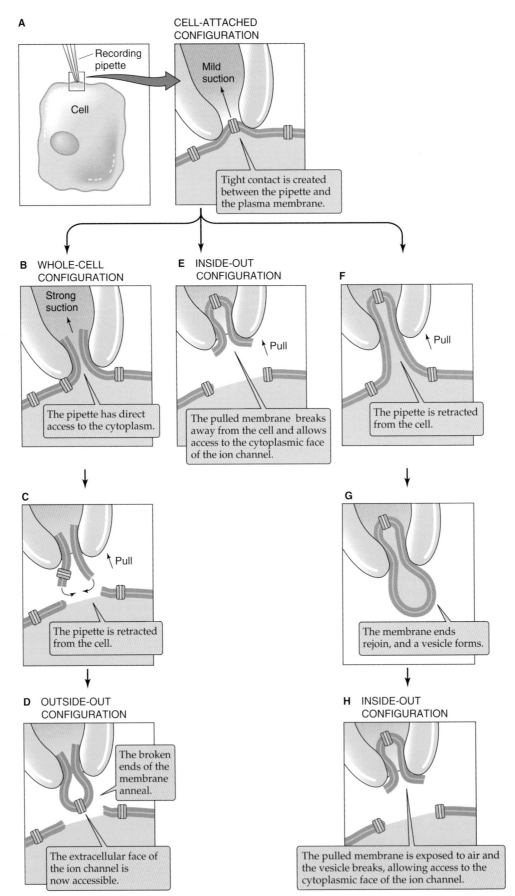

Figure 6.8 Patch-clamp methods. (Data from Hamill OP, Marty A, Neher E, et al. Improved patch-clamp techniques for high-resolution current recording from cells and cell-free membrane patches. *Pflugers Arch.* 1981;391:85–100.)

arrive at the opposite orientation of the patch of membrane by starting in the cell-attached configuration (Fig. 6.8A), rupturing the cell-attached patch to produce a whole-cell configuration (Fig. 6.8B), and then pulling the pipette away from the cell (Fig. 6.8C). When the membranes reseal, the result is an **outside-out patch configuration** in which the *extracellular* patch surface faces the bath solution (Fig. 6.8D).

The different patch configurations summarized in Fig. 6.8 are useful for studying drug channel interactions, receptor-mediated processes, and biochemical regulatory mechanisms that take place at either the inner or external surface of cell membranes.

Single-channel currents sum to produce macroscopic membrane currents

Fig. 6.9 illustrates the results of a patch-clamp experiment that are analogous to the macroscopic experiment results on the right-hand side of Fig. 6.7B. Under the diagram of the voltage step in Fig. 6.9A are eight current records, each of which is the response to an identical step of depolarization lasting 45 ms. The smallest, nearly rectangular transitions of current correspond to the opening and closing of a single Na^+ channel. When two or three channels in the patch are open simultaneously, the measured current level is an integral multiple of the single channel or "unitary" transition.

The opening and closing process of ion channels is called **gating.** Patch-clamp experiments have demonstrated that macroscopic ionic currents represent the gating of single channels that have discrete unitary currents. Averaging consecutive microscopic Na^+ current records produces a time-dependent current (Fig. 6.9B) that has the same shape as the macroscopic I_m shown in Fig. 6.7B. If one does the experiment in the same way but blocks Na^+ channels with tetrodotoxin, the averaged current is equivalent to the zero current level, which indicates that Na^+ channels are the only channels present within the membrane patch.

Measuring the current from a single channel in a patch at different clamp voltages reveals that the size of the discrete current steps depends on voltage (Fig. 6.10A). Plotting the **unitary current** (i) of single channels versus the voltage at which they were measured yields a single channel *I-V* relationship (Fig. 6.10B). This single channel *I-V* relationship reverses direction at a certain potential (V_{rev}), just like a macroscopic current does. If a channel is permeable to only one type of ion present in the solution, the V_{rev} equals the equilibrium potential for that ion (E_X). However, if the channel is permeable to more than one ion, the single channel reversal potential depends on the relative permeabilities of the various ions, as described by the GHK voltage equation (see Equation 6.7).

The slope of a single channel *I-V* relationship is a measure of the conductance of a single channel, the **unitary conductance** (g). Every type of ion channel has a characteristic value of g under a defined set of ionic conditions. The single channel conductance of most known channel proteins is in the range of 1 to 500 picosiemens (pS), where 1 pS is equal to 10^{-12} Ω^{-1}.

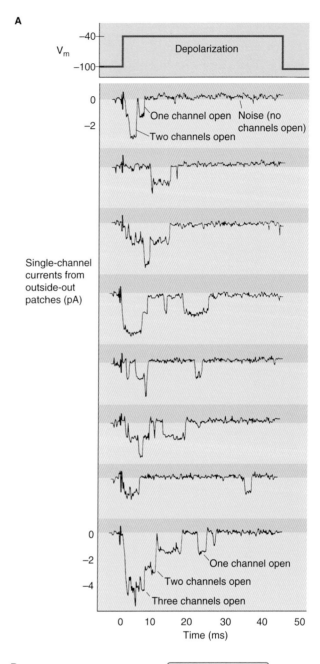

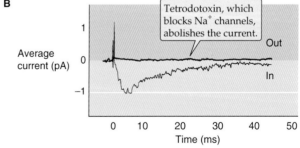

Figure 6.9 Outside-out patch recordings of Na^+ channels. (Data from Weiss RE, Horn R. Single-channel studies of TTX-sensitive and TTX-resistant sodium channels in developing rat muscle reveal different open channel properties. *Ann N Y Acad Sci.* 1986;479:152–161.)

A SINGLE-CHANNEL Cl⁻ CURRENTS

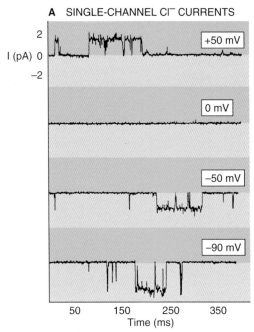

B I-V PLOT OF SINGLE Cl⁻ CHANNEL

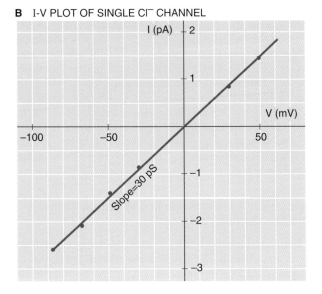

Figure 6.10 Voltage dependence of currents through single Cl⁻ channels in outside-out patches. (Data from Bormann J, Hamill OP, Sakmann B. Mechanism of anion permeation through channels gated by glycine and γ-aminobutyric acid in mouse cultured spinal neurones. *J Physiol.* 1987;385:243–286.)

Single channels can fluctuate between open and closed states

When a channel has opened from the **closed state** (zero current) to its full unitary conductance value, the channel is said to be in the **open state.** Channel gating thus represents the transition between closed and open states. A single channel record is actually a record of the conformational changes of a single protein molecule as monitored by the duration of opening and closing events.

Examination of the consecutive records of a patch recording, such as that in Fig. 6.9A, shows that the gating of a single channel is a probabilistic process. On average, there is a certain probability that a channel will open at any given time, but such openings occur randomly. For example, the average record in Fig. 6.9B indicates that the probability that the channels will open is highest ~4 ms after the start of the depolarization.

⊙ 6-4 The process of channel gating can be represented by kinetic models that are similar to the following hypothetical two-state scheme.

$$C \underset{k_c}{\overset{k_o}{\rightleftarrows}} O \qquad (6.17)$$

This scheme indicates that a channel can reversibly change its conformation between closed (C) and open (O) states according to first-order reactions that are determined by an opening rate constant (k_o) and a closing rate constant (k_c). The **probability of channel opening (P_o)** is the fraction of total time that the channel is in the open state.

We already have seen in Fig. 6.9 that the *average* of many single channel records from a given patch produces a time course that is similar to a macroscopic current recorded from the same cell. The same is true for the *sum* of the individual single channel current records. This conclusion leads to an important relationship: macroscopic ionic current is equal to the product of the **number of channels (N)** within the membrane area, the unitary current of single channels, and the probability of channel opening:

$$I = NP_o i \qquad (6.18)$$

Comparison of the magnitude of macroscopic currents recorded from large areas of voltage-clamped membrane with the magnitude of unitary current measured by patch techniques indicates that the surface density of ion channels typically falls into the range of 1 to 1000 channels per square micrometer of cell membrane, depending on the channel and cell type.

MOLECULAR PHYSIOLOGY OF ION CHANNELS

Classes of ion channels can be distinguished on the basis of electrophysiology, pharmacological and physiological ligands, intracellular messengers, and sequence homology

Mammalian cells express a remarkable array of ion channels. One way of making sense of this diversity is to classify channels according to their functional characteristics. Among these characteristics are electrophysiological behavior, inhibition or stimulation by various pharmacological agents, activation by extracellular agonists, and modulation by intracellular regulatory molecules. In addition, we can classify channels by structural characteristics, such as amino-acid sequence homology and the kinds of subunits of which they are composed.

Electrophysiology The electrophysiological approach consists of analyzing ionic currents by voltage-clamp techniques and then characterizing channels on the basis of ionic selectivity, dependence of gating on membrane potential, and kinetics of opening and closing.

One of the most striking differences among channels is their **selectivity** for various ions. Indeed, channels are generally named according to which ion they are most permeable to—for example, Na^+ channels, Ca^{2+} channels, K^+ channels, and Cl^- channels.

Another major electrophysiological characteristic of channels is their **voltage dependence.** In electrically excitable cells (e.g., nerve, skeletal muscle, heart), a major class of channels becomes activated—and often inactivated—as a steep function of V_m. For example, the opening probability of the Na^+ channel in nerve and muscle cells increases steeply as V_m becomes more positive (see Fig. 7.7B). Such voltage-gated channels are generally highly selective for Na^+, Ca^{2+}, or K^+.

Channels are also distinguished by the kinetics of **gating** behavior.

Pharmacological Ligands Currents that are virtually indistinguishable by electrophysiological criteria can sometimes be distinguished pharmacologically. For example, subtypes of voltage-gated Na^+ channels can be distinguished by their sensitivity to the peptide toxin µ-conotoxin, which is produced by *Conus geographus,* a member of a family of venomous marine mollusks called cone snails. This toxin strongly inhibits the Na^+ channels of adult rat skeletal muscle but has little effect on the Na^+ channels of neurons and cardiac myocytes. Another conotoxin (ω-conotoxin) from a different *Conus* species specifically inhibits voltage-gated Ca^{2+} channels in the spinal cord. A synthetic version of this conotoxin (ziconotide) is available for treatment of neuropathic pain in patients.

Physiological Ligands Some channels are characterized by their unique ability to be activated by the binding of a particular molecule termed an **agonist.** For example, at the vertebrate neuromuscular junction, a channel called the nicotinic acetylcholine (ACh) receptor opens in response to the binding of ACh released from a presynaptic nerve terminal.

This ACh receptor is an example of the pentameric Cys-loop superfamily of **ligand-gated channels** or agonist-gated channels (see ⊙ 8-6). Other agonist-gated channels are activated directly by neurotransmitters such as glutamate, serotonin (5-hydroxytryptamine [5-HT]), gamma-aminobutyric acid (GABA), and glycine.

Intracellular Messengers Regulation by intracellular messengers is another basis for classifying channels. For example, increases in $[Ca^{2+}]_i$ stimulate Ca^{2+}-gated K^+ channels. Another example is seen in the plasma membrane of light-sensitive rod cells of the retina, in which a particular type of channel is directly activated by intracellular cGMP.

Sequence Homology The diversity of channels implied by functional criteria ultimately requires a molecular biological approach to channel classification. On the basis of amino-acid sequences of mammalian channel proteins, we now can identify ~20 distinct families of channel proteins, subclassified into a larger number of gene subfamilies. The three-dimensional structures of channels are now being revealed by x-ray crystallographic analysis and cryoelectron microscopy.

Many channels are formed by a radially symmetric arrangement of subunits or domains around a central pore

The essential function of a channel is to facilitate the passive flow of ions across the hydrophobic membrane bilayer according to the electrochemical gradient. This task requires the channel protein to form an aqueous pore.

For the majority of eukaryotic channels, the aqueous pores are located at the center of an oligomeric rosette-like arrangement of homologous subunits in the plane of the membrane (Fig. 6.11). Channels can have three, four, five, or six of these subunits, each of which is a polypeptide that weaves through the membrane several times. In some cases (e.g., voltage-gated Na^+ and Ca^{2+} channels), the channel is not a true homo-oligomer or hetero-oligomer but rather a pseudo-oligomer in which a single polypeptide contains repetitive, homologous domains. In these channels, the rosette-like arrangement of repetitive domains—rather than distinct subunits—surrounds a central pore.

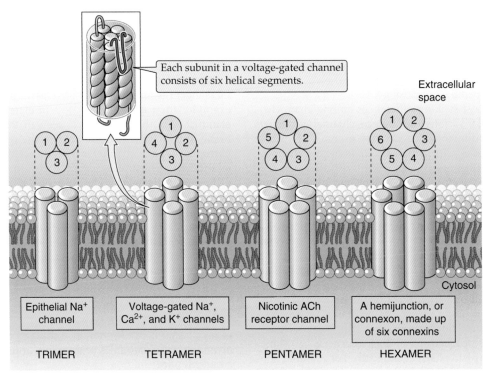

Each subunit in a voltage-gated channel consists of six helical segments.

Extracellular space

Cytosol

Epithelial Na⁺ channel	Voltage-gated Na⁺, Ca²⁺, and K⁺ channels	Nicotinic ACh receptor channel	A hemijunction, or connexon, made up of six connexins
TRIMER	TETRAMER	PENTAMER	HEXAMER

Figure 6.11   Structure of ion channels.

CHAPTER 7

ELECTRICAL EXCITABILITY AND ACTION POTENTIALS

Edward G. Moczydlowski

Cellular communication in the nervous system is based on electrical and chemical signaling events that are mediated by ion channels. Certain types of cells, including neurons and myocytes, have a remarkable property called **electrical excitability.** In cells with this property, depolarization of the membrane above a certain **threshold** voltage triggers a spontaneous all-or-none response called an **action potential.** This action potential is a transient, regenerative electrical impulse in which the membrane potential (V_m) rapidly rises to a peak that is ~100 mV more positive than the normal, negative resting voltage (V_{rest}). Such signals, also called spikes, can propagate for long distances along nerve or muscle fibers. Conduction of action potentials allows information from sensory organs to be transmitted along afferent nerves leading to the brain. Conversely, the brain exerts voluntary and involuntary control over muscles and other effector organs by efferent nerves leading away from it.

In the first part of this chapter, we examine the biophysical and molecular basis of action potentials and the mechanisms that underlie their genesis and propagation. The second part deals with the structure and function of voltage-gated ion channel proteins. Finally, we examine the conduction properties of neurons—called cable properties—and how they determine the spread of action potentials along the axon.

MECHANISMS OF NERVE AND MUSCLE ACTION POTENTIALS

⦿ 7-1 An action potential is a transient depolarization triggered by a depolarization beyond a threshold

The change in membrane potential that occurs during an action potential can be accurately measured by recording V_m with an intracellular microelectrode. Fig. 7.1A is a diagram illustrating various features of a typical action potential recorded from a nerve or muscle cell stimulated with an electrode. If the depolarizing stimulus causes V_m to become more positive than a threshold voltage, the depolarization triggers an action potential. The initial depolarizing (positive-going) phase of an action potential consists of a rapid and smooth increase in V_m from the negative resting potential (V_{rest}) to a maximum positive value that typically lies between +10 and +40 mV. This sharp rise in V_m to the peak voltage of the action potential is then followed by a slower repolarizing (negative-going) phase. The part of the action potential that lies above 0 mV is called

the **overshoot.** As we will see, the time course and shape of the repolarization phase vary considerably among different excitable tissues and cells. The repolarization phase may lead directly back to V_{rest}, or it may undershoot and give rise to a voltage minimum that is more negative than V_{rest} before relaxing back to V_{rest}. Such an undershoot is an example of an **afterhyperpolarization.**

The threshold, amplitude, time course, and duration of the action potential depend on the following factors:
1. The gating (opening and closing) and permeability properties of specific types of ion channels—these properties depend on both V_m and time
2. The intracellular and extracellular concentrations of the ions that pass through these channels, such as Na^+, K^+, Ca^{2+}, and Cl^-
3. Membrane properties such as capacitance, resistance, and the geometry of the cell

The shape of the action potential in a given cell reflects the specialized functions of that cell. For example, the brief action potentials of a nerve axon permit rapid signaling, whereas the prolonged, repetitive action potentials of cardiac and certain types of smooth-muscle cells mediate the slower, rhythmic contractions of these tissues. Fig. 7.1B compares action potentials recorded from an invertebrate nerve fiber (unmyelinated squid axon), a vertebrate nerve fiber (myelinated rabbit axon), a skeletal muscle fiber, and a cardiac atrial myocyte. This comparison illustrates the diversity in the duration and shape of the repolarizing phase of action potentials.

In contrast to an action potential, a graded response is proportional to stimulus intensity and decays with distance along the axon

Not all electrical activity in nerve or muscle cells is characterized by an all-or-none response. When we apply a small square pulse of hyperpolarizing current to a cell membrane, V_m gradually becomes more negative and then stabilizes (Fig. 7.2A). In such an experiment, the observed change in V_m approximates an exponential time course, with a time constant (see ⦿ 6-2) that is determined by the product of membrane resistance and capacitance ($\tau = RC$). Fig. 7.2A also shows that progressively greater hyperpolarizing currents produce progressively larger V_m responses, but the time constant is always the same. The size of the **graded voltage change** (i.e., the steady-state ΔV_m) is proportional to the

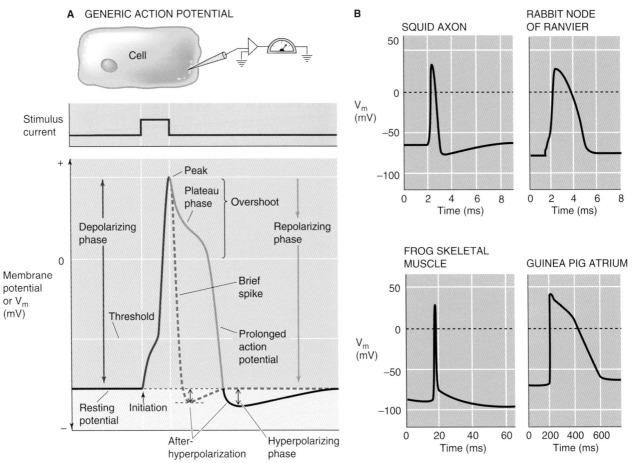

Figure 7.1   The action potential.

strength of the stimulus (i.e., the current), in accord with Ohm's law.

If instead of imposing a hyperpolarizing stimulus we impose a small *depolarizing* stimulus, V_m changes to the same extent and with the same time course as we described for the hyperpolarizing stimulus, but in the opposite direction (Fig. 7.2A). The size of ΔV_m is also proportional to the size of the depolarizing stimulus—up to a point. If the membrane is excitable, a square-wave depolarization above the threshold triggers an action potential, or voltage spike. Smaller or **subthreshold depolarizations** do not elicit an action potential. *Hyperpolarizations* are ineffective. Thus, both hyperpolarizations and subthreshold depolarizations behave like graded voltage changes. That is, the magnitude of a cell's voltage change increases proportionally with the size of the stimulus. Such graded responses can be seen in the response of certain cells to synaptic transmitters, to sensory stimuli (e.g., light), or, in the laboratory, to the injection of current into cells through a microelectrode.

Why do excitable cells exhibit threshold behavior? As V_m becomes progressively more and more positive, the **gating** process (i.e., transitions from closed to open states) of certain types of voltage-gated ion channels becomes activated. When V_m passes the threshold, opening of these voltage-gated channels initiates the runaway depolarization that characterizes the rising phase of the action potential. Thus, the firing

of an action potential is a binary, all-or-none event; that is, the spike has a constant, nongraded voltage peak that occurs only if the depolarizing stimulus exceeds the threshold.

Thus far we have seen that graded responses and action potentials differ markedly from one another if we examine the cell at one particular site. However, graded responses and action potentials also behave very differently in the way that they spread along the membrane from the site of origin. Fig. 7.2B illustrates how a graded hyperpolarizing response spreads along the axon of a neuron or along a skeletal muscle fiber. As the graded response spreads, its magnitude decays exponentially with the distance from the site of stimulation because of passive loss of electrical current to the medium. This decay is called **electrotonic conduction.** We see the same kind of electrotonic spread for a subthreshold, depolarizing stimulus.

Active propagation of an action potential signal is very different from the passive spread of a graded signal. In a healthy axon or muscle fiber, action potentials propagate at a constant velocity (up to ~130 m/s), without change in amplitude or shape. The amplitude of a propagating action potential does not diminish with distance, as would a graded, subthreshold response, because excitation of voltage-gated channels in adjacent regions of the excitable membrane progressively regenerates the original response. Because the action potential in a given nerve fiber propagates at a constant velocity, the time delay between the stimulus and the

A RESPONSE TO GRADED CURRENT STIMULI

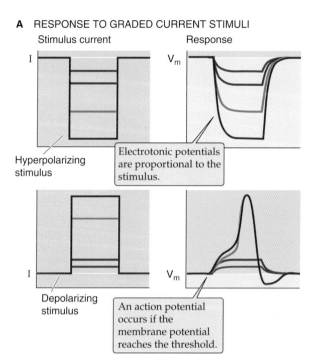

Stimulus current   Response

I V_m

Hyperpolarizing
stimulus

Electrotonic potentials
are proportional to the
stimulus.

I V_m

Depolarizing
stimulus

An action potential
occurs if the
membrane potential
reaches the threshold.

B RESPONSE TO STIMULI AS A FUNCTION OF DISTANCE

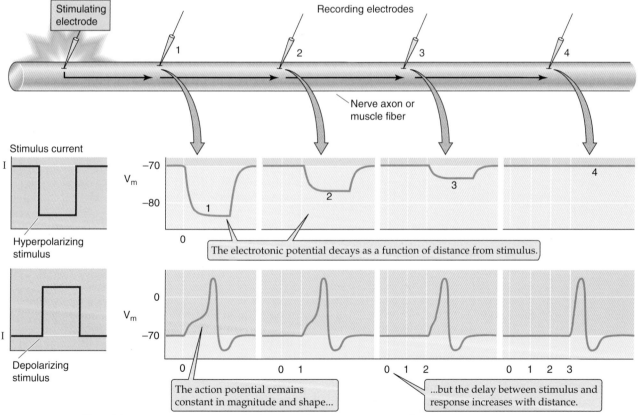

Stimulating
electrode

Recording electrodes

1   2   3   4

Nerve axon or
muscle fiber

Stimulus current

I V_m −70

−80   1   2   3   4

0

Hyperpolarizing
stimulus

The electrotonic potential decays as a function of distance from stimulus.

I V_m 0   −70

Depolarizing
stimulus

0   0 1   0 1 2   0 1 2 3

The action potential remains
constant in magnitude and shape...

...but the delay between stimulus and
response increases with distance.

Figure 7.2   Basic properties of action potentials. (A) The upper panels show four graded hyperpolarizing stimuli and the V_m responses. The lower panels show four graded depolarizing stimuli and the V_m responses. Note
that the two largest stimuli evoke identical action potentials. (B) A stimulating electrode injects current at the
extreme left of the cell. If the stimulus is hyperpolarizing, the graded V_m responses decay with distance from
the stimulus site. If the stimulus is depolarizing and large enough to evoke an action potential, a full action
potential appears at each of the recording sites.

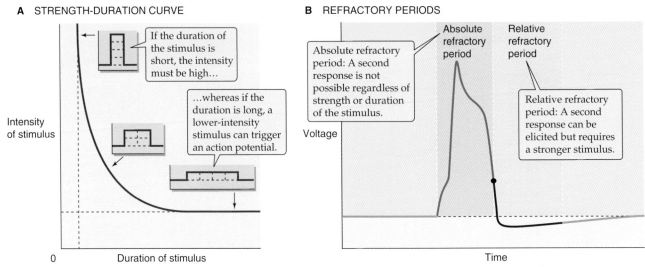

Figure 7.3 Determinants of nerve and muscle excitability. The curve in (A) represents the combination of the minimum stimulus intensity and duration that is required to reach threshold and to evoke an action potential. (B) A typical action potential with corresponding refractory periods.

peak of the action potential increases linearly with distance from the point of the stimulus.

Excitation of a nerve or muscle depends on the product (strength × duration) of the stimulus and on the refractory period

In the preceding section, the importance of the *magnitude* of the depolarizing stimulus emerged as a critical factor for firing of an action potential. However, the *duration* of the stimulus pulse is also important. A large stimulus is effective in triggering an action potential even at short duration, and a small stimulus may be effective at long duration (Fig. 7.3A). This strength-duration relationship arises because the same minimum electrical charge necessary to excite an action potential can come from a current that is either brief but large or prolonged but small. It is the *product* of strength and duration that determines excitability, and thus these two parameters are inversely related in their effectiveness. However, regardless of the stimulus duration, successful stimulation requires a minimum strength (horizontal asymptote in Fig. 7.3A).

An important feature of excitable cells is their ability to fire repetitive action potentials. Once a cell fires an action potential, how quickly can it fire a second? Suppose we inject a small step of current to produce a graded voltage response and then add a second current step while maintaining the first step. As long as V_m does not exceed the threshold, the resulting voltage response would be a simple algebraic and instantaneous summation of the two graded responses. The situation for action potentials is quite different. First, action potentials never summate. Second, after one action potential fires, a finite time must elapse before it is possible to trigger a second. The interval after initiation of an action potential when it is impossible or more difficult to produce a second spike is the **refractory period** (Fig. 7.3B). The refractory period consists of two distinct phases. The initial phase—the **absolute refractory period**—lasts from initiation of the spike to a time after the peak when repolarization is almost complete. Throughout this first phase, a second action potential cannot be elicited, regardless of the stimulus strength or duration. During the second phase—the **relative refractory period**—the minimal stimulus necessary for activation is stronger or longer than predicted by the strength-duration curve for the first action potential. The two phases of the refractory period arise from the gating properties of particular Na^+ and K^+ channels and the overlapping time course of their currents. The refractory periods determine the upper limit of firing frequency.

The action potential arises from changes in membrane conductance to Na^+ and K^+

The nerve action potential results from voltage-dependent currents of Na^+ and K^+ that flow through distinct molecular pathways called Na^+ channels and K^+ channels (Fig. 7.4). Ionic permeability changes underlying a nerve action potential can be interpreted with a form of the constant-field equation (see Equation 6.7) that includes only Na^+ and K^+:

$$V_{rev} = \frac{RT}{F} \ln\left(\frac{P_K[K^+]_o + P_{Na}[Na^+]_o}{P_K[K^+]_i + P_{Na}[Na^+]_i}\right) \tag{7.1}$$

According to Equation 7.1, V_{rev} would correspond to a resting V_m of −60 mV for a K^+/Na^+ permeability ratio (P_K/P_{Na}) of ~14:1. The change in V_m to a value near +40 mV at the peak of the action potential involves a transient and selective increase in the permeability to Na^+ because E_{Na} is positive (see Fig. 6.4). If $[Na^+]_o$ is reduced, the nerve action potential decreases in amplitude.

The time course of the action potential (Fig. 7.4) can be dissected into an initial, transient increase in Na^+ conductance (and thus permeability), followed by a similar but delayed increase in K^+ conductance. Thus, the depolarizing and repolarizing phases of the action potential reflect a transient reversal of the ratio of K^+/Na^+ conductances.

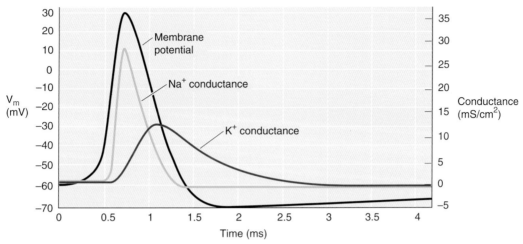

Figure 7.4 Changes in ionic conductance that underlie the action potential in a squid giant axon. Data from Hodgkin AL, Huxley AF: A quantitative description of membrane current and its application to conduction and excitation in nerve. *J Physiol.* 1952;117:500–544.

Macroscopic Na⁺ and K⁺ currents result from the opening and closing of many channels

The pore of an open channel is expected to have a linear or ohmic *I-V* relationship:

$$i_X = gx\,(V_m - E_X) \tag{7.2}$$

Here, i_x is the single channel current and g_x is the single channel conductance. We already introduced a similar relationship as Equation 6.12. Fig. 7.5A illustrates the predicted linear behavior of single channel currents as a function of V_m for hypothetical Na⁺ and K⁺ channels. Assuming an Na⁺ reversal potential (E_{Na}) of +50 mV, the Na⁺ current is zero at a V_m of +50 mV. Similarly, with an E_K of −80 mV, the K⁺ current is zero at a V_m of −80 mV. Assuming a unitary conductance of 20 picosiemens (pS) for each channel, the two *I-V* relationships have the same slope.

However, in the negative voltage range, the macroscopic peak *I-V* relationships for Na⁺ and K⁺ deviate from the linear (or ohmic) behavior in Fig. 7.5A. The reason for this deviation is that the probability that the Na⁺ and K⁺ channels are "open" (P_o)—and therefore able to conduct current—depends on voltage. To see why V_m might affect P_o, we consider a simplified model.

⊙ **7-2** Assume that a channel protein molecule may exist in either of two conformational states, closed (C) and open (O), and that these two conformational states are in equilibrium with one another:

$$C \rightleftarrows O$$

The equilibrium constant K_{eq} for this reaction is the ratio of the concentrations of open to closed channels, which can also be expressed as the ratio of the probability that the channel is open (P_o) to the probability that the channel is closed (P_c):

$$K_{eq} = \frac{[\text{Open}]}{[\text{Closed}]} = \frac{P_o}{P_c} \tag{7.3}$$

In the case of voltage-gated channel proteins, V_m changes affect K_{eq} and thus the distribution of channels between the open and closed states. The probability of a channel's being open depends on V_m according to a Boltzmann distribution (Fig. 7.5B). Accordingly, if the valence (*z*) of the voltage-sensing part of the channel protein (i.e., the "gating charge") is positive, the probability of channel opening should increase from 0 to 1 in a sigmoid fashion as V_m becomes more positive. Fig. 7.5B shows the behavior of P_o for hypothetical Na⁺ and K⁺ channels that simulate Na⁺ and K⁺ channels in real cells.

To summarize, Fig. 7.5A shows that once a single channel is open, the current flowing through the open channel is linearly related to V_m. Fig. 7.5B shows that the likelihood that the channel is open depends on V_m in a sigmoid fashion. The actual macroscopic current (I_X) depends on the number of channels (*N*) in the area of membrane being sampled, the open probability, and the single channel current, as we already pointed out in Equation 6.18:

$$I_X = NP_o i_X \tag{7.4}$$

Thus, we can use Equation 7.4 to compute the macroscopic currents *(I)* contributed by our hypothetical Na⁺ and K⁺ channels. We merely multiply the number of channels (which we assume to be 100 for both cations), the open probability for Na⁺ and K⁺ channels in Fig. 7.5B, and the single channel currents for Na⁺ and K⁺ in Fig. 7.5A. This result provides a reasonable description of voltage-sensitive ionic currents.

The properties of Na⁺ and K⁺ channels are responsible for the action-potential threshold and refractory periods

Fig. 7.4 shows an action potential in a squid giant axon. An increase in Na⁺ conductance causes the upswing or depolarizing phase of the action potential as V_m rapidly approaches E_{Na}, whereas **inactivation** of Na⁺ conductance and **delayed activation** of K⁺ conductance underlie the repolarization of V_m to its resting value near E_K.

A SINGLE-CHANNEL I-V RELATIONSHIPS

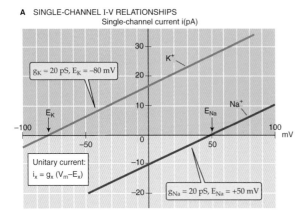

B VOLTAGE DEPENDENCE OF
SINGLE-CHANNEL OPEN PROBABILITIES

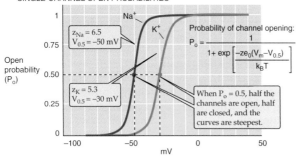

C MACROSCOPIC I-V RELATIONSHIPS

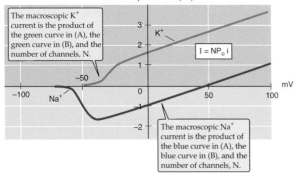

Figure 7.5 Microscopic basis of macroscopic *I-V* relationships. (A) The blue line represents the *I-V* relationship of an idealized open Na^+ channel. The green line represents the *I-V* relationship of an idealized open K^+ channel. Because the channels are assumed always to be fully open, the current through them is linear or ohmic. When positive charges move into the cell, the "inward current" is, by convention, negative and plotted beneath the x-axis. Conversely, when positive charges move out of the cell, the "outward current" is, by convention, positive and plotted above the x-axis. (B) The *blue curve* shows the open probability of Na^+ channels. The *green curve* shows the open probability of K^+ channels. (C) We can obtain a reasonable estimate for the macroscopic Na^+ current and the macroscopic K^+ current by multiplying the single channel current in (A), the P_o in (B), and the number of channels *(N)*. We assume that there are 100 Na^+ and 100 K^+ channels.

For an action potential to fire, an external stimulus must depolarize the membrane above threshold to activate a sufficient number of Na^+ channels. The external stimulus can come from an electrode, a synaptic event, or propagation of a depolarizing wave along the cell membrane. What determines whether a stimulus will be sufficient to reach the threshold V_m for firing of an action potential? The local depolarization

produced by the current flowing through Na^+ channels is opposed by current through K^+ channels and current that spreads to excite distant portions of axonal membrane. Thus, the **threshold** is the level of depolarization where the **inward current** through the open Na^+ channels exceeds the **outward current** through open K^+ channels. The net inward current depolarizes the cell, which opens more Na^+ channels—*positive feedback*. Once threshold is reached, further activation of Na^+ channels rapidly drives V_m toward E_{Na}.

The basis of the **absolute refractory period,** the time during which a second action potential cannot occur under any circumstances, is *Na^+ channel inactivation.* In other words, it is impossible to recruit a sufficient number of Na^+ channels to generate a second spike unless previously activated Na^+ channels have recovered from inactivation, a process that takes several milliseconds. The **relative refractory period,** during which a stronger-than-normal stimulus is required to elicit a second action potential, depends largely on delayed *K^+ channel opening.* In other words, for a certain period after the peak of the action potential, the increased K^+ conductance tends to hyperpolarize the membrane, so a stronger depolarizing stimulus is required to activate the population of Na^+ channels that in the meantime have recovered from inactivation.

⊙ 7-3 PHYSIOLOGY OF VOLTAGE-GATED CHANNELS AND THEIR RELATIVES

A large superfamily of structurally related membrane proteins includes voltage-gated and related channels

Voltage-gated Na^+ channels, Ca^{2+} channels, and K^+ channels are part of a superfamily of channel proteins called the **voltage-gated–like (VGL) ion channel superfamily**. This superfamily also includes structurally related channels that are not strictly activated by voltage. Fig. 7.6 shows a dendrogram based on an analysis of evolutionary relationships of the minimal pore regions of 143 human channels belonging to the VGL superfamily. Major branches of the tree define groups of related channel genes present in the human genome. In this section, we discuss how structural relationships among these proteins determine their physiological functions.

Voltage-gated K^+ channels typically have six transmembrane segments, S1 to S6—a conserved structural feature of all Kv channels. Transmembrane segments S1 to S6 have an α-helical secondary structure and are connected by cytoplasmic and extracellular linker regions (Fig. 7.7).

Extensive mutagenesis studies on cloned channel genes have associated various channel functions and binding properties with particular domains. The amino-terminal part of the channel, including the S1 to S4 transmembrane segments, forms a **voltage-sensing domain** (Fig. 7.7). The **S4 segment** has four to seven arginine or lysine residues that occur at every third S4 residue in voltage-gated K^+, Na^+, and Ca^{2+} channels. The positively charged S4 segment acts as the **voltage sensor** for channel activation by moving outward when the membrane depolarizes. This movement causes the four S6 helices—which form the inner lining of the pore—to bend away from the pore axis, thereby opening the channel.

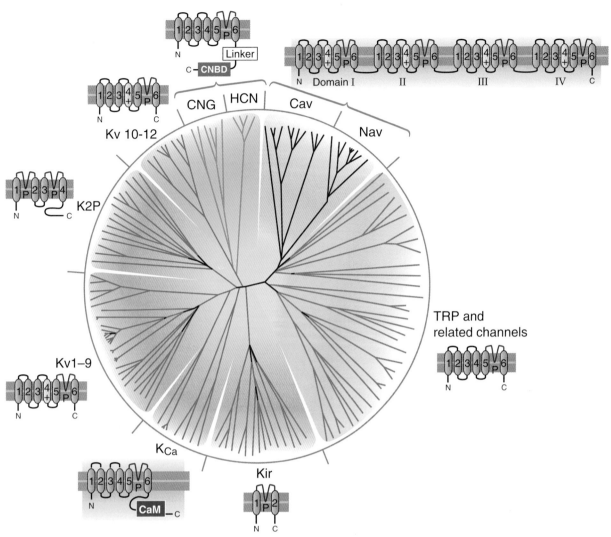

Figure 7.6 Dendrogram of the superfamily of VGL channels. Data from Yu FH, Catterall WA: The VGL-chanome: A protein superfamily specialized for electrical signaling and ionic homeostasis. *Sci STKE*. 2004; 253:re15.

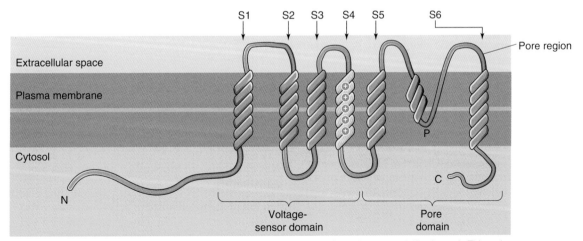

Figure 7.7 Membrane topology model of a single subunit of a voltage-gated K$^+$ channel. This voltage-dependent K$^+$ channel, a member of the Shaker family (Kv1.1), has six transmembrane segments (S1 to S6). The S4 segment *(highlighted in yellow)* has a large number of positively charged lysine and arginine residues and is part of the voltage-sensing domain that comprises the entire S1 to S4 region. S5 and S6—as well as the intervening P region—comprise the S5-P-S6 pore domain (Fig. 7.8).

A TOP VIEW OF TETRAMER

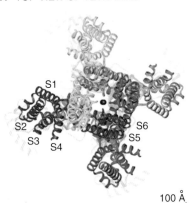

B LATERAL VIEW OF TETRAMER

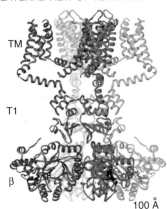

C LATERAL VIEW OF ONE MONOMER

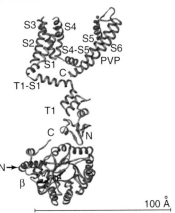

Figure 7.8   Crystal structure of the mammalian K^+ channel, Kv1.2, at a resolution of 2.9 Å. (A) Four α subunits of the channel (each analogous to the model in Fig. 7.7), each in a different color, viewed from the extracellular side. A K^+ ion is shown in the central open pore. (B) Side view of the four α and four β subunits of the channel, each in a different color, with extracellular solution on the top and intracellular solution on the bottom. The transmembrane domain (TM) of each α subunit is preceded by an –NH₂ terminus (T1 domain). The T1 domain is located over the intracellular entryway to the pore but allows access of K^+ ions to the pore through side portals. The T1 domain is also a docking platform for the oxidoreductase β subunit. Each β subunit is colored according to the α subunit it contacts. (C) Side view of one α subunit and adjacent β subunit. Transmembrane segments are labeled S1 to S6. From Long SB, Campbell EB, MacKinnon R: Crystal structure of a mammalian voltage-dependent Shaker family K^+ channel. *Science.* 2005;309:897–903.

The extracellular linker region between the S5 and S6 segments is termed the **P region** (for pore region) and contains residues that form the binding sites for toxins and external blocking molecules such as TEA. The **pore domain** formed by S5-P-S6 is the minimal structure required to form an ion-conducting pore for this class of channels (Fig. 7.7). The P region also contains conserved residues that form the **selectivity filter,** which determines the ionic selectivity for permeant cations.

Since the discovery and recognition of diverse genes belonging to the voltage-gated channel superfamily, structural-biological studies have substantially advanced our understanding of the three-dimensional structure of certain channel proteins. Fig. 7.8 shows the structure of a voltage-gated K^+ channel.

Fig. 7.9 shows a comparison of the predicted membrane-folding diagrams of three families of voltage-gated channels: Na^+, Ca^{2+}, and K^+ channels. The channel-forming subunit of each type of channel is called the α subunit for Na^+ and K^+ channels and the $α_1$ subunit for Ca^{2+} channels. Accessory subunits include $β_1$ and $β_2$ for Na^+ channels; $α_2$, δ, β, and γ, for Ca^{2+} channels; and β for K^+ channels.

The α subunit of Na^+ channels (Fig. 7.9A) and the $α_1$ subunit of Ca^{2+} channels (Fig. 7.9B) consist of four internally homologous repeats—domains I, II, III, and IV—each containing an S1 to S6 motif composed of the S1 to S4 voltage-sensing domain and the S5-P-S6 pore domain. In contrast, voltage-gated K^+ channels (Fig. 7.9C) are tetramers of four α subunits, whereas Na^+ and Ca^{2+} channels are pseudotetramers. Molecular evolution of the pseudotetrameric I to IV domain structure of Na^+ and Ca^{2+} channels is believed to have occurred by consecutive gene duplication of a primordial gene encoding a structure similar to the basic S1 to S6 motif of K^+ channels.

Na^+ channels generate the rapid initial depolarization of the action potential

Because the equilibrium potential for Na^+ and Ca^{2+} is in the positive voltage range for normal cellular ionic gradients, channels that are selectively permeable to these ions mediate electrical depolarization. However, prolonged cellular depolarization is an adverse condition inasmuch as it results in sustained contraction and rigor of muscle fibers, cardiac dysfunction, and abnormally elevated levels of intracellular Ca^{2+}, which leads to cell death. Thus, it is critical that Na^+ and Ca^{2+} channels normally reside in a closed conformation at the resting membrane potential. Their opening is an intrinsically transient process that is determined by the kinetics of channel activation and inactivation.

The primary role of voltage-gated Na^+ channels is to produce the initial depolarizing phase of fast action potentials in neurons and skeletal and cardiac muscle. The selectivity of Na^+ channels for Na^+ is high, with a permeability ratio of Na^+ relative to K^+ (P_{Na}/P_K) of 11 to 20. Voltage-gated Na^+ channels are virtually impermeable to Ca^{2+} and other divalent cations under normal physiological conditions.

Humans have 10 homologous genes that encode the pore-forming α subunit of **voltage-gated Na^+ channels (Navs)**. The isoforms encoded by these genes are expressed in different excitable tissues and can be partially discriminated on the basis of their sensitivity to TTX.

Na^+ channels are blocked by neurotoxins and local anesthetics

Studies of the mechanism of action of neurotoxins have provided important insight into channel function and structure. The guanidinium **toxins** tetrodotoxin (TTX) and saxitoxin (STX) are specific blocking agents of Na^+ channels that act on the extracellular side of the cell membrane.

Other neurotoxins from animals, plants, and microorganisms also act on Na^+ channels. Some of these neurotoxins are stimulatory, acting primarily by altering gating kinetics, so

A Na$^+$ CHANNEL

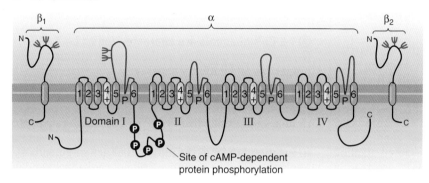

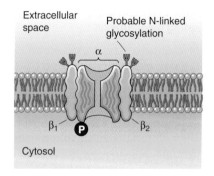

B Ca^{2+} CHANNEL

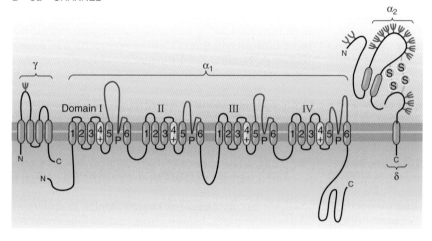

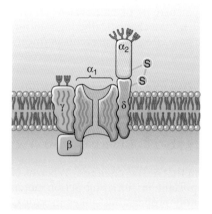

C K$^+$ CHANNEL

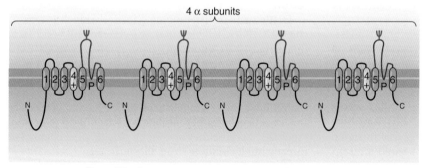

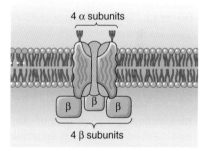

Figure 7.9 Subunit structure and membrane-folding models of voltage-gated channels. (A) A voltage-gated Na$^+$ channel (Nav) is made up of a pseudo-oligomeric α subunit as well as membrane-spanning β$_1$ and β$_2$ subunits. (B) A voltage-gated Ca^{2+} channel (Cav) is made up of a pseudo-oligomeric α$_1$ subunit as well as an extracellular α$_2$ subunit, a cytoplasmic β subunit (not shown in left panel), and membrane-spanning γ and δ subunits. Note that the domains I to IV of the Nav and Cav α subunits are homologous to a single subunit of a voltage-gated K$^+$ channel (see C). (C) A voltage-gated K$^+$ channel is made up of four α subunits as well as four cytoplasmic β subunits (not shown in left panel). Data from Isom LL, De Jongh KS, Catterall WA: Auxiliary subunits of voltage-gated ion channels. *Neuron.* 1994;12:1183–1194.

the Na$^+$ channels are open at voltages in which Na$^+$ channels are normally closed or inactivated. Others block the channel by stabilizing the voltage sensor in the resting (i.e., channel-closed) conformation.

Local anesthetics are a large group of synthetic drugs. Local anesthetics that are used clinically, such as procaine, **lidocaine,** and **tetracaine,** reversibly block nerve impulse generation and propagation by inhibiting voltage-gated Na$^+$ channels. The action of these drugs is "use dependent," which

means that inhibition of Na$^+$ current progresses in a time-dependent manner with increasing repetitive stimulation or firing of action potentials. **Use dependence** occurs because the drug binds most effectively only after the Na$^+$ channel has already opened. This use-dependent action of the drug further enhances inhibition of nerve impulses at sites where repetitive firing of action potentials takes place. Local anesthetics are widely used to control pain during dental procedures, many types of minor surgery, and labor in childbirth.

⊙ 7-4 Ca²⁺ channels contribute to action potentials in some cells and function in electrical and chemical coupling mechanisms

Ca^{2+} channels play important roles in the depolarization phase of certain action potentials, in coupling electrical excitation to secretion or muscle contraction, and in other signal-transduction processes. Because $[Ca^{2+}]_o$ is ~1.2 mM, whereas resting $[Ca^{2+}]_i$ is only ~10^{-7} M, a huge gradient favors the passive influx of Ca^{2+} into cells. At physiological $[Ca^{2+}]_o$, voltage-gated Ca^{2+} channels are ~1000-fold selective for Ca^{2+} over Na^+. Other alkaline earth divalent cations such as Sr^{2+} and Ba^{2+} also readily permeate Ca^{2+} channels. However, if $[Ca^{2+}]_o$ is experimentally reduced to a *nonphysiological* level of <10^{-6} M with the use of chelating agents, Ca^{2+} channels can also conduct large currents of monovalent alkali cations, such as Na^+ and K^+. Mechanistically, high-affinity binding of Ca^{2+} in the pore effectively prevents permeation of all other physiological ions.

The mechanism of this extraordinary selectivity behavior is based on ion-ion interactions within the selectivity filter of the pore. For the Ca^{2+} channel to conduct current, at least two Ca^{2+} ions must bind simultaneously.

Voltage-gated Ca^{2+} channels contribute to the depolarizing phase of **action potentials** in certain cell types. Notably, the gating of voltage-gated Ca^{2+} channels is slower than that of Na^+ channels. Whereas Na^+ channels are most important in initiating action potentials and generating rapidly propagating spikes in axons, Ca^{2+} channels often give rise to a more sustained depolarizing current, which is the basis for the long-lived action potentials in cardiac cells, smooth-muscle cells, secretory cells, and many types of neurons.

The exquisite selectivity of Ca^{2+} channels under physiological conditions endows them with special roles in **cellular regulation.** When activated by a depolarizing electrical stimulus or a signal-transduction cascade, these Ca^{2+} channels mediate an influx of Ca^{2+} that raises $[Ca^{2+}]_i$. Thus, in serving as a major gateway for Ca^{2+} influx across the plasma membrane, Ca^{2+} channels not only contribute to membrane depolarization but also play a role in signal transduction because Ca^{2+} is an important second messenger (see ⊙ **3-15**).

Ca^{2+} channels also play a pivotal role in a special subset of signal-transduction processes known as excitation-contraction coupling and excitation-secretion coupling. **Excitation-contraction (EC) coupling** refers to the process by which an electrical depolarization at the cell membrane leads to cell contraction, such as the contraction of a skeletal muscle fiber (see ⊙ **9-2**).

Excitation-secretion (ES) coupling is the process by which depolarization of the plasma membrane causes release of neurotransmitters in the nervous system and the secretion of hormones in the endocrine system. Such processes require an increase in $[Ca^{2+}]_i$ to trigger exocytosis of synaptic and secretory vesicles.

In keeping with the diverse roles of Ca^{2+} channels, the human genome contains 10 distinct genes for the channel-forming α_1 subunit of **voltage-gated Ca^{2+} channels (Cavs).**

Molecular studies have also identified four accessory subunits of Ca^{2+} channels: α_2, δ, β, and γ (Fig. 7.9B).

⊙ 7-5 Ca²⁺ channels are characterized as L-, T-, P/Q-, N-, and R-type channels on the basis of kinetic properties and inhibitor sensitivity

T-type channels are activated at a lower voltage threshold (more negative than −30 mV) than are other types of Ca^{2+} channels and are also inactivated over a more negative voltage range. These characteristics of T-type channels permit them to function briefly in the initiation of action potentials and to play a role in the repetitive firing of cardiac cells and neurons. Other types of Ca^{2+} channels, including L-, N-, P/Q-, and R-type channels, which are activated at a higher voltage threshold (more positive than −30 mV), mediate the long-lived plateau phase of slow action potentials, and provide a more substantial influx of Ca^{2+} for contractile and secretory responses. N-, P/Q-, and R-type Ca^{2+} channels mediate the entry of Ca^{2+} into presynaptic nerve terminals and thus play an important role in the release of neurotransmitters.

In addition to discrimination on the basis of gating behavior, Ca^{2+} channel isoforms can also be distinguished by their sensitivity to different drugs and toxins. **Ca²⁺ channel blockers** are an important group of therapeutic agents. Three important classes of Ca^{2+} channel blockers are the 1,4-dihydropyridines (DHPs), the phenylalkylamines, and the benzothiazepines. These synthetic compounds are available for treatment of cardiovascular disorders such as angina pectoris, hypertension, and various arrhythmias and also have potential applications in the treatment of CNS conditions such as cerebral vasospasm and epileptic seizure.

DHPs such as nitrendipine selectively block L-type Ca^{2+} channels. Phenylalkylamines (e.g., verapamil) and benzothiazepines (e.g., diltiazem) also inhibit L-type Ca^{2+} channels; however, these other two classes of drugs act at sites that are distinct from the site that binds DHPs. Particular DHP derivatives, such as Bay K8644, actually *enhance* rather than inhibit Ca^{2+} channel currents. DHPs can have the contrasting effects of either inhibitors (antagonists) or activators (agonists) because they act not by plugging the channel pore directly but by binding to an allosteric site.

⊙ **7-6** Other molecules useful in discriminating Ca^{2+} channel isoforms are present in the venom of the marine snail *Conus geographus* and the funnel web spider *Agelenopsis aperta.* The snail produces a peptide called ω-conotoxin GVIA, which selectively blocks N-type Ca^{2+} channels. The spider produces the peptide ω-agatoxin IVA, which selectively blocks P/Q-type Ca^{2+} channels. In contrast, an R-type neuronal Ca^{2+} channel is resistant to these two peptide toxins.

K⁺ channels determine resting potential and regulate the frequency and termination of action potentials

K^+ channels are the largest and most diverse family of voltage-gated ion channels. Humans have at least 79 distinct genes encoding K^+ channels, characterized by a K^+-selective S5-P-S6 pore domain (Fig. 7.7). Ion conduction through most types of K$^+$ channels is very selective for K$^+$ according to the permeability sequence K$^+$ > Rb$^+$ > NH$_4^+$ ≫ Cs$^+$ > Li$^+$, Na$^+$, Ca^{2+}. Under normal physiological conditions, the permeability ratio P_K/P_{Na} is >100, and Na$^+$ can block many K$^+$ channels.

Given such strong K$^+$ selectivity and an equilibrium potential near −80 mV, the primary role of K$^+$ channels in excitable cells is to oppose the action of excitatory Na$^+$ and Ca^{2+} channels and stabilize the resting state. Whereas some K$^+$ channels are major determinants of the resting potential, other K$^+$ channels mediate the repolarizing phase and shape of action potentials, control firing frequency, and define the bursting behavior of rhythmic firing. Such functions are broadly important in regulating the strength and frequency of all types of muscle contraction, in terminating transmitter release at nerve terminals, in attenuating the strength of synaptic connections, and in coding the intensity of sensory stimuli. Finally, in epithelia, K$^+$ channels also function in K$^+$ absorption and secretion.

Before understanding the molecular nature of K$^+$ channels, electrophysiologists classified K$^+$ currents according to their functional properties and gating behavior, grouping macroscopic K$^+$ currents into four major types:
1. Delayed outward rectifiers
2. Transient outward rectifiers (A-type currents)
3. Ca^{2+}-activated K$^+$ currents
4. Inward rectifiers

These four fundamental K$^+$ currents are the macroscopic manifestation of five distinct families of genes:
1. **Kv channels** (voltage-gated K$^+$ channels related to the Shaker family)
2. **Small- and intermediate-conductance K$_{Ca}$ channels** (Ca^{2+}-calmodulin–activated K$^+$ channels), including SK$_{Ca}$ and IK$_{Ca}$ channels
3. **Large-conductance K$_{Ca}$ channels** (Ca^{2+}-activated BK$_{Ca}$ channels and related Na$^+$- and H$^+$- activated K$^+$ channels)
4. **Kir channels** (inward-rectifier K$^+$ channels)
5. **K2P channels** (two-pore K$^+$ channels)

In the next three sections, we discuss the various families of K$^+$ channels and their associated macroscopic currents.

The Kv (or Shaker-related) family of K$^+$ channels mediates both the delayed outward-rectifier current and the transient A-type current

The K$^+$ current in the squid giant axon (Fig. 7.4) is an example of a **delayed outward rectifier.** This current activates with a lag phase (i.e., it is *delayed* in time). This current is said to be outwardly rectifying because its I-V curve in a real cell slopes upward toward more positive values of V_m.

A second variety of K$^+$ current that is also outwardly rectifying is the **transient A-type** K$^+$ current. A-type currents are activated and inactivated over a relatively rapid time scale. In neurons that spike repetitively, this A-type current can be very important in determining the interval between successive spikes and thus the timing of repetitive action potentials.

The channels responsible for both the delayed outward-rectifier and the transient A-type currents belong to the **Kv channel family** (where v stands for voltage-gated). All channels belonging to this family contain the conserved S1 to S6 core that is characteristic of the Shaker channel (Fig. 7.7).

The Kv channel family has multiple subclasses and vary widely in rates of activation and inactivation. Thus, these currents can modulate action potential duration by either keeping it *short* (e.g., in nerve and skeletal muscle) when the delayed rectifier turns on quickly or keeping it *long* (e.g., in heart) when the delayed rectifier turns on slowly.

⊙ 7-7 Two families of K$_{Ca}$ K$^+$ channels mediate Ca^{2+}-activated K$^+$ currents

Ca^{2+}-activated K$^+$ channels—K$_{Ca}$ channels—are present in the plasma membrane of cells in many different tissues. Both **BK$_{Ca}$** and **SK$_{Ca}$** channels (named for their "Big" vs. "Small" single channel conductances) are activated by increases in cytoplasmic Ca^{2+}, while BK$_{Ca}$ channels are synergistically activated by depolarization.

K$_{Ca}$ channels provide a stabilizing mechanism to counteract repetitive excitation and intracellular Ca^{2+} loading. K$_{Ca}$ channels mediate the afterhyperpolarizing phase of action potentials (Fig. 7.1A) in cell bodies of various neurons. They have also been implicated in terminating bursts of action potentials in bursting neuronal pacemaker cells.

The Kir K$^+$ channels mediate inward-rectifier K$^+$ currents, and K2P channels help set the resting potential

In contrast to the delayed rectifiers and A-type currents—which are *outwardly* rectifying K$^+$ currents—the inward-rectifier K$^+$ current (also known as the anomalous rectifier) actually conducts more K$^+$ current in the *inward* direction than in the outward direction. Such inwardly rectifying, steady-state K$^+$ currents have been recorded in many types of cells, including heart, skeletal muscle, and epithelia. Physiologically, since V_m is positive to E_K, these channels pass outward current to help clamp the resting membrane potential close to E_K. In epithelial cells, these inwardly rectifying K$^+$ currents are important because they stabilize V_m in the face of electrogenic ion transporters that tend to depolarize the cell (see Chapter 5).

⊙ **7-8** The channel-forming subunits of the **inward-rectifier (Kir)** K$^+$ channel family are relatively small proteins that lack the S1-S4 voltage sensing domain but have a conserved pore domain.

⊙ **7-9** The Kir family of K$^+$ channels exhibits various modes of regulation. One Kir subfamily (the G protein–activated inwardly rectifying K$^+$ channels, or **GIRKs**) is regulated by the βγ subunits of heterotrimeric **G proteins** (see ⊙ 3-3).

⊙ **7-10** Another subfamily of Kir K$^+$ channels known as **K$_{ATP}$ channels** are directly regulated by adenine nucleotides. K$_{ATP}$ channels are present in the plasma membrane of many cell types, including skeletal muscle, heart, neurons, insulin-secreting β cell of the pancreas, and renal tubule. These channels are inhibited by intracellular ATP and activated by ADP.

They provide a direct link between cellular metabolism and membrane excitability. For example, if cellular ATP levels fall because of oxygen deprivation, opening of such channels hyperpolarizes the cell to suppress Ca^{2+} influx and firing of action potentials and further reduce energy expenditure. Pancreatic β cells respond to an increase in plasma [glucose] by elevating their uptake of glucose and, thus, glucose metabolism and the cytoplasmic ATP/ADP ratio. This increased ratio inhibits enough K_{ATP} channels to cause a small depolarization, which in turn activates voltage-gated Ca^{2+} channels, resulting in Ca^{2+}-dependent insulin secretion (see ⊙ 51-3).

K_{ATP} channels are the target of a group of antidiabetic drugs called **sulfonylureas** that include tolbutamide and glibenclamide. Sulfonylureas are used in the treatment of type 2 (or non–insulin-dependent) diabetes mellitus because they inhibit pancreatic K_{ATP} channels and stimulate insulin release.

The two-pore K^+ channels—or **K2P channels**—consist of a tandem repeat of the basic Kir topology. Because the monomeric subunit of K2P channels contains two linked S5-P-S6 pore domains, a dimer of the monomer contains four S5-P-S6 pores and thereby forms a functional channel. K2P channels have been implicated in the genesis of the resting membrane potential. K^+ channels encoded by the 15 human genes for K2P channels may be activated by various chemical and physical signals including PIP_2, membrane stretch, heat, high intracellular pH, and general anesthetics.

PROPAGATION OF ACTION POTENTIALS

The propagation of electrical signals in the nervous system involves local current loops

The **electrotonic spread** of voltage changes along the cell occurs by the flow of electrical current that is carried by ions in the intracellular and extracellular medium along pathways of the least electrical resistance. Both depolarizations and hyperpolarizations of a small area of membrane produce **local circuit currents**. Fig. 7.10A illustrates how the transient voltage change that occurs during an action potential at a particular active site results in local current flow. The cytosol of the active region, where the membrane is depolarized, has a slight excess of positive charge compared with the adjacent inactive regions of the cytosol, which have a slight excess of negative charge. This charge imbalance within the cytosol causes currents of ions to flow from the electrically excited region to adjacent regions of the cytoplasm. Because current always flows in a complete circuit along pathways of least resistance, the current spreads longitudinally from positive to negative regions along the cytoplasm, moves outward across membrane conductance pathways ("leak channels"), and flows along the extracellular medium back to the site of origin, thereby closing the current loop. Because of this flow of current (i.e., positive charge), the region of membrane immediately adjacent to the active region becomes more depolarized, and V_m eventually reaches threshold. Thus, an action potential is generated in this adjacent region as well. Nerve and muscle fibers conduct impulses in both directions if an inactive fiber is excited at a central location, as in this example. However, if an action potential is initiated at one end of a nerve fiber, it will travel only to the opposite end and

stop because the refractory period prevents backward movement of the impulse (see ⊙ 12-1).

Likewise, currents generated by subthreshold responses migrate equally in both directions.

⊙ 7-11 Myelin improves the efficiency with which axons conduct action potentials

Animal nervous systems use two basic strategies to improve the conduction properties of nerve fibers: (1) increasing the diameter of the axon, thus decreasing the internal resistance of the cable; and (2) myelinating the fibers, which increases the electrical insulation around the cable. As **axon diameter** increases, the conduction velocity of action potentials increases because the internal resistance of the axoplasm is inversely related to the internal cross-sectional area of the axon. Unmyelinated nerve fibers of the invertebrate squid giant axon (as large as ~1000 μm in diameter) are a good example of this type of size adaptation. These nerve axons mediate the escape response of the squid from its predators and can propagate action potentials at a velocity of ~25 m/s.

⊙ **7-12** In vertebrates, **myelination** of smaller-diameter (~1- to 5-μm) nerve axons improves the efficiency of impulse propagation, especially over the long distances that nerves traverse between the brain and the extremities. Axons are literally embedded in myelin, which consists of concentrically wound wrappings of the membranes of certain glial cells (see ⊙ 11-8).

The glial cells that produce myelin are called Schwann cells in the periphery and oligodendrocytes in the brain. Because resistors in series add directly and capacitors in series add as the sum of the reciprocal, the insulating resistance of a myelinated fiber with 300 membrane layers is increased by a factor of 300, and the capacitance is decreased to 1/300 that of a single membrane. This large increase in membrane resistance minimizes loss of current across the leaky axonal membrane and forces the current to flow longitudinally along the inside of the fiber.

⊙ **7-13** In myelinated peripheral nerves, the myelin sheath is interrupted at regular intervals, forming short (~1 μm) uncovered regions called **nodes of Ranvier.** The length of the myelinated axon segments between adjacent unmyelinated nodes ranges from 0.2 to 2 mm. In mammalian axons, the density of voltage-gated Na^+ channels is very high at the nodal membrane, whereas K^+ channels are localized in the paranodal regions flanking each node. The unique anatomy of myelinated axons results in a mode of impulse propagation known as **saltatory conduction.** Current flow that is initiated at an excited node flows directly to adjacent nodes with little loss of transmembrane current through the internode region (Fig. 7.10B). In other words, the high membrane resistance in the internode region effectively forces the current to travel from node to node.

The high efficiency of impulse conduction in such axons allows several adjacent nodes in the same fiber to fire an action potential quickly as it propagates. Thus, saltatory conduction in a myelinated nerve can reach a very high velocity, up to 130 m/s. The action potential velocity in a

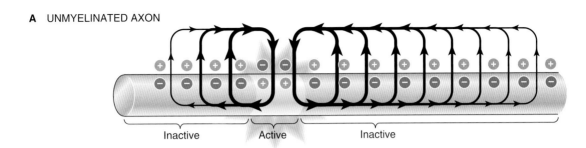

A   UNMYELINATED AXON

Inactive   Active   Inactive

B   MYELINATED AXON

Myelin sheath

A myelin sheath can have up to 300 layers of membrane.

Active

Figure 7.10   Local current loops during action potential propagation. (A) In an unmyelinated axon, the ionic currents flow at one instant in time as a result of the action potential ("active" zone). In the "inactive" zones that are adjacent to the active zone, the outward currents lead to a depolarization. (B) In this example, the "active" zone consists of a single node of Ranvier. As an action potential conducts along a myelinated axon, the ionic current flows only through the nodes, which lack myelin and have a very high density of Na⁺ channels. As an action potential fires at a *node,* the current flowing down the axon is conserved, and the current density at the nodes is very high, triggering an action potential at the next node.

myelinated nerve fiber can thus be several-fold greater than that in a giant unmyelinated axon, even though the axon diameter in the myelinated fiber may be more than two orders of magnitude smaller. During conduction of an action potential in a myelinated axon, the intracellular regions between nodes also transiently depolarize as a result of capacitative current. However, no transmembrane current flows in these internodal regions, and therefore no dissipation of ion gradients occurs. The nodal localization of Na⁺ channels conserves ionic concentration gradients that must be maintained at the expense of ATP hydrolysis by the Na-K pump.

⊙ 7-14 The cable properties of the membrane and cytoplasm determine the velocity of signal propagation

Fig. 7.11A illustrates the equivalent circuit diagram of a cylindrical membrane that is filled and bathed in a conductive electrolyte solution.

⊙ **7-15** How do the various electrical components of the cable model influence the electrotonic spread of current along an axon? To answer this question, we inject a steady electrical current into an axon with a microelectrode to produce a constant voltage (V_0) at a particular point ($x = 0$) along the length of the axon (Fig. 7.11B). This injection of current results in the longitudinal spread of current in both directions from point $x = 0$. The voltage (V) at various points along the axon decays exponentially with distance (x) from the point of current injection (Fig. 7.11C), according to the following equation:

$$V = V_0 e^{-x/\lambda} \tag{7.5}$$

The parameter λ has units of *distance* and is referred to as the **length constant** or the **space constant.** One length constant away from the point of current injection, V is $1/e$, or ~37% of the maximum value of V_0. The decaying *currents* that spread away from the location of a current-passing electrode are called **electrotonic currents.** Similarly, the passive spread of subthreshold *voltage* changes away from a site of origin is referred to as electrotonic spread, unlike the regenerative propagation of action potentials.

How does the diameter of an axon affect the length constant? Using the **specific resistances** R_m and R_i (expressed in terms of the area of axon membrane or cross-sectional area of axoplasm):

$$\lambda = \sqrt{\frac{aR_m}{2R_i}} \tag{7.6}$$

Thus, the length constant (λ) is directly proportional to the square root of the axon radius *(a)*. Equation 7.6 confirms basic intuitive notions about what makes an efficiently conducting electrical cable:

1. The greater the specific membrane resistance (R_m) and cable radius, the greater the length constant and the less the loss of signal.
2. The greater the resistance of the internal conductor (R_i), the smaller the length constant and the greater the loss of signal.

These relationships also confirm measurements of length constants in different biological preparations. For example, the length constant of a squid axon with a diameter of ~1 mm

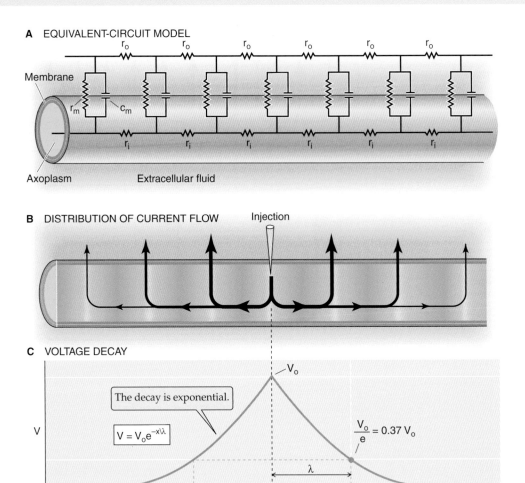

A EQUIVALENT-CIRCUIT MODEL

Membrane

Axoplasm   Extracellular fluid

B DISTRIBUTION OF CURRENT FLOW   Injection

C VOLTAGE DECAY

The decay is exponential.

$V = V_0 e^{-x/\lambda}$

V_0

$\dfrac{V_0}{e} = 0.37\,V_0$

λ

0   X

Figure 7.11 Passive cable properties of an axon. (A) The axon is represented as a hollow, cylindrical "cable" that is filled with an electrolyte solution. (B) When current is injected into the axon, the current flows away from the injection site in both directions. (C) Because the current density decreases with distance from the site of current injection in (B), the electrotonic potential *(V)* also decays exponentially with distance in both directions.

is ~13 mm, whereas that of a mammalian nerve fiber with a diameter of ~1 μm is ~0.2 mm.

So far, we have been discussing the *spatial* spread of voltage changes that are stable in *time*. In other words, we assumed that the amount of injected current was steady. What happens if the current is not steady? For example, what happens at the beginning of a stimulus when we (or a physiological receptor) first turn the current "on"? To answer these questions, we need to know how rapidly V_m changes in time at a particular site, which is described by a second cable parameter called the membrane **time constant (τ_m)**. The time constant influences the spread of voltage changes in *time* and thus the *velocity* of signal propagation. We previously discussed the time constant with respect to the time course of the change in V_m caused by a stepwise pulse of current (see Fig. 6.6A). Because the membrane behaves like an RC circuit, the voltage response to a square current pulse across a small piece of membrane follows an exponential time course with a time constant that is equal to the product of membrane resistance and capacitance:

$$\tau_m = R_m \cdot C_m \qquad (7.7)$$

We introduced this expression above as Equation 6.14. The shorter the time constant, the more quickly a neighboring region of membrane will be brought to threshold and the sooner the region will fire an action potential. Thus, the shorter the time constant, the faster the speed of impulse propagation and vice versa. In contrast, conduction velocity is directly proportional to the length constant. The greater the length constant, the further a signal can spread before decaying below threshold and the greater the area of membrane that the stimulus can excite. These relationships explain why, in terms of relative conduction velocity, a high-resistance, low-capacitance *myelinated* axon has a distinct advantage over an *unmyelinated* axon of the same diameter for all but the smallest axons.

In summary, the cable parameters of length constant and time constant determine the way in which graded potentials and action potentials propagate over space and time in biological tissue. These parameters are in turn a function of material properties that include resistance, capacitance, and geometric considerations. For *unmyelinated* axons, conduction velocity increases roughly with the square root of the axon's diameter, just as the length constant does (see Equation 7.6). In contrast, the conduction velocity of *myelinated* fibers is a linear function of diameter and increases ~6 m/s per 1-μm increase in outer diameter. Thus, a mammalian myelinated axon with an outer diameter of ~4 μm has roughly the same impulse velocity as a squid giant axon with a diameter of 500 μm!

The physiological importance of myelin in action potential propagation is most dramatically illustrated in the pathology that underlies human demyelinating diseases such as **multiple sclerosis.** This disease is an autoimmune disorder in which the myelin sheath surrounding CNS axons is progressively lost. Gradual demyelination is responsible for an array of neurological symptoms that involve various degrees of paralysis and altered or lost sensation. As myelin is eliminated, the loss of membrane resistance and increased capacitance mean that propagated action potentials may ultimately fail to reach the next node of Ranvier and thus result in nerve blockage.

CHAPTER 8

SYNAPTIC TRANSMISSION AND THE NEUROMUSCULAR JUNCTION

Edward G. Moczydlowski

The ionic gradients that cells maintain across their membranes provide a form of stored electrochemical energy that cells can use for electrical signaling. The combination of a resting membrane potential of −60 to −90 mV and a diverse array of voltage-gated ion channels allows excitable cells to generate action potentials that propagate over long distances along the surface membrane of a *single* nerve axon or muscle fiber. However, another class of mechanisms is necessary to transmit such electrical information from cell to cell throughout the neuronal networks that link the brain with sensory and effector organs. Electrical signals must pass across the specialized gap region between two apposing cell membranes that is called a **synapse.** The process underlying this cell-to-cell transfer of electrical signals is termed **synaptic transmission.** Communication between cells at a synapse can be either electrical or chemical. Electrical synapses provide direct electrical continuity between cells by means of gap junctions, whereas chemical synapses link two cells together by a chemical **neurotransmitter** that is released from one cell and diffuses to another.

In this chapter, we introduce the general principles of synaptic transmission and then focus on synaptic transmission between a motor neuron and a skeletal muscle fiber. This interface between the motor neuron and the muscle cell is called the neuromuscular junction. In Chapter 13, we expand upon this topic with a focus on synaptic transmission between neurons in the central nervous system (CNS).

MECHANISMS OF SYNAPTIC TRANSMISSION

Electrical continuity between cells is established by electrical or chemical synapses

⊙ **8-1** Electrical and chemical synapses have unique morphological features, distinguishable by electron microscopy. One major distinction is the distance of separation between the two apposing cell membranes. At **electrical synapses,** the adjacent cell membranes are separated by ~3 nm and appear to be nearly sealed together by a plate-like structure that is a fraction of a micrometer in diameter. Freeze-fracture images of the intramembrane plane in this region reveal a cluster of closely packed intramembranous particles that represent a **gap junction.** A gap junction corresponds to planar arrays of connexons, each of which is made up of six connexin monomers. The multiple connexons from apposing cells physically connect the two cells together via multiple aqueous channels (Fig. 8.1).

In contrast to those of the gap junction, the apposing cell membranes of the **chemical synapse** are separated by a much larger distance of ~30 nm at a neuronal chemical synapse

and up to 50 nm at the vertebrate nerve-muscle synapse. An additional characteristic of a chemical synapse is the presence of numerous synaptic vesicles on the side of the synapse that initiates the signal transmission, termed the **presynaptic** side. These vesicles are sealed, spherical membrane-bound structures that range in diameter from 40 to 200 nm and contain a high concentration of chemical neurotransmitter. The side of the synapse that receives the signal transmission is termed the **postsynaptic** side.

⊙ **8-2** The contrasting morphological characteristics of electrical and chemical synapses underline the contrasting mechanisms by which they function (Table 8.1). Electrical synapses pass voltage changes directly from one cell to another across the low-resistance continuity that is provided by the connexon channels. On the other hand, chemical synapses link two cells by the diffusion of a chemical transmitter across the large gap separating them. Key steps in chemical neurotransmission include release of transmitter from synaptic vesicles into the synaptic space, diffusion of transmitter across the cleft of the synapse, and activation of the postsynaptic cell by binding of transmitter to a specific receptor protein on the postsynaptic cell membrane.

⊙ 8-3 Chemical synapses use neurotransmitters to communicate between adjacent cells

By their very nature, chemical synapses are inherently rectifying or polarized. They propagate current in one direction: from the presynaptic cell that releases the transmitter to the postsynaptic cell that contains the receptors that recognize and bind the transmitter.

Fig. 8.2 summarizes the process of chemical transmission in a series of seven steps.

The molecular nature of chemical synapses permits functional diversity at the level of the transmitter substance, receptor protein, postsynaptic response, and subsequent electrical and biochemical processes. Many different small molecules serve as neurotransmitters (see ⊙ **13-5**).

These molecules include both small organic molecules, such as norepinephrine, ACh, serotonin (5-hydroxytryptamine [5-HT]), glutamate, gamma-aminobutyric acid (GABA), and glycine, and peptides such as endorphins and enkephalins.

Neurotransmitters can activate ionotropic or metabotropic receptors

Neurotransmitter receptors transduce information by two molecular mechanisms: some are ligand-gated ion channels and others are G protein–coupled receptors (see ⊙ **3-3**).

Several neurotransmitter molecules—such as ACh, glutamate, serotonin, GABA, and glycine—serve as ligands (agonists) for both types of receptors. Agonist-gated receptors that are also ion channels are known as **ionotropic receptors.** Receptors coupled to G proteins are called **metabotropic receptors** because their activation initiates a metabolic process.

Ionotropic and metabotropic receptors determine the functional response to transmitter release. Activation of an ionotropic receptor causes rapid opening of ion channels. This channel activation, in turn, results in depolarization or hyperpolarization of the postsynaptic membrane, depending on the ionic selectivity of the conductance change. Activation of a metabotropic G protein–linked receptor results in the production of active α and βγ subunits, which initiate a wide variety of cellular responses by direct interaction with either ion channel proteins or other second-messenger effector proteins. By their very nature, ionotropic receptors mediate fast ionic synaptic responses that occur on a millisecond time scale, whereas metabotropic receptors mediate slow, biochemically mediated synaptic responses in the range of seconds to minutes.

Fig. 8.3 compares the basic processes mediated by two prototypic ACh receptors (AChRs): (1) the ACh-activated ion channel at the neuromuscular junction of skeletal muscle, an ionotropic receptor also known as the **nicotinic** AChR (Fig. 8.3A), and (2) the G protein–linked AChR at the atrial parasympathetic synapse of the heart, a metabotropic receptor also known as the **muscarinic** AChR (Fig. 8.3B).

SYNAPTIC TRANSMISSION AT THE NEUROMUSCULAR JUNCTION

Neuromuscular junctions are specialized synapses between motor neurons and skeletal muscle

Motor neurons with cell bodies located in the ventral horn of the spinal cord have long axons that branch extensively near the point of contact with the target muscle (Fig. 8.4). Each axon process innervates a separate fiber of skeletal muscle. The whole assembly of muscle fibers innervated by the axon from one motor neuron is called a **motor unit.**

Typically, an axon makes a single point of synaptic contact with a skeletal muscle fiber, midway along the length of the muscle fiber. This specialized synaptic region is called the **neuromuscular junction** or the **end plate** (Fig. 8.4). An individual end plate consists of a small tree-like patch of unmyelinated nerve processes that are referred to as terminal arborizations. The bulb-shaped endings that finally contact the muscle fiber are called **boutons.** Schwann cells are intimately associated with the nerve terminal and form a cap over the face of the nerve membrane that is located away from the muscle membrane. The postsynaptic membrane of the skeletal muscle fiber lying directly under the nerve terminal is characterized by extensive invaginations known as **postjunctional folds.** These membrane infoldings greatly increase the surface area of the muscle plasma membrane in the postsynaptic region. The intervening space of the **synaptic cleft,** which is ~50 nm wide, is filled with a meshwork of proteins and proteoglycans that are part of the extracellular matrix. The synaptic basal lamina also contains a high concentration of the enzyme **acetylcholinesterase (AChE),** which ultimately terminates synaptic transmission by rapidly hydrolyzing free ACh to choline and acetate.

Electron micrographs of the bouton region demonstrate the presence of numerous spherical synaptic vesicles, each with a diameter of 50 to 60 nm. The cell bodies of motor neurons in the spinal cord produce these vesicles, and the microtubule-mediated process of fast axonal transport translocates them to the nerve terminal. The quantal nature of

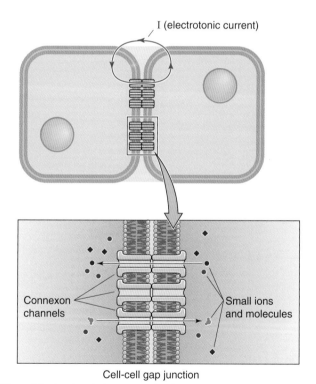

Figure 8.1 An electrical synapse. An electrical synapse consists of one or more gap junction channels permeable to small ions and molecules.

TABLE 8-1 Summary of Properties of Electrical and Chemical Synapses

| | **ELECTRICAL** | **CHEMICAL** | |
		IONOTROPIC	**METABOTROPIC**
Agonist	None	e.g., ACh	e.g., Ach
Membrane protein	Connexon	Receptor/channel	Receptor/G protein
Delay in transmission	Instantaneous	~1 ms	Seconds to minutes

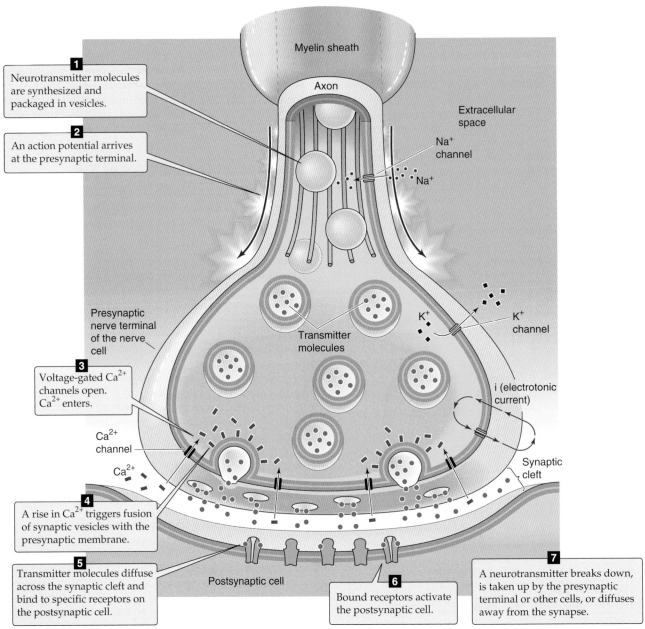

Figure 8.2 A chemical synapse. Synaptic transmission at a chemical synapse can be thought of as occurring in seven steps as shown.

The labeled callouts in the figure:

1 Neurotransmitter molecules are synthesized and packaged in vesicles.

2 An action potential arrives at the presynaptic terminal.

3 Voltage-gated Ca²⁺ channels open. Ca²⁺ enters.

4 A rise in Ca²⁺ triggers fusion of synaptic vesicles with the presynaptic membrane.

5 Transmitter molecules diffuse across the synaptic cleft and bind to specific receptors on the postsynaptic cell.

6 Bound receptors activate the postsynaptic cell.

7 A neurotransmitter breaks down, is taken up by the presynaptic terminal or other cells, or diffuses away from the synapse.

Myelin sheath — Axon — Extracellular space — Na⁺ channel — Na⁺ — K⁺ channel — K⁺ — Transmitter molecules — i (electrotonic current) — Presynaptic nerve terminal of the nerve cell — Synaptic cleft — Ca²⁺ channel — Ca²⁺ — Postsynaptic cell

transmitter release (described below in more detail) reflects the fusion of individual synaptic vesicles with the plasma membrane of the presynaptic terminal. Each synaptic vesicle contains 6000 to 10,000 molecules of ACh. The ACh concentration in synaptic vesicles is ~150 mM. ACh is synthesized in the nerve terminal—outside the vesicle—from choline and acetyl coenzyme A by the enzyme **choline acetyltransferase.** The ACh moves into the synaptic vesicle via a specific ACh-H exchanger, which couples the inward transport of ACh to the efflux of H⁺. Energetically, this process is driven by the vesicular proton electrochemical gradient (positive voltage and low pH inside), which in turn is produced by a vacuolar-type H⁺ pump fueled by ATP. The nerve terminal also contains numerous mitochondria that produce the ATP required to fuel energy metabolism.

⊙ **8-4** The process of fusion of synaptic vesicles and release of ACh occurs at differentiated regions of the presynaptic membrane called **active zones.** In electron micrographs, active zones appear as dense spots over which synaptic vesicles are closely clustered in apposition to the membrane. High-resolution images of active zones reveal a double linear array of synaptic vesicles and intramembranous particles. These zones are oriented directly over secondary *post*synaptic clefts that lie between adjacent postjunctional folds. The density of ionotropic (nicotinic) AChRs is very high at the crests of postjunctional folds. The microarchitecture of the neuromuscular synapse thus reveals a highly specialized structure for delivery of neurotransmitter molecules to a precise location on the postsynaptic membrane.

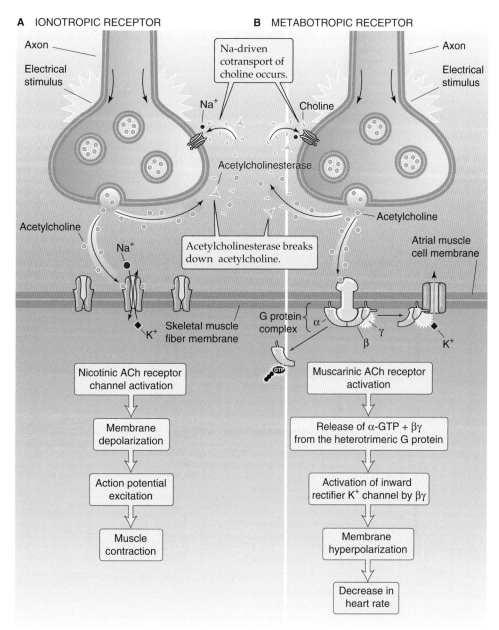

A IONOTROPIC RECEPTOR

B METABOTROPIC RECEPTOR

Axon

Electrical stimulus

Na-driven cotransport of choline occurs.

Na⁺

Choline

Axon

Electrical stimulus

Acetylcholinesterase

Acetylcholine

Na⁺

Acetylcholinesterase breaks down acetylcholine.

Acetylcholine

Atrial muscle cell membrane

G protein complex

α

β

γ

K⁺

Skeletal muscle fiber membrane

K⁺

GTP

Nicotinic ACh receptor channel activation

Muscarinic ACh receptor activation

Membrane depolarization

Release of α-GTP + βγ from the heterotrimeric G protein

Action potential excitation

Activation of inward rectifier K⁺ channel by βγ

Muscle contraction

Membrane hyperpolarization

Decrease in heart rate

Figure 8.3 Ionotropic and metabotropic AChRs.

ACh activates nicotinic AChRs to produce an excitatory end-plate current

Nerve stimulation normally drives the V_m of the muscle above threshold and elicits an action potential (see ⊙ 7-1).

⊙ **8-5** But if most of the AChRs are blocked by curare (a competitive antagonist), there is a transient depolarization in the muscle membrane after a delay of ~1 ms. The delay represents the time required for the release of ACh, its diffusion across the synapse, and activation of postsynaptic AChRs. This signal, known as the **end-plate potential (EPP),** is an example of an **excitatory postsynaptic potential.** It is produced by the transient opening of AChR channels, which are selectively permeable to monovalent cations such as Na⁺ and K⁺. The increase in Na⁺ conductance drives V_m to a more positive value in the vicinity of the end-plate

region. If the EPP does not reach the threshold to produce an action potential, the amplitude of the EPP diminishes with distance from the end-plate region according to the passive cable properties (see ⊙ 7-14) of the muscle fiber. This is an example of a graded response.

What ions pass through the AChR channels during generation of the EPP? This question can be answered by a voltage-clamp experiment, in which the motor nerve is stimulated while the muscle fiber in the region of its end plate is voltage-clamped to a chosen V_m. The recorded current, which is proportional to the conductance change at the muscle end plate, is called the **end-plate current (EPC).** The time course of the EPC corresponds to the opening and closing of a population of AChR channels, governed by the rapid binding and disappearance of ACh as it diffuses to the postsynaptic membrane and is hydrolyzed by AChE.

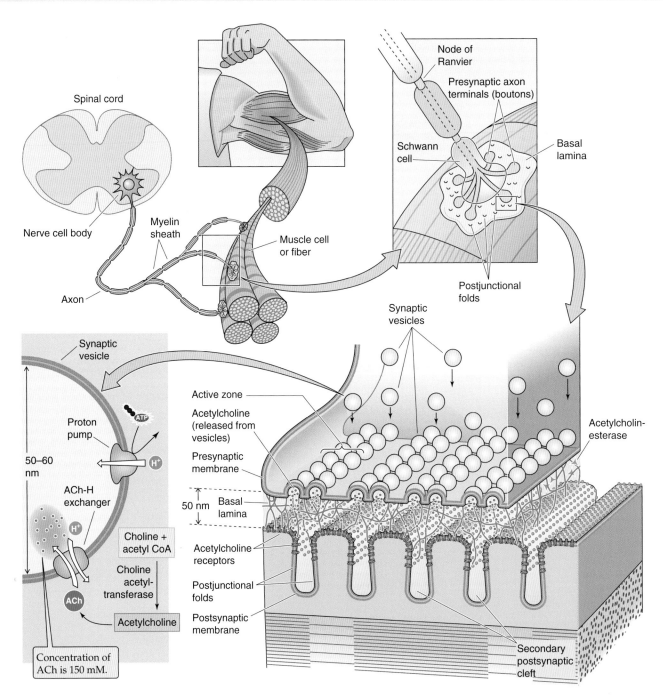

Figure 8.4   Vertebrate neuromuscular junction or motor end plate.

The reversal potential for the EPC is close to 0 mV. Because the EPC specifically corresponds to current through AChR channels, this reversal potential reflects the ionic selectivity of the AChR channels.

The AChR channel is permeable to several cations—Na$^+$, K$^+$, and Ca^{2+}—but not to anions such as Cl$^-$. The current attributable to Ca^{2+} is small under physiological conditions. On this basis, the AChR channel at the muscle end plate is often classified as a **nonselective cation channel.** Nevertheless, AChR opening is excitatory, because its reversal potential (near 0 mV) is positive to the threshold of about −50 mV, which is necessary for firing of an action potential.

When the nicotinic AChR channel at the muscle end plate opens, the normally high resting permeability of the muscle plasma membrane for K$^+$ relative to Na$^+$ falls so that Na$^+$ and K$^+$ become equally permeant and V_m shifts to a value between E_K (approximately −80 mV) and E_{Na} (approximately +50 mV).

Similar principles hold for the generation of postsynaptic currents by other types of agonist-gated channels. For example, the receptor-gated channels for serotonin and glutamate are cation selective and give rise to *depolarizing* **excitatory postsynaptic potentials.** In contrast, the receptor-gated channels for glycine and GABA are anion selective and drive

V_m in the hyperpolarizing direction, toward the equilibrium potential for Cl^-. These *hyperpolarizing* postsynaptic responses are called **inhibitory postsynaptic potentials.**

The nicotinic AChR is a member of the pentameric Cys-loop receptor family of ligand-gated ion channels

The neuromuscular AChR consists of four subunits (α, β, γ or ε, and δ) in a pentameric stoichiometry of 2α:1β:1γ (or ε):1δ (Fig. 8.5). Each subunit has a molecular mass of ~50 kDa and is homologous to the other subunits.

The α, β, γ, and δ subunits each have four distinct hydrophobic regions known as M1 to M4, which correspond to membrane-spanning segments. For each of the subunits, the M2 transmembrane segment lines the aqueous pore through which Na^+ and K^+ cross the membrane.

The pentameric complex has two agonist binding sites. The two ACh binding sites are located at the extracellular α/γ interface of one α subunit and the α/δ interface of the other α subunit.

⊙ 8-6 The nicotinic AChRs belong to the **pentameric Cys-loop receptor family** of ligand-gated ion channels, so named because they contain a highly conserved pair of disulfide-bonded cysteine residues. This family also contains three other classes of agonist-activated channels, those activated by **serotonin** (5-HT_3 receptor), **glycine** (GlyR), and **GABA** ($GABA_A$ receptor). As is the case for the AChRs, the 5-HT_3 receptor channels are permeable to cations and thus produce excitatory currents. In contrast, glycine-activated and $GABA_A$ channels are permeable to anions such as Cl^- and produce inhibitory currents (Chapter 13).

Activation of AChR channels requires binding of two ACh molecules

The EPC is the sum of many single-channel currents, each representing the opening of a single AChR channel at the neuromuscular junction. Above we described the random opening and closing of an idealized channel in a two-state model in which the channel could be either closed or open (see ⊙ 7-2):

$$C \rightleftarrows O \qquad (8.1)$$

However, binding of *two* molecules of ACh is required for channel opening:

$$C \rightleftarrows A_1C \rightleftarrows A_2C \rightleftarrows A_2O \qquad (8.2)$$

Closed   1 agonist   2 agonists   Open

Miniature EPPs reveal the quantal nature of transmitter release from the presynaptic terminals

Under physiological conditions, an action potential in a presynaptic motor nerve axon produces a depolarizing postsynaptic EPP that peaks at a level ~40 mV more positive than the resting V_m. This large signal results from the release of ACh from about 200 synaptic vesicles, each containing 6000 to 10,000 molecules of ACh. The neuromuscular junction is clearly designed for excess capacity inasmuch as a single end plate is composed of numerous synaptic contacts (~1000 at the frog muscle end plate), each with an active zone that is lined with dozens of mature synaptic vesicles. Thus, a large

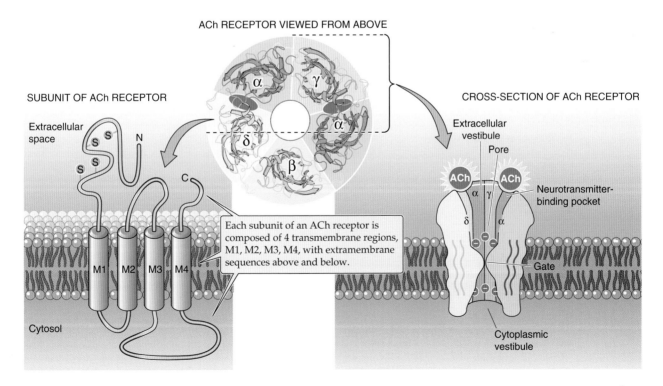

ACh RECEPTOR VIEWED FROM ABOVE

SUBUNIT OF ACh RECEPTOR

CROSS-SECTION OF ACh RECEPTOR

Each subunit of an ACh receptor is composed of 4 transmembrane regions, M1, M2, M3, M4, with extramembrane sequences above and below.

Figure 8.5 Structure of the *Torpedo* nicotinic AChR. For view from above, data from Unwin N. Refined structure of the nicotinic receptor at 4 Å resolution. *J Mol Biol.* 2005;346:968–989.)

inventory of ready vesicles ($>10^4$), together with the ability to synthesize ACh and to package it into new vesicles, allows the neuromuscular junction to maintain a high rate of successful transmission without significant loss of function as a result of presynaptic depletion of vesicles or ACh.

An intracellular recording from a muscle fiber at the end-plate reveals a curious electrical "noise," tiny depolarizations of ~0.4 mV that appear at random intervals. These small depolarizations were blocked by the AChR antagonist curare and they increased in size and duration with application of the AChE inhibitor neostigmine. Because the spontaneous V_m fluctuations also exhibited a time course similar to that of the normal EPP, they were named **miniature end-plate potentials** (also known as MEPPs). These observations suggested that even in the absence of nerve stimulation, there is a certain low probability of transmitter release at the presynaptic terminal, resulting in the opening of a small number of AChRs in the postsynaptic membrane. This finding led to the notion that ACh release is *quantized,* with the quantal event corresponding to ACh release from one synaptic vesicle.

Fig. 8.6A shows superimposed records of EPPs that were recorded from a frog muscle fiber during seven repetitive trials of nerve stimulation. The amplitudes of the peak responses occur in discrete multiples of ~0.4 mV. Among the seven records were one "nonresponse," two responses of ~0.4 mV, three responses of ~0.8 mV, and one response of ~1.2 mV. One of the recordings also revealed a spontaneous MEPP with a quantal amplitude of ~0.4 mV that appeared later in the trace. The EPP is the sum of many unitary events, each having a magnitude of ~0.4 mV (Fig. 8.6B). Microscopic observation of numerous vesicles in the synaptic terminal naturally led to the hypothesis that a single vesicle releases a relatively fixed amount of ACh and thereby produces a unitary MEPP. According to this view, EPPs correspond to the fusion of discrete numbers of synaptic vesicles: 0, 1, 2, 3, and so on.

Neuromuscular transmission exhibits synaptic plasticity

Short-term or long-term changes in the relative efficiency of neurotransmitter release can increase or decrease the

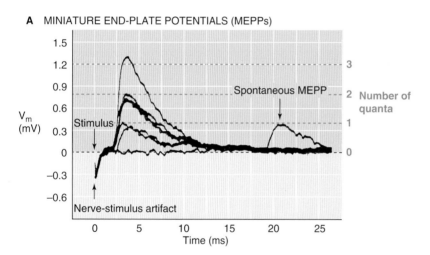

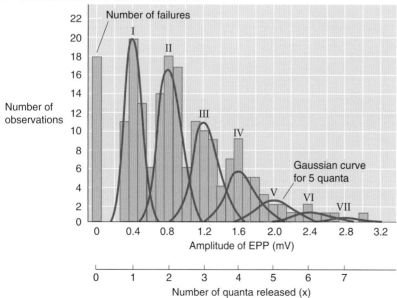

Figure 8.6 Evoked and spontaneous MEPPs. (A) Recordings of V_m in frog skeletal muscle fibers under conditions that minimize transmitter release, and thus make it possible to resolve the smallest possible MEPPs. (B) Histogram summarizing data from 198 trials on a cat neuromuscular junction. The distribution has eight peaks. The first represents stimuli that evoked no responses. The other seven represent stimuli that evoked MEPPs that were roughly integral multiples of the smallest MEPP. (Data from Magleby KL. Neuromuscular transmission. In Engel AG, Franzini-Armstrong C, eds. *Myology: Basic and Clinical,* 2nd ed. New York: McGraw-Hill; 1994:442–463.)

strength of a particular synapse and thereby give rise to an alteration in behavior. Three types of synaptic modulation occur at the neuromuscular junction, and they differ in how they affect the quantal release of neurotransmitter:

Facilitation is a *short-lived* enhancement of the EPP in response to a *brief* increase in the frequency of nerve stimulation. One way that facilitation may occur is by a transient increase in the mean number of quanta per nerve stimulus. This may be caused by "residual calcium," where the calcium entering the nerve terminal in response to one action potential is not completely removed before a second action potential arrives. Because vesicle fusion depends cooperatively on Ca^{2+}, a small increase in $[Ca^{2+}]_i$ can produce a large increase in transmitter release.

Potentiation (or post-tetanic potentiation) is a *long-lived* and pronounced increase in transmitter release that occurs after a *long* period of high-frequency nerve stimulation. This effect can last for minutes after the conditioning stimulus. Potentiation may be caused by a period of intense nerve firing, which increases $[Ca^{2+}]_i$ in the presynaptic terminal and thus increases the probability of exocytosis.

Synaptic **depression** is a *transient* decrease in the efficiency of transmitter release and, consequently, a reduction in the EPP in response to a period of frequent nerve stimulation. Depression may result from temporary depletion of transmitter-loaded vesicles from the presynaptic terminal, that is, a reduction in the number of available quanta. Thus, these three temporal changes in synaptic strength and efficiency appear to reflect changes at different steps of synaptic transmission. At the neuromuscular junction, the EPP is normally far above threshold, so depression normally does not produce failure of transmission or muscle weakness. However, neuromuscular diseases can reduce this "safety factor" and reveal underlying synaptic plasticity. Modulation of synaptic strength is critical in the CNS (Chapter 13).

Synaptic vesicles package, store, and deliver neurotransmitters

The physiology of synaptic vesicles in the nervous system is a variation on the universal theme used by endocrine or secretory cells in animals from the most primitive invertebrates up to mammals. Many proteins involved in synaptic vesicle movement and turnover are related to those involved in intracellular membrane trafficking in almost all eukaryotic cells.

As shown in Fig. 8.7, **nascent synaptic vesicles** are produced in the neuronal cell body by a process similar to that in the **secretory pathway.** The membrane proteins of synaptic vesicles are synthesized in the rough endoplasmic reticulum and are then directed to the Golgi network, where processing, maturation, and sorting occur. Nascent synaptic vesicles—which are, in fact, secretory vesicles—are then transported to the nerve terminal by **fast axonal transport.**

Vesicles destined to contain *peptide* neurotransmitters travel down the axon with the presynthesized peptides or peptide precursors already inside. On arrival at the nerve terminal (Fig. 8.7), the vesicles—now called **dense-core secretory granules** (100 to 200 nm in diameter)—become randomly distributed in the cytoplasm of the terminal (see ◉ 13-1).

Vesicles destined to contain *nonpeptide* neurotransmitters (e.g., ACh) travel down the axon with no transmitter inside. On arrival at the nerve terminal (Fig. 8.7), the vesicles take up the nonpeptide neurotransmitter, which is synthesized locally in the nerve terminal. These nonpeptide **clear synaptic vesicles** (40 to 50 nm in diameter) then attach to the actin-based cytoskeletal network. At this point, the mature clear synaptic vesicles are functionally ready for Ca^{2+}-dependent transmitter release and become docked at specific release sites in the **active zones** of the presynaptic membrane. After exocytotic fusion of the clear synaptic

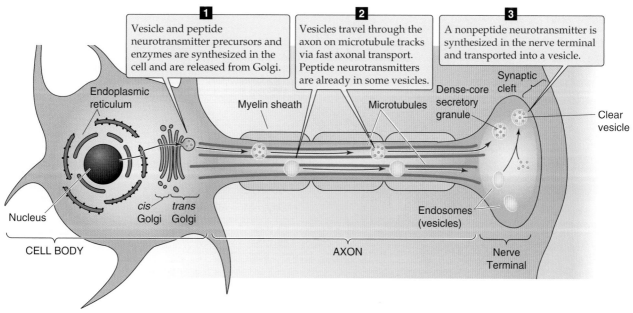

Figure 8.7 Synthesis and recycling of synaptic vesicles and their content.

vesicles, endocytosis via clathrin-coated vesicles recovers membrane components and recycles them to an endosome compartment in the terminal. Synaptic vesicles may then be re-formed within the terminal for reuse in neurotransmission, or they may be transported back to the cell body for turnover and degradation.

The uptake of nonpeptide neurotransmitters into clear synaptic vesicles is accomplished by the combination of a vacuolar-type H-ATPase and various neurotransmitter transport proteins.

Many proteins are involved in the fusion and recycling of synaptic vesicles. The **SNARE proteins,** which also participate in the secretory pathway, comprise the force-generating molecular machinery for membrane-membrane fusion.

Synaptotagmin is a synaptic vesicle protein that is the Ca^{2+}-sensor for exocytosis.

Re-uptake or cleavage of the neurotransmitter terminates its action

Effective transmission across chemical synapses requires not only release of the neurotransmitter and activation of the receptor on the postsynaptic membrane but also rapid and efficient mechanisms for removal of the transmitter. At synapses where ACh is released, this removal is accomplished by enzymatic destruction of the neurotransmitter. However, the more general mechanism in the nervous system involves re-uptake of the neurotransmitter mediated by specific

high-affinity transport systems located in the presynaptic plasma membrane and surrounding glial cells.

The enzyme AChE rapidly hydrolyzes ACh to choline and acetate in a two-step process:

$$\text{AChE} + \text{ACh} \underset{\text{choline}}{\rightarrow} \text{acetyl-AChE} \rightarrow \text{acetate} + \text{AChE} \qquad (8.3)$$

In the first step of the reaction, the enzyme cleaves choline from ACh, which results in the formation of a transient intermediate in which the acetate group is covalently coupled to a serine group on the enzyme. The second step is the hydrolysis and release of this acetate as well as the recovery of free enzyme. The nerve terminal recovers the extracellular choline via a high-affinity Na^+-coupled uptake system and uses it for the synthesis of ACh.

TOXINS AND DRUGS AFFECTING SYNAPTIC TRANSMISSION

Much of our knowledge of the synaptic physiology of the neuromuscular junction and the identities of its various molecular components have been derived from experiments using specific pharmacological agents and toxins that permit functional dissection of the system. Fig. 8.8 illustrates the relative synaptic location and corresponding pharmacology of AChE as well as several ion channels and proteins involved in exocytosis.

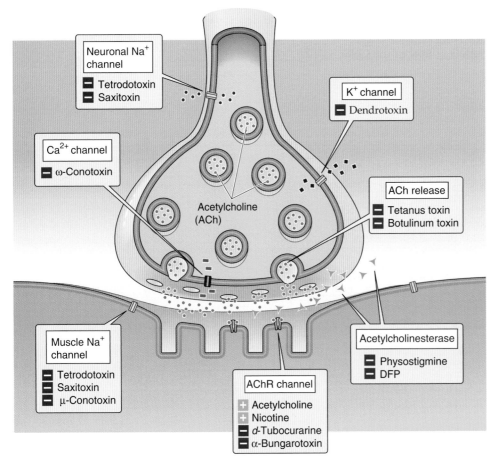

Figure 8.8 Pharmacology of the vertebrate neuromuscular junction. Many of the proteins that are involved in synaptic transmission at the mammalian neuromuscular junction are the targets of naturally occurring or synthetic drugs. The antagonists are shown as minus signs highlighted in *red*. The agonists are shown as plus signs highlighted in *green.*

Guanidinium neurotoxins such as tetrodotoxin prevent depolarization of the nerve terminal, whereas dendrotoxins inhibit repolarization

The action potential is the first step in transmission: a nerve action potential arriving at the terminal initiates the entire process. As discussed in Chapter 7, the depolarizing phase of the action potential is mediated by voltage-dependent Na^+ channels that are specifically blocked by nanomolar concentrations of the small guanidinium neurotoxins **tetrodotoxin** and **saxitoxin**.

The mamba snake toxin **dendrotoxin** has an effect that is precisely opposite that of tetrodotoxin: it facilitates the release of ACh that is evoked by nerve stimulation. Blockade of presynaptic K^+ channels by dendrotoxin inhibits repolarization of the presynaptic membrane, thereby prolonging the duration of the action potential and facilitating the release of transmitter in response to the entry of extra Ca^{2+} into the nerve terminal.

ω-Conotoxin blocks Ca^{2+} channels that mediate Ca^{2+} influx into nerve terminals, inhibiting synaptic transmission

Molluscan peptide toxins called **ω-conotoxins** (see ⊙ 7-6) block presynaptic Ca^{2+} currents in a virtually irreversible fashion. This effect is manifested as an abolition of muscle EPP when the preparation is stimulated via the nerve. Ca^{2+} channels are located precisely at the active zones of synaptic vesicle fusion. This arrangement provides for focal entry and short-range diffusion of Ca^{2+} entering the nerve terminal to the exact sites involved in promoting Ca^{2+}-dependent transmitter release.

Bacterial toxins such as tetanus and botulinum toxins cleave proteins involved in exocytosis, preventing fusion of synaptic vesicles

Another class of neurotoxins that specifically inhibits neurotransmitter release includes the tetanus and botulinum toxins. These large-protein toxins (~150 kDa) are respectively produced by the bacteria *Clostridium tetani* and *Clostridium botulinum*. *C. tetani* is the causative agent of **tetanus** (lockjaw), which is characterized by a general increase in muscle tension and muscle rigidity, beginning most often with the muscles of mastication. The reason for this paradoxical enhancement of muscle action is that the greatest effect of these toxins is to *inhibit* synaptic transmission by inhibitory neurons in the spinal cord, neurons that would normally *inhibit* muscle contraction. The result is hyperstimulation of skeletal muscle contraction. *C. botulinum* causes **botulism,** which is characterized by weakness and paralysis of skeletal muscle as well as by a variety of symptoms that are related to inhibition of cholinergic nerve endings in the autonomic nervous system.

Both agonists and antagonists of the nicotinic AChR can prevent synaptic transmission

The ionotropic (nicotinic) AChR channel located in the postsynaptic muscle membrane also has a rich and diverse pharmacology (Fig. 8.8) that can be exploited for clinical applications. These agents are classified as agonists or antagonists according to whether they activate opening of the channel or prevent its activation.

The agonist succinylcholine is used to produce sustained muscle relaxation or "flaccid paralysis," which is useful in surgery in which it is important to prevent excitation and contraction of skeletal muscles. This paralytic action occurs because succinylcholine prolongs the opening of AChR channels and thereby depolarizes the muscle membrane in the vicinity of the end plate. Such depolarization results in initial repetitive muscle excitation and tremors, followed by relaxation secondary to **inactivation of Na^+ channels** in the vicinity of the end plate. This effect prevents the spread of muscle action potentials beyond the end-plate region. On a longer time scale, such agents also lead to **desensitization of the AChR** to agonist, which further inhibits neuromuscular transmission.

Another important *agonist* acting on AChRs is **nicotine.** A classic example of a nicotinic AChR **antagonist** is *d*-tubocurarine, the active ingredient of curare. The indigenous tribes of the Amazon region used curare to poison arrows for hunting. *d*-**Tubocurarine** is a competitive inhibitor of ACh binding. This action leads to a *nondepolarizing* flaccid paralysis of skeletal muscle. A hallmark of the action of *d*-tubocurarine is that it can be reversed by an increase in ACh by binding competition, which can be produced indirectly by an inhibitor of AChE such as neostigmine (see ⊙ 8-7).

Another class of nicotinic AChR inhibitors is a family of ~8-kDa proteins present in the venom of Elapidae snakes (e.g., cobras). These toxins include **α-bungarotoxin** (α-Bgt) and homologous α toxins, which bind very strongly to nicotinic receptors.

Inhibitors of AChE prolong and magnify the EPP

Inhibition of AChE generally increases the amplitude and prolongs the duration of the postsynaptic response to ACh; thus the enzyme plays an important role in limiting the excitatory action of ACh under normal physiological conditions. In the absence of ACh breakdown by AChE, the prolonged decay of the EPP reflects slow depletion of the agonist in the vicinity of the junctional folds by diffusion of ACh.

⊙ 8-7 The plant alkaloid **physostigmine** (also known as eserine) is the prototypic anticholinesterase. **Neostigmine** (Prostigmin), a synthetic anti-AChE drug with chemical similarity to physostigmine, is used to treat myasthenia gravis.

CHAPTER 9

CELLULAR PHYSIOLOGY OF SKELETAL, CARDIAC, AND SMOOTH MUSCLE

Edward G. Moczydlowski

The primary function of muscle is to generate force or movement in response to a physiological stimulus. The human body contains three fundamentally different types of muscle adapted to specialized functions. Skeletal muscle is responsible for the voluntary movement of bones that underlies locomotion and work production. Cardiac muscle is specific to the heart as the biomechanical pump driving the delivery of blood to the lungs and tissues. Smooth muscle provides mechanical control of organ systems such as the digestive, urinary, and reproductive tracts as well as the blood vessels of the circulatory system and the airway passages of the respiratory system.

Contraction of muscles is initiated either by a chemical neurotransmitter or paracrine factor or by direct electrical excitation. All muscles transduce chemical energy released by hydrolysis of ATP into mechanical work. The unique physiological role of each of the three basic muscle types dictates inherent differences in the rate and duration of contraction, metabolism, fatigability, and ability to regulate contractile strength. Despite these differences, the trigger for muscle contraction is the same for all three types of muscle: a rise in the free cytosolic Ca^{2+} concentration ($[Ca^{2+}]_i$).

This chapter describes the fundamental physiology of muscle excitation, the coupling of excitation to contraction, the molecular mechanism of contraction, the regulation of contraction, and the related issues of muscle diversity. We describe general molecular mechanisms shared by all muscle cells and contrast the unique features of skeletal, cardiac, and smooth muscle. Because molecular mechanisms specific to cardiac myocytes are best understood in the unique context of the heart as a pump, we discuss details of cardiac muscle physiology in greater depth in Chapter 22.

SKELETAL MUSCLE

Contraction of skeletal muscle is initiated by motor neurons that innervate motor units

The smallest contractile unit of skeletal muscle is a multinucleated, elongated cell called a **muscle fiber** or **myofiber** (Fig. 9.1). A bundle of linearly aligned muscle fibers forms a **fascicle.** In turn, bundles of fascicles form a muscle, such as the biceps. Surrounding each muscle fiber is the plasma membrane of the muscle cell called the **sarcolemma.** An individual skeletal muscle cell contains a densely arranged

parallel array of cylindrical elements called **myofibrils.** Each myofibril is essentially an end-to-end chain of regular repeating units—or **sarcomeres**—that consist of smaller interdigitating filaments called **myofilaments;** these myofilaments contain both thin filaments and thick filaments.

Ⓩ 9-1 All skeletal muscle is under voluntary or reflex control by **motor neurons** of the somatic motor system. Somatic motor neurons are efferent neurons with cell bodies located in the central nervous system (CNS). A single muscle cell responds to only a single motor neuron whose cell body—except for cranial nerves—resides in the ventral horn of the spinal cord. However, the axon of a motor neuron typically branches near its termination to innervate a few or many individual muscle cells. The group of muscle fibers innervated by all of the collateral branches of a single motor neuron is referred to as a **motor unit.** A whole muscle can produce a wide range of forces and a graded range of shortening by varying the number of motor units excited within the muscle. The **innervation ratio** of a whole skeletal muscle is defined as the number of muscle fibers innervated by a single motor neuron. Muscles with a small innervation ratio control fine movements involving small forces. For example, fine, high-precision movements of the extraocular muscles that control positioning movements of the eye are achieved via an innervation ratio of as little as ~3 muscle fibers per neuron. Conversely, muscles with a large innervation ratio control coarse movement requiring development of large forces. Postural control by the soleus muscle uses an innervation ratio of ~200. The gastrocnemius muscle, which is capable of developing large forces required in athletic activities such as jumping, has innervation ratios that vary from ~100 to ~1000.

A motor nerve axon contacts each muscle fiber near the middle of the fiber to form a synapse called the **neuromuscular junction.** The specialized region of sarcolemma in closest contact with the presynaptic nerve terminal is called the **motor end plate.** Physiological excitation of skeletal muscle always involves chemical activation by release of acetylcholine (ACh) from the motor nerve terminal. Binding of ACh to the nicotinic receptor gives rise to a graded, depolarizing **end-plate potential.** An end-plate potential of sufficient magnitude raises the membrane potential to the firing threshold and activates voltage-gated Na^+ channels (Navs) in the vicinity of the end plate, triggering an action potential that propagates along the surface membrane.

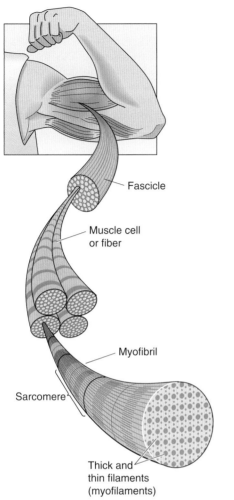

Figure 9.1 Structure of skeletal muscle, from muscle to myofilament.

Labels (top to bottom): Fascicle; Muscle cell or fiber; Myofibril; Sarcomere; Thick and thin filaments (myofilaments)

Action potentials propagate from the sarcolemma to the interior of muscle fibers along the transverse tubule network

As action potentials propagate along the surface membrane of skeletal and cardiac muscle fibers, they penetrate into the cell interior via radially oriented, tubular invaginations of the plasma membrane called **transverse tubules** or **T tubules** (Fig. 9.2). T tubules plunge into the muscle fiber and surround the myofibrils at two points in each sarcomere: at the junctions of the A and the I bands. Along its length the tubule associates with two **terminal cisternae,** which are specialized regions of the **sarcoplasmic reticulum (SR),** which serves as a storage organelle for intracellular Ca^{2+}. The combination of the T-tubule membrane and its two neighboring cisternae is called a **triad junction,** or simply a **triad.**

⊙ 9-2 Depolarization of the T-tubule membrane results in Ca^{2+} release from the SR at the triad

The ultimate intracellular signal that triggers and sustains contraction of skeletal muscle cells is a rise in $[Ca^{2+}]_i$. Ca^{2+} can enter the cytoplasm from the extracellular space through voltage-gated ion channels or, alternatively, Ca^{2+} can be released into the cytoplasm from the intracellular Ca^{2+} storage reservoir of the SR. Thus, both extracellular and intracellular sources may contribute to the increase in $[Ca^{2+}]_i$. The process by which electrical "excitation" of the surface membrane triggers an increase of $[Ca^{2+}]_i$ in muscle is known as **excitation-contraction coupling,** or EC coupling.

The propagation of the action potential into the T tubules of the myofiber depolarizes the triad region of the T tubules, as discussed in the above section, thereby activating **L-type Ca^{2+} channels.** These voltage-gated channels cluster in groups of four called tetrads (Fig. 9.3) and have a pivotal role

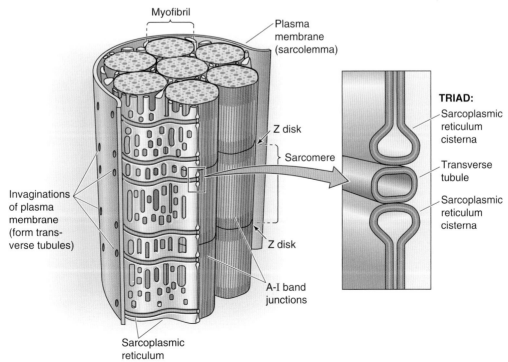

Labels: Myofibril; Plasma membrane (sarcolemma); Z disk; Sarcomere; Z disk; A-I band junctions; Invaginations of plasma membrane (form transverse tubules); Sarcoplasmic reticulum; **TRIAD:** Sarcoplasmic reticulum cisterna; Transverse tubule; Sarcoplasmic reticulum cisterna

Figure 9.2 Transverse tubules and SR in skeletal muscle.

as the **voltage sensor** in EC coupling. The L-type Ca^{2+} channel is also often referred to as the **DHP receptor** because it is inhibited by a class of antihypertensive and antiarrhythmic drugs known as dihydropyridines or calcium channel blockers. Depolarization of the T-tubule membrane produces conformational changes in each of the four Cav1.1 channels of the tetrad, resulting in two major effects. First, the conformational changes open the Cav1.1 channel pore, which allows electrodiffusive Ca^{2+} entry. Second, and more importantly in skeletal muscle, the voltage-driven conformational changes in the four Cav1.1 channels mechanically activate each of the four directly coupled subunits of another channel—the Ca^{2+}-release channel located in the portion of the terminal cisternae of the SR membrane that faces the T tubule (Fig. 9.3).

◉ **9-3** The SR **Ca^{2+}-release channel** is also known as the **ryanodine receptor (RYR)** because it is inhibited by the plant alkaloid *ryanodine*. Each of the four subunits of the RYR channel has a large extension—also known as a foot—that projects into the cytosol (Fig. 9.3).

In skeletal muscle, where the Ca^{2+}-release channels are of the RYR1 subtype, the monomer foot domain of each of the four RYR1 subunits is complementary to the cytoplasmic projection of one of the four Cav1.1 channels in a tetrad on the T tubule (Fig. 9.3).

Following activation of the L-type Ca^{2+} channel on the T-tubule membrane and mechanical activation of the Ca^{2+}-release channel in the SR, Ca^{2+} stored in the SR rapidly leaves through the Ca^{2+}-release channel. This increase in $[Ca^{2+}]_i$ activates troponin C, initiating formation of cross-bridges between myofilaments, as described below. EC coupling in skeletal muscle thus includes the entire process we have just described, beginning with the depolarization of the T-tubule membrane to the initiation of the cross-bridge cycle of contraction.

◉ 9-4 Striations of skeletal muscle fibers correspond to ordered arrays of thick and thin filaments within myofibrils

Myofilaments are of two types: thick filaments composed primarily of a protein called myosin and thin filaments largely composed of a protein called **actin**. The **sarcomere** is defined as the repeating unit between adjacent Z disks or Z lines (Fig. 9.4A and B). A myofibril is thus a linear array of sarcomeres stacked end to end. The highly organized sarcomeres within skeletal and cardiac muscle are responsible for the striped or striated appearance of muscle fibers of these tissues as visualized by various microscopic imaging techniques. Thus, both

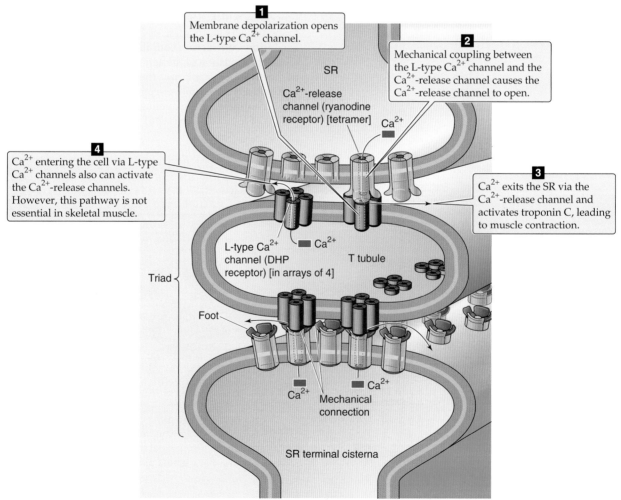

1 Membrane depolarization opens the L-type Ca^{2+} channel.

2 Mechanical coupling between the L-type Ca^{2+} channel and the Ca^{2+}-release channel causes the Ca^{2+}-release channel to open.

4 Ca^{2+} entering the cell via L-type Ca^{2+} channels also can activate the Ca^{2+}-release channels. However, this pathway is not essential in skeletal muscle.

3 Ca^{2+} exits the SR via the Ca^{2+}-release channel and activates troponin C, leading to muscle contraction.

SR

Ca^{2+}-release channel (ryanodine receptor) [tetramer]

Ca^{2+}

L-type Ca^{2+} channel (DHP receptor) [in arrays of 4]

Ca^{2+}

T tubule

Triad

Foot

Ca^{2+}

Ca^{2+}

Mechanical connection

SR terminal cisterna

Figure 9.3   EC coupling in skeletal muscle.

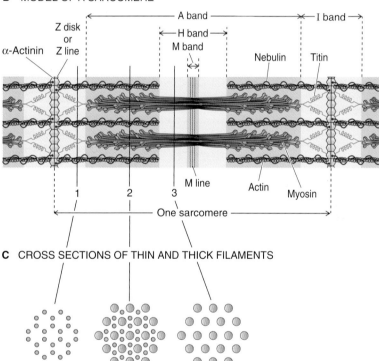

Figure 9.4   Structure of the sarcomere.

skeletal muscle and cardiac muscle are referred to as **striated muscle.** In contrast, smooth muscle lacks striations because actin and myosin have a less regular pattern of organization in these myocytes.

In striated muscle, **thin filaments**—composed of actin—are 5 to 8 nm in diameter and 1 μm in length. The plus end of the thin filaments attach to opposite faces of a dense disk known as the **Z disk** (Fig. 9.4B), which is perpendicular to the axis of the myofibril and has the diameter of the myofibril. Cross-linking the thin filaments at the Z disk are α-**actinin** proteins. Two large proteins, titin and nebulin, are

also tethered at the Z disks. Connections between the Z disks also tether each myofibril to its neighbors and align the Z disks and thus the sarcomeres.

The **thick filaments**—composed of myosin—are 10 to 15 nm in diameter and, in striated muscle, 1.6 μm in length (Fig. 9.4B). They lie between and partially interdigitate with the thin filaments. This partial interdigitation results in alternating light and dark bands along the axis of the myofibril. The light bands, which represent regions of the thin filament that do not overlap with thick filaments, are known as **I bands**. The Z disk is visible as a dark perpendicular line at

A F-ACTIN, TROPOMYOSIN, AND TROPONIN

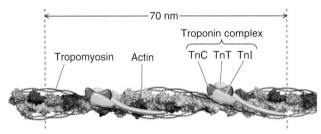

B MYOSIN MOLECULE

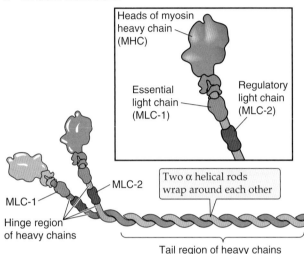

Figure 9.5 Structure of thin and thick filaments. (A, Courtesy of Roberto Dominguez, University of Pennsylvania).

the center of the I band. The dark bands, which represent the myosin filaments, are known as **A bands**. When the A band is viewed in cross section where the thick and thin filaments overlap, six thin filaments (actin) are seen to surround each thick filament (myosin) in a tightly packed hexagonal array (Fig. 9.4C). During contraction, the I bands (nonoverlapping region of actin) shorten, while the A bands (myosin) do not change in length. This observation led to the idea that the thick and thin filaments slide past each other—the **sliding filament model** of muscle contraction.

Thin and thick filaments are supramolecular assemblies of protein subunits

Thin Filaments The backbone of the thin filament is a two-stranded helix of noncovalently polymerized **actin** molecules, and two important regulatory actin-binding proteins: tropomyosin and the troponin complex (Fig. 9.5A).

The **tropomyosin** monomer of striated muscle is an α-helical protein that binds to seven actin monomers along the thin filament. Two tropomyosin monomers form a dimer aligned in parallel and wound about each other in a coiled-coil structure. Two such tropomyosin dimers flank each supramolecular helix of actin (Fig. 9.5A). Overlapping head-to-tail contacts between two tropomyosin dimers produce two nearly continuous double-helical filaments that shadow the actin double helix. As we describe below, tropomyosin acts as a gatekeeper in regulating the binding of myosin head groups to actin.

Troponin or the **troponin complex** is a heterotrimer consisting of the following:
1. **Troponin T** (TnT or TNNT), which binds to a single molecule of tropomyosin
2. ⊙ **9-5 Troponin C** (TnC or TNNC), which binds Ca^{2+}
3. **Troponin I** (TnI or TNNI), which binds to actin and inhibits contraction

Each troponin heterotrimer interacts with a single tropomyosin molecule, which in turn interacts with seven actin monomers. The troponin complex also interacts directly with the actin filaments. The coordinated interactions of troponin, tropomyosin, and actin allow the binding of actin and myosin to be regulated by changes in $[Ca^{2+}]_i$.

Thick Filaments ⊙ **9-6** Thick filaments are also an intertwined complex of proteins (Fig. 9.5B). In fast skeletal muscle, the thick filament is a bipolar superassembly of several hundred **myosin II** molecules. Myosin II is responsible for ATP-dependent force generation in all types of myocytes. The myosin II molecule is a pair of identical heterotrimers, each composed of a *myosin heavy chain* (MHC), and two myosin light chains (MLCs). One MLC is *an essential light chain* (ELC or MLC-1), and the other is a *regulatory light chain* (RLC or MLC-2). Both the MHCs and MLCs vary among muscle types.

The **essential light chain and regulatory light chain** bind to and mechanically stabilize the myosin neck region. Phosphorylation of RLC by **myosin light-chain kinases (MLCKs)** enhances myosin cross-bridge interactions. Phosphatases have the opposite effect. In smooth muscle, this phosphorylation plays an essential role in the initiation of contraction.

⊙ **9-7** Running alongside the thick filaments of skeletal muscle is a protein named **titin**—the **elastic filament** of sarcomeres. Titin includes ~300 immunoglobulin-like domains that appear to unfold reversibly upon stretch.

Nebulin is another large protein of muscle that runs from the Z disk along the actin thin filaments. Nebulin interacts with actin and controls the length of the thin filament; it also appears to function in sarcomere assembly by contributing to the structural integrity of myofibrils.

⊙ 9-8 During the cross-bridge cycle, contractile proteins convert the energy of ATP hydrolysis into mechanical energy

The fundamental process of skeletal muscle contraction involves a biochemical cycle, called the cross-bridge cycle, that occurs in six steps (Fig. 9.6): (1) ATP binding, (2) ATP hydrolysis, (3) weak cross-bridge formation, (4) release of P_i from myosin, (5) power stroke, and (6) ADP release. In Fig. 9.6, we start the cycle in the absence of both ATP and ADP, with the myosin head rigidly attached to an actin filament. In a corpse soon after death, the lack of ATP prevents the cycle from proceeding further; this leads to an extreme example of muscle rigidity—called rigor mortis—that is limited only by protein decomposition.

An increase in [Ca²⁺]ᵢ triggers contraction by removing the inhibition of cross-bridge cycling

In skeletal, cardiac, and smooth muscle, an increase in $[Ca^{2+}]_i$ initiates and allows cross-bridge cycling to continue. During

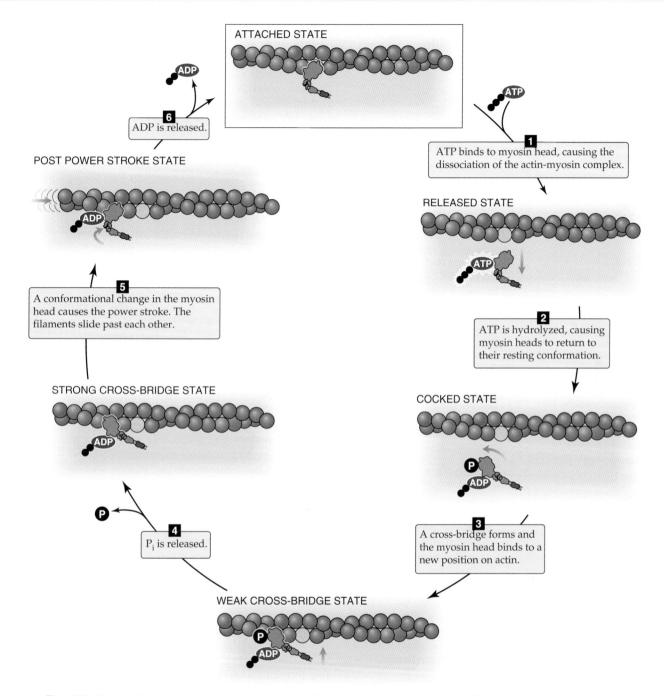

Figure 9.6   Cross-bridge cycle in skeletal and cardiac muscle. Each cycle advances the myosin head by two actin monomers, or ~11 nm.

this excitatory increase, $[Ca^{2+}]_i$ may rise from its resting level of $<10^{-7}$ M to $>10^{-5}$ M. The subsequent decrease in $[Ca^{2+}]_i$—discussed in the next section—is the signal to cease cross-bridge cycling and relax.

Regardless of the muscle type, Ca^{2+} exerts its effect by binding to *regulatory* proteins rather than directly interacting with contractile proteins. In the absence of Ca^{2+}, these regulatory proteins act in concert to inhibit actin-myosin interactions, thus inhibiting the contractile process. When Ca^{2+} binds to one or more of these proteins, a conformational change takes place in the regulatory complex that releases the inhibition of contraction. In both skeletal and cardiac muscle, the regulatory proteins form the **troponin complex,** which is composed of troponin C, troponin I, and troponin T. The **troponin T (TnT)** binds to tropomyosin, establishing the linkage between the troponin complex and tropomyosin.

⊙ **9-9** At high $[Ca^{2+}]_i$, **troponin C (TnC)** interacts with **troponin I (TnI)** in such a way as to cause tropomyosin to translocate on the F-actin surface, which allows the cocked myosin head group to interact weakly with actin (Fig. 9.6, step 3 of the cross-bridge cycle). As long as $[Ca^{2+}]_i$ remains high and the tropomyosin is out of the way, cross-bridge cycling will continue indefinitely.

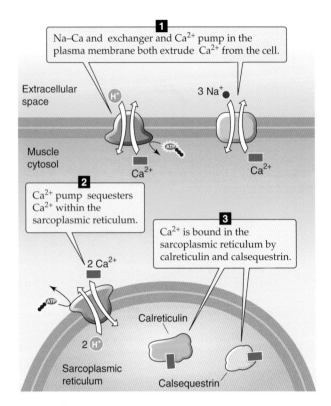

1 Na–Ca and exchanger and Ca²⁺ pump in the plasma membrane both extrude Ca²⁺ from the cell.

Extracellular space

3 Na⁺

Muscle cytosol

Ca²⁺

Ca²⁺

2 Ca²⁺ pump sequesters Ca²⁺ within the sarcoplasmic reticulum.

3 Ca²⁺ is bound in the sarcoplasmic reticulum by calreticulin and calsequestrin.

2 Ca²⁺

Calreticulin

2 H⁺

Sarcoplasmic reticulum

Calsequestrin

Figure 9.7 Mechanisms of Ca²⁺ removal from the cytoplasm.

Termination of contraction requires re-uptake of Ca²⁺ into the SR

After the action potential in the skeletal muscle has subsided, Ca²⁺ must be removed from the **sarcoplasm** for contraction actually to cease and for relaxation to occur. Removal of Ca²⁺ from the sarcoplasm occurs by two mechanisms. Ca²⁺ may be extruded across the cell plasma membrane or sequestered within intracellular compartments (Fig. 9.7).

The cell may extrude Ca²⁺ by use of either an **NCX** (Na-Ca exchanger) or **PMCA** (plasma membrane Ca-ATPase or pump). In skeletal muscle, Ca²⁺ re-uptake into the SR is the most important mechanism by which the cell returns [Ca²⁺]ᵢ to resting levels. Ca²⁺ re-uptake by the SR is mediated by a **SERCA** (sarcoplasmic and endoplasmic reticulum Ca-ATPase or pump.

Ca²⁺-binding proteins buffer the [Ca²⁺] increase in the SR during Ca²⁺ re-uptake and thus markedly increase the Ca²⁺ storage capacity of the SR.

Muscle contractions produce force under isometric conditions and force with shortening under isotonic conditions

The total force generated by a muscle—referred to as **tension**—is the sum of the forces generated by many independently cycling actin-myosin cross-bridges. The number of simultaneously cycling cross-bridges depends on the initial length of the muscle fiber and on the pattern or frequency of muscle cell stimulation. When muscle is stimulated to contract, it exerts a force tending to pull the attachment points at either end toward each other.

Two mechanical—and artificial—arrangements can be used to study force and length relationships in muscle contraction. In one, the attachment points are immobile, so that the muscle *length* is fixed. Here, stimulation causes an increase in tension, but no shortening. Because these contractions occur at constant length, they are referred to as **isometric contractions** (Fig. 9.8A). In the second arrangement, one of the two attachment points is mobile and tethered to a variable load, which tends to pull this mobile point away from the fixed one. Here, stimulation causes shortening, provided the tension developed by the muscle is greater than the opposing load. Because these shortenings occur at constant load, they are referred to as **isotonic contractions** (Fig. 9.8B). Physical activity involves various combinations of isometric and isotonic contractions.

Muscle length influences tension development by determining the degree of overlap between actin and myosin filaments

⊙ **9-10** The iso*metric* force of contractions depends on the initial length of the muscle fiber. The tension measured before muscle contraction is referred to as **passive tension** (Fig. 9.8C). Because muscle gets stiffer as it is distended, it takes increasing amounts of passive tension to progressively elongate the muscle cell. If at any fixed length (i.e., isometric conditions) the muscle is stimulated to contract, an additional **active tension** develops because of cross-bridge cycling. The total measured tension is thus the sum of the passive and active tension. This incremental or *active* tension—the difference between total tension and passive tension—is quite small when the muscle is less than ~70% of its normal resting length (Fig. 9.8D). As muscle length increases toward its normal length, active tension increases. Active tension is maximal at an **optimal length** (*blue point* in Fig. 9.8D). Active tension decreases with further lengthening; thus active tension is again small when the muscle is stretched beyond 150% of its normal resting length. Although the relationship between muscle length and tension has been best characterized for skeletal muscle, the tension of cardiac and smooth muscle also appears to depend on length in a similar manner.

This length-tension relationship is a direct result of the anatomy of the thick and thin filaments within individual sarcomeres (Fig. 9.8D). As muscle length increases, the ends of the actin filaments arising from neighboring Z disks are pulled away from each other. When length is increased beyond 150% of the resting sarcomere length, the ends of the actin filaments are pulled beyond the ends of the myosin filaments. Under this condition, no interaction occurs between actin and myosin filaments and hence no active tension develops. As muscle length shortens from this point, actin and myosin filaments begin to overlap and tension can develop; the amount of tension developed corresponds to the degree of overlap between the actin and the myosin filaments. As the muscle shortens further, opposing actin filaments slide over one another and the ends of the myosin filaments and—with extreme degrees of shortening—eventually butt up against the opposing Z disks. Under these conditions, the spatial relationship between actin and myosin is distorted and active tension falls. The maximal degree of overlap between actin and myosin filaments, and

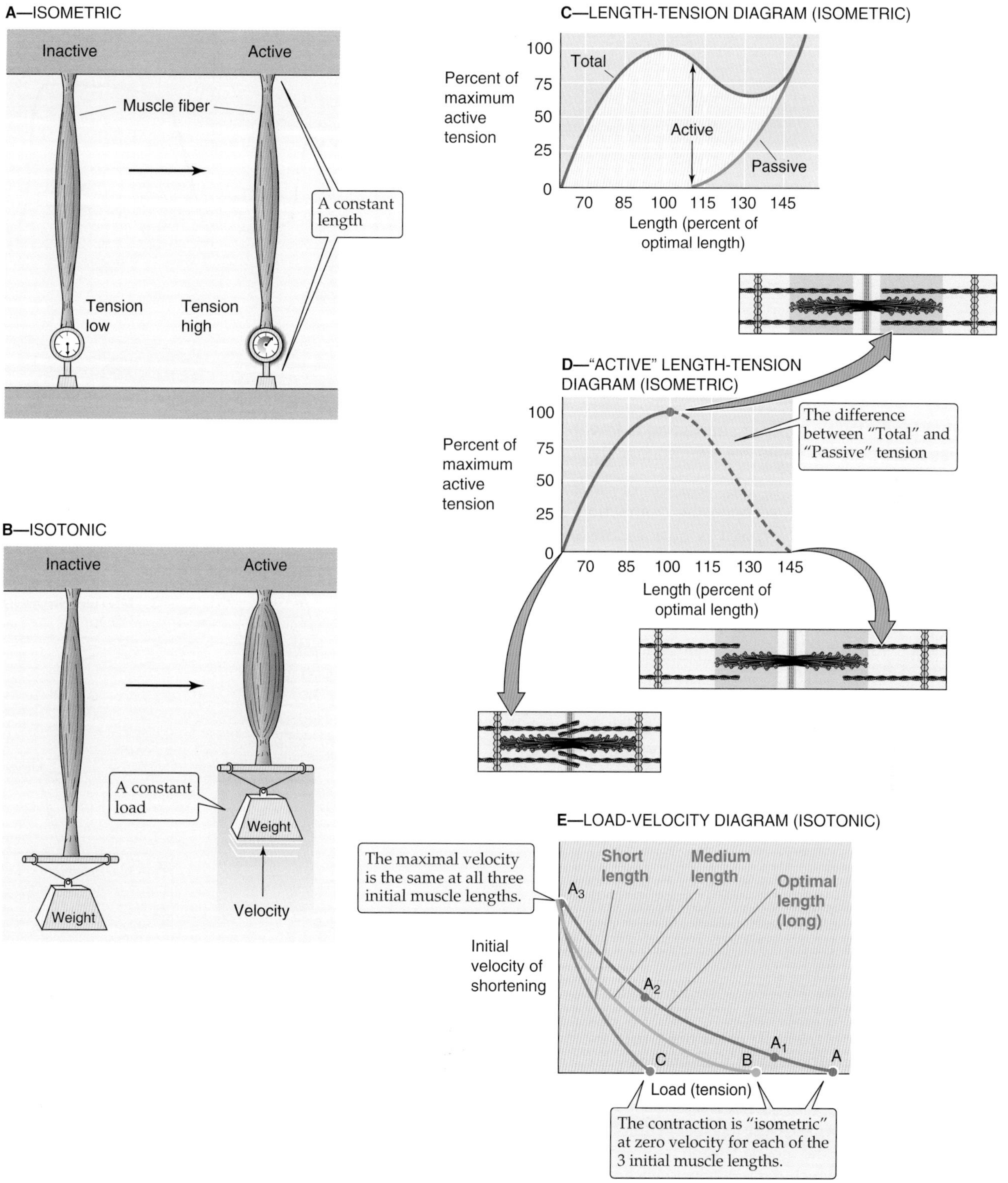

A—ISOMETRIC

B—ISOTONIC

C—LENGTH-TENSION DIAGRAM (ISOMETRIC)

D—"ACTIVE" LENGTH-TENSION DIAGRAM (ISOMETRIC)

E—LOAD-VELOCITY DIAGRAM (ISOTONIC)

Figure 9.8 Isometric and isotonic contraction. (A) Experimental preparation for study of muscle contraction under *isometric* conditions. (B) Experimental preparation for study of muscle contraction under *isotonic* conditions. (C) The *"Passive"* curve represents the tension that is measured at various muscle lengths before muscle contraction. The *"Total"* curve represents the tension that is measured at various muscle lengths during muscle contraction. (D) The active tension is the difference between the total and the passive tensions in (C). (E) The velocity of muscle shortening is greater if the muscle lifts a lighter weight. The *blue, green,* and *gold curves* also show that for any given velocity of shortening, a longer muscle can develop a greater tension than can a shorter muscle.

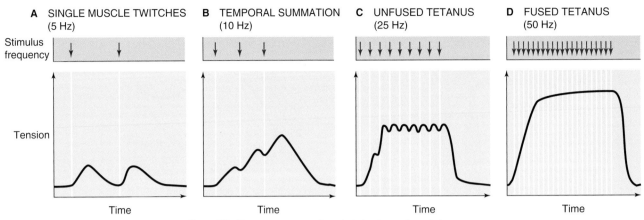

Figure 9.9 Frequency summation of skeletal muscle twitches.

hence maximal active tension, corresponds to a sarcomere length that is near its normal resting length.

At higher loads, the velocity of shortening is lower because more cross-bridges are simultaneously active

Under iso*tonic* conditions, the velocity of shortening decreases as the applied load opposing contraction of the muscle fiber increases. This point is obvious; anyone can lift a single French fry much faster than a sack of potatoes. As shown for any of the three downward-sloping curves in Fig. 9.8E—each of which represents a different initial length of muscle—there is an inverse relationship between velocity and load. Note that for isotonic contractions, the applied load is the same as the tension in the muscle.

In a single skeletal muscle fiber, the force developed may be increased by summing multiple twitches in time

At sufficiently low stimulation frequencies, the tension developed falls to the resting level between individual twitches (Fig. 9.9A). Single skeletal muscle twitches last between 25 and 200 ms, depending on the type of muscle. Although each twitch is elicited by a single muscle action potential, the duration of contraction is long compared with the duration of the exciting action potential, which lasts only several milliseconds. Because the muscle twitch far exceeds the duration of the action potential, it is possible to initiate a second action potential before a first contraction has fully subsided. When this situation occurs, the second action potential stimulates a twitch that is superimposed on the residual tension of the first twitch and thereby achieves greater isometric tension than the first (compare Fig. 9.9A and B). This effect is known as **frequency summation.**

When the stimulation frequency is increased sufficiently, the individual twitches occur so close together in time that they fuse (Fig. 9.9D) and cause the muscle tension to remain at a steady plateau. The state in which the individual twitches are no longer distinguishable from each other is referred to as **tetanus.** Tetanus arises when the time between successive action potentials is insufficient to return enough Ca^{2+} to the SR to lower $[Ca^{2+}]_i$ below a level that initiates relaxation. In fact, a sustained increase in $[Ca^{2+}]_i$ persists until the tetanic stimulus ceases. At stimulation frequencies above the **fusion frequency** that causes tetanus, muscle fiber tension increases very little.

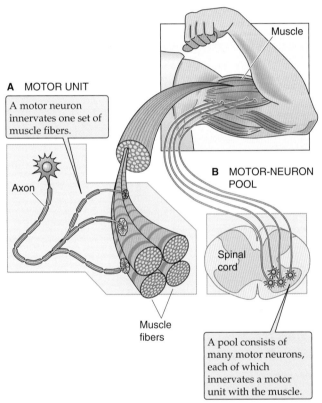

Figure 9.10 The motor unit and the motor-neuron pool.

In a whole skeletal muscle, the force developed may be increased by summing the contractions of multiple fibers

The CNS can control muscle force by determining the number of individual muscle fibers that it stimulates at a given time. As each additional motor-neuron cell body within the spinal cord is excited, those muscle fibers that are part of the *motor unit* of that motor neuron are added to the contracting pool of fibers (Fig. 9.10). This effect is known as **multiple-fiber summation.** The group of all motor neurons innervating a single muscle is called a **motor-neuron pool.**

Multiple-fiber summation, sometimes referred to as **spatial summation,** is an important mechanism that allows the force developed by a whole muscle to be relatively constant in time.

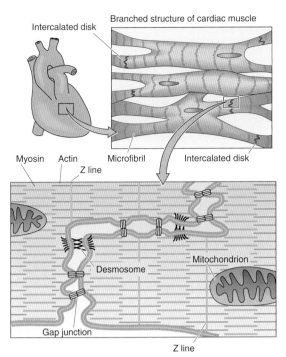

Figure 9.11 Electrical coupling of cardiac myocytes.

CARDIAC MUSCLE

Action potentials propagate between adjacent cardiac myocytes through gap junctions

Cardiac muscle and its individual myocytes have a morphological character different from that of skeletal muscle and its cells (Fig. 9.11). Cardiac myocytes are shorter, branched, and interconnected from end to end by structures called **intercalated disks,** visible as dark lines in the light microscope. The intercalated disks connecting the ends of adjoining cardiac myocytes contain **desmosomes** (see ◉ 2-20) that link adjacent cells mechanically and **gap junctions** that link cells electrically. Cardiac muscle thus acts as a mechanical and electrical syncytium of coupled cells, unlike skeletal muscle fibers, which are separate cells bundled together by connective tissue. Like skeletal muscle, cardiac muscle is striated (see ◉ 9-4), and its sarcomeres contain similar arrays of thin and thick filaments.

Contraction of cardiac muscle cells is not initiated by neurons as in skeletal muscle but by electrical excitation originating from the heart's own **pacemaker,** the sinoatrial node. When an action potential is initiated in one cell, current flows through the gap junctions and depolarizes neighboring cells, producing self-propagating action potentials.

However, cardiac myocytes do receive synaptic input from the sympathetic and parasympathetic divisions of the autonomic nervous system (see Chapter 14), which *modulate* rather than *initiate* electrical activity and contractile force.

Cardiac contraction requires Ca²⁺ entry through L-type Ca²⁺ channels

◉ **9-11** Whereas EC coupling in skeletal muscle does not require Ca^{2+} influx through L-type Ca^{2+} channels (see ◉ 7-5), cardiac contraction has an *absolute requirement* for

Ca^{2+} influx through these channels during the action potential. Cardiac myocytes have a T-tubule network similar to that of skeletal muscle myofibers except that a single terminal cisterna of the SR forms a **dyad junction** with the T-tubule rather than a triad junction. Furthermore, T-tubules of cardiac myocytes are located at the Z lines separating sarcomeres rather than at the A-I band junctions. Because the T-tubule lumen is an extension of the extracellular space, it facilitates the diffusion of Ca^{2+} from bulk extracellular fluid to the site of the L-type Ca^{2+} channels on the T-tubule membrane. Thus, the extracellular Ca^{2+} can simultaneously reach superficial and deep regions of the muscle. The increase in $[Ca^{2+}]_i$ resulting from Ca^{2+} influx through the L-type Ca^{2+} channels alone is not, however, sufficient to initiate contraction. Rather, this increase in $[Ca^{2+}]_i$ leads to an opening of the RYR Ca^{2+}-release channels through a process known as **Ca²⁺-induced Ca²⁺ release (CICR).** Indeed, because the Ca^{2+}-release channels remain open for a longer period than do L-type Ca^{2+} channels, the contribution of CICR to the rise in $[Ca^{2+}]_i$ is greater than the flux contributed by the L-type Ca^{2+} channels of the T tubules.

Cross-bridge cycling and termination of cardiac muscle contraction are similar to the events in skeletal muscle

Cardiac muscle is similar to skeletal muscle in the interaction of the actin and myosin during cross-bridge cycling, the resynthesis of ATP, and the termination of contraction. However, in cardiac muscle, SR Ca-pump activity is inhibited by the regulatory protein **phospholamban (PLN).** When PLN is phosphorylated by cAMP-dependent PKA, its ability to inhibit the SR Ca pump is lost. Thus, activators of PKA, such as the neurotransmitter epinephrine, may enhance the rate of cardiac myocyte relaxation.

In cardiac muscle, increasing the entry of Ca²⁺ enhances the contractile force

Whereas frequency summation and multiple-fiber summation are important mechanisms for regulating the strength of skeletal muscle contractions, the contractile function in cardiac muscle is regulated either by modulating the magnitude of the rise in $[Ca^{2+}]_i$ or by altering the Ca^{2+} sensitivity of the regulatory proteins.

SMOOTH MUSCLE

Smooth muscles may contract in response to synaptic transmission or electrical coupling

Like skeletal muscle, smooth muscle receives synaptic input. However, the synaptic input to smooth muscle differs from that of skeletal muscle in two ways. First, the neurons are part of the autonomic nervous system rather than the somatic nervous system (see Chapter 14). Second, the neuron makes multiple synaptic contacts with a smooth-muscle cell in the form of a series of swellings called **varicosities** (see ◉ 14-4) that contain the presynaptic machinery for vesicular release of transmitter.

◉ **9-12** The mechanisms of intercellular communication between smooth-muscle cells vary more widely among

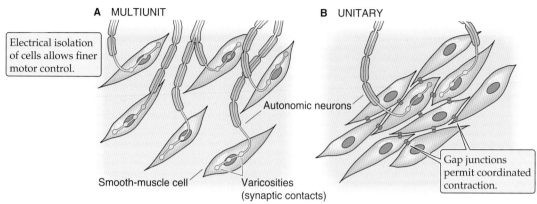

A MULTIUNIT

Electrical isolation of cells allows finer motor control.

B UNITARY

Autonomic neurons

Smooth-muscle cell

Varicosities (synaptic contacts)

Gap junctions permit coordinated contraction.

Figure 9.12 Smooth-muscle organization.

tissues. There are two basic types of smooth-muscle tissues, known as multiunit and single-unit smooth muscle. In **multiunit smooth muscle,** each smooth-muscle cell receives synaptic input but there is little intercellular electrical coupling between cells (i.e., few gap junctions). As a result, each smooth-muscle cell may contract independently of its neighbor. Thus, the term *multiunit* describes smooth muscle that behaves like multiple, independent cells or groups of cells (Fig. 9.12A). Multiunit smooth muscles are capable of fine control. Indeed, multiunit smooth muscle is found in the iris and ciliary body of the eye as well as the piloerector muscles of the skin.

Unitary or single-unit smooth muscle (Fig. 9.12B) is a group of cells that work as a syncytium because gap junctions provide electrical and chemical communication between neighboring cells. Direct electrical coupling allows coordinated contraction of many cells. Gap junctions also allow ions and small molecules to diffuse between cells, which gives rise to phenomena such as spreading **Ca^{2+} waves** among coupled cells. Unitary smooth muscle is the predominant smooth-muscle type within the walls of visceral organs such as the gastrointestinal and urinary tracts, the uterus, and many blood vessels. Thus, unitary smooth muscle is often referred to as **visceral smooth muscle.** Electrical coupling of smooth-muscle units exhibits a tissue-specific continuum from multiunit to unitary coupling.

Action potentials of smooth muscles may be brief or prolonged

Although action potentials initiate contraction in both skeletal and cardiac muscle, diverse changes in membrane potential (V_m) can either initiate or modulate contraction in smooth-muscle cells. The stimuli that produce a **graded response** of V_m include many circulating and local humoral factors as well as mechanical stimuli such as stretching of the cell. These graded V_m changes may be either hyperpolarizing or depolarizing; they sum temporally as well as spatially. If the summation of graded depolarizations brings V_m above threshold, action potentials will fire in electrically excitable smooth-muscle cells.

Action potentials—characteristic responses of unitary (visceral) smooth muscle—typically have a slower upstroke and longer duration (up to ~100 ms) than do skeletal muscle action potentials (~2 ms). The action potential in a smooth-muscle cell can be a simple spike, a spike followed by a plateau, or a series of spikes on top of slow waves of V_m (Fig. 9.13A). In any case, the depolarizing phase of the action potential reflects opening of L-type voltage-gated Ca^{2+} channels. Repolarization of the smooth-muscle cell is relatively slow because L-type Cav Ca^{2+} channels exhibit prolonged openings and inactivate slowly. In addition, the slow repolarization reflects the delayed activation of voltage-gated K^+ channels and, in many cases, Ca^{2+}-activated K^+ channels, which depend on significant elevation of $[Ca^{2+}]_i$.

Some smooth-muscle cells spontaneously generate either pacemaker currents or slow waves

Although smooth-muscle cells undergo changes in V_m in response to neural, hormonal, or mechanical stimulation, many smooth-muscle cells are capable of initiating spontaneous electrical activity. In some tissues, this spontaneous activity results from **pacemaker currents.** In the intestine, for example, special pacemaker cells called **interstitial cells of Cajal** initiate and control rhythmic contractions of the smooth-muscle layers. Pacemaker electrical activity arises from time- and voltage-dependent properties of ion channels that spontaneously produce either an increase in inward depolarizing currents (e.g., voltage-gated Ca^{2+} currents) or a decrease in outward hyperpolarizing currents (e.g., voltage-gated K^+ currents). If V_m reaches threshold, an action potential fires.

⊙ **9-13** In other smooth-muscle cells, this spontaneous electrical activity results in regular, repetitive oscillations in V_m—and contractions—that occur at a frequency of several cycles per minute. These are referred to as **slow waves** (Fig. 9.13B). One hypothesis regarding the origin of slow-wave potentials suggests that voltage-gated Ca^{2+} channels—active at the resting V_m—depolarize the cell enough to activate more voltage-gated Ca^{2+} channels. This activation results in progressive depolarization and Ca^{2+} influx. The increase in $[Ca^{2+}]_i$ activates Ca^{2+}-dependent K^+ channels, which leads

A—TYPES OF SMOOTH-MUSCLE ACTION POTENTIALS

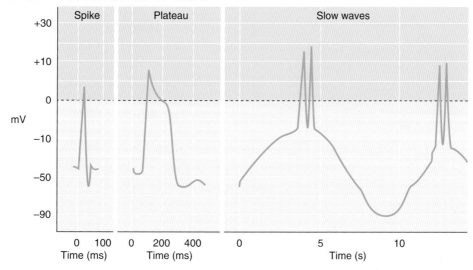

B—GENERATION OF SLOW WAVES

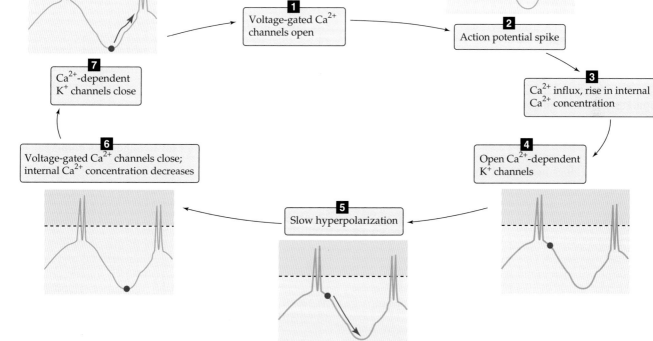

Figure 9.13 Action potentials and slow waves in smooth muscle.

to progressive hyperpolarization and eventual termination of the depolarization. These periodic depolarizations and $[Ca^{2+}]_i$ increases cause periodic tonic contractions of the smooth muscle. When the amplitude of the slow V_m waves is sufficient to depolarize the cell to threshold, the ensuing action potentials lead to further Ca^{2+} influx and phasic contractions.

Some smooth muscles contract without action potentials

Whereas generation of an action potential is essential for initiating contraction of skeletal and cardiac muscle, many smooth-muscle cells contract despite being unable to generate an action potential.

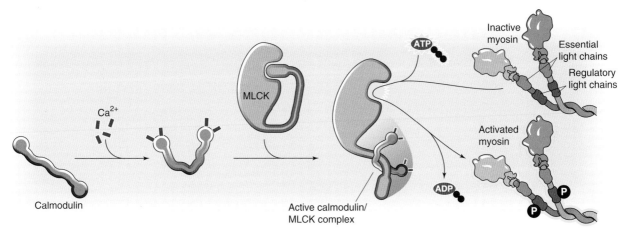

Figure 9.14 Role of Ca^{2+} in triggering the contraction of smooth muscle.

Some smooth-muscle cells contract simply in response to extracellular agonists, with minimal depolarization and negligible Ca^{2+} entry from the outside. For example, a neurotransmitter can bind to a receptor, activate a G protein, and—via phospholipase C—lead to the generation of IP_3, binding to IP_3R, and Ca^{2+} release from the SR.

Sarcoplasmic Ca^{2+} release—if sufficiently robust—may occur by either of two mechanisms in smooth muscle: (1) Ca^{2+} entry through small clusters of the L-type Cav channels, activating the RYR3 subtype of ryanodine receptors and causing CICR—a robust amplification of the Ca^{2+} signal and (2) IP_3 activation of IP_3R. Whereas the rise of $[Ca^{2+}]_i$ via CICR is a prominent aspect of cardiac muscle, the receptor-mediated IP_3 pathway is particularly significant for SR Ca^{2+} release in smooth muscle.

Ca^{2+}-dependent phosphorylation of the myosin regulatory light chain activates cross-bridge cycling in smooth muscle

As we noted above, because smooth-muscle actin and myosin are not as highly organized as in skeletal and cardiac muscle, smooth muscle does not exhibit striations characteristic of skeletal and cardiac muscle. The actin filaments of smooth muscle are oriented mainly parallel or oblique to the long axis of the cell. Multiple actin filaments are joined at specialized locations in the cell called **dense bodies,** which contain α-actinin and are analogous to the filament-organizing Z lines of striated muscle. Dense bodies are found immediately beneath the cell membrane as well as within the interior of the myocyte. Thick filaments are interspersed among the thin filaments in smooth muscle and are far less abundant than in skeletal or cardiac muscle.

⊙ **9-14** In contrast to the mechanism in striated muscle, an entirely different mechanism controls cross-bridge turnover in smooth muscle (Fig. 9.14). The first step is the binding of four Ca^{2+} ions to **calmodulin (CaM).** Next, the Ca^{2+}-CaM complex activates the enzyme **MLCK,** which in turn phosphorylates the regulatory light chain that is associated with each neck of the dimeric myosin II heavy chain (see ⊙ **9-6**). Phosphorylation of the light chain causes a conformational change of the myosin head, which increases the angle between the head and neck domain of myosin

and also increases its ATPase activity, allowing it to interact efficiently with actin and act as a molecular motor. Thus, in smooth muscle, CaM rather than troponin C is the Ca^{2+}-binding protein responsible for transducing the contraction-triggering increases in $[Ca^{2+}]_i$. Note that in smooth muscle, contraction cannot begin until MLCK increases the ATPase activity of myosin.

Termination of smooth-muscle contraction requires dephosphorylation of myosin light chain

Because Ca^{2+} triggers smooth-muscle contraction by inducing phosphorylation of the myosin regulatory light chain rather than by simple binding to troponin C as in striated muscle, merely restoring $[Ca^{2+}]_i$ to its low resting value does not produce muscle relaxation. Rather, relaxation of smooth muscle requires dephosphorylation of the MLCs by **myosin light-chain phosphatase (MLCP).**

In smooth muscle, increases in both $[Ca^{2+}]_i$ and the Ca^{2+} sensitivity of the contractile apparatus enhance contractile force

Contractile force in smooth muscle largely depends on the relative balance between the phosphorylation and dephosphorylation of MLCs. The rate of MLC phosphorylation is regulated by the Ca^{2+}-CaM complex, which in turn depends on *levels of intracellular Ca^{2+}.* Smooth-muscle cells can regulate $[Ca^{2+}]_i$ over a wider range than skeletal and cardiac muscle for several reasons. First, smooth-muscle cells that do not generate action potentials—but rather exhibit graded V_m responses to neurotransmitters or hormones—are able to fine-tune Ca^{2+} influx via voltage-gated channels. Second, release of Ca^{2+} from intracellular stores may be modulated via neurotransmitter-induced generation of intracellular second messengers such as IP_3. This modulation allows finer control of Ca^{2+} release than occurs in the SR Ca^{2+}-release channel by L-type Ca^{2+} channels in skeletal and cardiac muscle.

A second level of control over contractile force occurs by regulation of the *Ca^{2+} sensitivity* of proteins that regulate contraction. For example, inhibiting MLCP alters the balance between phosphorylation and dephosphorylation, in effect allowing a greater contraction at a lower $[Ca^{2+}]_i$. Some neurotransmitters act by inhibiting the phosphatase, which appears to occur via activation of G protein–coupled receptors. Another mechanism for governing the Ca^{2+} sensitivity of proteins that regulate contraction is alteration of the Ca^{2+} sensitivity of the MLCK. Phosphorylation of MLCK by several protein kinases—including PKA, PKC, and CaMK—decreases the sensitivity of MLCK to activation by the Ca^{2+}-CaM complex.

DIVERSITY AMONG MUSCLES

As we have seen, each muscle type (skeletal, cardiac, and smooth) is distinguishable on the basis of its unique histological features, EC coupling mechanisms, and regulation of contractile function. However, even within each of the three categories, muscle in different locations must serve markedly different purposes, with different demands for strength, speed, and fatigability. This diversity is possible because of differences in the expression of specific isoforms of various contractile and regulatory proteins.

Skeletal muscle is composed of slow-twitch and fast-twitch fibers

Some skeletal muscles must be resistant to fatigue and be able to maintain tension for relatively long periods, although they need not contract rapidly. Examples are muscles that maintain body posture, such as the soleus muscle of the lower part of the leg. In contrast, some muscles need to contract rapidly, yet infrequently. Examples are the extraocular muscles, which must contract rapidly to redirect the eye as an object of visual interest moves about.

Individual muscle fibers are classified as *slow twitch (type I)* or *fast twitch (type II)*, depending on their rate of force development. These fiber types are also distinguished by their histological appearance and their ability to resist fatigue.

Slow-twitch fibers (Table 9.1) are generally thinner and have a denser capillary network surrounding them. These **type I** fibers also appear red because of a large amount of the oxygen-binding protein **myoglobin** (see ⊙ 29-2) within the cytoplasm. This rich capillary network together with myoglobin facilitates oxygen transport to the slow-twitch fibers, which mostly rely on oxidative metabolism for energy. The metabolic machinery of the slow-twitch fiber also favors oxidative metabolism because it has low glycogen content and glycolytic-enzyme activity but a rich mitochondrial and oxidative-enzyme content. Oxidative metabolism is slow but efficient, which makes these fibers resistant to fatigue.

Fast-twitch fibers differ among themselves with respect to fatigability. Some fast-twitch fibers are fatigue resistant **(type IIa)**; they rely on oxidative metabolism and are quite similar to slow-twitch fibers with respect to myoglobin content (indeed, they are red) and metabolic machinery. One important difference is that fast-twitch oxidative fibers contain abundant glycogen and have a greater number of mitochondria than slow-twitch fibers do. These features ensure adequate ATP generation to compensate for the increased rate of ATP hydrolysis in fast-twitch fibers.

Other fast-twitch fibers are not capable of sufficient oxidative metabolism to sustain contraction. Because these fibers must rely on the energy that is stored within glycogen (and phosphocreatine), they are more easily fatigable. Fatigable fast-twitch fibers **(type IIx/IIb)** have fewer mitochondria and lower concentrations of myoglobin and oxidative enzymes. Because of their low myoglobin content, type IIb muscle fibers appear white. They are, however, richer in glycolytic-enzyme activity than other fiber types are.

In reality, slow- and fast-twitch fibers represent the extremes of a continuum of muscle fiber characteristics. Moreover, each whole muscle is composed of fibers of each twitch type, with one twitch type predominating.

One particularly interesting feature of muscle differentiation is that fiber-type determination is not static. Through exercise training or changes in patterns of neuronal stimulation, alterations in contractile and regulatory protein isoform expression may occur. For example, it is possible for a greater proportion of fast-twitch fibers to develop in a specific muscle with repetitive training. It is even possible to induce cardiac-specific isoforms in skeletal muscle, given appropriate stimulation patterns.

Skeletal, cardiac, and smooth-muscle cells have characteristic differences in structure and function

A summary comparison among muscle types is presented in Table 9.2.

TABLE 9-1 Properties of Fast- and Slow-Twitch Muscle Fibers

	SLOW-TWITCH	FAST-TWITCH	FAST-TWITCH
Synonym	Type I	Type IIa	Type IIx/IIb
Fatigue	Resistant	Resistant	Fatigable
Color	Red (myoglobin)	Red (myoglobin)	White (low myoglobin)
Metabolism	Oxidative	Oxidative	Glycolytic
Mitochondria	High number	Higher	Fewer
Glycogen	Low	Abundant	High

TABLE 9-2 **Comparison of Properties Among Muscle Types**

	SKELETAL	CARDIAC	SMOOTH
Mechanism of excitation	Neuromuscular transmission (release of ACh, activating nicotinic ACh receptor)	Pacemaker depolarization, spread electrotonically via gap junctions	Synaptic transmission Agonist-activated receptors Electrical coupling Pacemaker potentials
Electrical activity of muscle cell	Action potential spikes	Action potential plateaus	Action potential spikes, plateaus Graded membrane potential changes Slow waves
Ca^{2+} sensor	Troponin C	Troponin C	CaM
EC coupling	L-type Ca^{2+} channel (Cav1.1, DHP receptor) in T-tubule membrane mechanically activates Ca^{2+}-release channel (RYR1) in SR membrane	Ca^{2+} entry via L-type Ca^{2+} channel (Cav1.2, DHP receptor) triggers Ca^{2+}-induced Ca^{2+} release (sparks) via RYR2 in SR membrane	Ca^{2+} entry via voltage-gated Ca^{2+} channel, Cav1.2 Ca^{2+}- or IP_3-mediated Ca^{2+} release via RYR3 or IP_3R1, IP_3R2, IP_3R3 in SR membrane
Terminator of contraction	Breakdown of ACh by acetylcholinesterase SR Ca^{2+} uptake	Action potential repolarization SR Ca^{2+} uptake	MLCP SR Ca^{2+} uptake
Twitch duration	20–200 ms	200–400 ms	200 ms—sustained
Regulation of force	Frequency and multifiber summation	Regulation of calcium entry	Balance between MLCK phosphorylation and dephosphorylation
Metabolism	Oxidative, glycolytic	Oxidative	Oxidative

THE NERVOUS SYSTEM

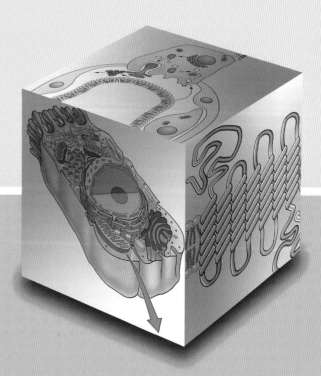

CHAPTER 10

ORGANIZATION OF THE NERVOUS SYSTEM

Bruce R. Ransom

The human brain is the most complex tissue in the body. It mediates behavior ranging from simple movements and sensory perception to learning, memory, and consciousness. It is the organ of the mind and accounts for the human capacity for invention, discovery, and language. Many of the brain's functions are poorly understood.

In this part of the book, we present the physiology of the nervous system in a manner that is intended to be complementary to texts on neurobiology and neuroanatomy. In this chapter, we review the basic cellular and gross anatomy of the nervous system. In Chapter 11, we discuss the fluid environment of the neurons in the brain, how this environment interacts with the rest of the extracellular fluid of the body, and the role of glial cells. Chapter 12 and Chapter 13 focus on the broad physiological principles that underlie how the brain's cellular elements operate. In Chapter 14, we discuss the autonomic nervous system, which controls viscera such as the heart, lungs, and gastrointestinal tract. Finally, in Chapter 15 and Chapter 16, we discuss the special senses and simple neuronal circuits.

The nervous system can be divided into central, peripheral, and autonomic nervous systems

All elements of the nervous system work closely together in a way that has no clear boundaries. Nevertheless, the traditional definitions of the subdivisions provide a useful framework.

The **central nervous system (CNS)** consists of the brain and spinal cord (Table 10.1). It is covered by three layers of "membranes"—the meninges. Within the CNS, some neurons are grouped into aggregations called **nuclei.** The CNS can also be divided into gray matter, which contains neuron cell bodies, and white matter, which is rich in myelin (see ◉ 7-11).

The **peripheral nervous system (PNS)** consists of those parts of the nervous system that lie outside the meninges (Table 10.1). These elements include sensory receptors for various kinds of stimuli, the peripheral portions of spinal and cranial nerves, and all the peripheral portions of the autonomic nervous system. The **sensory** nerves that carry messages from the periphery to the CNS are termed **afferent nerves.** Conversely, the peripheral **motor** nerves that carry messages from the CNS to peripheral tissues are called **efferent nerves.** **Peripheral ganglia** are groups of nerve cells concentrated into small knots or clumps that are located outside the CNS.

The **autonomic nervous system (ANS)** is that portion of the nervous system that regulates and controls visceral functions. The ANS is anatomically composed of parts of the CNS and PNS (Table 10.1). Visceral control is achieved by reflex arcs that consist of visceral afferent (i.e., sensory) neurons that send messages from the periphery to the CNS, control centers in the CNS that receive this input, and visceral motor output.

Each area of the nervous system has unique nerve cells and a different function

Nervous tissue is composed of neurons and neuroglial cells. **Neurons** vary greatly in their structure throughout the nervous system (see Chapter 12). Neuroglial cells, often simply called **glia,** are not primary signaling cells (see Chapter 11).

The human brain contains ~10^{11} neurons and slightly more glial cells. Each of these neurons may interact with thousands of other neurons.

Few, if any, of the receptors, ion channels, or cells in the human brain are unique to humans. The unparalleled capabilities of the human brain are presumed to result from its unique patterns of connectivity and its large size.

The brain's diverse functions are the result of tremendous regional specialization. Any compensation of neural function by a patient with a brain lesion (e.g., a stroke) reflects enhancement of existing circuits or recruitment of latent circuits. A corollary is that damage to a specific part of the brain causes predictable symptoms that enable a clinician to establish the anatomical location of the problem, a key step in diagnosis of neurological diseases.

CELLS OF THE NERVOUS SYSTEM

Nerve cells have four specialized regions: cell body, dendrites, axon, and presynaptic terminals

Neurons are specialized for sending and receiving signals, a purpose reflected in their unique shapes and physiological adaptations. The structure of a typical neuron can generally be divided into four distinct domains: (1) the cell body, also called the soma or perikaryon; (2) the dendrites; (3) the axon; and (4) the presynaptic terminals (Fig. 10.1). The shape and organelle composition of these domains depends strongly on their cytoskeleton, which consists of three fibrillary structures: neurofilaments (i.e., intermediate filaments), microtubules, and thin filaments (see Table 2.2). The cytoskeleton—especially the microtubules and thin filaments, is dynamic and imbues axons and dendrites with the capacity to change shape, a plasticity believed to participate in the synaptic alterations associated with learning and memory.

TABLE 10.1 Subdivisions of the Nervous System

SUBDIVISION	COMPONENTS	SPECIAL FEATURES
Central	Brain (including CN II and retina) and spinal cord	Oligodendrocytes provide myelin Axons cannot regenerate
Peripheral	Peripheral ganglia (including cell bodies); sensory receptors; peripheral portions of spinal and cranial nerves (except CN II), both afferent and efferent	Schwann cells provide myelin Axons can regenerate
Autonomic	Selected portions of the CNS and PNS	Functionally distinct system

CN, Cranial nerve.

Cell Body The cell body is the portion of the cell surrounding the nucleus. It contains much of the cell's complement of endoplasmic reticular membranes as well as the Golgi complex. The cell body is responsible for many of the neuronal housekeeping functions, including the synthesis and processing of proteins.

Dendrites These structures are tapering processes that arise from the cell body. Dendrites, and to a lesser extent the cell body, are the main areas for receiving information. Thus, their membranes are endowed with **receptors** that bind and respond to the neurotransmitters released by neighboring cells. The chemical message is translated by membrane receptors into an electrical or a biochemical event that influences the state of excitability or function of the receiving neuron.

Axon Perhaps the most remarkable feature of the neuron, the axon is a projection that arises from the cell body, like the dendrites. Its point of origin is a tapered region known as the **axon hillock.** Just distal to the cone-shaped hillock is an untapered, unmyelinated region known as the **initial segment.** This area is also called the spike initiation zone because it is where an action potential normally arises as the result of the electrical events that have occurred in the cell body and dendrites. In contrast to the dendrites, the axon is thin, does not taper, and can extend for more than a meter. Because of its length, the typical axon contains much more cytoplasm than does the cell body, up to 1000 times as much. The neuron uses special metabolic mechanisms to sustain this unique structural component. The cytoplasm of the axon, the axoplasm, is packed with parallel arrays of microtubules and neurofilaments that provide structural stability and a means to rapidly convey materials back and forth between the cell body and the axon terminus. Axons are self-reliant in energy metabolism, taking up glucose and oxygen from their immediate environment to produce ATP. Specialized glial cells called oligodendrocytes contribute in complex ways to axon integrity (see ⊙ 11-8).

Axons are the message-sending portion of the neuron. The axon carries the neuron's signal, the action potential, to a specific target, such as another neuron or a muscle. Some axons have a special electrical insulation, called **myelin,** that consists of the coiled cell membranes of glial cells that wrap themselves around the nerve axon (see ⊙ 11-8).

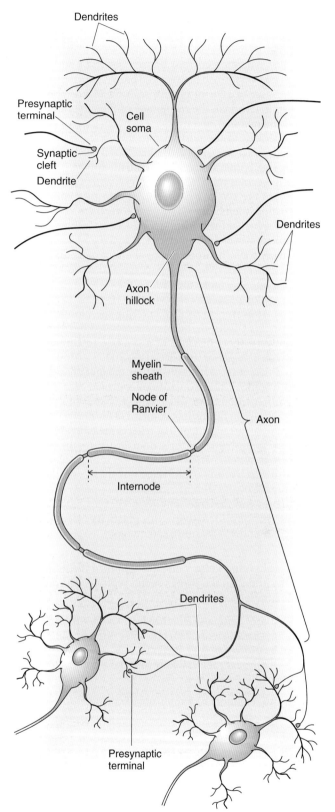

Figure 10.1 Morphology of a typical neuron.

Presynaptic Terminals   At its target, the axon terminates in multiple endings—the presynaptic terminals. When the action potential reaches the presynaptic terminal, it causes the release of chemical signaling molecules in a complex process called synaptic transmission (see Chapter 8 and 13).

The junction formed between the presynaptic terminal and its target is called a chemical synapse. A synapse comprises the presynaptic terminal, the membrane of the target cell (postsynaptic membrane), and the space between the two (synaptic cleft). The area of the postsynaptic membrane is frequently amplified to increase the surface that is available for receptors, often by small projections called **dendritic spines.**

The molecules released by the presynaptic terminals diffuse across the synaptic cleft and bind to receptors on the postsynaptic membrane. The receptors then convert the chemical signal of the transmitter molecules—either directly or indirectly—back into an electrical signal.

In many ways, neurons can be thought of as highly specialized *endocrine cells.* They package and store hormones and hormone-like molecules, which they release rapidly into the extracellular space by exocytosis in response to an action potential. However, instead of entering the bloodstream to exert *systemic* effects, the substances secreted by neurons act over the very short distance of a synapse to communicate *locally* with a neighboring cell (see ◉ 3-1).

In a different sense, neurons can be thought of as *polarized cells* with some of the properties of epithelial cells. Like epithelial cells, neurons have different populations of membrane proteins at each of the distinct domains of the neuronal plasma membrane, an arrangement that reflects the individual physiological responsibilities of these domains. Thus, the design of the nervous system permits information transfer across synapses in a selective and coordinated way that serves the needs of the organism and summates to produce complex behavior.

Synapses can undergo long-term changes based on certain patterns of prior activity. This **plasticity** (see ◉ 13-8) is believed to underlie learning and memory.

The cytoskeleton helps compartmentalize the neuron and also provides the tracks along which material travels between different parts of the neuron

Neurons are compartmentalized in both structure and function. *Dendrites* are tapered, have limited length, and contain neurotransmitter receptor proteins in their membranes. *Axons* can be very long and have a high density of

Na^+ channels. *Dendrites* and the *cell body* contain messenger RNA, ribosomes, and a Golgi apparatus.

How does this compartmentalization come about? The molecular orientation of **microtubules** (see Table 2.2) together with **microtubule-associated proteins (MAPs)** play important roles in dictating the vectorial transport of organelles and proteins. **Tau proteins** are confined to axons; their suppression in cultured neurons prevents formation of the axon without altering formation of the dendrites. Hyperphosphorylated tau proteins can assemble into pathological aggregates called neurofibrillary tangles, which are a hallmark of **Alzheimer disease.**

The polarization of microtubules helps to create remarkable morphological and functional divisions in neurons. In axons, microtubules assemble with their plus ends pointed away from the cell body; this orientation polarizes the flow of material into and out of the axon. The cytoskeletal "order" provided by the microtubules and the MAPs helps define what should or should not be in the axonal cytoplasm. In dendrites, microtubules do not have a consistent orientation.

The neuron cell body is the main manufacturing site for the membrane proteins and membranous organelles that are necessary for the structural integrity and function of its processes. Axons have little or no intrinsic protein synthetic ability, whereas dendrites have some free ribosomes and are able to engage in limited protein production. The transport of proteins from the cell body all the way to the end of long axons is a challenging task. The neuron also has a second task: moving various material in the opposite direction, from presynaptic terminals at the end of the axon to the cell body. The neuron solves these problems by using two distinct mechanisms for moving material to the presynaptic terminals in an "anterograde" direction and a third mechanism for transport in the opposite or "retrograde" direction (Table 10.2).

Fast Axoplasmic Transport   If the flow of materials from the soma to the distant axon terminus were left to diffusion, it could take months for needed proteins to diffuse to the end of an axon. To overcome this difficulty, neurons exploit a rapid, Pony Express–style system of conveyance known as **fast axoplasmic transport** (Table 10.2). Membranous organelles, including vesicles and mitochondria, are the principal freight of fast axoplasmic transport. The proteins (some associated with RNA), lipids, and polysaccharides that move at fast rates in axons do so because they have caught a ride with a membranous organelle (i.e., they are sequestered inside the organelle or bound to or inserted into the organellar membrane). The

TABLE 10.2 Features of Axoplasmic Transport

TRANSPORT TYPE	SPEED (mm/DAY)	MECHANISM	MATERIAL TRANSPORTED
Fast anterograde	~400	Saltatory movement along microtubules via the motor molecule kinesin (ATP dependent)	Mitochondria Vesicles containing peptides and other neurotransmitters, some degradative enzymes
Fast retrograde	~200–300	Saltatory movement along microtubules via the motor molecule MAP-1C (brain dynein, ATP dependent)	Degraded vesicular membrane Absorbed exogenous material (toxins, viruses, growth factors)
Slow (anterograde only)	0.2–8	Not clear; requires intact microtubules (ATP dependent)	Cytoskeletal elements (e.g., neurofilament and microtubule subunits) Soluble proteins of intermediary metabolism Actin

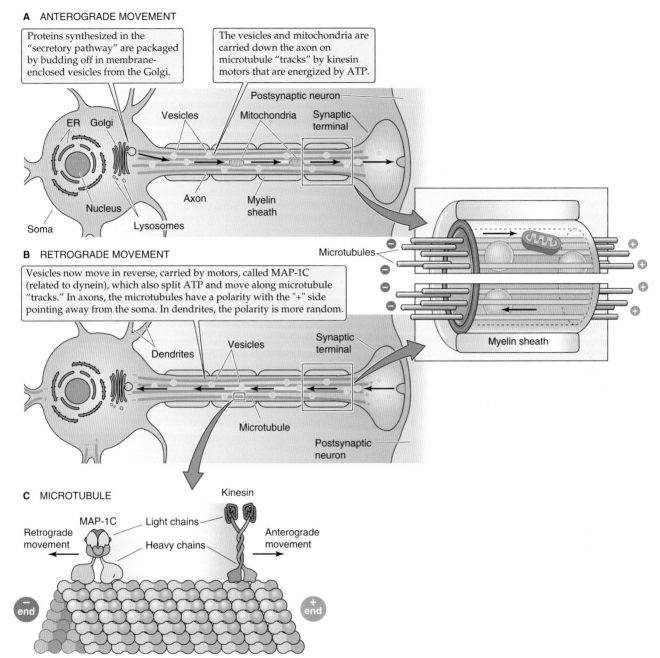

A ANTEROGRADE MOVEMENT

Proteins synthesized in the "secretory pathway" are packaged by budding off in membrane-enclosed vesicles from the Golgi.

The vesicles and mitochondria are carried down the axon on microtubule "tracks" by kinesin motors that are energized by ATP.

Postsynaptic neuron

ER Golgi Vesicles Mitochondria Synaptic terminal

Nucleus Axon Myelin sheath

Soma Lysosomes

Microtubules

B RETROGRADE MOVEMENT

Vesicles now move in reverse, carried by motors, called MAP-1C (related to dynein), which also split ATP and move along microtubule "tracks." In axons, the microtubules have a polarity with the "+" side pointing away from the soma. In dendrites, the polarity is more random.

Dendrites Vesicles Synaptic terminal

Microtubule

Myelin sheath

Postsynaptic neuron

C MICROTUBULE

Kinesin

MAP-1C Light chains

Retrograde movement Heavy chains Anterograde movement

− end + end

Figure 10.2 Fast axoplasmic transport. *ER*, Endoplasmic reticulum.

peptide and protein contents of dense-core secretory granules, which are found in the presynaptic axonal terminals, are synthesized as standard secretory proteins and are shipped to the axon in the lumens of Golgi-derived carrier vesicles.

Organelles and vesicles, and their macromolecule payloads, move along **microtubules** with the help of a microtubule-dependent motor protein called **kinesin** (Fig. 10.2A). The kinesin motor is an ATPase that produces vectorial movement of its payload along the microtubule. This system can move vesicles down the axon at rates of up to 400 mm/day; variations in cargo speed simply reflect more frequent pauses during the journey. Kinesins always move toward the plus end of microtubules (i.e., away from the cell body), and transport function is lost if the microtubules are disrupted.

Fast Retrograde Transport Axons move material back toward the cell body via a different ATPase motor protein called **brain dynein** or **MAP-1C** (Fig. 10.2B). MAP-1C moves along microtubules in the opposite direction to kinesin (Fig. 10.2C), at a slightly slower pace. Retrograde transport provides a mechanism for target-derived growth factors, like nerve growth factor, to reach the nucleus of a neuron where they can influence survival. How this signal is transmitted up the axon has been a persistent question. It may be endocytosed at the axon's terminal and transported to the cell body in a "signaling endosome." The loss of ATP production in axons, as occurs with blockade of oxidative metabolism, causes fast axonal transport in both the antero-grade and retrograde directions to fail.

Slow Axoplasmic Transport Axons also have a need for hundreds of other proteins, including cytoskeletal proteins and soluble proteins that are used as enzymes for intermediary metabolism. These proteins are delivered by a slow anterograde axoplasmic transport mechanism that moves material at a mere 0.2 to 8 mm/day, the nervous system's equivalent of snail mail. The slowest-moving proteins are neurofilament and microtubule subunits (0.2 to 1 mm/day). The mechanism of slow axoplasmic transport is not well understood, but molecular motors operating on microtubule tracks appear to be involved. In fact, the difference between slow and fast axonal transport may primarily be the number of transport *interruptions* during the long axonal journey.

Neurons can be classified on the basis of their axonal projection, their dendritic geometry, and the number of processes emanating from the cell body

The trillions of nerve cells in the CNS have great structural diversity. Typically, neurons are classified on the basis of where their axons go (i.e., where they "project"), the geometry of their dendrites, and the number of processes that emanate from the cell body (Fig. 10.3), properties with functional implications.

Axonal Projection Neurons with long axons that connect with other parts of the nervous system are called **projection neurons.** Each of these cells has a clearly defined axon, which can be 1 m long. All the other processes that a projection neuron has are dendrites. In contrast, **interneurons** have processes confined to one region of the brain. Some of these cells have very short axons, whereas others seem to lack a conventional axon altogether and may be referred to as *anaxonal.*

Dendritic Geometry A roughly pyramid-shaped set of dendritic branches characterizes **pyramidal cells,** whereas a radial pattern of dendritic branches defines **stellate cells.** All pyramidal cells appear to have dendritic spines, but stellate cells may have them (spiny) or may not (aspiny).

Number of Processes ⊙ **10-1** Neurons can also be classified by the number of processes that extend from their cell bodies. The dorsal root ganglion cell is the classic **unipolar** neuron. The process that extends into the CNS from this unipolar neuron is easily recognized as an axon because it carries information *away* from the cell body. The process that extends to sensory receptors in the skin and elsewhere is a typical axon in the sense that it can conduct an action potential, has myelin, and is characterized by an axonal cytoskeleton. However, it conveys information *toward* the cell body. **Bipolar** neurons, such as the retinal bipolar cell, have two processes extending from opposite sides of the cell body. Most neurons in the brain are **multipolar.** Cells with many dendritic processes are designed to receive large numbers of synaptic inputs.

Glial cells provide a physiological environment for neurons Glial cells lack axons, action potentials, and synaptic potentials. They are more numerous than neurons and are diverse in structure and function. The main types of CNS glial cells are oligodendrocytes, astrocytes, and microglial cells. In the PNS, the main types of glial cells are satellite cells in autonomic and sensory ganglia, Schwann cells, and enteric glial cells. Glial function is discussed in Chapter 11. Oligodendrocytes form the myelin sheaths of CNS axons, and Schwann cells myelinate peripheral nerves. Glial cells are involved in nearly every function of the brain and are far more than simply "nerve glue."

Glia fills in almost all the space around neurons, with a narrow extracellular space left between neurons and glial cells that has an average width of only ~0.02 μm. Glial cells have a major impact on the composition of the extracellular fluid, which in turn has a major impact on brain function, as we will see in Chapter 11.

Neurons do not regenerate

Neurons Most human neurons arise in about the first 4 months of intrauterine life. After birth, neurons do not divide, and if a neuron is lost for any reason, it is generally not replaced, which is the main reason for the relatively limited recovery from serious brain and spinal cord injuries. It has been argued that this lack of regenerative ability is a design principle to ensure that learned behavior and memories are preserved in stable populations of neurons throughout life. A notable exception to this rule is olfactory bulb neurons, which are continually renewed throughout adult life by a population of stem cells or neuronal progenitor cells. Learning how to make functional new CNS neurons after severe neural injury is the holy grail of regeneration research.

Axons Another reason that relatively little recovery follows severe brain and spinal cord injury is that axons within the CNS do not regenerate effectively. This lack of axon regeneration in the CNS is in sharp contrast to the behavior of axons in the PNS, which can regrow and reconnect to appropriate end organs, either muscle or sensory receptors. For example, if the median nerve of the forearm is crushed by blunt trauma, the distal axon segments die off in a process called wallerian degeneration because the sustaining relationship with their proximal cell bodies is lost. These PNS axons can slowly regenerate and connect to muscles and sensory receptors in the hand. It is believed that the inability of CNS axons to regenerate is the fault of the local environment more than it is an intrinsic property of these axons. The remarkable ability of damaged peripheral nerves to regenerate has encouraged hope that CNS axons might, under the right conditions, be able to perform this same feat. It would mean that victims of spinal cord injury might walk again.

Glia Unlike neurons, glial cells can be replaced from progenitor cells if they are lost or injured in an adult. The most typical reaction of mammalian brains to a wide range of injuries is the formation of an **astrocytic glial scar.** This scar is produced primarily by an enlargement of individual astrocytes (*hypertrophy*). Only a small degree of astrocytic *proliferation* (i.e., an increase in cell number) accompanies this reaction. **Microglial cells,** which derive from cells related to the monocyte-macrophage lineage in blood, also react strongly to brain injury and are the main cells that proliferate at the injury site.

SUBDIVISIONS OF THE NERVOUS SYSTEM

This section provides an overview of nervous system anatomy. We in turn consider the CNS, PNS, and ANS (Table 10.1).

Fig. 10.4A shows the directional terms used to describe brain structures.

Basis for classification	Example	Functional implication	Structure
1. Axonal projection			
Goes to a distant brain area	Projection neuron or Principal neuron or Golgi type I cell (cortical motor neuron)	Affects different brain areas	Dorsal root ganglion cell 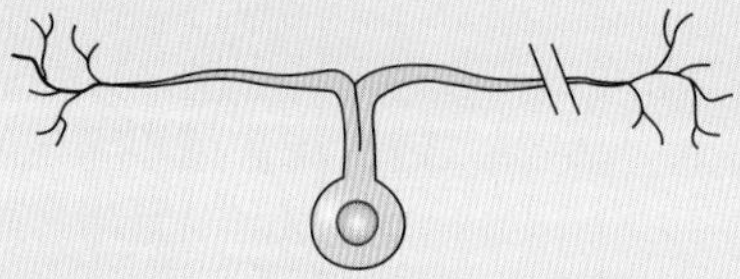
Stays in a local brain area	Intrinsic neuron or Interneuron or Golgi type II cell (cortical inhibitory neuron)	Affects only nearby neurons	Retinal bipolar cell 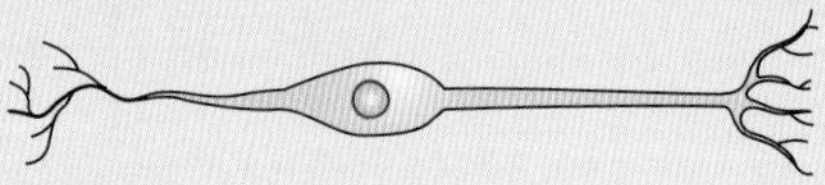
2. Dendritic pattern			
Pyramid-shaped spread of dendrites	Pyramidal cell (hippocampal pyramidal neuron)	Large area for receiving synaptic input; determines the pattern of incoming axons that can interact with the cell (i.e., pyramid-shaped)	Pyramidal cell 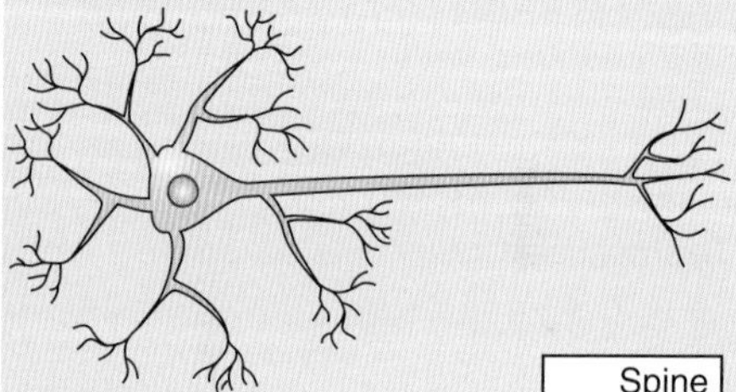
Radial-shaped spread of dendrites	Stellate cell (cortical stellate cell)	Large area for receiving synaptic input; determines pattern of incoming axons that can interact with the cell (i.e., star-shaped)	Stellate cell 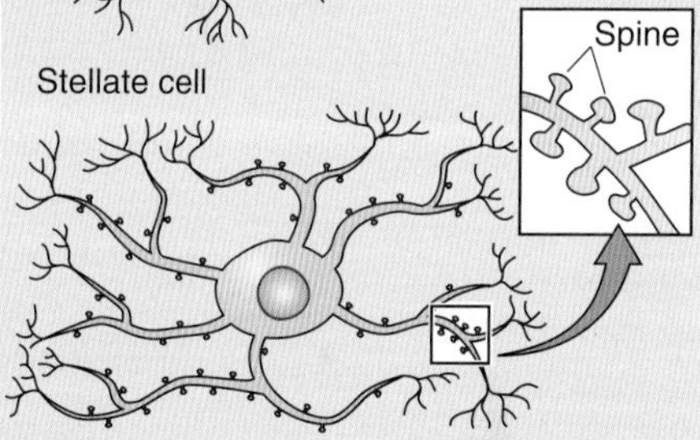 — Spine
3. Number of processes			
One process exits the cell body	Unipolar neuron (dorsal root ganglion cell)	Small area for receiving synaptic input; highly specialized function	Unipolar 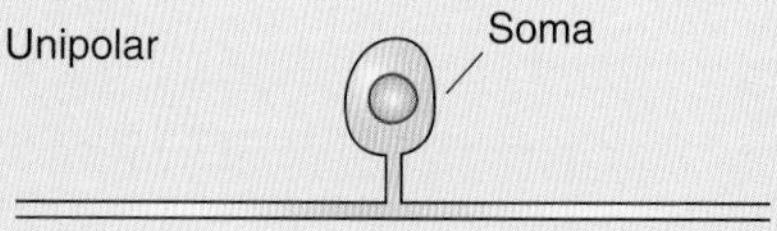 — Soma
Two processes exit the cell body	Bipolar neuron (retinal bipolar cell)	Small area for receiving synaptic input; highly specialized function	Bipolar 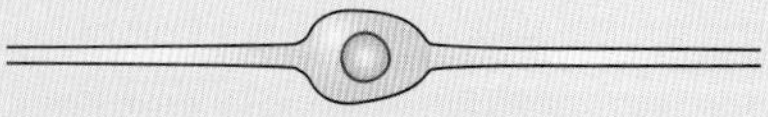
Many processes exit the cell body	Multipolar neuron (spinal motor neuron)	Large area for receiving synaptic input; determines the pattern of incoming axons that can interact with the cell	Multipolar 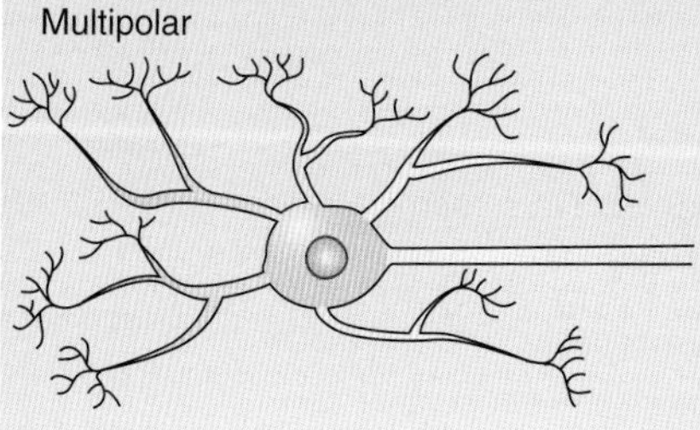

Figure 10.3 Classification of neurons based on their structure.

A AXES OF THE CNS

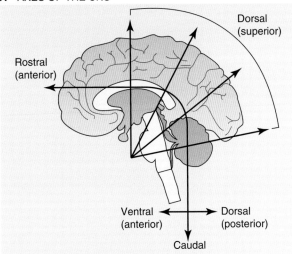

B MAJOR COMPONENTS OF THE CNS

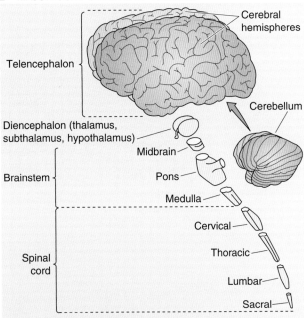

C SURFACE ANATOMY OF THE CEREBRAL CORTEX

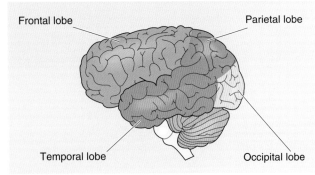

Figure 10.4 Gross anatomy of the CNS.

The CNS consists of the telencephalon, cerebellum, diencephalon, midbrain, pons, medulla, and spinal cord

The CNS can be conveniently divided into five major areas: (1) telencephalon, (2) cerebellum, (3) diencephalon, (4) brainstem (consisting of the midbrain, pons, and medulla), and (5) spinal cord (Fig. 10.4B). Each of these areas has symmetrical right and left sides.

Telencephalon One of the crowning glories of evolution is the human **cerebral cortex,** the most conspicuous part of the paired cerebral hemispheres. The human cerebral cortex has a surface area of ~2200 cm² and is estimated to contain 1.5 to 2×10^{10} neurons. The number of synaptic contacts between these cells is $\sim 3 \times 10^{14}$. The cortical surface area of mammals increases massively from mouse to monkey to humans in a ratio of 1:100:1000. The capacity for information processing by this neural machine includes a remarkable range of functions: thinking, learning, memory, and consciousness.

The cortex is topographically organized in two ways. First, certain areas of the cortex mediate specific functions. For example, the area that mediates motor control is a well-defined strip of cortex located in the frontal lobe (Fig. 10.4C). Second, within a portion of cortex that manages a specific function (e.g., motor control, somatic sensation, hearing, or vision), the parts of the body spatially map onto this cortex in an orderly way. We discuss this principle of **somatotopy** in Chapter 16 (see ⊙ 16-4).

⊙ **10-2** Another part of the telencephalon is the great mass of axons that stream into and out of the cerebral cortex and connect it with other regions. The **corpus callosum** and smaller white matter tracts interconnect the two cerebral hemispheres. The final parts of the telencephalon are the **basal ganglia,** a functionally related group of neuron clusters consisting of the striatum (caudate nucleus and putamen), globus pallidus, amygdala, and hippocampal formation. These are all paired structures. The basal ganglia have indirect connections with motor portions of the cerebral cortex and are involved in motor control. The **amygdala** participates in the expression of emotion, and the **hippocampal formation** is crucial in the formation of new memories. Indeed, injury to both hippocampal formations can cause a severe amnestic disorder.

Cerebellum This brain region lies immediately dorsal to the brainstem. Although the cerebellum represents only ~10% of the CNS by volume, it contains ~50% of all CNS neurons. The exceedingly large number of input connections to the cerebellum conveys information from nearly every type of receptor in the nervous system, including visual and auditory input. Combined, these afferent fibers outnumber the efferent projections by an estimated ratio of 40:1.

Diencephalon This brain region consists of the thalamus, the subthalamus, and the hypothalamus. The **thalamus** is the main integrating station for sensory information that is bound for the cerebral cortex, where it will reach the level of conscious perception. Along with the **subthalamus,** the thalamus receives projections from the basal ganglia that are important for motor function. Input to the thalamus from the cerebellum is important for normal motor control. Patients with **Parkinson disease,** a severe movement disorder, gradually lose the ability to make voluntary movements; in some of these patients, it is possible to improve movement by stimulating certain areas of the subthalamus.

The **hypothalamus** is the CNS structure that most affects the ANS. It acts through strong, direct connections with autonomic nuclei in the brainstem and spinal cord. It also acts as part of the endocrine system in two major ways. First, specialized neurons in the hypothalamus synthesize hormones and transport them down their axons to the posterior pituitary gland, where the hormones are secreted into the blood. Second, other specialized neurons in other nuclei synthesize "releasing hormones" and release them into a plexus of veins, called a portal system, that carries the releasing hormones to cells in the anterior pituitary. There, the releasing hormones stimulate cells to secrete hormones into the bloodstream. We discuss these principles in Chapter 47 (see ◉ 47-1). The hypothalamus also has specialized centers that play important roles in controlling body temperature (see ◉ 59-9), hunger (see ◉ 48-10), thirst (see ◉ 40-10), and the cardiovascular system. It is the main control center of the ANS.

Brainstem (Midbrain, Pons, and Medulla) The brainstem lies immediately above, or rostral to, the spinal cord. Like the spinal cord, the midbrain, pons, and medulla have a segmental organization, receive sensory (afferent) information, and send out motor (efferent) signals through paired nerves that are called **cranial nerves.** The midbrain, pons, and medulla also contain important control centers for the ANS (see Chapter 14). Not only are motor neurons, autonomic neurons, and sensory neurons present at each level, but the caudal brainstem serves as a conduit for a large volume of axons traveling from higher CNS centers to the spinal cord (descending pathways) and vice versa (ascending pathways). Additionally, this portion of the brainstem contains a loosely organized interconnected collection of neurons and fibers called the **reticular formation.** This neuronal network has diffuse connections with the cortex and other brain regions and affects the level of consciousness or arousal.

The **midbrain** has somatic motor neurons that control eye movement. These neurons reside in the nuclei for cranial nerve III (CN III) and CN IV. Other midbrain neurons are part of a system, along with the cerebellum and cortex, for motor control. The midbrain also contains groups of neurons that are involved in relaying signals related to hearing and vision.

Just caudal to the midbrain is the **pons,** which contains the somatic motor neurons that control mastication (nucleus for CN V), eye movement (nucleus for CN VI), and facial muscles (nucleus for CN VII). The pons also receives somatic sensory information from the face, scalp, mouth, and nose (portion of the nucleus for CN V). It is also involved in processing information that is related to hearing and equilibrium (nucleus for CN VIII). Neurons in the ventral pons receive input from the cortex, and these neurons in turn form a massive direct connection with the cerebellum (see above) that is crucial for coordinating motor movements.

The most caudal portion of the brainstem is the **medulla.** The organization of the medulla is most similar to that of the spinal cord. The medulla contains somatic motor neurons that innervate the muscles of the neck (nucleus of CN XI) and tongue (nucleus of CN XII). Along with the pons, the medulla is involved in controlling blood pressure, heart rate, respiration, and digestion (nuclei of CN IX and X). The medulla is the first CNS way station for information traveling from the special senses of hearing and equilibrium.

Spinal Cord Continuous with the caudal portion of the medulla is the spinal cord. The spinal cord runs from the base of the skull to the end of the body of the first lumbar vertebra (L1).

The spinal cord consists of 31 segments that each have a motor and sensory nerve root. These nerve roots combine to form 31 bilaterally symmetrical pairs of spinal nerves. The spinal roots, nerves, and ganglia are part of the PNS.

Sensory information from the skin, muscle, and visceral organs enters the spinal cord through fascicles of axons called dorsal roots (Fig. 10.5A). Dorsal root axons have their cell bodies of origin in the spinal ganglia (i.e., **dorsal root ganglia**) associated with that spinal segment.

Ventral roots contain strictly efferent fibers (Fig. 10.5B). Most of the efferent fibers are somatic efferents that innervate skeletal muscle to mediate voluntary movement. The other fibers are visceral efferents that synapse with postganglionic autonomic neurons, which in turn innervate visceral smooth muscle or glandular tissue.

If sensory fibers enter the spinal cord and synapse directly on motor neurons in that same segment, this connection underlies a simple **segmental reflex** or interaction. If the incoming fibers synapse with neurons in other spinal segments, they can participate in an **intersegmental reflex** or interaction. Finally, if the incoming signals travel rostrally to the brainstem before they synapse, they constitute a **suprasegmental interaction.**

The PNS comprises the cranial and spinal nerves, their associated sensory ganglia, and various sensory receptors

The PNS serves four main purposes: (1) it transduces stimuli both from the external environment and from within the body into sensory information through receptors; (2) it conveys sensory information to the CNS along axon pathways; (3) it conveys motor signals from the CNS along axon pathways to target organs, primarily skeletal and smooth muscle; and (4) it converts the motor signals to chemical signals at synapses on target tissues in the periphery. Fig. 10.5B summarizes these four functions for a simple reflex arc in which a painful stimulus to the foot results in retraction of the foot from the source of the pain.

Like the CNS, the PNS can be divided into *somatic* and *autonomic* parts. The somatic division includes the sensory neurons and axons that innervate the skin, joints, and muscle as well as the motor axons that innervate skeletal muscle. The somatic division of the PNS primarily deals with the body's *external environment,* either to gather information about this environment or to interact with it through voluntary motor behavior. The autonomic portion of the PNS consists of the motor axons that innervate smooth muscle, the exocrine glands, and other viscera. This division mainly deals with the body's *internal environment.*

Axons in the PNS are organized into bundles called **peripheral nerves** (Fig. 10.6). These nerves contain, in a large nerve such as the sciatic nerve, tens of thousands of axons. Axons range in diameter from <1 to 20 μm. Because axons are extremely fragile, adaptations that enhance

A   SPINAL CORD AND NERVE ROOTS

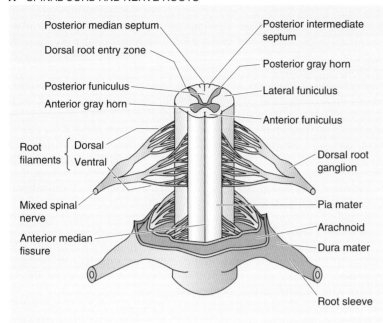

B   A SPINAL REFLEX ARC

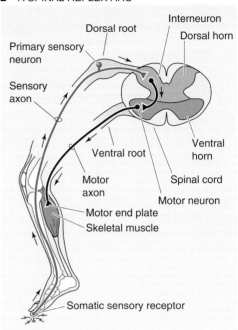

Figure 10.5   Spinal cord. (A) Each spinal segment has dorsal and ventral nerve roots that carry sensory and motor nerve fibers, respectively. (B) The simple "flexor" reflex arc is an illustration of the four functions of the PNS: (1) a receptor transduces a painful stimulus into an action potential, (2) a primary sensory neuron conveys the information to the CNS, (3) the CNS conveys information to the target organ via a motor neuron, and (4) the electrical signals are converted to signals at the motor end plate.

mechanical stability are very important. Nervous tissue in the PNS is designed to be much tougher, physically, than that in the CNS. The PNS must be mechanically flexible, tolerant of minor physical trauma, and sustainable by a blood supply that is less dependable than the one providing for the CNS. A spinal cord transplanted to the lower part of the leg would not survive the running of a 100-m dash.

Axons in peripheral nerves are closely associated with Schwann cells. In the case of a myelinated axon, a Schwann cell forms a myelinated wrap around a single adjacent axon, a single internodal myelin segment between 250 and 1000 μm in length. Many such internodal myelin segments, and thus many Schwann cells, are necessary to myelinate the entire length of the axon. In an unmyelinated nerve, the Schwann cell surrounds but does not wrap multiple times around axons. Unmyelinated axons outnumber myelinated axons by about 2:1 in typical human nerves. Diseases that affect the PNS can disrupt nerve function by causing either loss of myelin or axonal injury.

The functional organization of a peripheral nerve is best illustrated by a typical thoracic spinal nerve and its branches. Every spinal nerve is formed by the dorsal and ventral roots joining together and emerging from the spinal cord at that segmental level (Fig. 10.5A). The dorsal roots coalesce and display a spindle-shaped swelling called the spinal or dorsal root ganglion, which contains the cell bodies of the sensory axons in the dorsal roots. Individual neurons called dorsal root ganglion cells are unipolar neurons with a single process that bifurcates in a T-like manner into a peripheral and central branch (Fig. 10.3). The central branch carries sensory information into the CNS and the peripheral branch terminates as a sensory ending.

Spinal nerves divide into several branches that distribute motor and sensory axons to the parts of the body associated with that segment. Axons conveying autonomic motor or autonomic sensory signals also travel in these branches. These branches are said to be "mixed" because they contain both efferent and afferent axons.

The ANS innervates effectors that are not under voluntary control

The nervous system regulates some physiological mechanisms in a way that is independent or *autonomous* of voluntary control. Control of body temperature is an example of a fundamental process that most individuals cannot consciously regulate. Other examples include blood pressure and heart rate. The absence of voluntary control means that the ANS has little cortical representation.

The ANS has three divisions: sympathetic, parasympathetic, and enteric. The sympathetic and parasympathetic divisions have both CNS and PNS parts. The enteric division lies entirely within the PNS. The **parasympathetic** and **sympathetic** efferent systems are composed of two-neuron pathways. The cell body of the first neuron is located in the CNS and that of the second in the PNS. The sympathetic and parasympathetic divisions innervate most visceral organs and have a yin-yang functional relationship. The **enteric** division regulates the rhythmic contraction of intestinal smooth muscle and also regulates the secretory functions of intestinal epithelial cells. It receives afferent input from the gut wall and is subject to modulation by the two other divisions of the ANS.

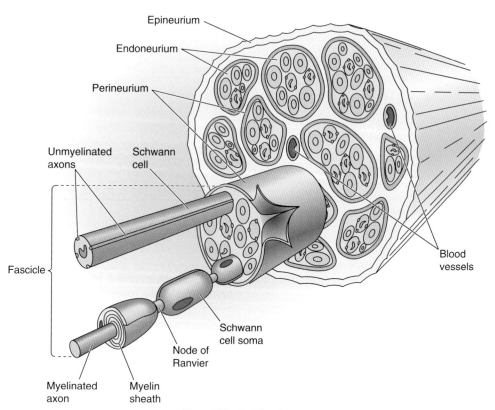

Figure 10.6   Peripheral nerve.

CHAPTER 11

THE NEURONAL MICROENVIRONMENT

Bruce R. Ransom

Extracellular fluid in the brain provides a highly regulated environment for central nervous system neurons

Everything that surrounds individual neurons can be considered part of the **neuronal microenvironment:** the extracellular fluid (ECF), capillaries, glial cells, and adjacent neurons. How the microenvironment interacts with neurons and how the brain stabilizes it to provide constancy for neuronal function are the subjects of this discussion.

The concentrations of solutes in **brain extracellular fluid (BECF)** fluctuate with neural activity, and conversely, changes in ECF composition can influence nerve cell behavior. The brain carefully controls the composition of this important compartment in three major ways. First, the brain uses the **blood-brain barrier (BBB)** to protect the BECF from fluctuations in blood composition. Second, the **cerebrospinal fluid (CSF),** produced by choroid plexus epithelial cells, strongly influences the composition of the BECF. Third, the surrounding glial cells "condition" the BECF.

The brain is physically and metabolically fragile

The ratio of brain weight to body weight in humans is the highest in the animal kingdom. The average adult brain weight is ~1400 g—approximately the same weight as the liver. This large and vital structure, which has the consistency of thick pudding, is protected from mechanical injury by a surrounding layer of bone and by the CSF in which it floats.

The brain is also *metabolically* fragile. This fragility arises from its high rate of energy consumption, absence of significant stored fuel in the form of glycogen (~5% of the amount in the liver), and rapid development of cellular damage when ATP is depleted. The brain is not the greediest of the body's organs; both the heart and kidney cortex have higher metabolic rates. Nevertheless, although it constitutes only 2% of the body by weight, the brain receives ~15% of resting blood flow. More than half of the energy consumed by the brain is directed to maintain ion gradients, primarily through operation of the Na-K pump (see ⊙ 5-6). An interruption of the continuous supply of oxygen or glucose to the brain results in rapid depletion of energy stores and disruption of ion gradients. Because of falling ATP levels in the brain, consciousness is lost within 10 seconds of a blockade in cerebral blood flow. Irreversible nerve cell injury can occur after only 5 to 10 minutes of interrupted blood flow.

CEREBROSPINAL FLUID

CSF is a colorless, watery liquid. It fills the ventricles of the brain and forms a thin layer around the outside of the brain and spinal cord in the subarachnoid space. CSF is secreted within the brain by a highly vascularized epithelial structure called the **choroid plexus** and circulates to sites in the subarachnoid space, where it enters the venous blood system. The composition of CSF is highly regulated, and because it directly mixes with BECF, it helps regulate the composition of BECF. The choroid plexus can be thought of as the brain's "kidney" in that it stabilizes the composition of CSF, just as the kidney stabilizes the composition of blood plasma.

CSF fills the ventricles and subarachnoid space

⊙ 11-1 The **ventricles** of the brain are four small compartments located within the brain (Fig. 11.1A). Each ventricle contains a choroid plexus and is filled with CSF. The ventricles are linked together by channels, or foramina, that allow CSF to move easily between them. The fourth ventricle is continuous with the central canal of the spinal cord. CSF escapes from the fourth ventricle and flows into the subarachnoid space through foramina. We shall see below how CSF circulates throughout the subarachnoid space of the brain and spinal cord, and how it moves through brain tissue itself.

The brain and spinal cord are covered by three membranous tissue layers called the **meninges.** The innermost of these three layers is the pia mater; the middle is the arachnoid mater; and the outermost layer is the dura mater (Fig. 11.1B). Between the arachnoid mater and pia mater is the **subarachnoid space,** which is filled with CSF that flows from the fourth ventricle. The CSF in the subarachnoid space completely surrounds the brain and spinal cord. In adults, the subarachnoid space and the ventricles with which they are continuous contain ~150 mL of CSF, 30 mL in the ventricles and 120 mL in the subarachnoid spaces of the brain and spinal cord.

The **pia mater** is a thin layer of connective tissue cells that is very closely applied to the surface of the brain and covers blood vessels as they plunge through the arachnoid into the brain. A nearly complete layer of astrocytic endfeet (see ⊙ 11-5)—the **glia limitans**—abuts the pia from the brain side and is separated from the pia by a basement membrane.

A VENTRICLES OF THE BRAIN

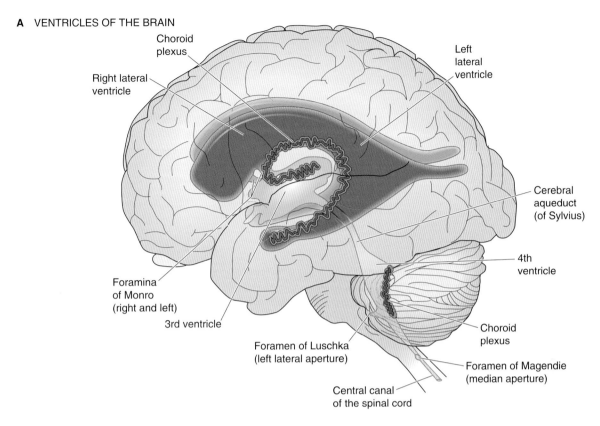

B CSF CIRCULATION

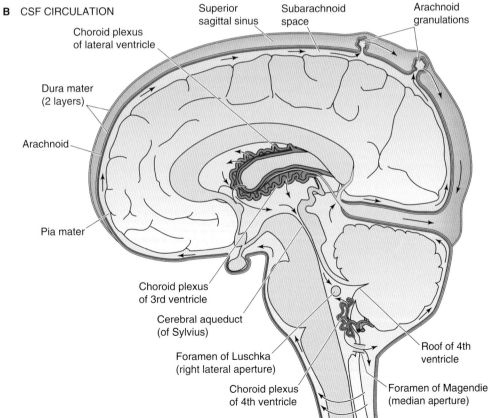

Figure 11.1 The brain ventricles and the CSF. (A) This is a transparent view, looking from the left side of the brain. The two lateral ventricles communicate with the third ventricle, which in turn communicates with the fourth ventricle. (B) Each ventricle contains a choroid plexus, which secretes CSF. The CSF escapes from the fourth ventricle and into the subarachnoid space through foramina.

The **arachnoid mater** is composed of layers of cells, resembling those that make up the pia, linked together by *tight junctions.* The arachnoid isolates the CSF in the subarachnoid space from blood in the overlying vessels of the dura mater. Arachnoid cells can phagocytose foreign material in the subarachnoid space.

The **dura mater** forms an outer protective envelope around the brain. Blood vessels between the endosteal and meningeal layer of the dura mater are outside the BBB, and the blood-CSF barrier created by the arachnoid prevents diffusion from dural capillaries to the CSF.

The brain floats in CSF, which acts as a shock absorber

An important function of CSF is to buffer the brain from mechanical injury. The CSF that surrounds the brain reduces the effective weight of the brain from ~1400 g to <50 g. This buoyancy is a consequence of the difference in the specific gravities of brain tissue (1.040) and CSF (1.007). The mechanical buffering that the CSF provides greatly diminishes the risk of acceleration-deceleration injuries in the same way that wearing a bicycle helmet reduces the risk of head injury. As you strike a tree, the foam insulation of the helmet gradually compresses and reduces the velocity of your head. The importance of this fluid suspension system is underscored by the consequences of reduced CSF pressure, which sometimes happens transiently after the diagnostic procedure of removal of CSF from the spinal subarachnoid space. Patients with reduced CSF pressure experience severe pain when they try to sit up or stand because the brain is no longer cushioned by shock-absorbing fluid. Fortunately, the puncture hole easily heals itself, with prompt resolution of all symptoms.

The choroid plexuses secrete CSF into the ventricles, and the arachnoid granulations absorb it

Total CSF production is ~500 mL/day. Because the entire volume of CSF is ~150 mL, the CSF "turns over" about three times each day. Most of the CSF is produced by the **choroid plexuses,** which lie along the roofs of the ventricles (Fig. 11.1). The capillaries within the brain appear to form as much as 30% of the CSF.

Secretion of new CSF creates a slight pressure gradient, which drives the circulation of CSF from its ventricular sites of origin into the subarachnoid space. CSF percolates throughout the subarachnoid space and is finally absorbed into venous blood. The sites of absorption are specialized evaginations of the arachnoid membrane into the venous sinus. These structures act as pressure-sensitive one-way valves for bulk CSF clearance; CSF can cross into venous blood but venous blood cannot enter CSF.

The pressure of the CSF, which is higher than that of the venous blood, promotes net CSF movement into venous blood. When intracranial pressure (equivalent to CSF pressure) exceeds ~70 mm H_2O, absorption commences and increases in a graded fashion with further intracranial pressure (Fig. 11.2). In contrast to CSF absorption, CSF formation is not sensitive to intracranial pressure. Thus, if intracranial pressure increases, CSF absorption increases, so absorption exceeds formation, decreasing CSF volume and counteracting the increased intracranial pressure. However,

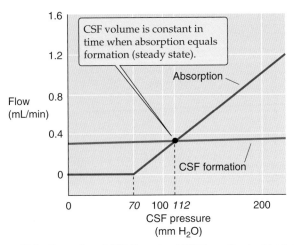

Figure 11.2 Absorption of CSF. The rate of CSF formation is virtually insensitive to changes in the pressure of the CSF. On the other hand, the absorption of CSF increases steeply at CSF pressures above ~70 mm H_2O.

if absorption of CSF is impaired even at an initially normal intracranial pressure, CSF volume increases and causes an increase in intracranial pressure, which can lead to a disturbance in brain function.

Some subarachnoid CSF flows into "sleeves" around arteries. This CSF appears to exit the sleeve by flowing across the pia/glia limitans and into **brain extracellular space (BECS),** where it mixes with BECF. Moving by convection, the BECF eventually appears to cross the pia/glia limitans that surrounds veins, and return to the subarachnoid space. This parenchymal CSF circuit—termed the **glymphatic system**—may be an efficient pathway to rid the brain of extracellular debris, including glutamate and potentially dangerous peptides such as amyloid beta.

⊙ 11-2 The epithelial cells of the choroid plexus secrete the CSF

The choroid epithelial cells are specialized ependymal cells. Blood flow to the plexuses—per unit mass of tissue—is ~10-fold greater than the average cerebral blood flow. Sympathetic and parasympathetic nerves innervate each plexus, and sympathetic input appears to inhibit CSF formation. A high density of relatively leaky capillaries is present within each plexus; these capillaries are outside the BBB. The choroid epithelial cells are bound to one another by tight junctions that completely encircle each cell, an arrangement that makes the epithelium an effective barrier to free diffusion. Thus, although the choroid capillaries are outside the BBB, the choroid epithelium insulates the ECF around these capillaries from the CSF.

The composition of CSF differs considerably from that of plasma; thus CSF is not just an ultrafiltrate of plasma (Table 11.1). For example, CSF has lower concentrations of K^+ and amino acids than plasma does, and it contains almost no protein. Moreover, the choroid plexuses rigidly maintain the concentration of ions in CSF in the face of large swings in ion concentration in plasma. The neuronal microenvironment is so well protected from the blood by the choroid plexuses and the rest of the BBB that essential **micronutrients,** such as vitamins and trace elements that are needed in very small amounts, must be selectively transported into the brain.

TABLE 11.1 Composition of CSF

SOLUTE	PLASMA (mM OF PROTEIN-FREE PLASMA)	CSF (mM)	CSF/PLASMA RATIO
Na^+	153	147	0.96
K^+	4.7	2.9	0.62
Ca^{2+}	1.3 (ionized)	1.1 (ionized)	0.85
Mg^{2+}	0.6 (ionized)	1.1 (ionized)	1.8
Cl^-	110	113	1.03
HCO_3^-	24	22	0.92
$H_2PO_4^-$ and HPO_4^{2-}	0.75 (ionized)	0.9	1.2
pH	7.40	7.33	
Amino acids	2.6	0.7	0.27
Proteins	7 g/dL	0.03 g/dL	0.004
Osmolality	290 mOsm	290 mOsm	1.00

CSF forms in two sequential stages. First, ultrafiltration of plasma occurs across the fenestrated capillary wall (see ◉ 20-3) into the ECF beneath the basolateral membrane of the choroid epithelial cell. Second, choroid epithelial cells secrete fluid into the ventricle.

BRAIN EXTRACELLULAR SPACE

Neurons, glia, and capillaries pack tightly together in the CNS

The average width of the space between brain cells is ~20 nm. However, because the surface membranes of neurons and glial cells are highly folded (i.e., have a large surface-to-volume ratio), the BECF in toto has a sizeable volume fraction, ~20%, of total brain volume. The fraction of the brain occupied by BECF varies somewhat in different areas of the CNS and increases during sleep. Moreover, because brain cells can increase volume rapidly during intense neural activity, the BECF fraction can reversibly decrease within seconds from ~20% to ~17% of brain volume.

A particle that diffuses through the BECF from one side of a neuron to the other must take a circuitous route that is described by a parameter called **tortuosity.** Tortuosity normally slows diffusion by ~60% compared with movement in free solution. Decreases in cell-to-cell spacing can further slow diffusion. For example, brain cells, especially glial cells, swell under certain pathological conditions and sometimes with intense neural activity. Cell swelling is associated with a reduction in BECF because water moves from the BECF into cells. The intense cell swelling associated with acute anoxia, for example, can reduce BECF volume from ~20% to ~5% of total brain volume. By definition, this reduced extracellular volume translates to reduced cell-to-cell spacing, which further slows the extracellular movement of solutes between the blood and brain cells.

The BECF is the route by which important molecules such as oxygen, glucose, and amino acids reach brain cells and by which the products of metabolism, including CO_2 and catabolized neurotransmitters, leave the brain. The BECF also permits molecules that are released by brain cells to diffuse to adjacent cells. Neurotransmitter molecules released at synaptic sites can spill over from the synaptic cleft and contact nearby glial cells and neurons, in addition to their target postsynaptic cell. Glial cells express neurotransmitter receptors, and neurons have **extrajunctional receptors;** therefore, these cells are capable of receiving "messages" sent through the BECF. Numerous trophic molecules (see ◉ 11-7) secreted by brain cells diffuse in the BECF to their targets. Intercellular communication by way of the BECF is especially well suited for the transmission of tonic signals for longer-term modulation of the behavior of aggregates of neurons and glial cells.

The CSF communicates freely with the BECF, which stabilizes the composition of the neuronal microenvironment

CSF in the ventricles and the subarachnoid space can exchange freely with BECF across two borders, the pia mater and ependymal cells. Thus, macromolecules and ions can also easily pass through this cellular layer through paracellular openings (some notable exceptions to this rule are considered below) and equilibrate between the CSF in the ventricle and the BECF.

CSF and BECF have a similar chemical composition. For example, $[K^+]$ is ~3.3 mM in freshly secreted CSF and ~3 mM in both the CSF of the subarachnoid space (Table 11.1) and BECF. The $[K^+]$ of blood is ~4.5 mM. However, changes in the composition of CSF are reflected slowly in the BECF and probably incompletely.

CSF is an efficient waste-management system because of its high rate of production, its circulation over the surface of the brain, and the free exchange between CSF and BECF. Products of metabolism and other substances released by cells can diffuse into the CSF and ultimately be removed either by bulk resorption or by active transport.

The ion fluxes that accompany neural activity alter extracellular ion concentrations

As discussed in Chapter 7, ionic currents through cell membranes underlie the synaptic and action potentials by which neurons communicate. These currents lead to changes in the ion concentrations of the BECF. It is estimated that even a single action potential can transiently lower $[Na^+]_o$ by ~0.75 mM and increase $[K^+]_o$ by a similar amount. Repetitive neuronal activity causes larger perturbations. Because ambient $[K^+]_o$ is much lower than $[Na^+]_o$, activity-induced changes in $[K^+]_o$ are proportionately larger. For example, K^+ accumulation in the vicinity of active neurons depolarizes nearby glial cells. In this way, neurons signal to glial cells the pattern and extent of their activity. Even small changes in $[K^+]_o$ can alter metabolism and ionic transport in glial cells. Glial cells and neurons both function to prevent excessive extracellular accumulation of K^+ and neurotransmitters.

⊙ 11-3 THE BLOOD-BRAIN BARRIER

The blood-brain barrier prevents some blood constituents from entering the brain extracellular space

Blood is not a suitable environment for neurons. Blood contains a large variety of solutes, some of which can vary greatly in concentration, depending on factors such as diet, metabolism, illness, and age. For example, the concentration of many amino acids increases significantly after a protein-rich meal. Some of these amino acids act as neurotransmitters within the brain, and if these molecules could move freely from the blood into the neuronal microenvironment, they would nonselectively activate receptors and disturb normal neurotransmission. The BBB helps protect the brain from such influences.

⊙ **11-4** The choroid plexus and several restricted areas of the brain lack a BBB. The BECF in the vicinity of these leaky capillaries is more similar to blood plasma than to normal BECF. The small brain areas that lack a BBB are called the **circumventricular organs** because they surround the ventricular system (Fig. 11.3). The ependymal cells that overlie the leaky capillaries in some of these regions (e.g., the choroid plexus) are linked together by tight junctions that form a barrier between the local BECF and the CSF.

Neurons within the circumventricular organs are directly exposed to blood solutes and macromolecules, enabling a neuroendocrine control system for maintaining such parameters as osmolality. Humoral signals are integrated by connections of circumventricular organ neurons to endocrine, autonomic, and behavioral centers within the CNS. In the median eminence, neurons discharge "releasing hormones," which diffuse into leaky capillaries for carriage through the pituitary portal system to the anterior pituitary (see ⊙ **47-1**). The lack of a BBB in the posterior pituitary is necessary to allow hormones that are released there to enter the general circulation (see ⊙ **47-3**).

Continuous tight junctions link brain capillary endothelial cells

The BBB is both a physical barrier to diffusion from blood to BECF and as a selective set of transport mechanisms that determine how organic solutes move between the blood and brain. Thus, the BBB facilitates the entry of needed substances, removes waste metabolites, and excludes toxic or disruptive substances.

The structure of brain capillaries differs from that of capillaries in other organs (Fig. 11.4A). Capillaries in other organs generally have simple openings between their endothelial cells. In most capillaries outside the CNS, solutes can easily diffuse through the clefts and fenestrae. The physical barrier to solute diffusion in *brain* capillaries (Fig. 11.4B) is provided by the capillary endothelial cells, which are fused to each other by continuous **tight junctions.** The tight junctions prevent water-soluble ions and molecules from passing from the blood into the brain through the paracellular route.

Elsewhere in the systemic circulation, molecules may traverse the endothelial cell by the process of **transcytosis** (see ⊙ **20-9**). In cerebral capillaries, transcytosis is uncommon, and brain endothelial cells have fewer endocytic vesicles than do systemic capillaries.

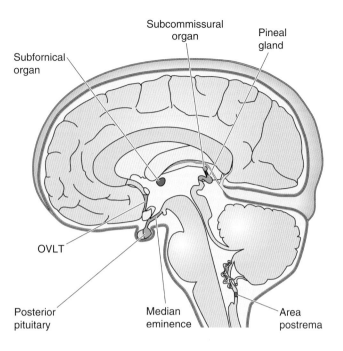

Figure 11.3 The circumventricular organs. The capillaries of the brain are leaky in several areas: the area postrema, the posterior pituitary, the subfornical organ, the median eminence, the pineal gland, and the organum vasculosum laminae terminalis (OVLT).

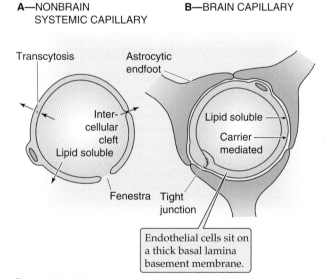

Figure 11.4 BBB function of brain capillaries. (A) Capillaries from most other organs often have interendothelial clefts or fenestrae, which makes them relatively leaky. (B) Brain capillaries are not leaky and have reduced transcytosis.

⊙ **11-5** Other interesting features of brain capillaries are the thick **basement membrane** that underlies the endothelial cells, the presence of occasional **pericytes** within the basement membrane sheath, and the **astrocytic endfeet** (or processes) that provide a nearly continuous covering of the capillaries and other blood vessels. The close apposition of the astrocyte endfoot to the capillary also could facilitate transport of substances between these cells and blood.

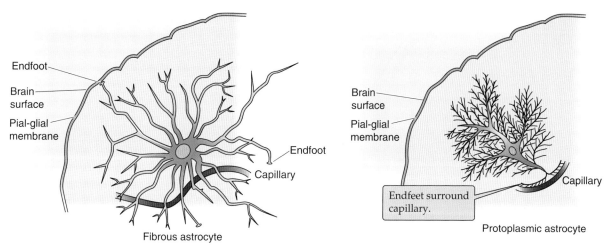

Figure 11.5 Astrocytes. The endfeet of both fibrous and protoplasmic astrocytes abut the pia mater (Fig. 11.1B) and the capillaries (Fig. 11.4B).

◉ 11-6 Uncharged and lipid-soluble molecules more readily pass through the blood-brain barrier

The capacity of the brain capillaries to exclude large molecules is strongly related to the molecular mass of the molecule and its hydrated diameter. Diffusion of a solute is also generally limited by ionization at physiological pH, by low lipid solubility, and by binding to plasma proteins. For example, gases such as CO_2 and O_2 and drugs such as ethanol, caffeine, nicotine, heroin, and methadone readily cross the BBB. However, ions such as K^+ or Mg^{2+} and protein-bound metabolites such as bilirubin have restricted access to the brain. Finally, the BBB is permeable to water mainly because of the presence of AQP4 in the astrocytic endfeet (Fig. 11.4B). Thus, water moves across the BBB in response to changes in plasma osmolality. When dehydration raises the osmolality of blood plasma, the increased osmolality of the CSF and BECF can affect the behavior of brain cells.

Cerebral capillaries also express enzymes that can affect the movement of substances from blood to brain and vice versa. Peptidases and other enzymes are present in CNS endothelial cells and can degrade a range of biologically active molecules. Orally administered dopamine is not an effective treatment of Parkinson disease (see ◉ 13-4), a condition in which CNS dopamine is depleted, because dopamine is rapidly broken down by monoamine oxidase in the capillaries. Fortunately, the dopamine precursor l-dopa is effective for this condition. Neutral amino-acid transporters in capillary endothelial cells move l-dopa to the BECF, where presynaptic terminals take up the l-dopa and convert it to dopamine.

Transport by capillary endothelial cells contributes to the blood-brain barrier

Two classes of substances can pass readily between blood and brain. The first consists of the small neutral molecules discussed in the preceding section. The second group consists of water-soluble compounds (e.g., glucose) that traverse the BBB by specific transporters.

As noted above, brain endothelial cells secrete interstitial fluid at a rate equivalent to ~30% of that of CSF.

GLIAL CELLS

Glial cells constitute half the volume of the brain and outnumber neurons

The three major types of glial cells in the CNS are astrocytes, oligodendrocytes, and microglial cells (Fig. 11.5). As discussed in Chapter 10, the peripheral nervous system (PNS) contains other, distinctive types of glial cells, including satellite cells, Schwann cells, and enteric glia. Glial cells represent about half the volume of the brain and are more numerous than neurons. Unlike neurons, which have little capacity to replace themselves when lost, glial cells can proliferate throughout life. An injury to the nervous system is the usual stimulus for proliferation. Glial cells are intimate partners with neurons in virtually every function of the brain.

Astrocytes supply fuel to neurons in the form of lactic acid

Astrocytes have elaborate processes that closely approach both blood vessels and neurons. This arrangement led to the idea that astrocytes transport substances between the blood and neurons. Throughout the brain, astrocytes envelop neurons, and both cells bathe in a common BECF. Therefore, astrocytes are ideally positioned to modify and to control the immediate environment of neurons. Most astrocytes in the brain are traditionally subdivided into fibrous and protoplasmic types (Fig. 11.5). In cortical regions, the dense processes of an individual astrocyte define its spatial domain, into which adjacent astrocytes do not encroach. The cytoskeleton of astrocytes contains an identifying intermediate filament protein called **glial fibrillar acidic protein (GFAP).**

Astrocytes store virtually all the **glycogen** present in the adult brain. They also contain all the enzymes needed for metabolizing glycogen. The brain's high metabolic needs are primarily met by glucose transferred from blood; in the

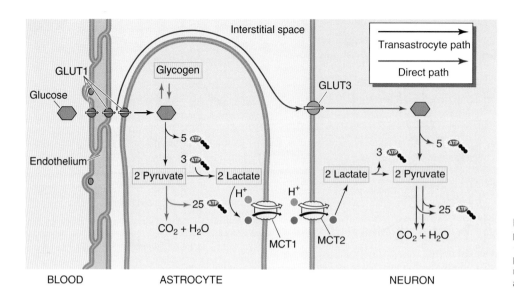

Figure 11.6 Role of astrocytes in providing lactate as fuel for neurons. *GLUT1* and *GLUT3*, Glucose transporters 1 and 3; *MCT1* and *MCT2*, monocarboxylate cotransporters 1 and 2.

absence of glucose, astrocytic glycogen could sustain the brain for only 5 to 10 minutes. Astrocytes share with neurons the energy stored in glycogen by releasing not glucose, but lactate (Fig. 11.6). This may be important during periods of intense neuronal activity, when the demand for glucose exceeds the supply from blood.

Glucose may be preferentially taken up by astrocytes and shuttled through astrocytic glycolysis to lactic acid, a significant portion of which is excreted into the BECF surrounding neurons. The two molecules of lactate derived from the breakdown of one molecule of glucose provide nearly as much ATP (28 molecules) as the complete oxidation of glucose itself (30 molecules of ATP). This is **substrate buffering.** The availability of *glucose* in the neuronal microenvironment depends on moment-to-moment supply from the blood and varies as a result of changes in neural activity. The concentration of extracellular *lactate*, however, is buffered against such variability by the surrounding astrocytes, which continuously shuttle lactate to the BECF by metabolizing glucose or by breaking down glycogen.

Astrocytes are predominantly permeable to K$^+$ and also help regulate [K$^+$]$_o$

The membrane potential of glial cells is more negative than that of neurons. For example, astrocytes have a V_m of about −85 mV, whereas the resting neuronal V_m is about −65 mV, because glial membranes have higher K$^+$ selectivity than neuronal membranes do (see ⊚ 6-1). Astrocytes express a few Na$^+$ and Ca^{2+} channels but are not capable of generating action potentials.

One consequence of the higher K$^+$ selectivity of astrocytes is that the V_m of astrocytes is far more sensitive than that of neurons to changes in [K$^+$]$_o$. For example, when [K$^+$]$_o$ is raised from 4 to 20 mM, astrocytes depolarize by ~25 mV versus only ~5 mV for neurons. This relative insensitivity of neuronal resting potential to changes in [K$^+$]$_o$ in the "physiological" range stabilizes the resting potential of *neurons* in the face of the transient increases in [K$^+$]$_o$ that accompany neuronal activity. In contrast, neural stimulation, can cause

depolarizations of up to 10 mV in *astrocytes.* Small increases in [K$^+$]$_o$ also cause astrocytes to increase their glucose metabolism and to provide more lactate for active neurons.

Not only do astrocytes respond to changes in [K$^+$]$_o$, they also help regulate it (Fig. 11.7A). Active neurons lose K$^+$ into the BECF, and the resulting increased [K$^+$]$_o$ tends to act as a positive-feedback signal that increases excitability by further depolarizing neurons. This potentially unstable situation is opposed by efficient mechanisms that expedite K$^+$ removal and limit its accumulation to a maximum level of 10 to 12 mM, the so-called ceiling level. Neurons and blood vessels can contribute to K$^+$ homeostasis, but glial mechanisms are probably most important. Conversely, when neural activity decreases, K$^+$ and Cl$^−$ leave the astrocytes through ion channels.

Gap junctions couple astrocytes to one another, allowing diffusion of small solutes

The anatomical substrate for cell-cell coupling among astrocytes is the **gap junction.** Coupling between astrocytes is strong. Ions and organic molecules that are up to 1 kDa in size, regardless of charge, can diffuse from one cell into another through these large channels. Thus, a broad range of biologically important molecules have access to this pathway.

Gap junctions may coordinate the metabolic and electrical activities of cell populations, amplify the consequences of signal transduction, and control intrinsic proliferative capacity. Thus, the network of astrocytes functionally behaves like a **syncytium,** much like the myocytes in the heart (see ⊚ 21-1).

The coupling among astrocytes may also play an important role in controlling [K$^+$]$_o$ by a mechanism known as **spatial buffering.** The selective K$^+$ permeability of glia, together with their low-resistance cell-cell connections, permits them to transport K$^+$ from focal areas of high [K$^+$]$_o$, where a portion of the glial syncytium would be depolarized, to areas of normal [K$^+$]$_o$, where the glial syncytium would be more normally polarized (Fig. 11.7B). Redistribution of K$^+$ proceeds by way of a current loop in which K$^+$ enters glial cells at the

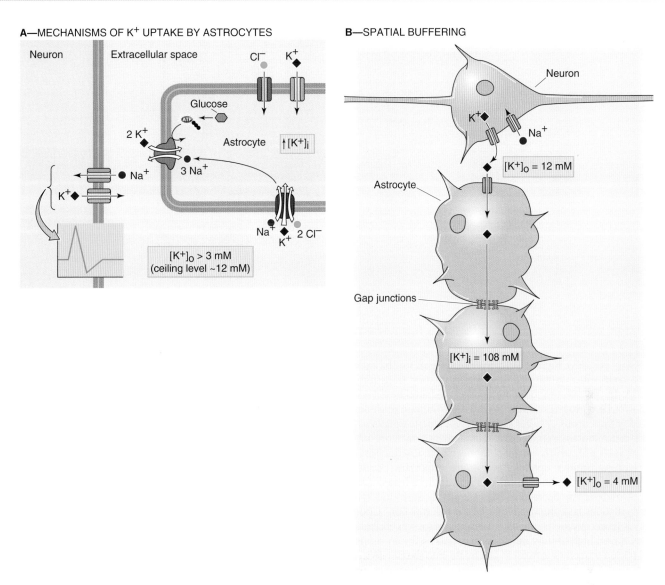

Figure 11.7 K+ handling by astrocytes.

point of high $[K^+]_o$ and leaves them at sites of normal $[K^+]_o$, with the extracellular flow of Na^+ completing this circuit. At a site of high neuronal activity, $[K^+]_o$ might rise to 12 mM, which would produce a very large depolarization of an isolated, uncoupled astrocyte. However, because of the electrical coupling among astrocytes, the V_m of the affected astrocyte remains more negative than the equilibrium potential for K^+ (E_K) predicted for a $[K^+]_o$ of 12 mM. Thus, K^+ would tend to passively enter coupled astrocytes through channels at sites of high $[K^+]_o$.

Astrocytes synthesize neurotransmitters, take them up from the extracellular space, and have neurotransmitter receptors

Astrocytes synthesize at least 20 neuroactive compounds, including both glutamate and gamma-aminobutyric acid (GABA). Neurons can manufacture glutamate from glucose or from the immediate precursor molecule glutamine (Fig. 11.8). The glutamine pathway appears to be the primary one in the synthesis of synaptically released glutamate. Glutamine, however, is manufactured only in astrocytes by use of the astrocyte-specific enzyme **glutamine synthetase** to convert glutamate to glutamine. Astrocytes release this glutamine into the BECF through the SNAT3 and SNAT5 transporters for uptake by neurons via SNAT1 and SNAT2. Consistent with its role in the synthesis of glutamate for neurotransmission, glutamine synthetase is localized to astrocytic processes surrounding glutamatergic synapses. In the presynaptic terminals of neurons, glutaminase converts the glutamine to glutamate for release into the synaptic cleft. Finally, astrocytes take up much of the synaptically released glutamate to complete this **glutamate-glutamine cycle.**

Glutamine derived from astrocytes is also important for synthesis of the brain's most prevalent inhibitory neurotransmitter, GABA. In the neuron, the enzyme **glutamic acid decarboxylase** converts glutamate (generated from glutamine) to GABA (Fig. 13.6A). Because astrocytes play such an important role in the synthesis of synaptic transmitters, these glial cells are in a position to modulate synaptic efficacy.

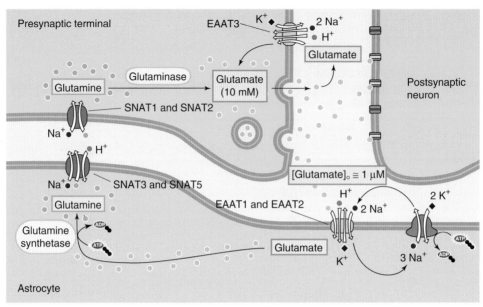

Figure 11.8   Role of astrocytes in the glutamate-glutamine cycle.

Astrocytes have **high-affinity uptake systems** for the excitatory transmitter glutamate and the inhibitory transmitter GABA. In the case of glutamate uptake, mediated by EAAT1 and EAAT2, astrocytes appear to play the dominant role compared with neurons or other glial cells. Glutamate uptake systems can maintain extracellular glutamate at concentrations as low as ~1 µM, which is crucial for normal brain function.

Neurotransmitter uptake systems are important because they help terminate the action of synaptically released neurotransmitters. Astrocyte processes frequently surround synaptic junctions and are ideally placed for this function. Under pathological conditions in which transmembrane ion gradients break down, high-affinity uptake systems may work in reverse and release transmitters, such as glutamate, into the BECF.

Astrocytes express a wide variety of ionotropic and metabotropic **neurotransmitter receptors** that are similar or identical to those present on neuronal membranes. As in neurons, activation of these receptors can open ion channels or generate second messengers. In most astrocytes, glutamate produces depolarization by increasing Na^+ permeability, whereas GABA hyperpolarizes cells by opening Cl^- channels, similar to the situation in neurons (see ⊙ **13-6**). Transmitter substances released by neurons at synapses can diffuse in the BECF to activate nearby receptors on astrocytes, thus providing, at least theoretically, a form of neuronal-glial signaling.

Astrocytes apparently can actively enhance or depress neuronal discharge and synaptic transmission by releasing neurotransmitters that they have taken up or synthesized. The release mechanisms are diverse and include stimulation by certain neurotransmitters, a fall in $[Ca^{2+}]_o$, or depolarization by elevated $[K^+]_o$.

⊙ 11-7 Astrocytes secrete trophic factors that promote neuronal survival and synaptogenesis

Astrocytes, and other glial cell types, are a source of important trophic factors and cytokines. The development of fully functional excitatory synapses in the brain requires the presence of astrocytes. In the absence of astrocytes, only ~20% of the normal number of synapses form.

Astrocytic endfeet modulate cerebral blood flow

Astrocytic endfeet (see ⊙ 11-5) surround not only capillaries but also small arteries. Neuronal activity can lead to astrocytic $[Ca^{2+}]_i$ waves that spread to the astrocytic endfeet, or to isolated $[Ca^{2+}]_i$ increases in the endfoot. In either case, the result is a rapid increase in blood vessel diameter and thus in local blood flow. This is one mechanism of neuronvascular coupling—a local increase in neuronal activity that leads to a local increase in blood flow. Radiologists exploit this physiological principle in a form of **functional magnetic resonance imaging (fMRI)** called blood oxygen level–dependent (BOLD) MRI, which uses blood flow as an index of neuronal activity.

⊙ 11-8 Oligodendrocytes and Schwann cells make and sustain myelin

The primary function of oligodendrocytes is to provide and to maintain myelin sheaths on axons of the central nervous systems. As discussed earlier (see ⊙ 7-11), myelin is the insulating "electrical tape" of the nervous system (see Fig. 7.10B). **Oligodendrocytes** are present in all areas of the CNS. In white matter, the oligodendrocytes responsible for myelination have (Fig. 11.9A) 15 to 30 processes, each of which connects a myelin sheath to the oligodendrocyte's cell body. Each myelin sheath, which is up to 250 µm wide, wraps many times around the long axis of one axon. The small exposed area of axon between adjacent myelin sheaths is called the **node of Ranvier** (see ⊙ 7-13). In gray matter, oligodendrocytes do not produce myelin and exist as perineuronal satellite cells.

During the myelination process, the leading edge of one of the processes of the oligodendrocyte cytoplasm wraps around the axon many times (Fig. 11.9A, upper axon). The

A OLIGODENDROCYTE

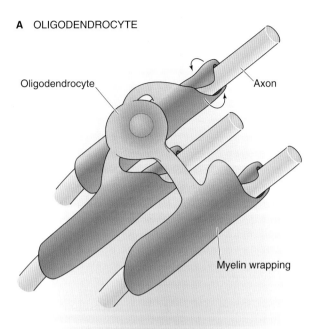

Oligodendrocyte

Axon

Myelin wrapping

B SCHWANN CELL

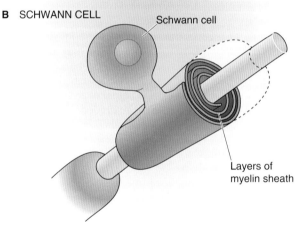

Schwann cell

Layers of
myelin sheath

Figure 11.9 Myelination of axons by oligodendrocytes and Schwann cells.

cytoplasm is then squeezed out of the many cell layers surrounding the axon in a process called **compaction.** This process creates layer upon layer of tightly compressed membranes that is called **myelin.** The myelin sheaths remain continuous with the parent glial cells, which nourish them.

In the PNS, a single **Schwann cell** provides a single myelin segment to a single axon of a myelinated nerve (Fig. 11.9B). In contrast, one oligodendrocyte myelinates many axons. The process of myelination that occurs in the PNS is analogous to that outlined for oligodendrocytes.

Myelin has a biochemical composition different from that of the oligodendrocyte or Schwann cell plasma membrane from which it arose.

Myelination greatly enhances conduction of the action potential down the axon because it allows the regenerative electrical event to skip from one node to the next rather than gradually spreading down the whole extent of the axon. This process is called **saltatory conduction** (see ⊙ 7-13). Oligodendrocytes induce the clustering of Na^+ channels at the nodes (see Fig. 12.4B), which is essential for saltatory conduction.

It is well known that severed axons in the PNS can regenerate with restoration of lost function. Severed axons in the CNS do not show functional regrowth.

Microglial cells are the macrophages of the CNS

Microglial cells are of mesodermal origin and derive from cells related to the monocyte-macrophage lineage. Microglia represent ~20% of the total glial cells within the mature CNS. These cells are rapidly activated by injury to the brain, which causes them to proliferate, to change shape, and to become phagocytic (Fig. 11.10). When activated, they are capable of releasing substances that are toxic to neurons, including free radicals and nitric oxide. It is believed that microglia are involved in most brain diseases, not as initiators but as highly reactive cells that shape the brain's response to any insult.

Microglia are also the most effective antigen-presenting cells within the brain. Activated T lymphocytes are able to breech the BBB and enter the brain. To become mediators of tissue-specific disease or to destroy an invading infectious agent, T lymphocytes must recognize specific antigenic targets. Such recognition is accomplished through the process of antigen presentation, which is a function of the microglia.

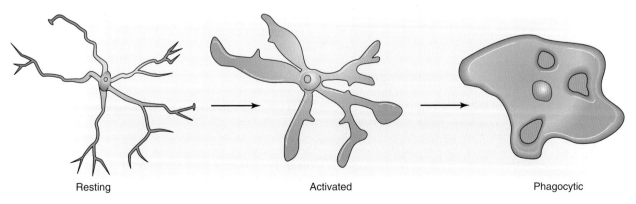

Resting

Activated

Phagocytic

Figure 11.10 Microglial cells. Resting microglial cells become activated by injury to the brain, which causes them to proliferate and to become phagocytic.

CHAPTER 12

PHYSIOLOGY OF NEURONS

Barry W. Connors

Neurons receive, combine, transform, store, and send information

Neurons have arguably the most complex job of any cell in the body. Consequently, they have an elaborate morphology and physiology. Each neuron is an intricate computing device. A single neuron may receive chemical input from tens of thousands of other neurons. It then transmits a *single new message* through its axon, which itself may contact and inform hundreds of other neurons. Under the right circumstances, neurons also possess the property of *memory*; some of the information coursing through a neuron's synapses may be stored for periods as long as years.

Neural information flows from dendrite to soma to axon to synapse

Numerous dendrites converge on a central cell body, from which an axon emerges and branches (see Fig. 10.1). Each branch culminates at a presynaptic terminal that contacts another cell. In most neurons, dendrites are the principal synaptic input sites, although synapses may also be found on the soma, on the axon hillock (the region of the soma neighboring the axon), or even on the axons. In some primary sensory neurons, the dendrites themselves are transducers of environmental energy. Signals—voltage changes across the membrane—typically flow from dendrites to soma to axon and finally to synapses on the next set of cells.

Excitatory input to a neuron generates an inward flow of positive charge (i.e., an inward current) across the dendritic membrane. This inward current **depolarizes** the cell. Conversely, inhibitory input to a neuron generates an outward current and hyperpolarization.

Through a chemical synapse, neurotransmitters trigger currents by activating ion channels. The change in membrane potential (V_m) caused by the flow of charge is called a **postsynaptic potential (PSP).** The postsynaptic V_m changes may be either positive or negative. Excitatory transmitters produce a depolarizing PSPs, called an **excitatory postsynaptic potential (EPSP),** while inhibitory neurotransmitters produce a *hyperpolarizing* **inhibitory postsynaptic potential (IPSP).** The V_m change is *graded*. More synapses activated together generate larger PSPs. A graded response is one form of neural coding whereby the size and duration of the input are encoded as the size and duration of the change in the dendritic V_m.

The synaptic potentials generated at the ends of a dendrite are communicated to the soma, usually with substantial attenuation of the signal (Fig. 12.1A). Extended cellular processes such as dendrites behave like leaky electrical cables (see ◉ 7-14). As a consequence, dendritic potentials usually decline in amplitude before reaching the soma. As an EPSP reaches the soma, it may also combine with EPSPs arriving via other dendrites on the cell; this behavior is a type of **spatial summation** and can lead to EPSPs that are substantially larger than those generated by any single synapse (Fig. 12.1B and C). **Temporal summation** occurs when EPSPs arrive rapidly in succession; when the first EPSP has not yet dissipated, a subsequent EPSP tends to add its amplitude to the residual of the preceding EPSP (Fig. 12.1D).

If the V_m change in the soma is large enough to reach the threshold voltage, the depolarization may trigger one or more action potentials between the soma and axon, as shown in Fig. 12.1 B through D. As described in Chapter 7, an action potential can carry a signal over long distances. Notice that the neuron converts the graded-voltage code of the dendrites (the PSPs) to a temporal code of action potentials in the axon.

Action potentials are fixed in amplitude, not graded, and have uniform shape. So how is information encoded by action potentials? Because one axonal spike looks like another, neurons vary the number of spikes and their timing. For a single axon, information may be encoded by the average rate of action potential firing, the total number of action potentials, their temporal pattern, or some combination of these mechanisms. Fig. 12.1 illustrates that as the synaptic potential in the soma increases in size, the resultant action potentials occur more frequently, and the burst of action potentials in the axon lasts longer. By the time the signal has propagated down the axon, the graded potential has vanished, whereas the action potentials have retained their size, number, and temporal pattern. The final output of the neuron is entirely encoded by these action potentials. When action potentials reach axonal terminals, they may trigger the release of a neurotransmitter at the next set of synapses, and the cycle begins again.

SIGNAL CONDUCTION IN DENDRITES

Dendrites arborize through a volume of brain tissue so that they can collect *information* in the form of synaptic input. Dendrites exhibit a great diversity of shapes. The dendrites of a single neuron may receive as many as 200,000 synaptic inputs. The electrical and biochemical properties of dendrites have a profound influence on the transfer of information from synapse to soma.

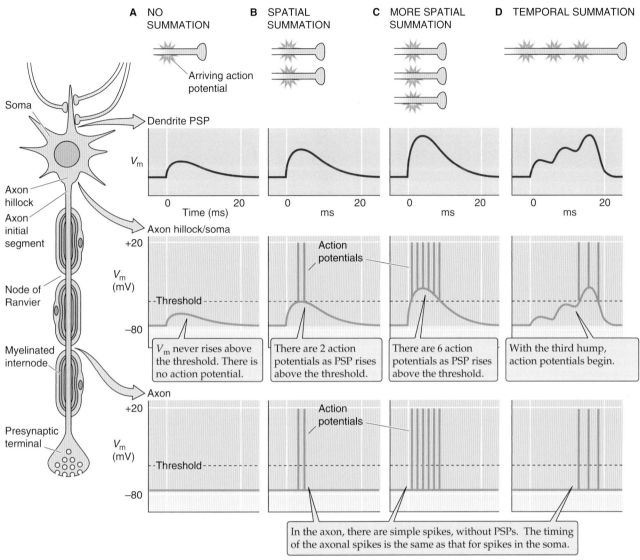

Figure 12.1   Spatial versus temporal summation of EPSPs.

Dendrites attenuate synaptic potentials

Dendrites tend to be long and thin. Their cytoplasm has relatively low electrical resistivity, and their membrane has relatively high resistivity. These are the properties of a *leaky electrical cable*, that predict how much current flows down the length of the dendrite through the cytoplasm and how much of it leaks out of the dendrite across the membrane. Thick dendrites let more current flow toward the soma than thin dendrites do. The transmembrane voltage generated by the current falls off exponentially with distance from the site of current injection, according to the length constant (λ; see ⊚ 7-15). For example, assuming the same cellular properties, a thin dendrite with a radius of 0.1 μm would have a λ of only 354 μm, whereas a thick one with a radius of 5 μm would have a λ of 2500 μm. Thus, the graded signal voltage spreads farther in a thick dendrite.

Branching *increases* attenuation because current has more paths to follow. An increased diameter increases λ and thus *decreases* attenuation. In the working brain, cable properties are not constant but may vary dynamically with ongoing brain activity. In summary, *voltage signals are attenuated as they travel down a dendrite.*

So far, we have described how a dendrite might attenuate a *sustained* voltage change. Indeed, the definition of length constant applies only to a *steady-state* voltage shift. However, signal attenuation along a cable depends on the *frequency* components of that signal—how rapidly voltage changes over time. When V_m varies over time, some current is lost to membrane capacitance (see Fig. 6.5), and less current is carried along the dendrite downstream from the source of the current. Because action potentials and EPSPs are rapid, they are attenuated much more strongly than the steady-state λ implies. Thus, *dendrites attenuate high-frequency (i.e., rapidly changing) signals more than low-frequency or steady signals.* Dendrites are **low-pass filters** that let slowly changing signals pass more easily than rapidly changing ones.

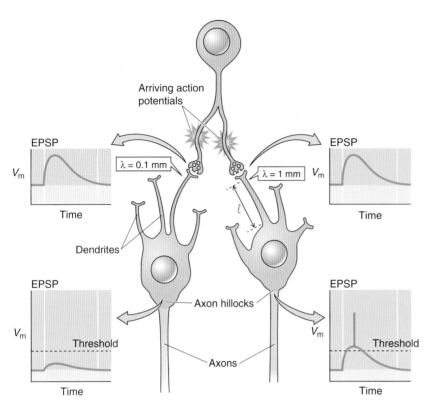

Arriving action
potentials

EPSP

V_m

Time

$\lambda = 0.1$ mm

$\lambda = 1$ mm

EPSP

V_m

Time

Dendrites

EPSP

V_m

Threshold

Time

Axon hillocks

Axons

EPSP

V_m

Threshold

Time

Figure 12.2 Attenuation of EPSPs in dendrites. The neuron at the top fires an action potential that reaches the left and right neurons below, each at a single synapse. The EPSPs are identical. However, the left neuron has a thin dendrite and therefore a small length constant ($\lambda = 0.1$ mm). As a result, the signal is almost completely attenuated by the time it reaches the axon hillock, and there is no action potential. In the right neuron, the dendrite is thicker and therefore has a larger length constant ($\lambda = 1$ mm). As a result, the signal that reaches the axon hillock is large enough to trigger an action potential.

Fig. 12.2 shows how an EPSP propagates along two different dendrites with very different length constants. If we assume the synapses trigger EPSPs of similar size in the end of each dendrite, then the dendrites with the longer λ deliver a larger signal to the axon hillock.

Dendritic membranes have voltage-gated ion channels

All mammalian dendrites have voltage-gated ion channels that influence their signaling properties. Most dendrites have a relatively low density of voltage-gated channels (see ⊙ 7-3) that may amplify synaptic signals by adding additional inward current as the signals propagate from distal dendrites toward the soma. If the membrane has voltage-gated channels that are able to carry more inward current (Na$^+$ or Ca^{2+}) under depolarized conditions, a sufficiently strong EPSP would drive V_m into the activation range of the voltage-gated channels. Their additional inward current would add to that generated initially by the synaptic channels. Thus, the synaptic signal would fall off much less steeply with distance than in a passive dendrite. Voltage-gated channels can be distributed all along the dendrite and thus amplify the signal along the entire dendritic length, or they can be clustered at particular sites. In either case, voltage-gated channels can boost the synaptic signal considerably.

CONTROL OF SPIKING PATTERNS IN THE SOMA

Electrical signals from dendrites converge and summate at the soma. Ion channels in the soma modulate the temporal patterns of action potentials that ultimately course down the axon.

Neurons can transform a simple input into a variety of output patterns

Most neurons within the CNS generate action potentials in the conventional way (see Fig. 7.4), with fast voltage-gated Na$^+$ channels and slower K$^+$ channels. However, neurons produce spikes with a range of shapes. Although a fast Na$^+$ current invariably drives the fast upstroke of neuronal action potentials, an additional fast Ca^{2+} current (see ⊙ 7-4) can frequently occur and, if it is large enough, broaden the spike duration. The greatest variability occurs in the repolarization phase of the spike. Many neurons are repolarized by several other voltage-gated K$^+$ currents in addition to the delayed outward-rectifier K$^+$ current, and some also have K$^+$ currents carried by channels that are rapidly activated by the combination of membrane depolarization and a rise in [Ca^{2+}]$_i$ (see ⊙ 7-7).

More dramatic variations occur in the **repetitive spiking patterns** of neurons. One way to illustrate this is to apply a simple continuous stimulus and to measure the neuron's output (the number and pattern of action potentials fired at its soma). The current pulse is similar to a steady, strong input of excitatory synaptic currents. Some examples are shown in Fig. 12.3, which illustrates recordings from three types of neurons in the cerebral cortex. In response to a sustained current stimulus, some cells generate a rapid train of action potentials that *do not adapt* (Fig. 12.3A); that is, the spikes occur at a regular interval throughout the current pulse. Other cells fire rapidly at first but then *adapt strongly* (Fig. 12.3B); that

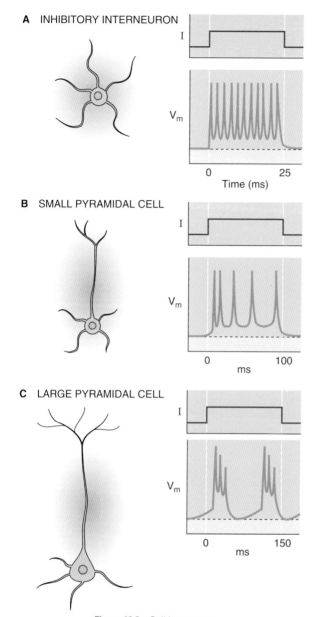

Figure 12.3 Spiking patterns.

is, the spikes gradually become less frequent during the current pulse. Some cells fire a burst of action potentials and then stop firing altogether, and still others generate *rhythmic bursts* of action potentials that continue as long as the stimulus (Fig. 12.3C). These varied behaviors are not arbitrary but are characteristic of each neuron type. A neuron's firing patterns are determined by the interaction of its intrinsic membrane properties and synaptic inputs.

Rhythmically bursting cells are particularly interesting and occur in a variety of places in the brain. As described later (see ⊙ 16-3), they may participate in the central circuits that generate rhythmic motor output for behavior such as locomotion and respiration.

Intrinsic firing patterns are determined by a variety of ion currents with relatively slow kinetics

What determines the variety of spiking patterns in each type of neuron, and why do neurons differ in their intrinsic

patterns? The key is a large set of ion channel types that have variable and often relatively *slow* kinetics compared with the *quick* Na^+ and K^+ channels that shape the spike. Each neuron expresses a different complement of these slow channels and has a unique spatial arrangement of them on its dendrites, soma, and axon initial segment. The channels are gated primarily by membrane voltage and $[Ca^{2+}]_i$, and a neuron's ultimate spiking pattern is determined by the net effects of the slow currents that it generates. We provide three examples.

1. A neuron with only fast voltage-gated Na^+ channels and delayed-rectifier K^+ channels will generate repetitive spikes when it is presented with a long stimulus. The pattern of those spikes will be quite regular over time, as in Fig. 12.3A.
2. If the neuron also has another set of K^+ channels that activate very slowly, the spiking pattern becomes more time dependent: the spiking frequency may initially be very high, but it adapts to progressively lower rates as a slow K^+ current turns on to counteract the stimulus, as shown for the small pyramidal cell in Fig. 12.3B.
3. A neuron, by exploiting the interplay between two or more voltage-gated currents with relatively slow kinetics, can generate spontaneous rhythmic bursting—as in the case of the large pyramidal neuron in Fig. 12.3C—even without ongoing synaptic activity to drive it.

AXONAL CONDUCTION

Axons are specialized for rapid, reliable, and efficient transmission of electrical signals

The axon has the relatively simple job of carrying the computed signal—a sequence of action potentials—from one place in the brain to another without changing it significantly. Some axons are thin, unmyelinated, and slow; these properties are sufficient to achieve their functions. However, the axon can be exquisitely optimized, with myelin and nodes of Ranvier, for fast and reliable saltatory conduction of action potentials over very long distances (see ⊙ 7-13). Consider the sensory endings in the skin of your foot, which must send their signals to your lumbar spinal cord 1 m away (see Fig. 10.5B). The axon of such a sensory cell transmits its message in just a few tens of milliseconds! As we see in our discussion of spinal reflexes (see ⊙ 16-1), axons of similar length carry signals in the opposite direction, from your spinal cord to the muscles within your feet, and they do it even faster than most of the sensory axons. Axons within the CNS can also be very long; examples include the corticospinal axons that originate in the cerebral cortex and terminate in the lumbar spinal cord. Alternatively, many central axons are quite short, only tens of micrometers in length, and they transmit their messages locally between neurons. The spinal interneuron between a sensory neuron and a motor neuron (see Fig. 10.5B) is an example. Some axons target their signal precisely, from one soma to only a few other cells, whereas others may branch profusely to target thousands of postsynaptic cells.

Without myelinated axons, the large, complex brains necessary to control warm, fast mammalian bodies could not exist. For *un*myelinated axons to conduct action potentials sufficiently fast for many purposes, their diameters

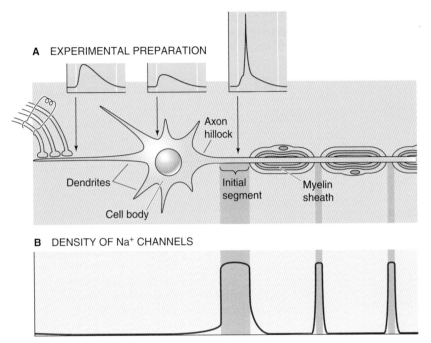

A   EXPERIMENTAL PREPARATION

Axon
hillock

Dendrites

Initial
segment

Myelin
sheath

Cell body

B   DENSITY OF Na⁺ CHANNELS

Figure 12.4 Simultaneous recording of action potentials from different parts of a neuron. (A) An excitatory synapse on a dendrite is stimulated and the response near that dendrite is recorded in the soma and at the initial segment. The EPSP attenuates in the soma and the initial segment, but the EPSP is large enough to trigger an action potential at the initial segment. (B) The density of Na⁺ channels is high only at the initial segment and at each node of Ranvier.

would have to be so large that the axons alone would take up far too much space and use impossibly large amounts of energy.

12-1 Action potentials usually initiate at the initial segment

The soma, axon hillock, and initial segment of the axon together serve as a kind of focal point in most neurons. EPSPs evoked in the dendrites propagate down to and through the soma and trigger an action potential in a myelin-free zone of axon ~15 to 50 μm from the soma (Fig. 12.4A). The action potential then propagates in two directions: forward—**orthodromic** conduction—into the axon, with no loss of amplitude, and backward—**antidromic** conduction—into the soma and dendrites, with strong attenuation. Orthodromic propagation carries the signal to the next set of neurons. The function of antidromic propagation is not completely understood. It is very likely that backwardly propagating spikes trigger biochemical changes in the neuron's dendrites and synapses, and they may have a role in plasticity of synapses and intrinsic membrane properties.

The axon achieves a uniquely *low threshold* in its initial segment by a combination of large numbers of Na⁺ channels (Fig. 12.4B) and their opening at relatively negative voltage.

Conduction velocity of a myelinated axon increases linearly with diameter

The larger the diameter of an axon, the faster its conduction velocity, other things remaining equal. However, conduction velocity is usually much faster in myelinated axons than it is in unmyelinated axons (see ⊙ 7-12).

Unmyelinated axons still have a role in vertebrates. At diameters less than ~1 μm, unmyelinated axons in the PNS conduct more rapidly than myelinated ones do. In a

testament to evolutionary frugality, the thinnest axons of the peripheral sensory nerves, called **C fibers,** are ~1 μm wide or less, and all are unmyelinated. Axons larger than ~1 μm in diameter are all myelinated. Every axon has its biological price: the largest axons obviously take up the most room and are the most expensive to synthesize and to maintain metabolically. The largest, swiftest axons are therefore used sparingly. They are used only to carry sensory information about the most rapidly changing stimuli over the longest distances, or to control finely coordinated contractions of muscles. The thinnest, slowest C fibers in the periphery are mainly sensory axons related to chronic pain and temperature sensation, for which the speed of the message is not as critical.

In normal central axons, Na⁺ channels populate nodes of Ranvier at a density of 1000 to 2000 channels per square micrometer (Fig. 12.4B). The same axonal membrane in the internodal regions, under the myelin, has <25 channels per square micrometer (versus between 2 and 200 channels per square micrometer in unmyelinated axons). K⁺ channels are relatively less important in myelinated axons than they are in most other excitable membranes. Very few of these channels are present in the nodal membrane, and fast K⁺ currents contribute little to repolarization of the action potential in mature myelinated axons. However, some K⁺ channels are located in the axonal membrane under the myelin, particularly in the paranodal region; they may set the resting V_m of the internodes and help stabilize the firing properties of the axon.

Demyelinated axons conduct action potentials slowly, unreliably, or not at all

Numerous clinical disorders selectively damage or destroy myelin sheaths and leave the axonal membranes intact but bare. These **demyelinating diseases** may affect either peripheral or central axons and can lead to severely impaired conduction. The most common demyelinating disease of the CNS is **multiple sclerosis**, a progressive disorder characterized by distributed zones of demyelination in the brain and spinal cord. The specific clinical signs of these disorders vary and depend on the particular sets of axons affected.

In a normal, myelinated axon, the action currents generated at a node can effectively charge the adjacent node and bring it to threshold within ~20 μsec (Fig. 12.5A), because myelin increases the resistance and reduces the capacitance of the pathways between the axoplasm and the extracellular fluid (see ⊙ 7-11). The inward membrane current flowing across each node is actually 5-fold to 7-fold higher than necessary to initiate an action potential at the adjacent node. Removal of the insulating myelin, however, means that the same nodal action current is distributed across a much longer, leakier, higher-capacitance stretch of axonal membrane (Fig. 12.5B). Several consequences are possible. Compared with normal conduction, conduction in a demyelinated axon may continue, but at a *lower velocity,* if the demyelination is not too severe (Fig. 12.5B, record 1). In experimental studies, the internodal conduction time through demyelinated fibers can be as slow as 500 μs, 25 times longer than normal. The ability of axons to transmit *high-frequency* trains of impulses may also be impaired (Fig. 12.5B, record 2). Extensive demyelination of an axon causes *total blockade* of conduction (Fig. 12.5B, record 3). Clinical studies indicate that the blockade of action potentials is more closely related to symptoms than is the simple slowing of conduction. Demyelinated axons can also become the source of spontaneous, **ectopically generated action potentials** because of changes in their intrinsic excitability (Fig. 12.5B, record 4) or mechanosensitivity (Fig. 12.5B, record 5). Moreover, the signal from one demyelinated axon can excite an adjacent demyelinated axon and induce **crosstalk** (Fig. 12.5C), which may cause action potentials to be conducted in both directions in the adjacent axon.

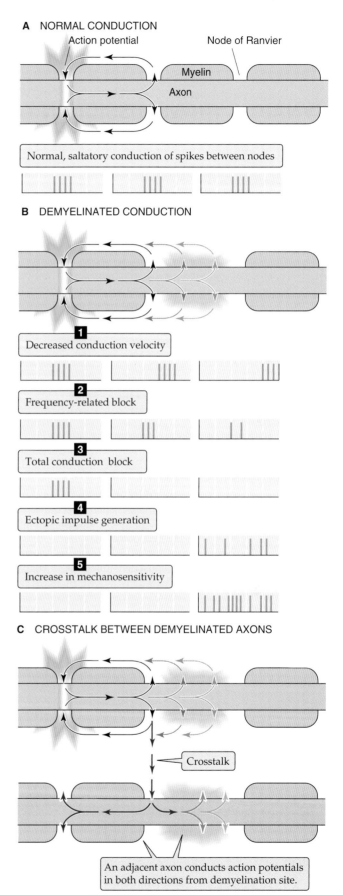

A NORMAL CONDUCTION

Normal, saltatory conduction of spikes between nodes

B DEMYELINATED CONDUCTION

1 Decreased conduction velocity

2 Frequency-related block

3 Total conduction block

4 Ectopic impulse generation

5 Increase in mechanosensitivity

C CROSSTALK BETWEEN DEMYELINATED AXONS

Crosstalk

An adjacent axon conducts action potentials in both directions from demyelination site.

Figure 12.5 Effects of demyelination.

CHAPTER 13

SYNAPTIC TRANSMISSION IN THE NERVOUS SYSTEM

Barry W. Connors

Neurons come very close together at chemical synapses (see ⊙ 8-3), but their membranes and cytoplasm remain distinct. At electrical synapses (see ⊙ 8-2), which are less common than chemical synapses, the membranes remain distinct, but ions and other small solutes can diffuse through the gap junctions.

NEURONAL SYNAPSES

The molecular mechanisms of neuronal synapses are similar but not identical to those of the neuromuscular junction

Chemical synapses use diffusible **transmitter molecules** to communicate messages between two cells. The first chemical synapse to be understood in detail was the neuromuscular junction in vertebrate skeletal muscle, which is described in Chapter 8. In this chapter, we are concerned with the properties of the synapses that occur. Synapses share certain basic biochemical and physiological mechanisms, and thus many basic insights gained from the neuromuscular junction are also applicable to synapses in the brain. However, neuronal synapses differ from neuromuscular junctions in many important ways; they also differ widely among themselves, and it is the diverse properties of synapses that help make each part of the brain unique.

Synaptic transmission at chemical synapses occurs in seven steps:

Step 1: Neurotransmitter molecules are packaged into membranous vesicles, and the vesicles docked at the presynaptic terminal.

Step 2: The presynaptic membrane depolarizes, usually as the result of an action potential.

Step 3: The depolarization causes voltage-gated Ca^{2+} channels to open and allows Ca^{2+} ions to flow into the terminal.

Step 4: The resulting increase in intracellular $[Ca^{2+}]$ triggers fusion of vesicles with the presynaptic membrane (see ⊙ 8-4), and the rate of transmitter release increases ~100,000-fold. The Ca^{2+} dependence of fusion is conferred by proteins called synaptotagmins. The fusion events require only a fraction of a millisecond.

Step 5: The transmitter is released into the extracellular space and diffuses across the synaptic cleft.

Step 6: Some of the transmitter molecules bind to receptors in the postsynaptic membrane, and the activated receptors trigger some postsynaptic event, usually the opening of an ion channel or the activation of a G protein–coupled signal cascade.

Step 7: Transmitter molecules diffuse away from postsynaptic receptors and are cleared away by diffusion, enzymatic degradation, or active uptake into cells. In addition, the presynaptic machinery retrieves the membrane of the exocytosed synaptic vesicle.

The molecular machinery of synapses is closely related to components that are universal in eukaryotic cells. Ligand-gated ion channels and G protein–coupled receptors (GPCRs), the receptors on the postsynaptic membrane, are also present in all eukaryotic cells. Most neurotransmitters are simple molecules, identical or similar to those used in general cellular metabolism. However, neuronal synapses vary widely in the size of the synaptic contact, the identity of the neurotransmitter, the nature of the postsynaptic receptors, the efficiency of synaptic transmission, the mechanism used for terminating transmitter action, and the degree and modes of synaptic plasticity.

A major difference between the neuromuscular junction and most neuronal synapses is the type of neurotransmitter used. All skeletal neuromuscular junctions use acetylcholine (ACh). In contrast, neuronal synapses use many transmitters. The most ubiquitous are amino acids: glutamate and aspartate excite, whereas gamma-aminobutyric acid (GABA) and glycine inhibit. Other transmitters include simple amines (e.g., ACh, norepinephrine, serotonin, and histamine), ATP, adenosine, and a wide array of peptides.

Even more varied than the neuronal transmitters are their receptors. Whereas skeletal muscle manufactures a few modest variants of its ACh receptors, the nervous system typically has several major receptor variants for each neurotransmitter. Transmitter systems in the brain generate responses with widely varying durations that range from a few milliseconds to days (Fig. 13.1).

Presynaptic terminals may contact neurons at the dendrite, soma, or axon and may contain both clear vesicles and dense-core granules

Chemical synapses between neurons are generally small, often <1 μm in diameter, which means that their detailed

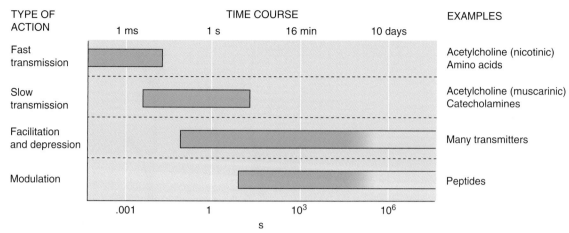

TYPE OF ACTION	TIME COURSE				EXAMPLES
	1 ms	1 s	16 min	10 days	
Fast transmission					Acetylcholine (nicotinic) Amino acids
Slow transmission					Acetylcholine (muscarinic) Catecholamines
Facilitation and depression					Many transmitters
Modulation					Peptides
	.001	1	10^3	10^6	
		s			

Figure. 13.1 Time courses of synaptic events in the nervous system. Note the logarithmic time axis. (Data from Shepherd GM: Neurobiology, 3rd ed. New York, Oxford University Press, 1994.)

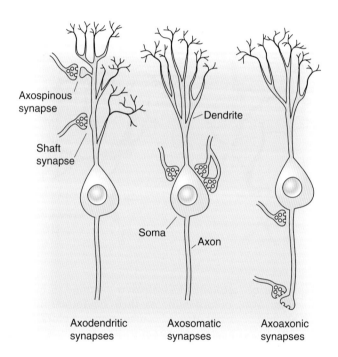

Figure. 13.2 The most common synaptic arrangements in the CNS.

structure can be seen only with an electron microscope; under the light microscope, brain synapses are usually visible only as swellings along or at the termination of the axons. These swellings are actually the **bouton terminals**—the presynaptic terminals. Most presynaptic terminals arise from axons, and they can form synapses on virtually any part of a neuron. The contact site and direction of communication determine the way in which a synapse is named: typically, **axodendritic, axosomatic,** and **axoaxonic** synapses (Fig. 13.2). In many cases, synapses occur on small outpockets of the dendritic membrane called **spines** and are termed **axospinous** synapses. However, not all synapses arise from axons, and **dendrodendritic, somatosomatic,** and even **somatodendritic** synapses may be found in the mammalian brain.

⊙ **13-1** Most synapses transmit information primarily in one direction. The presynaptic side contains numerous **clear vesicles,** 40 to 50 nm in diameter, that appear empty

when viewed by transmission electron microscopy. Synaptic termini may also contain large (100 to 200 nm in diameter) **dense-core secretory granules** that are morphologically quite similar to the secretory granules of endocrine cells. These granules contain neuropeptides; that is, peptides or small proteins that act as neurotransmitters and for which receptors exist in the postsynaptic membranes.

The clear synaptic vesicles are anchored and shifted about by a dense network of cytoskeletal proteins. Some vesicles are clustered close to the part of the presynaptic membrane that apposes the synaptic contact; these vesicle attachment sites are called **active zones.** Synaptic vesicles are lined up several deep along the active zones, which are the regions of actual exocytosis. Most synapses in the central nervous system (CNS) have relatively few active zones, often only 1 but occasionally as many as 10 or 20 (versus the hundreds in the neuromuscular junction).

Unlike the clear synaptic vesicles containing nonpeptide transmitters, dense-core secretory granules are distributed randomly throughout the cytoplasm of the synaptic terminus. They are not concentrated at the presynaptic density, and they do not appear to release their contents at the active zone.

The postsynaptic membrane contains transmitter receptors and numerous proteins clustered in the postsynaptic density

The postsynaptic membrane lies parallel to the presynaptic membrane, separated by a narrow **synaptic cleft** (~30 nm wide) that is filled with extracellular fluid. The most characteristic anatomical feature of the postsynaptic side is the **postsynaptic density,** which includes the receptors embedded within the postsynaptic membrane. Dendritic spines increase dendritic area and may act as electrical or chemical compartments distinct from dendritic shafts. In particular, spines may localize postsynaptic $[Ca^{2+}]_i$ and downstream signaling molecules to individual synapses. In >90% of all excitatory synapses in the CNS, the postsynaptic site is a **dendritic spine** (Fig. 13.3). Dendritic spines increase dendritic area and may act as electrical or chemical compartments distinct from dendritic shafts. In particular, spines

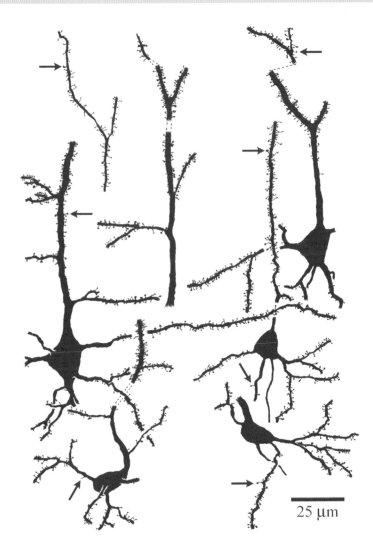

Figure. 13.3 Drawings of various dendrites in the neocortex, made from Golgi-stained material. The numerous protrusions are spines. (From Feldman ML: In Peters A, Jones EG [eds]: Cerebral Cortex: Cellular Components of the Cerebral Cortex, vol 1. New York, Plenum, 1984, pp 123–200.)

25 μm

may localize postsynaptic $[Ca^{2+}]_i$ and downstream signaling molecules to individual synapses.

Some transmitters are used by diffusely distributed systems of neurons to modulate the general excitability of the brain

The brain carries out many sensory, motor, and cognitive functions that require fast, specific, spatially organized neural connections and operations. Consider the detailed neural mapping that allows you to read this sentence or the precise timing required to play the piano. These functions require *spatially focused* networks (Fig. 13.4A).

Other functions, such as falling asleep, waking up, becoming attentive, or changing mood, involve more general alterations of the brain. Several **modulatory systems,** using different neurotransmitters, make diffuse synaptic connections to carry a simple message to vast regions of the brain, a *widely divergent* network (Fig. 13.4B). Both the activity of psychoactive drugs and the pathological processes of most psychiatric disorders seem to involve alterations in one or more of the modulatory systems.

The main modulatory systems of the brain are distinct anatomically and biochemically. Separate systems use norepinephrine, serotonin (5-hydroxytryptamine [5-HT]), dopamine, ACh, or histamine as their neurotransmitter. They all involve **metabotropic transmitter receptors** (see Fig. 8.3B). For example, the brain has 10 to 100 times more metabotropic muscarinic ACh receptors than ionotropic nicotinic ACh receptors. We briefly describe the anatomy and possible functions of each major system (Fig. 13.5).

⊚ **13-2 Norepinephrine**-containing neurons are in the tiny **locus coeruleus,** located bilaterally in the brainstem (Fig. 13.5A). Each human locus coeruleus has ~12,000 neurons. Axons from the locus coeruleus innervate just about every part of the brain: the entire cerebral cortex, the thalamus and hypothalamus, the olfactory bulb, the cerebellum, the midbrain, and the spinal cord. Just one of its neurons can make >250,000 synapses, and that cell can have one axon branch in the *cerebral* cortex and another in the *cerebellar* cortex! Locus coeruleus cells seem to be involved in the regulation of attention, arousal, and sleep-wake cycles as well as in learning and memory, anxiety and pain, mood, and brain metabolism. Locus coeruleus neurons are best activated by new, unexpected, nonpainful sensory stimuli in the animal's environment. The locus coeruleus may participate in general arousal of the brain during interesting events in the outside world.

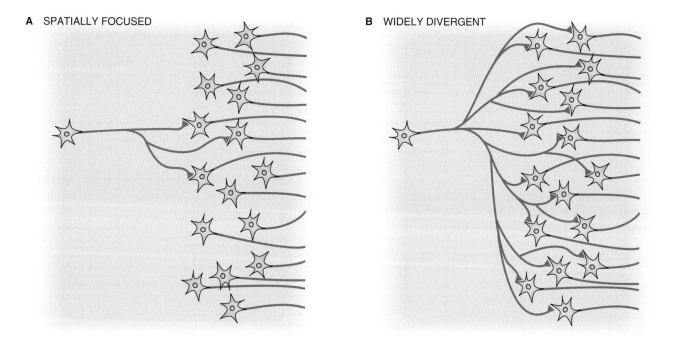

A SPATIALLY FOCUSED

B WIDELY DIVERGENT

Figure. 13.4 Synaptic connections.

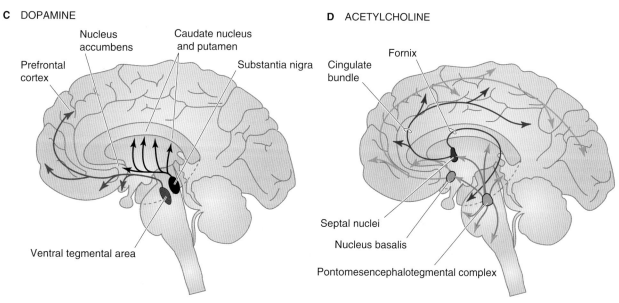

A NOREPINEPHRINE

Neocortex

Thalamus

Hypothalamus

Amygdala

Hippocampus

Locus coeruleus

To spinal cord

Cerebellum

B SEROTONIN

Basal ganglia

Raphé nuclei

C DOPAMINE

Prefrontal cortex

Nucleus accumbens

Caudate nucleus and putamen

Substantia nigra

Ventral tegmental area

D ACETYLCHOLINE

Fornix

Cingulate bundle

Septal nuclei

Nucleus basalis

Pontomesencephalotegmental complex

Figure. 13.5 Four diffusely connected systems of central neurons using modulatory transmitters.

⊙ **13-3 Serotonin**-containing neurons are mostly clustered within the nine **raphé nuclei** (Fig. 13.5B). Together they innervate most of the CNS in the same diffuse way as the locus coeruleus neurons. Similar to neurons of the locus coeruleus, cells of the raphé nuclei fire most rapidly during wakefulness, when an animal is aroused and active. The locus coeruleus and the raphé nuclei are part of the **ascending reticular activating system,** which arouses and awakens the forebrain. Raphé neurons seem to be intimately involved in the control of sleep-wake cycles as well as the different stages of sleep. Serotonergic raphé neurons have also been implicated in the control of mood and certain types of emotional behavior. Many hallucinogenic drugs, such as lysergic acid diethylamide (LSD), apparently exert their effects through interaction with serotonin receptors. Serotonin may also be involved in clinical depression; some of the most effective drugs now used to treat depression (e.g., fluoxetine [Prozac]) are potent blockers of serotonin reuptake and thus prolong its action in the brain.

⊙ **13-4** Although **dopamine**-containing neurons are scattered throughout the CNS, two closely related groups of dopaminergic cells have characteristics of the diffuse modulatory systems (Fig. 13.5C). One of these groups is the **substantia nigra** in the midbrain. Its cells project axons to the striatum, a part of the basal ganglia, and they facilitate the initiation of voluntary movement. Degeneration of the dopamine-containing cells in the substantia nigra produces the progressively worsening motor dysfunction of **Parkinson disease**. Another set of dopaminergic neurons lies in the **ventral tegmental area** of the midbrain; these neurons innervate the prefrontal cortex and parts of the limbic system. They have been implicated in reinforcement or reward as well as in aspects of drug addiction and psychiatric disorders, most notably schizophrenia. Antipsychotic drugs called neuroleptics are antagonists of certain dopamine receptors.

Acetylcholine is the familiar transmitter of the neuromuscular junction and the autonomic nervous system. Within the brain are two major diffuse modulatory cholinergic systems: the **basal forebrain complex** (which innervates the hippocampus and all of the neocortex) and the **pontomesencephalotegmental cholinergic complex** (which innervates the dorsal thalamus and parts of the forebrain) (Fig. 13.5D). They are involved in the regulation of general brain excitability during arousal and sleep-wake cycles, and in learning and memory formation.

Collectively, the diffuse modulatory systems may be viewed as providing general regulation of brain function. Because their axons spread so widely within the CNS, the few modulatory neurons can have an inordinately strong influence on behavior.

Electrical synapses serve specialized functions in the mammalian nervous system

Many cells are coupled to one another through gap junctions. If the first cell generates an action potential, current will flow through the gap junction channels and depolarize the second cell, as in the conduction of excitation across cardiac muscle. When gap junctions interconnect neurons, we describe them as electrical synapses.

Electrical synapses are extremely fast, are highly reliable, and can be bidirectional. However, electrical synapses tend to be outnumbered by chemical synapses.

Why are chemical synapses, as complex and relatively slow as they are, more prevalent than electrical synapses in the mature brain? One reason is **amplification.** Electrical synapses do not amplify the signal passed from one cell to the next; they can only diminish it. Thus, "synaptic strength" will be low. By contrast, a chemical synapse can trigger an amplifying cascade of molecular events and a relatively large postsynaptic change.

A second advantage of chemical synapses is their ability to either **excite** or **inhibit postsynaptic neurons selectively.** At an electrical synapse, a presynaptic depolarization can only depolarize the postsynaptic cell.

A third advantage of chemical synapses is that they can transmit information over a **broad time domain.** Chemical synapses can produce postsynaptic effects with time courses ranging from a few milliseconds to minutes and even hours.

Electrical synapses serve important but specialized functions in the nervous system. They seem to be most prevalent in neural circuits in which speed or a high degree of synchrony is at a premium. Gap junctions are also effective in diffusely spreading current through large networks of cells, which appears to be their function in photoreceptors and glia.

⊙ 13-5 NEUROTRANSMITTER SYSTEMS OF THE BRAIN

It is not enough to know the identity of a transmitter to predict its effect—one must also know the nature of the components that it interacts with, and these components may vary from one part of the brain to another and even between parts of a single neuron. This subchapter introduces the intricate and vital web of neurotransmitters. The clinical importance of the subject is difficult to overstate. Most drugs that alter mental function do so by interacting with neurotransmitter systems in the brain. Disorders of neurotransmitter systems are also implicated in many devastating brain disorders, such as schizophrenia, depression, epilepsy, Parkinson disease, the damage of stroke, and drug addiction.

Most of the brain's transmitters are common biochemicals

Most neurotransmitters are the standard chemicals of metabolism. Examples are the **amino acids** glutamate, aspartate, GABA, and glycine (Fig. 13.6A). Another important class of small neurotransmitters is the amines, including the **monoamines** (e.g., ACh, serotonin, and histamine) listed in Fig. 13.6B and the **catecholamines** (e.g., dopamine, norepinephrine, and epinephrine) listed in Fig. 13.6C. Neurons synthesize these small transmitters by adding only a few chemical steps to pathways that are present in every cell. **Purine derivatives** can also be important transmitters, notably ATP, the major chemical intermediate of energy metabolism. ATP acts on a variety of nucleotide receptors, both ionotropic and metabotropic. Adenosine is also a transmitter in the CNS.

The large-molecule transmitters, which constitute a much more numerous group, are proteins or small bits of protein called **neuroactive peptides.** A few of the better-studied neuropeptides are shown in Fig. 13.7. Among the neuroactive peptides are the **endorphins** (*endo*genous substances with *morphine*-like actions), which include small peptides called enkephalins. The term *opioids* refers to all substances with

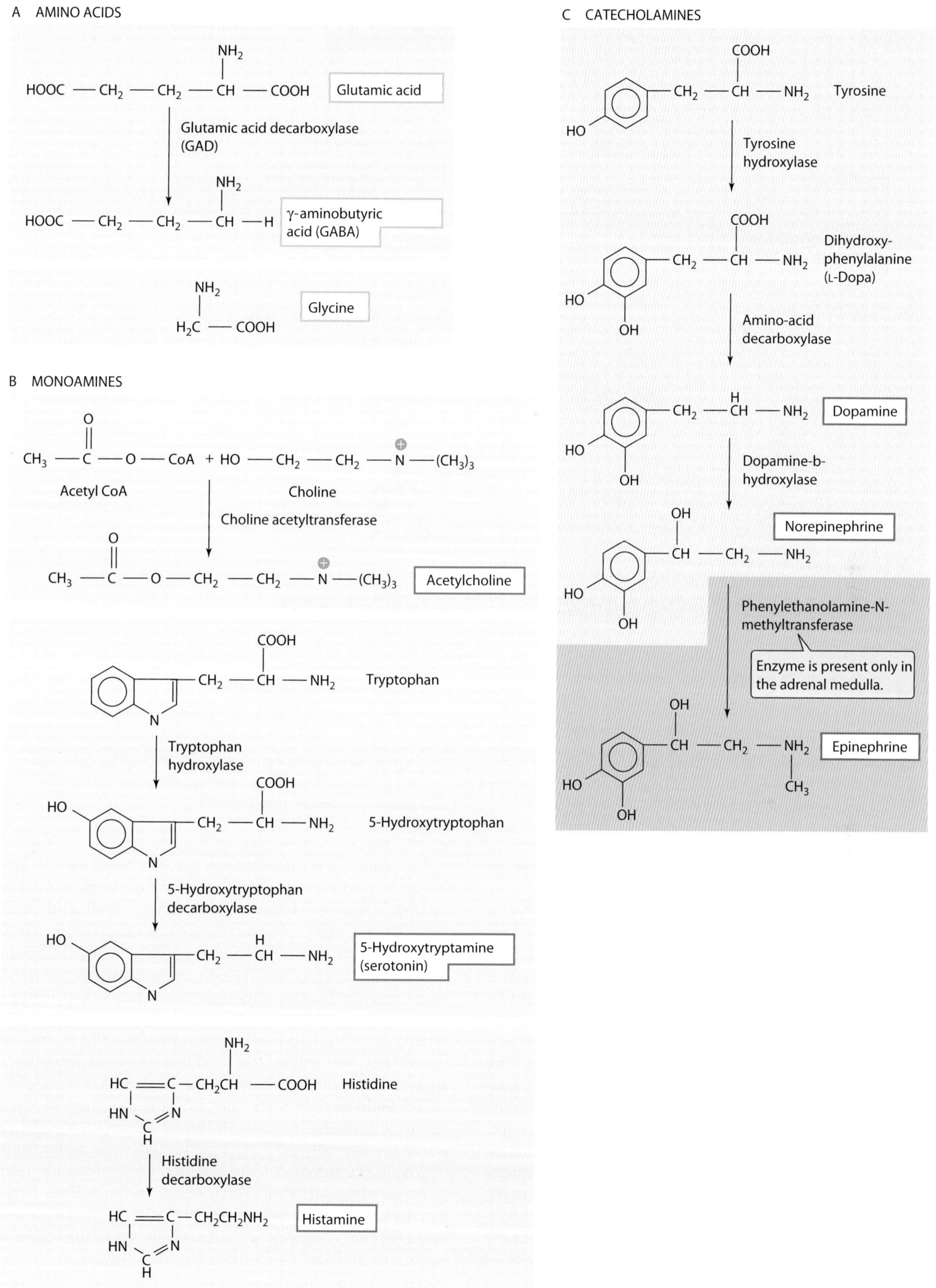

A AMINO ACIDS

C CATECHOLAMINES

B MONOAMINES

Figure. 13.6 Biosynthesis of some common small transmitter molecules. *CoA*, Coenzyme A.

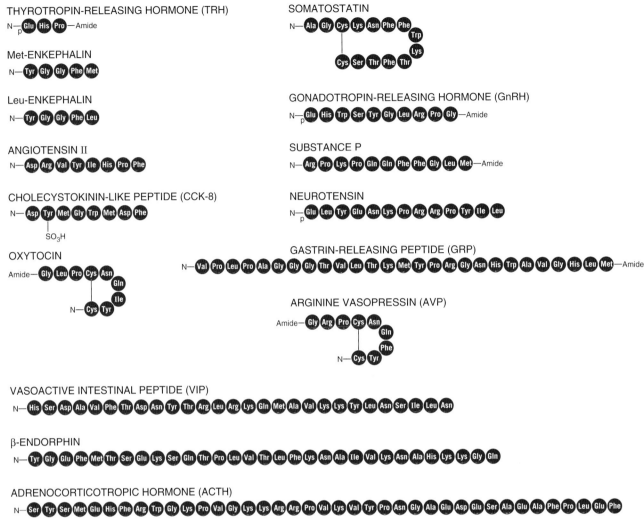

Figure. 13.7 Structure of some neuroactive peptides. All peptides are presented with their NH₂ termini to the left. The *p* on the amino-terminal glutamate on some of these peptides stands for pyroglutamate.

a morphine-like pharmacology—the endorphins (endogenous) as well as morphine and heroin (exogenous).

The synthesis of most neuropeptides begins like that of any other secretory protein, with the ribosome-directed assembly of a large **prehormone.** The prehormone is then cleaved to form a smaller **prohormone** in the Golgi apparatus and further reduced into small active neuropeptides that are packaged into vesicles. Thus, the synthesis of neuropeptides differs significantly from that of the small transmitters.

In summary, then, the neurotransmitters consist of both small molecules and peptides. The small transmitters are usually stored and released by separate sets of neurons, although some types of neurons do use two or more small transmitters. The peptides, however, are usually stored and released from the same neurons that use one of the small transmitters, an arrangement called **colocalization** of neurotransmitters. Thus, GABA may be paired with somatostatin in some synapses, serotonin and enkephalin in others, and so on. The colocalized transmitters may be released together, but of course each acts on its own receptors. In addition, both clear and dense-core vesicles contain ATP as well as their primary transmitter.

One unusual transmitter is a gaseous molecule, the labile free radical **nitric oxide (NO). Carbon monoxide (CO)** and hydrogen sulfide (H_2S) may also serve as transmitters. NO and CO can exert powerful biological effects by activating guanylyl cyclase, which converts GTP to cGMP. Because NO is *not* packaged into vesicles, its release does not require an increase in $[Ca^{2+}]_i$, although its synthesis does. NO may sometimes act as a retrograde messenger, that is, from postsynaptic to presynaptic structures. Because NO is small and membrane permeable, it can diffuse beyond immediately adjacent cells. On the other hand, NO breaks down rapidly.

The **endocannabinoids** are another unusual group of putative neurotransmitters. They include the endogenous lipophilic molecules anandamide and 2-arachidonoyl glycerol (2-AG), both of which are arachidonic acid metabolites. These substances mimic Δ^9-tetrahydrocannabinol (THC), the active ingredient in marijuana, by binding to and activating specific G protein–coupled "cannabinoid" receptors. Certain neurons synthesize and release endocannabinoids, which move readily across membranes to presynaptic terminals and modulate release of conventional transmitters. Activation of cannabinoid receptors with low doses of THC leads to euphoria, relaxed sensations, decreased pain,

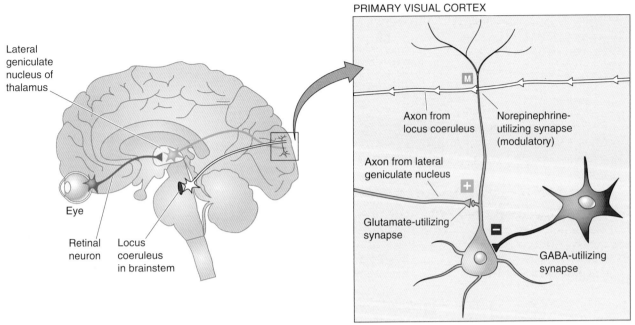

Figure. 13.8 Synaptic circuitry of the visual cortex. Visual pathways that originate in the retina activate neurons in the lateral geniculate nucleus of the thalamus. These glutamate-containing neurons in turn synapse on cortical pyramidal neurons and produce some *excitation*. Also within the primary visual cortex, a GABA-containing neuron mediates localized *inhibition*. Small cells in the locus coeruleus, a brainstem nucleus, make widely divergent connections onto cortical neurons and release norepinephrine and thus produce *modulation*.

and increased hunger; it can also impair problem-solving ability, short-term memory, and motor skills. High doses can alter personality and sometimes trigger hallucinations. THC and related drugs have promise for treatment of the nausea and vomiting of cancer patients undergoing chemotherapy, suppression of chronic pain, and stimulation of appetite in some patients with acquired immunodeficiency syndrome (AIDS).

Synaptic transmitters can stimulate, inhibit, or modulate the postsynaptic neuron

Each neuromuscular junction has a simple and stereotyped job: when an action potential fires in the motor neuron, the junction must reliably excite its muscle cell to fire an action potential and contract. Decisions about muscle contractions (where, when, and how much) are made within the CNS, and the neuromuscular junction exists simply to communicate that decision to the muscle unambiguously and reliably. To perform this function, neuromuscular transmission is failsafe under even the most extreme of physiological conditions.

Like neuromuscular junctions, some neuron-neuron synapses (**excitatory**) can rapidly excite. However, **inhibitory** synapses decrease postsynaptic excitability. In a third broad class of synapse (**modulatory**), the synapse often has little or no direct effect of its own but instead regulates or modifies the effect of other excitatory or inhibitory synapses by acting on either presynaptic or postsynaptic membranes. Typically, excitatory and inhibitory synapses act via ligand-gated ion channels, and modulatory synapses via GPCRs.

These three basic types of neural synapses are exemplified by their input to the *pyramidal neuron* of the cerebral cortex. In the example shown in Fig. 13.8, a pyramidal neuron in the visual cortex receives an excitatory synaptic input from the

thalamus (with glutamate as the neurotransmitter), an inhibitory synaptic input from an interneuron (with GABA as the neurotransmitter), and a modulatory input from the locus coeruleus (with norepinephrine as the neurotransmitter).

Excitatory Synapses Pyramidal cells receive excitatory inputs from many sources, including the axons of the thalamus. Most fast *excitatory synapses* in the brain use **glutamate** as their transmitter, and the thalamus–to–cerebral cortex synapses are no exception (Fig. 13.8). Such synapses are called **glutamatergic**. Glutamate-gated channels generate an **excitatory postsynaptic potential (EPSP)** that is very similar to the one produced by ACh at the neuromuscular junction (see ⦿ 8-5), except that it is usually much smaller than the EPSP in muscle. An EPSP from the activation of a *single* glutamatergic synapse in the cerebral cortex is typically ~1 mV, whereas one neuromuscular EPSP reaches a peak of ~40 mV. It takes the summation of EPSPs from many typical glutamatergic synapses to depolarize a postsynaptic neuron to the threshold for triggering an action potential.

Inhibitory Synapses Virtually all central neurons have numerous excitatory and inhibitory synapses. Thus, the excitability of neurons at any moment is governed by the dynamic balance of excitation and inhibition. **GABA** and **glycine** are the transmitters at the large majority of inhibitory synapses. Indeed, the inhibitory synapse between the interneuron and the pyramidal cell in Fig. 13.8 uses GABA. Both GABA and glycine bind to receptors that gate Cl^--selective channels (see ⦿ 13-6). Thus, the **reversal potential** for the Cl^--mediated **inhibitory postsynaptic potential (IPSP)** is the same as the E_{Cl}. If Cl^- conductance increases, the V_m has a tendency to move toward E_{Cl}. The effect is inhibitory because it tends to oppose other factors (mainly EPSPs) that might otherwise move the V_m toward or above the threshold for an action potential.

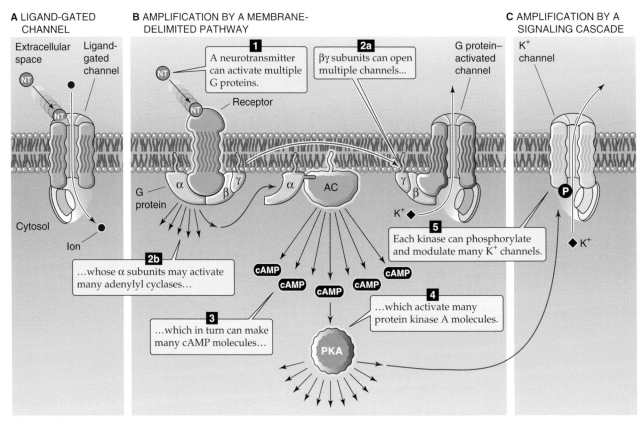

A LIGAND-GATED CHANNEL

B AMPLIFICATION BY A MEMBRANE-DELIMITED PATHWAY

C AMPLIFICATION BY A SIGNALING CASCADE

Figure. 13.9 Benefits of signal amplification. (A) The neurotransmitter (NT) binds directly to a channel, thereby activating it. (B) The neurotransmitter binds to a receptor that in turn activates 10 to 20 G proteins. In this example, each βγ subunit directly activates a K+ channel. In addition, each α subunit activates an adenylyl cyclase (AC) molecule, and each AC molecule produces many cAMP molecules that activate protein kinase A (PKA). (C) Each activated PKA molecule can phosphorylate and thereby modulate many channels.

Modulatory Synapses Many forms of *synaptic modulation* influence the nervous system (see ⊙ 13-8). As an example, consider the axons arising from the *locus coeruleus,* which synapse widely on pyramidal cells in the cerebral cortex (Fig. 13.5A). These axons release the transmitter **norepinephrine.** Norepinephrine acts on β adrenergic receptors in the pyramidal cell membrane. This effect of norepinephrine by itself has little influence on the activity of a resting neuron. However, a cell exposed to norepinephrine will react more powerfully when it is stimulated by a strong excitatory input (usually by glutamatergic synapses). Thus, norepinephrine *modulates* the cell's response to other inputs.

The molecular mechanisms of **neuromodulators** begin with a GPCR that activates an intracellular signal cascade (see ⊙ 3-3). Binding of norepinephrine to the β adrenergic receptor stimulates the intracellular enzyme adenylyl cyclase, which increases intracellular levels of cAMP (the second messenger), which in turn stimulates other enzymes to increase their rates of phosphorylation. Within the cortical neuron, phosphorylation of one or more types of K+ channel decreases the probability of the channels' being open (see ⊙ 6-4). Fewer open K+ channels mean higher membrane resistance, greater excitability, and less adaptation of spike firing rates during prolonged stimuli. Other effects are generated when norepinephrine activates other subtypes of adrenergic receptors and thus different second-messenger systems. Modulatory transmitters allow the nervous system to vary its state of excitability.

G proteins may affect ion channels directly, or indirectly through second messengers

GPCRs exist in every cell (see ⊙ 3-3). In the preceding section we described one example, the receptor for norepinephrine and its second messenger–mediated effect on certain K+ channels. However, norepinephrine alone has at least five major receptor types—two α receptors and three β receptors—that act on numerous effectors (see Table 14.2). In fact, each transmitter has multiple GPCRs, and their effects engage almost all aspects of cell function through several intracellular messenger systems. GPCRs can recognize a wide range of transmitter types, from small molecules to peptides.

The first—and simplest—G-protein cascade involves a direct linkage from the receptor to the G protein to the channel and is sometimes called the **membrane-delimited pathway.** For example, in heart muscle, ACh binds to a muscarinic ACh receptor (M_2) that activates a G protein, the βγ subunits of which in turn cause a K+ channel to open (Fig. 13.9B). Other receptors in various cells can modulate other K+ and Ca²⁺ channels in a similar way.

The membrane-delimited pathway is relatively fast, beginning within 30 to 100 ms—not quite as fast as a ligand-gated channel, but faster than the many-messenger cascades described next. The membrane-delimited pathway is also localized in comparison to the other cascades. Because the G protein cannot diffuse very far within the membrane, only channels nearby can be affected.

The other general type of G-protein signaling involves enzyme systems and second messengers, often diffusing through the cytoplasm, to influence an ion channel. Two or more cascades, each with different types of messengers, may sometimes be activated by one type of receptor (an example of *divergence*).

In Chapter 3, we discussed three of these longer, and slower, G-protein signal cascades: (1) the adenylyl cyclase pathway, (2) the phospholipase C pathway, and (3) the phospholipase A_2 pathway. Some of these messengers dissolve in the watery cytoplasm, whereas others diffuse within the fatty lipid bilayer. The final link in most of the messenger cascades is a **kinase.**

Protein phosphatases act rapidly to remove phosphate groups, and thus the degree of phosphorylation depends on the dynamic balance of phosphorylation and dephosphorylation.

Signaling cascades allow amplification, regulation, and a long duration of transmitter responses

At this point you may be wondering about the perversity of such complex, interconnected, indirect messenger cascades. Do these long chains of command have any benefit? Why not use simple, fast, ligand-gated channels (Fig. 13.9A) for all transmitter purposes? In fact, complex messenger cascades seem to have advantages.

One important advantage is *amplification*. When activated, one ligand-gated channel is just that: one ion channel in one place. However, when activated, one GPCR potentially influences many channels. Signal amplification can occur at several places in the cascade. One stimulated receptor can activate perhaps 10 to 20 G proteins, each of which can activate a channel by a membrane-delimited pathway such as the $\beta\gamma$ pathway (Fig. 13.9B). Alternatively, the α subunit of one G protein can activate an adenylyl cyclase, which can make many cAMP molecules, and the cAMP molecules can spread to activate many kinases; each kinase can then phosphorylate many channels (Fig. 13.9C). The use of small messengers that can diffuse quickly also allows signaling at a distance, over a wide stretch of cell membrane. Signaling cascades also provide many sites for further *regulation* as well as interaction between cascades. Finally, signal cascades can generate *long-lasting chemical changes* in cells, which may form the basis for, among other things, a lifetime of memories.

Neurotransmitters may have both convergent and divergent effects

Divergence means that one transmitter can affect different neurons (or even different parts of the same neuron) in very different ways, using different receptors or different downstream signaling pathways (Fig. 13.10A). Divergence may occur at any stage in the cascade of transmitter effects.

Neurotransmitters can also exhibit **convergence** of effects. This means that multiple transmitters, each activating its own receptor type, converge on a single type of ion channel in a single cell (Fig. 13.10B). Analogous to divergence, the molecular site of convergence may occur at a common second-messenger system, or different second messengers may converge on the same ion channel.

A DIVERGENT TRANSMITTER ACTIONS

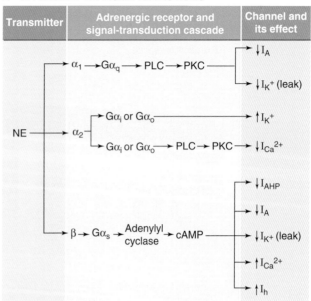

B CONVERGENT TRANSMITTER ACTIONS

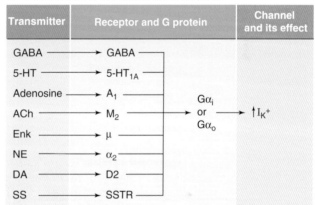

Figure. 13.10 Divergence and convergence of transmitter effects on channels. *DA,* Dopamine; *Enk,* enkephalin; *PKC,* protein kinase C; *PLC,* phospholipase C; *SS,* somatostatin; *SSTR,* somatostatin receptor.

FAST AMINO ACID–MEDIATED SYNAPSES IN THE CNS

Fast amino acid–mediated synapses account for most of the neural activity that we associate with specific information processing in the brain: events directly responsible for sensory perception, motor control, and cognition, for example. Glutamate-mediated excitation and GABA-mediated inhibition are the best understood of the brain's synapses.

Most EPSPs in the brain are mediated by two types of glutamate-gated channels

Glutamate can act on two major classes of receptors: GPCRs or *metabotropic* receptors, and ion channels or *ionotropic* receptors. As noted above, **metabotropic glutamate receptors (mGluRs**—the *m* stands for metabotropic) have seven membrane-spanning segments and are linked to heterotrimeric G proteins (Fig. 13.11A).

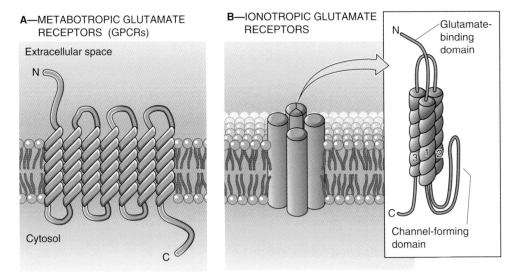

A—METABOTROPIC GLUTAMATE RECEPTORS (GPCRs)

Extracellular space

N

Cytosol

C

B—IONOTROPIC GLUTAMATE RECEPTORS

N

Glutamate-binding domain

3 1 2

C

Channel-forming domain

Figure. 13.11 Comparison of ionotropic and metabotropic glutamate receptors. In (B) the *inset* shows a prototypic subunit, with a large extracellular glutamate-binding domain, a membrane-spanning segment, a short loop that partially re-enters the membrane from the cytosolic side, and two more membrane-spanning segments. Four of these subunits appear to come together to form a single channel/receptor with a central pore.

TABLE 13.1 Ionotropic Glutamate Receptors

CLASS OF RECEPTOR	AGONIST	ANTAGONIST	KINETICS	PERMEABILITY
AMPA Genes: *GRIA* Proteins: GluA	α-amino-3-hydroxy-5-methyl-4-isoxazole propionic acid	CNQX (6-cyano-7-nitroquinoxaline-2,3-dione) GYKI 53655 (2,3-benzodiazepine derivatives)	Fast	Na^+, K^+ (Ca^{2+} in a few cases)
Kainate Genes: *GRIK* Proteins: GluK	Kainic acid Domoic acid	CNQX UBP 296 [(RS)-1-(2-amino-2-carboxyethyl)-3-(2-carboxybenzyl)pyrimidine-2,4-dione]	Fast	Na^+, K^+
NMDA Genes: *GRIN* Proteins: GluN	*N*-methyl-D-aspartate	APV (2-amino-5-phosphonovaleric acid)	Slow	Na^+, K^+, Ca^{2+}

The three classes of **ionotropic glutamate receptors** are the AMPA, NMDA, and kainate receptors (Table 13.1). They are activated by binding glutamate, but their pharmacology and functions differ. The receptor names are derived from their relatively specific agonists and can also be distinguished by selective antagonists.

Ionotropic glutamate receptors are constructed from ~14 different subunits. Each of these has a large extracellular glutamate-binding domain, followed by a transmembrane segment, a loop that partially enters the membrane from the cytosolic side, and then two more transmembrane segments (Fig. 13.11B). The loop appears to line the channel pore. The receptors are heterotetramers, with four subunits arranged around a central channel.

Most glutamate-mediated synapses generate an EPSP with two temporal components (Fig. 13.12A and C). The two phases have different pharmacological profiles, kinetics, voltage dependencies, ion dependencies, and permeabilities, and serve distinct functions in the brain. The faster phase is mediated by an AMPA-type glutamate receptor and the slower phase by an NMDA-type glutamate receptor. Both AMPA and NMDA receptors have nearly equal permeability to Na^+ and K^+.

AMPA-gated channels are found in most excitatory synapses in the brain, and they mediate fast excitation, with most types of AMPA channels normally letting very little Ca^{2+} into cells. They show little voltage dependence.

NMDA-gated channels have more complex behavior and slower kinetics. The ion selectivity of NMDA channels is the key to their functions: permeability to Na^+ and K^+ causes depolarization and thus excitation of a cell, but their high permeability to Ca^{2+} allows them to influence $[Ca^{2+}]_i$ significantly. It is difficult to overstate the importance of intracellular $[Ca^{2+}]$. Ca^{2+} can activate many enzymes, regulate the opening of a variety of channels, and affect the expression of genes. Excess Ca^{2+} can even precipitate the death of a cell.

The gating of NMDA channels is unusual: at normal resting voltage (about −70 mV), the channel is clogged by Mg^{2+}, and few ions pass through it; the Mg^{2+} pops out only when the membrane is depolarized above about −60 mV. Thus, the NMDA channel is **voltage dependent** in addition to being ligand gated; both glutamate and a relatively

A EPSP AT –80 mV

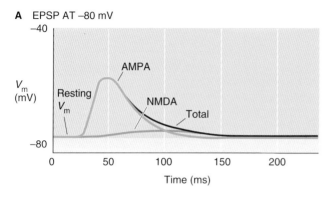

C EPSP AT –40 mV

B ONLY AMPA RECEPTOR CHANNEL OPEN

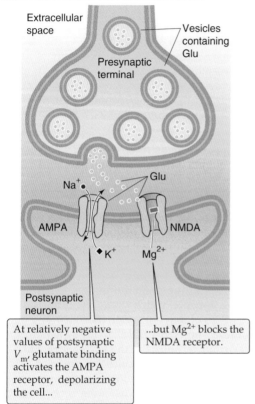

At relatively negative values of postsynaptic V_m, glutamate binding activates the AMPA receptor, depolarizing the cell...

...but Mg^{2+} blocks the NMDA receptor.

D AMPA AND NMDA RECEPTOR CHANNELS OPEN

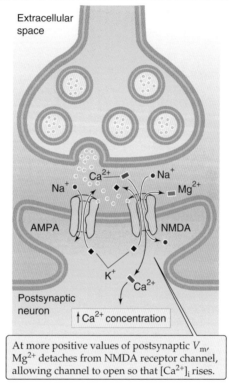

At more positive values of postsynaptic V_m, Mg^{2+} detaches from NMDA receptor channel, allowing channel to open so that [Ca^{2+}]$_i$ rises.

Figure. 13.12 Glutamate-gated channels. (A) At most glutamate-mediated synapses, the EPSP (*red curve*) is the sum of two components: (1) a rapid component that is mediated by an AMPA receptor (*green curve*) and (2) a slow component that is mediated by an NMDA receptor (*orange curve*). In this example, in which the postsynaptic V_m is relatively negative, the contribution of the NMDA receptor is very small. (B) At a relatively negative initial V_m in the postsynaptic cell, as in (A), the NMDA receptor does not open. The AMPA receptor, which is independent of postsynaptic V_m, opens. The result is a fast depolarization. (C) In this example, in which the postsynaptic V_m is relatively positive, the contribution of the NMDA receptor is fairly large. (D) At a relatively positive initial V_m in the postsynaptic cell, as in (C), glutamate activates both the AMPA and the NMDA receptors. The recruitment of the NMDA receptors is important because, unlike most AMPA receptors, they allow the entry of Ca^{2+} and have slower kinetics.

positive V_m are necessary for the channel to open. How do the NMDA-gated channels open? NMDA-gated channels coexist with AMPA-gated channels in many synapses of the brain. When the postsynaptic cell is at a relatively negative resting potential (Fig. 13.12A and B), the glutamate released from a synaptic terminal can open the AMPA-gated channel, which is voltage independent, but not the NMDA-gated channel. However, when the postsynaptic cell is more depolarized because of the action of other synapses (Fig. 13.12C and D), the larger depolarization of the

postsynaptic membrane allows the NMDA-gated channel to open by relieving its Mg^{2+} block. NMDA channels open only after the membrane has been sufficiently depolarized by the action of the faster AMPA channels from many simultaneously active synapses.

Kainate-gated channels may contribute to glutamate-mediated EPSPs in specific neuron types. The kainate receptor channels also exist on presynaptic GABAergic and glutamatergic terminals, where they regulate transmitter release.

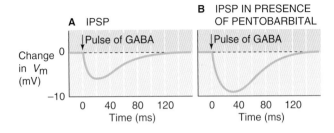

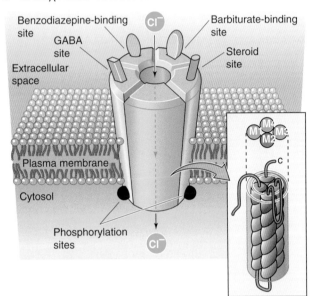

Figure. 13.13 Physiology and structure of the GABA$_A$ receptor channel. (A) When a pulse of GABA is released from a synapse, it elicits a small IPSP. (B) In the presence of a low dose of pentobarbital, the pulse of synaptic GABA elicits a much larger IPSP. Thus, the barbiturate enhances inhibition. (C) The channel receptor is a heteropentamer. It has not only a pore for Cl$^-$ but also separate binding sites for GABA and several classes of channel modulators. The *inset* shows the presumed structure of one of the five monomers. The M2 domain of each of the five subunits presumably lines the central channel pore.

Most IPSPs in the brain are mediated by the GABA$_A$ receptor, which is activated by several classes of drugs

GABA mediates the bulk of fast synaptic inhibition in the CNS, and glycine mediates most of the rest. Both the GABA$_A$ receptor and the glycine receptor are ionotropic receptors that are Cl$^-$-selective channels. GABA can also activate the GABA$_B$ receptor, which is a GPCR or *metabotropic* receptor.

Synaptic inhibition must be tightly regulated in the brain. Too much inhibition causes sedation, loss of consciousness, and coma, whereas too little leads to anxiety, hyperexcitability, and seizures. The need to control inhibition may explain why the GABA$_A$ receptor channel has, in addition to its GABA binding site, several other sites where chemicals can bind and thus dramatically modulate the function of the GABA$_A$ receptor channel. For example, two classes of drugs, **benzodiazepines** (one of which is the tranquilizer diazepam [Valium]) and **barbiturates** (e.g., the sedative phenobarbital), each bind to their own specific sites on the outside face of the GABA$_A$ receptor channel. By themselves, these drugs do very little to the channel's activity. However, when GABA is around,

benzodiazepines increase the *frequency* of channel opening, whereas barbiturates increase the *duration* of channel opening. Fig. 13.13 shows the effects of barbiturates on the IPSP.

Some steroids modulate the GABA$_A$ receptor in a manner similar to barbiturates—directly, through binding sites that are distinct from the other drug-binding sites on the GABA$_A$ receptor.

◉ 13-6 The ionotropic receptors for ACh, serotonin, GABA, and glycine belong to the superfamily of ligand-gated/pentameric channels

Even though the receptors for ACh, serotonin, GABA, and glycine are gated by such different ligands and have such different permeabilities, they have the same overall structure: five protein subunits, with each subunit being made up of four membrane-spanning segments.

Not *all* ligand-gated channels belong to the same superfamily. We have already seen that the family of ionotropic glutamate receptors is distinct from the family of ligand-gated/pentameric channels. P2X purinergic receptors for ATP have only two membrane-spanning segments, and a full channel comprises just three subunits.

Most neuronal synapses release a very small number of transmitter quanta with each action potential

A single neuromuscular junction has ~1000 active zones (see ◉ 8-4). A single presynaptic impulse releases 100 to 200 quanta of transmitter molecules, which generates an EPSP of >40 mV. The total number of quanta is far more than necessary to cause the muscle cell to fire an action potential and contract. Evolution has designed a neuromuscular junction that works every time, with a large margin of excess for safety. Synapses in the brain are quite different. A typical glutamatergic synapse, which has as few as one active zone, generates EPSPs of only ~1 mV. In most neurons, one EPSP does not cause a postsynaptic cell to fire an action potential.

Most synaptic terminals in the CNS release only a small number of transmitter molecules per impulse, often just those contained in a single quantum. Furthermore, the probability of release of that single quantum is often less than 1; in other words, a presynaptic action potential often results in the release of no transmitter at all.

Because most glutamatergic synapses in the brain contribute such a weak excitatory effect, it may require the nearly simultaneous action of many synapses (and the summation of their EPSPs) to bring the postsynaptic membrane potential above the threshold for an action potential. *The threshold number of synapses varies greatly among neurons, but it is roughly in the range of 10 to 100.*

◉ 13-7 When multiple transmitters colocalize to the same synapse, the exocytosis of large vesicles requires high-frequency stimulation

Some presynaptic terminals have two or more transmitters colocalized within them. In these cases, the small transmitters are packaged into relatively small vesicles (~40 nm in diameter), whereas neuropeptides are in larger dense-core vesicles (100 to 200 nm in diameter), as noted above. This dual-packaging scheme allows the neuron some control over

B LOW-FREQUENCY STIMULATION

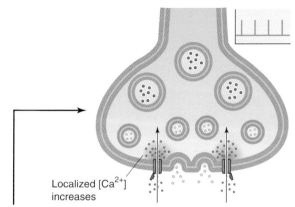

Localized [Ca^{2+}]
increases

A PRESYNAPTIC TERMINAL AT REST

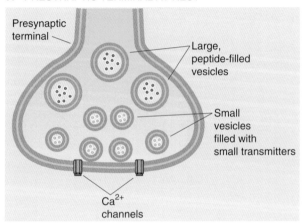

Presynaptic
terminal

Large,
peptide-filled
vesicles

Small
vesicles
filled with
small transmitters

Ca^{2+}
channels

C HIGH-FREQUENCY STIMULATION

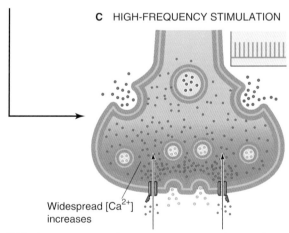

Widespread [Ca^{2+}]
increases

Figure. 13.14 Selective release of colocalized small transmitters and neuroactive peptides. (A) The presynaptic terminal at rest is filled with small vesicles (containing small transmitter molecules) and large dense-core vesicles (containing neuroactive peptides). (B) Fusion of small vesicles containing small transmitters. (C) Fusion of large, dense-core vesicles.

the relative release rates of its two types of transmitters (Fig. 13.14A). In general, **low-frequency stimulation** of the presynaptic terminal triggers the release of only the small transmitter (Fig. 13.14B); co-release of both transmitters requires bursts of **high-frequency stimulation** (Fig. 13.14C). Larger peptide-filled vesicles are farther from active zones, and high-frequency stimulation may be necessary to achieve higher, more distributed elevations of [Ca^{2+}]$_i$.

A RESPONSE TO HIGH-FREQUENCY STIMULATION

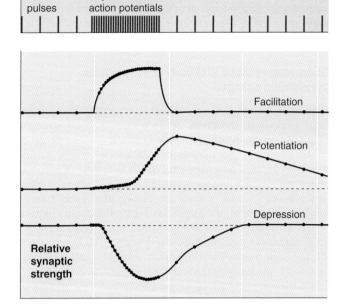

Test
pulses

Rapid train of
action potentials

Facilitation

Potentiation

Depression

**Relative
synaptic
strength**

B RESPONSE TO LOW-FREQUENCY STIMULATION

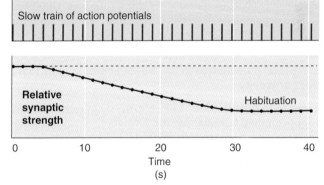

Slow train of action potentials

**Relative
synaptic
strength**

Habituation

0   10   20   30   40
Time
(s)

Figure. 13.15 Facilitation, potentiation, depression, and habituation. (Data from Levitan IB, Kaczmarek LK: The Neuron: Cell and Molecular Biology, 2nd ed. New York, Oxford University Press, 1997.)

PLASTICITY OF CENTRAL SYNAPSES

Use-dependent changes in synaptic strength underlie many forms of learning

⊙ **13-8** Arguably the greatest achievement of a brain is its ability to learn and to store the experience and events of the past so that it is better adapted to deal with the future. No single mechanism can explain all forms of memory. However, synapses are the physical site of many if not most forms of memory storage in the brain. The **synaptic strength** of many synapses may depend on their previous activity. This is all we need to build memory into a neural circuit.

Some forms of memory last just a few seconds or minutes, only to be lost or replaced by new memories. **Working memory** is an example. It is the continual series of fleeting memories that we use during the course of a day to remember facts and events, what was just spoken to us, where we put the phone down, whether we are coming or going—things that are useful for the moment but need not be stored longer. Other forms of memory may last for hours to decades and strongly resist disruption and replacement. Such **long-term memory** allows the accumulation of knowledge over a lifetime. Some memories may be formed after only a single trial (recall a particularly dramatic but unique event in your life), whereas others form only with repeated practice (examples include speaking a language or playing a guitar).

Short-term synaptic plasticity usually reflects presynaptic changes

Repetitive stimulation of neuronal synapses often yields brief periods of increased or decreased synaptic strength (Fig. 13.15): **facilitation** (which lasts tens to hundreds of milliseconds), **augmentation** (which lasts several seconds), and **post-tetanic potentiation** (which lasts tens of seconds to several minutes and outlasts the period of high-frequency stimulation). Not all of them are expressed at every type of synapse. In general, the longer-lasting modifications require longer periods of conditioning stimuli. Short-term *decreases* in synaptic strength include **depression,** which can occur during high-frequency stimulation, and **habituation,** which is a slowly progressing decrease that occurs during relatively low-frequency activation.

In principle, synaptic plasticity could result from either presynaptic changes (e.g., transmitter release), postsynaptic chances (e.g., sensitivity to the neurotransmitter), or both. Presynaptic changes appear to be more common. The cooperative dependence of transmitter release on $[Ca^{2+}]_i$ allows small changes in $[Ca^{2+}]_i$ to have large effects on release.

Long-term potentiation in the hippocampus may last for days or weeks

Long-term potentiation (LTP) is easily demonstrated in the **hippocampus,** essential for the formation of certain long-term memories. The induction of LTP has several interesting features that enhance its candidacy as a memory mechanism. First, it is **input specific,** which means that only the activated set of synapses onto a particular cell will be potentiated, whereas unactivated synapses to that same neuron remain unpotentiated. Second, induction of LTP requires coincident activity of the presynaptic terminals plus significant depolarization of the postsynaptic membrane—**cooperativity.**

The molecular mechanisms of one form of LTP in a particular region of the hippocampus have been partially elucidated. The synapse uses glutamate as its transmitter, and both AMPA and NMDA receptors are activated to generate an EPSP. Induction of LTP depends on an increase in *post*synaptic $[Ca^{2+}]_i$ levels beyond a critical level and lasting for about 1 to 2 seconds. Postsynaptic $[Ca^{2+}]_i$ levels rise during a tetanic stimulus because of the activation of NMDA receptors, the only type of glutamate-activated channel that is usually permeable to Ca^{2+} (Fig. 13.12). Recall also that the NMDA-type glutamate receptor channel is voltage dependent. If activation is strong (as it is when multiple inputs cooperate or when tetanus occurs), V_m becomes positive enough to allow NMDA channels to open. The stimulus-induced rise in postsynaptic $[Ca^{2+}]_i$ activates at least one essential kinase: **CaMKII** (see ⊙ 3-16). Expression of LTP involves the recruitment of more AMPA receptors to the postsynaptic membrane. LTP can be observed in some but not all other synapses, sometimes involving different molecular mechanisms.

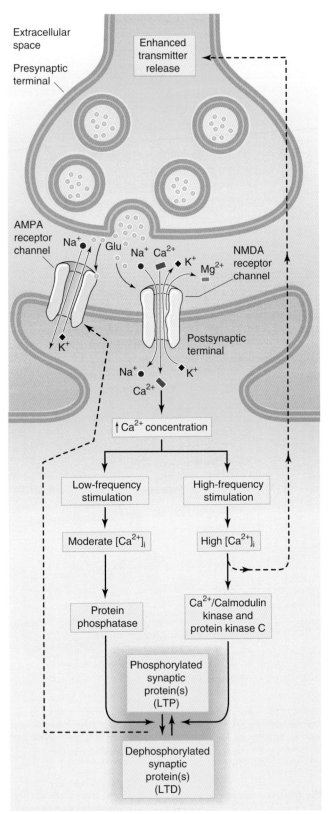

Figure. 13.16 Proposed molecular mechanism for LTP and LTD in one type of hippocampal synapse. Glutamate release from the presynaptic terminal activates NMDA receptor channels, which allow Ca^{2+} to enter the postsynaptic cell as well as AMPA receptor channels. One hypothetical pathway has the phosphorylated/dephosphorylated synaptic proteins modulating the AMPA receptor channel.

One form of long-term depression operates on the same hippocampal synapse as LTP

Memory systems may have mechanisms not only to increase synaptic strength but also to decrease it. In fact, **long-term depression (LTD)** can be induced in the same synapses within the hippocampus that generate the $[Ca^{2+}]_i$-dependent LTP described in the preceding section. The critical feature is the frequency of stimulation. For example, several hundred stimuli delivered at 50 Hz produce LTP, the same number delivered at 10 Hz has little effect, and at 1 Hz they produce LTD. One set of synapses can be strengthened or weakened repeatedly, which suggests that each process (LTP and LTD) acts on the same molecular component of the synapses.

LTD induced in this way shows the same input specificity as LTP—only the stimulated synapses onto a cell are depressed.

The key determinant of whether a tetanic stimulus induces LTP or LTD may be the level to which postsynaptic $[Ca^{2+}]_i$ rises. Fig. 13.16 illustrates a simple model of the induction mechanisms for LTD and LTP. Synaptic activation releases glutamate, which activates NMDA receptors, which in turn allow Ca^{2+} to enter the postsynaptic cell. In the case of high-frequency stimulation, postsynaptic $[Ca^{2+}]_i$ rises to very high levels; if stimulation is of low frequency, the rise in postsynaptic $[Ca^{2+}]_i$ is more modest. High levels of $[Ca^{2+}]_i$ lead to a net activation of protein *kinases,* whereas modest levels of $[Ca^{2+}]_i$ preferentially activate protein *phosphatases,* perhaps calcineurin.

CHAPTER 14

THE AUTONOMIC NERVOUS SYSTEM

George B. Richerson

The conscious and discontinuous nature of cortical brain function stands in sharp contrast to that of those parts of the nervous system responsible for control of our internal environment. These "autonomic" processes never stop attending to the wide range of metabolic, cardiopulmonary, and other visceral requirements of our body. Autonomic control continues whether we are awake and attentive, preoccupied with other activities, or asleep. We are unaware of most visceral sensory input, and we avoid any conscious effort to act on it unless it induces distress. In most cases, we have no awareness of motor commands to the viscera, and most individuals can exert voluntary control over visceral motor output in only minor ways. Consciousness and memory are frequently considered the most important functions of the human nervous system, but it is the visceral control system—including the **autonomic nervous system (ANS)**—that makes life and higher cortical function possible.

ORGANIZATION OF THE VISCERAL CONTROL SYSTEM

The ANS has sympathetic, parasympathetic, and enteric divisions

Output from the central nervous system (CNS) travels along two anatomically and functionally distinct pathways: the **somatic motor neurons,** which innervate striated skeletal muscle; and the **autonomic motor neurons,** which innervate smooth muscle, cardiac muscle, secretory epithelia, and glands. All viscera are richly supplied by efferent axons from the ANS that constantly adjust organ function.

The autonomic nervous system is the local nervous system of the gut and the efferent neurons innervating glands and involuntary muscle. In addition, the ANS includes visceral *afferents* as well as from those parts of the CNS that control the motor output of the ANS.

The ANS has three divisions: sympathetic, parasympathetic, and enteric. The **sympathetic** and **parasympathetic divisions** of the ANS are the two major efferent pathways controlling targets other than skeletal muscle. Each innervates target tissue by a two-synapse pathway (Fig. 14.1). The cell bodies of the first neurons lie within the CNS. These **preganglionic neurons** are found in columns of cells in the brainstem and spinal cord, and send axons out of the CNS to make synapses with **postganglionic neurons** in peripheral ganglia interposed between the CNS and their target cells. Axons from these postganglionic neurons then project to

their targets. The sympathetic and parasympathetic divisions often act in opposite ways, like an accelerator and brake to regulate visceral function. An increase in output of the sympathetic division occurs under conditions such as stress, anxiety, physical activity, fear, or excitement, whereas parasympathetic output increases during sedentary activity, eating, or other "vegetative" behavior.

⊙ **14-1** The **enteric division** of the ANS is a collection of afferent neurons, interneurons, and motor neurons that form networks of neurons called **plexuses** that surround the gastrointestinal (GI) tract. The enteric division is under the control of the CNS through sympathetic and parasympathetic fibers.

Sympathetic preganglionic neurons originate from spinal segments T1 to L3 and synapse with postganglionic neurons in paravertebral or prevertebral ganglia

Preganglionic Neurons The cell bodies of preganglionic sympathetic motor neurons are located in the thoracic and upper lumbar spinal cord between levels T1 and L3. At these spinal levels, autonomic neurons lie in the **intermediolateral cell column,** or lateral horn, between the dorsal and ventral horns (Fig. 14.2). Axons from preganglionic sympathetic neurons exit the spinal cord through the ventral roots along with axons from *somatic* motor neurons. After entering the spinal nerves, sympathetic efferents diverge from somatic motor axons to enter the white **rami communicantes.** These rami, or branches, are white because most preganglionic sympathetic axons are myelinated.

Paravertebral Ganglia Axons from preganglionic neurons enter the nearest sympathetic paravertebral ganglion through a white ramus. These ganglia lie adjacent to the vertebral column. Although preganglionic sympathetic fibers emerge only from levels T1 to L3, the chain of sympathetic ganglia extends all the way from the upper part of the neck to the coccyx. In general, one ganglion is positioned at the level of each spinal root, but adjacent ganglia are fused in some cases. The most rostral ganglion, the **superior cervical ganglion,** arises from fusion of C1 to C4 and supplies the head and neck. The next two ganglia are the **middle cervical ganglion,** which arises from fusion of C5 and C6, and the **inferior cervical ganglion** (C7 and C8), which is usually fused with the first thoracic ganglion to form the **stellate ganglion.**

After entering a paravertebral ganglion, a preganglionic sympathetic axon has one or more of three fates. It may

(1) synapse within that segmental paravertebral ganglion, (2) travel up or down the sympathetic chain to synapse within a neighboring paravertebral ganglion, or (3) enter the greater or lesser splanchnic nerve to synapse within one of the ganglia of the *pre*vertebral plexus.

Prevertebral Ganglia The **prevertebral plexus** lies in front of the aorta and along its major arterial branches, and includes the prevertebral ganglia and interconnected fibers (Fig. 14.3).

Each *pre*ganglionic sympathetic fiber synapses on ~200 *post*ganglionic sympathetic neurons in paravertebral or prevertebral ganglia.

Postganglionic Neurons The cell bodies of postganglionic sympathetic neurons that are located within *para*vertebral ganglia send out their axons through the nearest **gray rami communicantes,** which rejoin the spinal nerves (Fig. 14.2). These rami are gray because most postganglionic axons are unmyelinated. Because the paravertebral and prevertebral sympathetic ganglia lie near the spinal cord and thus relatively far from their target organs, the postganglionic axons of the sympathetic division tend to be long. On their way to reach their targets, some postganglionic sympathetic axons travel through *para*sympathetic terminal ganglia or cranial nerve ganglia without synapsing.

Parasympathetic preganglionic neurons originate from the brainstem and sacral spinal cord and synapse with postganglionic neurons in ganglia located near target organs.

The cell bodies of preganglionic parasympathetic neurons are located in the medulla, pons, and midbrain and in the S2 through S4 levels of the spinal cord (Fig. 14.4, right panel). Thus, unlike the sympathetic—or **thoracolumbar**—division, whose preganglionic cell bodies are in the thoracic and lumbar spinal cord, the parasympathetic—or **craniosacral**—division's preganglionic cell bodies are cranial and sacral. The preganglionic parasympathetic fibers originating in the brain distribute with four cranial nerves (III, VII, IX, and X).

Postganglionic parasympathetic neurons are located in **terminal ganglia** that are more peripherally located and more widely distributed than are the sympathetic ganglia. Terminal

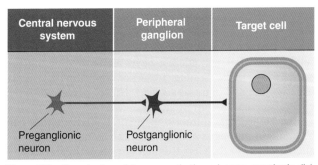

Figure 14.1 Organization of the sympathetic and parasympathetic divisions of the ANS.

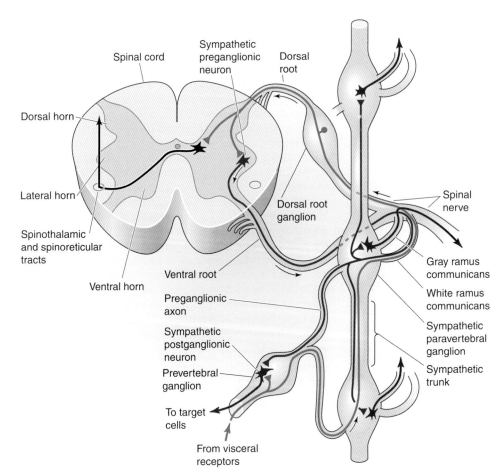

Figure 14.2 Anatomy of the sympathetic division of the ANS. The figure shows a cross section of the thoracic spinal cord and the nearby paravertebral ganglia as well as a prevertebral ganglion. Sympathetic preganglionic neurons are shown in *red* and postganglionic neurons in *dark blue-violet*. Afferent (sensory) pathways are in *blue*. Interneurons are shown in *black*.

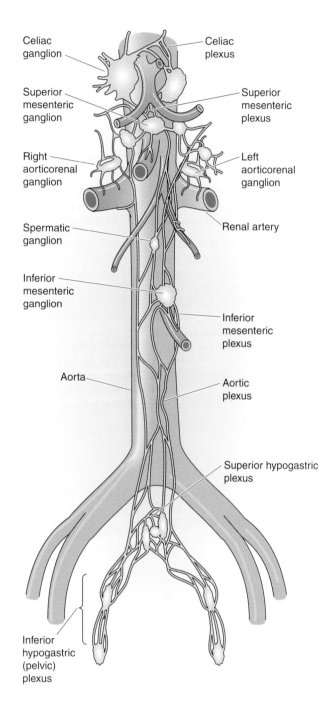

Celiac ganglion

Celiac plexus

Superior mesenteric ganglion

Superior mesenteric plexus

Right aorticorenal ganglion

Left aorticorenal ganglion

Spermatic ganglion

Renal artery

Inferior mesenteric ganglion

Inferior mesenteric plexus

Aorta

Aortic plexus

Superior hypogastric plexus

Inferior hypogastric (pelvic) plexus

Figure 14.3 Anatomy of the sympathetic *prevertebral* plexuses. Each ganglion and its associated plexus are named after the artery with which they are associated.

ganglia often lie within the walls of their target organs. Thus, postganglionic fibers of the parasympathetic division are short.

Cranial Nerves III, VII, and IX The preganglionic parasympathetic neurons that are distributed with CN III, CN VII, and CN IX originate in three groups of nuclei in the midbrain or medulla.

Cranial Nerve X ◉ 14-2 Most parasympathetic output occurs through the **vagus nerve** (CN X). Cell bodies of vagal preganglionic parasympathetic neurons are found in the medulla. This nerve supplies parasympathetic innervation to all the viscera of the thorax and abdomen, including the GI tract between the pharynx and distal end of the colon (Fig. 14.4, right panel).

Sacral Nerves The cell bodies of preganglionic parasympathetic neurons in the sacral spinal cord (S2 to S4) are located in a position similar to that of the preganglionic *sympathetic* neurons. Their axons leave through ventral roots and travel with the pelvic splanchnic nerves to their terminal ganglia in the descending colon and rectum, as well as to the bladder and the reproductive organs of the male and female.

The visceral control system also has an important afferent limb

All internal organs are densely innervated by visceral afferents. Some of these receptors monitor nociceptive (painful) input. Others are sensitive to a variety of mechanical and chemical stimuli. As is the case with somatic afferents, the cell bodies of visceral afferent fibers are located within the dorsal root ganglia (see Fig. 10.8A) or cranial nerve ganglia (e.g., nodose and petrosal ganglia). Ninety percent of these visceral afferents are unmyelinated.

The largest concentration of visceral afferent axons can be found in the **vagus nerve,** which carries non-nociceptive afferent input to the CNS from all viscera of the thorax and abdomen. Most fibers in the vagus nerve are *afferents,* even though all parasympathetic preganglionic output (i.e., *efferents*) to the abdominal and thoracic viscera also travels in the vagus nerve. Vagal afferents, whose cell bodies are located in the nodose ganglion, carry information about the distention of hollow organs (e.g., blood vessels, cardiac chambers, stomach, bronchioles), blood gases (e.g., P_{O_2}, P_{CO_2}, pH from the aortic bodies), and body chemistry (e.g., glucose concentration) to the medulla.

◉ 14-3 Internal organs also have nociceptive receptors that are sensitive to excessive stretch, noxious chemical irritants, and very large decreases in pH. In the CNS, this visceral pain input is mapped (see ◉ 16-4) *viscerotopically* at the level of the spinal cord and brainstem but not at the level of the cerebral cortex. Thus, awareness of visceral pain is not usually localized to a specific organ but is instead "referred" to the **dermatome** that is innervated by the same spinal nerve (see Fig. 10.8A). This **referred pain** results from lack of precision in the central organization of visceral pain pathways. Thus, you know that the pain is associated with a particular spinal nerve, but you do not know where the pain is coming from. For example, nociceptive input from the left ventricle of the heart is referred to the left T1 to T5 dermatomes and leads to discomfort in the left arm and left side of the chest. This visceral pain is often felt as a vague burning or pressure sensation.

The enteric division is a self-contained nervous system of the GI tract and receives sympathetic and parasympathetic input

The **enteric nervous system (ENS)** is a collection of nerve plexuses that surround the GI tract, including the pancreas and biliary system. Although it is entirely peripheral, the ENS receives input from the sympathetic and parasympathetic divisions of the ANS. The ENS is estimated to contain >100 million neurons. Enteric neurons contain many different

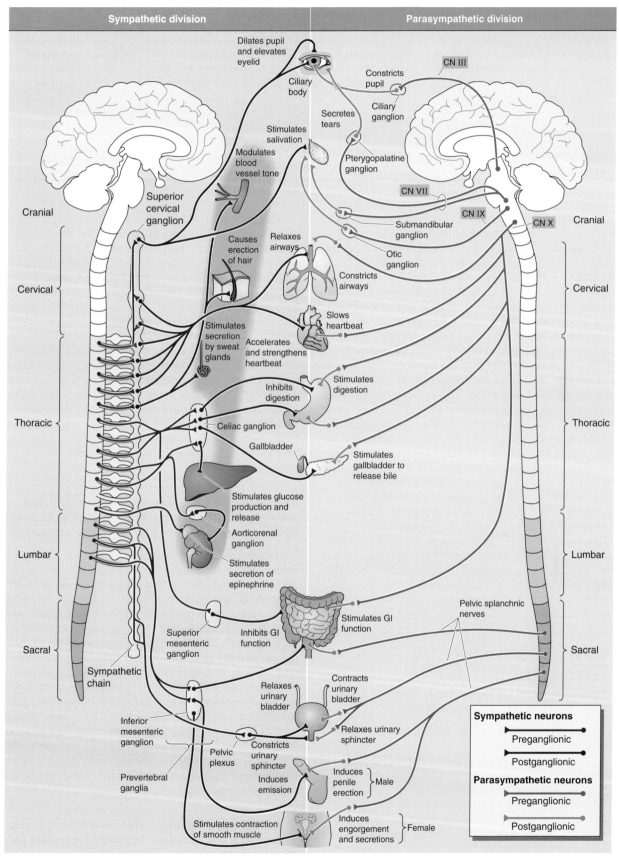

Figure 14.4 Organization of the sympathetic and parasympathetic divisions of the ANS. The *left panel* shows the sympathetic division. The cell bodies of sympathetic preganglionic neurons (*red*) are in the intermediolateral column of the thoracic and lumbar spinal cord (T1–L3). Their axons project to paravertebral ganglia (the sympathetic chain) and prevertebral ganglia. Postganglionic neurons (*blue*) therefore have long projections to their targets. The *right panel* shows the parasympathetic division. The cell bodies of parasympathetic preganglionic neurons (*orange*) are either in the brain (midbrain, pons, medulla) or in the sacral spinal cord (S2–S4). Their axons project to ganglia very near (or even inside) the end organs. Postganglionic neurons (*green*) therefore have short projections to their targets.

TABLE 14.1 **Properties of the Sympathetic and Parasympathetic Divisions**

	SYMPATHETIC PREGANGLIONIC	SYMPATHETIC POSTGANGLIONIC	PARASYMPATHETIC PREGANGLIONIC	PARASYMPATHETIC POSTGANGLIONIC
Location of neuron cell bodies	Intermediolateral cell column in the spinal cord (T1–L3)	Prevertebral and paravertebral ganglia	Brainstem and sacral spinal cord (S2–S4)	Terminal ganglia in or near target organ
Myelination	Yes	No	Yes	No
Primary neurotransmitter	ACh	Norepinephrine	ACh	ACh
Primary postsynaptic receptor	Nicotinic	Adrenergic	Nicotinic	Muscarinic

neurotransmitters and neuromodulators. Thus, not only does the total number of neurons in the enteric division exceed that of the spinal cord, but the neurochemical complexity of the ENS also approaches that of the CNS. We discuss the anatomy of the ENS as well as its role in controlling GI function later (see ◉ 41-1). The plexuses of the ENS are a system of ganglia sandwiched between the layers of the gut and connected by a dense meshwork of nerve fibers. The **myenteric** or Auerbach's plexus lies between the outer longitudinal and the inner circular layers of smooth muscle, whereas the **submucosal** or Meissner's plexus lies between the inner circular layer of smooth muscle and the most internal layer of smooth muscle, the muscularis mucosae (see Fig. 41.3). In the intestinal wall, the myenteric plexus is involved primarily in the control of motility, whereas the submucosal plexus is involved in the control of ion and fluid transport. Both the myenteric and the submucosal plexuses receive *preganglionic parasympathetic* innervation from the vagus nerve (or sacral nerves in the case of the distal portion of colon and rectum). The other major input to the ENS is from *postganglionic sympathetic* neurons. Thus, the ENS can be thought of as "postganglionic" or as a "terminal organ" with respect to the parasympathetic division, and "post-postganglionic" with respect to the sympathetic division. The isolated ENS can respond appropriately to local stimuli and control most aspects of gut function, including initiating peristaltic activity in response to gastric distention, controlling secretory and absorptive functions, and triggering biliary contractions.

SYNAPTIC PHYSIOLOGY OF THE AUTONOMIC NERVOUS SYSTEM

The sympathetic and parasympathetic divisions have opposite effects on most visceral targets

Many visceral targets receive both inhibitory and excitatory synaptic inputs. These antagonistic inputs arise from the two opposing divisions of the ANS, the sympathetic and the parasympathetic.

In organs that are stimulated during physical activity, the sympathetic division is excitatory and the parasympathetic division is inhibitory. For example, sympathetic input increases the heart rate, whereas parasympathetic input decreases it. In organs whose activity increases while the body is at rest, the opposite is true. For example, the parasympathetic division stimulates peristalsis of the gut, whereas the sympathetic division inhibits it.

Although antagonistic effects of the sympathetic and parasympathetic divisions of the ANS are the general rule for most end organs, exceptions exist. For example, the salivary glands are stimulated by both divisions. In addition, some organs receive innervation from only one of these two divisions of the ANS. For example, sweat glands, piloerector muscles, and most peripheral blood vessels receive input from only the sympathetic division.

◉ **14-4** Synapses of the ANS are specialized for their function. Rather than possessing synaptic terminals that are typical of somatic motor axons, many postganglionic autonomic neurons have bulbous expansions, or **varicosities,** that are distributed along their axons within their target organ. At each varicosity, autonomic axons form an *"en passant"* synapse with their end-organ target. This arrangement results in an increase in the number of targets that a single axonal branch can influence, with wider distribution of autonomic output.

All preganglionic neurons—both sympathetic and parasympathetic—release acetylcholine and stimulate N_2 nicotinic receptors on postganglionic neurons

At synapses between postganglionic neurons and target cells, the two major divisions of the ANS use different neurotransmitters and receptors (Table 14.1). However, in both the sympathetic and parasympathetic divisions, synaptic transmission between preganglionic and postganglionic neurons is mediated by **acetylcholine (ACh)** acting on nicotinic receptors (Fig. 14.5). Nicotinic receptors are ligand-gated channels (i.e., ionotropic receptors) with a pentameric structure (see ◉ 8-6). Table 14.2 summarizes some of the properties of nicotinic receptors. The nicotinic receptors on postganglionic autonomic neurons are of a molecular subtype (N_2) different from that found at the neuromuscular junction (N_1). Both are ligand-gated ion channels activated by ACh or nicotine. When activated, N_1 and N_2 receptors are both permeable to Na^+ and K^+. Thus, nicotinic transmission triggered by stimulation of preganglionic neurons leads to rapid depolarization of postganglionic neurons.

◉ 14-5 All postganglionic parasympathetic neurons release ACh and stimulate muscarinic receptors on visceral targets

All postganglionic *para*sympathetic neurons act through muscarinic ACh receptors on the postsynaptic target (Fig. 14.5).

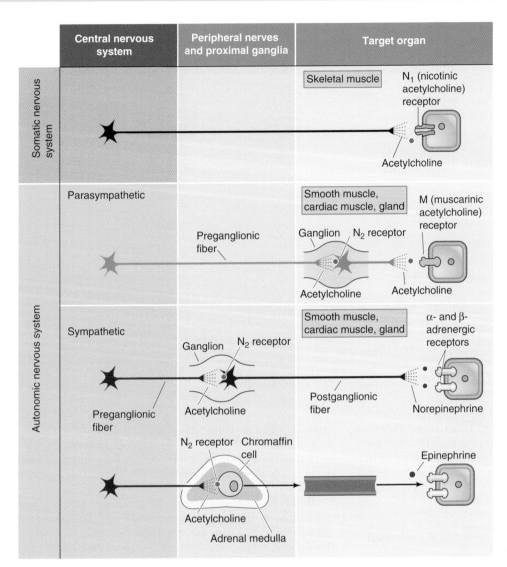

| Central nervous system | Peripheral nerves and proximal ganglia | Target organ |

Figure 14.5 Major neurotransmitters of the ANS.

Activation of this receptor can either stimulate or inhibit function of the target cell. **Muscarinic receptors** are G protein–coupled receptors (GPCRs; see ⊙ **3-3**) that (1) stimulate the hydrolysis of phosphoinositide and thus increase $[Ca^{2+}]_i$ and activate protein kinase C, (2) inhibit adenylyl cyclase and thus decrease cAMP levels, or (3) directly modulate K^+ channels through the G-protein βγ complex (see ⊙ **23-12**). Because they are mediated by second messengers, muscarinic responses, unlike the rapid responses evoked by nicotine receptors, are slow and prolonged.

Most postganglionic sympathetic neurons release norepinephrine onto visceral targets

⊙ **14-6** Most postganglionic sympathetic neurons release **norepinephrine** (Fig. 14.5), which acts on target cells through adrenergic receptors. The sympathetic innervation of sweat glands is an exception to this rule. Sweat glands are innervated by sympathetic neurons that release ACh and act via muscarinic receptors. The adrenergic receptors are all GPCRs and are highly homologous to the muscarinic receptors. Two major types of adrenergic receptors are recognized,

α and β, each of which exists in multiple subtypes (Table 14.2).

Adrenergic receptor subtypes have a tissue-specific distribution. α_1 receptors predominate on blood vessels, α_2 on presynaptic terminals, β_1 in the heart, β_2 in the bronchial muscle of the lungs, and β_3 in fat cells. This distribution has permitted the development of many clinically useful agents that are selective for different subtypes and tissues. For example, α_1 agonists are effective as nasal decongestants, and α_2 antagonists have been used to treat impotence. β_1 agonists increase cardiac output in congestive heart failure, whereas β_1 antagonists are useful antihypertensive agents. β_2 agonists are used as bronchodilators in patients with asthma and chronic lung disease.

⊙ **14-7** The adrenal medulla (see ⊙ **50-8**) is a special adaptation of the sympathetic division, homologous to a postganglionic sympathetic neuron (Fig. 14.5). It is innervated by preganglionic sympathetic neurons, and the postsynaptic target cells, which are called **chromaffin cells,** have nicotinic ACh receptors. However, rather than possessing axons that release norepinephrine onto a specific target organ, the chromaffin cells reside near blood vessels

TABLE 14.2 Signaling Pathways for Nicotinic, Muscarinic, Adrenergic, and Dopaminergic Receptors

RECEPTOR TYPE	AGONISTS[a]	ANTAGONISTS	G PROTEIN	LINKED ENZYME	SECOND MESSENGER
N_1 nicotinic ACh	ACh (nicotine, decamethonium)	d-Tubocurarine, α-bungarotoxin	—	—	—
N_2 nicotinic ACh	ACh (nicotine, TMA)	Hexamethonium	—	—	—
$M_1/M_3/M_5$ muscarinic ACh	ACh (muscarine)	Atropine, pirenzepine (M_1)	$G\alpha_q$	PLC	IP_3 and DAG
M_2/M_4 muscarinic ACh	ACh (muscarine)	Atropine, methoctramine (M_2)	$G\alpha_i$ and $G\alpha_o$	Adenylyl cyclase	↓ $[cAMP]_i$
α_1 adrenergic	NE ≥ Epi (phenylephrine)	Phentolamine	$G\alpha_q$	PLC	IP_3 and DAG
α_2 adrenergic	NE ≥ Epi (clonidine)	Yohimbine	$G\alpha_i$	Adenylyl cyclase	↓ $[cAMP]_i$
β_1 adrenergic	Epi > NE (dobutamine, isoproterenol)	Metoprolol	$G\alpha_s$	Adenylyl cyclase	↑ $[cAMP]_i$
β_2 adrenergic	Epi > NE (terbutaline, isoproterenol)	Butoxamine	$G\alpha_s$	Adenylyl cyclase	↑ $[cAMP]_i$
β_3 adrenergic	Epi > NE (isoproterenol)	SR59230A	$G\alpha_s$	Adenylyl cyclase	↑ $[cAMP]_i$
D1	Dopamine (fenoldopam)	LE 300	$G\alpha_s$	Adenylyl cyclase	↑ $[cAMP]_i$
D2	Dopamine (quinpirole)	Thioridazine	$G\alpha_i$	Adenylyl cyclase	↓ $[cAMP]_i$

[a]Selective agonists are in parentheses.
DAG, Diacylglycerol; *Epi,* epinephrine; *NE,* norepinephrine; *PLC,* phospholipase C; *TMA,* tetramethylammonium.

and release **epinephrine** into the bloodstream. This neuroendocrine component of sympathetic output enhances the ability of the sympathetic division to broadcast its output throughout the body. Norepinephrine and epinephrine both activate all five subtypes of adrenergic receptor, but with different affinities (Table 14.2).

Nonclassic transmitters can be released at each level of the ANS

Some neurotransmission in the ANS involves neither adrenergic nor cholinergic pathways. Moreover, many neuronal synapses use more than a single neurotransmitter. Such **cotransmission** is now known to be common in the ANS. As many as eight different neurotransmitters may be found within some neurons, a phenomenon known as **colocalization.**

⦿ **14-8** Nonadrenergic, noncholinergic (NANC) **transmitters** are found at every level of autonomic control, where they can cause a wide range of postsynaptic responses.

In some cases, the proportion of neurotransmitters released depends on the level of neuronal activity (see ⦿ 13-7). Such frequency-dependent modulation of synaptic transmission provides a mechanism for enhancing the versatility of the ANS.

Two nonclassic neurotransmitters are ATP and nitric oxide

ATP ATP is colocalized with norepinephrine in postganglionic sympathetic vasoconstrictor neurons. It is contained in synaptic vesicles, is released on electrical stimulation, and induces vascular constriction when it is applied directly to vascular smooth muscle. The effect of ATP results from activation of P_2 **purinoceptors** on smooth muscle, which include ligand-gated ion channels (P2X) and GPCRs (P2Y and P2U).

Nitric Oxide ⦿ **14-9** NO is produced locally from L-arginine by the enzyme nitric oxide synthase (NOS; see ⦿ 3-23). The NO then diffuses a short distance to a neighboring cell, where its effects are primarily mediated by the activation of guanylyl cyclase.

NOS is found in the preganglionic and postganglionic neurons of both the sympathetic and parasympathetic divisions as well as in vascular endothelial cells. It is not specific for any type of neuron inasmuch as it is found in both norepinephrine- and ACh-containing cells.

CENTRAL NERVOUS SYSTEM CONTROL OF THE VISCERA

Sympathetic output can be massive and nonspecific, as in the fight-or-flight response, or selective for specific target organs

⦿ **14-10** Generalized sympathetic activation readies the body for life-threatening situations—the **fight-or-flight** response. This response includes increases in heart rate, cardiac contractility, blood pressure, and ventilation of the lungs; bronchial dilatation; sweating; piloerection; liberation of glucose into the blood; inhibition of insulin secretion; reduction in blood clotting time; mobilization of blood cells by contraction of the spleen; and decreased GI activity. This mass response is a primitive mechanism for survival. In some people, such a response can be triggered spontaneously or with minimal provocation; each individual episode is then called a panic attack.

Under normal nonstressful conditions, output of the sympathetic division can also be more discrete and organ specific. This permits the sympathetic division to produce different effects on targets with different functions.

Parasympathetic neurons participate in many simple involuntary reflexes

As opposed to sympathetic neurons, parasympathetic neurons function only in a discrete, organ-specific, and reflexive manner. Together with visceral afferents, parasympathetic neurons mediate simple reflexes involving target organs. For example, the baroreceptor reflex is mediated by preganglionic parasympathetic neurons in the dorsal motor nucleus of the vagus (see ◉ 23-7). The pupillary light reflex is an example of an involuntary parasympathetic reflex that can be tested at the bedside (see ◉ 15-5).

A variety of brainstem nuclei provide basic control of the ANS

In addition to nuclei that contain parasympathetic preganglionic neurons, a variety of other brainstem structures are also involved in visceral control. These nuclei control specific autonomic functions or modulate the general level of autonomic tone.

◉ **14-11** One of the most important lower brainstem structures is the **nucleus tractus solitarii (NTS)** in the medulla. The NTS contains second-order sensory neurons that receive input from peripheral chemoreceptors (see ◉ 32-3) and baroreceptors (see ◉ 23-5), as well as non-nociceptive afferent input from every organ of the thorax and abdomen. Visceral afferents from the vagus nerve make their first synapse within the NTS, where they combine with other visceral afferent impulses. The NTS also receives input and sends output to many other CNS regions, including the brainstem nuclei as well as the hypothalamus and the forebrain. Thus, the NTS is the major lower brainstem command center for visceral control, participating in autonomic reflexes that maintain the homeostasis of many basic visceral functions.

The forebrain can modulate autonomic output and, reciprocally, visceral sensory input can influence the forebrain

Only a subset of the nervous system is necessary to maintain autonomic body homeostasis. The necessary structures include (1) the brainstem nuclei discussed in the preceding section, (2) the brainstem nuclei that contain the parasympathetic preganglionic neurons, (3) the spinal cord, and (4) the peripheral ANS. These components are capable of acting autonomously, even without input from forebrain regions. However, rostral CNS centers influence autonomic output.

◉ **14-12** The **hypothalamus,** especially the paraventricular nucleus, is the most important brain region for

TABLE 14.3 **Interactions Between Cortical and Autonomic Function**

Examples of Descending Cortical Control of Autonomic Output

Fear—initiates fight-or-flight response

Panic attacks—initiate activation of sympathetic division, increased breathing, and feeling of suffocation

Emotional stress (e.g., first day in gross anatomy lab) or painful stimuli—lead to massive vasodilation and hypotension, i.e., vasovagal syncope (fainting)

Seizures—can induce sudden cardiac death from massive sympathetic output and arrhythmias or sudden respiratory death from apnea

Chronic stress—can lead to peptic ulcers from increased gastric acid secretion

Sleep deprivation—in rats leads to death from loss of thermoregulation and cardiovascular control

Cognitive activity—can initiate sexual arousal

Nervousness (e.g., before an exam)—can lead to diarrhea

Examples in Which Visceral Afferents Overwhelm Cortical Function (i.e., Nothing Else Seems to Matter)

Hunger

Nausea

Dyspnea

Visceral pain

Bladder and bowel distention

Hypothermia/hyperthermia

coordination of autonomic output. The hypothalamus can initiate and coordinate an integrated response to the body's needs, including modulation of autonomic output as well as control of neuroendocrine function by the pituitary gland (see ◉ 47-1). The hypothalamus plays a dominant role in the integration of higher cortical and limbic systems with autonomic control. The hypothalamus can also initiate the fight-or-flight response.

The hypothalamus often mediates interactions between the forebrain and the brainstem. However, a number of forebrain regions also have direct connections to brainstem nuclei involved in autonomic control. Most of these forebrain regions are part of the **limbic system** rather than the neocortex. Even though we have minimal *conscious* control of autonomic output, cortical processes can strongly modulate the ANS. Emotions, mood, anxiety, stress, and fear can all alter autonomic output (Table 14.3, top section).

Not only does forebrain function influence the ANS, visceral activity also influences forebrain function. Visceral input can modulate the excitability of cortical neurons and, in some cases, can result in such overpowering sensory stimuli that it is not possible to focus cortical activity on anything else (Table 14.3, bottom section).

⊙ 14-13 CNS control centers oversee visceral feedback loops and orchestrate a feed-forward response to meet anticipated needs

The ANS maintains physiological parameters within an optimal range by means of **feedback loops** made up of sensors, afferent fibers, central autonomic control centers, and effector systems. These feedback loops achieve homeostasis by monitoring input from visceral receptors and adjusting the output of the sympathetic and parasympathetic divisions to specific organs so that they maintain activity at a set-point. Blood pressure control is an example of a visceral feedback loop in which the CNS monitors current blood pressure through afferents from baroreceptors, compares it with an internally determined set-point, and appropriately adjusts output to the heart, blood vessels, adrenal gland, and other targets. An increase in blood pressure (see ⊙ 23-7) causes a reflex decrease in sympathetic output to the heart and an increase in parasympathetic output.

Instead of merely responding through feedback loops, the ANS also anticipates the future needs of the individual. For example, when a person begins to exercise, sympathetic output increases before the increase in metabolic need to prevent an exercise debt from occurring. Because of this anticipatory response, alveolar ventilation rises to such an extent that blood levels of CO_2 (a byproduct of exercise) actually drop at the onset of exercise. This anticipation of future activity, or **feed-forward** stimulation prior to (and during) exercise, is a key component of the regulation of homeostasis during stress because it prevents large changes in physiological parameters that could be detrimental to optimal function.

The ANS has multiple levels of reflex loops

The human nervous system has a hierarchy that mirrors phylogenetic evolution. The **enteric nervous system** of humans is homologous to the most primitive nervous system, the neural net of jellyfish. In both cases, the component neurons control motility and nutrient absorption and respond appropriately to external stimuli.

The **autonomic ganglia** integrate afferent input from the viscera and have substantial independent control mechanisms. The largest of the sympathetic ganglia, the superior cervical ganglion, contains about 1 million neurons. In addition to postganglionic cell bodies, autonomic ganglia also contain interneurons. Axons from interneurons, sensory receptors located in the end organs, and preganglionic neurons converge with postganglionic neuron dendrites to form a dense network of nerve fibers, or a **neuropil,** within the ganglion. This neuropil confers considerable computational capability on the ganglia. Whereas feedback from skeletal muscle occurs only in the CNS, the peripheral synapses of visceral afferents result in substantial integration of autonomic activity at peripheral sites. Thus, although fast neurotransmission from preganglionic neurons to postganglionic neurons is an important role of the autonomic ganglia, the ganglia are not simply relays.

The **spinal cord** coordinates activity among different root levels. In humans who experience transection of the low cervical spinal cord—and in whom the outflow of the respiratory system is spared (see Chapter 32)—the caudal spinal cord and lower autonomic ganglia can still continue to maintain homeostasis. However, these individuals are incapable of more complex responses that require reflexes mediated by the cranial nerve afferents and cranial parasympathetic outflow. In many patients, this situation can lead to maladaptive reflexes such as autonomic hyper-reflexia, in which a full bladder results in hypertension and sweating.

The **medulla** coordinates all visceral control and optimizes it for survival. In humans, normal body homeostasis can continue indefinitely with only a medulla, spinal cord, and peripheral ANS.

The hypothalamus, limbic system, and cortex coordinate activity of the ANS with complex behaviors, motivations, and desires, but they are not required for normal homeostasis. Impulses from most visceral afferents never reach the cortex, and we are not usually conscious of them. Instead, they make synapses within the enteric plexuses, autonomic ganglia, spinal cord, and brainstem, and they close reflex loops that regulate visceral output at each of these levels.

CHAPTER 15

SENSORY TRANSDUCTION

Barry W. Connors

Sensory receptors convert environmental energy into neural signals

Sensation begins with sensory receptors that use energy from the environment to trigger electrochemical signals that can be transmitted to the brain—a process called **sensory transduction.** Transduction sets the basic limits of perception.

Senses are tuned to particular types of environmental energy. These **sensory modalities** include seeing, hearing, touching, smelling, and tasting, as well as our senses of pain, balance, body position, and movement. In addition, other sensory systems of which we are not conscious monitor the internal milieu and report on the body's chemical and metabolic state.

Sensory transduction uses adaptations of common molecular signaling mechanisms

Sensory processes are closely related to ubiquitous signaling molecules. Some modalities begin with G protein–coupled receptors (GPCRs). Other sensory systems use membrane ion channels in the primary transduction process.

To achieve a specificity for certain stimulus energies, many sensory receptors must use specialized cellular structures. Various receptors are slightly modified epithelial cells. Many are neurons alone, often just bare axons with no specialization visible by microscopy. Most sensory transduction cells lack their own axon to communicate with the CNS, instead using Ca^{2+}-dependent synaptic transmission onto a primary sensory neuron.

Sensory transduction requires detection and amplification, usually followed by a local receptor potential

⊙ **15-1** Sensory transducers must detect stimulus energy with selectivity and speed. In most cases, transduction involves signal amplification so that the sensory cell can reliably detect small stimuli in an environment with much sensory noise. The sensory cell must then convert the amplified signal into an electrical change by altering the gating of some ion channel, producing a voltage change called a **receptor potential.** The receptor potential is a graded electrotonic event. Very often, the receptor potential regulates the flux of Ca^{2+} into the cell and thus controls the release of some synaptic transmitter molecule onto the sensory afferent neuron.

Ultimately, receptor potentials determine the rate and pattern of action potential firing in a sensory neuron. This firing pattern is the signal that is actually communicated to the CNS. Useful information may be encoded in many features of the firing, including its rate and its temporal pattern.

CHEMORECEPTION

Chemoreceptors are ubiquitous, diverse, and evolutionarily ancient

Every cell is bathed in chemicals. Molecules can be food or poison, or they may serve as signals. The ability to recognize and respond to environmental chemicals can allow cells to find nutrients, avoid harm, attract a mate, navigate, or regulate a physiological process. In this chapter, we restrict ourselves to chemoreception as a *sensory* system.

The most familiar chemoreceptors are the sensory organs of taste (**gustation)** and smell (**olfaction).** However, chemoreception is widespread throughout the body. Chemoreceptors in the skin, mucous membranes, respiratory tract, and gut warn against irritating substances, and chemoreceptors in the carotid bodies (see ⊙ **32-5)** measure blood levels of O_2, CO_2, and $[H^+]$.

Taste receptors are modified epithelial cells, whereas olfactory receptors are neurons

Gustatory and olfactory receptors recognize the concentration and identity of dissolved molecules and communicate this information to the CNS. The two systems operate in parallel during eating, and the flavors of most foods are strongly dependent on both taste *and* smell. However, the receptor cells of gustation and olfaction are quite different. Olfactory receptors are neurons. Each olfactory cell has small dendrites at one end that are specialized to identify chemical stimuli, and at the other end an axon projects directly into the brain. Taste receptor cells are not neurons but synapse onto the axons of sensory neurons that communicate with the CNS.

Taste Receptor Cells Taste receptors are located mainly on the dorsal surface of the tongue (Fig. 15.1A), concentrated within projections called **papillae** (Fig. 15.1B). Papillae are a few millimeters in diameter. Each papilla in turn has numerous **taste buds** (Fig. 15.1C). One taste bud contains 50 to 150 taste receptor cells, basal and supporting cells, plus sensory afferent axons. Most people have 2000 to 5000 taste buds. The chemically sensitive part of a taste receptor cell is a small apical membrane region near the surface of the tongue. The apical ends have thin extensions called **microvilli** that

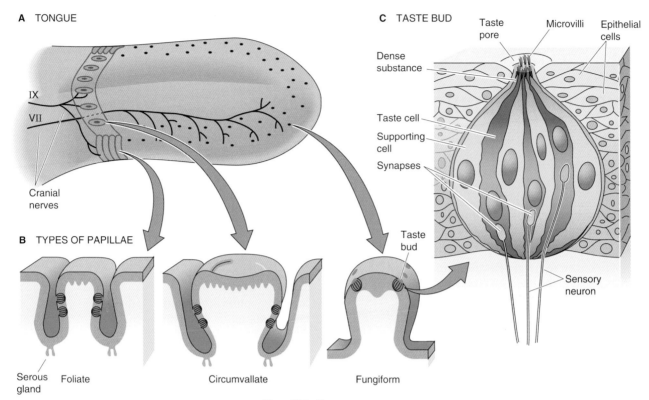

A   TONGUE

IX

VII

Cranial
nerves

B   TYPES OF PAPILLAE

Serous
gland   Foliate

Circumvallate

Fungiform

C   TASTE BUD

Taste
pore   Microvilli   Epithelial
cells

Dense
substance

Taste cell

Supporting
cell

Synapses

Taste
bud

Sensory
neuron

Figure 15.1   Taste receptors.

project into the **taste pore,** a small opening on the surface of the tongue where the taste cells are exposed to the contents of the mouth. Taste cells form synapses with the primary sensory axons near the bottom of the taste bud.

Cells of the taste bud undergo a ~2-week cycle of growth, death, and regeneration.

Olfactory Receptor Cells ⊙ **15-2** We smell with receptor cells in the thin **main olfactory epithelium,** which is placed high in the nasal cavity (Fig. 15.2A). The main olfactory epithelium has three primary cell types: **olfactory receptor cells** are the site of transduction; **support cells** are similar to glia and, among other things, help produce mucus; and stem cells, called **basal cells,** are the source of new receptor cells (Fig. 15.2B). Olfactory receptors die, regenerate, and grow in a cycle that lasts ~4 to 8 weeks. Olfactory receptor cells are one of the very few types of neurons in the mammalian nervous system that are regularly replaced throughout life.

The normal olfactory epithelium exudes a mucous layer 20 to 50 μm thick. Mucus contains antibodies, which are critical because olfactory cells offer a direct route for viruses or bacteria to enter the brain.

Complex flavors are derived from a few basic types of taste receptors, with contributions from sensory receptors of smell, temperature, texture, and pain

⊙ **15-3** We can distinguish among 4000 to 10,000 different chemicals with our taste buds. However, these discriminations represent only five primary taste qualities: **bitter, salty, sweet, sour,** and **umami.** Umami is the taste of certain L-amino acids, epitomized by L-glutamate (monosodium glutamate [MSG]).

In many cases, there is an obvious correlation between the chemistry of **tastants** (i.e., chemicals being tasted) and the quality of their taste. Most acids taste sour and most salts taste salty. However, for many other tastants, the linkage between taste and chemical structure is not clear. The familiar sugars (e.g., sucrose and fructose) are sweet, but certain proteins (e.g., monellin) and artificial sweeteners are 10,000 to 100,000 times sweeter by weight. Bitter substances are also chemically diverse. They include simple ions such as K^+ (KCl actually simultaneously evokes both bitter and salty tastes), larger metal ions such as Mg^{2+}, and complex organic molecules such as quinine.

If the tongue has only four or five primary taste qualities available to it, how does it discriminate complex flavors? First, the tongue's response to each tastant reflects distinct proportions of each of the primary taste qualities. Second, flavor is determined not only by taste but also by smell. Third, the mouth is filled with other types of sensory receptors that are sensitive to texture, temperature, and pain. The spiciness of hot peppers is generated by the chemical **capsaicin** by stimulation of heat-sensitive pain receptors in the mouth.

Taste transduction involves many types of molecular signaling systems

The receptor potentials of taste cells are usually depolarizing. Sour and salty taste cells use a conventional Ca^{2+}-triggered vesicular mechanism to release serotonin onto gustatory axons, whereas sweet-, bitter-, and umami-selective taste

A NASAL CAVITY AND OLFACTORY BULB

B OLFACTORY EPITHELIUM

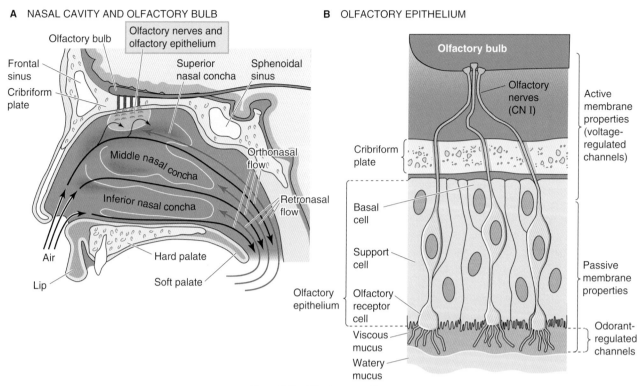

Figure 15.2 Olfactory reception.

cells use a Ca^{2+}-triggered nonvesicular mechanism to release ATP as their transmitter.

Each taste receptor cell responds to only one of the five basic taste modalities. Each of the taste receptor cells is, in turn, hard-wired to the CNS to convey a particular taste quality.

Salty The most common salty-tasting chemical is NaCl, or table salt. The taste of salt is mainly the taste of the cation Na^+. At relatively low concentrations (10 to 150 mM), NaCl is usually attractive to animals. Salt-sensitive taste cells detect low [NaCl] using the epithelial Na^+ channel ENaC. The taste channels are relatively insensitive to voltage and stay open at rest. When [Na^+] rises outside the receptor cell, Na^+ diffuses down its electrochemical gradient into the cell), and the membrane depolarizes, producing a receptor potential.

High concentrations of NaCl and other salts taste bad, because they activate bitter and sour taste cells. Anions may affect the taste of salts by modulating the saltiness of the cation or by adding a taste of their own.

Sour Sourness is evoked by protons (H^+ ions). One acid-sensitive channel is the nonselective cation channel TRPP3. Protons may also affect the gating of other cation-selective channels such as the hyperpolarization-activated channels (HCNs) and the acid-sensitive channels (ASICs) that would lead to depolarization of taste cells.

Carbonation—high levels of dissolved CO_2—can activate the gustatory, olfactory, and somatosensory neurons. Sour taste cells seem to be critical for the gustatory features of CO_2.

Sweet, Bitter, and Unami Taste receptors (T1R and T2R families) account for sweet, bitter, and umami transduction. These taste receptors are GPCRs, and use the same basic second-messenger pathway. The activated receptor activates a G protein that stimulates phospholipase C (PLC), which in turn increases its production of inositol 1,4,5-trisphosphate. IP_3 triggers the release of Ca^{2+} from internal stores, and the rise in [Ca^{2+}]$_i$ then activates a relatively nonselective cation channel called TRPM5, which is specific for taste cells. Opening TRPM5 depolarizes the taste cell, triggering the release of neurotransmitter onto the primary gustatory axon (Fig. 15.3B).

Bitter Bitterness often warns of poison. Perhaps because poisons are so chemically diverse, we have about 25 different types of bitter receptors to sense them. Each bitter taste cell expresses most or all of the 25 T2Rs. It may be more important to recognize that something is bitter, and potentially poisonous, than it is to recognize precisely what type of poison it may be.

Amino Acids Although many amino acids taste good, some taste bitter. The **umami** taste, which is characteristic of some Asian cuisines, is triggered by a mechanism very similar to that for sweet taste. The umami receptor is a heterodimer comprising two members of the T1R family, T1R1 and T1R3. The umami receptor activates the same signaling mechanisms that sweet and bitter receptors do.

The CNS can distinguish the various tastes from one another by somehow knowing which taste cell connects to a particular gustatory axon.

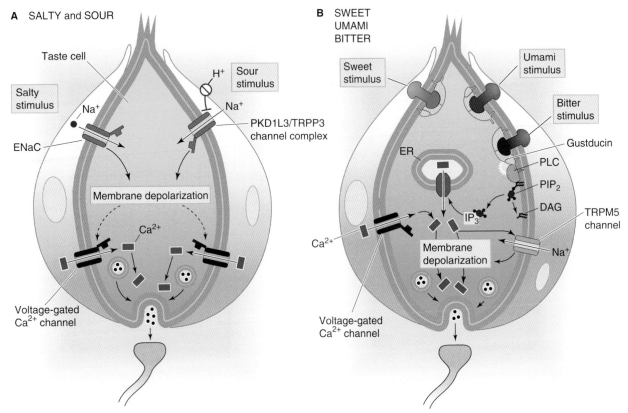

A SALTY and SOUR

Taste cell

Salty
stimulus

H⁺ → Sour
stimulus

Na⁺

Na⁺

ENaC

PKD1L3/TRPP3
channel complex

Membrane depolarization

Ca²⁺

Voltage-gated
Ca²⁺ channel

**B SWEET
UMAMI
BITTER**

Sweet
stimulus

Umami
stimulus

Bitter
stimulus

ER

Gustducin

PLC

PIP₂

DAG

IP₃

TRPM5
channel

Ca²⁺

Membrane
depolarization

Na⁺

Voltage-gated
Ca²⁺ channel

Figure 15.3 Cellular basis of taste transduction. Although, for convenience, we show two taste modalities in (A) and three in (B), individual taste cells do not express more than one of the taste mechanisms. *ER,* Endoplasmic reticulum; *PIP₂,* phosphatidylinositol 4,5-bisphosphate; *PLC,* phospholipase C.

Olfactory transduction involves specific receptors, G protein–coupled signaling, and a cyclic nucleotide–gated ion channel

We can smell >400,000 different substances. The *main* olfactory receptors use only one second-messenger mechanism. Fig. 15.4 summarizes the chain of events in the main olfactory receptor cells that leads to action potentials in the olfactory nerve (i.e., cranial nerve I [CN I]).

Step 1: The odorant binds to a specific **olfactory receptor protein** in the cell membrane of a cilium of an olfactory receptor cell.

Step 2: Receptor activation stimulates a heterotrimeric G protein called **G$_{olf}$**.

Step 3: The α subunit of G$_{olf}$ activates an **adenylyl cyclase**, which produces cAMP.

Step 4: The cAMP binds to a **cyclic nucleotide–gated (CNG)** cation channel.

Step 5: Opening of this channel increases permeability to Na⁺, K⁺, and Ca²⁺.

Step 6: The net inward current leads to membrane depolarization and increased [Ca²⁺]$_i$.

Step 7: The increased [Ca²⁺]$_i$ opens Ca²⁺-activated Cl⁻ channels called **anoctamin2.** Opening of these channels produces more depolarization because of the relatively high [Cl⁻]$_i$ of olfactory receptor neurons.

Step 8: If the receptor potential exceeds the threshold, it triggers action potentials in the soma that travel down the axon and into the brain.

All this molecular machinery, with the exception of the action potential mechanism, is squeezed into the thin cilia of olfactory receptor cells.

Olfactory receptor cells express a huge family of receptor proteins. Humans have ~350 genes that encode functional receptor proteins. This family of olfactory receptor proteins belongs to the superfamily of GPCRs.

Each receptor cell seems to express only a single odorant receptor gene. Because each odorant may activate a large proportion of the different receptor types, the central olfactory system's task is to decode the patterns of receptor cell activity that signals the identity of each smell.

VISUAL TRANSDUCTION

Light is an exceptionally useful source of information about the world because it is nearly ubiquitous and can travel far and fast and in straight lines with relatively little dispersion of its energy. The vertebrate eye has two major components: an **optical** part to gather light and to focus it to form an image and a **neural** part (the retina) to convert the optical image into a neural code.

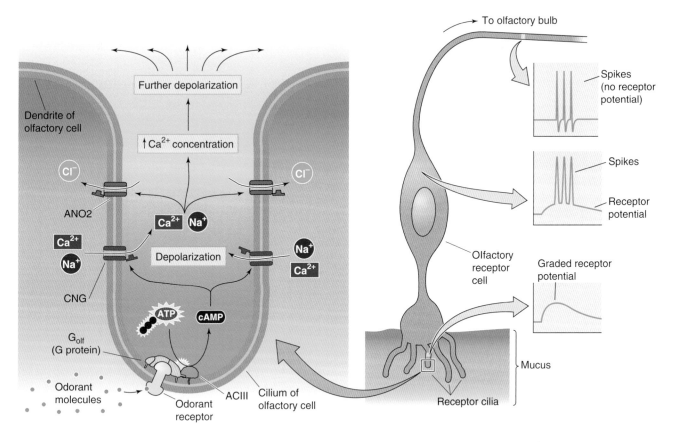

Figure 15.4   Cellular mechanism of odor sensation.

The optical components of the eye collect light and focus it onto the retina

The eye has systems to focus automatically, adjust its sensitivity for widely different light levels, move to track and stabilize a target, and even keep its surface washed and clear.

Fig. 15.5A shows a cross section through the human eye. A ray of light entering the eye passes through several relatively transparent elements to reach the retina; these elements include a thin film of tears and then the cornea, the aqueous humor, the lens, and finally the vitreous humor. **Tears** bathe the cornea and allow O_2 to diffuse from the air to the corneal cells. The **cornea** is a thin, transparent transporting epithelium that is devoid of blood vessels. The **ciliary epithelium,** a part of the ciliary body, constantly secretes **aqueous humor,** a protein-free ultrafiltrate of blood plasma, into the posterior chamber of the eye. The aqueous humor then flows between the iris and the anterior surface of the lens and reaches the **anterior chamber** through the pupil. This aqueous humor keeps the anterior portion of the eye slightly pressurized (~20 mm Hg), which helps maintain the eye's shape. Excess pressure in the anterior chamber produces a disease called **glaucoma.** The cells of the **lens** have a high concentration of proteins called α-crystallins, which help increase the density of the lens and enhance its focusing power. The **posterior chamber,** which is filled with a gelatinous substance called **vitreous humor,** is also kept pressurized by aqueous humor.

The light must be focused to generate a clear optical image on the retina. This is accomplished by the cornea and, to a lesser extent, the lens. Focusing requires the path of the light to bend, or refract, which occurs when light passes from a medium with one **index of refraction** to a medium with another.

Most of the focusing takes place at the interface between the air and the tear-covered anterior surface of the cornea because this region is where light encounters the greatest disparity in refractive indices on its path to the retina (Fig. 15.5B). The summed focal power of the optics of the relaxed eye allows it to focus light from distant objects onto the retina, ~24 mm behind the surface of the cornea (Fig. 15.6A).

⊙ 15-4 A normal *resting* eye is focused on distant objects, beyond ~7 m. To focus objects that are closer, the eye needs to increase its focal power, a process called **accommodation.** The eye achieves this goal by changing the shape of the lens (Fig. 15.5A). To accommodate, the ciliary muscle fibers contract and the lens becomes rounder. This increased curvature means increased focal power and a shift of the focal point closer to the eye.

With age, the lens becomes stiffer and less able to round up and accommodate. Additional refractive flaws may be caused by an eye that is too long or short for its focusing power or by aberrations in the refracting surfaces of the eye. **Myopia,** or nearsightedness, occurs when the eye is too long; distant objects focus in front of the retina and appear blurred (Fig. 15.6B). **Hyperopia** or farsightedness, is a feature of eyes that are too short; even with the lens fully accommodated, a near object

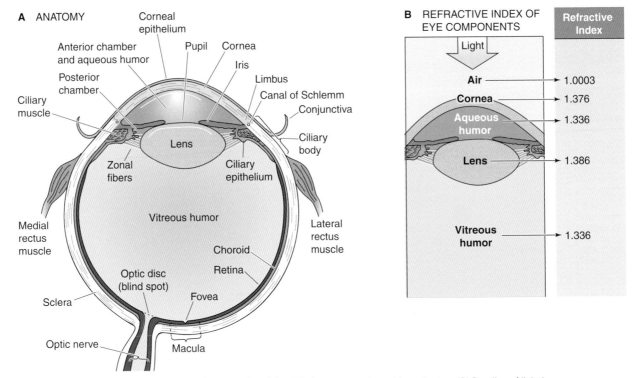

Figure 15.5   The eye. (A) Cross section of the right human eye, viewed from the top. (B) Bending of light by a structure depends not only on the radius of curvature but also on the difference in the indices of refraction of the two adjoining media.

focuses behind the retina and appears blurry (Fig. 15.6C). **Astigmatism** is caused by uneven curvature of the refractive surfaces of the eye (Fig. 15.6D). As a result, a point source of light cannot be brought to a precise focus on the retina.

⊙ **15-5** The **iris** is the colored structure visible through the window of the cornea. The iris's function is to create and to adjust the round opening that it encircles—the **pupil.** The pupil is like the aperture of the camera, and the iris is the diaphragm that regulates the amount of light allowed to enter the eye. The iris has sphincter muscles, innervated by postganglionic *parasympathetic* fibers that allow it to constrict **(miosis).** The iris also has radially oriented muscles, innervated by postganglionic *sympathetic* fibers from the superior cervical ganglion (see Fig. 14.4), that allow it to dilate **(mydriasis).** Pupil size depends on the balance of the two autonomic inputs. The regulation of pupillary size by ambient light levels is called the **pupillary light reflex.** Pupillary responses regulate the total amount of light that enters the eye (over a range of ~16-fold), and affect the quality of the retinal image (a smaller pupil diameter gives a greater depth of focus).

Other peripheral structures are also essential to proper visual function. The most important are the extraocular muscles that control eye movements. Fig. 15.5A shows two such muscles, the lateral and medial rectus muscles. The extraocular muscles determine the direction of gaze, the tracking of objects, and the coordination of the two eyes to keep their retinal images aligned as the eye, head, and visual world move about. Nuclei in the brainstem also control these tracking functions.

The retina is a small, displaced part of the CNS

The retina is a thin (~200 μm) sheet of tissue that lines the back of the eye and contains the light-sensitive cells, the **photoreceptors.** Photoreceptors capture photons, convert their light energy into chemical free energy, and generate a synaptic signal for relay to other visual neurons in the retina.

The retina is, histologically and embryologically, a part of the CNS. In addition to the photoreceptor cells, the retina has four additional types of neurons that form an orderly neural circuit (Fig. 15.7). One type, the **ganglion cell,** generates the sole output of the retina by sending its axons to the thalamus through the optic nerve (CN II).

The photoreceptors of the vertebrate eye—rods and cones—are on the *outer* surface of the retina, that is, the side facing *away* from the vitreous humor and incoming light. This causes only minor distortion of image quality because of the thinness and transparency of the neural layers. Because they face the back of the eye, these photoreceptors are close to the **pigment epithelium** (which aids the renewal process) and the blood vessels that supply the retina.

Each human eye has >100 × 10^6 photoreceptors but only 1 × 10^6 ganglion cells. Some of this convergence is mediated by **bipolar** cells, which directly connect photoreceptors and ganglion cells in a mainly radial direction (Fig. 15.7). The two remaining types of retinal neurons, horizontal cells and amacrine cells, are interneurons that mainly spread horizontally. **Horizontal cells** synapse within the outer layer of the retina and interconnect photoreceptors and bipolar cells to themselves and to each other. Horizontal cells often mediate interactions over a wide area of retina. **Amacrine cells** synapse within the inner layer of the retina and interconnect both bipolar cells and ganglion cells.

Because signaling distances are so short in the retina, synaptic potentials can spread effectively without action potentials. The main exceptions are the ganglion cells, which use action potentials to speed visual information along their axons to the brain.

A NORMAL VISION

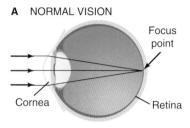

Focus
point

Cornea

Retina

Images out
of focus

B NEARSIGHTED (MYOPIA)

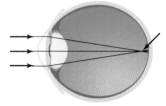

C FARSIGHTED (HYPEROPIA)

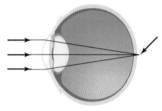

D ASTIGMATISM

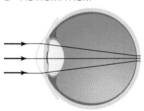

Figure 15.6 How the eye focuses incoming parallel light rays from a distant source.

There are three primary types of photoreceptors: rods, cones, and intrinsically photosensitive ganglion cells

The two main types of photoreceptors, **rods** and **cones,** are named for their characteristic shapes (Fig. 15.7). The human retina has only one type of rod, responsible for our monochromatic dark-adapted vision, and three subtypes of cones, responsible for color-sensitive vision. Rods outnumber cones by at least 16:1.

The mammalian retina has a third type of light-sensitive cell, the **intrinsically photosensitive retinal ganglion cell (ipRGC).** This rare subtype of ganglion cell expresses its own photopigment. Unlike the vast majority of ganglion cells, ipRGCs can respond to bright light even in the absence of input from rods and cones. The ipRGCs are involved in several nonimaging functions of the visual system.

In the central area of the primate retina is a small pit 300 to 700 µm in diameter called the **fovea,** which collects light from the center of our gaze (Fig. 15.5). Most foveal photoreceptors synapse on only one bipolar cell, which synapses on

only one ganglion cell, so central vision has high resolution. In other words, the **receptive field** of a foveal ganglion cell is small. At the periphery, the ratio of receptors to ganglion cells is high. The large receptive field reduces the spatial resolution of the peripheral portion of the retina but increases its sensitivity because more photoreceptors collect light for a ganglion cell. Foveal vision is purely cone mediated, small cones packed at the highest density (~0.3 µm from the center of one cone to another). Cone density falls to very low levels outside the fovea, and rod density rises. Both rods and cones mediate peripheral vision.

Rods and cones are elongated cells with synaptic terminals, an inner segment, and an outer segment (Fig. 15.7). The **synaptic terminals** connect to the inner segment by a short axon. The **inner segment** contains the nucleus and metabolic machinery. A thin ciliary stalk connects the inner segment to the outer segment. The **outer segment** is the transduction site. Structurally, the outer segment is a highly modified cilium. Each rod outer segment has ~1000 tightly packed stacks of *disk membranes,* which are flattened, membrane-bound intracellular organelles that have pinched off from the outer membrane. Cone outer segments have similarly stacked membranes, except that they are infolded and remain continuous with the outer membrane. The disk membranes contain the photopigments—**rhodopsin** in rods and molecules related to rhodopsin in cones.

Rods and cones hyperpolarize in response to light

Five to seven photons, each acting on only a single rod, are sufficient to evoke a sensation of light in humans. Thus, the rod is performing at the edge of its physical limits.

Photoreceptors use electrical events (receptor potentials) to carry the visual signal rapidly from the outer segment to their synapses. Light causes the cell's V_m to become *more negative* than the resting potential that it maintains in the dark.

Hyperpolarization reduces transmitter release from the photoreceptor onto its postsynaptic neurons. Thus, a flash of light causes a *decrease* in transmitter secretion. In the dark, each photoreceptor produces an ionic current that flows steadily into the outer segment and out of the inner segment. This **dark current** is carried mainly by inwardly directed Na^+ ions in the outer segment and by outwardly directed K^+ ions from the inner segment (Fig. 15.8A). Na^+ flows through a nonselective cation channel of the outer segment, which light indirectly regulates, and K^+ flows through a K^+ channel in the inner segment, which light does not regulate. Na^+ carries ~90% of the dark current in the outer segment, and Ca^{2+} ~10%. In the dark, V_m is about −40 mV.

Absorption of photons leads to closure of the nonselective cation channels in the outer segment. The total conductance of the cell membrane decreases. Because the K^+ channels of the inner segment remain open, K^+ continues to flow out of the cell, and this outward current causes the cell to hyperpolarize (Fig. 15.8B). The number of cation channels that close depends on the number of photons that are absorbed. The range of one rod's sensitivity is 1 to ~1000 photons.

Absorption of 1 photon suppresses entry of >10^6 Na^+ ions, an enormous amplification of energy. Cones respond similarly to single photons, but they are inherently noisier

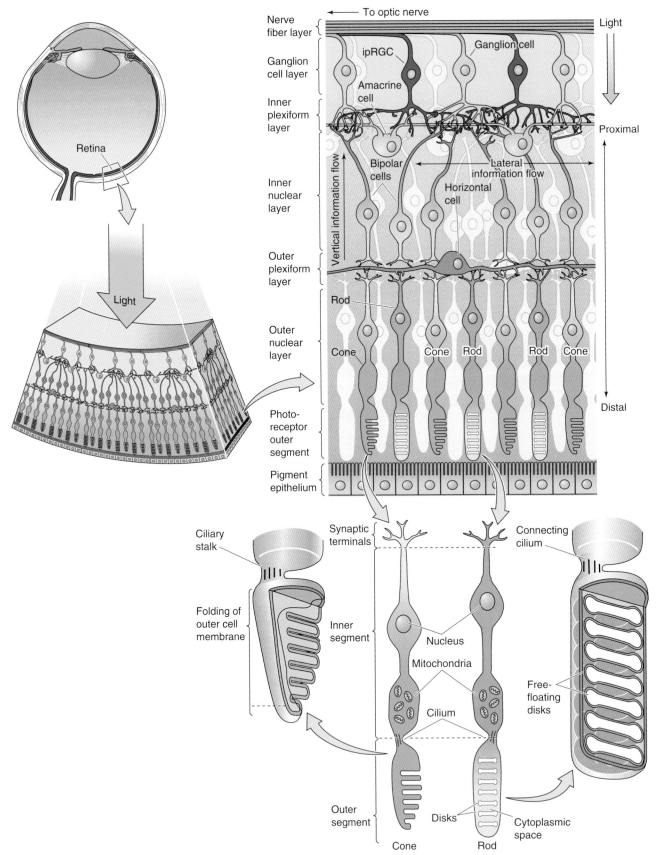

Figure 15.7 Neural circuits in the primate retina.

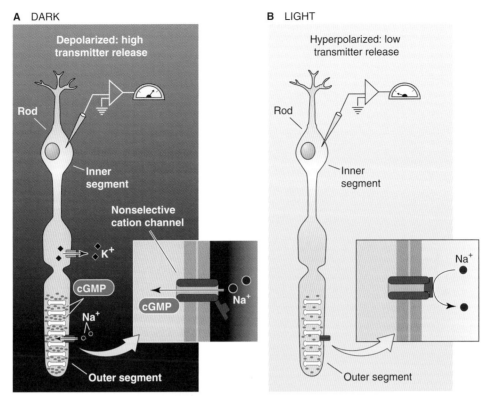

Figure 15.8 Phototransduction.

and their response is only ~1/50 the size of that in the rod. Cone responses do not saturate, even at the brightest levels of natural light. Cones also respond faster than rods.

Rhodopsin is a G protein–coupled "receptor" for light

How can a single photon stop the flow of 1 million Na^+ ions across the membrane of a rod cell? The process begins when the photon is absorbed by **rhodopsin,** the light receptor molecule (Fig. 15.9). One rod contains ~10^9 rhodopsin molecules. Rhodopsin has two key components: retinal and the protein opsin. Retinal is the aldehyde of **vitamin A,** or retinol (~500 Da). **Opsin** is a single polypeptide (~41 kDa) with seven membrane-spanning segments. It is a member of the superfamily of GPCRs.

Photons are absorbed by **11**-cis **retinal,** which isomerizes within 1 ps to a straighter and more stable version called **all-trans retinal.** This isomerization in turn triggers a conformational change in the opsin to **metarhodopsin II,** which can activate an attached molecule called transducin. Transducin carries the signal forward in the cascade and causes a reduction in Na^+ conductance.

Soon after isomerization, all-*trans* retinal and opsin separate in a process called **bleaching;** this separation causes the color to change from the rosy red of rhodopsin to the pale yellow of opsin. The photoreceptor cell converts all-*trans* retinal to retinol, which then translocates to the pigment epithelium and becomes 11-*cis* retinal. This compound makes its way back to the outer segment, where it recombines with opsin. This cycle of rhodopsin regeneration takes a few minutes.

15-6 Transducin is so named because it transduces the light-activated signal from rhodopsin into the photoreceptor membrane's response (Fig. 15.9). When it is activated by metarhodopsin, the α subunit of transducin exchanges a bound GDP for a GTP and then diffuses within the plane of the membrane to stimulate a **phosphodiesterase** that hydrolyzes cGMP to 5′-guanylate monophosphate.

cGMP is the diffusible second messenger that links the light-activated events of the disk membranes to the electrical events of the outer membrane. In the dark, a **constitutively active guanylyl cyclase** (Fig. 15.9) keeps cGMP levels high within the photoreceptor cytoplasm. This high [cGMP]$_i$ causes the cGMP-gated cation channels to open and accounts for the dark current. Because light stimulates the phosphodiesterase and decreases [cGMP]$_i$, light reduces the number of open cGMP-gated cation channels. The photoreceptor then hyperpolarizes, transmitter release falls, and a visual signal is passed to retinal neurons.

Strong amplification occurs along the phototransduction pathway. The absorption of 1 photon activates 1 metarhodopsin molecule, which can activate ~700 transducin molecules within ~100 ms. These transducin molecules activate phosphodiesterase, which increases the rate of cGMP hydrolysis by ~100-fold. One photon leads to the hydrolysis of ~1400 cGMP molecules by the peak of the response, thus reducing [cGMP] by ~8% in the cytoplasm around the activated disk. This decrease in [cGMP]$_i$ closes ~230 of the 11,000 cGMP-gated channels that are open in the dark. As a result, the dark current falls by ~2%.

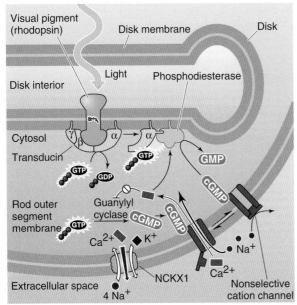

Figure 15.9 Rhodopsin, transducin, and signal transduction at the molecular level.

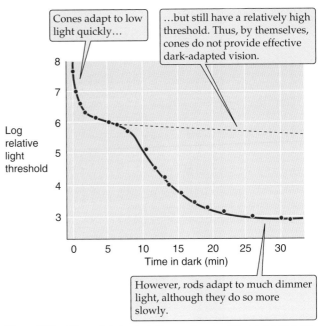

Figure 15.10 Effect of dark adaptation on the visual threshold. The subject was exposed to light at a level of 1600 millilumens and then switched to the dark. The graph is a plot of the time course of the subject's relative threshold (on a log scale) for detecting a light stimulus. (Data from Hecht S, Shlaer S, Smith EL, et al: The visual functions of the complete color blind. J Gen Physiol 31:459–472, 1948.)

The eye uses a variety of mechanisms to adapt to a wide range of light levels

⊙ **15-7** The human eye can operate effectively over a 10^{10}-fold range of light intensities, which is the equivalent of going from almost total darkness to bright sunlight on snow. However, moving from a bright to a dark environment, or vice versa, requires time for adaptation. Regulation of the size of the pupil by the iris can change light sensitivity by ~16-fold. During **dark adaptation,** two additional mechanisms are evident (Fig. 15.10). The first phase of adaptation is finished within ~10 minutes and is a property of the cones; the second takes at least 30 minutes and is attributed to the rods. When dark adapted, the rods can respond to the lowest light levels, but cones are available to respond when brighter stimuli appear.

Adaptation has both neural and photoreceptor mechanisms. The *neural* mechanisms are relatively fast, operate at relatively low ambient light levels, and involve multiple mechanisms within the neuronal network of the retina. The *photoreceptor* mechanisms include bleaching of rhodopsin, and consequences of decreased $[Ca^{2+}]_i$ as cGMP channels close. Low $[Ca^{2+}]_i$ increases guanylyl cyclase and inhibits phosphodiesterase, limiting the light-induced decrease in $[cGMP]_i$. In other words, the photoreceptor adapts to the increased background light intensity and remains responsive to small changes.

Color vision depends on the different spectral sensitivities of the three types of cones

The human eye responds only to a small region of the electromagnetic spectrum, but within it, we are exquisitely sensitive to the light's wavelength. We see colors because objects absorb some wavelengths while reflecting, refracting, or transmitting others.

The spectral sensitivity of the light-adapted eye depends on the photopigments in the cones. Each cone expresses a photopigment with a different absorbance spectrum (Fig. 15.11). The three cones and their pigments were historically called blue, green, and red, respectively. They are now more commonly called S, M, and L (for short, medium, and long wavelengths); we use this terminology here.

Single cones do not encode the wavelength of a light stimulus. If a cone responds to a photon, it generates the same response regardless of the wavelength of that photon. The pigment in a cone is more likely to absorb photons when their wavelength is at its peak absorbance, but light hitting the cone on the fringe of its absorbance range can still generate a large response if the light's intensity is sufficiently high. Because the nervous system can compare the *relative* stimulation of the three cone types to decode the wavelength, it can also distinguish changes in the intensity (luminance) of the light from changes in its wavelength.

The fovea has only M and L cones, which limits its color discrimination in comparison to the peripheral portions of the retina but leaves it best adapted to discriminate fine spatial detail.

The four different human visual pigments, including the rod pigment, have a similar structure. The presence of retinal and the mechanisms of its photoisomerization are essentially identical in each. Apparently, the amino-acid structures of the different opsins affect the absorption spectrum of 11-*cis* retinal.

The ipRGCs have unique properties and functions

The ipRGC, the third retinal photoreceptor, uses a light-sensitive protein called **melanopsin** that is most sensitive in the blue part of the spectrum (~475 nm; Fig. 15.11). IpRGCs

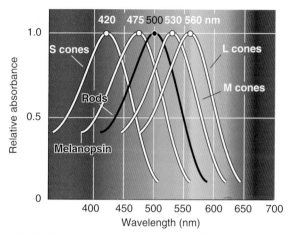

Figure 15.11 Sensitivity of photoreceptors at different wavelengths of light. The spectral sensitivity of rods (obtained with a spectrophotometer) peaks at ~500 nm; that of the three types of cones peaks at ~420 nm for the S *(blue)* cone, ~530 nm for the M *(green)* cone, and ~560 nm for the L *(red)* cone; and that of melanopsin peaks at ~475 nm. Each absorbance spectrum has been normalized to its peak sensitivity. (Rhodopsin data from Dartnell HJ, Bowmaker JK, Mollon JD: Microspectrophotometry of human photoreceptors. In Mollon JD, Sharpe LT [eds]: Colour Vision. London, Academic Press, 1983, pp 69–80; melanopsin data from Matsuyama T, Yamashita T, Imamoto Y, Shichida Y: Photochemical properties of mammalian melanopsin. Biochemistry 51:5454–5462, 2012.)

depolarize in response to light and can generate action potentials. The ipRGCs require bright light—orders of magnitude stronger than the threshold for cone responses. IpRGCs take seconds to respond, and they quite faithfully maintain their responses even when light levels are sustained for hours.

Melanopsin seems to activate a G protein of the G_q family, which stimulates PLC to produce IP_3 and diacylglycerol (DAG); this causes TRP channels to open and depolarizes the neuron. IpRGCs also receive some input from rods and cones via synapses of bipolar cells and amacrine cells.

IpRGCs can respond to ambient daytime illumination. IpRGCs send axons to the suprachiasmatic nuclei in the hypothalamus to ensure synchronization of its circadian clock with the light-dark cycles of day and night. The ipRGCs mediate the pupillary light reflex, inhibit production of melatonin by the pineal gland, and provide photic information to some of the brain's sleep-wake regulatory systems.

VESTIBULAR AND AUDITORY TRANSDUCTION: HAIR CELLS

Sensation in both the vestibular and auditory systems begins with the inner ear, and both use a receptor called the **hair cell.**

A VESTIBULAR HAIR BUNDLES

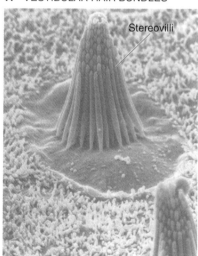

B VESTIBULAR HAIR CELLS

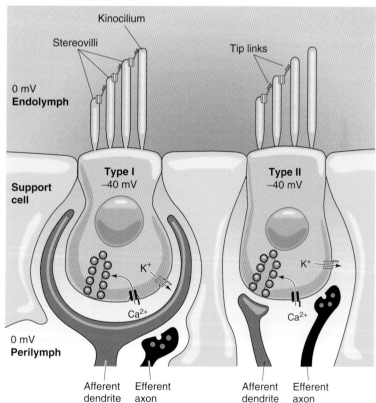

Figure 15.12 Vestibular hair cells. (A) Scanning electron micrograph of a bullfrog hair cell from the sensory epithelium of the saccule. (B) Type I and type II cells. (A, From Corey DP, Assad JA: In Corey DP, Roper SD [eds]: Sensory Transduction. New York, Rockefeller University Press, 1992; B, data from Philine Wangemann, Kansas State University.)

A POSITIVE MECHANICAL
DEFORMATION

B NEGATIVE MECHANICAL
DEFORMATION

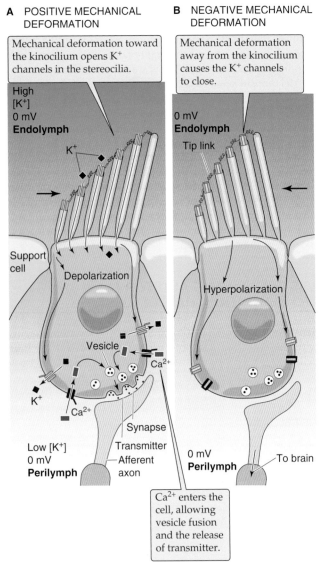

Figure 15.13 Mechanotransduction in the hair cell. Both panels portray a vestibular hair cell, with an endolymph voltage of 0 mV. In all hair cells except the auditory outer hair cells, the depolarization activates voltage-sensitive Ca^{2+} channels on the basal membrane, causing release of synaptic vesicles and stimulating the postsynaptic membrane of the accompanying sensory neuron.

The vestibular system generates our sense of balance and the auditory system provides our sense of hearing. **Vestibular sensation** operates constantly while we are awake and communicates to the brain the head's orientation and changes in the head's motion.

Auditory sensation is often at the forefront of our conscious experience, unlike vestibular information, which we rarely notice unless something goes wrong.

Bending the stereovilli of hair cells along one axis causes cation channels to open or to close

Hair cells are mechanoreceptors that are specialized to detect minuscule movement. The hair cell is an epithelial cell; the hair bundles project from the apical end, whereas synaptic

contacts occur at the basal end. In this section, we illustrate concepts mainly with the vestibular hair cell (Fig. 15.12A).

Both vestibular and auditory hair cells have 50 to 150 **stereovilli**. The stereovilli—often called stereocilia, although they lack the typical 9 + 2 pattern of true cilia—are 0.2 to 0.8 μm in diameter and are generally 4 to 10 μm in height. In the *vestibular* system, the kinocilium stands tallest along one side of the bundle, and the stereovilli fall away in height to the opposite side (Fig. 15.12B). Within the bundle, stereovilli are connected one to the next, but they can slide with respect to each other as the bundle is deflected side to side. The ends of the stereovilli are interconnected with very fine strands called **tip links.**

The epithelium of which the hair cells are a part separates perilymph from endolymph. The **perilymph** bathes the basolateral side of the hair cells. Perilymph is similar to CSF. Its voltage is zero. The basolateral resting potential of vestibular hair cells and auditory inner hair cells is about −40 mV (Fig. 15.12B). The **endolymph** bathing the stereovilli is singular in composition. It has a very high $[K^+]$ (150 mM) and a very low $[Na^+]$ (1 mM), more like cytoplasm than extracellular fluid. The voltage of the vestibular endolymph is ~0 mV relative to perilymph. Across the apical membrane of vestibular hair cells, the *chemical* gradient for K^+ is small. However, the *electrical* gradient is ~40 mV. Thus, a substantial force tends to drive K^+ into the vestibular hair cell across the apical membrane.

The appropriate stimulus for a hair cell is the bending of its hairs. Bending of the hair bundle *toward* the longer stereovilli (Fig. 15.13A) excites the cell and causes a depolarizing **receptor potential**. Bending of the hair bundle *away from* the longer stereovilli (Fig. 15.13B) hyperpolarizes the cell. Only tiny movements are needed. If the hairs are bent along the axis 90 degrees to their preferred direction, they are less than one tenth as responsive.

Mechanotransduction in hair cells seems to be accomplished by directly linking the movement of the stereovilli to the gating of apical mechanosensitive cation channels. The transduction channels are located near the tips of the stereovilli. The latency of channel opening is extremely short, <40 μs, suggesting a direct, physical coupling, likely a spring-like molecular linkage between the movement of stereovilli and channel gating. The tip links may be the tethers between stereovilli and the channels.

The mechanosensitive channels at the tips of the stereovilli are nonselective cation channels, allowing monovalent and some divalent cations, including Ca^{2+}, to pass easily. Each stereovillus has no more than two channels. Under physiological conditions, K^+ carries most of the current through the transduction channels. When the cell is at rest—hairs straight up—a small but steady leak of depolarizing K^+ current flows through the cell. This leak allows the hair cell to respond to both positive and negative deflections of its stereovilli. A positive deflection—toward the tallest stereovilli—further opens the apical channels, leading to *influx* of K^+ and thus *depolarization*. K^+ leaves the cell through mechano*insensitive* K^+ channels on the basolateral side (Fig. 15.13A), along a favorable electrochemical gradient. A negative deflection closes the apical channels and thus leads to *hyperpolarization* (Fig. 15.13B).

A hair cell is not a neuron. Instead the membrane near the presynaptic face of the cell has voltage-gated Ca^{2+} channels

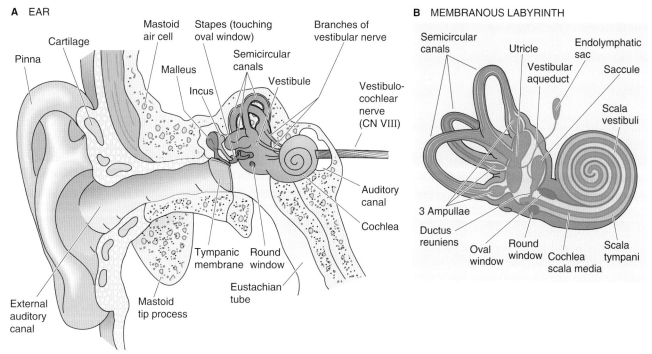

Figure 15.14 The ear, cochlea, and semicircular canals. (A) This section through the right ear of a human shows the outer, middle, and inner ear. (B) The labyrinth consists of an auditory and a vestibular portion. The auditory portion is the cochlea. The vestibular portion includes the two otolithic organs (the utricle and saccule) and the three semicircular canals.

that are somewhat active at rest but more active during mechanically induced depolarization. The Ca^{2+} that enters the hair cell through these channels triggers the graded release of glutamate as well as aspartate in the case of vestibular hair cells. These excitatory transmitters stimulate the postsynaptic terminal of sensory neurons that transmit information to the brain.

Hair cells are contained within bilateral sets of interconnected tubes and chambers called the **membranous labyrinth** (Fig. 15.14). The **vestibular** portion has five sensory structures: two **otolithic organs,** which detect gravity (i.e., head position) and linear head movements, and three **semicircular canals,** which detect head rotation. The **auditory** portion of the labyrinth is the spiraling **cochlea,** which detects rapid vibrations (sound) transmitted to it from the surrounding air.

The otolithic organs (saccule and utricle) detect the orientation and linear acceleration of the head

The **otolithic organs** are a pair of chambers—the **saccule** and the **utricle**—near the center of the labyrinth (Fig. 15.14B). These otolithic organs as well as the semicircular canals are (1) lined by epithelial cells, (2) filled with endolymph, (3) surrounded by perilymph, and (4) encased in the temporal bone. Within the epithelium, specialized **vestibular dark cells** secrete K^+ and are responsible for the high $[K^+]$ of the endolymph.

The saccule and utricle each have a sensory epithelium called the **macula,** which contains the hair cells. The stereovilli project into the gelatinous **otolithic membrane,** a

mass of mucopolysaccharides that is studded with otoliths or otoconia. **Otoconia** are crystals of calcium carbonate, 1 to 5 μm in diameter, that give the otolithic membrane a higher density than the surrounding endolymph. With either a change in the angle of the head or a linear acceleration, the inertia of the otoconia causes the otolithic membrane to move slightly, deflecting the stereovilli.

The hair cells of the saccule and utricle respond well to changes in head angle and to acceleration. Any tilt or linear acceleration of the head will enhance the stimulation of some hair cells, reduce the stimulation of others, and have no effect on the rest.

Each hair cell synapses on the ending of a primary sensory axon that is part of the **vestibular nerve,** which in turn is a branch of the vestibulocochlear nerve (CN VIII). The axons project to the ipsilateral vestibular nucleus in the brainstem.

The semicircular canals detect the angular acceleration of the head

Semicircular canals (Fig. 15.14B) also sense acceleration, but not the linear acceleration that the otolithic organs prefer. *Angular acceleration* generated by sudden head rotations is the primary stimulus for the semicircular canals.

In each canal, the hair cells are clustered within a sensory epithelium. The hair bundles project into a gelatinous, dome-shaped structure called the **cupula.** The cupula contains no otoconia. Thus, the cupula is not sensitive to *linear* acceleration. However, with a sudden rotation of the canal, the endolymph tends to stay behind because of its inertia. The endolymph exerts a force on the movable cupula, which bends the hairs and excites or suppresses the release of transmitter from the hair cells onto the sensory axons of the vestibular nerve. This arrangement makes the semicircular canals very sensitive to angular acceleration of the head.

Each side of the head has three semicircular canals that lie in approximately orthogonal planes. Because each canal best senses rotation about a particular axis, the three together give a good representation of all possible angles of head rotation. This complete representation is further ensured because each canal is paired with another on the opposite side of the head.

The outer and middle ears collect and condition air pressure waves for transduction within the inner ear

Sound waves vary in frequency, amplitude, and direction; our auditory systems are specialized to discriminate all three. Encoding of sound frequency and amplitude begins in the cochlea, followed by further analysis in the CNS. To distinguish the direction of a sound along the horizontal plane, the brain compares signals from the two ears.

The ear is traditionally divided into outer, middle, and inner components (Fig. 15.14A). The inner ear consists of the membranous labyrinth, with both its vestibular and auditory components.

Outer Ear   The most visible part of the ear is the **pinna,** a skin-covered flap of cartilage, and its small extension, the **tragus.** Together, they funnel sound waves into the **external auditory canal.** These structures focus sound waves on the tympanic membrane. The external ear parts in humans are essential for localization of sounds in the vertical plane. Sound enters the auditory canal both directly and after being reflected; the sound that we hear is a combination of the two. Thus, we hear a sound coming from above our head slightly differently than a sound coming from straight in front of us.

The external auditory canal is lined with skin and penetrates ~2.5 cm into the temporal bone, where it ends blindly at the eardrum (or **tympanic membrane**). Sound causes the tympanic membrane to vibrate, much like the head of a drum.

Middle Ear   The air-filled chamber between the tympanic membrane on one side and the **oval window** on the other is the middle ear (Fig. 15.14A). The **eustachian tube** connects the middle ear to the nasopharynx and makes it possible to equalize the air pressure on opposite sides of the tympanic membrane. The eustachian tube can also provide a path for throat infections and epithelial inflammation to invade the middle ear and lead to otitis media. The primary function of the middle ear is to transfer vibrations of the tympanic membrane to the oval window (Fig. 15.15). The key to accomplishing this task is a chain of three delicate bones called **ossicles:** the **malleus** (or hammer), **incus** (anvil), and **stapes** (stirrup).

Sound starts as a set of pressure waves in the air and ends up as pressure waves in a watery cochlear fluid within the inner ear. Sound traveling directly from air to water has insufficient pressure to move the dense water molecules. The middle ear saves most of the energy by two primary methods. First, the tympanic membrane has an area that is ~20-fold larger than that of the oval window, so a given pressure at the air side (the tympanic membrane) is amplified as it is transferred to the water

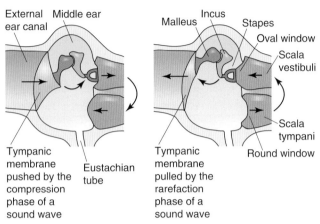

A   INWARD MOVEMENT OF TYMPANIC MEMBRANE

B   OUTWARD MOVEMENT OF TYMPANIC MEMBRANE

Figure 15.15   The middle ear. Displacement of the stapes and the oval window moves fluid in the scala vestibuli, causing opposite fluid movement in the scala tympani and thus an opposite displacement of the round window. (Data from Philine Wangemann, Kansas State University.)

side (the footplate of the stapes). Second, the malleus and incus act as a lever system, which again amplifies the pressure of the wave. Most of the energy is successfully transferred to the liquids of the inner ear.

Two tiny muscles of the middle ear insert onto the malleus and the stapes. These muscles control the stiffness of the ossicular chain, and their contraction serves to dampen the transfer of sound to the inner ear. They are reflexively activated when ambient sound levels become high.

The cochlea is a spiral of three parallel, fluid-filled tubes

The auditory portion of the inner ear is mainly the **cochlea,** a tubular structure that is ~35 mm long and is coiled 2.5 times into a snail shape about the size of a large pea (Fig. 15.16).

The cut through the cochlea in the lower left drawing in Fig. 15.16 reveals five cross sections of the spiral. In each cross section, two membranes divide the cochlea into three fluid-filled compartments. On one side is the compartment called the **scala vestibuli** (Fig. 15.16, right side), which begins at its large end near the oval window—where vibrations enter the inner ear. **Reissner's membrane** separates the scala vestibuli from the middle compartment, the **scala media.** The other boundary of the scala media is the **basilar membrane,** on which rides the **organ of Corti** and its hair cells. Below the basilar membrane is the **scala tympani,** which terminates at its basal or large end at the round window. Both the oval and round windows look into the middle ear (Fig. 15.15B).

Auditory endolymph has high K^+ and has a voltage of +80 mV relative to the perilymph. This **endocochlear potential** is the main driving force for sensory transduction in both inner and outer hair cells. Moreover, loss of the endocochlear potential is a frequent cause of hearing loss. A highly vascularized tissue called the stria vascularis secretes the K^+ into the scala media, and the resulting K^+ gradient between endolymph and perilymph generates the strong endocochlear potential.

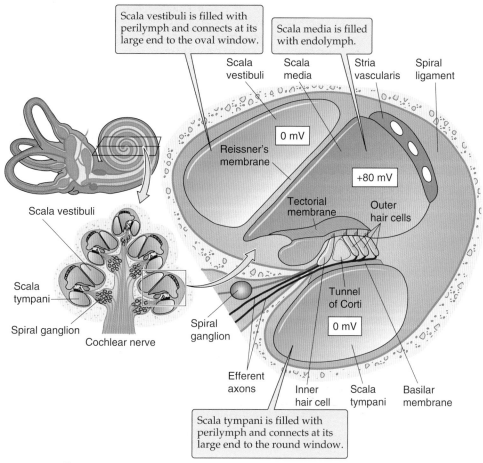

Figure 15.16 The cochlea. Data from Philine Wangemann, Kansas State University.

Inner hair cells transduce sound, whereas the active movements of outer hair cells amplify the signal

The business end of the cochlea is the **organ of Corti,** the portion of the basilar membrane that contains the hair cells. The organ of Corti has one row of ~3500 **inner hair cells** and three rows with a total of ~16,000 **outer hair cells** (Fig. 15.17A). The stereovilli of *inner* hair cells (Fig. 15.17B) float freely in the endolymph. The stereovilli of the *outer* hair cells (Fig. 15.17C) project into the gelatinous, collagen-containing **tectorial membrane.**

How do air pressure waves actually stimulate the auditory hair cells? Movements of the stapes against the oval window create traveling pressure waves within the cochlear fluids. Consider, for example, what happens as sound pressure falls in the outer ear.

Step 1: **Stapes moves outward.** As a result, the oval window moves *outward,* causing pressure in the scala vestibuli to decrease. The round window moves *inward* (Fig. 15.15B).

Step 2: **Scala vestibuli pressure falls below scala tympani pressure.**

Step 3: **Basilar membrane bows upward** (Fig. 15.17A).

Step 4: **Organ of Corti shears toward hinge of tectorial membrane.** The upward bowing of the basilar mem-brane creates a shear force between the hair bundle of the outer hair cells and the attached tectorial membrane.

Step 5: **Hair bundles of *outer* hair cells tilt toward their longer stereovilli.**

Step 6: **Transduction channels open in outer hair cells.** Because K+ is the major ion, the result is *depolarization* of the outer hair cells (Fig. 15.13A). The transduction-induced changes in membrane potential are **receptor potentials.** The molecular mechanisms are basically the same as in vestibular hair cells.

Step 7: **Depolarization contracts the motor protein prestin.** Outer hair cells express **prestin** (Fig. 15.17C). The con-traction of prestin molecules causes the outer hair cell to contract; this phenomenon is unique to outer hair cells and is called **electrical to mechanical transduction** or **electro-motility.** The change in shape is fast, beginning within 100 µs. The mechanical response of the outer hair cell does not depend on ATP, microtubule or actin systems, extracellular Ca^{2+}, or changes in cell volume.

Step 8: **Contraction of outer hair cells accentuates *upward* movement of the basilar membrane.** Outer hair cells act as a **cochlear amplifier**—sensing and then rapidly accentuating movements of the basilar membrane.

Step 9: **Endolymph moves beneath the tectorial mem-brane.** The upward movement of the basilar mem-brane—accentuated by the cochlear amplifier—forces

A   UPWARD BOWING OF BASILAR MEMBRANE

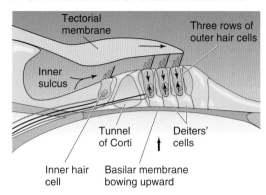

B   INNER HAIR CELL   **C**   OUTER HAIR CELL

D   DOWNWARD BOWING OF BASILAR MEMBRANE

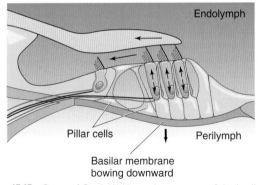

Figure 15.17   Organ of Corti. (A) Upward movement of the basilar membrane tilts the hair bundles *toward* the longer stereovilli, *opening* transduction channels. (B) In inner hair cells, depolarization causes enhanced transmitter release. (C) In outer hair cells, depolarization causes prestin to contract. (D) Downward movement of the basilar membrane tilts the hair bundles *away from* the longer stereovilli, *closing* transduction channels. (Data from Philine Wangemann, Kansas State University.)

endolymph to flow out from beneath the tectorial membrane, toward its tip.

Step 10: **Inner hair cell hair bundles bend toward longer stereovilli.** The flow of endolymph now causes the free-floating hair bundles of the inner hair cells to bend.

Step 11: **Transduction channels open in inner hair cells.** As in the outer hair cells, the result is a *depolarization*.

Step 12: **Depolarization opens voltage-gated Ca^{2+} channels. $[Ca^{2+}]_i$ rises in the inner hair cells.**

Step 13: **Synaptic vesicles fuse, releasing glutamate.** The neurotransmitter triggers action potentials in afferent neurons, relaying auditory signals to the brainstem. Note that the main response to depolarization is very different in the two types of hair cells. The outer hair cell contracts and thereby amplifies the movement of the basilar membrane. The inner hair cell releases neurotransmitter.

When the stapes reverses direction and moves inward, all of these processes reverse as well (Fig. 15.17D). The basilar membrane bows downward. In the outer hair cells, transduction channels close, causing *hyperpolarization* and cell elongation. The accentuated downward movement of the basilar membrane causes endolymph to move back under the tectorial membrane. In inner hair cells, transduction channels close, causing hyperpolarization and reduced neurotransmitter release.

The cochlea receives sensory and motor innervation from the **auditory or cochlear nerve,** a branch of CN VIII. The cell bodies of the sensory or *afferent* neurons of the cochlear nerve lie within the spiral ganglion. The dendrites of these neurons contact nearby hair cells, whereas the axons project to the cochlear nucleus in the brainstem (see Fig. 16.12). About 95% of the roughly 30,000 sensory neurons of each cochlear nerve innervate inner hair cells.

The frequency sensitivity of auditory hair cells depends on their position along the basilar membrane of the cochlea

Young humans can hear sounds with frequencies from ~20 to 20,000 Hz.

A continuous pure tone produces a wave that travels along the basilar membrane and has different amplitudes at different points along the base-apex axis (Fig. 15.18A). Increases in sound *amplitude* cause an increase in the *rate* of action potentials in auditory nerve axons—**rate coding.** The *frequency* of the sound determines *where* along the cochlea the cochlear membranes vibrate most—high frequencies at one end and low at the other—and thus which hair cells are stimulated. This selectivity is the basis for **place coding** in the auditory system; that is, the frequency selectivity of a hair cell depends mainly on its longitudinal position along the cochlear membranes. The cochlea is essentially a spectral analyzer that evaluates a complex sound according to its pure tonal components, with each pure tone stimulating a specific region of the cochlea.

Sounds of a particular frequency generate relatively localized waves in the basilar membrane and the envelope of these waves changes position according to the frequency of the sound (Fig. 15.18B). Low frequencies generate their maximal amplitudes near the apex. As sound frequency increases, the envelope shifts progressively toward the basal end (i.e., near the oval and round windows).

A ENVELOPE OF MAXIMUM WAVE AMPLITUDES

B EFFECT OF FREQUENCY ON ENVELOPE POSITION

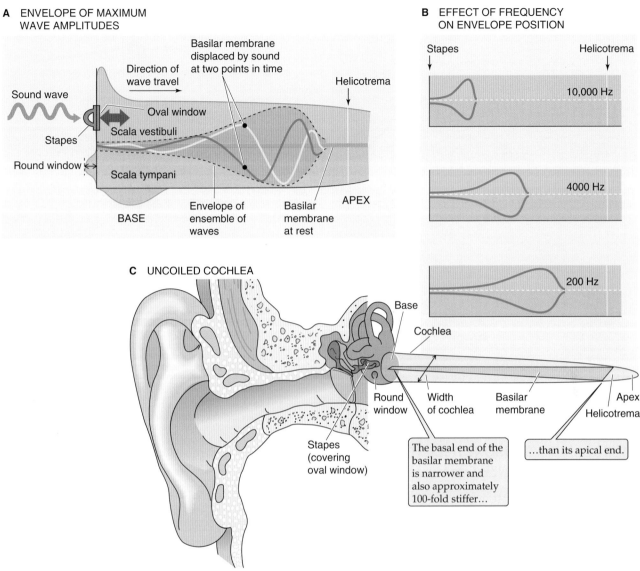

C UNCOILED COCHLEA

Figure 15.18   Waves along the basilar membrane of the cochlea. (A) As a wave generated by a sound of a single frequency travels along the basilar membrane, its amplitude changes. The *upper* and *lower broken lines* (i.e., the envelope) encompass all maximum amplitudes of all waves, at all points in time. (B) For a pure tone of 10,000 Hz, the envelope is confined to a short region of the basilar membrane near the stapes. For pure tones of 4000 Hz and 200 Hz, the widest part of the envelope moves closer to the helicotrema. (C) The cochlea narrows in diameter from base to apex, whereas the basilar membrane tapers in the opposite direction.

Two properties of the basilar membrane underlie the low-apical to high-basal gradient of resonance: taper and stiffness (Fig. 15.18C). The *basilar membrane* is wider at the apex, narrower at the base. More important, the narrow basal end is ~100-fold stiffer. Thus, the basilar membrane resembles a harp. At one end—the base, near the oval and round windows—it has short, taut strings that vibrate at high frequencies. At the other end—the apex—it has longer, looser strings that vibrate at low frequencies.

Some enhancement of tuning comes from the structure of the inner hair cells themselves. Those near the base have shorter, stiffer stereovilli, which makes them resonate to higher frequencies than possible with the longer, floppier stereovilli on cells near the apex.

The brain can control the tuning of hair cells. Axons that arise in the superior olivary complex in the brainstem synapse mainly on the outer hair cells and, sparsely, on the afferent axons that innervate the inner hair cells. Stimulation of these olivocochlear efferent fibers suppresses the responsiveness of the cochlea to sound and is thought to provide **auditory focus** by suppressing responsiveness to unwanted sounds—allowing us to hear better in noisy environments. The main efferent neurotransmitter is acetylcholine (ACh), which activates ionotropic ACh receptors and triggers an entry of Ca^{2+}. The influx of Ca^{2+} activates Ca^{2+}-activated K^+ channels, causing a hyperpolarization that suppresses the electromotility of outer hair cells and action potentials in afferent dendrites. Thus, the efferent axons allow the brain to control the gain of the inner ear.

A GLABROUS (HAIRLESS) SKIN

B PACINI'S CORPUSCLE

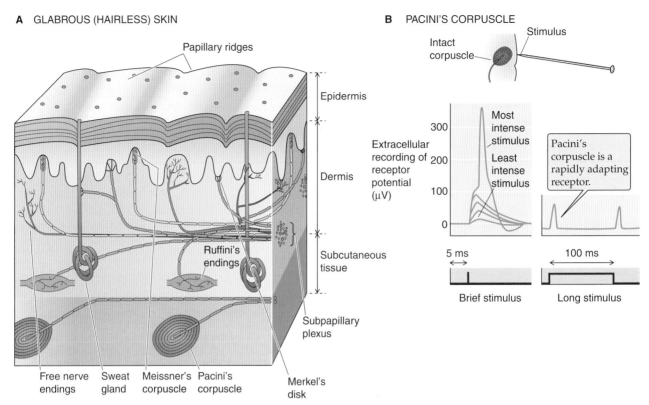

Figure 15.19 Sensors in the skin. (Data from Mendelson M, Loewenstein WR: Mechanisms of receptor adaptation. Science 144:554–555, 1964.)

⊙ 15-8 SOMATIC SENSORY RECEPTORS, PROPRIOCEPTION, AND PAIN

Somatic receptors are distributed throughout the body. Somatic sensation includes at least four sensory modalities: touch, temperature, pain (nociception), and body position (proprioception).

A variety of sensory endings in the skin transduce mechanical, thermal, and chemical stimuli

Somatic sensory receptors range from simple bare nerve endings to complex combinations of nerve, muscle, connective tissue, and supporting cells.

Mechanoreceptors are sensitive to physical distortion such as bending or stretching. They monitor physical contact with the skin, blood pressure in the heart and vessels, stretching of the gut and bladder, and pressure on the teeth. The transduction site of these mechanoreceptors is one or more unmyelinated axon branches. Similar to the transduction process in hair cells, cutaneous mechanoreceptive nerve endings probably gate ion channels.

Thermoreceptors respond best to changes in temperature, whereas **chemoreceptors** are sensitive to various kinds of chemical alterations. In the next three sections, we discuss mechanoreceptors, thermoreceptors, and chemoreceptors that are located in the skin.

Mechanoreceptors in the skin provide sensitivity to specific stimuli such as vibration and steady pressure

Skin protects us from our environment by preventing evaporation of body fluids, invasion by microbes, abrasion, and damage from sunlight. However, skin also provides our most direct contact with the world. The receptors in the skin respond when the skin is vibrated, pressed, pricked, or stroked, or when its hairs are bent or pulled. These are quite different kinds of mechanical energy, yet we can feel them all and easily tell them apart.

The largest mechanoreceptor is **Pacini's corpuscle,** which is up to 2 mm long and almost 1 mm in diameter (Fig. 15.19A). Pacini's corpuscle has an ovoid capsule with 20 to 70 onion-like, concentric layers of connective tissue and a nerve terminal in the middle. The capsule is responsible for the rapidly adapting response. When the capsule is compressed, energy is transferred to the nerve terminal, its membrane is deformed, and mechanosensitive channels open. Current flowing through the channels generates a depolarizing receptor potential that, if large enough, causes the axon to fire an action potential (Fig. 15.19B, *left panel*). However, the capsule layers are slick, with viscous fluid between them. If the stimulus pressure is maintained, the layers slip past one another and transfer the stimulus energy away so that the underlying axon terminal is no longer deformed and the receptor potential dissipates (Fig. 15.19B, *right panel*). When pressure is released, the events reverse themselves and the terminal is depolarized again. In this way, the non-neural covering of Pacini's corpuscle specializes the corpuscle for sensing of vibrations and makes it almost unresponsive to steady pressure. Pacini's corpuscle is most sensitive to vibrations of 200 to 300 Hz.

Several other types of encapsulated mechanoreceptors are located in the dermis. **Meissner's corpuscles** (Fig. 15.19A) are located in the ridges of glabrous skin and are about one tenth the size of Pacini's corpuscles. They are

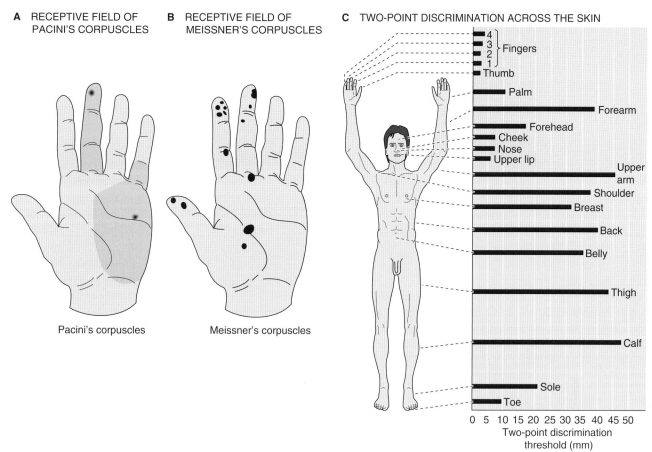

A RECEPTIVE FIELD OF PACINI'S CORPUSCLES

B RECEPTIVE FIELD OF MEISSNER'S CORPUSCLES

C TWO-POINT DISCRIMINATION ACROSS THE SKIN

Pacini's corpuscles

Meissner's corpuscles

4
3
2 } Fingers
1
Thumb
Palm
Forearm
Forehead
Cheek
Nose
Upper lip
Upper arm
Shoulder
Breast
Back
Belly
Thigh
Calf
Sole
Toe

0 5 10 15 20 25 30 35 40 45 50
Two-point discrimination threshold (mm)

Figure 15.20 Receptive fields and spatial discrimination of skin mechanoreceptors. (A) Each of the two *black dots* indicates an area of *maximal sensitivity* of a single Pacini's corpuscle. Each *blue-green area* is the receptive field of the corresponding corpuscle. (B) Each *dot* represents the entire (much smaller) receptive field of a single Meissner's corpuscle. (C) The *horizontal bars* represent the minimum distance at which two points can be perceived as distinct at various locations over the body. (A and B, Data from Vallbo AB, Johansson RS: Properties of cutaneous mechanoreceptors in the human hand related to touch sensation. Hum Neurobiol 3:3–14, 1984; C, data from Weinstein S: Intensive and extensive aspects of tactile sensitivity as a function of body part, sex and laterality. In Kenshalo DR [ed]: The Skin Senses. Springfield, IL, Charles C Thomas, 1968.)

rapidly adapting. **Ruffini's corpuscles** are *slowly* adapting receptors, so they respond best to low frequencies. **Merkel's disks** are also slowly adapting receptors made from a flattened epithelial cell that synapses on a nerve terminal. They lie at the border of the dermis and epidermis of glabrous skin. The nerve terminals of **Krause's end bulbs** appear knotted. They innervate the border areas of dry skin and mucous membranes (e.g., around the lips and external genitalia) and are probably rapidly adapting mechanoreceptors.

The **receptive fields** of different types of skin receptors vary greatly in size. Pacini's corpuscles have extremely broad receptive fields (Fig. 15.20A), whereas those of Meissner's corpuscles (Fig. 15.20B) and Merkel's disks are very small. The last two seem to be responsible for the ability of the fingertips to make very fine tactile discriminations. Spatial discrimination depends both on receptive field size and on receptor density (Fig. 15.20C).

TRPC channels appear to be involved in sensitivity to light touch. A non-TRP protein named **Piezo2** is associated with rapidly adapting mechanosensory currents in sensory neurons. Other mechanosensory channels are expressed in some sensory neurons, but their roles are still controversial.

Mechanosensory channels often need to be associated with other cellular components in order to be sensitive to mechanical stimuli.

Hair is a sensitive part of our somatic sensory system. Bending of the hair causes deformation of the follicle and surrounding tissue, which stretches, bends, or flattens the nerve endings and increases or decreases their firing frequency. Various mechanoreceptors innervate hair follicles, and they may be either slowly or rapidly adapting.

Separate thermoreceptors detect warmth and cold

Although many temperature-sensitive neurons are present in the skin, they are also clustered in the hypothalamus and the spinal cord (see ⊚ 59-8). The hypothalamic temperature sensors, like their cutaneous counterparts, are important for regulation of the physiological responses that maintain stable body temperature.

Fig. 15.21 shows how the steady (or tonic) discharge rate of both types of receptors varies with temperature. **Warmth receptors** begin firing above ~30°C and increase their firing rate until 44°C to 46°C, beyond which the rate falls off steeply and a sensation of pain begins, presumably mediated

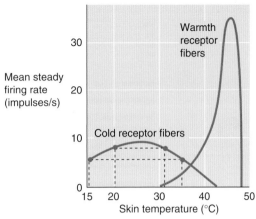

Figure 15.21 Temperature sensitivity of cutaneous thermoreceptors. (Data from Somjen GG: Sensory Coding in the Mammalian Nervous System. New York, Appleton-Century-Crofts, 1972.)

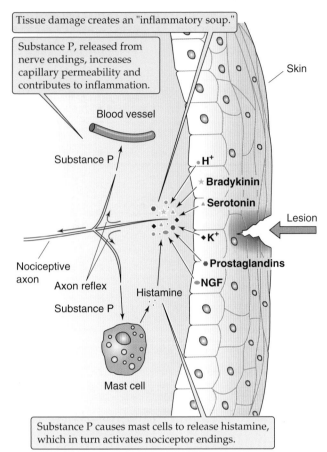

Figure 15.22 Hyperalgesia of inflammation.

by nociceptive endings. **Cold receptors** are relatively quiet at skin temperatures of ~40°C, but their steady discharge rate increases as the temperature falls to 24°C to 28°C, then decreases until the temperature falls to ~10°C.

Cold receptors also have a *phasic* response that enables them to report *changes* in temperature. Sudden decreases in temperature cause transient increases in activity, then a new steady-state rate of firing.

The transduction of relatively warm temperatures is carried out by several types of TRPV channels expressed in thermoreceptors. TRPV1 is activated by capsaicin, the ingredient that gives spicy foods their burning quality. Chili peppers taste "hot" because they activate some of the same ion channels that heat itself activates! TRPV1 and TRPV2 channels have painfully high temperature thresholds (~43°C and ~50°C, respectively) and thus help mediate the noxious aspects of thermoreception. Other TRPV channels (TRPV3 and TRPV4) are activated at more moderate temperatures and presumably provide our sensations of warmth.

Yet another TRP channel, TRPM8, mediates sensations of moderate cold. TRPM8 channels begin to open at temperatures below ~27°C and are maximally activated at 8°C. The cool-sensitive TRPM8 channel is a menthol receptor. Menthol evokes sensations of cold because it activates the same ion channel that is opened by cold temperatures.

Nociceptors are specialized sensory endings that transduce painful stimuli

Nociceptors mediate acutely painful feelings to warn us that body tissue is being damaged or is at risk of being damaged. The pain-sensing system has its own peripheral receptors and central circuits. Nociceptors are free nerve endings, widely distributed throughout the body, but are generally absent from the brain.

Nociceptors vary in their selectivity. **Mechanical nociceptors** respond to pressure from sharp objects. TRPA1 channels are involved in some forms of pain-related mechanosensation.

Thermal nociceptors signal either burning heat (above ~45°C, when tissues begin to be destroyed) or unhealthy cold; the heat-sensitive nociceptive neurons express the TRPV1 and TRPV2 channels, whereas the cold-sensitive nociceptors

express TRPA1 and TRPM8 channels. A uniquely cold-resistant Na⁺ channel, Nav1.8, allows cold-sensitive nociceptors to continue firing action potentials even at temperatures low enough to silence other neurons.

Chemical nociceptors respond to a variety of agents, including K⁺, extremes of pH, neuroactive substances such as histamine and bradykinin from the body itself, and various irritants from the environment. Some chemosensitive nociceptors express TRP channels that respond to plant-derived irritants such as capsaicin (TRPV1), menthol (TRPM8), and the pungent derivatives of mustard and garlic (TRPA1).

Finally, **polymodal nociceptors** are single nerve endings that are sensitive to combinations of mechanical, thermal, and chemical stimuli. Nociceptive axons include both fast **Aδ fibers** and slow, unmyelinated **C fibers**. Aδ axons mediate sensations of sharp, intense pain; C fibers elicit more persistent feelings of dull, burning pain.

Skin, joints, or muscles that have been damaged or inflamed are unusually sensitive to further stimuli. This phenomenon is called **hyperalgesia,** and it can be manifested as a reduced threshold for pain, an increase in perceived intensity of painful stimuli, or spontaneous pain. **Primary hyperalgesia** occurs within the area of damaged tissue, but within ~20 minutes after an injury, tissues surrounding a damaged area may become supersensitive by a process called **secondary hyperalgesia.** Hyperalgesia seems to involve processes near peripheral receptors (Fig. 15.22) as well as mechanisms in the CNS.

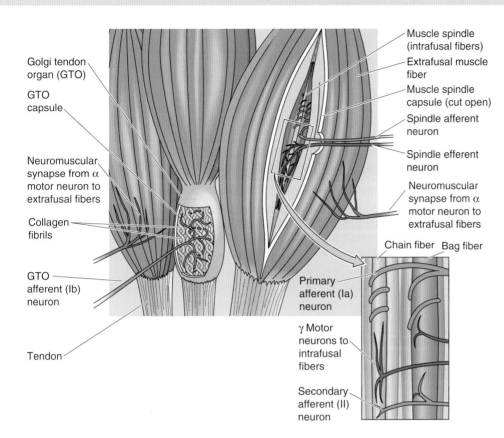

Golgi tendon organ (GTO)

GTO capsule

Neuromuscular synapse from α motor neuron to extrafusal fibers

Collagen fibrils

GTO afferent (Ib) neuron

Tendon

Muscle spindle (intrafusal fibers)

Extrafusal muscle fiber

Muscle spindle capsule (cut open)

Spindle afferent neuron

Spindle efferent neuron

Neuromuscular synapse from α motor neuron to extrafusal fibers

Chain fiber   Bag fiber

Primary afferent (Ia) neuron

γ Motor neurons to intrafusal fibers

Secondary afferent (II) neuron

Figure 15.23 Golgi tendon organ and muscle spindle fibers. A muscle contains two kinds of muscle fibers, extrafusal fibers (ordinary muscle fibers that cause contraction) and intrafusal fibers (aligned in parallel with the extrafusal fibers). Some of the extrafusal fibers have Golgi tendon organs located in series between the end of the muscle fiber and the macroscopic tendon. The intrafusal fibers contain muscle spindles, which receive both afferent (sensory) and efferent (motor) innervation. The spindle *(inset)* contains both bag fibers, with nuclei bunched together, and chain fibers, with nuclei in a row.

Damaged skin releases a variety of chemical substances from its many cell types, blood cells, and nerve endings. These substances—sometimes called the *inflammatory soup*—include neurotransmitters (e.g., glutamate, serotonin, adenosine, ATP), peptides (e.g., substance P, bradykinin), various lipids (e.g., prostaglandins, endocannabinoids), proteases, neurotrophins, cytokines, and chemokines, K^+, H^+, and others; they trigger the set of local responses that we know as **inflammation.** As a result, blood vessels become more leaky and cause tissue swelling (or edema) and redness. Nearby mast cells release the chemical histamine, which directly excites nociceptors.

By a mechanism called the **axon reflex,** action potentials can propagate along nociceptive axons from the site of an injury into side branches of the same axon that innervate neighboring regions of skin. The spreading axon branches of the nociceptors themselves may release substances that sensitize nociceptive terminals and make them responsive to previously nonpainful stimuli. Such "silent" nociceptors among our small Aδ and C fibers are normally unresponsive to stimuli—even destructive ones. Only after sensitization do they become responsive to mechanical or chemical stimuli and contribute greatly to hyperalgesia. For example, the neurotrophin nerve growth factor (NGF)—part of the inflammatory soup—triggers strong hypersensitivity to heat and mechanical stimuli by modulating TRPV1 channels. Activation of TRPA1 and ASICs are also important in hyperalgesia. The cytokine tumor necrosis factor-alpha (TNF-α) potentiates the inflammatory response directly and enhances release of substances that sensitize nociceptors. Drugs that interfere with neurotrophin and cytokine actions can be effective treatments for the pain of inflammatory diseases.

The cognitive sensations of pain are under remarkably potent control by the brain, more so than other sensory systems. In some cases, nociceptors may fire wildly, although perceptions of pain are absent; on the other hand, pain may be crippling although nociceptors are silent. Chronic activation of nociceptors can lead to central sensitization, a chronic enhancement of central pain-processing circuits. Prolonged activity in nociceptive axons and their spinal cord synapses causes increased glutamate release, strong activation of glutamate receptors, and eventually a form of long-term potentiation.

Nonpainful sensory input and neural activity from various nuclei within the brain can modify pain. For example, pain evoked by activity in nociceptors (Aδ and C fibers) can be reduced by simultaneous gentle massage or rubbing, which generates activity in low-threshold mechanoreceptors, which transmit signals via other fibers. A circuit in the spinal cord can "gate" the transmission of nociceptive information to the brain, by other sensory information, or by descending control from the brain.

A second mechanism for modifying the sensation of pain involves endorphins, acting through **opioid receptors.**

Muscle spindles sense changes in the length of skeletal muscle fibers, whereas Golgi tendon organs gauge the muscle's force

The somatic sensory receptors described thus far provide information about the *external* environment. **Proprioception** provides a sense of self, helping us judge the identity of external objects, and guiding many movements.

Skeletal muscles have two mechanosensitive proprioceptors: the muscle spindles (or stretch receptors) and Golgi tendon organs (Fig. 15.23). Muscle spindles measure the length and rate of stretch of the muscles, whereas the Golgi tendon organs gauge the force generated by a muscle by measuring the tension in its tendon. Together, they provide a full description of the dynamic state of each muscle. The different sensitivities of the spindle and the tendon organ are due partly to their structures but also to their placement: spindles are located in modified muscle fibers called *intrafusal* muscle fibers, which are aligned in *parallel* with the "ordinary" force-generating or *extrafusal* skeletal muscle fibers. On the other hand, Golgi tendon organs are aligned in *series* with the extrafusal fibers.

The **Golgi tendon organ** consists of bare nerve endings of axons. When tension develops in the muscle, distortion of the mechanosensitive nerve endings triggers action potentials.

The mammalian **muscle spindle** is a complex of modified skeletal muscle fibers **(intrafusal fibers)** combined with both afferent and efferent innervation. The spindle serves a purely sensory function. The muscle spindle contains intrafusal muscle fibers with sensory endings entwined about them. The discharge rate of afferent neurons increases when the whole muscle—and therefore the spindle—is stretched.

What is the function of the motor innervation of the muscle spindle? When the muscle contracts, the spindle (connected in parallel) would go slack. But γ motor neurons cause the intrafusal muscle fibers to contract, which greatly increases the range of lengths over which the spindle can work.

In addition to the muscle receptors, various mechanoreceptors are found in the connective tissues of **joints,** especially within the capsules and ligaments. Many resemble Ruffini, Golgi, and Pacini end organs; others are free nerve endings. They respond to changes in the angle, direction, and velocity of movement in a joint. Most are rapidly adapting, which means that sensory information about a *moving* joint is rich. It seems that information from joint receptors is combined with that from muscle spindles and Golgi tendon organs, and probably from cutaneous receptors as well, to estimate joint angle.

CHAPTER 16

CIRCUITS OF THE CENTRAL NERVOUS SYSTEM

Barry W. Connors

ELEMENTS OF NEURAL CIRCUITS

Neural circuits process sensory information, generate motor output, and create spontaneous activity

A neuron never works alone. Neurons participate in synaptically interconnected networks called **circuits.**

By the interconnection of various specialized neurons, even a simple neuronal circuit may accomplish astonishingly intricate functions. Some neural circuits may be primarily sensory (e.g., the retina) or motor (e.g., the ventral horns of the spinal cord). Many circuits combine both, with some neurons dedicated to providing and processing **sensory input,** others to commanding **motor output,** and many neurons doing both. Neural circuits may also generate their own intrinsic signals, with no need for any sensory or central input to activate them. The brain does more than just respond reflexively to sensory input. Some neural functions—such as walking, running, talking, and piano playing—require precise timing, with coordination of rhythmic temporal patterns across hundreds of outputs. These basic rhythms may be generated by neurons and neural circuits called **pacemakers** because of their clock-like capabilities. The patterns and rhythms generated by a pacemaking circuit can always be modulated—stopped, started, or altered—by input from sensory or central pathways.

This chapter introduces the basic principles of neural circuits in the mammalian central nervous system (CNS). We describe a few examples of specific systems in detail to illuminate general principles as well as the diversity of neural solutions to life's complex problems. However, this topic is enormous, and we have necessarily been selective and somewhat arbitrary in our presentation.

Nervous systems have several levels of organization

Many regions of the brain are composed of a large number of stereotyped **local circuits,** almost modular in their interchangeability, that are themselves interconnected. Within the local circuits are finer arrangements of neurons and synapses sometimes called **microcircuits.** At even finer resolution, neural systems can be understood by the properties of their individual neurons, **synapses,** membranes, **molecules** (e.g., neurotransmitters and neuromodulators), and ions as well as the **genes** that encode and control the system's molecular biology.

Most local circuits have three elements: input axons, interneurons, and projection (output) neurons

We will illustrate the general properties of local circuits with two examples: the ventral horn of the spinal cord and the cerebral neocortex. All local circuits have some form of **input,** usually axons that originate elsewhere and terminate in synapses within the local circuit. A major input to the spinal cord (Fig. 16.1) is the afferent sensory axons in the dorsal roots. These axons carry information from somatic sensory receptors in the skin, connective tissue, and muscles (see ⊙ **15-8**). However, local circuits in the spinal cord also have many other sources of input, including descending input from the brain and input from the spinal cord itself, both from the contralateral side and from spinal segments above and below. Input to the local circuits of the neocortex (Fig. 16.2) is also easily identified; relay neurons of the thalamus send axons into particular layers of the cortex to bring a range of information about sensation, motor systems, and the body's internal state. By far, the most numerous type of input to the local circuits of the neocortex comes from the neocortex itself—from adjacent local circuits, distant areas of cortex, and the contralateral hemisphere. These two systems illustrate a basic principle: local circuits receive multiple types of input.

Output is usually achieved with a subset of cells known as *projection neurons,* or *principal neurons,* which send axons to one or more targets. The most obvious spinal output comes from the α motor neurons, which send their axons out through the ventral roots to innervate skeletal muscle fibers. Output axons from the neocortex come mainly from large pyramidal neurons in layer V, which innervate many targets in the brainstem, spinal cord, and other structures, as well as from neurons in layer VI, which make their synapses back onto the cells of the thalamus. However, as was true with inputs, most local circuits have multiple types of outputs. Thus, spinal neurons innervate other regions of the spinal cord and the brain, whereas neocortical circuits make most of their connections to other neocortical circuits.

Rare, indeed, is the neural circuit that has only input and output cells. **Local processing** is achieved by additional neurons whose axonal connections remain within the local circuit. These neurons are usually called *interneurons* or *intrinsic neurons.* Interneurons vary widely in structure and function, and a single local circuit may have many different

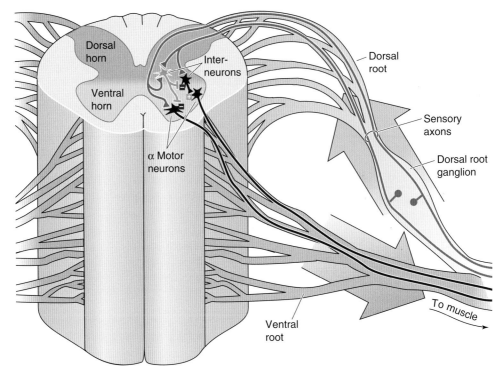

Figure 16.1 Local circuits in the spinal cord. A basic local circuit in the spinal cord consists of inputs (e.g., sensory axons of the dorsal roots), interneurons (both excitatory and inhibitory), and output neurons (e.g., α motor neurons that send their axons through the ventral roots).

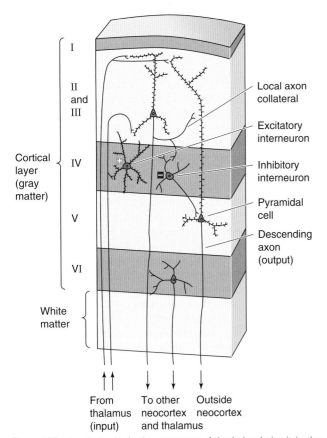

Figure 16.2 Local circuits in the neocortex. A basic local circuit in the neocortex consists of inputs (e.g., afferent axons from the thalamus), excitatory and inhibitory interneurons, and output neurons (e.g., pyramidal cells).

types. Both the spinal cord and neocortex have excitatory and inhibitory interneurons, interneurons that make very specific or widely divergent connections, and interneurons that either receive direct contact from input axons or process only information from other interneurons. In many parts of the brain, interneurons vastly outnumber output neurons.

The "principles" of local circuits outlined here have many variations. For example, a projection cell may also synapse within the local circuit. Some interneurons may entirely lack an axon and instead make their local synaptic connections through very short neurites or even dendrites. Although the main neurons within a generic local circuit are wired in *series* (Figs. 16.1 and 16.2), local circuits, often in massive numbers, operate in *parallel* with one another. Furthermore, these circuits usually demonstrate *crosstalk*; information from each circuit is shared, and each circuit influences neighboring circuits.

⊙ 16-1 SIMPLE, STEREOTYPED RESPONSES: SPINAL REFLEX CIRCUITS

Passive stretching of a skeletal muscle causes a reflexive contraction of that same muscle and relaxation of the antagonist muscles

Reflexes are among the most basic of neural functions and involve some of the simplest neuronal circuits. A motor *reflex* is a rapid, stereotyped motor response to a particular sensory stimulus.

Reflexes are essential, if rudimentary, elements of behavior. However, intricate behaviors may be built up from sequences of simple reflexive responses. Neural circuits that generate reflexes almost always mediate or participate in

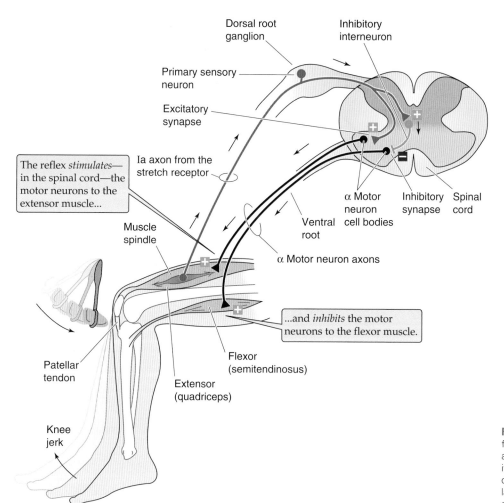

Dorsal root ganglion

Inhibitory interneuron

Primary sensory neuron

Excitatory synapse

The reflex *stimulates*— in the spinal cord—the motor neurons to the extensor muscle...

Ia axon from the stretch receptor

α Motor neuron cell bodies

Inhibitory synapse

Spinal cord

Muscle spindle

Ventral root

α Motor neuron axons

...and *inhibits* the motor neurons to the flexor muscle.

Patellar tendon

Flexor (semitendinosus)

Extensor (quadriceps)

Knee jerk

Figure 16.3 Knee-jerk (myotatic) reflex. Tapping the patellar tendon with a percussion hammer elicits a reflexive knee jerk caused by contraction of the quadriceps muscle and the relaxation of the semitendinosus muscle: the *stretch reflex*.

much more complex behaviors. Here we examine a relatively well understood example of reflex-mediating circuitry.

The CNS commands the body to move about by activating motor neurons, which excite skeletal muscles. Motor neurons receive synaptic input from many sources within the brain and spinal cord. However, in some circumstances, motor neurons can be commanded directly by a simple sensory stimulus—muscle stretch—with only the minimum of neural machinery intervening between the sensory cell and motor neuron: one synapse. Understanding of this simplest of reflexes, the **stretch reflex** or **myotatic reflex,** first requires knowledge of some anatomy.

Each motor neuron, with its soma in the spinal cord or brainstem, commands a group of skeletal muscle cells; a single motor neuron and the muscle cells that it synapses on are collectively called a **motor unit** (see Fig. 9.10A). Each muscle cell belongs to only one motor unit. The group of all motor neurons innervating a single muscle is called a **motor neuron pool** (see Fig. 9.10B).

When a skeletal muscle is abruptly stretched, a rapid, reflexive contraction of the same muscle often occurs. The contraction increases muscle tension and opposes the stretch. This stretch reflex is particularly strong in physiological extensor muscles—those that resist gravity. The most familiar version

is the knee jerk, which is elicited by a light tap on the patellar tendon. The tap deflects the tendon, which then pulls on and briefly stretches the quadriceps femoris muscle. A reflexive contraction of the quadriceps quickly follows (Fig. 16.3). The basic circuit for the stretch reflex begins with the primary sensory axons from the **muscle spindles** (see Fig. 15.23) in the muscle itself. Increasing the length of the muscle stimulates the spindle afferents, particularly the large group Ia axons from the primary sensory endings. In the spinal cord, these group Ia sensory axons terminate monosynaptically onto the α motor neurons that innervate the same muscle. Thus, stretching a muscle causes rapid feedback excitation of the same muscle through the minimum possible circuit: one sensory neuron, one central synapse, and one motor neuron.

At the same time the stretched muscle is being stimulated to contract, parallel circuits are inhibiting the α motor neurons of its *antagonist* muscles. Thus, as the knee-jerk reflex causes contraction of the quadriceps muscle, it simultaneously causes relaxation of its antagonists, including the semitendinosus muscle (Fig. 16.3). To achieve inhibition, branches of the group Ia sensory axons excite specific interneurons that *inhibit* the α motor neurons of the antagonists. This **reciprocal innervation** increases the effectiveness of the stretch reflex by minimizing the antagonistic forces of the antagonist muscles.

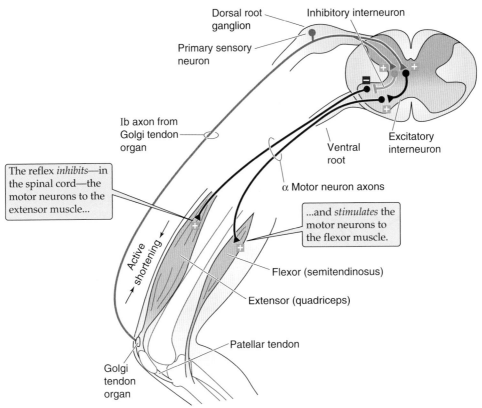

Figure 16.4   Golgi tendon organ reflex.

Force applied to the Golgi tendon organ regulates muscle contractile strength

Skeletal muscle contains another mechanosensory transducer in addition to the stretch receptor: the **Golgi tendon organ** (see Fig. 15.23). Tendon organs are aligned in series with the muscle; they are sensitive to the *tension* within a tendon and thus respond to the force generated by the muscle rather than to muscle length. Tendon organs are stimulated particularly well during active contractions of a muscle. The group Ib sensory axons of the tendon organs excite both excitatory and inhibitory interneurons within the spinal cord (Fig. 16.4). In some cases, this interneuron circuitry *inhibits* the muscle in which tension has increased and *excites* the antagonistic muscle; therefore, activity in the tendon organs can yield effects that are almost the opposite of the stretch reflex. Under other circumstances, particularly during rapid movements such as locomotion, sensory input from Golgi tendon organs actually excites the motor neurons activating the same muscle. In general, reflexes mediated by the Golgi tendon organs serve to control the force within muscles and the stability of particular joints.

Noxious stimuli can evoke complex reflexive movements

Sensations from the skin and connective tissue can also evoke strong spinal reflexes. Imagine walking on a beach and stepping on a sharp piece of shell. Your response is swift and coordinated and does not require thoughtful reflection: you rapidly withdraw the wounded foot by activating the leg flexors and inhibiting the extensors. To keep from falling, you also extend your opposite leg by activating its extensors and

inhibiting its flexors (Fig. 16.5). This response is an example of a **flexion-withdrawal reflex.** The original stimulus for the reflex came from fast pain afferent neurons in the skin.

This bilateral flexor reflex response is coordinated by sets of inhibitory and excitatory interneurons within the spinal gray matter. Note that this coordination requires circuitry not only on the side of the cord ipsilateral to the wounded side, but also on the contralateral side. That is, while you withdraw the foot that hurts, you must extend the opposite leg. Flexor reflexes can be activated by most of the various sensory afferents that detect noxious stimuli. Motor output spreads widely up and down the spinal cord, as it must to orchestrate so much of the body's musculature into an effective response. A remarkable feature of flexor reflexes is their specificity. Touching a hot surface, for example, elicits reflexive withdrawal of the hand in the direction opposite the side of the stimulus, and the strength of the reflex is related to the intensity of the stimulus. Unlike simple stretch reflexes, flexor reflexes coordinate the movement of entire limbs and even pairs of limbs. Such coordination requires precise and widespread wiring of the spinal interneurons.

RHYTHMIC ACTIVITY: CENTRAL PATTERN GENERATORS

Central pattern generators in the spinal cord can create a complex motor program even without sensory feedback

⊙ **16-2** A common feature of motor control is the **motor program,** a set of structured muscle commands that are determined by the nervous system before a movement begins and

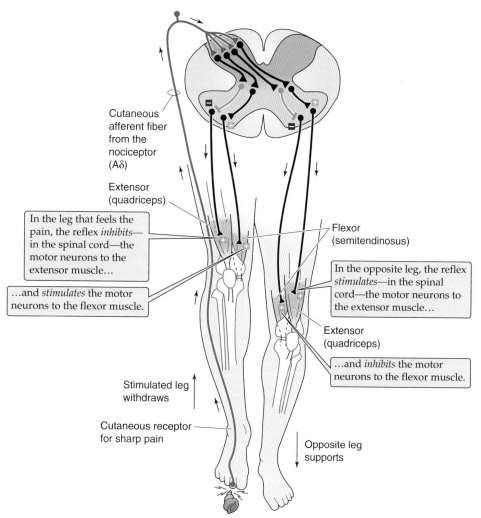

Figure 16.5   Flexion-withdrawal reflex.

Labels within figure:

Cutaneous afferent fiber from the nociceptor (Aδ)

Extensor (quadriceps)

In the leg that feels the pain, the reflex *inhibits*— in the spinal cord—the motor neurons to the extensor muscle...

...and *stimulates* the motor neurons to the flexor muscle.

Flexor (semitendinosus)

In the opposite leg, the reflex *stimulates*—in the spinal cord—the motor neurons to the extensor muscle...

Extensor (quadriceps)

...and *inhibits* the motor neurons to the flexor muscle.

Stimulated leg withdraws

Cutaneous receptor for sharp pain

Opposite leg supports

that can be sent to the muscles with the appropriate timing so that a sequence of movements occurs without any need for sensory feedback. The brain or spinal cord can command a variety of voluntary and automatic movements, such as walking, even in the complete absence of sensory feedback from the periphery. However, motor behavior without sensory feedback is always different from that with normal feedback. Here we focus on **central pattern generators (CPG)**, circuits that underlie many rhythmic motor activities.

Rhythmic behavior includes walking, running, swimming, breathing, chewing, certain eye movements, shivering, and even scratching. The CPGs driving each of these activities share certain basic properties. At their core is a set of cyclic, coordinated timing signals that are generated by a cluster of interconnected neurons. These basic signals command many muscles, each contracting or relaxing during a particular phase of the cycle; for example, with each walking step, the knee must first be flexed and then extended. Fig. 16.6 shows how the extensor and flexor muscles of the left hind limb of a cat contract rhythmically—and out of phase with one another—while the animal walks. Rhythms must also be coordinated; for humans to walk, one leg must move forward while the other thrusts backward. For four-footed animals, the rhythms are even more complicated and must

be able to accommodate changes in gait. For coordination to be achieved among the various limbs, sets of CPGs must be interconnected. The motor patterns must also have great flexibility so that they can be altered on a moment's notice—consider the adjustments necessary when one foot strikes an obstacle while walking or the changing motor patterns necessary to go from walking, to trotting, to running, to jumping. Finally, reliable methods must be available for regulating the speed of the patterns and for turning them on and off.

The CPGs for locomotion reside in the spinal cord itself. Even with the spinal cord transected so that the lumbar segments are isolated from all higher centers, cats on a treadmill can generate well-coordinated stepping movements. Furthermore, stimulation of sensory afferents or descending tracts can induce the spinal pattern generators in four-footed animals to switch rapidly from walking, to trotting, to galloping patterns by altering not only the frequency of motor commands but also their pattern and coordination. Each limb has at least one CPG. Under most circumstances, the various spinal CPGs are coupled to one another, although the nature of the coupling must change to explain, for example, the switch from trotting to galloping patterns.

⊙ 16-3 Pacemaker cells and synaptic interconnections both contribute to central pattern generation

How do neural circuits generate rhythmic patterns of activity? Different circuits use different mechanisms. The simplest pattern generators are single neurons whose membrane characteristics endow them with pacemaker properties, analogous to those of cardiac muscle cells. It is easy to imagine how intrinsic pacemaker neurons might act as the primary rhythmic driving force for sets of motor neurons that in turn command cyclic behavior. Most commonly, pacemakers are embedded within interconnected circuits, and it is the combination of intrinsic pacemaker properties and synaptic interconnections that generates rhythms.

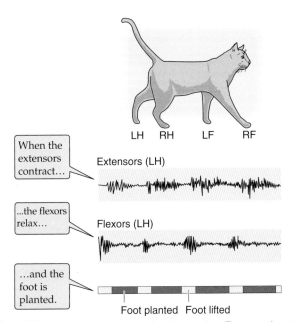

Figure 16.6 Rhythmic patterns during locomotion. The experimental tracings are electromyograms (EMGs)—extracellular recordings of the electrical activity of muscles—of a walking cat. The *pink bars* indicate that the foot is lifted; the *purple bars* indicate that the foot is planted. (Data from Pearson K: The control of walking. Sci Am 2:72–86, 1976.)

Neural circuits without pacemaker neurons can also generate rhythmic output. The **half-center model** is a set of excitatory and inhibitory interneurons arranged to inhibit one another reciprocally (Fig. 16.7). Each half-center commands one of a pair of antagonist muscles. For the circuit to work, a tonic (i.e., nonrhythmic) drive must be applied to the excitatory interneurons; this drive could come from axons originating outside the circuit (e.g., from neurons in the brain) or from the intrinsic excitability of the neurons themselves. Furthermore, some built-in mechanism must limit the duration of the inhibitory activity so that excitability can cyclically switch from one half-center to the other. Note that feedback from the muscles is not needed for the rhythms to proceed indefinitely.

Central pattern generators in the spinal cord take advantage of sensory feedback, interconnections among spinal segments, and interactions with brainstem control centers

CPGs in the lamprey spinal cord provide valuable insight into how more advanced circuits can operate. The lamprey pattern-generating circuit improves on the half-center model in three ways. The first is **sensory feedback.** As the lamprey swims, it activates stretch-receptor neurons on the side that is currently relaxed. Activated stretch receptors act via interneurons to facilitate contraction on the same side and inhibit contraction on the contralateral side.

The second improvement of the lamprey circuit over the half-center model is the **interconnection of spinal segments,** which ensures the smooth progression of contractions down the length of the body. Specifically, each segment must command its muscles to contract slightly later than the one anterior to it, with a lag of ~1% of a full activity cycle.

A third improvement over the half-center model is the **reciprocal communication** between the lamprey spinal pattern generators and control centers in the brainstem. Not only does the brainstem modulate the generators, but the spinal generators also inform the brainstem of their activity.

The features outlined for swimming lampreys are relevant to walking cats and humans. All use spinal pattern generators, sensory feedback, and reciprocal communication between spinal generators and brainstem control centers.

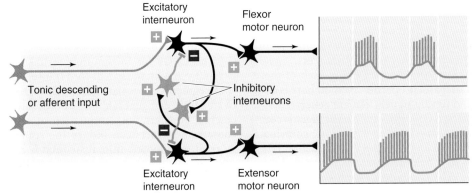

Figure 16.7   Half-center model for alternating rhythm generation in flexor and extensor motor neurons. Stimulating the upper excitatory interneuron has two effects. First, the stimulated excitatory interneuron excites the motor neuron to the flexor muscle. Second, the stimulated excitatory interneuron excites an inhibitory interneuron, which inhibits the lower pathway. Stimulating the lower excitatory interneuron has the opposite effects. Thus, when one motor neuron is active, the opposite one is inhibited.

A CORONAL SECTION SHOWING PROJECTION OF THE RETINA TO THE PRIMARY VISUAL CORTEX

B SAGITTAL SECTIONS SHOWING VISUOTOPY OF THE PRIMARY VISUAL CORTEX

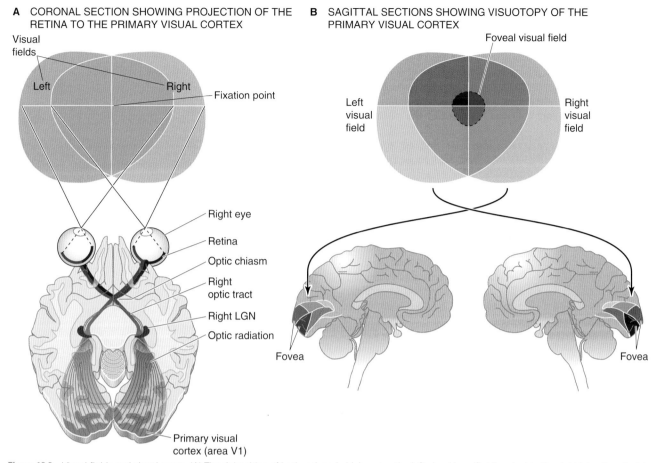

Figure 16.8   Visual fields and visual maps. (A) The right sides of both retinas (which sense the left visual hemifield) project to the right lateral geniculate nucleus (LGN), which in turn projects to the right primary visual cortex (area V1). (B) The upper parts of the visual fields project to lower parts of the contralateral visual cortex, and vice versa.

SPATIAL REPRESENTATIONS: SENSORY AND MOTOR MAPS IN THE BRAIN

How does the brain organize sensory input and motor output? In many cases, it organizes these functions spatially with neural maps. Maps in the brain represent selected aspects of our sensory information about the environment or the motor systems controlling our body.

The nervous system contains maps of sensory and motor information

In some cases, sensory receptors form straightforward **spatial maps** of the sensory environment that they encode. For example, the somatic sensory receptors of the skin literally form a map of the body surface. The topographies of other sensory receptors represent qualities other than spatial features of the sensory stimuli. For example, there are **chemical maps** for olfaction and taste. Each sensory surface may be mapped and remapped many times within the brain.

The cerebral cortex has multiple visuotopic maps

Some of the best examples of brain maps are those of the visual fields. Fig. 16.8A shows the basic anatomical

pathway extending from the retina to the lateral geniculate nucleus of the thalamus and on to the **primary visual cortex** (area V1). Note that area V1 actually maps the visual thalamus, which in turn maps the retina. Thus, the V1 map is a *retinotopic map.* Fig. 16.8B shows how the visual fields are mapped onto cortical area V1. The *left* half of the visual field is represented on the *right* cortex and the *upper* half of the visual field is represented on the *lower* portions of the cortex. This orientation is strictly determined by the system's anatomy. For example, all the retinal axons from the *left*-most halves of both eyes (which are stimulated by light from the *right* visual hemifield) project to the *left* half of the brain. Compare the red and blue pathways in Fig. 16.8A.

Scaling of the visual fields onto the visual cortex—the **magnification factor**—is not constant. In particular, the central region of the visual fields—the fovea—is greatly magnified on the cortical surface, since primates require vision of particularly high resolution in the center of their gaze.

Understanding a visual scene requires us to analyze many of its features simultaneously. Several features of a visual scene, such as motion, form, and color, are processed in parallel with strong and reciprocal interconnections between the visual maps in various areas of the brain.

Maps of somatic sensory information magnify some parts of the body more than others

⊙ 16-4 The human **somatotopic** map resembles a trapeze artist hanging upside down: the legs are hooked over the top of the postcentral gyrus and dangle into the medial cortex between the hemispheres, and the trunk, upper limbs, and head are draped over the lateral aspect of the postcentral gyrus.

Two interesting features should be noticed about the somatotopic map in Fig. 16.9A. First, mapping of the body surface is not always continuous. For example, the representation of the hand separates those of the head and face. Second, the map is not scaled like the human body. Instead, it looks like a cartoon character: the mouth, tongue, and fingers are very large, whereas the trunk, arms, and legs are tiny. As was the case for mapping of the visual fields onto the visual cortex, the magnification factor for the body surface varies. The relative size of cortex that is devoted to each body part is correlated with the *density* of sensory input received from that part, and 1 mm^2 of fingertip skin has many more sensory endings than a similar patch on the buttocks. Size on the map is also related to the *importance* of the sensory input from that part of the body.

⊙ 16-5 The cerebral cortex has a motor map that is adjacent to and well aligned with the somatosensory map

Neural maps are not limited to sensory systems. Motor maps (Fig. 16.9B) look remarkably like somatosensory maps, which lie in the adjacent cortical gyrus (Fig. 16.9A). Not surprisingly, there are myriad axonal interconnections between the primary motor and primary somatosensory areas. Rather than following an obvious somatotopic progression, it instead appears that neurons in the arm area of the motor cortex form distributed and cooperative networks that control collections of arm muscles. Somatotopic maps still suffice to describe the gross organization of the motor cortex.

In other parts of the brain, *motor and sensory functions may even occupy the same tissue*, and precise alignment of the motor and sensory maps is usually the case. Maps of different sensory modalities may be superimposed.

Sensory and motor maps are fuzzy and plastic

Maps may be the most efficient way of generating **nearest-neighbor relationships** between neurons that must be interconnected for proper function. Orderly mapping minimizes the length of axons necessary for interconnections. In addition, if brain structures are arranged topographically, neighboring neurons will be most likely to become activated synchronously. Neighboring neurons are very likely to be interconnected in structures such as the cortex, and their synchronous activity serves to reinforce the strength of their interconnections because of the inherent rules governing synaptic plasticity (see ⊙ 13-8).

An additional advantage of mapping is that it may simplify establishment of the proper connections between neurons during **development**. For example, it is easier for an axon from neuron A to find neuron B if distances are short. Maps may also facilitate the effectiveness of **inhibitory connections**. Perception of the edge of a stimulus (edge detection)

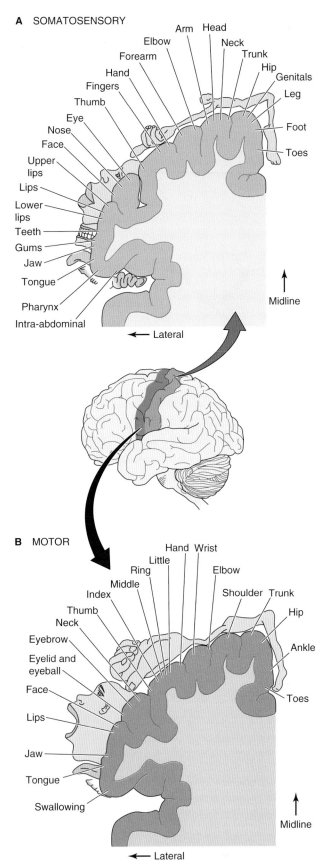

Figure 16.9 Somatosensory and motor maps. (A) The plane of section runs through the postcentral gyrus of the cerebral cortex, shown as a *blue band* on the image of the brain. (B) The plane of section runs through the precentral gyrus of the cerebral cortex, shown as a *violet band* on the image of the brain. (Data from Penfield W, Rasmussen T: The Cerebral Cortex of Man. New York, Macmillan, 1952.)

is heightened by lateral connections that suppress the activity of neurons representing the space slightly away from the edge. If sensory areas are mapped, it is a simple matter to arrange the inhibitory connections onto nearby neurons and thereby construct an edge-detector circuit.

Neuronal maps are not perfectly precise. For example, a point in sensory space (e.g., a spot of light) activates a relatively large group of neurons in a sensory region of the brain. This is not due to errors of connectivity; the spatial dissemination of activity is part of the mechanism used to encode and to process information. The *strength* of activation is most intense within the center of the activated neuronal group, but the population of more weakly activated neurons may encompass a large portion of an entire brain. A point in sensory space is not encoded by the activity of a single neuron, but by the distributed activity in a large population of neurons. Such a distributed code has computational advantages, and some redundancy also guards against errors.

Finally, maps may change with time. All sensory and motor maps are clearly dynamic and can be reorganized rapidly and substantially as a function of development, behavioral state, training, or damage to the brain or periphery. Such changes are referred to as **plasticity.** For example, severing a peripheral nerve causes the part of the map that normally relates to the body part served by this severed nerve to become remapped to another body part. Similar processes probably underlie our ability to learn sensorimotor skills with practice and to adjust and improve after neural damage from trauma or stroke.

TEMPORAL REPRESENTATIONS: TIME-MEASURING CIRCUITS

To localize sound, the brain compares the timing and intensity of input to the ears

Neural circuits are very good at resolving time intervals, in some cases down to microseconds or less. One of the most demanding tasks of timing is performed by the auditory system as it localizes the source of certain sounds. Sound localization is an important skill, whether you are prey, predator, or pedestrian. In this subchapter, we briefly review general strategies of sound localization, and then explain how a circuit measures the relative timing of low-frequency sounds to localize the source.

Sound localization along the **vertical plane** depends on the shape of the external ear, the *pinna*. Much of the sound that we hear enters the auditory canal directly, and its energy is transferred to the cochlea. However, some sound reflects off the curves and folds of the pinna before it enters the canal and thus takes slightly longer to reach the cochlea. Because of the arcing shape of the pinna, the reflected path of sounds coming from above is shorter than that of sounds from below (Fig. 16.10). The combined sound (direct + reflected) has spectral properties that are characteristic of the elevation of the sound source. This mechanism of vertical sound localization works well even with one ear at a time.

For humans, accurate determination of the direction of a sound along the **horizontal plane** requires two working ears. Sounds must first be processed by the cochlea in each ear

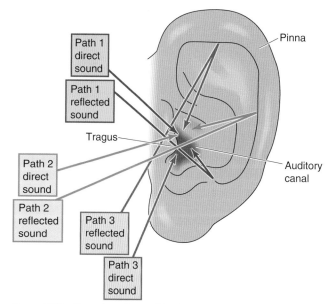

Figure 16.10 Detection of sound in the vertical plane. The detection of sound in the vertical plane requires only one ear. Regardless of the source of a sound, the sound reaches the auditory canal by both direct and reflected pathways. The brain localizes the source of the sound in the vertical plane by detecting differences in the combined sounds from the direct and reflected pathways.

and then compared by neurons within the CNS to estimate horizontal direction. For sounds that are relatively high in frequency (~2 to 20 kHz), the important measure is the *interaural* (i.e., ear-to-ear) *intensity difference*. The ear facing the sound hears it as louder than the ear facing away because the head casts a "sound shadow" (Fig. 16.11A). If the sound is directly to the right or left of the listener, this difference is maximal; if the sound is straight ahead, no difference is heard; and if the sound comes from an oblique direction, intensity differences are intermediate. Note that this system can be fooled. A sound source straight ahead gives the same intensity difference (i.e., none) as a sound source directly behind.

The interaural intensity difference is not helpful at lower frequencies. Sounds below ~2 kHz have a wavelength that is longer than the width of the head itself. At low frequencies, the nervous system measures *interaural delay* (Fig. 16.11B). Consider a 200-Hz sound coming directly from the right at the speed of sound in air of 343 m/s. Its peak-to-peak distance (i.e., the wavelength) is ~172 cm, which is considerably more than the 20-cm width of the head. Each sound wave peak will reach the right ear ~0.6 ms before it reaches the left ear. If the sound comes from a 45-degree angle ahead, the interaural delay is ~0.3 ms; if it comes from straight ahead (or directly behind), the delay is 0 ms. Delays of small fractions of a millisecond are well within the capabilities of certain brainstem auditory neurons to detect. Sound onset or offset, clicks, or any abrupt changes in the sound give opportunities for interaural time comparisons. Obviously, measurement of interaural delay is subject to the same front-back ambiguity as interaural intensity, and indeed, it is sometimes difficult to distinguish whether a sound is in front of or behind your head.

A HIGH-FREQUENCY SOUND

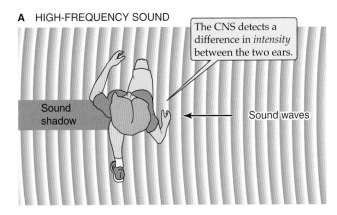

The CNS detects a difference in *intensity* between the two ears.

Sound shadow

Sound waves

B LOW-FREQUENCY SOUND

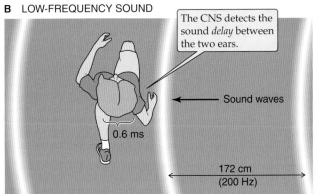

The CNS detects the sound *delay* between the two ears.

Sound waves

0.6 ms

172 cm
(200 Hz)

Figure 16.11 Sound detection in a horizontal plane. (A) Two ears are necessary for the detection of sound in a horizontal plane. For frequencies between 2 kHz and 20 kHz, the CNS detects the ear-to-ear *intensity* difference. (B) For frequencies <2 kHz, the CNS detects the ear-to-ear *delay*.

The brain measures interaural timing by a combination of neural delay lines and coincidence detectors

To detect very small *time* differences, the nervous system uses a precise arrangement of neurons in *space*. Neurons in each of the cochlear nuclei receive information from only the ear on that one side, whereas neurons from the **medial superior olivary (MSO) nucleus**—and higher CNS centers—receive abundant input from both ears (Fig. 16.12). When cochlear nucleus neurons are activated by auditory stimuli, their action potentials tend to fire with a particular phase relationship to the sound stimulus. That is, its firing is *phase locked* to the sound waves for relatively low frequencies. Hence, cochlear neurons preserve the timing information of sound stimuli. Neurons in the MSO nucleus receive synaptic input from axons originating in both cochlear nuclei, so they are well placed to compare the timing (the phase) of sounds arriving at the two ears. Recordings from MSO neurons demonstrate that they are exquisitely sensitive to interaural time delay, and the optimal delay for superior olivary neurons varies systematically across the nucleus. In other words, the MSO nucleus has a spatial map of *interaural delay*. The MSO also has a systematic map of sound *frequency*, so it simultaneously maps two qualities of sound stimuli.

The tuning of MSO neurons to interaural delay seems to depend on neural circuitry that combines "delay lines" with "coincidence detection." **Delay lines** are the axons from each cochlear nucleus; their length and conduction velocity determine how long it takes sound-activated action potentials to reach MSO neurons (Fig. 16.12). Axons from both the right and left cochlear nuclei converge and synapse onto a series of

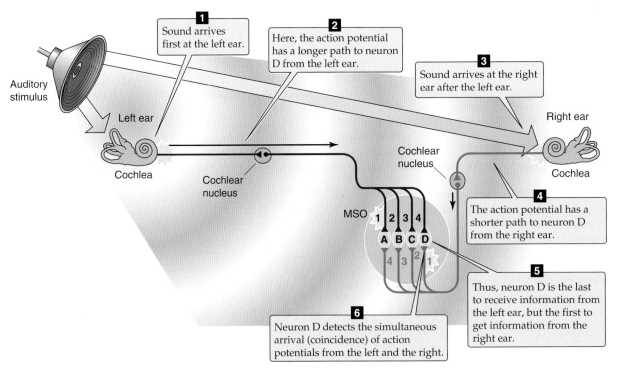

1 Sound arrives first at the left ear.

2 Here, the action potential has a longer path to neuron D from the left ear.

3 Sound arrives at the right ear after the left ear.

4 The action potential has a shorter path to neuron D from the right ear.

5 Thus, neuron D is the last to receive information from the left ear, but the first to get information from the right ear.

6 Neuron D detects the simultaneous arrival (coincidence) of action potentials from the left and the right.

Auditory stimulus

Left ear

Cochlea

Cochlear nucleus

Cochlear nucleus

Right ear

Cochlea

MSO 1 2 3 4
      A B C D
      4 3 2 1

Figure 16.12 Perception of interaural delay by coincidence detection. Neurons in the MSO nucleus are each tuned to a different interaural delay that provides information about the horizontal direction of sound sources. Only when action potentials from the right and left sides arrive at the MSO neuron simultaneously does the neuron fire an action potential (coincidence detection).

neurons in the MSO nucleus. The difference in conduction delay between the axon from the right side and that from the left side determines the optimal interaural delay for that particular olivary neuron. It is the olivary neuron that acts as the **coincidence detector:** only when action potentials from *both* the left- and right-ear axons reach the postsynaptic MSO neuron simultaneously (meaning that sound has reached the two ears at a particular interaural delay) is that neuron likely to fire an action potential. Because neurons arrayed across the olive are mapped so that the axons connecting them have different delays, each is **tuned** to a different interaural delay and a different sound locale. The orderly arrangement of delay lines across the olive leads to the orderly spatial mapping of sound direction.

Synaptic inhibition, and perhaps other neuronal properties, also contribute to the measurement of timing.

Neural maps of sound localization are an interesting example of a sensory map that the brain must *compute*. The cochlea does not have any map for sound location. Instead, the CNS localizes low-frequency sounds by calculating an interaural *time-delay* map, using information from both ears together. Other circuits can build a computed map of interaural *intensity differences,* which can be used for localization of high-frequency sounds (Fig. 16.11A). This combination of hierarchic (lower to higher centers) and parallel information processing is ubiquitous in the CNS and is a general strategy for the analysis of much more complex sensory problems than those described here.

THE CARDIOVASCULAR SYSTEM

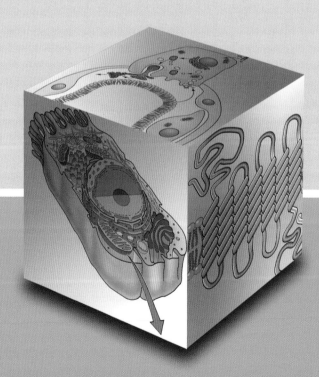

CHAPTER 17

ORGANIZATION OF THE CARDIOVASCULAR SYSTEM

Emile L. Boulpaep

ELEMENTS OF THE CARDIOVASCULAR SYSTEM

Circulation is an evolutionary consequence of body size

Isolated single cells and small organisms do not have a circulatory system as they can meet their metabolic needs by the simple processes of diffusion and convection of solutes from the *external* to the *internal milieu*. The requirement for a circulatory system is an evolutionary consequence of the increasing size and complexity of multicellular organisms.

In complex organisms, a circulatory system provides a steep concentration gradient from the blood to centrally located cells for nutrients and in the opposite direction for waste products. Maintenance of such steep intracellular-to-extracellular concentration gradients requires a fast convection system that rapidly circulates fluid between surfaces that equilibrate with the *external milieu* (e.g., the lung, gut, and kidney epithelia) and individual cells located deep inside the organism. In mammals and birds, the exchange of gases with the external milieu is so important that they have evolved a two-pump, dual circulatory system that delivers the full output of the "heart" to the lungs (see ⊙ 31-3).

The primary role of the **circulatory system** is the distribution of dissolved gases and other molecules for nutrition, growth, and repair. Secondary roles have also evolved: (1) fast chemical signaling to cells by means of circulating hormones or neurotransmitters, (2) dissipation of heat by delivery of heat from the core to the surface of the body, and (3) mediation of inflammatory and host defense responses against invading microorganisms.

The circulatory system of humans integrates three basic functional parts, or organs: a pump (the **heart**) that circulates a liquid (the **blood**) through a set of containers (the **vessels**). This integrated system is able to adapt to the changing circumstances of normal life. Demand on the circulation fluctuates widely between sleep and wakefulness, between rest and exercise, with acceleration/deceleration, during changes in body position or intrathoracic pressure, during digestion, and under emotional or thermal stress. To meet these variable demands, the entire system requires sophisticated and integrated regulation.

The heart is a dual pump that drives the blood in two serial circuits: the systemic and the pulmonary circulations

A remarkable pump, weighing ~300 g, drives the human circulation. The heart really consists of two pumps, the **left heart,** or main pump, and the **right heart,** or boost pump. These pumps operate in series and require a delicate equalization of their outputs. The output of each pump is ~5 L/min, but this can easily increase 5-fold during exercise.

With each heartbeat, the ventricles impart the energy necessary to circulate the blood by generating the pressure head that drives the flow of blood through the **vascular system.** On the basis of its anatomy, we can divide this system of tubes into two main circuits: the **systemic** and the **pulmonary** circulations. We could also divide the vascular system into a **high-pressure** part (extending from the contracting left ventricle to the systemic capillaries) and a **low-pressure** part (extending from the systemic capillaries, through the right heart, across the pulmonary circulation and left atrium, and into the left ventricle in its relaxed state). The vessels also respond to the changing metabolic demands of the tissues they supply by directing blood flow to (or away from) tissues as demands change. The circulatory system is also self-repairing/self-expanding. Endothelial cells lining vessels mend the surfaces of existing blood vessels and generate new vessels (**angiogenesis).**

Some of the most important life-threatening human diseases are caused by failure of the heart as a pump (e.g., congestive heart failure), failure of the blood as an effective liquid organ (e.g., thrombosis and embolism), or failure of the vasculature either as a competent container (e.g., hemorrhage) or as an efficient distribution system (e.g., atherosclerosis). Moreover, failure of the normal interactions among these three organs can by itself elicit or aggravate many human pathological processes.

HEMODYNAMICS

Blood flow is driven by a constant pressure head across variable resistances

To keep concepts simple, assume that blood flow throughout the circulation is steady or nonpulsatile.

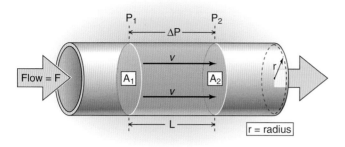

Figure 17.1 Flow through a straight tube. The flow *(F)* between a high-pressure point *(P₁)* and a low-pressure point *(P₂)* is proportional to the pressure difference (ΔP). *A₁* and *A₂* are cross-sectional areas at these two points. A cylindrical bolus of fluid—between the disks at *P₁* and *P₂*—moves down the tube with a linear velocity *v*.

To understand the *steady flow* of blood, driven by a *constant pressure* head, we can apply classical hydrodynamic laws analogous to Ohm's law of electricity:

$$\Delta V = I \cdot R \quad \text{for electricity}$$
$$\Delta P = F \cdot R \quad \text{for liquids} \tag{17.1}$$

That is, the pressure difference (ΔP) between an upstream point (pressure P_1) and a downstream site (pressure P_2) is equal to the product of the flow *(F)* and the resistance *(R)* between those two points (Fig. 17.1).

◉ **17-1** In reality, the **pressure difference** (ΔP) between the beginning and end points of the human systemic circulation—that is, between the high-pressure side (aorta) and the low-pressure side (vena cava)—turns out to be fairly constant over time. Thus, the heart behaves more like a generator of a constant pressure head than like a generator of constant flow, at least within physiological limits. Indeed, **flow** (F), the output of the left heart, is quite variable in time and depends greatly on the physiological circumstances (e.g., whether one is active or at rest). Like flow, **resistance** (R) varies with time; in addition, it varies with location within the body. The overall resistance of the circulation reflects the contributions of a complex network of vessels in both the systemic and pulmonary circuits.

As shown in Fig. 17.2, blood can take many different pathways *from the left heart to the right heart.*

The overall resistance (R_{total}) across a circulatory bed results from parallel and serial arrangements of branches and is governed by laws similar to those for the electrical resistance of DC circuits. For multiple resistance elements (R_1, R_2, R_3, …) arranged in series,

$$R_{\text{total}} = R_1 + R_2 + R_3 + \dots \tag{17.2}$$

For multiple elements arranged in parallel,

$$\frac{1}{R_{\text{total}}} = \frac{1}{R_1} + \frac{1}{R_2} + \frac{1}{R_3} + \dots \tag{17.3}$$

Blood pressure is always measured as a pressure difference between two points

Physicists measure pressure in the units of grams per square centimeter or dynes per square centimeter.

However, physiologists most often gauge blood pressure by the height it can drive a column of liquid. This pressure is

$$P = \rho g h \tag{17.4}$$

where ϱ is the density of the liquid in the column, *g* is the gravitational constant, and *h* is the height of the column. Therefore, if we neglect variations in *g* and know ϱ for the fluid in the column (usually water or mercury), we can take the height of the liquid column as a measure of blood pressure. Physiologists usually express this pressure in millimeters of mercury or centimeters of water. Clinicians use the classical blood pressure gauge (sphygmomanometer) to report arterial blood pressure in millimeters of mercury.

Pressure is never expressed in absolute terms but as a **pressure difference** ΔP relative to some "reference" pressure. We can make this concept intuitively clear by considering pressure as a force *F* applied to a surface area *A*.

$$P = F / A \tag{17.5}$$

We can define a movement or distortion of a mechanical system only by the *difference* between two forces. In hemodynamics, we compare the difference between two pressures.

Because a pressure difference is always between two points—and these two points are separated by some distance (Δ*x*) and have a spatial orientation to one another—we can define a pressure gradient (ΔP/Δ*x*) with a spatial orientation. Considering orientation, we can define three different kinds of pressure differences in the circulation:

1. **Driving pressure.** In Fig. 17.3, the ΔP between points x_1 and x_2 inside the vessel—along the axis of the vessel—is the axial pressure difference. Because this ΔP causes blood to flow from x_1 to x_2, it is also known as the driving pressure. In the circulation, the driving pressure is the ΔP between the arterial and venous ends of the systemic (or pulmonary) circulation, and it governs blood flow (Fig. 17.1).

2. **Transmural pressure.** ◉ **17-2** The ΔP in Fig. 17.3 between point r_1 (inside the vessel) and r_2 (just outside the vessel)—along the radial axis—is an example of a radial pressure difference. The ΔP between r_1 and r_2 is the transmural pressure; that is, the difference between the intravascular pressure and the tissue pressure. Because blood vessels are distensible, transmural pressure governs vessel diameter, which is in turn the major determinant of resistance.

3. **Hydrostatic pressure.** ◉ **17-3** Because of the density of blood and gravitational forces, a third pressure difference arises if the vessel does not lie in a horizontal plane, as was the case in Fig. 17.1. The ΔP in Fig. 17.3 between point h_1 (bottom of a liquid column) and h_2 (top of the column)—along the height axis—is the hydrostatic pressure difference $P_1 - P_2$. This ΔP is similar to the *P* in Equation 17.4 (here, ϱ is the density of blood), and it exists even in the absence of any blood flow. If we express increasing altitude in positive units of *h*, then hydrostatic ΔP = $-\varrho g(h_1 - h_2)$.

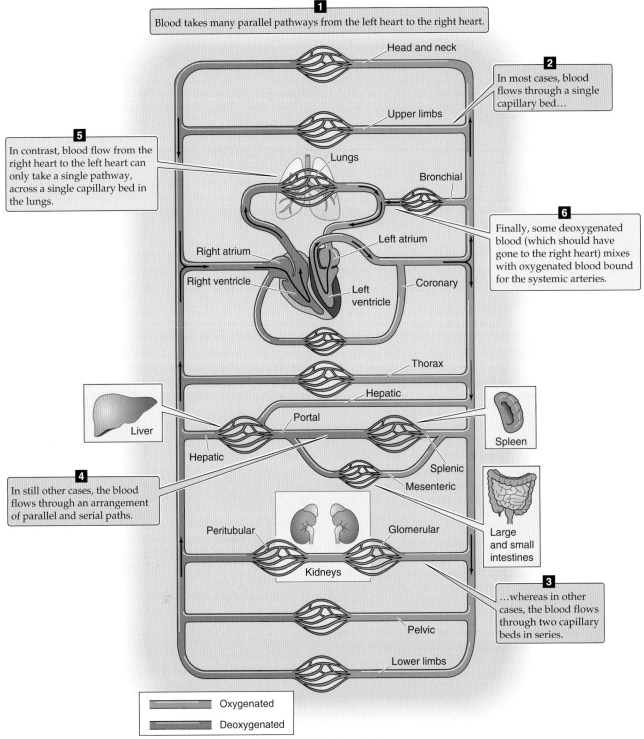

1 Blood takes many parallel pathways from the left heart to the right heart.

Head and neck

2 In most cases, blood flows through a single capillary bed...

Upper limbs

5 In contrast, blood flow from the right heart to the left heart can only take a single pathway, across a single capillary bed in the lungs.

Lungs

Bronchial

Left atrium

Right atrium

6 Finally, some deoxygenated blood (which should have gone to the right heart) mixes with oxygenated blood bound for the systemic arteries.

Right ventricle

Left ventricle

Coronary

Thorax

Hepatic

Liver

Portal

Spleen

Hepatic

4 In still other cases, the blood flows through an arrangement of parallel and serial paths.

Splenic

Mesenteric

Peritubular

Glomerular

Large and small intestines

Kidneys

3 ...whereas in other cases, the blood flows through two capillary beds in series.

Pelvic

Lower limbs

Oxygenated

Deoxygenated

Figure 17.2 Circulatory beds.

Total blood flow, or cardiac output, is the product (heart rate) × (stroke volume)

The flow of blood delivered by the heart, or the total mean flow in the circulation, is the **cardiac output (CO).** The output during a single heartbeat, from either the left or the right ventricle, is the stroke volume (SV). For a given **heart rate (HR),**

$$CO = F = HR \cdot SV \qquad (17.6)$$

The cardiac output is usually expressed in liters per minute; at rest, it is 5 L/min in a 70-kg human. Cardiac output depends on body size and is best normalized to body surface area. The cardiac index (*units:* liters per minute per square meter) is the cardiac output per square meter of body surface area. The normal adult cardiac index at rest is about 3.0 L/(min m²).

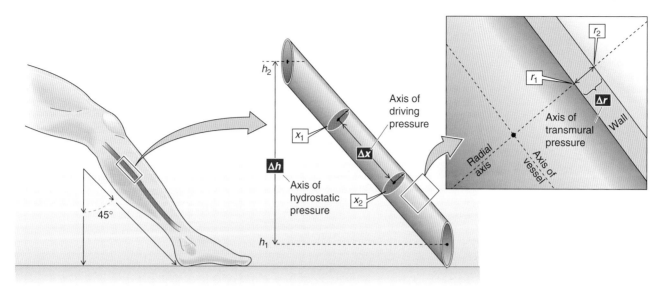

Figure 17.3   Three kinds of pressure differences, and their axes, in a blood vessel.

⊙ **17-4** The **principle of continuity of flow** is the principle of conservation of mass applied to flowing fluids. It requires that the volume entering the systemic or pulmonary circuit per unit time be equal to the volume leaving the circuit per unit time, assuming that no fluid has been added or subtracted in either circuit. Therefore, the flow of the right and left hearts (i.e., right and left cardiac outputs) must be equal in the steady state.

Flow in an idealized vessel increases with the fourth power of radius (Hagen-Poiseuille equation)

Flow (F) is the displacement of volume (ΔV) per unit time (Δt):

$$F = \frac{\Delta V}{\Delta t} \qquad (17.7)$$

In Fig. 17.1, we could be watching a bolus with a cross-sectional area A and a length L—move along the tube with a mean velocity $\bar{v}$. During a time interval Δt, the cylinder advances by Δx, so the volume passing some checkpoint (e.g., at P_2) is $(A \cdot \Delta x)$. Thus,

$$F = \overbrace{\frac{A \cdot \Delta x}{\Delta t}}^{\frac{\Delta V}{\Delta t}} = A \cdot \overbrace{\frac{\Delta x}{\Delta t}}^{\bar{v}} = A \cdot \bar{v} \qquad (17.8)$$

In a physically well-defined system, it is also possible to *predict* the flow from the geometry of the vessel and the properties of the fluid (Poiseuille's law):

$$F = \Delta P \cdot \underbrace{\frac{\pi r^4}{8 \eta l}}_{1/R} \qquad (17.9)$$

This is the Hagen-Poiseuille equation, where F is the flow, ΔP is the driving pressure, r is the inner radius of the tube, l is its length, and η is the viscosity. Equation 17.9 requires that both driving pressure and the resulting flow be constant.

Three implications of Poiseuille's law are as follows:
1. Flow is directly proportional to the axial pressure difference, ΔP. The proportionality constant—$(\pi r^4)/(8\eta l)$—is the reciprocal of resistance (R).
2. Flow is directly proportional to the fourth power of vessel radius.
3. Flow is inversely proportional to both the length of the vessel and the viscosity of the fluid.

Unlike Ohm's law of hydrodynamics $(F = \Delta P/R)$, which applies to *all* vessels no matter how complicated, the Hagen-Poiseuille equation applies only to rigid, cylindrical tubes.

Viscous resistance to flow is proportional to the viscosity of blood but does not depend on properties of the blood vessel walls

The simplest approach for expressing vascular resistance is to rearrange Ohm's law of hydrodynamics (see Equation 17.1):

$$R = \frac{\Delta P}{F} \qquad (17.10)$$

This approach is independent of geometry and is even applicable to very complex circuits, such as the entire peripheral circulation. The units of total peripheral resistance are millimeters of mercury/(milliliters per second)—also known as **peripheral resistance units (PRUs).**

Alternatively, if the flow through the tube fulfills Poiseuille's requirements, we can express "viscous" resistance in terms of the dimensions of the vessel and the *viscous* properties of the circulating fluid. Combining Equation 17.9 and Equation 17.10, we get

$$R = \frac{8}{\pi} \cdot \frac{\eta l}{r^4} \qquad (17.11)$$

Thus, *viscous* resistance is proportional to the *viscosity* of the fluid and the length of the tube but inversely proportional to the fourth power of the radius of the blood vessel. Note

A DEFINITION OF VISCOSITY

B VISCOUS FLOW IN A CYLINDER

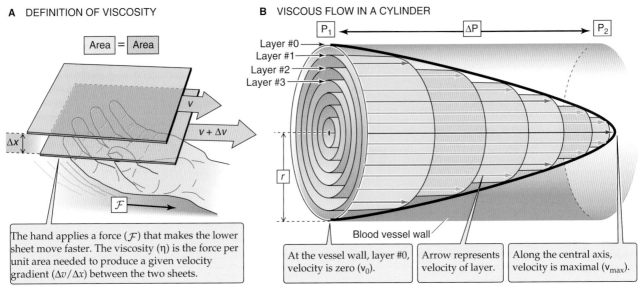

The hand applies a force ($\mathcal{F}$) that makes the lower sheet move faster. The viscosity (η) is the force per unit area needed to produce a given velocity gradient ($\Delta v / \Delta x$) between the two sheets.

At the vessel wall, layer #0, velocity is zero (v_0).

Arrow represents velocity of layer.

Along the central axis, velocity is maximal (v_{max}).

Figure 17.4 Viscosity.

that this equation makes no statement regarding the properties of the vessel wall per se. The resistance to flow results from the geometry of the fluid—as described by l and r—and the internal friction of the fluid, the **viscosity** (η). Viscosity is a property of the content (i.e., the fluid), unrelated to any property of the container (i.e., the vessel).

The viscosity of blood is a measure of the lack of internal slipperiness between two layers of fluid

Isaac Newton described the interaction as illustrated in Fig. 17.4A. Imagine that two parallel planes of fluid, each with an area A, are moving past one another. The velocity of the first is v, and the velocity of the slightly faster moving second plane is $v + \Delta v$. The difference in velocity between the moving planes is Δv and the separation between the two planes is Δx. Thus, the *velocity gradient* in a direction perpendicular to the plane of shear, $\Delta v / \Delta x$ (*units:* [centimeters/second]/centimeter = second^{-1}), is the **shear rate.** The additional *force* that we must apply to the second sheet to make it move faster than the first is the **shear stress.** The greater the area of the sheets, the greater the force needed to overcome the friction between them. Thus, shear stress is expressed as force per unit area *(F/A)*. The *shear stress* required to produce a particular *shear rate* Newton defined as the viscosity:

$$\eta = \frac{\text{shear stress}}{\text{shear rate}} = \frac{F/A}{\Delta v / \Delta x} \qquad (17.12)$$

Viscosity measures the resistance to sliding when layers of fluid are shearing against each other. The unit of viscosity is the **poise** (P). Whole blood has a viscosity of ~3 centipoise (cP).

If we apply a pressure head to the blood in a cylindrical vessel, each fluid lamina will move parallel to the long axis of the tube. Because of cohesive forces between the inner surface of the vessel wall and the blood, we can assume that an infinitesimally thin layer of blood close to the wall

of the tube (Fig. 17.4B, layer #0) cannot move. However, the adjacent concentric cylindrical layer, layer #1, moves in relation to the stationary outer layer #0, but slower than the next inner concentric cylinder, layer #2, and so on. Thus, the velocities of the layers or laminae increase from the wall to the center of the cylinder. The resulting velocity profile is a parabola with a maximum velocity, v_{max}, at the central axis. The lower the viscosity, the sharper the point of the bullet-shaped velocity profile.

HOW BLOOD FLOWS

Blood flow is laminar

From the law of hydrodynamics ($\Delta P = F \cdot R$), flow should increase linearly with driving pressure if resistance is constant. In cylindrical vessels, flow does indeed increase linearly with ΔP *up to a certain point* (Fig. 17.5A). However, at high flow rates—beyond a critical velocity—flow rises less steeply and is no longer proportional to ΔP but to roughly the square root of ΔP, because R apparently increases. Here, blood flow is no longer laminar but **turbulent.** Because turbulence causes substantial kinetic energy losses, it is energetically wasteful.

⊙ 17-5 The critical parameter that determines when flow becomes turbulent is a dimensionless quantity called the **Reynolds number *(Re),*** named after Osborne Reynolds:

$$Re = \frac{2r\bar{v}\rho}{\eta} \qquad (17.13)$$

Blood flow is laminar when Re is below ~2000 and is mostly turbulent when Re exceeds ~3000. The terms in the numerator reflect disruptive forces produced by the *inertial momentum* in the fluid. Thus, turbulent blood flow occurs when r is large (e.g., aorta) or when v is large (e.g., high cardiac output). Turbulent flow can also occur when a local decrease in vessel diameter (e.g., arterial stenosis) causes a local increase in v. The term in the denominator of Equation

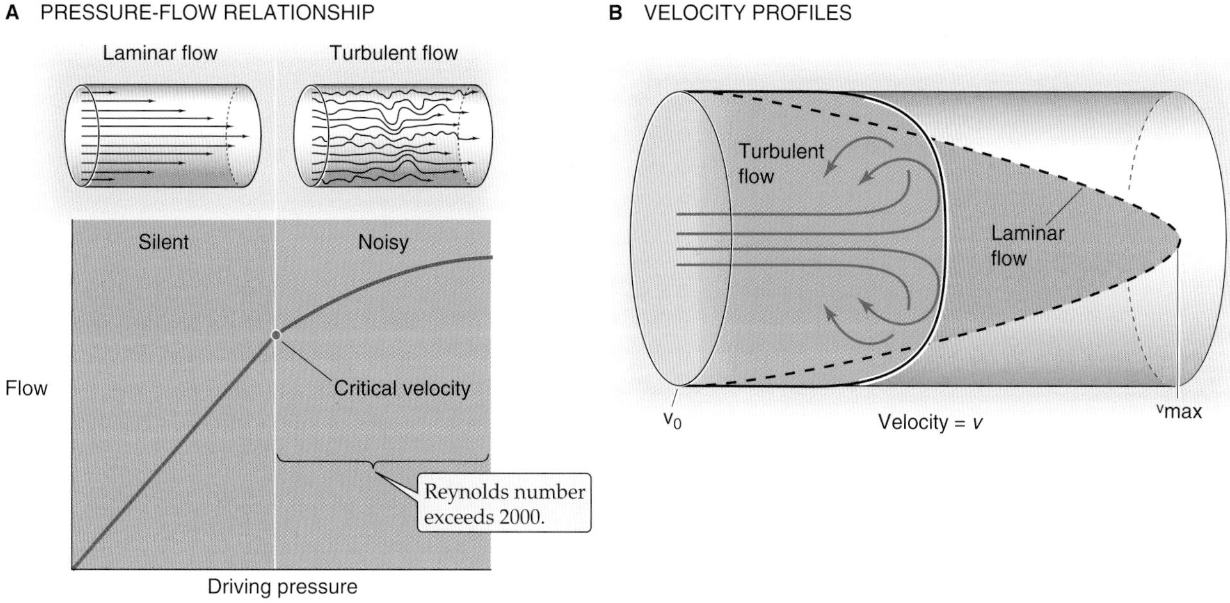

A PRESSURE-FLOW RELATIONSHIP

Laminar flow   Turbulent flow

B VELOCITY PROFILES

Turbulent flow

Laminar flow

v_0 Velocity = v v_{max}

Figure 17.5   Laminar versus turbulent flow.

17.13, viscosity, reflects the cohesive forces that tend to keep the layers well organized. Therefore, a low viscosity (e.g., in anemia—a low red blood cell count) predisposes to turbulence. When turbulence arises, the parabolic profile of the linear velocity across the radius of a cylinder becomes blunted (Fig. 17.5B).

The distinction between laminar and turbulent flow is clinically very significant. Laminar flow is silent, whereas vortex formation during turbulence sets up **murmurs.** These Korotkoff sounds are useful in assessing arterial blood flow in the traditional auscultatory method for determination of blood pressure. These murmurs are also important for diagnosis of vessel stenosis, vessel shunts, and cardiac valvular lesions. Intense forms of turbulence may be detected not only as loud acoustic murmurs but also as mechanical vibrations or **thrills** that can be felt by touch.

Pressure and flow oscillate with each heartbeat between maximum systolic and minimum diastolic values

Thus far, we have considered blood flow to be steady and driven by a constant pressure generator. That is, we have been working with a *mean* blood flow and a *mean* driving pressure (the difference between the mean arterial and venous pressures). However, we are all aware that the heart is a pump of the "two-stroke" variety, with a filling and an emptying phase. Because both the left and right hearts perform their work in a cyclic fashion, flow is pulsatile in both the systemic and pulmonary circulations.

⊙ **17-6** The mean blood pressure in the large systemic arteries is ~95 mm Hg. This is a single, time-averaged value. In reality, the blood pressure cycles between a maximal **systolic** arterial pressure (~120 mm Hg) that corresponds to the contraction of the ventricle and a minimal **diastolic** arterial pressure (~80 mm Hg) that corresponds to the relaxation of the ventricle. The difference between the systolic pressure and the diastolic pressure is the **pulse pressure.** Note that the

mean arterial pressure is not the arithmetic mean of systolic and diastolic values, which would be (120 + 80)/2 = 100 mm Hg in our example. A reasonable value for the mean arterial pressure is 95 mm Hg.

ORIGINS OF PRESSURE IN THE CIRCULATION

Four factors help generate pressure in the circulation: gravity, compliance of the vessels, viscous resistance, and inertia.

Gravity causes a hydrostatic pressure difference when there is a difference in height

Because gravity produces a hydrostatic pressure difference between two points whenever there is a *difference in height* (Δh; see Equation 17.4), one must always express pressure at h_1 relative to some reference h_2 level. In cardiovascular physiology, this reference h_2—zero height—is the level of the heart.

Whether the body is recumbent (i.e., horizontal) or upright (i.e., erect) has a tremendous effect on the intravascular pressure. In the horizontal position (Fig. 17.6A), where we assume that the entire body is at the level of the heart, we do not need to add a hydrostatic pressure component to the various intravascular pressures. Thus, the mean pressure in the aorta is 95 mm Hg, and—because it takes a driving pressure of ~5 mm Hg to pump blood into the end of the large arteries—the mean pressure at the end of the large arteries in the foot and head is 90 mm Hg. Similarly, the mean pressure in the large veins draining the foot and head is 5 mm Hg, and—because it takes a driving pressure of ~3 mm Hg to pump blood to the right atrium—the mean pressure in the right atrium is 2 mm Hg.

When a 180-cm tall person is standing (Fig. 17.6B), we must *add* a 130-cm column of blood (the Δh between the heart and large vessels in the foot) to the pressure prevailing in the large arteries and veins of the foot. Because a

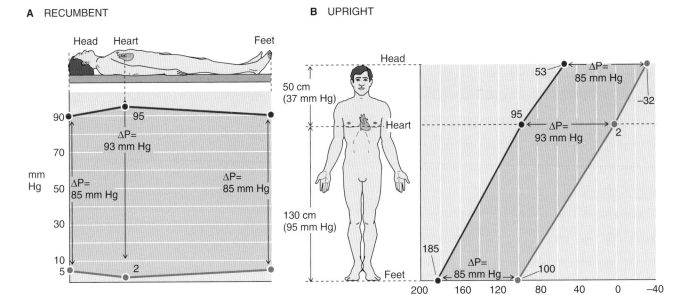

Figure 17.6 Arterial and venous pressures in the horizontal and upright positions. The pressures are different in (A) and (B), but the driving pressures (ΔP) between arteries and veins *(separation between red and blue lines, violet shading)* are the same.

water column of 130 cm is equivalent to 95 mm Hg, the mean pressure for a large artery in the foot will be 90 + 95 = 185 mm Hg, and the mean pressure for a large vein in the foot will be 5 + 95 = 100 mm Hg. On the other hand, in the head the Δh is negative. Thus, we must *subtract* a 50-cm column of blood from the pressure prevailing in the head. Because a water column of 50 cm is equivalent to 37 mm Hg, the mean pressure for a large artery in the head will be 90 − 37 = 53 mm Hg, and the mean pressure for a large vein in the head will be 5 − 37 = −32 mm Hg. Of course, this "negative" value really means that the pressure in a large vein in the head is 32 mm Hg lower than the pressure outside the vein.

⊙ **17-7** The veins of the limbs have a series of one-way valves that allow blood to flow only toward the heart. These valves act like a series of relay stations so that the contraction of skeletal muscle around the veins pushes blood from one valve to another (see ⊙ **22-1**). Thus, veins in the foot do not "see" the full hydrostatic column of 95 mm Hg when the leg muscles pump blood away from the foot veins.

Although the absolute arterial and venous pressures are much higher in the foot than in the head, the ΔP that *drives* blood flow is the same in the vascular beds of the foot and head. Thus, in the horizontal position, the ΔP across the vascular beds in the foot or head is 90 − 5 = 85 mm Hg. In the upright position, the ΔP for the foot is 185 − 100 = 85 mm Hg, and for the head, 53 − (−32) = 85 mm Hg. Thus, gravity does not affect the driving pressure that governs flow. On the other hand, in "dependent" areas of the body (i.e., vessels "below" the heart in a gravitational sense), the hydrostatic pressure does tend to increase the *transmural* pressure (intravascular versus extravascular "tissue" pressure) and

thus the diameter of distensible vessels. Because various anatomical barriers separate different tissue compartments, it is assumed that gravity does not appreciably affect this tissue pressure.

Low compliance of a vessel causes the transmural pressure to increase when the vessel blood volume is increased

Because blood vessels are distensible but have a finite compliance (see ⊙ **19-8**), if we were to inject a volume of blood into the vessel, the volume of the vessel would increase by the same amount (ΔV), and the intravascular pressure would also increase. The ΔP accompanying a given ΔV is greater if the compliance of the vessel is lower. The relationship between ΔP and ΔV is a *static* property of the vessel wall and holds whether or not there is flow in the vessel. Thus, if we were to infuse blood into a patient's blood vessels, the intravascular pressure would rise throughout the circulation, even if the heart were stopped.

The viscous resistance of blood causes an axial pressure difference when there is flow

As we saw in Ohm's law of hydrodynamics (see Equation 17.1), during steady flow down the axis of a tube (Fig. 17.1), the driving pressure (ΔP) is proportional to both flow and resistance. Viewed differently, if we want to achieve a constant flow, then the greater the resistance, the greater the ΔP that we must apply along the axis of flow. Of the four sources of pressure in the circulatory system, this ΔP due to viscous resistance is the only one that appears in Poiseuille's law (see Equation 17.9).

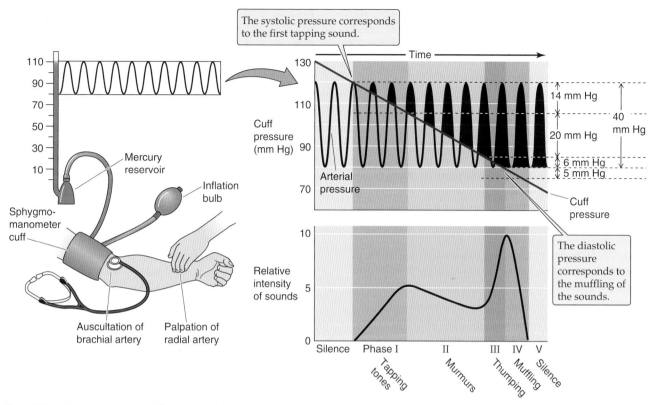

Figure 17.7 Sphygmomanometry. The clinician inflates the cuff to a pressure that is higher than the anticipated systolic pressure and then slowly releases the pressure in the cuff.

The inertia of the blood and vessels causes pressure to decrease when the velocity of blood flow increases

For the most part, we have been assuming that the flow of blood as well as its mean linear velocity is steady. However, blood flow in the circulation is not steady; the heart imparts its energy in a *pulsatile* manner, with each heartbeat. Therefore, v̄ in the aorta increases and reaches a maximum during systole and falls off during diastole. These *changes in velocity* lead to compensatory changes in intravascular *pressure.*

The tradeoff between velocity and pressure reflects the conversion between two forms of energy. Although we generally state that fluids flow from a higher to a lower *pressure,* it is more accurate to say that fluids flow from a higher to a lower *total energy.* This energy is made up of both the pressure or **potential energy** and the **kinetic energy** ($KE = \frac{1}{2}mv^2$). The impact of the interconversion between these two forms of energy is manifested by the familiar **Bernoulli effect.** As fluid flows along a horizontal tube with a narrow central region, which has a smaller diameter than that of the two ends, the pressure in the central region is lower—and the velocity is higher—than at the distal end of the tube. In other words, although the blood in the central region has a lower *potential energy* (lower pressure) than the blood at the distal end of the tube (higher pressure), it has a higher *kinetic energy.* Thus, the total energy of the fluid in the center exceeds that in the distal region, so the fluid does indeed flow down the *total energy gradient.*

HOW TO MEASURE BLOOD PRESSURE AND CARDIAC VOLUMES

Blood pressure can be measured indirectly by use of a sphygmomanometer

In clinical practice, one may measure arterial pressure indirectly by use of a manual sphygmomanometer (Fig. 17.7). An inextensible cuff containing an inflatable bag is wrapped around the arm (or occasionally, the thigh). Inflation of the bag by means of a rubber squeeze bulb to a pressure level above the expected systolic pressure occludes the underlying brachial artery and halts blood flow downstream. The pressure in the cuff, measured by means of a mercury or aneroid manometer, is then allowed to slowly decline (Fig. 17.7, *diagonal red line*). The physician can use either of two methods to monitor the blood flow downstream of the slowly deflating cuff. In the **palpatory method,** the physician detects the pulse as an indicator of flow by feeling the radial artery at the wrist. In the **auscultatory method,** the physician detects flow by using a stethoscope to detect the changing character of Korotkoff sounds over the brachial artery in the antecubital space.

The palpatory method permits determination of the systolic pressure; that is, the pressure in the cuff below which it is just possible to detect a radial pulse. Because of limited sensitivity of the finger, palpation probably slightly underestimates systolic pressure. The auscultatory method permits the detection of both systolic and diastolic pressure. The sounds heard during the slow deflation of the cuff can be divided into five phases (Fig. 17.7). During phase I, there is a sharp tapping sound, indicating that a spurt of blood is escaping under the cuff when cuff pressure is just below systolic pressure. The pressure at which these taps are first heard closely represents systolic pressure. In phase II, the sound becomes a blowing or swishing murmur. During phase III, the sound becomes a louder thumping. In phase IV, as the cuff pressure falls toward the diastolic level, the sound becomes muffled and softer. Finally, in phase V, the sound disappears. Although some debate persists about whether the point of muffling or the point of silence is the correct diastolic pressure, most favor the point of muffling as being more consistent. Actual diastolic pressure may be somewhat overestimated by the point of muffling but underestimated by the point of silence.

⊙ 17-8 Ventricular dimensions, ventricular volumes, and volume changes can be measured by angiography and echocardiography

Clinicians can use a variety of approaches to examine the cardiac chambers. **Gated radionuclide imaging** employs compounds of the gamma-emitting isotope ^{99m}Tc, which has a half-life of 6 hours. After ^{99m}Tc is injected, a gamma camera provides imaging of the cardiac chambers. Electrocardiogram (ECG) gating (i.e., synchronization to a particular spot on the ECG) allows the apparatus to snap a picture at a specific part of the cardiac cycle and to sum these pictures over many cycles. Because this method does not provide a high-resolution image, it yields only a *relative* ventricular volume. From the difference between the count at the maximally filled state (end-diastolic volume) and at its minimally filled state (end-systolic volume), the cardiologist can estimate the fraction of ventricular blood that is ejected during systole—**the ejection fraction**—which is an important measure of cardiac function.

Angiography can accurately provide the linear dimensions of the ventricle, allowing the cardiologist to calculate *absolute* ventricular volumes. A catheter is threaded into either the left or the right ventricle, and saline containing a contrast substance (i.e., a chemical opaque to x-rays) is injected into the ventricle. This approach provides a two-dimensional projection of the ventricular volume as a function of time.

⊙ **17-9 Echocardiography,** which exploits ultrasonic waves to visualize the heart and great vessels, can be used in two modes. In *M-mode echocardiography* (M is for motion), the technician places a single transducer in a fixed position on the chest wall and obtains a one-dimensional view of heart components. As shown in the upper portion of Fig. 17.8, the ultrasonic beam transects the anterior wall of the right ventricle, the right ventricle, the septum, the left ventricle, the leaflets of the mitral valve, and the posterior wall of the left ventricle. The lower portion of Fig. 17.8 shows the positions of the borders between these structures (x-axis) during a single cardiac cycle (y-axis) and thus how the size of the left ventricle—along the axis of the beam—changes with time. Of course, the technician can obtain other views by changing the orientation of the beam.

In *two-dimensional echocardiography,* the probe automatically and rapidly pivots, scanning the heart in a single

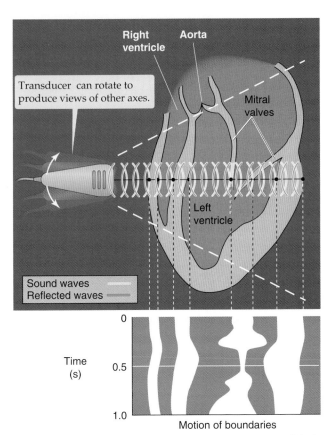

Figure 17.8   M-mode and two-dimensional echocardiography. With the transducer in a single position *(upper panel)*, one obtains the tracing in the *bottom panel*; this is an M-mode echocardiogram during one cardiac cycle. The waves represent motion (M) of heart boundaries transected by a stationary ultrasonic beam. In two-dimensional echocardiography (also shown in *upper panel*), the probe rapidly rotates between the two extremes *(broken lines)*, producing an image of a slice through the heart at one instant in time.

anatomical slice or plane (Fig. 17.8, area between the two broken lines) and providing a true cross section. This approach is therefore superior to angiography, which provides only a two-dimensional projection. Because cardiac output is the product of heart rate and stroke volume, one can calculate cardiac output from echocardiographic measurements of ventricular end-diastolic and end-systolic volume.

In addition to ultrasound methods and angiography, the technique of **magnetic resonance angiography,** an application of magnetic resonance tomography, is used to obtain two-dimensional images of slices of ventricular volumes or of blood vessels.

⊙ **17-10** In contrast to standard echocardiography, **Doppler echocardiography** provides information on the velocity, direction, and character of blood flow, just as police radar monitors traffic. In Doppler echocardiography, most information is obtained with the beam parallel to the flow of blood. In the simplest application of Doppler flow measurements, one can continuously monitor the velocity of flowing blood in a blood vessel or part of the heart. On such a record, the x-axis represents time, and the y-axis represents the spectrum of *velocities* of the moving red blood cells (i.e., different cells can be moving at different

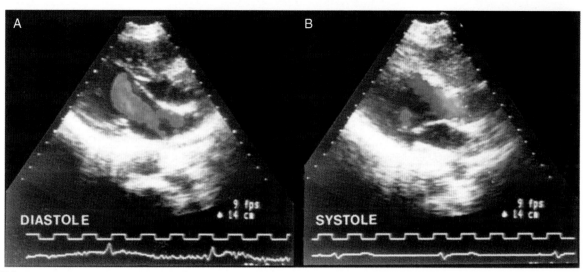

Figure 17.9   The colors, which encode the velocity of blood flow, are superimposed on a two-dimensional echocardiogram, which is shown in a gray scale. (A) Blood moves through the mitral valve and into the left ventricle during diastole. Because blood is flowing toward the transducer, its velocity is encoded as *red*. (B) Blood moves out of the ventricle and toward the aortic valve during systole. Because blood is flowing away from the transducer, its velocity is encoded as *blue*. (From Feigenbaum H. Echocardiography. In Braunwald E [ed]: Heart Disease: A Textbook of Cardiovascular Medicine, 5th ed. Philadelphia, WB Saunders, 1997.)

velocities). Flow toward the transducer appears above baseline, whereas flow away from the transducer appears below baseline. The intensity of the record at a single point on the y-axis (encoded by a gray scale or false color) represents the strength of the returning signal, which depends on the *number* of red blood cells moving at that velocity. Thus, Doppler echocardiography is able to distinguish the character of flow: laminar versus turbulent. Alternatively, at one instant in time, the Doppler technician can scan a region of a vessel or the heart, obtaining a two-dimensional, color-encoded map of blood velocities. If we overlay such two-dimensional Doppler data on a two-dimensional echocardiogram, which shows the position of the vessel or cardiac structures, the result is a color flow Doppler echocardiogram (Fig. 17.9).

Finally, a magnetic resonance scanner can also be used in two-dimensional phase-contrast mapping to yield quantitative measurements of blood flow velocity.

CHAPTER 18

BLOOD

Emile L. Boulpaep

Blood is a complex fluid consisting of **plasma**—extracellular fluid rich in proteins—and **formed elements**—RBCs (or erythrocytes), **WBCs** (leukocytes, which include granulocytes, lymphocytes, and monocytes), and **platelets** (thrombocytes). Total blood volume is ~70 mL/kg body weight in the adult woman and ~80 mL/kg body weight in the adult man (see Table 5.1).

BLOOD COMPOSITION

⊙ 18-1 Whole blood is a suspension of cellular elements in plasma

The **hematocrit** (see ⊙ 5-1) is the fraction of the total column occupied by RBCs. The normal hematocrit is ~40% for adult women and ~45% for adult men. The hematocrit in the newborn is ~55%. The hematocrit is a measure of concentration of RBCs, not of total body red cell mass. Total RBC volume is ~28 mL/kg body weight in the adult woman and ~36 mL/kg body weight in the adult man.

⊙ **18-2 Plasma** is a pale-white watery solution of electrolytes, plasma proteins, carbohydrates, and lipids. Pink-colored plasma suggests the presence of hemoglobin caused by **hemolysis** (lysis of RBCs) and release of hemoglobin into the plasma. The electrolyte composition of plasma differs only slightly from that of interstitial fluid on account of the volume occupied by proteins and their electrical charge (see Table 5.2).

Plasma proteins at a normal concentration of ~7.0 g/dL account for a colloid osmotic pressure or oncotic pressure of ~25 mm Hg (see ⊙ 20-15). Principal plasma proteins are albumin, fibrinogen, globulins, and other coagulation factors. The molecular weights of plasma proteins range up to 970 kDa. The plasma concentration of **albumin** ranges from 3.5 to 5.5 g/dL, which provides the body with a total plasma albumin pool of ~135 g. Albumin is synthesized by the liver at a rate of ~120 mg/kg body weight per day and, due to catabolism, has a half-life in the circulation of ~20 days. Urinary losses of albumin are normally negligible (<20 mg/day; see ⊙ 20-15).

⊙ **18-3** Many plasma proteins are involved in blood coagulation through coagulation cascades, the end point of which is the cleavage of **fibrinogen** into fibrin monomers that further assemble into a fibrin polymer. During clotting, the cross-linked polymers of fibrin form strands that trap red and white cells, platelets, and plasma inside the thrombus

(i.e., blood clot). When the clot shrinks to a plug, it expels a slightly yellow-tinged fluid called **serum,** which differs principally from plasma by the absence of fibrinogen and other coagulation factors.

Subtraction of the albumin and fibrinogen moiety from total protein concentration yields the concentration of all the proteins grouped as **globulins.**

Bone marrow is the source of most blood cells

If you spread a drop of anticoagulated blood thinly on a glass slide, you can detect under the microscope the cellular elements of blood. In such a **peripheral blood smear,** the following mature cell types are easily recognized: erythrocytes; granulocytes divided in neutrophils, eosinophils, and basophils; lymphocytes; monocytes; and platelets (Fig. 18.1).

Hematopoiesis is the process of generation of all the cell types present in blood. Pluripotent **long-term hematopoietic stem cells (LT-HSCs)** constitute a population of **adult stem cells** found in bone marrow that are multipotent and able to self-renew. The **short-term hematopoietic stem cells (ST-HSCs)** give rise to **committed stem cells** or progenitors, which after proliferation are able to differentiate into lineages that in turn give rise to **burst-forming units (BFUs)** or **colony-forming units (CFUs),** each of which ultimately will produce one or a limited number of mature cell types: erythrocytes, the megakaryocytes that give rise to platelets, eosinophils, basophils, neutrophils, monocytes-macrophages/dendritic cells, and B or T lymphocytes and natural killer cells (Fig. 18.2). Soluble factors known as **cytokines** guide the development of each lineage. **Colony-stimulating factors** are hematopoietic cytokines that stimulate colony formation by progenitor cells. The main colony-stimulating factors are granulocyte-macrophage colony-stimulating factor (GM-CSF; see ⊙ 3-27), granulocyte colony-stimulating factor (G-CSF), macrophage colony-stimulating factor (M-CSF), interleukin-3 (IL-3) and IL-5 (see ⊙ 3-27), thrombopoietin (TPO), and erythropoietin (EPO; see ⊙ 18-5).

GM-CSF stimulates proliferation of a common myeloid progenitor and promotes the production of neutrophils, eosinophils, and monocytes-macrophages.

⊙ **18-4 G-CSF and M-CSF** guide the ultimate development of granulocytes and monocytes-macrophages/dendritic cells, respectively. M-CSF is also required for osteoclast development (see Fig. 52.3).

A NEUTROPHIL

B EOSINOPHIL

C BASOPHIL

D LYMPHOCYTE

E MONOCYTE

F PLATELETS

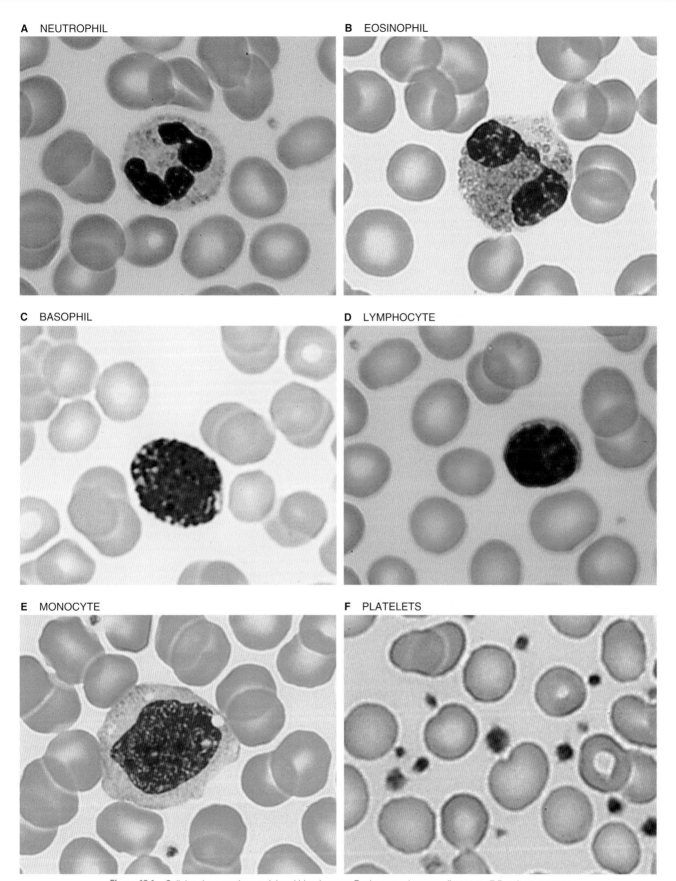

Figure 18.1 Cellular elements in a peripheral blood smear. Erythrocytes (average diameter, ~7.5 µm) are present in all panels. The cellular elements are not represented according to their abundance. From Goldman L, Ausiello D: Cecil's Textbook of Medicine, ed 22, Philadelphia, 2004, WB Saunders.

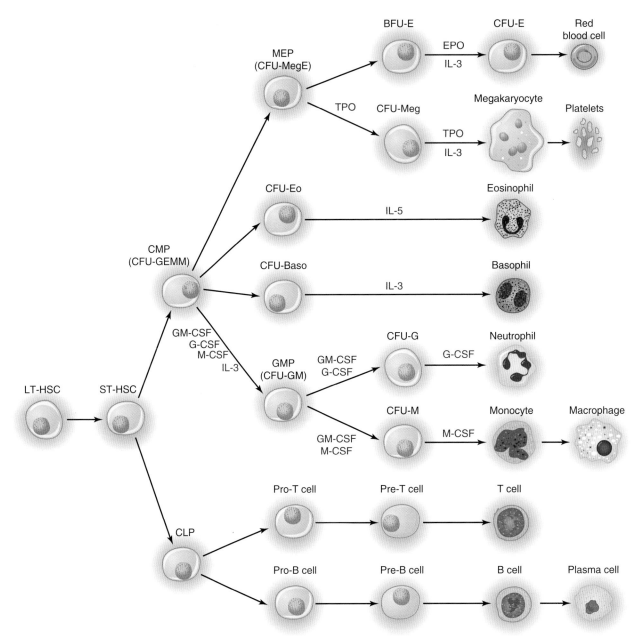

Figure 18.2 Hematopoietic lineages. Cytokines guiding a transition are shown in red. *BFU-E*, Burst form-ing unit-erythroid; *CFU*, Colony forming unit—with suffixes -*Baso* (basophilic), -*E* (erythroid), -*Eo* (eosino-phil), -*G* (granulocyte), -*GEMM* (granulocyte, erythrocyte, megakaryocyte, macrophage), -*GM* (granulocyte/macrophage), -*M* (macrophage), -*Meg* (megakaryocyte), -*MegE* (megakaryocyte/erythroid); *CMP*, common myeloid progenitor; *CLP*, common lymphoid progenitor; *GMP*, granulocyte-macrophage progenitor; *MEP*, megakaryocyte-erythroid progenitor.

IL-3 has a broad effect on multiple lineages. **IL-5** sustains the terminal differentiation of eosinophilic precursors.

TPO binds to a TPO receptor that induces an increase in the number and size of megakaryocytes—the cells that pro-duce platelets—which thereby greatly augments the number of circulating platelets.

⊙ **18-5 EPO** is produced by the kidney and to a lesser extent by the liver. This cytokine supports **erythropoiesis** or red cell development (Fig. 18.3). Hypoxia increases the abun-dance of the α subunit of hypoxia-inducible factor 1 (HIF-1α), which enhances production of EPO messenger RNA. EPO is essential for the differentiation of burst-forming unit–erythroid cells (BFU-Es) to colony-forming unit–erythroid

cells (CFU-Es) or **proerythroblasts** (also known as pronor-moblasts), which still lack hemoglobin. Hemoglobin first appears at the stage of **polychromatic erythroblasts** and is clearly evident in **orthochromatic erythroblasts.** The subse-quent exocytosis of the nucleus produces **reticulocytes** (Fig. 18.3), whereas the loss of ribosomes and mitochondria yields mature erythrocytes, which enter the circulation. The mature erythrocyte has a life span of ~120 days.

RBCs are mainly composed of hemoglobin

RBCs are the most abundant elements in blood. RBCs are non-nucleated biconcave cells with a diameter of ~7.5 μm

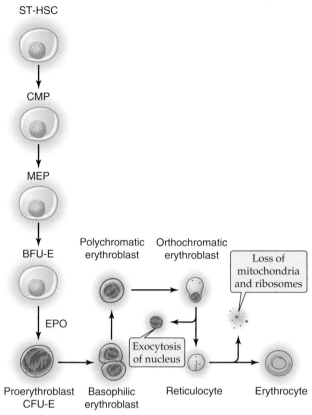

Figure 18.3 Erythropoiesis. *CMP*, Common myeloid progenitor; *MEP*, megakaryocyte-erythroid progenitor.

TABLE 18.1 Typical Blood Cell Parameters

RBC count ($10^6/\mu L$ blood)	4.0 (female); 4.5 (male)
Hematocrit (%)	40 (female); 45 (male)
Hemoglobin (g/dL blood)	14.0 (female); 15.5 (male)
Mean red cell volume, MCV (fL/cell)	90
Mean red cell hemoglobin, MCH (pg/cell)	30
Mean cell hemoglobin concentration, MCHC (g/dL RBCs)	35
Red cell distribution width, RDW (%)	13
WBC count ($10^3/\mu L$ blood)	8
Platelet count ($10^3/\mu L$ blood)	300

TABLE 18.2 Leukocytes[a]

	COUNT ($10^3/\mu L$ BLOOD)	DIFFERENTIAL COUNT (%)
Total leukocytes	7.4	100
Neutrophils	4.4	59 (56 segmented, 3 band)
Lymphocytes	2.5	34
Monocytes	0.3	4
Eosinophils	0.2	3
Basophils	0.04	0.5

[a]Listed in order of abundance.

and a volume of ~90 fL (90×10^{-15} L). Maintaining the shape of the RBC is a cytoskeleton that is anchored to the plasma membrane. The RBC performs three major tasks: (1) carrying O_2 from the lungs to the systemic tissues, (2) carrying CO_2 from tissues to the lungs, and (3) assisting in the buffering of acids and bases.

⊙ **18-6** Table 18.1 lists the properties of RBCs that are routinely determined in the clinical laboratory. The most important constituent of the RBC is **hemoglobin.** Normal blood hemoglobin content is ~14.0 g/dL in the adult female and ~15.5 g/dL in the adult male. The hemoglobin concentration in red cell cytosol is extremely high, **~5.5 mM.** The mean cell hemoglobin concentration is ~35 g/dL RBCs, or about five times the concentration of proteins in plasma.

Because the mature RBCs contain no nucleus or other organelles, they can neither synthesize proteins nor engage in oxidative metabolism. The RBC can engage in two metabolic pathways: glycolysis, which consumes 90% of glucose uptake; and the pentose shunt, which consumes the remaining 10% of glucose. The cell generates its ATP exclusively by glycolysis. An important constituent of the RBC—normally present at 4 to 5 mM—is **2,3-diphosphoglycerate (2,3-DPG),** which plays an important role in reducing the O_2 affinity of hemoglobin (see ⊙ 29-6).

Erythrocytes contain **glutathione** at ~2 mM. A high ratio of reduced glutathione (GSH) to oxidized glutathione (GSSG) protects the RBC against oxidant damage.

⊙ **18-7** RBCs carry two cytoplasmic isoforms of **carbonic anhydrase** (see ⊙ 28-2), CA I and CA II. These enzymes, which rapidly interconvert CO_2 and HCO_3^- play a critical

role in carrying metabolically produced CO_2 from the systemic tissues to the pulmonary capillaries for elimination in the exhaled air (see ⊙ 29-9).

CO_2 carriage also depends critically on the **Cl-HCO$_3$ exchanger AE1** (see Fig. 5.8D) in the RBC membrane. AE1 is the most abundant membrane protein in RBCs, with ~1 million copies per cell. One AE1 molecule can transport as many as 50,000 ions per second—it is one of the fastest known transporters.

The **water channel AQP1** (see ⊙ 5-13) is the second most abundant membrane protein in RBCs, with ~200,000 copies per cell. AQP1 appears to contribute more than half of the CO_2 permeability of the RBC membrane (see ⊙ 29-9).

Leukocytes defend against infections

Table 18.2 summarizes the relative abundance of various leukocytes in the blood. These WBCs are in two major groups: the granulocytes, and the lymphocytes and monocytes. **Granulocytes** (Fig. 18.1) are so named because of their cytoplasmic granules, which on a blood smear stained with Giemsa stain or Wright stain appear red (eosinophils), blue (basophils), or intermediate (neutrophils). The name *polymorphonuclear leukocytes* applies to all three types of granulocytes, but often is used to refer specifically to neutrophils. Granulocytes have a brief life span in the blood (<12 hours) but on activation can migrate into the tissues.

Neutrophils The most abundant leukocytes are neutrophils, which have two types of granules (specific and azurophilic) that contain lysosomal enzymes, peroxidase, collagenase, and other enzymes capable of digesting foreign material. In the presence of a chemotactic attractant, neutrophils approach foreign substances, such as bacteria, to phagocytose them within a phagocytic vacuole. By a process known as degranulation, granules merge with the vacuole and empty their contents into the vacuole. Bacteria are destroyed within the vacuole by the action of hydrogen peroxide (H_2O_2) and the superoxide anion radical (O_2^-; see Fig. 62.1).

Eosinophils The granules of eosinophils contain **major basic protein (MBP),** which is toxic to parasites, as well as other enzymes. These cells are important in the response to parasites and viruses. Eosinophils also play a role in allergic reactions.

Basophils Basophils, the least common granulocytes, are a major source of the cytokine IL-4, which in turn stimulates B lymphocytes to produce IgE antibodies. The granules contain histamine, heparin, and peroxidase. Like eosinophils, basophils also play a role in allergic reactions.

Lymphocytes Like the monocytes, lymphocytes do not have granules. Lymphocytes come in different classes.

T lymphocytes, or T cells, which represent 70% to 80% of peripheral lymphocytes in blood, undergo maturation primarily in the *thymus.* T lymphocytes are responsible for cell-mediated immunity.

B lymphocytes, or B cells, which represent 10% to 15% of peripheral lymphocytes in blood, undergo maturation in *bone* marrow and peripheral lymphoid tissue. When B cells interact with antigen in the presence of T cells and macrophages, B cells can transform into **plasma cells,** which abundantly make and secrete antibodies that are directed against specific antigens. Thus, B cells are responsible for humoral immunity.

Monocytes Because they migrate from the bone marrow to peripheral tissues, monocytes are not abundant in blood. Monocytes spend most of their long life in peripheral tissues, where they develop into larger macrophages (20 to 40 µm in diameter). The **macrophage** serves two functions: (1) the phagocytosis of pathogens or cellular debris and (2) the presentation of antigens to lymphocytes.

Platelets are nucleus-free fragments

Platelets form in the bone marrow by budding off from large cells called **megakaryocytes,** the maturation of which depends on TPO and IL-3. Each megakaryocyte can produce up to a few thousand platelets. Normal blood contains 150,000 to 450,000 platelets per microliter. A feedback mechanism operates between platelets and megakaryocytes, controlling platelet production. Platelets carry receptors for TPO that are able to bind and remove TPO from the plasma. A hypoplastic marrow generating few megakaryocytes leads to **thrombocytopenia** (platelet shortage) and thereby little removal of TPO, which in turn stimulates megakaryocyte production and corrects the lack of platelets. A hyperplastic marrow creating many megakaryocytes leads to **thrombocytosis** (platelet excess) and thereby greater TPO removal, which ultimately turns off megakaryocyte production.

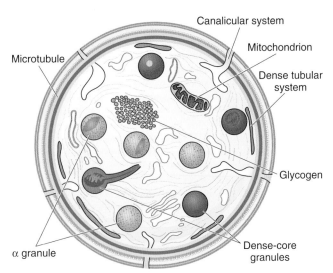

Figure 18.4   Discoid platelet.

The life span of platelets is about 10 days. In their unactivated state, these nucleus-free fragments are disk shaped and 2 to 3 µm in diameter (Fig. 18.4). Platelets have two types of special organelles: α granules and, less abundantly, dense core granules. The **α granules** store von Willebrand factor, platelet fibrinogen, and clotting factor V. The **dense-core granules** store ATP, ADP, serotonin and Ca^{2+}. As discussed later, platelets are essential for hemostasis (see ⊙ 18-8).

BLOOD VISCOSITY

Whole blood has an anomalous viscosity

Water and saline solutions are homogeneous or newtonian liquids. For these, the relationship between shear stress (force needed to move one lamina faster than its neighbor) and shear rate (velocity gradient between laminae) is linear and passes through the origin (Fig. 18.5, *blue line*). Viscosity (see Equation 17.12) is the slope of this line. Blood plasma (Fig. 18.5, *yellow line*) and serum are nearly newtonian. However, normal *whole blood is non-newtonian:* it has a nonlinear shear stress–to–shear rate relationship that intersects the y-axis above the origin (Fig. 18.5, *red curve*). In other words, one has to apply some threshold force (i.e., the yield shear stress) before the fluid will move at all. At lower forces, the fluid is immobile. However, at higher shear rates (such as those achieved physiologically after the velocity of blood flow has increased sufficiently), the relationship between shear stress and shear rate assumes the newtonian ideal, with a slope that corresponds to a viscosity of ~3.2 centipoise (cP).

Blood viscosity increases with the hematocrit and the fibrinogen plasma concentration

The viscosity of whole blood depends on several physiological factors: (1) fibrinogen concentration, (2) hematocrit, (3) vessel radius, (4) linear velocity, and (5) temperature. The viscosity of whole blood in the linear region of Fig. 18.5 is ~3.2 cP, assuming a typical fibrinogen concentration of 260 mg/dL, a hematocrit of 40%, and a temperature of 37°C.

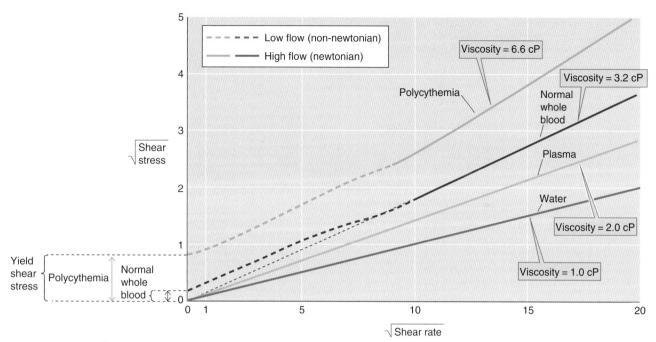

Figure 18.5 Anomalous viscosity of blood. To emphasize deviations from linearity, we plot the square roots of shear stress (force/area) and shear rate ($\Delta v/\Delta x$).

Fibrinogen Fibrinogen is a major protein component of human plasma (see ◉ 18-2) and is a key element in the coagulation cascade. The main reason for the non-newtonian behavior of blood is the interaction of this fibrinogen with RBCs. At normal hematocrits, fibrinogen and, perhaps, low-density lipoproteins (see ◉ 46-8), electrophoretically seen as β-lipoproteins, are the only plasma proteins capable of creating a yield shear stress.

At normal hematocrits, the absence of fibrinogen (in congenital afibrinogenemia) eliminates the yield shear stress altogether. Conversely, hyperfibrinogenemia elevates yield shear stress and, in the extreme, leads to a clustering of RBCs that increases their effective density. This increased effective density causes the RBCs to settle toward the bottom of a vertical tube—easily measured as an increased **erythrocyte sedimentation rate.**

Hematocrit Increases in hematocrit elevate blood viscosity by two mechanisms (Fig. 18.6). One prevails at physiological hematocrits, the other at higher hematocrits. Starting from values of 30%, raising the hematocrit increases the interactions among RBCs—both directly and by proteins such as fibrinogen—and thereby increases viscosity. At hematocrits >60%, the cells are so tightly packed that further increases lead to cell-cell interactions that increasingly deform the RBCs, thereby increasing viscosity. The combination of a high hematocrit and a high fibrinogen level can be expected to lead to extremely high viscosities.

Vessel Radius In reasonably large vessels (radius greater than ~1 mm), blood viscosity is independent of vessel radius (Fig. 18.7). However, the viscosity decreases steeply at lower radii. This Fahraeus-Lindqvist phenomenon has four major causes.

Poiseuille observed that RBCs move faster in the center of an arteriole or venule than at the periphery and that the *concentration* of RBCs is greater at the center. Very near the wall is present a "transparent space" occupied only by plasma (Fig. 18.8A). This axial accumulation of RBCs occurs because the plasma imparts a spin to an erythrocyte caught between two layers of plasma sliding past one another at different velocities (see Fig. 17.4B) that causes the cell to move toward the center of the vessel. One consequence of axial accumulation is that local viscosity is lowest in the cell-poor region near the vessel wall and greatest in the cell-enriched core. The net effect in smaller vessels is that the overall viscosity of the blood is *decreased* because the cell-poor plasma (low intrinsic viscosity) moves to the periphery where the shearing forces are the greatest, whereas the cell-enriched blood (high intrinsic viscosity) is left along the central axis where the shearing forces are least. A second consequence of axial accumulation is that branch vessels preferentially skim the plasma from the main stream of the parent vessel, which leads to a lower hematocrit in branch vessels.

In vessels (e.g., capillaries) so small that their diameter is about the size of a single erythrocyte, we can no longer speak of the friction between concentric laminae. Instead, in small capillaries, the RBC membrane rolls around the cytoplasm—tank treading—like the track of a bulldozer (Fig. 18.8C). As two treading erythrocytes shoot down a capillary, they spin the bolus of plasma trapped between them (bolus flow).

In vessels smaller than an erythrocyte, highly deformed—literally bullet-shaped—RBCs squeeze through the capillaries, so the effective viscosity falls even farther (Fig. 18.8D). Under these conditions, the cells automatically "focus" themselves to the centerline of the capillary and maintain a fixed distance between two successive cells.

At relatively low hematocrits, viscosity increases because of the stickiness of red blood cells.

At higher hematocrits, viscosity increases because of cell deformation.

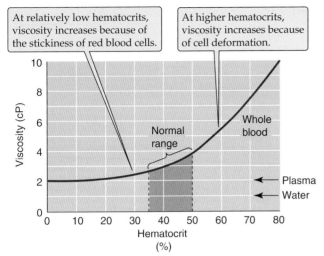

Figure 18.6   Dependence of viscosity on hematocrit.

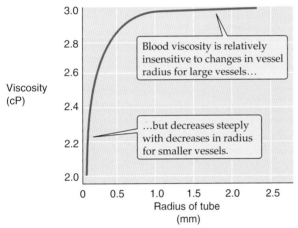

Blood viscosity is relatively insensitive to changes in vessel radius for large vessels…

…but decreases steeply with decreases in radius for smaller vessels.

Figure 18.7   Dependence of viscosity on vessel radius.

Velocity of Flow   The dependence of flow on pressure is linear for blood *plasma* (Fig. 18.9, gold curve). However, for *whole blood,* the pressure-flow relationship deviates slightly from linearity at velocities close to zero. These deviations at very low flows have two explanations. First, at low flows, the shear rate is also low, which causes the whole blood to behave in a non-newtonian manner (Fig. 18.5) and to have a high apparent viscosity. In fact, one must apply a threshold force to get the blood to move at all. The second reason for the nonlinear pressure-flow relationship is that the tendency for RBCs to move to the center of the stream—thereby lowering viscosity—requires a modest flow. After this axial accumulation "saturates," however, the relationship becomes linear.

Temperature   Cooling normal whole blood from 37°C to 0°C increases its viscosity ~2.5-fold. However, physiologically, this effect is negligible in humans except during intense cooling of the extremities. In some patients, the presence of **cryoglobulins** in the blood can cause an abnormal rise in viscosity even with less intense cooling of limbs.

A   AXIAL ACCUMULATION

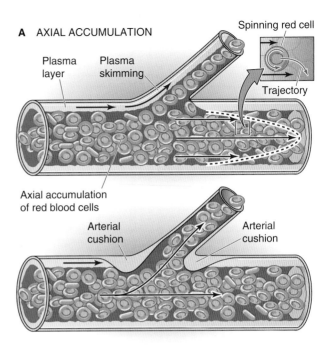

B   LIMITED NUMBER OF LAMINAE IN SMALL VESSEL

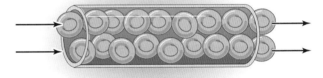

C   TANK TREADING OF RED BLOOD CELLS

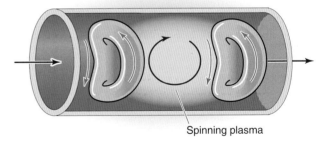

D   DEFORMATION OF RED BLOOD CELLS

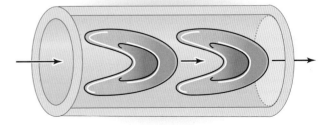

Figure 18.8   Flow of blood in small vessels.

HEMOSTASIS AND FIBRINOLYSIS

Blood is normally in a liquid state inside blood vessels because it does not come into contact with negatively charged surfaces (e.g., the collagen beneath endothelial cells) that activate an *intrinsic* coagulation pathway, nor does it contact tissue factors (e.g., released from damaged tissue) that activate an *extrinsic* pathway.

⊙ **18-8 Hemostasis** or the prevention of hemorrhage, can be achieved by four methods: (1) vasoconstriction, (2) increased tissue pressure, (3) formation of a platelet plug in the case of capillary bleeding, and (4) coagulation or clot formation.

Vasoconstriction contributes to hemostasis because it raises the critical closing pressure and thus collapses vessels that have an intravascular pressure below the critical closing pressure. Vessel constriction is also promoted by chemical byproducts of platelet plug formation and of coagulation. For example, activated platelets release the vasoconstrictors thromboxane A_2 (TXA$_2$; see ⊙ **3-18**) and serotonin (5-HT; see Fig. 13.8B). Moreover, thrombin, a major product of the clotting machinery, triggers the endothelium to generate endothelin 1 (ET-1; see ⊙ **20-20**), the most powerful physiological vasoconstrictor.

Increased tissue pressure contributes to hemostasis because it decreases transmural pressure (see ⊙ **17-2**) which is the difference between intravascular pressure and tissue pressure. Transmural pressure is the main determinant of blood vessel radius. Given the fourth-power relationship between flow and blood vessel radius (see Equation 17.9), an increase in tissue pressure that causes radius to decrease by a factor of 2 would diminish flow by a factor of 16.

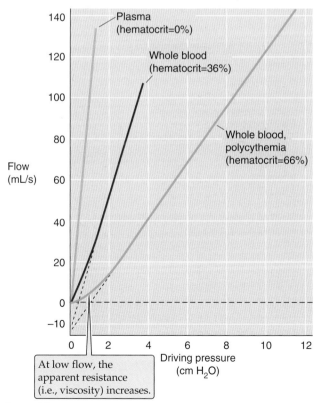

Figure 18.9 Pressure-flow relationships over a range of hematocrits. The slope of the linear portion of each curve is 1/resistance; resistance (or viscosity) increases from plasma to normal whole blood to polycythemic blood.

Platelets can plug holes in small vessels

In a highly controlled fashion, platelets plug small breaches in the vascular endothelium. Plug formation is a process that includes adhesion, activation, and aggregation.

Adhesion Platelets do not adhere to themselves, to other blood cells, or to endothelial membranes. One preventive factor may be the negative surface charge on both platelets and endothelial cells. In the case of endothelial cells, the negative surface charge reflects the presence of proteoglycans, mainly heparan sulfate. Platelet adhesion occurs in response to an increase in the shearing force at the surface of platelets or endothelial cells and in response to vessel injury or humoral signals.

Platelet adhesion is mediated by **platelet receptors** integral membrane proteins belonging to a class of matrix receptors known as integrins (see ⊙ **2-6**). One ligand naturally present in the blood plasma is **von Willebrand factor (vWF),** a glycoprotein made by endothelial cells and megakaryocytes. vWF is found in Weibel-Palade bodies of the endothelial cells and in α granules of platelets. High shear, certain cytokines, and hypoxia all trigger the release of vWF from endothelial cells. vWF binds to the platelet receptor known as glycoprotein Ib/Ia (Gp Ib/Ia).

A breach of the endothelium exposes platelet receptors to ligands that are components of the subendothelial matrix. These ligands include **collagen,** which binds to Gp Ia/IIa, and **fibronectin** and **laminin** (see ⊙ **2-6**), both of which bind to Gp Ic/IIa.

Activation The binding of these ligands triggers a conformational change in the platelet receptors that initiates an intracellular signaling cascade, which leads to an exocytotic event known as platelet activation. Activated platelets exocytose the contents of their **dense storage granules,** which include ATP, ADP, serotonin, and Ca^{2+}. Activated platelets also exocytose the contents of **α granules,** which contain several proteins, including growth factors and three hemostatic factors: vWF and two clotting factors, clotting factor V and fibrinogen. Activated platelets also use cyclooxygenase (see Fig. 3.9) to initiate the breakdown of arachidonic acid to thromboxane A_2. Platelet activation is also associated with marked cytoskeletal and morphological changes as the platelet extends first a broad lamellipodium and then many finger-like filopodia.

Aggregation Signaling molecules released by activated platelets amplify the platelet activation response. ADP, serotonin, and thromboxane A_2 all activate additional platelets, and this recruitment promotes platelet aggregation. As noted before, vWF released by activated platelets binds to the platelet receptor Gp Ib/Ia, thereby activating even more platelets and forming molecular bridges between platelets. Platelet activation also induces a conformational change in Gp IIb/IIIa, another platelet receptor, endowing it with the capacity to bind fibrinogen. Thus, as a result of the conformational change in Gp IIb/IIIa, the fibrinogen that is always present in blood forms bridges between platelets and participates in the formation of a platelet plug.

A controlled cascade of proteolysis creates a blood clot

A **blood clot** is a semisolid mass composed of both platelets and fibrin and—entrapped in the mesh of fibrin—erythrocytes, leukocytes, and serum. A **thrombus** is also a blood clot, but the term is usually reserved for an *intravascular* clot. The relative composition of thrombi varies with the site of **thrombosis** (i.e., thrombus formation). A higher proportion of platelets is present in clots of the arterial circulation, whereas a higher proportion of fibrin is present in clots of the venous circulation.

Platelet plug formation and blood clotting are related but distinct events that may occur in parallel or in the absence of one other. As we will see below, activated platelets can release small amounts of some of the factors (e.g., Ca^{2+}) that play a role in blood clotting. Conversely, some clotting factors (e.g., thrombin and fibrinogen) play a role in platelet plug formation. Thus, molecular crosstalk between the machinery involved in platelet plug formation and clot formation helps coordinate hemostasis.

The cardiovascular system normally maintains a precarious balance between two pathological states. On the one hand, inadequate clotting would lead to the leakage of blood from the vascular system and, ultimately, to hypovolemia. On the other hand, overactive clotting would lead to thrombosis and, ultimately, to cessation of blood flow. The cardiovascular system achieves this balance between an antithrombotic (anticoagulant) and a prothrombotic (procoagulant) state by a variety of components of the vascular wall and blood. Promoting an antithrombotic state is a normal layer of endothelial cells, which line all luminal surfaces of the vascular system. Promoting a prothrombotic state are events associated with vascular damage: (1) the failure of endothelial cells to produce the proper antithrombotic factors, and (2) the physical removal or injury of endothelial cells, which permits the blood to come into contact with thrombogenic factors that lie beneath the endothelium.

Two distinct sequences can precipitate coagulation: the intrinsic pathway and the extrinsic pathway. It is the **intrinsic pathway** that becomes activated when blood comes into contact with a negatively charged surface. The **extrinsic pathway** is activated when blood comes in contact with material from damaged cell membranes. In both cases, the precipitating event triggers a chain reaction that converts precursors into activated factors, which in turn catalyze the conversion of other precursors into other activated factors, and so on. Most of these "precursors" are zymogens that give rise to "activated factors" that are serine proteases. Thus, *controlled proteolysis* plays a central role in amplifying the clotting signals. In the case of the intrinsic pathway, the chain reaction occurs mainly at the membrane of activated platelets. In the case of the extrinsic pathway, the reactions occur mainly at a "tissue factor" that is membrane bound. Both pathways converge on a **common pathway** that culminates in generation of thrombin and, ultimately, "stable" fibrin. Table 18.3 provides the names, synonyms, and properties of

TABLE 18.3 Procoagulant Factors

NAME	ALTERNATE NAMES	PROPERTIES
Procoagulant Factors		
Factor I	Fibrinogen	Plasma globulin
Factor Ia	Fibrin	
Factor II	Prothrombin	Plasma α_2-globulin Synthesis in liver requires vitamin K*
Factor IIa	Thrombin	Serine protease
Factor III (cofactor)	Tissue factor Tissue thromboplastin	Integral membrane glycoprotein; member of type II cytokine receptor family Receptor for factor VIIa Must be present in a phospholipid membrane for procoagulant activity
Factor IV	Ca^{2+}	
Factor V	Labile factor Proaccelerin Accelerator globulin	Plasma protein synthesized by liver and stored in platelets Single-chain protein
Factor Va (cofactor)		Heterodimer held together by a single Ca^{2+} ion Highly homologous to factor VIIIa
Factor VII	Stable factor Serum prothrombin conversion accelerator (SPCA) Proconvertin	Plasma protein Synthesis in liver requires vitamin K*
Factor VIIa		Serine protease

Continued

TABLE 18.3 Procoagulant Factors—cont'd

NAME	ALTERNATE NAMES	PROPERTIES
Factor VIII	Antihemophilic factor (AHF) Factor VIII procoagulant component (FVIII:C)	Plasma protein with phospholipid-binding domain
Factor VIIIa (cofactor)		Highly homologous to factor Va
Factor IX	Christmas factor Plasma thromboplastin component (PTC)	Plasma protein Synthesis in liver requires vitamin K*
Factor IXa		Protease Disulfide-linked heterodimer
Factor X	Stuart factor	Plasma glycoprotein Synthesis in liver requires vitamin K*
Factor Xa		Protease
Factor XI	Plasma thromboplastin antecedent (PTA)	Plasma protein produced by megakaryocytes and stored in platelets
Factor XIa		Protease Disulfide-linked homodimer
Factor XII	Hageman factor (HAF)	Plasma glycoprotein
Factor XIIa		Protease
Factor XIII	Fibrin-stabilizing factor (FSF)	Plasma protein stored in platelets
Factor XIIIa		Transglutaminase Tetramer of two A chains and two B chains
High-molecular-weight kininogen	HMWK Fitzgerald factor	Plasma protein stored in platelets Kallikrein clips bradykinin from HMWK
Plasma prekallikrein	Fletcher factor Plasma kallikrein precursor	Plasma protein
Plasma kallikrein		Serine protease Kallikrein clips bradykinin from HMWK
von Willebrand factor	vWF	Plasma glycoprotein made by endothelial cells and megakaryocytes Stabilizes factor VIIIa Promotes platelet adhesion and aggregation

*See ● 46-10 for a discussion of vitamin K.

the procoagulant and anticoagulant factors in various parts of the clotting scheme.

Intrinsic Pathway (Surface Contact Activation) The left branch of Fig. 18.10 shows the intrinsic pathway, a cascade of protease reactions initiated by factors that are all present within blood. When in contact with a negatively charged surface such as glass or the membrane of an activated platelet, a plasma protein called factor XII (Hageman factor) can become **factor XIIa**—the suffix *a* indicates that this is the *activated* form of factor XII. A molecule called **high-molecular-weight kininogen (HMWK),** a product of platelets that may in fact be attached to the platelet membrane, helps anchor factor XII to the charged surface and thus serves as a cofactor. Once a small amount of factor XIIa accumulates, this protease converts prekallikrein to kallikrein, with HMWK as an anchor. In turn, the newly produced **kallikrein** accelerates the conversion of factor XII to factor XIIa—an example of positive feedback.

In addition to amplifying its own generation by forming kallikrein, factor XIIa (together with HMWK) proteolytically cleaves factor XI to factor XIa. In turn, factor XIa proteolytically cleaves factor IX (Christmas factor) to factor IXa. Factor IXa and two downstream products of the cascade—factors Xa and, most important, thrombin—proteolytically cleave factor VIII to factor VIIIa, a cofactor in the next reaction. Finally, factors IXa and VIIIa, together with Ca^{2+} (which may come largely from activated platelets) and negatively charged phospholipids, form a trimolecular complex called tenase. **Tenase** then converts factor X (Stuart factor) to factor Xa.

Extrinsic Pathway (Tissue Factor Activation) The right branch of Fig. 18.10 shows the extrinsic pathway, a cascade of protease reactions initiated by factors that are outside the vascular system. Nonvascular cells constitutively express an integral membrane protein called **tissue factor** (tissue thromboplastin, or factor III), which is a receptor for a plasma

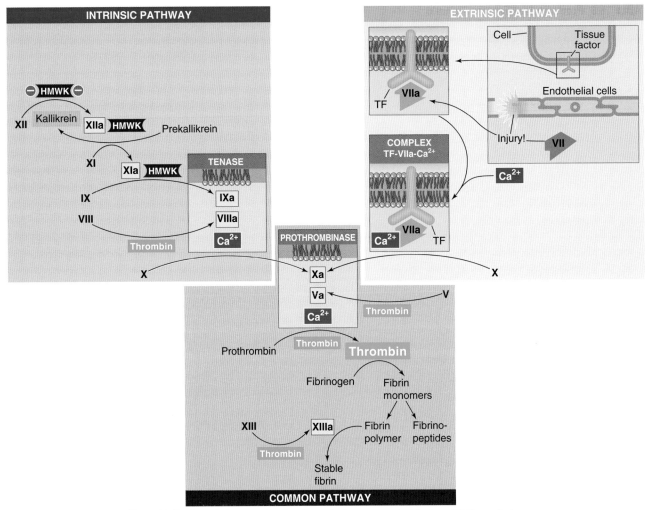

Figure 18.10 Coagulation cascade, showing only the procoagulant factors. *TF,* Tissue factor.

protein called factor VII. When an injury to the endothelium allows factor VII to come into contact with tissue factor, the tissue factor non-proteolytically activates factor VII to factor VIIa. Subsequently, tissue factor, factor VIIa, and Ca^{2+} form a trimolecular complex analogous to tenase. Like tenase, the trimolecular complex of [tissue factor + factor VIIa + Ca^{2+}] proteolytically cleaves the proenzyme factor X to factor Xa. An interesting feature is that when factor X binds to the trimolecular complex, factor VIIa undergoes a conformational change that prevents it from dissociating from tissue factor.

Regardless of whether factor Xa arises by the intrinsic or extrinsic pathway, the cascade proceeds along the common pathway.

Common Pathway Factor Xa from either the intrinsic or extrinsic pathway is the first protease of the common pathway (center of Fig. 18.10). Reminiscent of the conversion of factor VIII to the cofactor VIIIa in the intrinsic pathway, the downstream product thrombin clips factor V to form the cofactor Va. Factor V is highly homologous to factor VIII, and in both cases the proteolytic activation clips a single protein into two peptides that remain attached to one another. Factors Xa and Va, together with Ca^{2+} and phospholipids, form yet another trimolecular complex called **prothrombinase.**

Prothrombinase acts on a plasma protein called prothrombin to form thrombin.

Thrombin is the central protease of the coagulation cascade, responsible for three major kinds of actions:

1. **Activation of downstream components in the clotting cascade.** The main action of thrombin is to catalyze the proteolysis of fibrinogen (see ◉ 18-3), releasing fibrinopeptides. The release of the fibrinopeptide results in the formation of fibrin monomers that are still soluble. **Fibrin monomers** now composed of α, β, and γ chains spontaneously polymerize to form a *gel* of **fibrin polymers** that traps blood cells. Thrombin also activates factor XIII to factor XIIIa, which mediates the covalent cross-linking of the α and γ chains of fibrin polymers to form a *mesh* called **stable fibrin** that is even less soluble than fibrin.

2. **Positive feedback at several upstream levels of the cascade.** Thrombin can catalyze the formation of new thrombin from prothrombin and also the formation of the cofactors Va and VIIIa.

3. **Paracrine actions that influence hemostasis.** First, thrombin causes endothelial cells to release nitric oxide, prostaglandin I_2 (PGI_2), ADP, vWF, and tissue plasminogen activator. Second, thrombin can activate platelets

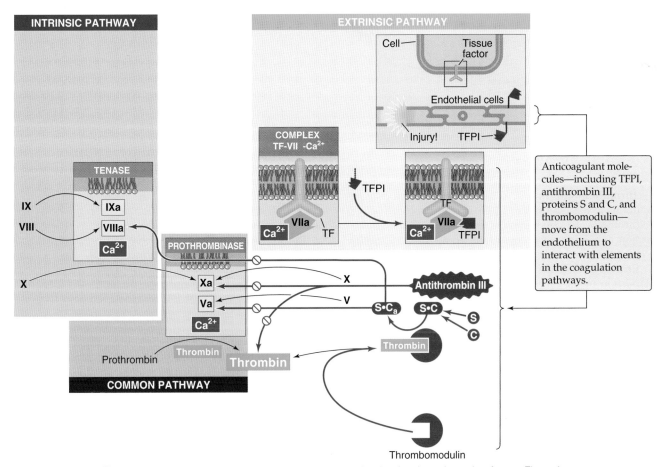

Figure 18.11 Abbreviated version of the coagulation cascade, showing the anticoagulant factors. The anticoagulant pathways are indicated in *red*. *TF*, Tissue factor.

through PAR-1, a protease-activated receptor that belongs to the family of G protein–coupled receptors (see ⊙ 3-3). Thus, thrombin is a key part of the molecular crosstalk introduced above between platelet activation and blood clotting, both of which are required for optimal clot formation.

Coagulation as a Connected Diagram The concept of independent intrinsic and extrinsic branches converging on a common pathway is becoming obsolete. However, coagulation is best conceptualized as a "connected diagram" (see Fig. 25.1C). One example of interconnections is thrombin's multiple actions just discussed. Another example is the trimolecular complex of [tissue factor + factor VIIa + Ca^{2+}] of the extrinsic pathway, which activates factors IX and XI of the intrinsic pathway. In the other direction, factors IXa and Xa of the intrinsic pathway can activate factor VII of the extrinsic pathway. Thus, the intrinsic pathway and extrinsic pathway are strongly interconnected to form a *network*.

Coagulation depends largely on the extrinsic pathway. Although tissue factor is normally absent from intravascular cells, inflammation can trigger peripheral blood monocytes and endothelial cells to express tissue factor, which increases the risk of coagulation.

Anticoagulants keep the clotting network in check

Endothelial cells are the main sources of the agents that help maintain normal blood fluidity. These agents are of two general types, paracrine factors and anticoagulant factors.

Paracrine Factors Endothelial cells generate prostacyclin (PGI$_2$; see ⊙ 3-19), which promotes vasodilation and thus blood flow and also inhibits platelet activation and thus clotting. Stimulated by thrombin, endothelial cells also produce nitric oxide (see ⊙ 3-23). Through cGMP, nitric oxide inhibits platelet adhesion and aggregation.

Anticoagulant Factors As summarized in Fig. 18.11, endothelial cells also generate anticoagulant factors that interfere with the clotting cascade that generates fibrin.

1. **Tissue factor pathway inhibitor (TFPI).** TFPI is a plasma protein that binds to the trimolecular complex [tissue factor + factor VIIa + Ca^{2+}] in the extrinsic pathway and blocks the protease activity of factor VIIa.

2. **Antithrombin III (AT III).** AT III binds to and inhibits factor Xa and thrombin. The sulfated glycosaminoglycans **heparan sulfate** and **heparin** enhance the binding of AT III to factor Xa or to thrombin, thus inhibiting coagulation. Heparan sulfate is present on the external surface of most cells, including endothelial surfaces. Mast cells and basophils release heparin.

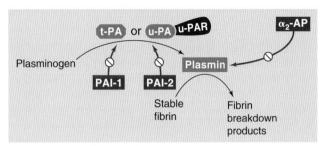

Figure 18.12 Fibrinolytic cascade.

3. **Thrombomodulin.** A glycosaminoglycan product of endothelial cells, thrombomodulin can form a complex with thrombin, thereby removing thrombin from the circulation and inhibiting coagulation. In addition, thrombomodulin also binds protein C.
4. **Protein C.** After protein C binds to the thrombomodulin portion of the thrombin-thrombomodulin complex, the thrombin activates protein C. Activated protein C (C_a) is a protease. Together with its cofactor protein S, activated protein C inactivates the cofactors Va and VIIIa, thus inhibiting coagulation.
5. **Protein S.** This is the cofactor of protein C and is thus an anticoagulant.

Finally, clearance of activated clotting factors by the Kupffer cells of the liver also keeps hemostasis under control.

Fibrinolysis breaks up clots

Through the interaction of actin and myosin in the platelets, a clot shrinks to a plug and thereby expels serum. After plug formation, fibrinolysis—the breakdown of stable fibrin—breaks up the clot in a more general process known as thrombolysis. As shown in Fig. 18.12, the process of fibrinolysis begins with the conversion of plasminogen to plasmin, catalyzed by one of two activators: tissue-type plasminogen activator or urokinase-type plasminogen activator.

The source of **tissue plasminogen activator (t-PA),** a serine protease, is endothelial cells. t-PA converts the plasma zymogen plasminogen to the active fibrinolytic protease plasmin. The presence of fibrin greatly accelerates the conversion of plasminogen to plasmin.

Besides t-PA, the other plasminogen activator, **urokinase-type plasminogen activator (u-PA),** is present in plasma either as a single-chain protein or as the two-chain product of a proteolytic cleavage. Like t-PA, u-PA converts plasminogen to the active protease plasmin. However, this proteolysis requires that u-PA attach to a receptor on the cell surface called urokinase plasminogen activator receptor (u-PAR).

Plasminogen, mainly made by the liver, is a large, single-chain glycoprotein that is composed of an N-terminal heavy chain (A chain) and a C-terminal light chain (B chain). The N-terminal heavy chain contains five kringles, and the C-terminal light chain contains the protease domain. t-PA cleaves plasminogen at the junction between the heavy and light chains, yielding plasmin.

Plasmin is a serine protease that can break down both fibrin and fibrinogen. Plasmin proteolytically cleaves stable fibrin to fibrin breakdown products. Plasmin can also cleave t-PA between the kringle and protease motifs of t-PA. The C terminus of single-chain t-PA nonetheless retains its protease activity.

The cardiovascular system regulates fibrinolysis at several levels, using both enhancing and inhibitory mechanisms. Catecholamines and bradykinin increase the levels of circulating t-PA. Two *serine protease inhibitors* (serpins) reduce the activity of the plasminogen activators: plasminogen activator inhibitor 1 (PAI-1) and plasminogen activator inhibitor 2 (PAI-2). **PAI-1** complexes with and inhibits both single-chain and two-chain t-PA as well as u-PA. PAI-1 is produced mainly by endothelial cells. **PAI-2** mainly inhibits u-PA. PAI-2 is important in pregnancy because it is produced by the placenta and may contribute to increased risk of thrombosis in pregnancy.

It is of interest that activated protein C, which inhibits coagulation Fig. 18.11, also inhibits PAI-1 and PAI-2, thereby facilitating fibrinolysis. α_2-**antiplasmin** (α_2-**AP**) made by liver, kidney, and other tissues, targets plasmin. When plasmin is not bound to fibrin, α_2-AP complexes with and thereby readily inactivates plasmin. However, when plasmin is attached to lysine residues on fibrin, the inhibition by α_2-AP is greatly reduced. In other words, the very presence of a clot (i.e., fibrin) promotes the breakdown of the clot (i.e., fibrinolysis).

CHAPTER 19

ARTERIES AND VEINS

Emile L. Boulpaep

ARTERIAL DISTRIBUTION AND VENOUS COLLECTION SYSTEMS

Hemodynamics is the study of the physical laws of blood circulation. It therefore addresses the properties of both the "content" (i.e., blood) and the "container" (i.e., blood vessels). The anatomy and functions of the various segments of the vasculature differ greatly from one to another. We can think of the **arteries** as a *distribution system,* the **microcirculation** as a *diffusion and filtration system,* and the **veins** as a *collection system.*

Physical properties of vessels closely follow the level of branching in the circuit

The aorta branches out into billions of capillaries that ultimately regroup into a single vena cava (Fig. 19.1, *panel 1*). At each level of arborization of the peripheral circulation, the values of several key parameters vary dramatically:

1. Number of vessels at each level of arborization
2. Radius of a typical individual vessel
3. Aggregate cross-sectional area of all vessels at that level
4. Mean linear velocity of blood flow within an individual vessel
5. Flow (i.e., volume per second) through a single vessel
6. Relative blood volume (i.e., the fraction of the body's total blood volume present in all vessels of a given level)
7. Circulation (i.e., transit) time between two points of the circuit
8. Pressure profile along that portion of the circuit
9. Structure of the vascular walls
10. Elastic properties of the vascular walls

The **number of vessels** at a particular level of arborization (Table 19.1) increases enormously from a single aorta to ~10^4 small arteries, ~10^7 arterioles, and finally ~4×10^{10} capillaries. Only about one fourth of all capillaries are normally open to flow at rest. All of the blood returns to a single vessel where the superior and inferior venae cavae join.

⊙ **19-1** The **radius of an individual vessel** (r_i; Table 19.1) declines as a result of the arborization, decreasing from 1.1 cm in the aorta to a minimum of ~3 μm in the smallest capillaries. Because the **cross-sectional area** of an individual vessel is proportional to the square of the radius, this parameter decreases even more precipitously.

The aggregate cross-sectional area (Table 19.1) at any level of branching is the sum of the single cross-sectional areas of all parallel vessels at that level of branching.

A fundamental law of vessel branching is that at each branch point, the combined cross-sectional area of daughter vessels exceeds the cross-sectional area of the parent vessel. In this process of bifurcation, the steepest increase in total cross-sectional area occurs in the microcirculation (Fig. 19.1, panel 2). Assuming that only a quarter of the capillaries are usually open (Table 19.1), we can estimate the peak aggregate cross-sectional area of the postcapillary venules can be ~1000-fold greater than the cross section of the parent artery (e.g., aorta), as shown in panel 2 of Fig. 19.1.

The profile of the **mean linear velocity** of flow ($\bar{v}$) along a vascular circuit (Fig. 19.1, panel 3) is roughly a mirror image of the profile of the total cross-sectional area. According to the principle of continuity, the **total volume flow** of blood must be the same at any level of arborization. Indeed, as we make multiple vertical slices along the x-axis of panel 1 in Fig. 19.1, the aggregate flow for each slice is the same:

$$F_{\text{total}} = \underbrace{A_1 \cdot \bar{v}_1}_{\text{Level 1}} = \underbrace{A_2 \cdot \bar{v}_2}_{\text{Level 2}} = \underbrace{A_3 \cdot \bar{v}_3}_{\text{Level 3}} = \ldots \qquad \textbf{(19.1)}$$

As a consequence, $\bar{v}$ must be minimal in the postcapillary venules (~0.03 cm/s), where A_{total} is maximal. Conversely, $\bar{v}$ is maximal in the aorta (~20 to 50 cm/s). Thus, both A_{total} and $\bar{v}$ values range ~1000-fold from the aorta to the capillaries, but are inversely related to one another. The vena cava, with a cross-sectional area ~50% larger than that of the aorta, has a mean linear velocity that is about one third less.

⊙ **19-2 Single-vessel flow,** in contrast to total flow, varies by ~10 orders of magnitude. In the aorta, the flow is ~83 mL/s, the same as the cardiac output (~5 L/min). When about 25% of the capillaries are open, a *typical* capillary has a mean linear velocity of 0.03 cm/s and a flow of 8×10^{-9} mL/s (8 pL/s)—10 orders of magnitude less than the flow in the aorta. Within the microcirculation, single-vessel flow has considerable range. At one extreme, a first-order arteriole (r_i ~ 30 μm) may have a flow of 20×10^{-6} mL/s. At the other, the capillaries that are closed at any given time have zero flow.

⊙ 19-3 Most of the blood volume resides in the systemic veins

The body's **total blood volume** (*V*) of about 5 L (see Table 5.1) is not uniformly distributed along the x-axis of panel 1 in Fig. 19.1. At any level of branching, the total blood volume is the sum of the volumes of all parallel branches. Table 19.2

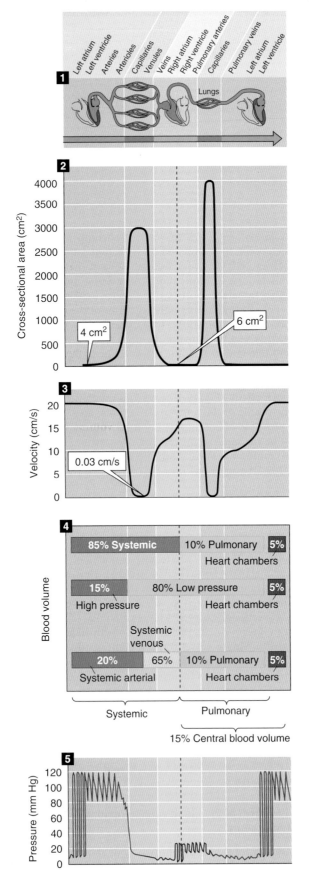

Figure 19.1 Profile of key parameters along the cardiovascular system.

summarizes—for a hypothetical 70-kg woman—the distribution of total blood volume expressed as both absolute blood volumes and **relative blood volumes** (percentage of total blood volume). Panel 4 in Fig. 19.1 summarizes four useful ways of grouping these volumes.

First, we can divide the blood volume into the *systemic* circulation (where ~85% of blood resides), the *pulmonary* circulation (~10%), and the *heart* chambers (~5%). The pulmonary blood volume is quite adjustable (i.e., it can be much higher than 10%) and is carefully regulated.

Second, we can divide blood volume into what is contained in the *high-pressure* system (~15%), the *low-pressure* system (~80%), and the heart chambers (~5%).

Third, we can group the blood volumes into those in the *systemic venous system* versus the remainder of the circulation. Of the 85% of the total blood volume that resides in the systemic circulation, about three fourths—or 65% of the total—is on the venous side, particularly in the smaller veins. Thus, the venous system acts as a volume reservoir. Changes in the diameters of veins have a major impact on the amount of blood they contain. For example, an abrupt increase in venous capacity causes pooling of blood in venous segments and may lead to **syncope** (i.e., fainting).

◉ **19-4** We can also use a fourth approach for grouping of blood volumes—divide the blood into the **central blood volume** (volumes of heart chambers and pulmonary circulation) versus the rest of the circulation. This central blood volume is very adjustable, and it constitutes the filling reservoir for the left heart. Left-sided heart failure can cause the normally careful regulation of the central blood volume to break down.

The **circulation time** is the time required for a bolus of blood to travel either across the entire length of the circulation or across a particular vascular bed. Total circulation time (the time to go from left to right across panel 1 in Fig. 19.1) is ~1 minute. Circulation time across a single vascular bed (e.g., coronary circulation) may be as short as 10 seconds.

The intravascular pressures along the systemic circuit are higher than those along the pulmonary circuit

Panel 5 in Fig. 19.1 shows the profile of pressure along the systemic and pulmonary circulations. Pressures are far higher in the systemic than in the pulmonary circulation. Although the cardiac outputs of the left and right hearts are the same in the steady state, the total resistance of the systemic circulation is far higher than that of the pulmonary circulation (see ◉ **31-3**). This difference explains why the upstream driving pressure averages ~95 mm Hg in the *systemic circulation* but only ~15 mm Hg in the *pulmonary circulation*. In both the systemic and pulmonary circulations, the systolic and diastolic pressures decay downstream from the ventricles (Fig. 19.2). The instantaneous pressures vary throughout each cardiac cycle for much of the circulatory system (Fig. 19.1, panel 5). In addition, the systemic venous and pulmonary pressures vary with the respiratory cycle, and venous pressure in the lower limbs varies with the contraction of skeletal muscle.

As noted above, the circulation can be divided into a high-pressure and a low-pressure system. The **high-pressure**

TABLE 19.1 Key Systemic Vascular Parameters That Vary with Arborization

PARAMETER	AORTA	SMALL ARTERIES[a]	ARTERIOLES[a]	CAPILLARIES[b]	VENA CAVA
Number of units (N)	1	8000	2×10^7	1×10^{10} open (4×10^{10} total)	1
Internal radius (r_i)	1.13 cm	0.5 mm	15 µm	3 µm	1.38 cm
Cross-sectional area ($A_i = \pi r_i^2$)	4 cm²	7.9×10^{-3} cm²	7.1×10^{-7} cm²	2.8×10^{-7} cm²	6 cm²
Aggregate cross-sectional area ($A_{total} = N\pi r_i^2$)	4 cm²	63 cm²	141 cm²	2827 cm²[c]	6 cm²
Aggregate flow (F_{total})	83 cm³/s (mL/s)	83 cm³/s	83 cm³/s	83 cm³/s	83 cm³/s
Mean linear velocity ($\bar{v} = F_{total}/A_{total}$)	21 cm/s	1.3 cm/s	0.6 cm/s	0.03 cm/s[c]	14 cm/s
Single-unit flow ($F_i = F_{total}/N = A_i \cdot \bar{v}$)	83 cm³/s (mL/s)	0.01 cm³/s	4×10^{-6} cm³/s	8×10^{-9} cm³/s[c]	83 cm³/s

[a]The values in this column are for a representative generation.
[b]The values in this column are for the smallest capillaries, at the highest level of branching.
[c]Assuming that only 25% of the capillaries are open.

TABLE 19.2 Distribution of Blood Volume[a]

REGION	ABSOLUTE VOLUME (mL)		RELATIVE VOLUME (%)
Systemic Circulation		4200	84
Aorta and large arteries	300		6.0
Small arteries	400		8.0
Capillaries	300		6.0
Small veins	2300		46.0
Large veins	900		18
Pulmonary Circulation		440	8.8
Arteries	130		2.6
Capillaries	110		2.2
Veins	200		4.0
Heart (End Diastole)	360	360	7.2 7.2
Total	5000	5000	100 100

[a]Values are for a 70-kg woman. For a 70-kg man, scale up the absolute values by 10%.

system extends from the left ventricle in the *contracted state* all the way to the systemic arterioles. The **low-pressure system** extends from the systemic capillaries, through the rest of the systemic circuit, into the right heart, and then through the pulmonary circuit into the left heart in the *relaxed state*. The pulmonary circuit, unlike the systemic circuit, is entirely a low-pressure system; mean arterial pressures normally do not exceed 15 mm Hg, and the capillary pressures do not rise above 10 mm Hg.

Under normal conditions, the steepest pressure drop in the systemic circulation occurs in arterioles, the site of greatest vascular resistance

If we assume that the left heart behaves like a constant pressure generator of 95 mm Hg and the right heart behaves like a constant pressure generator of 15 mm Hg, it is the resistance of each vascular segment that determines the profile of pressure fall between the upstream arterial and downstream venous ends of the circulation. The pressure difference between two points along the axis of the vessel (i.e., the driving pressure difference, ΔP) depends on flow and resistance: $\Delta P = F \cdot R$ (see ⊙ 17-1). According to Poiseuille's law (see Equation 17.9), the resistance (R_i) of an individual, unbranched vascular segment is inversely proportional to the fourth power of the radius. Thus, the *pressure drop between any two points along the circuit depends critically* on the *diameter of the vessels* between these two points. However, the steepest pressure drop ($\Delta P/\Delta x$) does *not* occur along the capillaries, where vessel diameters are smallest, but rather along the *precapillary arterioles* because the **aggregate resistance** of vessels of a particular order of arborization depends also on the *number* of vessels in parallel. The more vessels in parallel, the smaller the aggregate resistance. Although the resistance of a single capillary exceeds that of a single arteriole, capillaries far outnumber arterioles. The result is that the aggregate resistance is larger in the arterioles, and this is where the steepest ΔP occurs.

⊙ 19-5 Local intravascular pressure depends on the distribution of vascular resistance

The ΔP between an upstream checkpoint and a downstream checkpoint depends on the resistance between these points. The absolute pressure at some location *between* the two checkpoints depends on the upstream arterial and downstream venous pressures and the *distribution of resistance* between the two checkpoints. A good example to explain this concept is the distribution of resistance and pressure in the systemic microvasculature. Just how the upstream pressure in the arteriole and the downstream pressure in the venule affect the pressure at the midpoint of the capillary (P_c) depends on the relative size of the upstream and downstream resistances. For the simple circuit illustrated in Fig. 19.3A,

A   SYSTEMIC CIRCULATION

B   PULMONARY CIRCULATION

Figure 19.2   Pressure profiles along systemic and pulmonary circulations. In (A) and (B), the oscillations represent variations in time, not distance. *Boxed numbers* indicate mean pressures. *L*, Left; *Pulm.*, pulmonary; *R*, right.

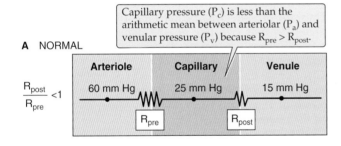

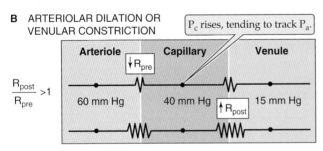

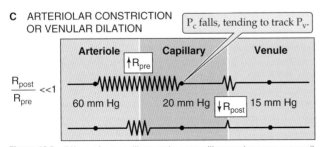

Figure 19.3   Effect of precapillary and postcapillary resistances on capillary pressure.

$$P_c = \frac{\left(R_{post}\, /\, R_{pre}\right) \cdot P_a + P_v}{1 + \left(R_{post}\, /\, R_{pre}\right)} \qquad (19.2)$$

where P_a is arteriolar pressure, P_v is venular pressure, R_{pre} is precapillary resistance upstream of the capillary bed, and R_{post} is postcapillary resistance downstream of the capillary.

⊙ **19-6** From this equation, we can draw three conclusions about local microvascular pressure. First, even though arteriolar pressure is 60 mm Hg and venular pressure is 15 mm Hg in our example, capillary pressure is not necessarily 37.5 mm Hg, the arithmetic mean. According to Equation 19.2, P_c would be the arithmetic mean only if the precapillary and postcapillary resistances were identical (i.e., $R_{post}/R_{pre} = 1$). The finding that P_c is ~25 mm Hg in most vascular beds (Fig. 19.3A) implies that R_{pre} exceeds R_{post} (i.e., $R_{post}/R_{pre} < 1$). Under normal conditions in most microvascular beds, R_{post}/R_{pre} ranges from 0.2 to 0.4.

The second implication of Equation 19.2 is that as long as the *sum* $(R_{pre} + R_{post})$ is constant, reciprocal changes in R_{pre} and R_{post} would not alter the total resistance of the circuit and would therefore leave both P_a and P_v constant. However, as R_{post}/R_{pre} increases, P_c would increase, thereby approaching P_a (Fig. 19.3B). Conversely, as R_{post}/R_{pre} decreases, P_c would decrease, approaching P_v (Fig. 19.3C). This conclusion is also intuitive. If we reduced R_{pre} to zero (but increased R_{post} to keep $R_{post} + R_{pre}$ constant), no pressure drop would occur along the precapillary vessels, and P_c would be the same as P_a. Conversely, if R_{post} were zero, P_c would be the same as P_v.

The third conclusion from Equation 19.2 is that, depending on the value of R_{post}/R_{pre}, P_c may be more sensitive to changes in arteriolar than in venular pressure, or vice versa.

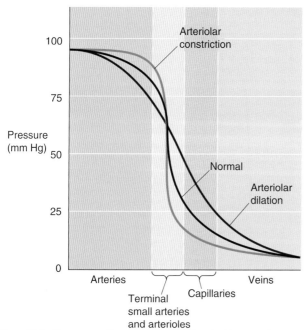

Figure 19.4   Pressure profiles during vasomotion. In this example, we assume that constriction or dilation of terminal arteries and arterioles does not affect the overall driving pressure (ΔP) between aorta and vena cava.

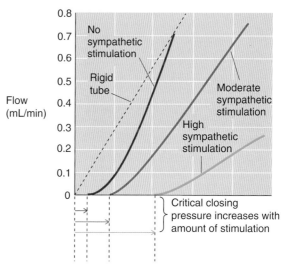

Figure 19.5   Nonlinear dependence of flow on pressure.

For example, when the ratio R_{post}/R_{pre} is low (i.e., $R_{pre} > R_{post}$, as in Fig. 19.3A or C), capillary pressure tends to follow the downstream pressure in large veins. This phenomenon explains why standing may cause the ankles to swell. The elevated pressure in large leg veins translates to an increased P_c, which leads to increased transudation of fluid from the capillaries into the interstitial spaces (see ⊙ 20-10). It also explains why elevation of the feet, which lowers the pressure in the large veins, reverses ankle edema.

Vascular resistance varies in time and depends critically on the action of vascular smooth-muscle cells. The *major site of control* of vascular resistance in the systemic circulation is the *terminal small arteries (or feed arteries) and arterioles*. Fig. 19.4 illustrates the effect of vasoconstriction or vasodilation on the pressure profile. Whereas the overall ΔP between source and end point may not vary appreciably during a change in vascular resistance, the *shape* of the local pressure profile may change appreciably. Thus, during arteriolar constriction, the pressure drop between two points along the circuit (i.e., axial pressure gradient, $\Delta P/\Delta x$) is steep and concentrated at the arteriolar site (Fig. 19.4, *green curve*). During arteriolar dilation, the gradient is shallow and more spread out (Fig. 19.4, *violet curve*).

ELASTIC PROPERTIES OF BLOOD VESSELS

Blood vessels are elastic tubes

The walls of blood vessels consist of three layers: the intima, the media, and the adventitia. Capillaries only have an intimal layer of endothelial cells resting on a basal lamina. Regardless of the organization of layers, four building blocks make up the vascular wall: endothelial cells, elastic fibers, collagen fibers, and smooth-muscle cells.

Endothelial cells form a single, continuous layer that lines all vascular segments. Junctional complexes keep the endothelial cells together in arteries but are less numerous in veins.

Elastic fibers are a rubber-like material that accounts for most of the stretch of vessels at normal pressures. Elastic fibers have two components: a core of **elastin** and a covering of **microfibrils**. The elastin assembles into a highly elastic network of fibers, capable of stretching more than 100%.

Collagen fibers constitute a jacket of far less extensible material than the elastic fibers, like the fabric woven inside the wall of a rubber hose. Collagen can be stretched only 3% to 4%.

⊙ **19-7 Vascular smooth-muscle cells (VSMCs)** are also present in all vascular segments except the capillaries. In *elastic* arteries, VSMCs are arranged in spirals with pitch varying from nearly longitudinal to nearly transverse-circular; whereas in *muscular* arteries, they are arranged either in concentric rings or as helices with a low pitch.

Because of the elastic properties of vessels, the pressure-flow relationship of passive vascular beds is nonlinear

Because blood vessels are elastic, we must revise our concept of blood flow, which was based on Poiseuille's law for rigid tubes (see Equation 17.9). Poiseuille's law predicts a linear pressure-flow relationship (Fig. 19.5, *broken line*). However, in reality, the *pressure-flow relationship is markedly nonlinear* in an in vivo preparation of a vascular bed (Fig. 19.5, *red curve*). Starting at the foot of the red curve at a driving pressure of about 6 mm Hg, we see that the curve rises more steeply as the driving pressure increases. The reason is that an increase of the driving pressure (i.e., axial pressure gradient) also increases the transmural pressure, causing the vessel to distend. Because radius increases, resistance falls and flow rises more than it would in a rigid tube. Thus, the plot curves upward. The *elastic properties* of vessels are the major cause of such nonlinear pressure-flow relationships in vascular beds exhibiting little or no "active tension."

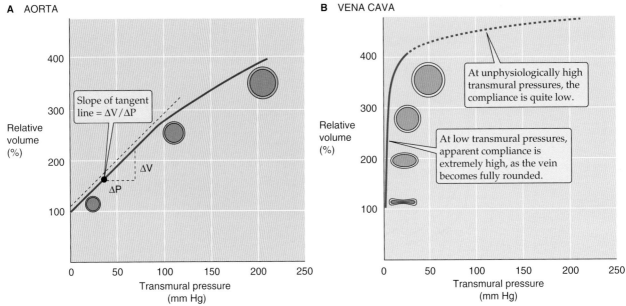

Figure 19.6 Compliance of blood vessels. In (A) and (B), a relative volume of 100% represents the volume in a fully relaxed vessel.

Contraction of smooth muscle halts blood flow when driving pressure falls below the critical closing pressure

At low values of driving pressure, flow totally ceases when the pressure falls below about 6 mm Hg, the critical closing pressure (Fig. 19.5, *red curve*). The stoppage of flow occurs because of the combined action of elastic fibers and *active tension* from VSMCs. Graded increases in active tension—produced, for example, by sympathetic stimulation—shift the pressure-flow relationship to the right and decrease the slope (Fig. 19.5, *blue* and *green curves*). The critical closing pressure also shifts upward with increasing degrees of vasomotor tone.

⊙ 19-8 Elastic and collagen fibers determine the distensibility and compliance of vessels

Arteries and veins must withstand very different transmural pressures in vivo. Moreover, their relative blood volumes respond in strikingly different ways to increases in transmural pressure (Fig. 19.6). Arteries have a low volume capacity but can withstand large transmural pressure differences. In contrast, veins have a large volume capacity (and are thus able to act as blood reservoirs) but can withstand only small transmural pressure differences.

The abundance of structural elements in the vascular walls also differs between arteries and veins. These disparities contribute to differences in the elastic behavior of arteries and veins.

The most useful index of distensibility is **compliance** *(C)*, which is the slope of the tangent to any point along the pressure-volume diagrams in Fig. 19.6:

$$C = \frac{\Delta V}{\Delta P} \tag{19.3}$$

Here, the ΔV and ΔP values are *minute* displacements. The steeper the slope of a pressure-volume diagram, the greater the compliance (i.e., the easier it is to increase volume). In

Fig. 19.6, the slope—and thus the compliance—decreases with increasing volumes. A compliance reading should always include the transmural pressure or the volume at which it was made (see ⊙ 27-3).

Differences in compliance cause arteries to act as resistors and veins to act as capacitors

The compliance of a relaxed elastic artery is substantial (Fig. 19.6A). Increasing the transmural pressure from 0 to 100 mm Hg (near the normal mean arterial pressure) increases relative volume by ~180%. With further increases in pressure and diameter, compliance decreases only modestly. For example, increase of transmural pressure from 100 to 200 mm Hg increases relative volume by a further ~100 percentage points. Thus, arteries are properly constituted for development and withstanding of high transmural pressures. Because muscular arteries have a rather stable resistance, they are sometimes referred to as **resistance vessels.**

Veins behave very differently. The pressure-volume diagram of a vein (Fig. 19.6B) shows that compliance is extremely high—far higher than for "elastic arteries"—at least in the low-pressure range. For a relaxed vein, a relatively small increase of transmural pressure from 0 to 10 mm Hg increases volume by ~200%. This high compliance in the low-pressure range is not due to a property of the elastic fibers. Rather, it reflects a change in geometry. At pressures <6 to 9 mm Hg, the vein's cross section is ellipsoidal. A small rise in pressure causes the vein to become circular, without an increase in perimeter but with a greatly increased cross-sectional area. Thus, in their normal pressure range, veins can accept relatively large volumes of blood with little buildup of pressure. Because they act as *volume reservoirs*, veins are sometimes referred to as **capacitance vessels.** The true distensibility or compliance of the venous wall—related to the increase in *perimeter* produced by pressures >10 mm Hg—is rather poor, as shown by the flat slope at higher pressures in Fig. 19.6B.

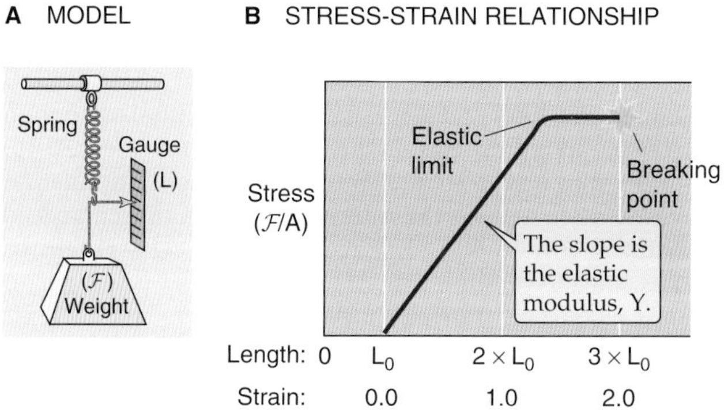

A MODEL

B STRESS-STRAIN RELATIONSHIP

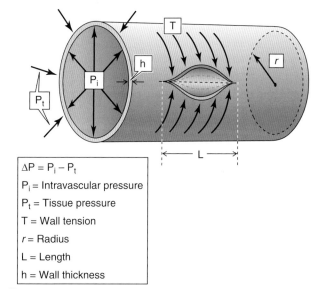

Figure 19.7 Elastic properties of a spring.

19-9 Laplace's law describes how tension in the vessel wall increases with transmural pressure

Because compliance depends on the elastic properties of the vessel wall, the discussion here focuses on how an external force F deforms elastic materials (Fig. 19.7A). When the force vanishes, the deformation vanishes, and the material returns to its original state.

If an elastic body requires a larger force to achieve a certain deformation, it is stiffer or less compliant. The largest stress that the material can withstand while remaining elastic is the **elastic limit.** If it is deformed beyond this limit, the material reaches its yield point and, eventually, its breaking point.

Stress is the force per unit cross-sectional area ($\mathcal{F}/A$). Thus, if we pull on an elastic band—stretching it from an initial length L_0 to a final length L—the stress is the force we apply, divided by the area of the band in cross section. **Strain** is the fractional increase in length, that is, $\Delta L/L_0$ or $(L - L_0)/L_0$ (Fig. 19.7B).

The proportionality factor, the Young **elastic modulus** *(Y)*, is the force per cross-sectional area required to stretch the material to twice its initial length and also the slope of the strain-stress diagram in Fig. 19.7B. Thus, the stiffer a material is, the steeper the slope, and the greater the elastic modulus. For example, collagen is >1000-fold stiffer than elastin.

We can describe the elastic properties of a vessel by considering only what happens along the circumference. The transmural pressure (ΔP) is the distending force that tends to increase the circumference of the vessel. Opposing this elongation is a force inside the vessel wall. It is convenient to express this wall **tension** *(T)* as the force that must be applied to bring together the two edges of an imaginary cut in the wall along the longitudinal axis of the vessel (Fig. 19.8).

The equilibrium between ΔP and T depends on the vessel radius and is expressed by a law derived independently by Thomas Young and the Marquis de Laplace in the early 1800s.

Thus, for a given transmural pressure, the wall tension in the vessel gets larger as the radius increases. This is known as **Laplace's law:**

$$T = \Delta P \cdot r \qquad \textbf{(19.4)}$$

Thus, for a given transmural pressure, the wall tension in the vessel gets larger as the radius increases.

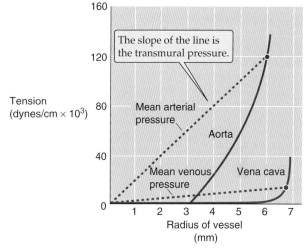

$\Delta P = P_i - P_t$

P_i = Intravascular pressure

P_t = Tissue pressure

T = Wall tension

r = Radius

L = Length

h = Wall thickness

Figure 19.8 Laplace's law. The circumferential arrows that attempt to bring together the edges of an imaginary slit along the length of the vessel represent the constricting force of the tension in the wall. The *radial arrows* that push the wall outward represent the distending force. At equilibrium, the two sets of forces balance. *h*, wall thickness.

Figure 19.9 Elastic diagram (tension versus radius) of blood vessels.

The vascular wall is adapted to withstand wall tension, not transmural pressure

With Laplace's law ($T = \Delta P \cdot r$), we can transform the pressure-volume relationship of Fig. 19.6 into the kind of "elastic diagram" that we used in Fig. 19.7B to understand the properties of a blood vessel as a rubber band.

Laplace's law (see Equation 19.4) allows us to plot wall tension versus radius for both the aorta and vena cava (Fig. 19.9). Comparing vessels of *similar size,* Laplace's law tells us that a high wall tension is required to withstand a high pressure.

Comparing two vessels of very *different size* reveals a disparity between wall tension and pressure. A large vein, such as the vena cava, must resist only 10 mm Hg in transmural pressure but is equipped with a fair amount of elastic tissue. A capillary, on the other hand, which must resist a transmural pressure of 25 mm Hg, does not have any elastic tissue at all. Why? The key concept is that what the vessel really has to withstand is not pressure but *wall tension*. The higher the tension that the vessel wall must bear, the greater is its complement of elastic tissue.

Elastin and collagen separately contribute to the wall tension of vessels

With increasing stretch, the vessel wall resists additional deformation more (Fig. 19.9); that is, the slope of the relationship becomes steeper due to the heterogeneity of the elastic material of the vascular wall. Elastic and collagen fibers have different elastic moduli. In the absence of elastin, the length-tension relationship is very steep (Fig. 19.10, *orange curve*). In the absence of collagen fibers, the length-tension relationship is fairly flat (Fig. 19.10, *violet curve*). The orange curve (collagen) is steeper than the violet curve (elastin) because collagen is stiffer than elastin. In a normal vessel (Fig. 19.10, *red curve*), modest degrees of stretch elongate primarily the elastin fibers along a relatively flat slope. Progressively greater degrees of stretch recruit collagen fibers, resulting in a steeper slope.

⊙ 19-10 Aging reduces the distensibility of arteries

With aging, important changes occur in the elastic properties of blood vessels, primarily arteries. The radius-tension diagrams in Fig. 19.11 show the effects of age on the elastic properties of blood vessels. Because of the progressive, diffuse fibrosis of vessel walls with age, and because of an increase in the amount of collagen, the maximal slope of the radius-tension diagram increases with age. In addition, with age, these curves start to bend upward at lower radii, as the same degree of stretch recruits a larger number of collagen fibers. Underlying this phenomenon is an increased cross-linking among collagen fibers (see ⊙ 62-4) and thus less slack in their connections to other elements in the arterial wall. Thus, even modest elongations challenge the stiffer collagen fibers to stretch.

Active tension from smooth-muscle activity adds to the elastic tension of vessels

Although we have been treating blood vessels as though their walls are purely elastic, the **active tension** (see ⊙ 9-10) from VSMCs also contributes to wall tension. Stimulation of VSMCs can reduce the internal radius of muscular feed arteries by 20% to 50%. Laplace's law ($T = \Delta P \cdot r$) tells us that as the VSMC shortens—thereby reducing vessel radius against a constant transmural pressure—there is a decrease in the tension that the muscle must exert to maintain that new, smaller radius.

For a blood vessel in which both passive elastic components and active smooth-muscle components contribute to the total tension, the radius-tension relationship reflects the contributions of each. The red curve in Fig. 19.12 shows such

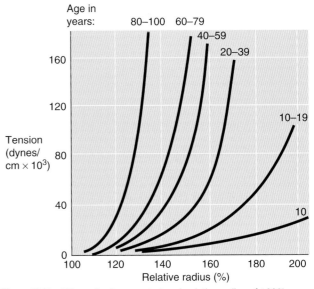

Figure 19.11   Effect of aging on arteries. A relative radius of 100% represents the fully relaxed value.

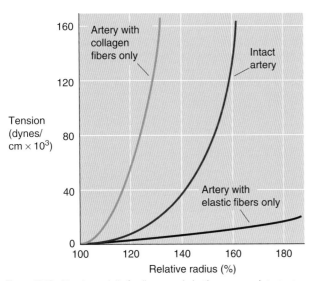

Figure 19.10   Elastic moduli of collagen and elastin versus an intact artery.

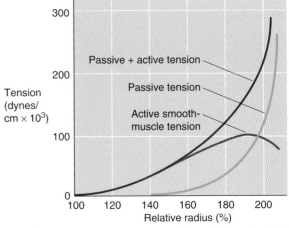

Figure 19.12   Active versus passive tension. The relative radius of 100% is that of an excised vessel maximally stimulated by norepinephrine (*red curve*, total tension) but not "stressed" (i.e., transmural pressure is 0). When the vessel is maximally poisoned with potassium cyanide, the baseline radius is ~150% (*green curve*, passive tension), which reflects its relaxed state. The *blue curve* is just the active (i.e., smooth-muscle) component of tension.

a compounded (passive + active) radius-tension diagram for an artery in which the sympathetic neurotransmitter norepinephrine (see ⊙ 14-6) has maximally stimulated the VSMCs. The green curve shows a passive radius-tension relationship for just the elastic component of the tension (i.e., in the absence of VSMCs). Of course, the green curve is the radius-tension diagram on which we have focused in the previous figures (e.g., Fig. 19.9). Subtraction of the green from the red curve in Fig. 19.12 yields the *active* length-tension diagram (blue curve) for the vascular smooth muscle.

CHAPTER 20

THE MICROCIRCULATION

Emile L. Boulpaep

The microcirculation serves both nutritional and non-nutritional roles

The primary function of the cardiovascular system is to maintain a suitable environment for the tissues. The microcirculation is the "business end" of the system. The capillary is the principal site for exchange of gases, water, nutrients, and waste products. In most tissues, capillary flow exclusively serves these **nutritional** needs. In a few tissues, however, a large portion of capillary flow is **non-nutritional.** For example, in the glomeruli of the kidneys, capillary flow forms the glomerular filtrate (see ⊙ 34-2). Blood flow through the skin, some of which may shunt through arteriovenous anastomoses, plays a key role in temperature regulation (see ⊙ 59-12). Capillaries also serve other non-nutritional roles, such as signaling (e.g., delivery of hormones) and host defense (e.g., delivery of platelets). The morphology and local regulatory mechanisms of the microcirculation are designed to meet the particular needs of each tissue.

⊙ 20-1 The microcirculation extends from the arterioles to the venules

The microcirculation is defined as the blood vessels from the first-order arteriole to the first-order venule. Although the details vary from organ to organ, the principal components of an idealized microcirculation include a single arteriole and venule, between which extends a network of true capillaries (Fig. 20.1). Sometimes a metarteriole —somewhat larger than a capillary—provides a shortcut through the network. Both the arteriole and the venule have vascular smooth-muscle cells (VSMCs). Precapillary sphincters—at the transition between a capillary and either an arteriole or a metarteriole—control the access of blood to particular segments of the network. Sphincter closure or opening creates small local pressure differences that may reverse the direction of blood flow in some segments of the network.

⊙ **20-2 Arteries** consist of an inner layer of endothelium, an internal elastic lamina, and a surrounding sheath of at least two continuous layers of innervated VSMCs (see ⊙ 19-7). The inner radius of **terminal arteries** may be as small as 25 μm. **Arterioles** (inner radius, 5 to 25 μm) are similar to arteries but have only a *single* continuous layer of VSMCs, which are innervated. **Metarterioles** are similar

to arterioles, but of shorter length. Moreover, their VSMCs are discontinuous and are usually not innervated. The **precapillary sphincter** is a small cuff of smooth muscle that usually is not innervated but is very responsive to local tissue conditions.

True capillaries (inner radius, 2 to 5 μm) consist of a single layer of endothelial cells surrounded by a basement membrane, a fine network of reticular collagen fibers, and—in some tissues—pericytes. The endothelial cells have a smooth surface and are extremely thin. The thickness and density of the capillary **basement membrane** vary among organs.

Linking endothelial cells together are **interendothelial junctions** where the two cell membranes are ~10 nm apart. **Tight junctions** (see ⊙ 2-17) may also be present in which the apposed cell membranes appear to fuse, and **claudins** as well as **occludin** seal the gap.

⊙ 20-3 Some endothelial cells have membrane-lined **fenestrations** that run completely through the cell, from the capillary lumen to the interstitial space. These fenestrations are 50 to 80 nm in diameter and are seen primarily in tissues with large fluid and solute fluxes across the capillary walls (e.g., intestine, choroid plexus, exocrine glands, and renal glomeruli). A thin diaphragm often closes the perforations of the fenestrae (e.g., in intestinal capillaries).

The endothelia of the sinusoidal capillaries in the liver, bone marrow, and spleen have very large fenestrations as well as **gaps** 100 to 1000 nm wide *between* adjacent cells.

Capillaries fall into three groups, based on their degree of leakiness (Fig. 20.2).
1. **Continuous capillary.** This is the most common form of capillary, with interendothelial junctions 10 to 15 nm wide (e.g., skeletal muscle).
2. **Fenestrated capillary.** In these capillaries, the endothelial cells are thin and perforated with fenestrations. These capillaries can be found in the small intestine and exocrine glands.
3. **Discontinuous capillary.** In addition to fenestrae, these capillaries have large gaps. Discontinuous capillaries are found in sinusoids (e.g., liver).

At their distal ends, true capillaries merge into **venules** (inner radius, 5 to 25 μm), which carry blood back into low-pressure veins that return blood to the heart. Venules have a discontinuous layer of VSMCs and therefore can control local blood flow. Venules may also exchange some solutes across their walls.

CAPILLARY EXCHANGE OF SOLUTES

The exchange of O_2 and CO_2 across capillaries depends on the diffusional properties of the surrounding tissue

Gases diffuse by a **transcellular route** across the two cell membranes and cytosol of the endothelial cells of the capillary with the same ease that they diffuse through the surrounding tissue. Arterial blood has a relatively high O_2 level. As blood traverses a systemic capillary, the principal site of gas exchange, O_2 diffuses across the capillary wall and into the tissue space, which includes the interstitial fluid and the neighboring cells.

◉ **20-4** The most frequently used model of gas exchange is **Krogh's tissue cylinder,** a volume of tissue surrounding a single capillary that supplies it with O_2 (Fig. 20.3). The radius of a tissue cylinder in an organ is typically half the average spacing from one capillary to the next. Capillary density and mean intercapillary distance vary greatly among tissues. Capillary density is highest in tissues with high O_2 consumption (e.g., myocardium) and lowest in tissues consuming little O_2 (e.g., joint cartilage). Capillary density is extraordinarily high in the lungs (see ◉ **31-5**).

Arteriole
Smooth muscle
Capillaries
Precapillary sphincters
Metarteriole
Venule

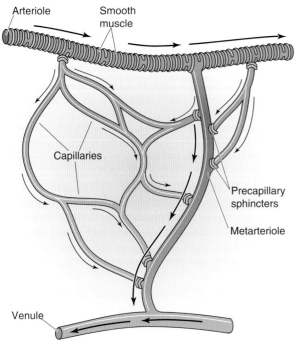

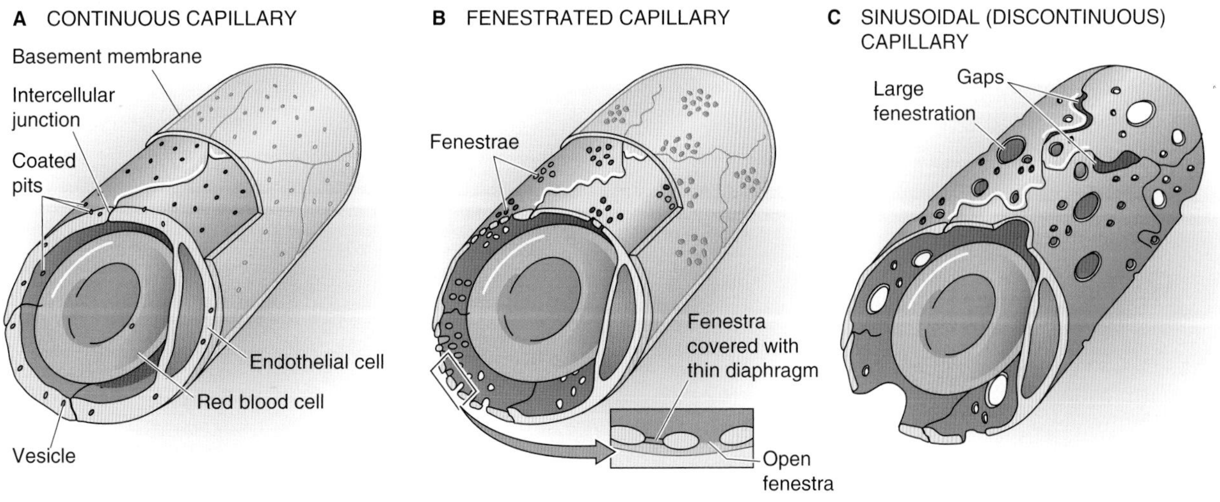

Figure 20.1 Idealized microcirculatory circuit.

◉ 20-5 The O_2 extraction ratio of a whole organ depends primarily on blood flow and metabolic demand

In principle, beginning with a model like Krogh's, one could sum up many capillary segments and then calculate gas exchange in an entire tissue. However, it is more convenient to pool all the capillaries in an organ and to focus on a single arterial inflow and single venous outflow. The difference in concentration of a substance in the arterial inflow and venous outflow of that organ is the **arteriovenous (a-v) difference** of that substance. For example, if the arterial O_2 *content* ($[O_2]_a$) entering the tissue is 20 mL O_2/dL blood and the venous O_2 content leaving it ($[O_2]_v$) is 15 mL O_2/dL blood, the O_2 a-v difference for that tissue is 5 mL O_2 gas/dL blood.

◉ **20-6** For a substance like O_2, which *exits* the capillaries, another way of expressing the amount that the tissues remove is the **extraction ratio.** This parameter is merely the a-v difference *normalized* to the arterial content of the substance.

$$E_{O_2} = \frac{[O_2]_a - [O_2]_v}{[O_2]_a} \qquad \textbf{(20.1)}$$

Thus, in our example,

$$E_{O_2} = \frac{20\text{mL } O_2/\text{dL} - 15\text{mL } O_2/\text{dL}}{20\text{mL } O_2/\text{dL}} = \frac{5}{20} = 25\% \qquad \textbf{(20.2)}$$

What are the factors that determine O_2 extraction? The two most important are capillary flow and metabolic demand). The O_2 extraction ratio decreases with increased

A CONTINUOUS CAPILLARY
Basement membrane
Intercellular junction
Coated pits
Endothelial cell
Red blood cell
Vesicle
B FENESTRATED CAPILLARY
Fenestrae
Fenestra covered with thin diaphragm
Open fenestra
C SINUSOIDAL (DISCONTINUOUS) CAPILLARY
Gaps
Large fenestration

Figure 20.2 Three types of capillaries.

flow but increases with increased O_2 consumption. Increased metabolic demands require that the tissue extract more of the incoming O_2.

$$\underbrace{[O_2]_a - [O_2]_v}_{\substack{\text{Related to} \\ \text{extraction ratio}}} = \frac{\dot{Q}_{O_2}}{F} \qquad \textbf{(20.3)}$$

⊙ 20-7 Equation 20.3 is a form of the **Fick Principle**, which states that the rate of O_2 consumption in the systemic tissues ($\dot{Q}_{O2}$) is the difference between the rate of O_2 delivery ($F \times [O_2]_a$) and the rate at which O_2 enters the systemic veins ($F \times [O_2]_v$).

Another important factor is that not all of the capillaries in a tissue may be active at any one time. For example, skeletal muscle contains roughly a half million capillaries per gram of tissue. However, only ~20% are perfused at rest. During exercise, when the O_2 consumption of the muscle increases, the resistance vessels and precapillary sphincters dilate to meet the increased demand. This vasodilation increases muscle blood flow and the density of perfused capillaries.

The velocity of blood flow in the capillaries also increases during exercise. This increased velocity would cause P_{O_2} to fall *less steeply* along the capillary lumen.

According to Fick's law, the diffusion of small water-soluble solutes across a capillary wall depends on both the permeability and the concentration gradient

Although the endothelial cell is freely permeable to O_2 and CO_2, it offers a significant barrier to the exchange of lipid-insoluble substances. Hydrophilic solutes that are smaller than albumin can traverse the capillary wall by **diffusion** via a paracellular route (i.e., through the clefts and interendothelial junctions as well as gaps and fenestrae, if these are present).

The amount of solute that crosses a particular surface area of a capillary per unit time is called a **flux**. The flux is proportional to the magnitude of the concentration difference across the capillary wall and is larger in leakier capillaries (Fig. 20.4), as described by **Fick's law** (see **⊙ 5-2**):

$$J_X = P_X \cdot \left([X]_c - [X]_{if}\right) \qquad \textbf{(20.4)}$$

Here, J_X is the flux of the solute X (*units:* moles/[cm^2 s]). $[X]_c$ and $[X]_{if}$ are the dissolved concentrations of the solute in the capillary and interstitial fluid, respectively. Because the capillary wall thickness a (*units:* cm) is difficult to determine, we combined the diffusion coefficient D_X (*units:* cm^2/s) and wall thickness into a single term (D_X/a) called P_X, the **permeability coefficient** (*units:* cm/s). Thus, P_X expresses the ease with which the solute crosses a capillary by diffusion.

Because, in practice, the surface area *(S)* of the capillary is often unknown, it is impossible to compute the *flux* of a solute, which is expressed per unit area. Rather, it is more common to compute the *mass flow* ($\dot{Q}$), which is simply the amount of solute transferred per unit time (*units:* moles/s):

$$\dot{Q} = S \cdot J_X = S \cdot P_X \cdot \left([X]_c - [X]_{if}\right) \qquad \textbf{(20.5)}$$

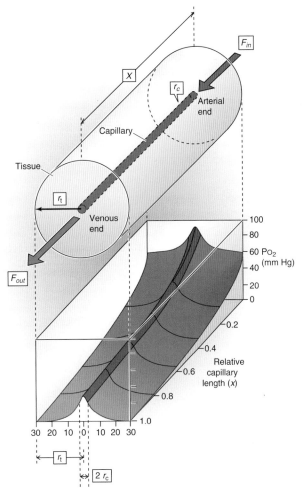

Figure 20.3 Delivery and diffusion of O_2 to systemic tissues, as represented by Krogh's tissue cylinder. The cylinder consists of a single capillary (radius r_c) surrounded by a concentric cylinder of tissue (radius r_t) that the capillary supplies with O_2 and other nutrients. Blood flow into the capillary is F_{in}, and blood flow out of the capillary is F_{out}. The lower panel shows the profile of partial pressure of O_2 (P_{O2}) along the longitudinal axis of the capillary and the radial axis of the tissue cylinder.

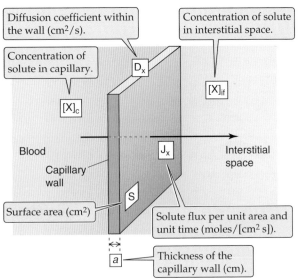

Figure 20.4 Diffusion of a solute across a capillary wall.

Small polar molecules have a relatively low permeability because they can traverse the capillary wall only by diffusing through water-filled pores (small-pore effect)

For substances such as CO_2 and O_2, the permeability is much larger than for more hydrophilic solutes like NaCl and glucose. Small water-soluble, polar molecules have a relatively low permeability because they can diffuse only by a paracellular path through interendothelial clefts or other water-filled pathways, which constitute only a fraction of the total capillary area. **Discontinuities** or gaps in tight-junction strands could form the basis for the small pores. Alternatively, the molecular sieving properties of the small pores may reside in a **fiber matrix** (Fig. 20.5) that consists of either a meshwork of glycoproteins in the paracellular clefts (on the abluminal side of the tight junctions) or the glycocalyx on the surface of the endothelial cell (on the luminal side of the tight junctions).

Interendothelial clefts are wider—and fenestrae are more common—at the venular end of the capillary than at its arteriolar end, so that P_X increases along the capillary. Therefore, if the transcapillary concentration difference ($[X]_c - [X]_{if}$) were the same, the solute flux would actually be larger at the venous end of the microcirculation.

Small proteins can also diffuse across interendothelial clefts or through fenestrae. In addition to molecular size, the *electrical charge* of proteins and other macromolecules is a major determinant of their apparent permeability coefficient. In general, the flux of negatively charged proteins is much smaller than that of neutral macromolecules of equivalent size, whereas positively charged macromolecules have the highest apparent permeability coefficient. Fixed negative charges in the endothelial glycocalyx exclude macromolecules with negative charge and favor the transit of macromolecules with positive charge. Selective permeability based on the electrical charge of the solute is a striking feature of the filtration of proteins across the glomerular barrier of the nephron (see ◉ 34-3).

◉ **20-8** The diffusive movement of solutes is the dominant mode of transcapillary exchange. However, the convective movement of water can also carry solutes. This **solvent drag** is the flux of a dissolved solute that is swept along by the bulk movement of the solvent. Compared with the diffusive flux of a small solute with a high permeability coefficient (e.g., glucose), the contribution of solvent drag is minor.

The exchange of macromolecules across capillaries can occur by transcytosis (large-pore effect)

◉ **20-9** Macromolecules with a radius >1 nm (e.g., plasma proteins) can cross the capillary, at a low rate, through wide intercellular clefts, fenestrations, and gaps—when these are present. However, **caveolae**—small vesicles distinguished by the presence of intrinsic membrane proteins called caveolins—are predominantly responsible for the large-pore effect that allows transcellular translocation of macromolecules. The **transcytosis** of very large macromolecules by vesicular transport involves (1) equilibration of dissolved macromolecules in the capillary lumen with the fluid phase inside the open vesicle; (2) pinching off of the vesicle; (3) vesicle shuttling to the cytoplasm and probably transient fusion with other vesicles within the cytoplasm, allowing intermixing of the vesicular content; (4) fusion of vesicles with the opposite plasma membrane; and (5) equilibration with the opposite extracellular fluid phase.

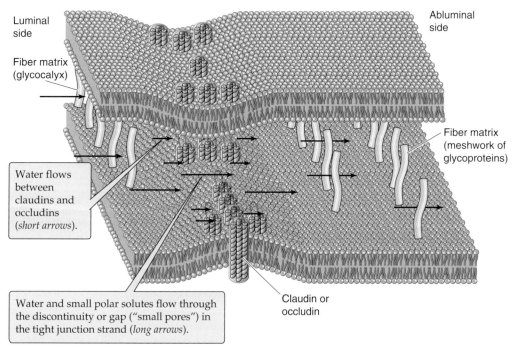

Luminal side

Abluminal side

Fiber matrix (glycocalyx)

Fiber matrix (meshwork of glycoproteins)

Water flows between claudins and occludins (*short arrows*).

Water and small polar solutes flow through the discontinuity or gap ("small pores") in the tight junction strand (*long arrows*).

Claudin or occludin

Figure 20.5 Model of endothelial junctional complexes. The figure shows two adjacent endothelial cell membranes at the tight junction, with a portion of the membrane of the upper cell cut away. (Data from Firth JA: Endothelial barriers: From hypothetical pores to membrane proteins. J Anat 200:541–548, 2002.)

The laws of diffusion (see Equation 20.4) do not govern transcytosis. The "apparent permeability" of typical capillaries to macromolecules reflects the total movement of the macromolecule, regardless of the pathway. The apparent permeability falls off steeply with increases in molecular radius, a feature called **sieving.** Both transcytosis and chains of fused vesicles are less prominent in brain capillaries. The presence of continuous tight junctions and the low level of transcytosis account for the blood-brain barrier's much lower apparent permeability to macromolecules.

CAPILLARY EXCHANGE OF WATER

⊙ 20-10 Fluid transfer across capillaries is convective and depends on net hydrostatic and osmotic forces (i.e., Starling forces)

The pathway for fluid movement across the capillary wall is a combination of transcellular and paracellular pathways. Endothelial cell membranes express constitutively active **aquaporin 1** (AQP1) water channels (see ⊙ 5-13). It is likely that AQP1 constitutes the principal *transcellular* pathway for water movement. The interendothelial clefts, fenestrae, or gaps may be the anatomical substrate of the *paracellular* pathway.

Whereas the main mechanism for the transfer of gases and other solutes is *diffusion,* the main mechanism for the net transfer of fluid across the capillary membrane is **convection.** The two driving forces for the convection of fluid across the capillary wall are the transcapillary hydrostatic pressure difference and *effective* osmotic pressure difference, also known as the colloid osmotic pressure or oncotic pressure difference (see ⊙ 5-14).

The **hydrostatic pressure difference** (ΔP) across the capillary wall is the difference between the intravascular pressure (i.e., capillary hydrostatic pressure, P_c) and the extravascular pressure (i.e., interstitial fluid hydrostatic pressure, P_{if}).

The **colloid osmotic pressure difference** ($\Delta \pi$) across the capillary wall is the difference between the intravascular colloid osmotic pressure caused by plasma proteins (π_c) and the extravascular colloid osmotic pressure caused by interstitial proteins and proteoglycans (π_{if}). A positive ΔP tends to drive water *out of* the capillary lumen, whereas a positive $\Delta \pi$ attracts water *into* the capillary lumen.

The description of the volume flow (F) or volume flux (J_V) of fluid across the capillary wall is embodied in **Starling's equation:**

$$J_V = L_p \left[\underbrace{(P_c - P_{if})}_{\substack{\Delta P \\ \text{Hydrostatic} \\ \text{pressure} \\ \text{difference}}} - \sigma \underbrace{(\pi_c - \pi_{if})}_{\substack{\Delta \pi \\ \text{Colloid osmotic} \\ \text{pressure} \\ \text{difference}}} \right] = F/S_f$$

$$\underbrace{\phantom{J_V = L_p [(P_c - P_{if}) - \sigma (\pi_c - \pi_{if})]}}_{\substack{\text{Net filtration pressure} \\ \text{(i.e., net driving force)}}}$$

(20.6)

Here, L_p is the **hydraulic conductivity,** the proportionality constant that relates the net driving force to J_V and expresses the total permeability provided by the ensemble of AQP1 channels and the paracellular pathway. P_c is the capillary hydrostatic pressure, P_{if} is the hydrostatic pressure of the interstitial fluid, σ is the reflection coefficient, π_c is the capillary colloid osmotic pressure caused by plasma proteins, π_{if} is the colloid osmotic pressure caused by interstitial proteins and proteoglycans, F is the flow of fluid across the capillary wall, and S_f is the functional surface area.

⊙ **20-11** According to van't Hoff's law of osmotic pressure, the theoretical colloid osmotic pressure difference ($\Delta \pi_{theory}$) is directly proportional to the protein concentration difference ($\Delta[X]$). However, because capillary walls exclude proteins *imperfectly,* the observed colloid osmotic pressure difference ($\Delta \pi_{obs}$) is less than the ideal. The ratio $\Delta \pi_{obs}/\Delta \pi_{theory}$ is the **reflection coefficient** (σ).

⊙ **20-12** The net driving force in Equation 20.8 is $[(P_c - P_{if}) - \sigma (\pi_c - \pi_{if})]$, and it has a special name—**net filtration pressure. Filtration** of fluid from the capillary into the tissue space occurs when the net filtration pressure (i.e., net driving force) is positive. Conversely, **absorption** of fluid from the tissue space into the vascular space occurs when the net filtration pressure is negative. At the arterial end of the capillary, the net filtration pressure is generally positive, so that filtration occurs. At the venous end, the net filtration pressure is generally negative, so that absorption occurs. However, as is discussed below, some organs do not adhere to this general rule.

In the next four sections, we examine each of the four Starling forces that constitute the net filtration pressure: P_c, P_{if}, π_c, and π_{if}.

⊙ 20-13 Capillary blood pressure (P_c) falls from ~35 mm Hg at the arteriolar end to ~15 mm Hg at the venular end

Capillary blood pressure is also loosely called the capillary *hydrostatic* pressure, to distinguish it from capillary *colloid osmotic* pressure.

When the arteriolar pressure is 60 mm Hg and the venular pressure is 15 mm Hg, the midcapillary pressure is not the mean value of 37.5 mm Hg but only 25 mm Hg. The explanation for the difference is that normally the precapillary upstream resistance exceeds the postcapillary downstream resistance (R_{post}/R_{pre} is typically 0.3; see ⊙ **19-6**). However, the midcapillary pressure is not a constant and uniform value. In the previous chapter, we saw that P_c varies with changes in R_{pre} and R_{post} (see Equation 19.2). P_c also varies with changes in four other parameters: (1) upstream and downstream pressure, (2) location, (3) time, and (4) gravity.

Arteriolar (P_a) and Venular (P_v) Pressure Because R_{post} is less than R_{pre}, P_c follows P_v more closely than P_a (see Equation 19.2). Thus, increasing P_a by 10 mm Hg—at a constant R_{post}/R_{pre} of 0.3—causes P_c to rise by only 2 mm Hg. On the other hand, increasing P_v by 10 mm Hg causes P_c to rise by 8 mm Hg.

Location Capillary pressure differs markedly among tissues. For example, the high P_c of glomerular capillaries in the kidney, ~50 mm Hg, is required for ultrafiltration. The retinal capillaries in the eye must also have a high P_c because they bathe in a vitreous humor that is under a pressure of ~20 mm Hg (see Fig. 15.5). A higher P_c is needed to keep the capillaries patent in the face of the external compressing force. The pulmonary capillaries have unusually *low* P_c values, 5 to 15 mm Hg, which minimizes the ultrafiltration that otherwise would lead to the accumulation of edema fluid in the alveolar air spaces (see ⊙ **31-4**).

Time Capillary blood pressure varies considerably from moment to moment at any given site, depending on the arteriolar diameter and tone of the precapillary sphincter (i.e., R_{pre}).

Gravity Finally, the effect of gravity on P_c is the same as that discussed for arterial and venous pressure. Thus, a capillary bed below the level of the heart has a higher P_c than a capillary bed at the level of the heart.

Interstitial fluid pressure (P_{if}) is slightly negative, except in encapsulated organs

The interstitium consists of both a solid and a liquid phase. The solid phase is made up of collagen fibers and proteoglycans. In the liquid phase, only a small fraction of interstitial water is totally "free" and capable of moving under the influence of convective forces.

Estimation of P_{if} is very difficult because the probe used to make the measurement is far larger than the interstitial space; thus, the measurement itself can alter P_{if}. If one inserts a probe percutaneously and immediately uses a null-point method to measure P_{if}, the values are +1 to +2 mm Hg. However, during the next 4 to 5 hours, the measured value drops to −1 to −2 mm Hg.

A value of −2 mm Hg is a reasonable average in *loose tissues,* such as the lung and subcutaneous tissue. P_{if} is slightly negative because of fluid removal by the lymphatics (see below). Inside *rigid enclosed compartments,* such as the bone marrow or brain, P_{if} is positive. It is also positive in *encapsulated organs* such as the kidney, where P_{if} is +1 to +3 mm Hg within the parenchyma. The same principle applies to skeletal muscle, which is surrounded by layers of fascia.

⊙ **20-14** P_{if} is also sensitive to the addition of fluid to the interstitial compartment. When small amounts of fluid are added to the interstitial compartment, the interstitium behaves like a low-compliance system, so that P_{if} rises steeply for the small amount of added fluid. Adding more fluid disrupts the solid phase of collagen fibers and the gel of proteoglycans, so that large volumes can now accumulate with only small additional pressure increases.

⊙ 20-15 Capillary colloid osmotic pressure (π_c), which reflects the presence of plasma proteins, is ~25 mm Hg

The colloid osmotic pressure difference across the capillary endothelium is due solely to the plasma proteins, such as albumin, globulins, and fibrinogen. Total plasma protein concentration is ~7.0 g/dL, which corresponds to ~1.5 mM of protein.

π_c does not vary appreciably along the length of the capillary. Indeed, most capillary beds filter <1% of the fluid entering at the arteriolar end. Thus, the loss of protein-free fluid does not measurably concentrate plasma proteins along the capillary and does not appreciably raise π_c.

Because clinical laboratories report plasma protein concentrations in grams per deciliter and not all proteins have the same molecular weight, a plasma protein concentration of 7 g/dL can produce different π_c values, depending on the protein *composition* of the plasma. Because albumin has a much lower molecular weight than γ-globulin, replacement of 1 g of the heavier γ-globulin with 1 g of the lighter albumin raises π_c.

Interstitial fluid colloid osmotic pressure (π_{if}) varies between 0 and 10 mm Hg among different organs

It is difficult to measure the interstitial fluid colloid osmotic pressure because it is virtually impossible to obtain uncontaminated samples. As a first approximation, we generally assume that π_{if} is the same as the colloid osmotic pressure of *lymph.* The protein content of lymph varies greatly from region to region; for example, it is 1 to 3 g/dL in the legs, 3 to 4 g/dL in the intestine, and 4 to 6 g/dL in the liver. Such lymph data predict that π_{if} ranges from 3 to 15 mm Hg. However, the protein concentration in the interstitial fluid is probably somewhat higher than in the lymph. A total-body average value for π_{if} is ~3 mm Hg, substantially less than the value of 25 mm Hg for π_c in the capillary lumen.

The π_{if} appears to increase along the axis of the capillary. The lowest values are near the arteriolar end, where the interstitium receives protein-free fluid from the capillary as the result of filtration. The highest values are near the venular end, where the interstitium loses protein-free fluid to the capillary as the result of absorption.

⊙ 20-16 The Starling principle predicts ultrafiltration at the arteriolar end and absorption at the venular end of most capillary beds

The idealized forces acting on fluid movement across a capillary are shown in Fig. 20.6A. Using the Starling equation and the values in Table 20.1, we can calculate the net transfer of fluid (J_V) at both the arteriolar and venular ends of a typical capillary:

$$J_v = L_p[(P_c - P_{if}) - (\sigma\pi_c - \sigma\pi_{if})]$$

$$\text{Arteriolar end: } J_v = L_p[(35 - (-2)) - (25 - 0.1)]$$

$$= L_p(+12\,\text{mm Hg}) \qquad \textbf{(20.7)}$$

$$\text{Venular end: } J_v = L_p[(15 - (-2)) - (25 - 3)]$$

$$= L_p(-5\,\text{mm Hg})$$

The net filtration pressure is thus positive (favoring filtration) at the arteriolar end, and it gradually makes the transition to negative (favoring absorption) at the venular end (see Fig. 20.6B). At the point where the filtration and reabsorptive forces balance each other, an equilibrium exists, and no net movement of water occurs across the capillary wall.

Net filtration pressure varies among tissues. For example, in the intestinal mucosa, P_c is so much lower than π_c that absorption occurs continually along the entire length of the capillary. On the other hand, in glomerular capillaries, P_c exceeds π_c throughout most of the network, so that filtration may occur along the entire capillary (see Equation 34.4). Hydraulic conductivity also can affect the filtration/absorption profile along the capillary. Because the interendothelial clefts become larger toward the venular end of the capillary, L_p increases along the capillary from the arteriolar to the venular end.

The *flow* of fluid across a group of capillaries *(F)* is the product of the *flux* (J_V) and the functional surface area (S_f):

TABLE 20.1 Typical Values of Transcapillary Driving Forces for Fluid Movement in Loose, Nonencapsulated Tissue

	CAPILLARY BLOOD PRESSURE (P_c)	INTERSTITIAL FLUID PRESSURE (P_{if})	EFFECTIVE CAPILLARY COLLOID OSMOTIC PRESSURE ($\sigma\Pi_c$)	EFFECTIVE INTERSTITIAL FLUID COLLOID OSMOTIC PRESSURE ($\sigma\Pi_{if}$)	NET FORCE
Arteriolar end	+35 mm Hg	−2 mm Hg	+25 mm Hg	+0.1 mm Hg	+12 mm Hg
Venular end	+15 mm Hg	−2 mm Hg	+25 mm Hg	+3 mm Hg	−5 mm Hg

$F = J_V \cdot S_f$. Thus, net filtration of fluid in an organ depends not only on the net filtration pressure and the hydraulic conductivity of the capillary wall (terms that contribute to J_V), but also on the surface area of capillaries that happen to be perfused.

LYMPHATICS

Lymphatics return excess interstitial fluid to the blood

Lymphatics arise in the interstitium as small, thin-walled channels of endothelial cells that then join together to form increasingly larger vessels (Fig. 20.7). The **initial lymphatics** are similar to capillaries but with many interendothelial junctions that behave like one-way microvalves, also called **primary lymph valves.** Anchoring filaments tether the initial lymphatics to surrounding connective tissue. The walls of the larger **collecting lymphatics** are similar to those of small veins, consisting of endothelium and sparse smooth muscle. The large lymphatic vessels, like the veins, have **secondary lymph valves** that restrict retrograde movement of lymph. Lymph nodes are located along the path of the collecting lymphatics. The large lymphatics ultimately drain into the left and right subclavian veins.

At the level of the initial lymphatics, interendothelial junctions have few tight junctions or adhesion molecules connecting neighboring endothelial cells. As a result, flaps of endothelial cells can overlap with each other and act as the microvalve discussed above. Although initial lymphatics may appear collapsed and show no contractile activity, a pressure gradient from the interstitial fluid to the lymphatic lumen deforms the endothelial cells so that the microvalves open and fluid enters the initial lymphatic during the expansion phase (Fig. 20.7A). During this time, the secondary lymph valves are closed.

External pressure (e.g., from skeletal muscle) shuts the microvalves and causes fluid to enter larger lymphatics through the now-open secondary lymph valves (Fig. 20.7B). Most organs contain both initial and collecting lymphatics, but skeletal muscle and intestine have only initial lymphatics within their tissue. True lymphatics are absent from the brain (see ◉ 11-1). They are most prevalent in the skin and the genitourinary, respiratory, and gastrointestinal tracts.

Filtration at the arteriolar end of capillaries is estimated to exceed absorption at the venular end by 2 to 4 L/day. However, fluid does not normally accumulate in the interstitium because this excess fluid and protein move into the lymphatics, maintaining a steady state.

Flow in Initial Lymphatics Hydrostatic pressure in the initial lymphatics (P_{lymph}) ranges from −1 mm Hg to +1 mm Hg. Inasmuch as the mean interstitial fluid pressure is somewhat more *negative* than these values, what provides the driving force for interstitial fluid to move into the terminal

A INDIVIDUAL HYDROSTATIC AND OSMOTIC PRESSURES

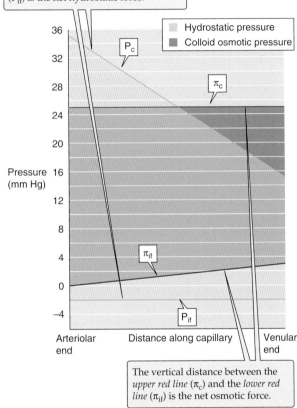

The vertical distance between the *upper yellow line* (P_c) and the *lower yellow line* (P_{if}) is the net hydrostatic force.

The vertical distance between the *upper red line* (π_c) and the *lower red line* (π_{if}) is the net osmotic force.

B NET FILTRATION PRESSURE

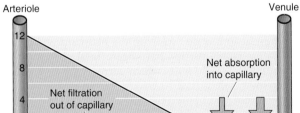

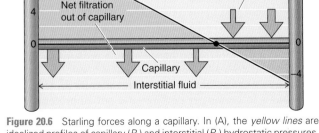

Figure 20.6 Starling forces along a capillary. In (A), the *yellow lines* are idealized profiles of capillary (P_c) and interstitial (P_{if}) hydrostatic pressures. The *red lines* are idealized capillary (π_c) and interstitial (π_{if}) colloid osmotic pressures. In (B), the net filtration pressure is ($P_c − P_{if}$) − $\sigma(\pi_c − \pi_{if})$.

A EXPANSION PHASE

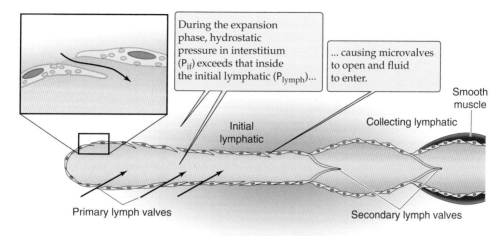

During the expansion phase, hydrostatic pressure in interstitium (P_{if}) exceeds that inside the initial lymphatic (P_{lymph})...

... causing microvalves to open and fluid to enter.

Smooth muscle

Collecting lymphatic

Initial lymphatic

Primary lymph valves

Secondary lymph valves

B COMPRESSION PHASE

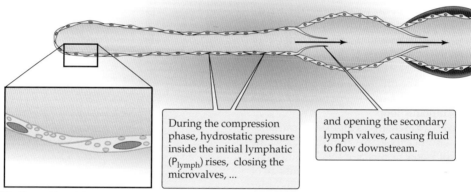

During the compression phase, hydrostatic pressure inside the initial lymphatic (P_{lymph}) rises, closing the microvalves, ...

and opening the secondary lymph valves, causing fluid to flow downstream.

Figure 20.7 Flow of lymph into initial and collecting lymphatics during the expansion phase (A) and the compression phase (B).

lymphatics? The answer is that transient increases in P_{if} temporarily raise P_{if} above P_{lymph}.

Because the interstitium exhibits a variable compliance (see ⊚ 20-14), fluid added to the interstitium in its low-compliance range raises the P_{if} substantially, providing the driving force for fluid to enter the lymphatics. In this same range of P_{if} values, lymphatic flow is especially sensitive to increases in P_{if}. Thus, lymphatic efflux nicely matches the excess capillary filtration, so that the interstitial fluid volume changes very little. The situation is very different if the interstitium is already expanded and in its high-compliance range. In this case, fluid added to the interstitium raises the already elevated P_{if} only moderately (e.g., from +2 to +4 mm Hg). In this range of P_{if} values, lymphatic uptake is not very responsive to increases in P_{if}. In this case, lymphatic return does not compensate well for the excess capillary filtration, so that interstitial fluid volume increases further (i.e., edema begets more edema).

Intermittent compression and relaxation of lymphatics occur during respiration, walking, and intestinal peristalsis. When P_{lymph} in a downstream segment falls below that in an upstream segment, fluid aspiration produces unidirectional flow. This suction may be largely responsible for the subatmospheric values of the P_{if} observed in many tissues.

Flow in Collecting Lymphatics Pressures in the collecting lymphatics range from +1 to +10 mm Hg, and they increase progressively with each valve along the vessel. As P_{lymph} rises in the collecting lymphatic vessels, smooth muscle in the lymphatic walls actively contracts by an intrinsic **myogenic** mechanism that also plays a role in blood vessels. Thus, downstream occlusion of a lymphatic vessel increases P_{lymph} and the frequency of smooth-muscle contractions, whereas an upstream occlusion does the opposite. Because of the presence of one-way valves, smooth-muscle contraction drives lymph toward the veins. The rhythmic contraction and relaxation of VSMCs—**vasomotion**—in lymphatics is essential for the propulsion of lymph.

In addition to vasomotion, passive processes also propel lymph toward the blood. As is the case for the initial lymphatics, skeletal muscle contraction, respiratory movements, and intestinal contractions all passively compress the collecting lymphatics. This intermittent pumping action moves lymph into the veins.

Transport of Proteins and Cells Proteins that entered interstitial fluid from the capillary cannot return to the circulation because of the adverse chemical gradient across the capillary endothelial wall. The buildup of these macromolecules in the interstitium creates a diffusional gradient from the interstitium to the lymph that complements the convective movement of these macromolecules (along with fluid) into the lymphatic system. In an average person, the lymphatics return 100 to 200 g of proteins to the circulation each day. Even before lymph reaches lymph nodes, it contains leukocytes—which had moved from the blood into the interstitium—but no RBCs or platelets. Cycles of lymphatic compression and relaxation not only enhance fluid movement but also greatly increase the leukocyte count of lymph.

The circulation of extracellular fluids involves three convective loops: blood, interstitial fluid, and lymph

Extracellular fluid moves in *three convective loops* (Fig. 20.8). The first is the **cardiovascular loop.** Assuming a cardiac output of 5 L/min, the convective flow of blood through the circulation at rest is 7200 L/day. The second is the **transvascular loop,** in which fluid moves out of the capillaries at their arteriolar end and into the capillaries at their venular end. Not counting the kidney, whose glomeruli filter a vast amount of fluid (see ⊙ 34-2), all the other tissues of the body filter ~20 L/day at the arteriolar end of their capillaries and reabsorb 16 to 18 L at the venular end. The difference between filtration and absorption, 2 to 4 L/day, is a reasonable estimate of the third fluid loop, the **lymphatic loop.**

In addition to convective exchange, a *diffusional exchange* of water and solutes also occurs across the capillaries. The diffusional exchange of **water** occurs at a much higher rate than does convective movement: ~80,000 L/day across all of the body's systemic capillaries. This value is about an order of magnitude greater than blood flow in the cardiovascular loop and three orders of magnitude larger than the convective flow in the transvascular filtration/absorption loop of the microcirculation. However, the diffusion of water molecules is an *exchange* process that does not contribute appreciably to the *net* movement of water. In other words, every day, 80,000 L of water diffuses out of the capillaries and 80,000 L diffuses back.

REGULATION OF THE MICROCIRCULATION

The active contraction of vascular smooth muscle regulates precapillary resistance, which controls capillary blood flow

Smooth-muscle tone in arterioles, metarterioles, and precapillary sphincters determines the access resistance to the capillary beds. This resistance upstream of the capillary bed is also known as the afferent or **precapillary resistance** (R_{pre}). The overall resistance of a microcirculatory bed is the sum of R_{pre}, the resistance of the capillary bed itself (R_{cap}), and the efferent or **postcapillary resistance** (R_{post}).

How do these resistances influence the flow of blood (F_{cap}) through a capillary bed? We can answer this question

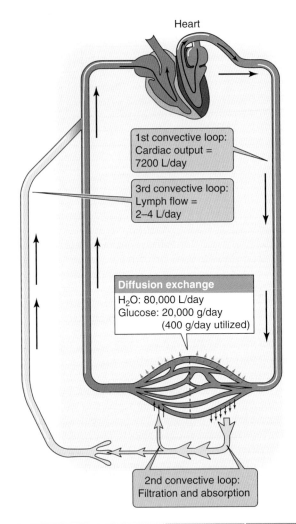

1st convective loop:
Cardiac output = 7200 L/day

3rd convective loop:
Lymph flow = 2–4 L/day

Diffusion exchange
H_2O: 80,000 L/day
Glucose: 20,000 g/day
(400 g/day utilized)

2nd convective loop:
Filtration and absorption

	Lymph flow (3rd loop)	Entry into capillary (2nd loop)	Exit from capillary (2nd loop)
FLUID	2–4 L/day	16–18 L/day	20 L/day
PROTEIN	95–195 g/day	5 g/day	100–200 g/day
GLUCOSE			20 g/day

Figure 20.8 Convective loops of extracellular fluid and protein.

by rearranging the Ohm's law–like expression that we introduced as Equation 17.1:

$$F_{cap} = \frac{\Delta P}{R_{total}} = \frac{P_a - P_v}{R_{pre} + R_{cap} + R_{post}} \tag{20.8}$$

P_a is the pressure just before the beginning of the precapillary resistance, and P_v is the pressure just after the end of the postcapillary resistance. Because the aggregate R_{cap} is small, and R_{post}/R_{pre} is usually ~0.3, R_{pre} is usually much greater than $R_{cap} + R_{post}$. Because R_{pre} is the principal determinant of total resistance, capillary flow is roughly inversely proportional to R_{pre}. Thus, modulating the contractility of VSMCs in *precapillary* vessels is the main mechanism for adjusting perfusion of a particular tissue.

Smooth-muscle cells can function as a syncytium when they are coupled through gap junctions (unitary smooth muscle), or they can function independently of one another as do skeletal muscle fibers (multiunit smooth muscle; see ⊙ 9-12). Most vascular smooth muscle has a multiunit organization. In contrast to skeletal muscle, VSMCs receive multiple excitatory as well as inhibitory inputs. Moreover, these inputs come not only from chemical synapses (i.e., neural control) but also from circulating chemicals (i.e., humoral control). The actual contraction of VSMCs may follow smooth-muscle electrical activity in the form of action potentials, slow waves of depolarization, or graded depolarizations without spikes. VSMCs can show spontaneous rhythmic variations in tension leading to periodic changes in vascular resistance and microcirculatory flow in a process called **vasomotion.** These spontaneous, rhythmic smooth-muscle contractions result either from pacemaker currents or from slow waves of depolarization and associated $[Ca^{2+}]_i$ increases in the VSMCs (see ⊙ 9-13). Humoral agents can also directly trigger contraction of VSMCs via increases in $[Ca^{2+}]_i$ without measurable fluctuations in membrane potential.

VSMCs rely on a different molecular mechanism of contraction than skeletal muscle does, although an increase in $[Ca^{2+}]_i$ is the principal trigger of contraction in both cases (see Fig. 9.14).

Contraction of Vascular Smooth Muscle The following changes promote contraction:

- ↑$[Ca^{2+}]_i$ → ↑Ca^{2+}-CaM → ↑MLCK activity → ↑phosphorylation of MLC → VSMC contraction.
- ↓$[cAMP]_i$ → ↓PKA → ↓phosphorylation of MLCK → ↑MLCK activity → ↑phosphorylation of MLC → VSMC contraction.
- ↓$[cGMP]_i$ → ↓PKG → ↓phosphorylation of MLCK → ↑MLCK activity → ↑phosphorylation of MLC → VSMC contraction.

Relaxation of Vascular Smooth Muscle The following changes promote relaxation:

- ↓$[Ca^{2+}]_i$ → ↓Ca^{2+}-CaM → ↓MLCK activity → ↓phosphorylation of MLC → VSMC relaxation.
- ↑$[cAMP]_i$ → ↑PKA → ↑phosphorylation of MLCK → ↓MLCK activity → ↓phosphorylation of MLC → VSMC relaxation.
- ↑$[cGMP]_i$ → ↑PKG → ↑phosphorylation of MLCK → ↓MLCK activity → ↓phosphorylation of MLC → VSMC relaxation.

⊙ 20-17 Tissue metabolites regulate local blood flow in specific vascular beds, independently of the systemic regulation

VSMCs not only control the resistance of arterioles (i.e., R_{pre}) and thus local blood flow, they also control the resistance of small terminal arteries and thereby play an important role in regulating systemic arterial blood pressure. The subject of the present discussion is *local regulatory mechanisms* that use the arterioles to regulate blood flow through specific vascular beds. These local control mechanisms can override any of the neural or systemic humoral influences.

⊙ **20-18** Mechanisms of local control involve (1) myogenic activity and (2) local chemical and humoral factors.

Myogenic regulation refers to an *intrinsic* mode of control of activity in which stretch of the VSMC membrane activates stretch-sensitive nonselective cation channels. The result is a depolarization that affects pacemaker activity, thereby eliciting contraction of the VSMC.

The most prominent **chemical factors** are interstitial P_{O_2}, P_{CO_2}, and pH as well as local concentrations of K^+, lactic acid, ATP, ADP, and adenosine. Total osmolality may also make a contribution. The local regulation of VSMCs by *interstitial* P_{O_2}, P_{CO_2}, and pH is distinct from the regulation of systemic blood pressure by the peripheral chemoreceptors, which respond to changes in *arterial* P_{O_2}, P_{CO_2}, and pH (see ⊙ 32-3) and initiate a complex neural reflex that modulates VSMC activity (see ⊙ 23-15). In the case of *local* control, chemical changes in interstitial fluid act *directly* on the VSMCs through one of the three principal second-messenger systems (i.e., intracellular Ca^{2+}, cAMP, cGMP). Changes that typically accompany increased metabolism (e.g., low P_{O_2}, high P_{CO_2}, and low pH) vasodilate vessels in the systemic circulation. Such local changes in P_{O_2}, P_{CO_2}, and pH have opposite effects in the pulmonary circulation (see ⊙ 31-6).

The endothelium of capillary beds is the source of several vasoactive compounds, including nitric oxide, endothelium-derived hyperpolarizing factor, and endothelin

Table 20.2 lists several endothelial factors that act on blood vessels.

Nitric Oxide ⊙ **20-19** Originally called endothelium-derived relaxing factor (EDRF), nitric oxide (NO) is a potent vasodilator. NO also inhibits platelet aggregation, induces platelet disaggregation, and inhibits platelet adhesion. Bradykinin and acetylcholine both stimulate the NO synthase III (NOS III, or eNOS) isoform of NOS (see ⊙ 3-23) that is constitutively present in endothelial cells. Increases in shear stress—the force acting on the endothelial cell along the axis of blood flow—can also stimulate the enzyme. NOS III, which depends on both Ca^{2+} and CaM for its activity, catalyzes the formation of NO from arginine. NO, a lipophilic gas with a short half-life, exits the endothelial cells, diffuses locally, and enters VSMCs. Inside the VSMC is the "receptor" for NO, a soluble guanylyl cyclase that converts GTP to cyclic GMP (cGMP). cGMP-dependent protein kinase (i.e., PKG) then phosphorylates MLCK (see ⊙ 9-14), SERCA Ca pumps (see ⊙ 5-11), and BK_{Ca} K^+ channels. Phosphorylation *inhibits* the MLCK, thus leading to a net decrease in the phosphorylation of MLC and a decrease in the interaction between myosin and actin. Phosphorylation *activates* SERCA, thereby decreasing $[Ca^{2+}]_i$. Finally, phosphorylation *activates* BK_{Ca}, causing hyperpolarization. By these three complementary effects, the NO released by endothelial cells relaxes VSMCs, producing vasodilation.

The NO-mediated cascade is one of the most important mechanisms for vasodilation in the circulatory system. Physicians have used exogenous organic nitrates (e.g., nitroglycerin) for decades to dilate peripheral vessels for relief of the pain of angina pectoris. These powerful vasodilators exert their activity by breaking down chemically, thereby releasing NO near VSMCs.

TABLE 20.2 Vasoactive Agents Produced by Endothelial Cells

VASODILATORS	VASOCONSTRICTORS
Nitric oxide (NO)	Endothelin (ET)
Endothelium-derived hyperpolarizing factor (EDHF)	Endothelium-derived constricting factor 1 (EDCF$_1$)
Prostacyclin (PGI$_2$)	Endothelium-derived constricting factor 2 (EDCF$_2$)

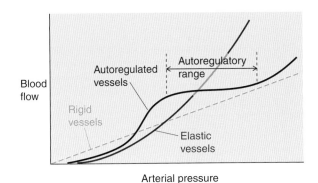

Figure 20.9   Autoregulation of blood flow.

Prostacyclin (Prostaglandin I$_2$)   Prostacyclin synthase (see Fig. 3.9) metabolizes arachidonic acid to the vasodilator prostacyclin (prostaglandin I$_2$, or PGI$_2$). This agent acts by increasing [cAMP]$_i$ and promoting the phosphorylation of MLCK, which ultimately decreases the phosphorylation of MLCs. PGI$_2$ is especially important for dilation of pulmonary vessels at birth (see ⊙ 57-2).

Endothelins ⊙ 20-20   Endothelial cells produce endothelin (ET), which causes an extremely potent and long-lasting **vasoconstriction** in most VSMCs. Endothelin exists as three isopeptides: ET-1, ET-2, and ET-3. The precursor of **ET-1** is *preproendothelin,* which the endothelial cell converts first to *proendothelin* and then to the mature *endothelin,* which it releases. The ET receptor subtype for vasoconstriction is ET$_A$. Other ET receptors also exist. ET$_{B1}$ mediates vasodilation, ET$_{B2}$ mediates vasoconstriction, and ET$_C$ has as yet no clearly defined function. ET$_A$ receptors predominate in high-pressure parts of the circulation, whereas ET$_B$ receptors predominate in low-pressure parts of the circulation.

The binding of an ET to any ET receptor subtype ultimately results in an increase in [Ca^{2+}]$_i$. In the *vasoconstriction* response, ET-1 binding to ET$_A$ receptors acts through the phospholipase C pathway to generate inositol trisphosphate, to release Ca^{2+} from intracellular stores, and to raise [Ca^{2+}]$_i$ (see ⊙ 3-14). In a second, delayed phase, which is not well understood, Ca^{2+} entering from the outside contributes to the increase in [Ca^{2+}]$_i$. The increased [Ca^{2+}]$_i$ activates Ca^{2+}-CaM, stimulating MLCK to phosphorylate MLCs and culminating in contraction.

Thromboxane A$_2$ Endothelial cells and platelets metabolize arachidonic acid via the cyclooxygenase pathway to produce thromboxane A$_2$ (TXA$_2$; see ⊙ 3-19). This agent activates TXA$_2$/prostaglandin H$_2$ (TP) receptors, which leads to opening of L-type Ca channels and a consequent increase in [Ca^{2+}]$_i$. In addition, TP activation increases the levels of superoxide anion radical O$_2^-$ (see Fig. 62.1A) in VSMCs. In turn, O$_2^-$ reacts with NO, thereby reducing the vasodilating effect of NO.

⊙ 20-21 Autoregulation stabilizes blood flow despite large fluctuations in systemic arterial pressure

As we saw in Chapter 17, the pressure-flow relationship of an idealized rigid vessel is linear (Fig. 20.9, *gray line*). In most real (i.e., elastic) vessels, however, increases in pressure cause a dilation that reduces resistance and leads to a steeper-than-linear flow (Fig. 20.9, *red curve*). However, some vascular beds behave very differently. Despite large changes in the

systemic arterial pressure—and thus large changes in the driving pressure—these special vascular beds maintain local blood flow within a narrow range. This phenomenon is called **autoregulation.** These vascular beds behave more or less like rigid tubes at very low and at very high perfusion pressures (Fig. 20.9, *purple curve*). However, in the physiological pressure range over which autoregulation occurs, changes in perfusion pressure have little effect on flow. Instead, increases in *pressure* lead to increases in *resistance* that keep blood flow within a carefully controlled range.

⊙ 20-22   Autoregulatory behavior takes time to develop and is due to an active process. If the perfusion pressure were to increase abruptly, we would see that immediately after the pressure increase, the pressure-flow diagram would look much like the one for the rigid tube in Fig. 20.9. However, the vascular arteriolar tone then slowly adjusts itself to produce the characteristic autoregulatory pressure-flow diagram. The contraction of VSMCs that underlies autoregulation is *autonomous;* that is, it is entirely local and independent of neural and endocrine mechanisms. Both myogenic and metabolic mechanisms play an important role in the adjustments of smooth-muscle tone during autoregulation. For example, the stretch of VSMCs that accompanies the increased perfusion pressure triggers a **myogenic contraction** that reduces blood flow. Also, the increase in P$_{O2}$ (or decrease in P$_{CO2}$, or increase in pH) that accompanies increased perfusion pressure triggers a metabolic vasoconstriction that reduces blood flow.

Autoregulation is useful for at least two reasons. First, with an increase in perfusion pressure, autoregulation avoids a waste of perfusion in organs in which the flow is already sufficient. Second, with a decrease in perfusion pressure, autoregulation maintains capillary flow and capillary pressure. Autoregulation is very important under these conditions for organs that are very sensitive to ischemia or hypoxia (particularly the heart, brain, and kidneys) and for organs whose job it is to filter the blood (again, the kidney).

⊙ 20-23 Blood vessels proliferate in response to growth factors by a process known as angiogenesis

In adults, the anatomy of the microcirculation remains rather constant. Increased capillary density is important in physical training (see ⊙ 60-6) and in acclimatization to altitude (see ⊙ 61-2).

TABLE 20.3 Agents That Affect Vascular Growth

PROMOTERS	INHIBITORS
Vascular endothelial growth factor (VEGF)	Endostatin
Fibroblast growth factors (FGFs)	Angiostatin
Angiopoietin 1 (ANGPT1)	Angiopoietin 2 (ANGPT2)

The development of new vessels is called **angiogenesis.** The first step is dissolution of the venular basement membrane at a specific site, followed by activation and proliferation of previously quiescent endothelial cells. The new cells, attracted by growth factors, migrate to form a tube. Eventually, the budding tubes connect with each other, allowing the flow of blood and the development of vascular smooth muscle as the new microvascular network establishes itself. Angiogenesis relies on a balance between positive and negative regulation. The body normally produces some factors that promote angiogenesis and others that inhibit it (Table 20.3).

CHAPTER 21

CARDIAC ELECTROPHYSIOLOGY AND THE ELECTROCARDIOGRAM

W. Jonathan Lederer

The heart's electrical signal originates in a group of cells high in the right atrium that depolarize spontaneously; it then spreads throughout the heart from cell to cell (Fig. 21.1). As this action potential propagates through the heart—carried by cells that form specialized conducting pathways and by the very cells that generate the force of contraction—it assumes different appearances (Fig. 21.2). Based on the speed of the upstroke, we can characterize action potentials as either **slow** (sinoatrial and atrioventricular nodes) or **fast** (atrial myocytes, Purkinje fibers, and ventricular myocytes).

Because the excitation of cardiac myocytes triggers contraction—a process called *excitation-contraction coupling* (see ◉ 9-2) —the propagation of action potentials must be carefully timed to synchronize ventricular contraction and optimize the ejection of blood.

ELECTROPHYSIOLOGY OF CARDIAC CELLS

◉ 21-1 The cardiac action potential starts in specialized muscle cells of the sinoatrial node and then propagates in an orderly fashion throughout the heart

The cardiac action potential originates in a group of cells called the **sinoatrial (SA) node** (Fig. 21.1), located in the right atrium. These cells depolarize spontaneously and fire action potentials at a regular, intrinsic rate that is usually between 60 and 100 times per minute for an individual at rest. Both parasympathetic and sympathetic neural input can modulate this intrinsic **pacemaker** activity, or *automaticity* (see ◉ 16-3).

Because cardiac cells are electrically coupled through gap junctions (Fig. 21.3), the action potential propagates from cell to cell. A spontaneous action potential originating in the SA node will conduct from cell to cell throughout the right atrial muscle and spread to the left atrium. About one tenth of a second after its origination, the signal arrives at the **atrioventricular (AV) node** (Fig. 21.1). The impulse cannot spread directly from the atria to the ventricles because of the presence of a fibrous **atrioventricular ring.** Instead, it must travel from the AV node to the **His-Purkinje fiber system,** a network of specialized conducting cells that carries the signal to the muscle of both ventricles.

The cardiac action potential conducts from cell to cell via gap junctions

◉ 21-2 The electrical influence of one cardiac cell on another depends on the voltage difference between the cells and on the resistance of the gap junction connecting them. A **gap junction** (see ◉ 8-1) is an **electrical synapse** (Fig. 21.3) that permits electrical current to flow between neighboring cells in a manner proportional to the voltage difference between the two cells but inversely proportional to the electrical resistance between them.

When the cells are tightly coupled, the gap junctions are minimal barriers to the flow of depolarizing current.

Imagine that several interconnected cells are initially all at their normal resting potentials. An action potential propagating from the left of cell A now injects depolarizing current into cell A. As a result, the cell depolarizes to V_A, which is now somewhat positive compared with V_B. Thus, a small depolarizing current (i.e., positive charges) will move from cell A to cell B and depolarize cell B. In turn, current flowing from cell B will then depolarize cell C. By this process, the cells closest to the current source undergo the greatest depolarization.

In principle, we could make the action potential propagate more rapidly down the chain of cells in two ways. First, we could allow more ion channels to open in the active region of the heart, so that depolarizing current is larger. Second, we could lower the threshold for the regenerative action potential ("more negative threshold"), so that even a smaller current is sufficient to trigger an action potential in cell B.

The intracellular and extracellular currents in heart muscle (Fig. 21.3) must be equal and opposite. Cells that have reached threshold and elicited action potentials provide the *source* of current that depolarizes cells that are approaching threshold. As cell A depolarizes to and beyond threshold, its Na^+ and Ca^{2+} channels open, enabling these cations to enter. The positive charge that enters cell A not only depolarizes cell A but also produces a flow of positive charge to cell B (i.e., **intracellular current**) that depolarizes cell B, releasing extracellular positive charges that were associated with the membrane. These extracellular positive charges constitute the **extracellular current.** The flow of intracellular current from cell A to cell B and the flow of extracellular current from around cell B to around cell A are equal and opposite. The flow of this *extracellular* current in the heart generates an instantaneous electrical vector, which changes with time. Each point on an **electrocardiogram (ECG)** is the sum of the many such electrical vectors, generated by the many cells of the heart.

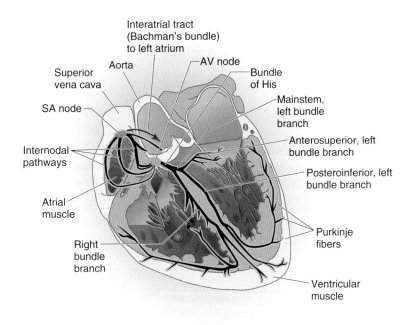

Figure 21.1 Conduction pathways through the heart. A section through the long axis of the heart is shown.

Cardiac action potentials have as many as five distinctive phases

The initiation time, shape, and duration of the action potential are distinctive for different parts of the heart, reflecting their different functions (Fig. 21.2). These distinctions arise because the myocytes in each region of the heart have a characteristic set of channels and anatomy. Underlying cardiac action potentials are four major time-dependent and voltage-gated membrane currents:

1. The **Na⁺ current** (I_{Na}) is responsible for the rapid **depolarizing** phase of the action potential in atrial and ventricular muscle and in Purkinje fibers.
2. The **Ca²⁺ current** (I_{Ca}) is responsible for the rapid **depolarizing** phase of the action potential in the SA node and AV node; it also triggers contraction in all cardiomyocytes.
3. The **K⁺ current** (I_K) is responsible for the **repolarizing** phase of the action potential in all cardiomyocytes.
4. The **pacemaker current** (I_f) is responsible, in part, for pacemaker activity in SA nodal cells, AV nodal cells, and Purkinje fibers.

Besides these four currents, channels carry numerous other currents in heart muscle. In addition, two *electrogenic* transporters carry current across plasma membranes: the type 1 Na-Ca exchanger (NCX1; see Fig. 5.8A) and the Na-K pump (see ◉ 5-6).

Traditionally, the changes in **membrane potential (V_m)** during the cardiac action potential are divided into separate phases, as illustrated in Fig. 21.4A for cardiac action potentials from the SA node and in Fig. 21.4B for those from ventricular muscle.

Phase 0 is the upstroke of the action potential. If the upstroke is due only to I_{Ca} (Fig. 21.4A), it will be slow. If the upstroke is due to both I_{Ca} and I_{Na} (Fig. 21.4B), it will be fast.

Phase 1 is the rapid repolarization component of the action potential (when it exists). This phase is due to almost total inactivation of I_{Na} or I_{Ca} and may also depend on the activation of a minor K⁺ current, called I_{to} (for *transient* outward current).

Phase 2 is the plateau phase of the action potential, which is prominent in ventricular muscle. It depends on the continued entry of Ca²⁺ or Na⁺ ions through their major channels and on a minor membrane current due to the Na-Ca exchanger NCX1.

Phase 3 is the repolarization component of the action potential. It depends on I_K.

Phase 4 constitutes the electrical diastolic phase of the action potential. V_m during phase 4 is termed the **diastolic potential;** the most *negative* V_m during phase 4 is the **maximum diastolic potential.** In SA and AV nodal cells, changes in I_K, I_{Ca}, and I_f produce pacemaker activity during phase 4. Purkinje fibers also exhibit pacemaker activity but use only I_f. Atrial and ventricular muscle have no time-dependent currents during phase 4.

The Na⁺ current is the largest current in the heart

The Na⁺ current is the largest current in heart muscle. Na⁺ channels are present only in ventricular and atrial muscle, in Purkinje fibers, and in specialized conduction pathways of the atria.

The channel that underlies I_{Na} is a classic voltage-gated Na⁺ channel, with both α and β₁ subunits (see Fig. 7.9A). The unique cardiac α subunit (Nav1.5) has several phosphorylation sites that make it sensitive to stimulation by cAMP-dependent protein kinase (see ◉ 3-9).

At the negative resting potentials of the ventricular muscle cells, the Na⁺ channels are closed. However, these channels rapidly activate (in 0.1 to 0.2 ms) in response to local

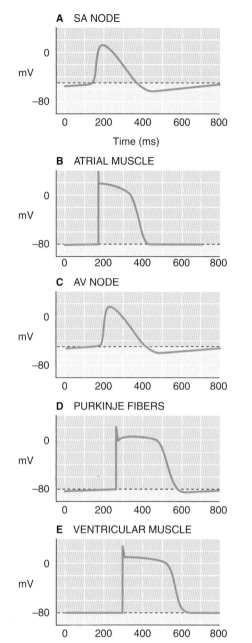

Figure 21.2 Cardiac action potentials. The distinctive shapes of action potentials at five sites along the spread of excitation are shown.

depolarization induced by action potentials and produce a massive inward current that underlies most of the rapid upstroke of the cardiac action potential (phase 0 in Fig. 21.4B). If V_m remains at a positive level, these channels close in a time-dependent process known as **inactivation.** This process is partly responsible for the rapid repolarization of the action potential (phase 1).

The depolarization produced by the Na^+ current not only activates I_{Na} in neighboring cells but also activates other membrane currents in the same cell, including I_{Ca} and I_K. For example, in cardiac myocytes the depolarization—initiated by Nav1.5—activates the L-type cardiac Ca^{2+} channel (Cav1.2; see next section), which greatly prolongs the depolarizing phase of the cardiac action potential. Local anesthetic **antiarrhythmic drugs,** such as lidocaine, work by partially blocking I_{Na}.

The Ca^{2+} current in the heart passes primarily through L-type Ca^{2+} channels

The Ca^{2+} current (I_{Ca}) is present in all cardiac myocytes. The L-type Ca^{2+} channel (Cav1.2; see ◉ 7-5) is the dominant one in the heart. T-type Ca^{2+} channels, with different biophysical and pharmacological properties, are also present but in smaller amounts.

In the SA node, the role of I_{Ca} is to contribute to pacemaker activity. In both the SA and AV nodes, I_{Ca} is the inward current source that is responsible for the upstrokes (phase 0) of the SA and AV nodal action potentials. Because the nodal cells lack the larger I_{Na}, their upstrokes are slower than those in atrial and ventricular muscle (compare A and B of Fig. 21.4). Therefore, the smaller I_{Ca} discharges the membrane capacitance of neighboring cells in the SA and AV nodes less rapidly, so that the speed of the conducted action potential is much slower than that of any other cardiac tissue. This feature in the AV node leads to an **electrical delay** between atrial contraction and ventricular contraction that permits more time for the atria to empty blood into the ventricles.

A small I_{Ca} remains during phase 2 of the action potential, helping to prolong the plateau. In atrial and ventricular muscle cells, the Ca^{2+} entering via L-type Ca^{2+} channels activates the release of Ca^{2+} from the sarcoplasmic reticulum (SR) by **calcium-induced Ca^{2+} release** (see ◉ 9-11). **Blockers of L-type Ca^{2+} channels**—therapeutic agents such as verapamil, diltiazem, and nifedipine (see ◉ 7-5)—act by inhibiting I_{Ca}.

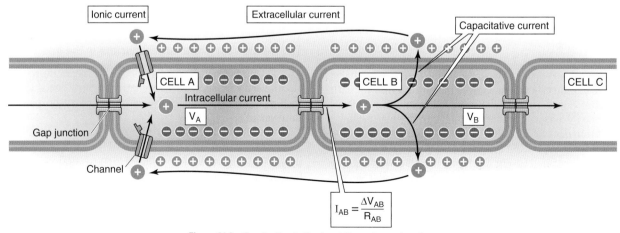

Figure 21.3 Conduction in the heart through gap junctions.

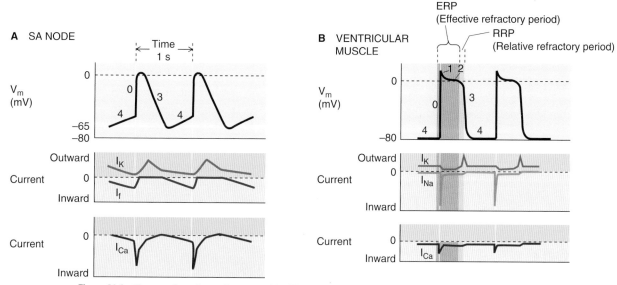

Figure 21.4 Phases of cardiac action potentials. The records in this figure are idealized. I_K, I_{Na}, I_{Ca}, and I_f are currents through K^+, Na^+, Ca^{2+}, and nonselective cation channels, respectively.

The repolarizing K⁺ current turns on slowly

Cardiac action potentials last two orders of magnitude longer than action potentials in skeletal muscle because the repolarizing K⁺ current turns on very slowly and—in the case of atrial myocytes, Purkinje fibers, and ventricular myocytes—with a considerable delay. The **repolarizing K⁺ current** (I_K) is found in all cardiac myocytes and is responsible for repolarizing the membrane at the end of the action potential (phase 3 in Fig. 21.4A and B). With depolarization, it slowly activates (20 to 100 ms) but does not inactivate. In SA and AV nodal cells, it contributes to pacemaker activity by slowly deactivating at the diastolic voltage.

Early Outward K⁺ Current (A-type Current) Atrial and ventricular muscle cells have some early *transient outward current* (I_{to}). This current is activated by depolarization but rapidly inactivates. It contributes to phase 1 repolarization.

G Protein–Activated K⁺ Current Acetylcholine activates muscarinic receptors and, activates an outward K⁺ current (see ⊙ 7-9). This current is prominent in SA and AV nodal cells, where it decreases pacemaker rate by cell hyperpolarization. When activated, this current also slows the conduction of the action potential through the AV node.

K_ATP Current ATP-sensitive K⁺ channels (K_ATP; see ⊙ 7-10), activated by low intracellular [ATP], are present in abundance and may play a role in electrical regulation of contractile behavior.

The I_f current is mediated by a nonselective cation channel

The pacemaker current (I_f) is found in SA and AV nodal cells and in Purkinje fibers (Fig. 21.4A, *blue curve*). The channel underlying this current is a nonspecific cation channel called **HCN** (for *h*yperpolarization activated, *c*yclic *n*ucleotide gated). Because the HCN channels conduct both K⁺ and Na⁺, the reversal potential of I_f is around −20 mV, between the Nernst potentials for K⁺ (about −90 mV) and Na⁺ (about

+50 mV). The HCN channels have the unusual property (hence the subscript *f*, for "funny" current) that they do not conduct at positive potentials but are activated by *hyperpolarization* at the end of phase 3. The activation is slow (100 ms), and the current does not inactivate. Thus, I_f produces an inward, *depolarizing* current as it slowly activates at the end of phase 3. In addition to the I_f current I_{Ca} and I_K also contribute significantly to the phase 4 depolarization and pacemaker activity of SA and AV nodal cells.

Different cardiac tissues uniquely combine ionic currents to produce distinctive action potentials

The shape of the action potential differs among different cardiac cells (Fig. 21.2) because of the unique combination of various currents—both the voltage-gated/time-dependent currents discussed in the preceding four sections and the "background" currents—present in each cell type.

Not only does each current *independently* affect the shape of the action potential, but the voltage- and time-dependent currents interact with one another because they affect—and are affected by—V_m.

⊙ 21-3 The SA node is the primary pacemaker of the heart

The Concept of Pacemaker Activity The normal heart has three intrinsic pacemaking tissues: the SA node, the AV node, and the Purkinje fibers. The term **pacemaker activity** refers to the spontaneous time-dependent depolarization of the cell membrane that leads to an action potential in an otherwise quiescent cell. The pacemaker with the highest frequency will be the one to trigger an action potential that will propagate throughout the heart. Inward or depolarizing membrane currents interact with outward or hyperpolarizing membrane currents to establish regular cycles of spontaneous depolarization and repolarization.

TABLE 21.1 Electrical Properties of Different Cardiac Tissues

TISSUE NAME	FUNCTION	PRINCIPAL TIME-DEPENDENT AND VOLTAGE-DEPENDENT CURRENTS	β-ADRENERGIC EFFECT (e.g., EPINEPHRINE)	CHOLINERGIC EFFECT (e.g., ACH)
SA node	Primary pacemaker	I_{Ca}, I_K, I_f	↑ Conduction velocity ↑ Pacemaker rate	↓ Pacemaker rate ↓ Conduction velocity
Atrial muscle	Expel blood from atria	I_{Na}, I_{Ca}, I_K	↑ Strength of contraction	Little effect
AV node	Secondary pacemaker	I_{Ca}, I_K, I_f	↑ Conduction velocity ↑ Pacemaker rate	↓ Pacemaker rate ↓ Conduction velocity
Purkinje fibers	Rapid conduction of action potential Tertiary pacemaker	I_{Na}, I_{Ca}, I_K, I_f	↑ Pacemaker rate	↓ Pacemaker rate
Ventricular muscle	Expel blood from ventricles	I_{Na}, I_{Ca}, I_K	↑ Contractility	Little effect

SA Node ⊙ 21-4 The SA node is found in the right atrium and is the primary site of origin of the electrical signal in the mammalian heart (Table 21.1). It is the smallest electrical region of the heart and constitutes the *fastest normal pacemaker,* with an intrinsic rate of about 60 beats/min, or faster in an individual at rest. The interactions among three time-dependent and voltage-gated membrane currents (I_{Ca}, I_K, and I_f) control the intrinsic rhythmicity of the SA node. The sum of a *decreasing outward* current (I_K; green curve in Fig. 21.4A) and two *increasing inward* currents (I_{Ca} and I_f; red and blue curves in Fig. 21.4A) produces the slow pacemaker depolarization (phase 4) associated with the SA node. The maximum diastolic potential (i.e., the most negative V_m) of the SA nodal cells, which occurs during phase 4 of the action potential, is between −60 and −70 mV. As V_m rises toward the threshold of about −55 mV, I_{Ca} becomes increasingly activated and eventually becomes regenerative, producing the upstroke of the action potential. This depolarization rapidly turns off (i.e., deactivates) I_f, and the whole process begins again.

AV Node The AV node, located just above the AV ring, is the secondary site of origin of the electrical signal in the mammalian heart. Normally, the AV node may be excited by an impulse reaching it by way of the specialized atrial conduction pathways (see below). Like that of the SA node, the intrinsic rhythmicity of the AV node depends on the interaction of three time-dependent and voltage-gated currents: I_K, I_{Ca}, and I_f. Electrically, the SA and AV nodes have similar action potentials, pacemaker mechanisms, and drug sensitivities and a similarly slow conduction of action potentials. Because the intrinsic pacemaker rate of the AV node is slower (~40 beats/min) than that of the SA node, it does not set the heart rate; its pacemaker activity is considered secondary. However, if the SA node should fail, the AV node can assume control of the heart and drive it successfully.

Purkinje Fibers The His-Purkinje fiber system originates at the AV node with the bundle of His and splits to form the left and right bundle branches (Fig. 21.1). The right bundle conducts the electrical signal to the right ventricle, and the left bundle, to the left ventricle.

Purkinje fiber cells have the slowest intrinsic pacemaker rate (20 beats/min or less). Thus, Purkinje fiber cells become functional pacemakers only if the SA and AV pacemakers fail, and are considered tertiary pacemakers. On the other hand, the bundle of His and the Purkinje fibers are an effective conduction system within the ventricles because they conduct action potentials more quickly than any other tissue within the heart.

The action potential of the Purkinje fibers depends on four time- and voltage-dependent membrane currents: I_{Na} (not present in the SA and AV nodal cells), I_{Ca}, I_K, and I_f. The maximum diastolic potential is a very negative V_m, and the pacemaker depolarization (phase 4) is very slow. As a result, V_m may not reach the threshold for triggering of an action potential, making Purkinje fiber cells unreliable pacemakers. Normally, the action potential passing through the AV node activates the Purkinje fiber cells, resulting in a rapid upstroke (phase 0), mediated by I_{Na} and I_{Ca}. Because I_{Na} is large, Purkinje fibers conduct action potentials rapidly.

Atrial and ventricular myocytes fire action potentials but do not have pacemaker activity

Atrial Muscle Within each atrium, the action potential spreads among cardiac myocytes via a direct cell-to-cell pathway. The atrial action potential depends on three primary time- and voltage-dependent membrane currents: I_{Na}, I_K, and I_{Ca}. There is no normal spontaneous (i.e., pacemaker) activity in atrial muscle. It has been proposed that atrial muscle has four special conducting bundles (Fig. 21.1).

Ventricular Muscle After the action potential reaches the AV node, it travels to the His-Purkinje fiber network and out into the ventricular muscle. Because of this single electrical connection between the atria and the ventricles, there is a well-defined and orderly sequence of electrical activity through the rapidly conducting His-Purkinje network to the ventricles. Within the ventricular muscle, the action potential conducts from cell to cell. Steps 2 to 6 in Fig. 21.5 summarize the sequence of events in ventricular activation, which is completed in ~100 ms.

Ventricular muscle has three major time- and voltage-gated membrane currents: I_{Na}, I_{Ca}, and I_K (Fig. 21.4B). Ventricular muscle has no I_f, and therefore show no pacemaker activity. Starting from a resting potential of −80 mV,

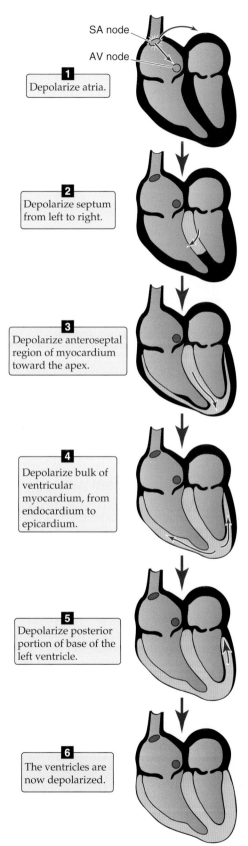

SA node
AV node

1
Depolarize atria.

2
Depolarize septum from left to right.

3
Depolarize anteroseptal region of myocardium toward the apex.

4
Depolarize bulk of ventricular myocardium, from endocardium to epicardium.

5
Depolarize posterior portion of base of the left ventricle.

6
The ventricles are now depolarized.

Figure 21.5 Sequence of depolarization in cardiac tissue.

the rapid upstroke of the ventricular action potential results from the activation of I_{Na} by an external stimulus (e.g., an impulse conducted to the muscle by a Purkinje fiber or by a neighboring ventricular muscle cell). The Ca^{2+} current provides the Ca^{2+} influx that activates the release of Ca^{2+} from the SR. The rapid repolarization (phase 1), the plateau (phase 2), and the repolarization (phase 3) all appear to be governed by mechanisms similar to those found in the Purkinje fibers.

⊙ **21-5** Once a ventricular muscle cell is activated electrically, it is refractory to additional activation. This **effective refractory period** arises because the inward currents (I_{Na} and I_{Ca}) that are responsible for activation are largely inactivated by the membrane depolarization (Fig. 21.4B). During the effective refractory period, an additional electrical stimulus has no effect on the action potential. At the end of the plateau, the cell begins to repolarize as I_K increases in magnitude. As I_{Ca} and I_{Na} begin to recover from inactivation, the **relative refractory period** begins. During this period, an additional electrical stimulus can produce an action potential, but a smaller one than usual. Refractoriness provides the heart with a measure of electrical safety because it prevents extraneous pacemakers (which may arise pathologically) from triggering **ectopic beats.** An extrasystolic contraction would make the heart a less efficient pump.

Acetylcholine and catecholamines modulate pacemaker activity, conduction velocity, and contractility

In principle, three mechanisms can slow the firing rate of the SA node (i.e., negative chronotropic effect). First, the steepness of the depolarization during phase 4 can decrease, thereby lengthening the time necessary for V_m to reach threshold (Fig. 21.6A, *blue curve*). In this way, diastole is longer and the heart rate falls. Second, the maximum diastolic potential can become more negative (Fig. 21.6B, *green curve*). In this case, V_m starts phase 4 at a more negative potential and thus takes longer to reach threshold, assuming that the steepness of the phase 4 depolarization has not changed. Third, the threshold for the action potential can become more positive (Fig. 21.6C, *purple curve*). Assuming no change in either the maximum diastolic potential (i.e., starting point) or the steepness of the phase 4 depolarization, V_m requires a longer time to reach a more positive threshold. A combination of these three mechanisms would have an enhanced effect. Conversely, the SA nodal cells can use each of these three mechanisms in the opposite sense to increase their firing rate (positive chronotropic effect).

Acetylcholine ⊙ **21-6** The vagus nerve, which is parasympathetic (see ⊙ **14-2**), releases acetylcholine (ACh) onto the SA and AV nodes and slows the intrinsic pacemaker activity by all three mechanisms discussed in the preceding paragraph. First, ACh decreases I_f in the SA node (Table 21.1), reducing the steepness of the phase 4 depolarization (Fig. 21.6A). Second, ACh opens GIRK channels, increasing relative K^+ conductance and making the maximum diastolic potential of SA nodal cells more negative (Fig. 21.6B). Third, ACh reduces I_{Ca} in the SA node, thereby reducing the steepness of the phase 4 depolarization (Fig. 21.6A) and also moving the threshold to more positive values (Fig. 21.6C). All three effects cooperate to

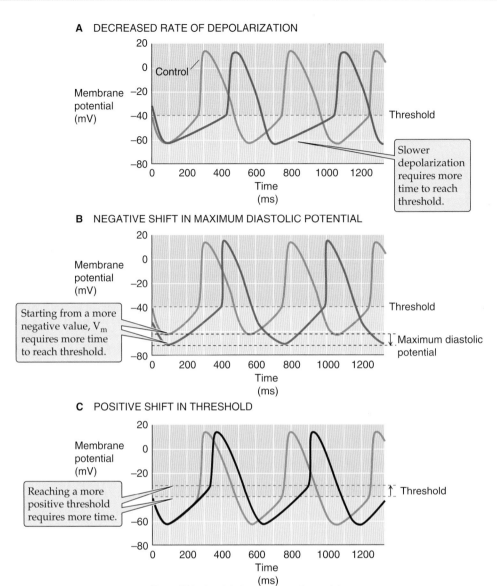

A DECREASED RATE OF DEPOLARIZATION

Membrane potential (mV)

Control

Threshold

Slower depolarization requires more time to reach threshold.

B NEGATIVE SHIFT IN MAXIMUM DIASTOLIC POTENTIAL

Membrane potential (mV)

Starting from a more negative value, V_m requires more time to reach threshold.

Threshold

Maximum diastolic potential

C POSITIVE SHIFT IN THRESHOLD

Membrane potential (mV)

Reaching a more positive threshold requires more time.

Threshold

Time (ms)

Figure 21.6 Modulation of pacemaker activity.

lengthen the time for the SA node to depolarize to threshold; the net effect is to lower the heart rate.

The effects of ACh on currents in the AV node are similar to its effects on those in the SA node. However, because the pacemaker normally does not reside in the AV node, the physiological effect of ACh on the AV node is to slow **conduction velocity** (Table 21.1).

Catecholamines Sympathetic innervation to the heart is plentiful, releasing mostly norepinephrine. In addition, the adrenal medulla releases epinephrine into the circulation. Catecholamines, which act through β_1-adrenergic receptors, produce an increase in heart rate (Table 21.1) by two mechanisms. First, catecholamines increase I_f in the nodal cells, thereby increasing the steepness of the phase 4 depolarization (i.e., opposite to the effect in Fig. 21.6A). Second, catecholamines increase I_{Ca} in all myocardial cells. The increase in I_{Ca} in the SA and AV nodal cells steepens the phase 4 depolarization (i.e., opposite to the effect in Fig. 21.6A) and also makes the threshold more negative (i.e., opposite to the effect in Fig. 21.6C). Note that catecholamines do not appear to change the maximum diastolic potential.

⊙ **21-7** In atrial and ventricular muscle, catecholamines cause an increase in the strength of contraction (Table 21.1)—the **positive inotropic effect**—for four reasons. First, the increased I_{Ca} (i.e., Ca^{2+} influx) leads to a greater local increase in $[Ca^{2+}]_i$ and also a greater Ca^{2+}-induced Ca^{2+} release (see ⊙ 9-11) from the SR. Second, the catecholamines increase the sensitivity of the SR Ca^{2+}-release channel to cytoplasmic Ca^{2+}. Third, catecholamines also enhance Ca pumping into the SR by stimulation of the SERCA Ca pump (see ⊙ 5-11), thereby increasing Ca^{2+} stores for later release. Fourth, the increased I_{Ca} presents more Ca^{2+} to SERCA, so that SR Ca^{2+} stores increase over time. The four mechanisms make more Ca^{2+} available to troponin C, enabling a more forceful contraction.

THE ELECTROCARDIOGRAM

An ECG generally includes five waves

⊙ **21-8** The electrocardiogram (ECG) is the standard clinical tool used to measure the electrical activity of the heart. It is a

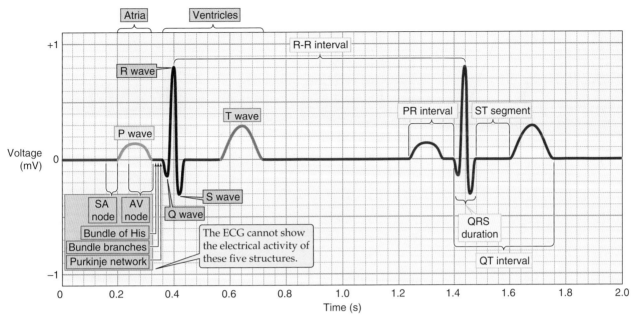

Figure 21.7   Components of the ECG recording.

recording of the small *extracellular* signals produced by the movement of action potentials through cardiac myocytes. To obtain a standard 12-lead ECG, one places two **electrodes** on the upper extremities, two on the lower extremities, and six on standard locations across the chest. In various combinations, the electrodes on the extremities generate the six limb leads (three standard and three augmented), and the chest electrodes produce the six precordial leads. Each lead looks at the heart from a unique angle and plane; that is, from what is essentially its own unique point of view.

⊙ **21-9** The fluctuations in extracellular voltage recorded by each lead vary from fractions of a millivolt to several millivolts. These fluctuations are called **waves** and are named with the letters of the alphabet (Fig. 21.7). The **P** wave reflects depolarization of the right and left atrial muscle. The **QRS** complex represents depolarization of ventricular muscle. The **T** wave represents repolarization of both ventricles. Finally, the rarely seen **U** wave may reflect repolarization of the papillary muscle. The shape and magnitude of these waves are different in each lead because each lead views the electrical activity of the heart from a unique position in space.

Because the movement of charge (i.e., the spreading wave of electrical activity in the heart) has both a three-dimensional **direction** and a **magnitude,** the signal measured on an ECG is a **vector.** The system that clinicians use to measure the heart's three-dimensional, time-dependent electrical vector is simple to understand and easy to implement, but it can be challenging to interpret.

A pair of ECG electrodes defines a lead

To record the complicated time-dependent electrical vector of the heart, the physician or ECG technician constructs a system of leads in two planes that are perpendicular to each other. One plane, the **frontal plane,** is defined by the six **limb leads** (Fig. 21.8A). A perpendicular **transverse plane** is defined by the six **precordial leads** (Fig. 21.8B). Each lead

is an axis in one of the two planes, onto which the heart projects its electrical activity. The ECG recording from a single lead shows how that lead views the time-dependent changes in voltage of the heart.

Recording from all 12 leads is extremely useful because a signal of interest may be easier to see in one lead than in another. For example, an acute myocardial infarction involving the inferior (diaphragmatic) portion of the heart might be easily visualized in leads II, III, and aVF but go completely undetected (or produce so-called reciprocal changes) in the other leads.

The Limb Leads One obtains a 12-lead ECG by having the patient relax in a supine position and connecting four electrodes to the limbs (Fig. 21.8A). Electrically, the torso and limbs are viewed as an equilateral triangle (Einthoven's triangle) with one vertex on the groin and the other two on the shoulder joints (Fig. 21.9A). Because the body is an electrical "volume conductor," an electrical attachment to an arm is electrically equivalent to a connection at the shoulder joint, and an attachment to either leg is equivalent to a connection at the groin. By convention, the left leg represents the groin. The fourth electrode, connected to the right leg, is used for electrical grounding. The three initial limb leads represent the difference between two of the limb electrodes:

- **I** (positive connection to left arm, negative connection to right arm). This lead defines an axis in the frontal plane at 0 degrees (Fig. 21.9A and B).
- **II** (positive to left leg, negative to right arm). This lead defines an axis in the frontal plane at 60 degrees.
- **III** (positive to left leg, negative to left arm). This lead defines an axis in the frontal plane at 120 degrees.

The three augmented unipolar limb leads compare one limb electrode to the average of the other two:

- **aVR** (positive connection to *right* arm, negative connection is electronically defined in the middle of the heart): The axis defined by this limb lead in the frontal plane is −150 degrees (Fig. 21.9B). The *a* stands for augmented, and the *V* represents unipolar.

A FRONTAL PLANE LEADS

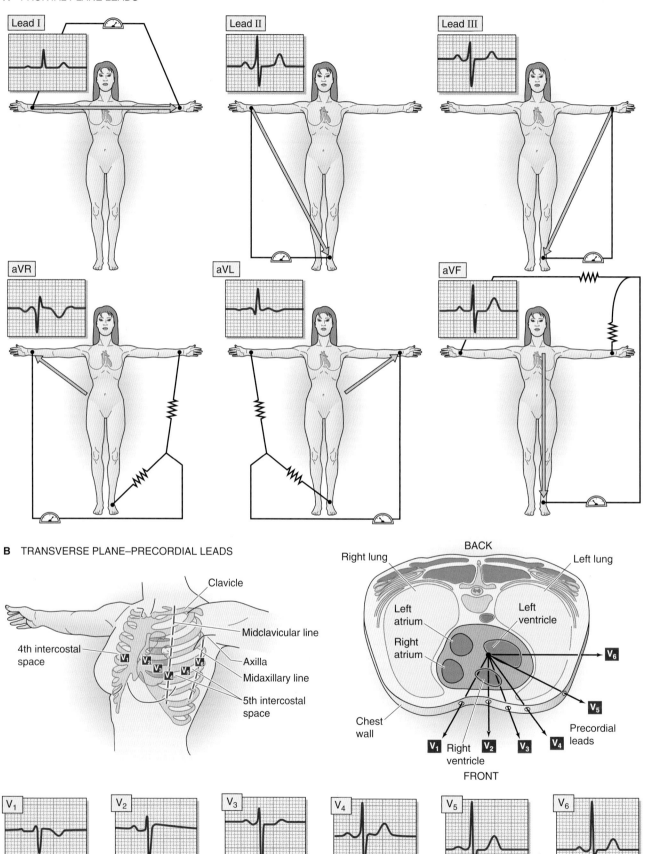

B TRANSVERSE PLANE–PRECORDIAL LEADS

Figure 21.8 The ECG leads.

A EINTHOVEN'S TRIANGLE

B CIRCLE OF AXES

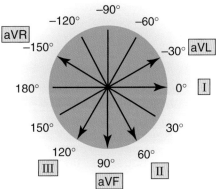

Figure 21.9 Axes of the limb leads. (A) The frontal plane limb leads behave as if they are located at the shoulders (RA [right arm] and LA [left arm]) and groin (LL [left leg]). Leads I, II, and III are separated from one another by 60 degrees. The augmented leads, referenced to the center of the heart, bisect each of the 60-degree angles formed by leads I, II, and III. (B) Translating each of the six frontal leads so that they pass through a common point defines a polar coordinate system, providing views of the heart at 30-degree intervals.

- **aVL** (positive to *left* arm, negative is middle of the heart): The axis defined by this limb lead in the frontal plane is −30 degrees.
- **aVF** (positive to left leg [*foot*], negative is middle of the heart): The axis defined by this limb lead in the frontal plane is +90 degrees.

Thus, the positive and negative ends of these six leads define axes every 30 degrees in the frontal plane (Fig. 21.9B).

The Precordial Leads The precordial leads lie in the transverse plane, perpendicular to the plane of the frontal leads. The positive connection is one of six different locations on the chest wall (Fig. 21.8B), and the negative connection is electronically defined in the middle of the heart by averaging of the three limb electrodes. The resultant leads are named V_1 to V_6, where the *V* stands for unipolar:

- V_1: fourth intercostal space to the right of the sternum
- V_2: fourth intercostal space to the left of the sternum
- V_4: fifth intercostal space at the midclavicular line
- V_3: halfway between V_2 and V_4
- V_6: fifth intercostal space at the midaxillary line
- V_5: halfway between V_4 and V_6

CARDIAC ARRHYTHMIAS

Any change in cardiac rhythm from the normal sinus rhythm is defined as an **arrhythmia.** Although some arrhythmias are pathological and even life-threatening, others are normal and appropriately adaptive, including sinus tachycardia and sinus arrhythmia.

Sinus tachycardia is a heart rate faster than normal, driven by the sinus node. This arrhythmia is seen in frightened or startled individuals or during normal exercise. Rarely, sinus tachycardia can be pathological—for example, in patients with acute hyperthyroidism (see Table 49.1).

Sinus arrhythmia is the name given to a normal phenomenon: a subtle change in heart rate that occurs with each respiratory cycle. Inspiration accelerates the heart rate (see ◉ 23-22); expiration slows it. Deepening of the respirations exaggerates these cyclic changes. The magnitude of the effect can vary significantly among individuals. The heart rate is still under the control of the SA node, but cyclic variations

in sympathetic and parasympathetic tone modulate the SA node's pacemaker rate. The loss of sinus arrhythmia can be a sign of autonomic system dysfunction, as may be seen in patients with diabetes.

Although the list of pathological arrhythmias is long, two basic problems are responsible for nearly all arrhythmias: altered conduction and altered automaticity.

Conduction abnormalities are a major cause of arrhythmias

Disturbances of conduction make up the first major category of cardiac arrhythmias. Conduction disturbances can have multiple causes and can occur at any point in the conduction pathway. Conduction disturbances can be partial or complete. The two major causes of conduction disturbances are depolarization and abnormal anatomy.

If a tissue is injured (e.g., by stretch or anoxia), an altered balance of ionic currents can lead to a **depolarization.** The depolarization, in turn, partially inactivates I_{Na} and I_{Ca}, slowing the spread of current (i.e., slowing conduction). As a result, the tissue may become less excitable (partial conduction block) or completely inexcitable (complete conduction block).

Another type of conduction disturbance is the presence of an aberrant conduction pathway, reflecting **abnormal anatomy.** One such example is an accessory conduction pathway that rapidly transmits the action potential from the atria to the ventricles, bypassing the AV node, which normally imposes a conduction delay.

Re-Entry An independent focus of pacemaker activity can develop as a consequence of a conduction disturbance. This class of conduction disturbance is called re-entry (or re-entrant excitation or circus movement) and is one of the major causes of clinical arrhythmias. It occurs when a wave of depolarization travels in an apparently endless circle. Re-entry has three requirements: (1) a closed conduction loop, (2) a region of unidirectional block (at least briefly), and (3) a sufficiently slow conduction of action potentials around the loop.

A conduction defect that is essential for re-entry is the unidirectional block. **Unidirectional block** is a type of partial

A NORMAL CONDUCTION IN BOTH DIRECTIONS

B UNIDIRECTIONAL BLOCK

C NORMAL CONDUCTION THROUGH A BIFURCATION

D RE-ENTRANT EXCITATION

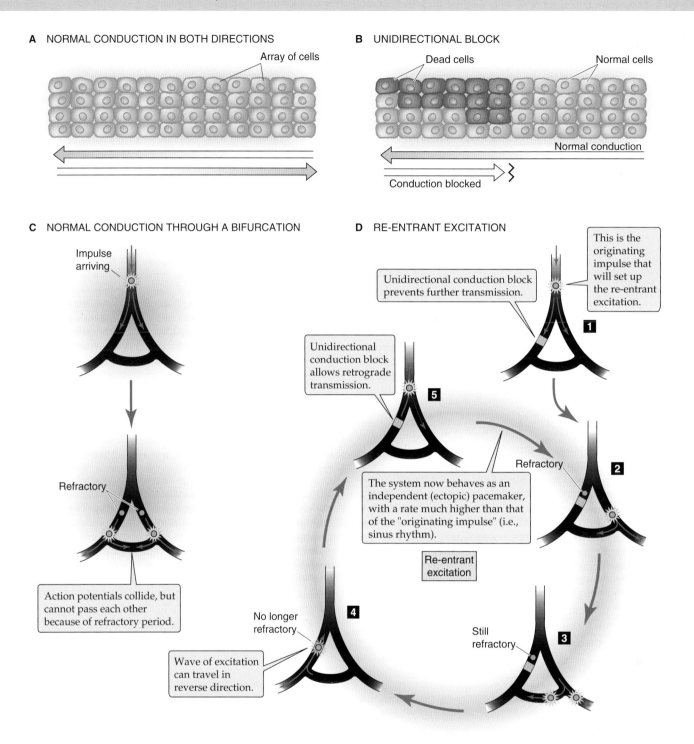

Figure 21.10 Abnormal conduction.

conduction block in which impulses travel in one direction but not in the opposite one. Unidirectional block may arise as a result of a local depolarization or may be due to pathological changes in functional anatomy. Normal cardiac tissue can conduct impulses in both directions (Fig. 21.10A). However, after an asymmetric anatomical lesion develops, many more healthy cells may remain on one side of the lesion than on the other. When conduction proceeds in the direction from the many healthy cells to the few healthy cells, the current from the many may be sufficient to excite the few

(right to left in Fig. 21.10B). On the other hand, when conduction proceeds in the opposite direction, the few healthy cells cannot generate enough current to excite the region of many healthy cells (left to right in Fig. 21.10B). The result is a unidirectional block.

Imagine that an impulse is traveling down a bifurcating Purkinje fiber and is about to reach a group of ventricular myocytes—a *closed conduction loop* (Fig. 21.10C). The refractory zones prevent the re-entry of impulses from the right to the left, and vice versa. In the presence of a lesion that causes a *unidirectional conduction block* in the left branch of the Purkinje fiber, when the impulse reaches the fork in the road, it spreads in both directions (Fig. 21.10D, step 1) but it cannot continue past the unidirectional block in the left branch. The impulse traveling down the right branch stimulates the distal conducting cells (Fig. 21.10D, step 2), leaving them in an effective refractory period (see ◉ 21-5). When the impulse reaches the ventricular muscle, it begins to travel back toward the damaged left branch (Fig. 21.10D, step 3). At this point, the cells in the normal right branch may still be refractory to excitation. The impulse finally reaches the damaged left branch and travels in a retrograde fashion up this branch, reaching and passing through the region of the unidirectional conduction block (Fig. 21.10D, step 4). Because enough time has elapsed for the cells at the bifurcation and in the right branch to recover from their refractory period, as the impulse reached the bifurcation (Fig. 21.10D, step 5), it can now travel retrograde up the main part of the Purkinje fiber as well as orthograde down the right branch—for a second time.

If this re-entrant movement (steps 2 → 5 → 2, and so on) continues, the frequency of re-entry will ultimately outpace the SA nodal pacemaker (frequency of step 1) and be responsible for tachyarrhythmias (e.g., atrial and ventricular tachycardia, atrial and ventricular fibrillation) because the fastest pacemaker sets the heart rate.

Fibrillation In fibrillation, many regions of re-entrant electrical activity are present, creating electrical chaos that is not associated with useful contraction. **Atrial fibrillation** is commonly found in elderly patients, sometimes with mitral valve or coronary artery disease, but often without any evidence of underlying cardiac disease. The re-entry loop within the atria moves wildly and rapidly, generating a rapid succession of action potentials—as many as 500 per minute. This wandering re-entry circuit easily becomes the fastest pacemaker in the heart, outpacing the SA node. As the AV node cannot repolarize fast enough to pass along all of these impulses only some reach the ventricles, resulting in the irregular appearance of QRS complexes without any detectable P waves. Although only some atrial impulses reach the ventricles, the ventricular rate can still be quite high.

Because the atria function mainly as a booster pump, many patients tolerate atrial fibrillation without harm and may even be unaware that they have it. Others may suffer greatly from the loss of a coordinated atrial contraction, particularly the elderly or those with coexisting cardiac disease. In most individuals, attempts should be made to convert the rhythm back to normal sinus rhythm if possible, by either electrical or chemical means (e.g., digitalis, β-adrenergic blockers, or Ca^{2+}-channel blockers).

Ventricular fibrillation is a life-threatening medical emergency. The heart cannot generate cardiac output because the ventricles are not able to pump blood without a coordinated ventricular depolarization.

Altered automaticity can originate from the sinus node or from an ectopic locus

Pacemaker cells can experience an alteration in or even a complete absence of automaticity. Conversely, other cells that normally have no automaticity (e.g., ventricular muscle) can become "ectopic" pacemakers. These disturbances of automaticity make up the second major category of cardiac arrhythmias.

Depolarization-Dependent Triggered Activity A positive shift in the maximum diastolic potential brings V_m closer to the threshold for an action potential and can induce automaticity in cardiac tissue that otherwise has no pacemaker activity. The development of depolarization-induced triggered activity depends on the interaction of the Ca^{2+} current (I_{Ca}) and the repolarizing K^+ current (I_K). This mechanism can produce a more rapid pacemaker depolarization in the SA or AV nodal cells, causing them to accelerate their pacemakers. It can also increase the intrinsic pacemaker rate in Purkinje fiber cells, which normally have a very slow pacemaker.

Depolarization-induced triggered activity is particularly dramatic in nonpacemaker tissues (e.g., ventricular muscle), which normally exhibit no diastolic depolarization. Factors that significantly prolong action potential duration can cause depolarization-dependent triggered activity. During the repolarization phase, I_{Na} remains inactivated because the cell is depolarized (Fig. 21.11A). On the other hand, I_{Ca} has had enough time to recover from inactivation and—because the cell is still depolarized—triggers a slow, positive deflection in V_m known as an **early afterdepolarization (EAD).** Eventually, I_K increases and returns V_m toward the resting potential. EADs that are large may trigger an extrasystole. Isolated ventricular extrasystoles may occur in normal individuals. Alterations in cellular Ca^{2+} metabolism (discussed in the next section) may increase the tendency of a prolonged action potential to produce an extrasystole. Drugs used to treat arrhythmias can become *arrhythmogenic* by producing EADs (e.g., quinidine presumably by inhibiting Na^+ channels and some K^+ channels and thus prolonging the ventricular muscle action potential).

More than one extrasystole—a **run of extrasystoles** (Fig. 21.11B)—is pathological. A run of three or more ventricular extrasystoles is the minimal requirement for diagnosis of **ventricular tachycardia.** This arrhythmia is life-threatening, because it can degenerate into ventricular fibrillation, which is associated with no meaningful cardiac output.

Long QT Syndrome Patients with long QT syndrome (LQTS) have a prolonged ventricular action potential and are prone to ventricular arrhythmias. The congenital form can involve mutations of cardiac Na^+ channels or K^+ channels. The acquired form of LQTS, which is much more common, can result from various electrolyte disturbances (especially hypokalemia and hypocalcemia) or from prescribed or over-the-counter medications (e.g., several antiarrhythmic drugs, tricyclic antidepressants, and some nonsedating antihistamines when they are taken together with certain antibiotics, notably erythromycin).

Ca^{2+} overload and metabolic changes can also cause arrhythmias

Ca^{2+} Overload Ca^{2+} overload in the heart has many potential causes. One frequent factor is digitalis intoxication. Another is injury-related cellular depolarization. Ca^{2+} overload occurs when $[Ca^{2+}]_i$ increases, causing the SR to sequester too much Ca^{2+}. Thus overloaded, the SR begins

A PROLONGED ACTION POTENTIAL LEADS
TO EARLY AFTERDEPOLARIZATION

B PROLONGED ACTION POTENTIAL LEADS
TO A "RUN" OF SPONTANEOUS ACTIVITY

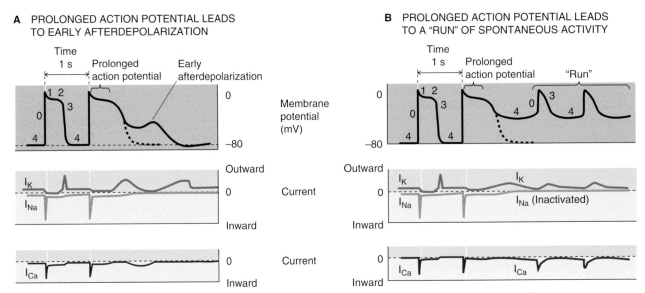

Figure 21.11 Abnormal automaticity in ventricular muscle. The records in this figure are idealized.

to cyclically—and spontaneously—dump Ca^{2+} and then take it back up. The Ca^{2+} release may be large enough to stimulate a Ca^{2+}-activated nonselective cation channel and the Na-Ca exchanger (see Fig. 5.8A). These current sources combine to produce I_{ti}, a **transient inward current** that produces a **delayed afterdepolarization (DAD).** When it is large enough, I_{ti} can depolarize the cell beyond threshold and produce a spontaneous action potential.

Metabolism-Dependent Conduction Changes During ischemia and anoxia, the fall in intracellular ATP levels activates the ATP-sensitive K^+ channel (K_{ATP}), present in cardiac myocytes. The activation of this channel may explain, in part, the slowing or blocking of conduction that may occur during ischemia or in the peri-infarction period.

CHAPTER 22

THE HEART AS A PUMP

Emile L. Boulpaep

THE CARDIAC CYCLE

The sequence of mechanical and electrical events that repeats with every heartbeat is called the **cardiac cycle.** The **duration** of the cardiac cycle is the reciprocal of the heart rate:

$$\text{Duration (s/beat)} = \frac{60\,(\text{s / min})}{\text{Heart rate (beats / min)}} \quad \textbf{(22.1)}$$

For example, for a heart rate of 75 beats/min, the cardiac cycle lasts 0.8 s or 800 ms.

The closing and opening of the cardiac valves define four phases of the cardiac cycle

Under normal circumstances, the electrical pacemaker in the sinoatrial node (see ⊙ 21-3) determines the duration of the cardiac cycle, and the electrical properties of the cardiac conduction system and cardiac myocytes determine the relative duration of contraction and relaxation.

The cardiac **atria** are small chambers. The right atrium receives deoxygenated systemic venous return from the inferior and superior venae cavae. The left atrium receives oxygenated blood from the lungs through the pulmonary circulation. Both atria operate more as passive reservoirs than as mechanical pumps.

The inlet valves of the ventricles are called the **AV (atrioventricular) valves.** They permit blood to flow in one direction only, from the atria to the ventricles. The valve located between the *right* atrium and the right ventricle is the **tricuspid valve** because it has three flaps, or cusps. The valve located between the *left* atrium and the left ventricle is the **mitral valve** because it has only two cusps.

The outlet valves of the ventricles are called **semilunar valves.** They also allow blood to flow in just a single direction, from each ventricle into a large outflow-tract vessel. Both the **pulmonary valve,** located between the right ventricle and pulmonary artery, and the **aortic valve,** located between the left ventricle and aorta, have three cusps.

Cardiac valves open passively when upstream pressure exceeds downstream pressure. They close passively when downstream pressure exceeds upstream pressure. The movement of the valve leaflets can be detected by echocardiography (see ⊙ 17-9); their closure makes **heart sounds** that can be heard with a stethoscope. During certain parts of the cardiac cycle, blood passing through either **regurgitant** or **stenotic** lesions makes characteristic sounds that are called **murmurs.**

From the point of view of the ventricles and the positions of their valves, we must consider a minimum of four distinct **phases:**

- *Inflow phase.* The inlet valve is open and the outlet valve is closed.
- *Isovolumetric contraction.* Both valves are closed, with no blood flow.
- *Outflow phase.* The outlet valve is open and the inlet valve is closed.
- *Isovolumetric relaxation.* Both valves are closed, with no blood flow.

Table 22.1 summarizes these four phases and the key events of the cardiac cycle. Note that the same events occur in the right heart as in the left heart.

It is common to separate these phases into two parts. **Systole** includes phases 2 and 3, when the ventricles are contracting, whereas **diastole** includes phases 4 and 1, when the ventricles are relaxing. At a heart rate of 75 beats/min (cycle duration = 800 ms), systole occupies ~300 ms, and diastole ~500 ms. With increasing heart rate, diastole shortens relatively more than systole does.

Fig. 22.1 illustrates the changes in pressure and volume that occur during the cardiac cycle. The four vertical lines indicate the timing of the four *valvular events* that terminate each of the four phases defined previously:

- AV valve closure terminates phase 1.
- Semilunar valve opening terminates phase 2.
- Semilunar valve closing terminates phase 3.
- AV valve opening terminates phase 4.

The shapes of pressure tracings for the right heart (Fig. 22.1A) and the left heart (Fig. 22.1B) are quite similar except that the pressures on the right are a scaled-down version of those on the left. In both cases, the tracings begin in the *middle* of phase 1; that is, the period of decreased filling toward the end of diastole called **diastasis.** Note that the volume changes in the left ventricle are exactly the same as those in the right ventricle because the cardiac outputs of the right and left hearts are virtually identical (see ⊙ 17-4).

Diastasis Period (Middle of Phase 1) During the diastasis, the mitral valve is open, but little blood flows from the left atrium to the left ventricle; ventricular volume slowly rises and approaches a plateau. The pressures in both the left atrium and the left ventricle rise slowly, driven by the

TABLE 22.1 Events in the Cardiac Cycle

VALVULAR EVENTS	CARDIAC CHAMBER EVENTS	PHASE	
Opening of AV valves (tricuspid and mitral)	Rapid ventricular filling	1	Diastole
	Decreased ventricular filling; diastasis	1	Diastole
	Atrial contraction (additional ventricular filling)	1	Diastole
Closing of AV valves (tricuspid and mitral)	Isovolumetric ventricular contraction (with all valves closed)	2	Systole
Opening of semilunar valves (pulmonary and aortic)	Rapid ventricular ejection (fast muscle shortening)	3	Systole
	Decreased ventricular ejection (slower muscle shortening)	3	Systole
Closing of semilunar valves (pulmonary and aortic)	Isovolumetric ventricular relaxation (with all valves closed)	4	Diastole
Opening of AV valves (tricuspid and mitral)			

pressure in the pulmonary veins, which is only slightly higher. The atrial pressure parallels the ventricular pressure because the mitral valve is wide open, and the flow between the two chambers is minimal. The P wave of the electrocardiogram (ECG; see ⊚ 21-9), which corresponds to atrial excitation, occurs at the end of this phase.

Atrial Contraction (End of Phase 1) Immediately following the P wave is the atrial contraction, which causes a variable amount of blood to enter the left ventricle. In a person at rest, the atrial contraction transfers into the left ventricle a volume of blood that represents <20% of the subsequent stroke. Atrial contraction causes a slight rise in intra-atrial pressure, and a comparable rise in ventricular pressure and volume. All during this period, the aortic pressure decreases as blood flows out to the periphery.

Isovolumetric Contraction (Phase 2) When the ventricles begin to depolarize, as evidenced by the QRS complex on the ECG, systole commences. The ventricles contract, and very soon the pressure in the left ventricle exceeds that in the left atrium (first crossover of *blue* and *orange pressure tracings* in Fig. 22.1B, *top*). As a result, the *mitral valve closes*. The aortic valve has been closed this entire time. Thus, the left ventricle contracts with both mitral and aortic valves closed. Because the blood has no place to go, the result is an isovolumetric contraction that causes the pressure in the left ventricle to rise rapidly, eventually exceeding the pressure in the aorta (first crossover of blue and red tracings) and causing the aortic valve to open.

Ejection or Outflow (Phase 3) As the *aortic valve opens*, the ejection phase begins. During the first part of phase 3—**rapid ejection**—ventricular pressure (*blue tracing* in Fig. 22.1B, *top*) continues to rise, closely followed by a rapid elevation of aortic pressure. Accompanying these rapid pressure increases is a precipitous reduction in ventricular volume (Fig. 22.1B, *bottom*), as blood flows into

the aorta. Aortic pressure continues to rise and eventually exceeds ventricular pressure (second crossover of *blue* and *red tracings* in Fig. 22.1B, *top*) just before both the aortic and ventricular pressures begin to fall. Despite the reversal of the pressure gradient across the aortic valve, the cusps of the aortic valve do not immediately snap shut because of the inertia of blood flow, which imparts considerable kinetic energy to the blood. During the latter part of phase 3—**decreased ejection**—the decrease in ventricular volume becomes less rapid, and both the ventricular and aortic pressures fall off. During the entire ejection phase, about 70 mL of blood flows into the aorta, leaving about 50 mL behind in the ventricle.

Isovolumetric Relaxation (Phase 4) Late in the ejection phase, blood flow across the aortic valve falls to extremely low values, until it actually reverses direction (i.e., retrograde or negative flow). At this point, the *aortic valve closes*, defining the onset of diastole. As blood flow in the aorta again becomes briefly positive (i.e., forward), there is a small upward deflection in the aortic pressure trace. The result is the **dicrotic notch**. Because both the aortic and mitral valves are closed, and no blood can enter the left ventricle, this is the period of isovolumetric relaxation. Pressure falls rapidly in the left ventricle.

Rapid Ventricular Filling Period (Beginning of Phase 1) When ventricular pressure falls below that in the left atrium (second crossover of *blue* and *orange tracings* in Fig. 22.1B), the *mitral valve opens*. Immediately following mitral valve opening, left ventricular volume begins to increase rapidly (Fig. 22.1B, *bottom*). During this period of rapid ventricular filling, the left atrial and ventricular pressures evolve in parallel because the mitral valve is wide open. A period of relatively decreased filling follows (i.e., the diastasis). Thus, diastole includes both the rapid ventricular filling period and diastasis.

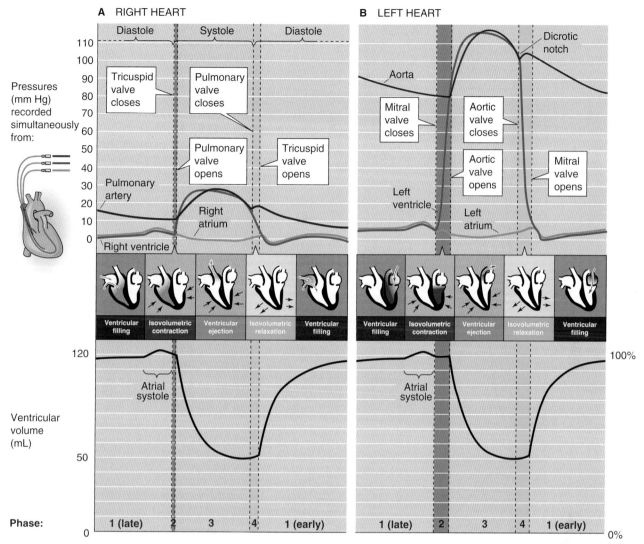

Figure 22.1 Pressures and ventricular volumes during the cardiac cycle. (A) Right heart. (B) Left heart. The *inset* shows the placement of catheters used for pressure measurements in the right heart.

During rapid ventricular filling, the aortic valve remains closed. Because blood continues to flow out to the periphery, owing to the recoil of the aorta's elastic wall, the aortic pressure falls. This fall continues during diastasis.

The electrocardiogram, phonocardiogram, and echocardiogram all follow the cyclic pattern of the cardiac cycle

Accompanying the basic cyclic pattern of cardiac pressure and volume changes are characteristic mechanical, electrical, acoustic, and echocardiographic changes. Fig. 22.2 illustrates these events for the left heart and the systemic circulation. Notice that the pressure records in the top panel of Fig. 22.2 start with the atrial contraction—that is, slightly later than in Fig. 22.1.

Aortic Blood Flow Blood flow from the left ventricle to the ascending aorta (Fig. 22.2, *second panel from top*) rises most rapidly during the rapid ejection phase of the left ventricle.

Jugular Venous Pulse The third panel of Fig. 22.2 includes the jugular venous pulse, for comparison with the timing of other events.

Electrocardiogram The ECG (Fig. 22.2, *fourth panel from top*, and ⊙ 21-8) begins with the middle of the P wave (atrial depolarization). The QRS complex (ventricular depolarization) is the prelude to the upswing in ventricular pressure. The T wave (ventricular repolarization) occurs in the decreased-ejection phase.

Phonocardiogram and Heart Sounds The opening and closing of the valves are accompanied by **heart sounds** (Fig. 22.2, *fifth panel from top*), easily heard through a stethoscope or recorded with a digital stethoscope and stored as a phonocardiogram. Each of the vertical dotted lines in Fig. 22.1 indicates the movement of two valves, one on the right heart and one on the left. Thus, two valves can contribute to a single heart sound, although the two components can often be separated by the ear. The phonocardiogram in Fig. 22.2

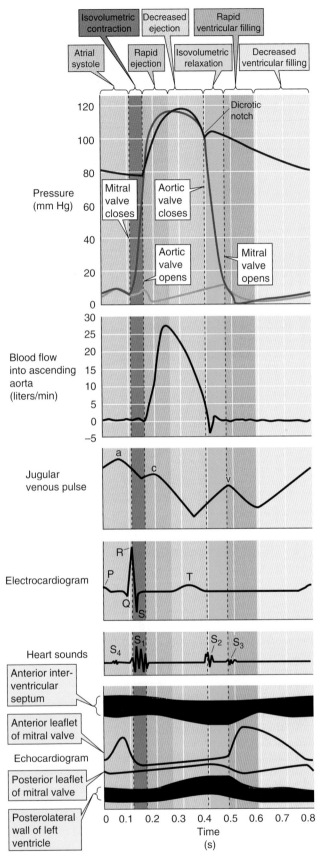

Figure 22.2 Mechanical, electrical, acoustic, and echocardiographic events in the cardiac cycle. *Top,* A repeat of Fig. 22.1B, with three modifications: (1) the cardiac cycle begins with atrial contraction; (2) phase 1 of the cardiac cycle has three subparts: rapid ventricular filling, decreased ventricular filling, and atrial systole; (3) phase 3 has two subparts: rapid and decreased ventricular ejection.

shows the timing of the two major, or physiological, heart sounds (S_1 and S_2), as well as two other sounds (S_3 and S_4) that are occasionally heard.

The physiological heart sounds S_1 and S_2 are heard following the closure of the cardiac valves: the mitral and tricuspid valves for S_1, and the aortic and pulmonary valves for S_2. Vibrations resulting from sudden tension in the AV valves and the adjacent ventricular walls produce the **first heart sound, S_1.** Similarly, vibrations of the large vessel walls and columns of blood produce the **second heart sound, S_2,** following closure of the semilunar valves.

Although the four vertical lines that define the four phases of the cardiac cycle are very similar for the right and left hearts, they do not line up perfectly with one another, as can be seen by comparing Fig. 22.1A and B.

A physiological **third heart sound, S_3,** is present in some normal individuals, particularly children. S_3 occurs in early diastole when rapid filling of the ventricles results in recoil of ventricular walls that have a limited distensibility. The addition of an S_3 to the physiological S_1 and S_2 creates a three-sound sequence, S_1-S_2-S_3, that is termed a **protodiastolic gallop** or ventricular gallop.

When present, a **fourth heart sound, S_4,** coincides with atrial contraction. It is usually heard in pathological conditions in which an unusually strong atrial contraction occurs in combination with low compliance of the left ventricle.

Echocardiogram We discussed echocardiography earlier (see ⊙ 17-9). The echocardiogram in the bottom panel of Fig. 22.2 shows that the separation between the anterior and posterior leaflets of the mitral valve increases during atrial contraction. During the decreased phase of ventricular filling, the leaflets once again move closer together, until the next atrial contraction.

The cardiac cycle causes flow waves in the aorta and peripheral vessels

With the closing and opening of the heart's exit valves (i.e., pulmonary and aortic valves), blood flow and blood velocity across these valves oscillate from near zero, when the valves are closed, to high values, when the valves are open. *Pressure* in the aortic arch typically oscillates between ~80 and ~120 mm Hg (Fig. 22.3B, *panel 1*) but varies greatly among individuals. Phasic changes in pressure and flow also occur in the peripheral arteries. Arterial pressure is usually measured in a large artery, such as the brachial artery (see Fig. 17.7). Because very little pressure drop occurs between the aorta and such a large, proximate artery, the measured **systolic** and **diastolic** arterial pressures, as well as the pulse pressure and mean arterial pressure (see ⊙ 17-6), closely approximate the corresponding aortic pressures.

The ratio $\Delta P/F$ is no longer resistance—a simple, time-*in*dependent quantity—but a *complex* quantity called the **mechanical impedance** that depends on the classical "resistance" as well as the compliance and inertial properties of the vessels and blood.

Because of these resistive, compliant, and inertial properties, the pressure and flow waves in vessels distal to the aorta are not quite the same as in the aorta.

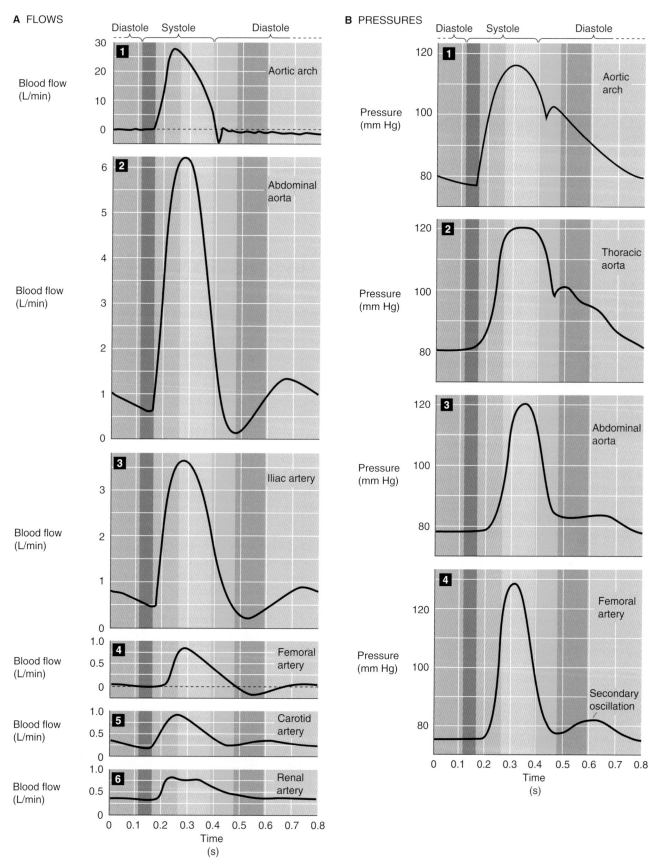

Figure 22.3 Flow (A) and pressure (B) profiles in the aorta and smaller vessels.

Aortic Arch During the rapid-ejection phase, peak *flow* through the aortic arch is remarkably high, ~30 L/min (dark beige band in Fig. 22.3A, *panel 1*). The peak linear velocity is ~100 cm/s, which makes it more likely that the blood will reach the critical Reynolds number value for turbulence (see Equation 17.13). The rapid ejection of blood also causes a rapid rise of the *pressure* in the aorta to above that in the ventricle (Fig. 22.3B, *panel 1*). As the aortic valve closes, it produces the dicrotic notch in the aortic pressure trace.

Thoracic-Abdominal Aorta and Large Arteries Just distal to the aortic arch, a transformation of the flow and pressure curves begins to occur. The records in panels 2 through 4 in Fig. 22.3A show the flow curves for the abdominal aorta and some of its large branches. Peak systolic flow becomes smaller as one moves from the aorta toward the periphery (i.e., iliac and femoral arteries). However, in the abdominal aorta, a new phenomenon is seen. As the elastic aorta—which stored blood during systole—releases blood during diastole, a second peak of flow appears. Of particular importance is the sizable diastolic flow in the carotid and renal arteries (Fig. 22.3A, *panels 5 and 6*).

The cardiac cycle also causes pressure waves in the aorta and peripheral vessels

The *pressure* curves in Fig. 22.3B show that, with increasing distance from the heart *(panels 1 to 4)*, the rising portion of the wave becomes steeper and the peak narrower. Because the peak gradually increases in height and the minimum pressure gradually decreases, the pulse pressure becomes greater. With increasing distance from the heart, an important secondary pressure oscillation appears during diastole (Fig. 22.3B, *panel 4*).

Terminal Arteries and Arterioles In the smallest arteries, the pulse wave gets damped out for two reasons. First, because we are dealing with many parallel vessels with a large aggregate wall area, the aggregate compliance increases, damping the pressure wave. Second, because these smaller arteries have a smaller radius and thus a far greater resistance, the mean arterial pressure must fall in proportion to the much higher resistance.

Capillaries By the time the blood reaches the capillaries, the damping is so severe that pulsations (i.e., pressure oscillations) do not normally occur—blood flow is continuous. The pulmonary capillaries are an exception; their upstream vessels are short, and they have low resistance and high compliance.

Distortion of pressure waves is the result of their propagation along the arterial tree Imagine that you are listening to a patient's heart with a stethoscope while simultaneously feeling the pulse of the radial artery near the wrist. For each heartbeat that you hear, you feel a radial pulse after a delay of only ~0.1 s. Red blood cells (RBCs) take several seconds to flow from the heart to the wrist (see ◉ **19-4**). The reason for this difference is that the blood vessels conduct the palpable pulse as a **pressure wave** (Fig. 22.3B) traveling at a velocity of 5 to 6 m/s in the aorta, and increasing to 10 to 15 m/s in the small arteries.

The downstream propagation of the wave through the larger arteries is accompanied by a serious *distortion* of

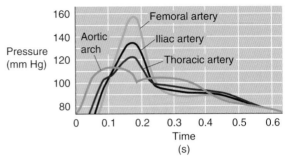

Figure 22.4 Arterial pressure waves. These simultaneous pressure records are from a dog, with catheters placed at 0, 10, 20, and 30 cm from the aortic arch. As the wave moves down the vessel, the upstroke is delayed, but the peak is higher.

the pressure profile: it gets narrower and taller as we move downstream (Fig. 22.4).

Effect of Frequency on Wave Velocity and Damping The pressure wave moving from the aorta to the periphery is actually an ensemble of many individual waves, each with its own frequency. Higher-frequency waves travel faster and undergo more damping than low-frequency waves (Fig. 22.5A).

Effect of Wall Stiffness on Wave Velocity As the pressure wave reaches vessels that have a stiffer wall (e.g., greater ratio of wall thickness to vessel diameter), the velocity of the wave increases (Fig. 22.5B). Conversely, with a more compliant vessel, some of the energy of the pressure pulse goes into dilation of the vessel, so that the pressure wave spreads out and slows down. Because aging causes a decrease in vessel compliance (i.e., distensibility), the velocity of propagation actually increases.

Pressure waves in veins do not originate from arterial waves

Flow in *capillaries* is usually not pulsatile. Nevertheless, blood flow in systemic capillaries can exhibit slow oscillations unrelated to the cardiac cycle. The action of upstream vasomotor control elements in arterioles and precapillary sphincters can cause fluctuations. In addition, changes in tissue pressure (e.g., caused by muscle contraction) can compress capillaries and cause further fluctuations in capillary flow. Pulmonary capillary flow is especially susceptible to changes in the surrounding alveolar pressure (see ◉ **31-8**).

Although systemic *veins* have pressure waves, these waves do not originate from arterial waves propagating through the capillary beds, which are nonpulsatile. Three mechanisms can contribute to the **venous pulse:** (1) retrograde action of the heartbeat during the cardiac cycle, (2) the respiratory cycle, and (3) the contraction of skeletal muscles.

Effect of the Cardiac Cycle A large vein close to the heart, such as the **jugular vein,** has a complex pulse wave (Fig. 22.6A) synchronized to the cardiac cycle. The three maxima, or peaks, in the jugular pulse wave are labeled *a, c,* and *v*. The three minima, or dips, are labeled *av, x,* and *y*. These pressure transients reflect events in the cardiac cycle:

- The *a* **peak** is caused by the contraction of the right atrium.
- The *av* **minimum** is due to relaxation of the right atrium and closure of the tricuspid valve.

A DISTORTION IN A VESSEL WITH UNIFORM DISTENSIBILITY

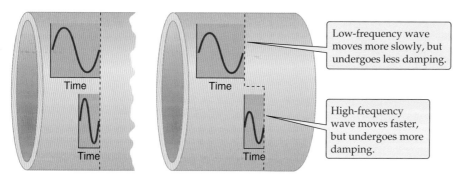

Low-frequency wave moves more slowly, but undergoes less damping.

High-frequency wave moves faster, but undergoes more damping.

B DISTORTION IN A VESSEL WITH DECREASING DOWNSTREAM DISTENSIBILITY

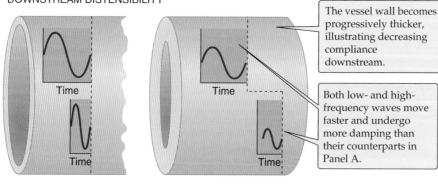

The vessel wall becomes progressively thicker, illustrating decreasing compliance downstream.

Both low- and high-frequency waves move faster and undergo more damping than their counterparts in Panel A.

Figure 22.5 Propagation of pressure waves. (A) Waveform changes along a vessel with uniform distensibility. (B) Waveform changes along a vessel with decreasing distensibility. In (A) and (B), the flow is from left to right. The left pair of pressure waves is at the same early time, whereas the right pair of pressure waves is at the same late time. If on the right (i.e., end of the vessel), we sum waves of different frequencies at the same instant in time, then the composite wave is distorted (like the green femoral artery curve in Fig. 22.4).

- The c **peak** reflects the pressure rise in the right ventricle early during systole and the resultant bulging of the tricuspid valve into the right atrium.
- The x **minimum** occurs as the ventricle contracts and shortens during the ejection phase later in systole.
- The v **peak** is related to filling of the right atrium against a closed tricuspid valve, which causes right atrial pressure to rise. As the tricuspid valve opens, the *v* peak begins to wane.
- The y **minimum** reflects a fall in right atrial pressure during rapid ventricular filling, as blood leaves the right atrium through an open tricuspid valve and enters the right ventricle.

Effect of the Respiratory Cycle The pressure in the jugular vein becomes negative during inspiration (Fig. 22.6B) as the diaphragm descends, causing intrathoracic pressure (and therefore the pressure inside the thoracic vessels) to decrease and intra-abdominal pressure to increase. Consequently, the venous return from the head and upper extremities transiently increases, as low-pressure vessels literally suck blood into the thoracic cavity. Simultaneously, the venous flow decreases from the lower extremities because of the relatively high pressure of the abdominal veins during inspiration. Therefore, during inspiration, pressure in the jugular vein falls while pressure in the femoral vein rises.

Effect of Skeletal Muscle Contraction ("Muscle Pump") ⊙ **22-1** The contraction of skeletal muscle can also affect pressure and flow in veins. Large veins in the lower limbs are equipped with valves that prevent retrograde movement of blood (see ⊙ **17-7**). When a person is at rest and in the recumbent position, all venous valves

are open and venous blood flow toward the heart is continuous. Standing causes the venous pressure in the foot to rise gradually to the hydrostatic pressure dictated by the vertical blood column from the foot to the heart (Fig. 22.6C). If the person begins to walk, the combination of the pumping action of the leg muscles on the leg veins and the action of the venous valves as hydrostatic relay stations causes the venous pressure in the foot to decrease.

CARDIAC DYNAMICS

The heart is a system of two pumps linked in series. The muscular wall of the left ventricle is thicker and more powerful than that of the right. The interventricular septum welding the two pumps together is even thicker. The thick muscular walls of the ventricles are responsible for exerting the heart's pumping action.

Pacemaker cells within the heart itself initiate cardiac excitation. When the heart is in a normal sinus rhythm, the pacemaker cells setting the rate are located in the sinoatrial (SA) node of the right atrium (see ⊙ 21-4). The action potential then spreads through atrial myocytes and specialized tracts or bundles. The impulse cannot cross from the atria to the ventricles except through the AV node. The AV node inserts a time delay into the conduction that is essential to allow the ventricles to finish filling with blood before contraction and ejection occur. From the AV node, the impulse spreads through the bundle of His and then the right and the left bundle branches, the latter of which divides in an anterior

A JUGULAR VENOUS PRESSURE CHANGES
CAUSED BY CARDIAC CYCLE

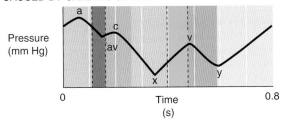

B JUGULAR VENOUS PRESSURE CHANGES
CAUSED BY RESPIRATORY CYCLE

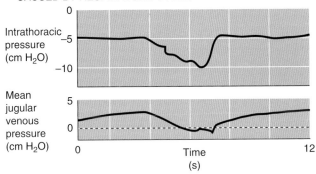

C VENOUS PRESSURE CHANGES IN FOOT
CAUSED BY MUSCLE CONTRACTION

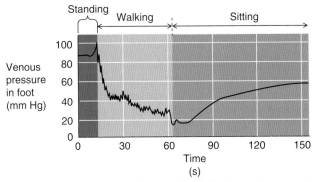

Figure 22.6 Venous pressure changes. In (A) the time scale is a single cardiac cycle. The relative heights of the peaks and valleys are variable. In (B) the time scale surrounds one protracted inspiration (i.e., several heartbeats); the y-axis in the lower panel shows the *mean* jugular venous pressure. (B, Data from Brecher GA: Venous Return. New York, Grune & Stratton, 1956; C, data from Pollack AA, Wood EH: Venous pressure in the saphenous vein at the ankle in man during exercise and changes in posture. J Appl Physiol 1:649–662, 1949.)

and posterior fascicle. Finally, the system of Purkinje fibers excites the ventricular myocytes, where the impulse propagates from cell to cell through gap junctions.

The right ventricle contracts like a bellows, whereas the left ventricle contracts like a hand squeezing a tube of toothpaste

The two ventricles share a common envelope of spiral and circular muscle layers. The arrangement of the spiral bundles ensures that ventricular contraction virtually wrings the blood out of the heart, although incompletely. The apex contracts before some of the basal portions of the ventricle,

a sequence that propels blood upward to the aortic and pulmonary valves.

The mechanical action of the **right ventricle** resembles that of a bellows used to fan a fire. Although the distance between the free wall and the septum is small, the free wall has such a large surface area that a small movement of the free wall toward the septum ejects a large volume.

The mechanical action of the **left ventricle** occurs by a dual motion: First, constriction of the *circular muscle layers* reduces the diameter of the chamber, progressing from apex to base, akin to squeezing a tube of toothpaste. Second, contraction of the *spiral muscles* pulls the mitral valve ring toward the apex, thereby shortening the long axis.

The contraction of the **atria** normally makes only a minor contribution to the filling of the two ventricles when the subject is at rest. However, the contraction of the atria is a useful safety factor during tachycardia, when the diastolic interval—and thus the time for passive filling—is short, the atrial contraction can provide a much-needed boost.

The right atrium contracts before the left, but the left ventricle contracts before the right

The timing of the events in the right and left heart is slightly different (Fig. 22.7).

Atrial Contraction Because the SA node is located in the right atrium, atrial contraction begins and ends earlier in the right atrium than in the left (Fig. 22.7, *"Contraction"* panel).

Initiation of Ventricular Contraction Ventricular contraction starts slightly earlier on the *left* side, and the mitral valve closes before the tricuspid valve (Fig. 22.7, *"Valve movements"* panel). On the other hand, the right ventricle has a briefer period of isovolumetric contraction because it does not need to build up as much pressure to open its semilunar (i.e., outflow) valve and to initiate ejection. Thus, the pulmonary valve opens slightly ahead of the aortic valve.

Ventricular Ejection Ejection from the right ventricle lasts longer than that from the left. The semilunar valves do not close simultaneously. The aortic valve, with its higher downstream pressure, closes before the pulmonary valve. Therefore, the pulmonary valve—with its lower downstream pressure—opens first and closes last. This timing difference in the closure of the semilunar valves explains the normal physiological splitting of S_2 (Fig. 22.7, *"Sounds"* panel).

Ventricular Relaxation Isovolumetric relaxation is briefer in the right heart than in the left. The pulmonary valve closes *after* the aortic valve, and the tricuspid valve opens *before* the mitral valve. Therefore, the right ventricle begins filling before the left.

Measurements of ventricular volumes, pressures, and flows allow clinicians to judge cardiac performance

Definitions of Cardiac Volumes The cardiac output is the product of heart rate and stroke volume (see Equation 17.6). The **stroke volume (SV)** is the difference between ventricular **end-diastolic volume (EDV)** and ventricular **end-systolic volume (ESV)**; that is, the difference between the maximal and minimal ventricular volumes. EDV is typically 120 mL, and ESV is 50 mL, so that

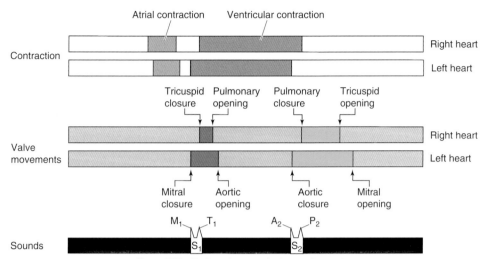

Figure 22.7 Timing of events in the cardiac cycle.

$$SV = EDV - ESV$$
$$= 120ml - 50ml$$
$$= 70ml \qquad \textbf{(22.2)}$$

◉ **22-2** The **ejection fraction (EF)** is a dimensionless value, defined as the SV normalized to the EDV:

$$EF = \frac{SV}{EDV} \qquad \textbf{(22.3)}$$

In our example, the EF is (70 mL)/(120 mL) or ~0.6. The value should exceed 55% in a healthy person.

Measurements of Cardiac Volumes Clinicians routinely measure the volumes of the cardiac chambers by means of angiography or echocardiography (see ◉ **17-8**). **One-dimensional (or M-mode) echocardiography** allows one to assess left ventricular performance in terms of linear dimensions and velocities by providing measurements of (1) velocity of the posterior left ventricular wall, (2) fractional shortening of the left ventricular circumference, and (3) rate of fractional circumferential shortening. **Two-dimensional echocardiography** makes it possible to determine several ventricular volumes:

- Left ventricular end-diastolic volume (LVEDV)
- Left ventricular end-systolic volume (LVESV)
- Stroke volume (SV = LVEDV – LVESV)
- Left ventricular ejection fraction (LVEF = SV/LVEDV)

Measurement of Ventricular Pressures For *right-sided heart catheterizations*, the physician advances the catheter percutaneously through a large systemic vein, into the right heart, and then into the pulmonary circulation, where the catheter tip literally *wedges* in a small pulmonary artery. Because a continuous and presumably closed column of blood connects the probe's end and the left atrium, the **wedge pressure** is taken as an index of left atrial pressure. For *left-sided heart catheterizations*, the physician inserts a catheter percutaneously into an artery and then advances the catheter tip upstream to the left heart.

Measurement of Flows The cardiologist can calculate flow from changes in ventricular volume, as measured by echocardiography and the Doppler ultrasound technique (see ◉ **17-10**), both of which measure the flow of blood in the outflow tract (i.e., aorta). Although the two ventricles expel on average the same *amount* of blood in a single cardiac cycle, the peak *velocity* is much higher in the left ventricle. In addition, the velocity rises far more rapidly in the left ventricle, which indicates greater acceleration of the blood during ejection. The *pressure* wave is about five times larger in the left ventricle than in the right, and the rate at which the pressure rises ($\Delta P/\Delta t$) is more rapid in the left ventricle.

The pressure-volume loop of a ventricle illustrates the ejection work of the ventricle

In Fig. 22.1, we saw separate plots of ventricular *pressure* against time and *volume* against time. If, at each point in time, we now plot pressure against volume, the result is a **pressure-volume loop,** as is shown in Fig. 22.8 for the left ventricle. This loop describes the relationship between left ventricular pressure and left ventricular volume during the cardiac cycle. Notice that, although *time* does not explicitly appear in this plot, as we make one complete counterclockwise cycle around the loop, we sequentially plot pressure and volume at all time points of one cardiac cycle—from point A to F and then back to A.

Segment AB Point A in Fig. 22.8 represents the instant at which the *mitral valve opens*. At this point, left ventricular volume is at its minimal value of ~50 mL, and left ventricular pressure is at the fairly low value of ~7 mm Hg. As the mitral valve opens, the ventricle begins to fill passively, because atrial pressure is higher than ventricular pressure. During interval AB, ventricular pressure falls slightly to ~5 mm Hg because the ventricular muscle is continuing to relax during diastole.

Segment BC During a second phase of ventricular filling, volume rises markedly from ~70 to ~120 mL, accompanied by a rather modest increase in pressure from ~5 to ~10 mm Hg. The modest rise in pressure, despite a doubling of ventricular volume ΔV, reflects the high compliance ($C = \Delta V/\Delta P$) of the ventricular wall during late diastole.

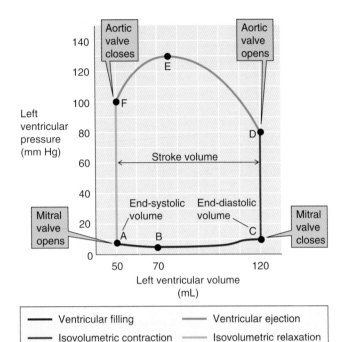

Figure 22.8 Pressure-volume loop of the left ventricle.

Segment CD Point C in Fig. 22.8 represents the *closure of the mitral valve.* At this point, ventricular filling has ended and **isovolumetric contraction**—represented by the vertical line CD—is about to begin. Thus, by the definition of *isovolumetric,* ventricular volume remains at 120 mL while left ventricular pressure rises to ~80 mm Hg, about equal to the aortic end-diastolic pressure.

Segment DE Point D in Fig. 22.8 represents the *opening of the aortic valve.* With the outlet to the aorta now open, the ventricular muscle can begin to shorten and to eject blood. During this period of rapid ejection, ventricular volume decreases from ~120 to ~75 mL. Notice that as contraction continues during interval DE, the ventricular pressure rises even farther, reaching a peak systolic value of ~130 mm Hg at point E.

Segment EF Point E in Fig. 22.8 represents the instant at which the ventricular muscle starts to relax. During this period of decreased ejection, ventricular pressure falls from ~130 to ~100 mm Hg. Nevertheless, blood continues to leave the ventricle, and ventricular volume falls from ~75 mL at point E to ~50 mL at point F. Point F represents end-systolic volume and pressure. Therefore, the stroke volume is substantially less than the maximum ventricular volume (i.e., EDV). The ejection fraction in this example is ~60%, which is in the normal range.

Segment FA Point F in Fig. 22.8 represents the *closing of the aortic valve.* At this point, ejection has ended and **isovolumetric relaxation** is about to begin. The ventricular volume remains at 50 mL, while left ventricular pressure falls from ~100 mm Hg at point F to ~7 mm Hg at point A. At the end of isovolumetric relaxation, the mitral valve opens and the cardiac cycle starts all over again with ventricular filling.

The six segments of the pressure-volume loop in Fig. 22.8 correspond to different phases of the cardiac cycle:
- *Phase 1,* the inflow phase, includes segments AB and BC.
- *Phase 2,* isovolumetric contraction, includes segment CD.
- *Phase 3,* the outflow phase, includes segments DE and EF.
- *Phase 4,* isovolumetric relaxation, includes segment FA.

Segments CDEF represent systole, whereas segments FABC represent diastole.

The "pumping work" done by the heart accounts for a small fraction of the total energy the heart consumes

The heart does its useful work as a pump by imparting momentum to the blood and propelling it against the resistance of the periphery.

Work, in its simplest definition, is the product of the force applied to an object and the distance the object moves ($W =$ force × distance). In considering **pressure-volume work,** the external work is

$$W = P \cdot \Delta V \qquad (22.4)$$

If the aortic pressure were constant, the work done with each heartbeat would be simply the product of the aortic pressure *(P)* and the stroke volume (ΔV = SV = EDV − ESV).

The pressure-volume relationships in Fig. 22.9 illustrate the pressure-volume work of the **left ventricle.** The surface below the *segment* ABC (i.e., filling phase) is the work done *by the blood.* The surface below DEF (i.e., ejection phase) is the work done *by the heart* on the blood during the ejection (Fig. 22.9B). The difference between the areas in Fig. 22.9A and B—that is, the area within the single-cycle loop—is the *net* external work done by the heart (Fig. 22.9C).

The pressure-volume diagram for the **right ventricle** has the same general shape. However, the area (i.e., *net* external work) is only about one fifth as large because the pressures are so much lower.

The area of the loop in Fig. 22.9C—that is, the pressure-volume work ($P \cdot V$)—ignores the speed at which the ventricle pumps the blood. The work per beat should also include the **kinetic energy** ($\frac{1}{2}mv^2$) that the heart imparts to the ejected blood:

$$\underbrace{W}_{\substack{\text{Total} \\ \text{external} \\ \text{work}}} = \underbrace{P \cdot V}_{\substack{\text{Pressure-} \\ \text{volume} \\ \text{work}}} + \underbrace{\frac{1}{2}mv^2}_{\substack{\text{Kinetic} \\ \text{energy}}} \qquad (22.5)$$

During the isovolumetric contraction, the ventricle develops and maintains a high pressure without performing any total external work, and the muscle breaks down ATP as long as it maintains isometric tension; the energy ends up as heat. This type of energy cost in heart muscle is called **tension heat,** which is proportional to the product of the tension of the ventricular wall *(T)* and the length of time (Δt) that the ventricle maintains this tension (i.e., tension-time integral). In the case of the heart, the pressure against which the ventricle must pump is a major determinant of the wall tension.

The total energy transformed in one cardiac cycle is the sum of the total external work done on the blood and the tension heat:

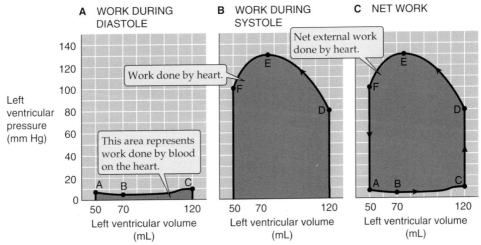

Figure 22.9 External work of the left ventricle.

$$E = \underbrace{P \cdot V}_{\substack{\text{Pressure-}\\\text{volume}\\\text{work}}} + \underbrace{\tfrac{1}{2}mv^2}_{\substack{\text{Kinetic}\\\text{energy}}} + \underbrace{k \cdot T \cdot \Delta t}_{\substack{\text{Tension}\\\text{heat}}} \qquad \textbf{(22.6)}$$

$$\underbrace{\phantom{P \cdot V + \tfrac{1}{2}mv^2 + k \cdot T \cdot \Delta t}}_{\text{Total external work}}$$

where k is a proportionality constant that converts $T \cdot \Delta t$ into units of energy. The tension heat is the *major* determinant of the total energy requirements of the heart.

The tension heat is not only far more costly for the heart than the pressure-volume work but also of considerable practical interest for the patient with coronary artery disease who wishes to step up cardiac output during increased physical activity. It is advantageous to the patient to have a low wall tension *(T)*—that is, a low blood pressure—and not to spend too much time (Δt) in systole. The heart spends a greater fraction of its time in systole when the heart rate is high. Thus, the cardiac patient is better off to increase cardiac output at low pressure and low heart rate (i.e., a low $T \cdot \Delta t$ product). The only option left is to increase stroke volume.

The ratio of the ventricle's total external work ($P \cdot V + \tfrac{1}{2}mv^2$) to the total energy cost (i.e., W/E) is the heart's **mechanical efficiency.** Note that the mechanical efficiency has nothing to do with how effective the ventricle is at expelling blood (i.e., ejection fraction).

FROM CONTRACTILE FILAMENTS TO A REGULATED PUMP

In Chapter 9, we examined the general features of muscle contraction and compared the properties of skeletal, cardiac, and smooth muscle. Here, we examine how some of the features of cardiac muscle underlie cardiac performance.

The entry of Ca²⁺ from the outside triggers Ca²⁺–induced Ca²⁺ release from the sarcoplasmic reticulum

Excitation-contraction (EC) coupling in cardiac ventricular myocytes (see ◉ 9-11) is similar to EC coupling in skeletal muscle (see ◉ 9-2). In the ventricular myocyte, action potentials in adjacent myocytes depolarize the target cell through gap junctions (see ◉ 21-2) and thereby generate an action potential.

The depolarization of the plasma membrane in the ventricular myocyte invades T tubules that run radially to the long axis of the myocyte, and *axial* T tubules that run parallel to the long axis of the cell and interconnect adjacent radial T tubules.

Ca^{2+} entry through the L-type Ca^{2+} channel Cav1.2 (Fig. 22.10, *black arrow No. 1*) in the cardiac plasma membrane is essential for raising $[Ca^{2+}]_i$ in the vicinity of the RYR2 Ca^{2+}-release channels on the sarcoplasmic reticulum (SR), and causing them to release Ca^{2+} locally into the cytoplasm by **Ca²⁺-induced Ca²⁺ release** (**CICR**; Fig. 22.10, *black arrow No. 2*). The CICR mechanism is a robust amplification system whereby the local influx of Ca^{2+} from small clusters of L-type Cav channels in the plasma membrane triggers the coordinated release of Ca^{2+} from the high-capacity Ca^{2+} stores of the SR. Such single CICR events can raise $[Ca^{2+}]_i$ to as high as 10 μM in microdomains of ~1 μm in diameter. These localized increases in $[Ca^{2+}]_i$ appear as **calcium sparks** when monitored with a Ca^{2+}-sensitive dye by confocal microscopy. If many L-type Ca^{2+} channels open simultaneously in ventricular myocytes, the spatial and temporal summation of many elementary Ca^{2+} sparks leads to a global increase in $[Ca^{2+}]_i$ that lasts longer than the action potential (compare *blue* and *gray curves* in inset in Fig. 22.10) because the RYR Ca^{2+}-release channels remain open for a longer time than L-type Ca^{2+} channels.

A global rise in [Ca²⁺]ᵢ initiates contraction of cardiac myocytes

After $[Ca^{2+}]_i$ increases, Ca^{2+} binds to the cardiac isoform of troponin C (TNNC1, see ◉ 9-5), and the Ca^{2+}-TNNC1 complex releases the inhibition of the cardiac isoform of troponin I (TNNI3) on actin. As a result, the tropomyosin (TPM1) filaments bound to cardiac troponin T (TNNT2) on the thin filament shift out of the way, allowing myosin to interact with active sites on the actin. ATP fuels the subsequent cross-bridge cycling (see Fig. 9.6). Because the heart can never rest, cardiac myocytes have a very high density of

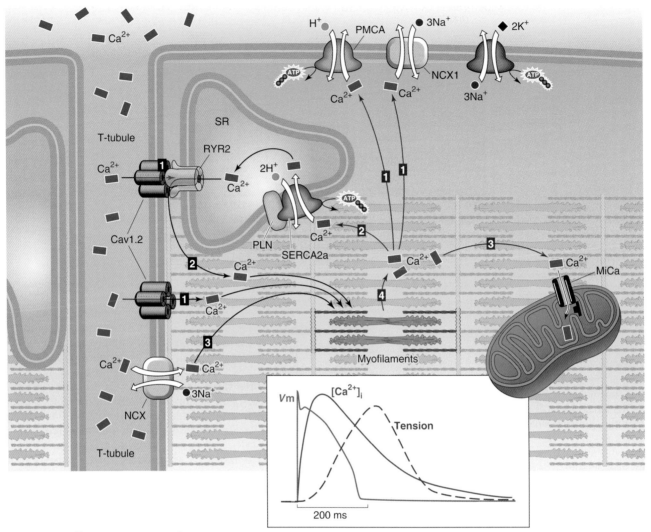

Figure 22.10 Role of Ca^{2+} in cardiac contraction. The *inset* pertains to ventricular myocytes. V_m, Membrane potential.

mitochondria and thus are capable of sustaining very high rates of ATP synthesis.

The cross-bridge cycling causes thick filaments to slide past thin filaments, generating tension. The time course of cardiac tension development is delayed relative to the time course of the global surge in $[Ca^{2+}]_i$ (compare *red* and *blue curves* in inset of Fig. 22.10).

For heart muscle, which wraps around the ventricle, the length parameter in a length-tension diagram can be either the ventricular volume, which is analogous to whole-muscle length, or the sarcomere length. The sarcomere, stretching from one Z line to another, is the functional unit in cardiac muscle.

⊙ 22-3 Phosphorylation of phospholamban and of troponin I speeds cardiac muscle relaxation

With the waning of the phase 2 plateau of the cardiac action potential (Fig. 21.4B, top panel), the influx of Ca^{2+} through L-type Ca^{2+} channels decreases, which lessens the release of Ca^{2+} by the SR. By itself, halting of Ca^{2+} entry and release can only prevent a further increase in $[Ca^{2+}]_i$. The actual relaxation

of the contractile proteins depends on four processes: (1) extrusion of Ca^{2+} into the extracellular fluid (ECF), (2) reuptake of Ca^{2+} from the cytosol by the SR, (3) uptake of Ca^{2+} from the cytosol into the mitochondria, and (4) dissociation of Ca^{2+} from troponin C. Processes 2 and 4 are highly regulated.

Extrusion of Ca^{2+} Into the ECF Even during the plateau of the action potential, the myocyte extrudes some Ca^{2+}. After the membrane potential returns to more negative values, Ca^{2+} extrusion (Fig. 22.10, *red arrow No. 1*) gains the upper hand and $[Ca^{2+}]_i$ falls. This extrusion of Ca^{2+} into the ECF occurs by two pathways: (1) a sarcolemmal Na-Ca exchanger (NCX1), which operates at relatively high levels of $[Ca^{2+}]_i$; and (2) a sarcolemmal Ca pump (cardiac subtypes 1, 2, and 4 of plasma-membrane Ca ATPase, or PMCA), which may function at even low levels of $[Ca^{2+}]_i$.

Reuptake of Ca^{2+} by the SR Even during the plateau of the action potential, some of the Ca^{2+} accumulating in the cytoplasm is sequestered into the SR (Fig. 22.10, *red arrow No. 2*) by the cardiac subtype of the sarcoplasmic and endoplasmic reticulum Ca pump SERCA2a (see ⊙ 5-11). **Phospholamban (PLN),** an integral SR membrane protein with a single transmembrane segment, is an important regulator of SERCA2a.

In SR membranes of cardiac, smooth, and slow-twitch skeletal muscle, unphosphorylated PLN can exist as a homopentamer. The dissociation of the pentamer allows the hydrophilic cytoplasmic domain of PLN monomers to inhibit SERCA2a. However, phosphorylation of PLN by any of several kinases relieves PLN's inhibition of SERCA2a, allowing Ca^{2+} resequestration to accelerate. The net effect of phosphorylation is an increase in the rate of cardiac muscle relaxation.

Phosphorylation of PLN by protein kinase A (PKA) explains why β_1-adrenergic agonists (e.g., epinephrine), which act through the PKA pathway (see ⊙ 3-9), speed up the relaxation of cardiac muscle. Phosphoprotein phosphatase 1 (PP1) dephosphorylates PLN, thereby terminating Ca^{2+} reuptake.

Uptake of Ca^{2+} by Mitochondria The mitochondria take up a minor fraction of the Ca^{2+} accumulating in the cytoplasm (Fig. 22.10, *red arrow No. 3*). The inner mitochondrial membrane contains large-conductance, highly selective Ca^{2+} channels (MiCas) that are inwardly rectifying. At potentials of –160 mV, which are typical for energized mitochondria, the MiCa channels carry a substantial Ca^{2+} current. Unlike many other Ca^{2+} channels, MiCa does not inactivate as intramitochondrial $[Ca^{2+}]$ rises to micromolar concentrations.

Dissociation of Ca^{2+} from Troponin C As $[Ca^{2+}]_i$ falls, Ca^{2+} dissociates from troponin C (Fig. 22.10, *red arrow No. 4*; see ⊙ 9-5), blocking actin-myosin interactions and causing relaxation. β_1-adrenergic agonists accelerate relaxation by promoting phosphorylation of troponin I, which in turn enhances the dissociation of Ca^{2+} from troponin C.

The overlap of thick and thin filaments cannot explain the unusual shape of the cardiac length-tension diagram

The **passive length-tension diagrams** for skeletal and cardiac muscle are quite different. The passive tension of cardiac muscle (Fig. 22.11A, *violet curve*) begins to rise at much lower sarcomere lengths and rises much more steeply. As a result, cardiac muscle will break if it is stretched beyond a sarcomere length of 2.6 μm.

The reason for the higher passive tension is that the noncontractile (i.e., elastic) components of cardiac muscle are less distensible. The most important elastic component is the giant protein **titin** (see ⊙ 9-7), which acts as a spring that provides the opposing force during stretch and the restoring force during shortening (see Fig. 9.9C).

The **active length-tension diagrams** also differ between skeletal and cardiac muscle. In cardiac muscle (Fig. 22.11A, *brown curve*), active tension has a relatively sharp peak when the muscle is prestretched to an initial sarcomere length of ~2.4 μm. As the prestretched sarcomere length increases from 1.8 to 2.4 μm, active tension rises steeply. The rise in tension at longer sarcomere lengths in cardiac muscle probably has two general causes: (1) Raising the sarcomere length above 1.8 μm increases the Ca^{2+} sensitivity of the myofilaments. One mechanism controlling the Ca^{2+} sensitivity may be interfilament spacing between thick and thin filaments. As we stretch the muscle to greater sarcomere lengths, the lateral filament lattice spacing is less than in an unstretched fiber so that the probability of cross-bridge interaction increases. Increased cross-bridge formation in turn increases the Ca^{2+} affinity of TNNC1, thereby recruiting more cross-bridges

and therefore producing greater force. Another mechanism could be that, as the muscle elongates, increased strain on titin either alters lattice spacing or alters the packing of myosin molecules within the thick filament. (2) Raising the sarcomere length above 1.8 μm increases tension on stretch-activated Ca^{2+} channels, thereby increasing Ca^{2+} entry from the ECF and thus enhancing Ca^{2+}-induced Ca^{2+} release.

As cardiac sarcomere length increases above 2.4 μm, active tension declines precipitously. This fall-off does not reflect a problem in the overlap of thin and thick filaments. Instead, titin increases the passive *stiffness* of cardiac muscle and may also impede development of *active tension* at high sarcomere lengths.

Starling's law states that a greater fiber length (i.e., greater ventricular volume) causes the heart to deliver more mechanical energy

⊙ **22-4 Starling's Law** states that "the mechanical energy set free on passage from the resting to the contracted state depends on the area of 'chemically active surfaces,' i.e., on the length of the fibers." Therefore, the initial length of myocardial fibers determines the work done during the cardiac cycle. Starling assumed that the initial *length* of the myocardial fibers is proportional to the end-diastolic volume, and that *tension* in the myocardial fibers is proportional to the systolic pressure. Fig. 22.11B shows how end-diastolic volume (length) determines systolic pressure (tension).

Starling's diagram for *systole* (Fig. 22.11B, *red curve*) is more or less equivalent to the ascending phase of the *active* length-tension diagram for cardiac muscle (Fig. 22.11A, *brown curve*). Therefore, Starling's systole curve shows that the heart is able to generate more pressure (i.e., deliver more blood) when more is presented to it.

A **ventricular performance curve** (Fig. 22.11C) is another representation of Starling's length-tension diagram, but it is one a clinician can obtain for a patient. The curve shows stroke work ($P \cdot \Delta V$, see Equation 22.4, which includes Starling's systolic pressure (itself an estimate of muscle tension) on the y-axis, plotted against left atrial pressure, which corresponds to Starling's end-diastolic volume (itself an estimate of muscle length), on the x-axis. The Starling's law *is not a fixed relationship*. For instance, the norepinephrine released during sympathetic stimulation—which increases myocardial contractility (as we will see below in this chapter)—steepens the performance curve and shifts it upward and to the left (see *brown arrow* in Fig. 22.11C). Similar shifts occur with other **positive inotropic** agents (e.g., cardiac glycosides), that is, drugs that increase myocardial contractility. Note also that ventricular performance curves show no descending component because sarcomere length does not increase beyond 2.2 to 2.4 μm in healthy hearts.

The velocity of cardiac muscle shortening falls when the contraction occurs against a greater opposing force (or pressure) or at a shorter muscle length (or lower volume)

The functional properties of cardiac muscle—how much tension it can develop, how rapidly it can contract—depend on

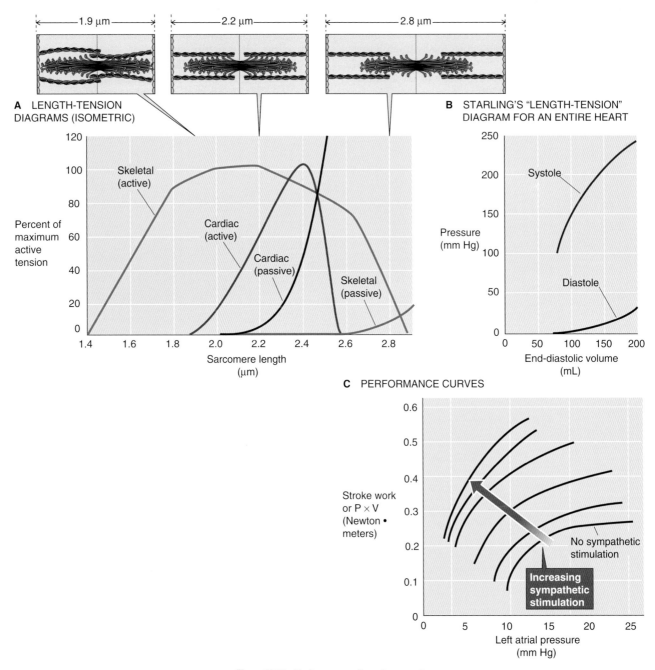

A LENGTH-TENSION DIAGRAMS (ISOMETRIC)

B STARLING'S "LENGTH-TENSION" DIAGRAM FOR AN ENTIRE HEART

C PERFORMANCE CURVES

Figure 22.11 Performance of cardiac muscle.

many factors, but especially on two properties intrinsic to the cardiac myocyte.

1. *Initial sarcomere length.* For the beating heart, a convenient index of initial sarcomere length is *EDV*. Both initial sarcomere length and EDV are measures of the **preload** imposed on the cardiac muscle *just before* it ejects blood from the ventricle during systole. *Starling's law,* in which the independent variable is EDV, focuses on preload.

2. ⊙ **22-5** *Force that the contracting myocytes must overcome.* In the beating heart, a convenient index of opposing force is the *arterial pressure* that opposes the outflow of blood from the ventricle. Both opposing force and arterial

pressure are measures of the **afterload** the ventricular muscle must overcome *as* it ejects blood during systole.

In Fig. 22.12A, we plot the velocities of muscle shortening as a function of afterload. The purple, blue, and red points on the load-velocity curve represent three different degrees of afterload. The velocity of muscle shortening corresponds to the outflow velocity of the ventricle. Thus, at higher opposing arterial pressures (afterload) the outflow velocity should decrease. The *black curve* in Fig. 22.12A applies to a muscle that we stretched only slightly in the preload phase (i.e., low preload). The *red curve* shows a similar load-velocity relationship for a muscle that we stretched greatly in the preload

A LOAD-VELOCITY DIAGRAM

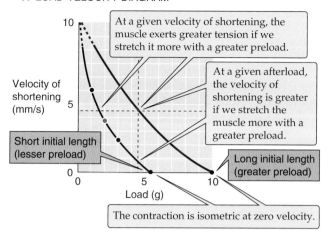

At a given velocity of shortening, the muscle exerts greater tension if we stretch it more with a greater preload.

At a given afterload, the velocity of shortening is greater if we stretch the muscle more with a greater preload.

Velocity of shortening (mm/s)

Short initial length (lesser preload)

Long initial length (greater preload)

Load (g)

The contraction is isometric at zero velocity.

B VELOCITY-LENGTH DIAGRAM

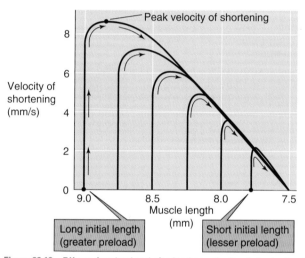

Peak velocity of shortening

Velocity of shortening (mm/s)

Muscle length (mm)

Long initial length (greater preload)

Short initial length (lesser preload)

Figure 22.12 Effect of preload and afterload on velocity of shortening. (A) Velocity as a function of load. (B) Velocity as a function of muscle length.

phase (i.e., high preload). In both cases, the velocity of shortening increases as the tension (i.e., afterload) falls.

When the afterload is so large that no shortening ever occurs, that afterload is the **isometric tension,** shown as the point of zero velocity on the x-axis of Fig. 22.12A. As expected from Starling's law, the greater the initial stretch (i.e., preload), the greater the isometric tension. In fact, at *any* velocity (*dashed horizontal line*), the tension is greater in the muscle that was stretched more in the preload phase (*red curve*)—a restatement of Starling's law.

In summary, at a given preload (i.e., walking up the *black curve* in Fig. 22.12A), the velocity of shortening for cardiac muscle becomes greater with lower afterloads (i.e., opposing pressure). Conversely, at a given afterload—that is, comparing the black and red curves for any common *x* value (dashed vertical line)—the velocity of shortening for cardiac muscle becomes greater with a greater preload (i.e., sarcomere length).

Finally, the curves in Fig. 22.12A do not represent a fixed set of relationships. Positive inotropic agents shift all curves up and to the right. Thus, a positive inotropic agent allows

the heart to achieve a given velocity against a greater load, or to push a given load with a greater velocity.

Another way of representing how velocity of shortening depends on the initial muscle length (i.e., preload) is to monitor velocity of shortening during a single isotonic contraction. If we first apply a large preload to stretch a piece of muscle to an initial length of 9.0 mm (Fig. 22.12B) and then stimulate it, the velocity instantly rises to a peak value of ~8.5 mm/s; it then gradually falls to zero as the muscle shortens to 7.5 mm. If we start by applying a smaller preload, thereby stretching the muscle to an initial length of 8.5 or 8.0 mm, the peak velocity falls. Thus, initial length determines not only the tension that cardiac muscle can generate, but also the speed with which the muscle can shorten.

Increases in heart rate enhance myocardial tension

⊙ **22-6** Heart muscle tension has a special dependence on the frequency of contraction. If we stimulate isolated heart muscle only a few times per minute, the tension developed is much smaller than if we stimulate it at a physiological rate of 70 times per minute. The progressive rise of tension after an increase in rate is defined as positive **staircase phenomenon.** Underlying the staircase phenomenon is an increase in SR Ca^{2+} content and release. The larger SR Ca^{2+} content has three causes. First, during each action potential plateau, more Ca^{2+} enters the cell through Cav1.2 L-type Ca^{2+} channels, and the larger number of action potentials per minute provides a longer aggregate period of Ca^{2+} entry through these channels. Second, the depolarization during the plateau of an action potential causes the Na-Ca exchanger NCX1 to operate in the reverse mode, allowing Ca^{2+} to enter the cell. At higher heart rates, these depolarizations occur more frequently and are accompanied by an increase in $[Na^+]_i$, which accentuates the reversal of NCX1, both of which enhance Ca^{2+} uptake. Third, the increased heart rate stimulates SERCA2a, thereby sequestering in the SR the Ca^{2+} that entered the cell because of the first two mechanisms. The mechanism of this stimulation is that the rising $[Ca^{2+}]_i$, through calmodulin (CaM), activates CaM kinase II, which leads to phosphorylation of PLN; phosphorylation of PLN in turn enhances SERCA2a.

Contractility is an intrinsic measure of cardiac performance

Now that we know that the performance of the heart depends on such factors as degree of filling (i.e., preload), arterial pressure (i.e., afterload), and heart rate, it would be useful to have a measure of the heart's *intrinsic* contractile performance, independent of these *extrinsic* factors. **Contractility** is such a measure. Clinically, it is a useful term to distinguish a better-performing heart from a poorly performing one. In a patient, one clinically useful measure of contractility is the ejection fraction (see ⊙ **22-2**). However, according to Starling's law, ejection depends on EDV (i.e., preload), which is *external* to the heart. Two somewhat better gauges of contractility are the **rate of pressure development** during ejection ($\Delta P/\Delta t$) and the **velocity of ejection.** Both correlate well with velocity of shortening in Fig. 22.12A and B, and they are very sensitive guides to the effect of inotropic interventions.

Positive inotropic agents increase myocardial contractility by raising [Ca^{2+}]$_i$

⊙ **22-7** Modifiers of contractility can affect the dynamics of cardiac muscle contraction independent of preload or afterload. These factors have in common their ability to change [Ca^{2+}]$_i$. When these factors increase myocardial contractility, they are called positive inotropic agents. When they decrease myocardial contractility, they are called negative inotropic agents.

Positive Inotropic Agents Factors that increase myocardial contractility increase [Ca^{2+}]$_i$, either by opening Ca^{2+} channels, inhibiting Na-Ca exchange, or inhibiting the Ca pump—all at the plasma membrane.

1. *Adrenergic agonists.* Catecholamines (e.g., epinephrine, norepinephrine) act on β_1 adrenoceptors to activate the α subunit of G_s-type heterotrimeric G proteins. The activated α_s subunits produce effects by two pathways. First, α_s raises intracellular levels of cAMP and stimulates PKA (see ⊙ **3-9**), which can phosphorylate several targets and thereby increase contractility and speed relaxation. Second, α_s can directly open L-type Ca^{2+} channels in the plasma membrane, which leads to an increased Ca^{2+} influx during action potentials, increased [Ca^{2+}]$_i$, and enhanced contractility.

2. *Cardiac glycosides.* Digitalis derivatives inhibit the Na-K pump on the plasma membrane (see ⊙ **5-7**) and therefore raise [Na^+]$_i$. The increased [Na^+]$_i$ will slow down the Na-Ca exchanger NCX1, to raise steady-state [Ca^{2+}]$_i$, and to enhance contractility. In addition, cardiac glycosides may also increase [Ca^{2+}]$_i$ by a novel pathway—increasing the Ca^{2+} permeability of Na^+ channels in the plasma membrane.

3. *High extracellular [Ca^{2+}].* Acting in two ways, elevated [Ca^{2+}]$_o$ increases [Ca^{2+}]$_i$ and thereby enhances contractility. First, it decreases the exchange of external Na^+ for internal Ca^{2+}. Second, more Ca^{2+} enters the myocardial cell through L-type Ca^{2+} channels during the action potential.

4. *Low extracellular [Na^+].* Reducing the Na^+ gradient decreases Ca^{2+} extrusion through NCX1, raising [Ca^{2+}]$_i$ and enhancing contractility.

5. *Increased heart rate.* ⊙ **22-8** As we noted in introducing the staircase phenomenon (see ⊙ **22-6**), an increased heart rate increases SR stores of Ca^{2+} and also increases Ca^{2+} influx during the action potential.

Negative Inotropic Agents Factors that decrease myocardial contractility all decrease [Ca^{2+}]$_i$.

1. *Ca^{2+}-channel blockers.* Inhibitors of L-type Ca^{2+} channels (see ⊙ **7-5**)—such as verapamil, diltiazem, and nifedipine—reduce Ca^{2+} entry during the plateau of the cardiac action potential. By reducing [Ca^{2+}]$_i$, they decrease contractility.

2. *Low extracellular [Ca^{2+}].* Depressed [Ca^{2+}]$_o$ lowers [Ca^{2+}]$_i$, both by increasing Ca^{2+} extrusion through NCX1 and by reducing Ca^{2+} entry through L-type Ca^{2+} channels during the plateau of the cardiac action potential.

3. *High extracellular [Na^+].* Elevated [Na^+]$_o$ increases Ca^{2+} extrusion through NCX1, thereby decreasing [Ca^{2+}]$_i$.

CHAPTER 23

REGULATION OF ARTERIAL PRESSURE AND CARDIAC OUTPUT

Emile L. Boulpaep

In this chapter, we focus on blood pressure, a critical hemo-dynamic factor necessary for proper organ perfusion. Too low, and we say that the patient is in shock. Too high, and we say that the patient is hypertensive; an acute and profound elevation of the blood pressure can be just as dangerous as a sudden plummeting of blood pressure. Here, we examine both the short- and long-term mechanisms that the body uses to regulate arterial blood pressure.

SHORT-TERM REGULATION OF ARTERIAL PRESSURE

Systemic mean arterial blood pressure is the principal variable that the cardiovascular system controls

Because of the anatomy of the circulatory system, all organs, whether close to or distant from the heart, receive the same mean arterial pressure. Each organ, in turn, controls local blood flow by increasing or decreasing local arteriolar resistance. Hence, a change in blood flow in one vascular bed does not affect blood flow in other beds—as long as the heart can maintain the mean arterial pressure. However, the circulatory system must keep mean arterial pressure not only *constant* but also *high enough* for glomerular filtration to occur in the kidneys or to overcome high tissue pressures in organs such as the eye.

The short-term regulation of arterial pressure—on a time scale of seconds to minutes—occurs via neural pathways and targets the heart, vessels, and adrenal medulla. This short-term regulation is the topic of the present discussion. The long-term regulation of arterial pressure—on a time scale of hours or days—occurs via pathways that target the blood vessels, as well as the kidneys, in their control of extracellular fluid (ECF) volume.

Neural reflexes mediate the short-term regulation of mean arterial blood pressure

The neural reflex systems that regulate mean arterial pressure operate as a series of negative-feedback loops. All such loops are composed of the following elements:

1. **A detector.** A sensor or receptor quantitates the controlled variable and transduces it into an electrical signal that is a measure of the controlled variable.
2. **Afferent neural pathways.** These convey the message away from the detector, to the central nervous system (CNS).

3. **A coordinating center.** A control center in the CNS compares the signal detected in the periphery to a set-point, generates an error signal, processes the information, and generates a message that encodes the appropriate response.
4. **Efferent neural pathways.** These convey the message from the coordinating center to the periphery.
5. **Effectors.** These elements execute the appropriate response and alter the controlled variable, thereby correcting its deviation from the set-point.

A dual system of sensors and neural reflexes controls mean arterial pressure. The primary sensors are baroreceptors, which detect distention of the vascular walls. The secondary sensors are chemoreceptors that detect changes in blood P_{O_2}, P_{CO_2}, and pH. The control centers are located within the CNS, mostly in the medulla, but also within the cerebral cortex and hypothalamus. The effectors include the pacemaker and muscle cells in the heart, the vascular smooth-muscle cells (VSMCs) in arteries and veins, and the adrenal medulla.

We all know from common experience that the CNS influences the circulation. Emotional stress can cause blushing of the skin or an increase in heart rate, pain or stress can elicit fainting because of a profound, generalized vasodilation and a decrease in heart rate (i.e., bradycardia). Similarly, stimulation of peripheral sympathetic nerves causes vasoconstriction, whereas interruption of the spinal cord in the lower cervical region drastically reduces blood pressure (i.e., produces hypotension). On the other hand, stimulation of the central (i.e., cranial) end of the vagus nerve or the central end of the sinus nerve (nerve of Hering), which innervates the carotid sinus—causes bradycardia and hypotension. These observations suggest that the depressor and sinus nerves carry sensory information to the brain and the brain uses this information to control cardiovascular function.

⊙ 23-1 High-pressure baroreceptors at the carotid sinus and aortic arch are stretch receptors that sense changes in arterial pressure

The entire control process, known as the **baroreceptor control of arterial pressure** (Fig. 23.1), consists of baroreceptors (i.e., the detectors), afferent neuronal pathways, control centers in the medulla, efferent neuronal pathways, and the heart and blood vessels (i.e., the effectors). The negative-feedback

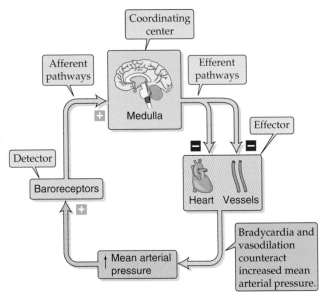

Figure 23.1 Baroreceptor control of arterial pressure. Here, we assume that an increase in mean arterial pressure *(violet box)* is the primary insult.

loop is designed so that *increased mean arterial pressure causes vasodilation and bradycardia,* whereas *decreased mean arterial pressure causes vasoconstriction and tachycardia* (i.e., increased heart rate).

⊙ 23-2 The sensor component consists of a set of mechanoreceptors located at strategic *high-pressure sites* within the cardiovascular system. The cardiovascular system also has *low-pressure* sensors that detect changes in venous pressure. The two most important high-pressure loci are the carotid sinus and the aortic arch. Stretching of the vessel walls at either of these sites causes vasodilation and bradycardia. The **carotid sinus** (Fig. 23.2A) is a very distensible portion of the wall of the internal carotid artery located just above the branching of the common carotid artery into the external and internal carotid arteries. The **aortic arch** (Fig. 23.2B) is also a highly compliant portion of the arterial tree that distends during each left ventricular ejection.

The baroreceptors in both the carotid sinus and the aortic arch are the branched and varicose (or coiled) terminals of myelinated and unmyelinated sensory nerve fibers, which are intermeshed within the elastic layers. An increase in the transmural pressure difference enlarges the vessel and thereby deforms the receptors. Baroreceptors are *stretch sensitive.* Direct stretching of the receptor results in increased firing of the baroreceptor's sensory nerve.

As shown by the red records in the upper two panels of Fig. 23.3A, a step increase in transmural pressure (i.e., stretch) produces an inward current that depolarizes the receptor, generating a **receptor potential** (see ⊙ **15-1**).

These sensory neurons are *bipolar neurons* (see ⊙ **10-1**) whose cell bodies are located in ganglia near the brainstem. The central ends of these neurons project to the medulla. The cell bodies of the aortic baroreceptor neurons are located in the nodose ganglion (a sensory ganglion of the vagus nerve.

⊙ 23-3 Increased arterial pressure raises the firing rate of afferent baroreceptor nerves

Graded increases in pressure produce graded depolarizations, resulting in graded increases in the spike frequency (Fig. 23.3A, *lower two panels*). Graded *decreases* in pressure gradually diminish receptor activity until the firing falls to vanishingly low frequencies at pressures around 40 to 60 mm Hg. Therefore, the baroreceptor encodes the mechanical response as a frequency-modulated signal.

A step increase in pressure generates a large initial depolarization, accompanied by a transient high-frequency discharge. The smaller steady depolarization is accompanied by a steady but lower spike frequency. Because baroreceptors have both a dynamic and a static response, they are sensitive to both the *waveform* and the *amplitude* of a pressure oscillation. Therefore, bursts of action potentials occurring in phase with the cardiac cycle encode information on the pulse pressure (i.e., difference between the peak systolic and lowest diastolic pressures). The **static** pressure-activity curve in Fig. 23.3B shows that the spike frequency rises sigmoidally with increases in *steady* blood pressure. The **pulsatile** pressure-activity curve in Fig. 23.3B shows that when the pressure is *oscillating,* the mean discharge frequency at low mean pressures is higher than when pressure is steady.

Not all arterial receptors have the same properties. As we gradually increase intravascular pressure, different single units in the isolated carotid sinus begin to fire at different static pressures. Thus, the overall baroreceptor response to a pressure increase includes both an increased firing rate of active units and the **recruitment** of more units, until a saturation level is reached at ~200 mm Hg.

Once a change in the arterial pressure has produced a change in the firing rate of the sensory nerve, the signal travels to the medulla. The afferent pathway for the carotid sinus reflex is the **sinus nerve,** which then joins the **glossopharyngeal** trunk (cranial nerve [CN] IX; see Fig. 23.2A). The cell bodies of the carotid baroreceptors are located in the petrosal (or inferior) ganglion of the glossopharyngeal nerve. The afferent pathways for the aortic arch reflex are sensory fibers in the **depressor branch** of the **vagus nerve** (CN X; Fig. 23.2B). After joining the superior laryngeal nerves, the sensory fibers run cranially to their cell bodies in the nodose (or inferior) ganglion of the vagus.

The medulla coordinates afferent baroreceptor signals

⊙ **23-4** The entire complex of medullary nuclei involved in cardiovascular regulation is called the medullary cardiovascular center. Within this center, broad subdivisions can be distinguished, such as a vasomotor area and a cardioinhibitory area. The medullary cardiovascular center receives all important information from the baroreceptors and is the major coordinating center for cardiovascular homeostasis.

⊙ **23-5** Most afferent fibers from the two high-pressure baroreceptors project to the **nucleus tractus solitarii (NTS),** one of which is located on each side of the dorsal medulla (Fig. 23.4).

⊙ **23-6** *Inhibitory* interneurons project from the NTS onto the **vasomotor area** in the ventrolateral medulla (Fig. 23.4).

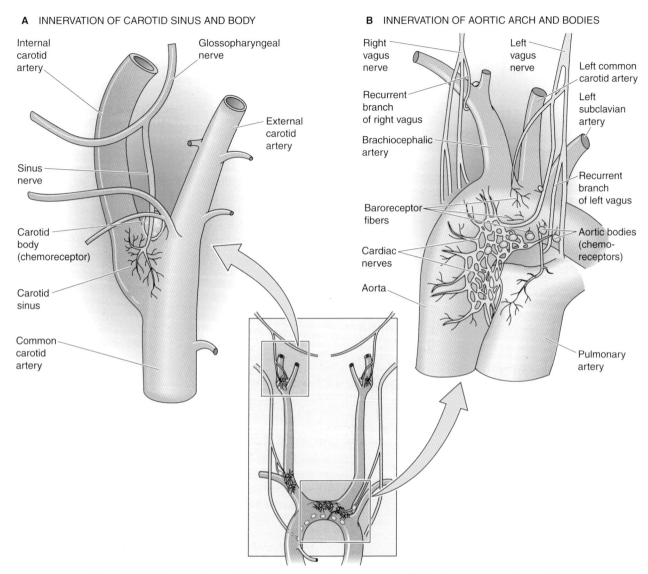

A INNERVATION OF CAROTID SINUS AND BODY

Internal carotid artery

Glossopharyngeal nerve

External carotid artery

Sinus nerve

Carotid body (chemoreceptor)

Carotid sinus

Common carotid artery

B INNERVATION OF AORTIC ARCH AND BODIES

Right vagus nerve

Left vagus nerve

Left common carotid artery

Recurrent branch of right vagus

Brachiocephalic artery

Left subclavian artery

Baroreceptor fibers

Recurrent branch of left vagus

Cardiac nerves

Aortic bodies (chemo-receptors)

Aorta

Pulmonary artery

Figure 23.2 Afferent pathways of the high-pressure baroreceptors. In (B) the chemoreceptors (i.e., aortic bodies) are located on the underside of the aortic arch as well as—on the right side of the body—at the bifurcation of the right brachiocephalic artery. On the left side of the body, aortic bodies, if present, are in a notch between the left common carotid artery and the left subclavian artery.

This vasomotor area includes the A1 and C1 areas in the rostral ventrolateral medulla, as well as the inferior olivary complex and other nuclei. Stimulation of the neurons in the **C1 area** produces a vasoconstrictor response. Unless inhibited by output from the NTS interneurons, neurons within the C1 area produce a tonic output that promotes vasoconstriction. Therefore, an increase in pressure stimulates baroreceptor firing, which, in turn, causes NTS interneurons to inhibit C1 neurons, resulting in vaso*dilation*. This C1 pathway largely accounts for the *vascular* component of the baroreceptor reflex. The bursting pattern of C1 neurons is locked to the cardiac cycle.

Excitatory interneurons project from the NTS onto a **cardioinhibitory area,** which includes the **nucleus ambiguus** and the **dorsal motor nucleus of the vagus** (Fig. 23.4). Neurons in the dorsal motor nucleus of the vagus largely account for the *cardiac* component of the baroreceptor

reflex (i.e., bradycardia). Some *inhibitory* interneurons probably project from the NTS onto a **cardioacceleratory** area, also located in the dorsal medulla. Stimulation of neurons in this area causes heart rate and cardiac contractility to increase.

⊙ 23-7 The efferent pathways of the baroreceptor response include both sympathetic and parasympathetic divisions of the autonomic nervous system

After the medullary cardiovascular center has processed the information from the afferent baroreceptor pathways and integrated it with data coming from other pathways, this center must send signals back to the periphery via efferent (i.e., motor) pathways. The baroreceptor response has two major efferent pathways: the sympathetic and parasympathetic divisions of the autonomic nervous system.

A RESPONSE TO INCREASED PRESSURE

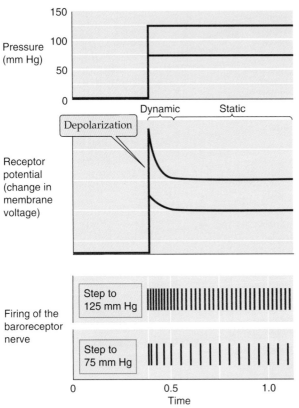

B PRESSURE-ACTIVITY RELATIONSHIPS

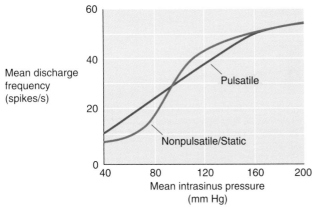

Figure 23.3 Afferent pathways of the high-pressure baroreceptors. In (A) the records refer to hypothetical experiments on a baroreceptor in which one suddenly raises blood pressure to 75 mm Hg *(purple)* or to 125 mm Hg *(red)*. In (B) the records refer to results from the carotid sinus nerve. Data from Chapleau MW, Abboud FM: Contrasting effects of static and pulsatile pressure on carotid baroreceptor activity in dogs. Circ Res 61:648–658, 1987.

Sympathetic Efferents Increased baroreceptor activity instructs the NTS to *inhibit* the C1 (i.e., vasomotor) and cardioacceleratory areas of the medulla. Functionally diverse bulbospinal neurons in both areas send axons down the spinal cord to synapse on and to stimulate preganglionic sympathetic neurons in the intermediolateral column of the spinal cord. The synapse can be adrenergic (in the case of the C1 neurons), peptidergic (e.g., neuropeptide Y), or glutamatergic. The glutamatergic synapses are the most important for the vasomotor response; the released glutamate acts on both NMDA (*N*-methyl-D-aspartate) and non-NMDA receptors on the preganglionic sympathetic neurons.

The cell bodies of the preganglionic sympathetic neurons are located in the intermediolateral gray matter of the spinal cord, between levels T1 and L3 (see Fig. 14.4). Most of the axons from these preganglionic neurons synapse with postganglionic sympathetic neurons located within ganglia of the paravertebral sympathetic chain as well as within prevertebral ganglia (see Figs. 14.2 and 14.3). The neurotransmitter between the preganglionic and postganglionic sympathetic neurons is acetylcholine (ACh). Sympathetic output does not distribute according to dermatomes (see ⊙ 14-3). Postganglionic sympathetic fibers control a wide range of functions (see Fig. 14.4). Those that control blood pressure run with the large blood vessels and innervate both *muscular arteries and arterioles and veins.*

Increased sympathetic activity produces vasoconstriction. Indeed, the baroreceptor reflex produces *vasodilation* because it *inhibits* the tonic stimulatory output of the vasomotor C1 neurons. Because the bulbospinal neurons synapse with preganglionic sympathetic neurons between T1 and L3, severing of the spinal cord above T1 causes a severe fall in blood pressure. Sectioning of the cord below L3 produces no fall in blood pressure.

Another important target of postganglionic neurons with a cardiovascular mission is the heart. Output from the middle cervical, stellate, and several upper thoracic ganglia (see Fig. 14.4) forms the cardiac nerves. Thus, severing of the spinal cord above T1 would block the input to the preganglionic sympathetic fibers to the heart. In addition, some preganglionic fibers do not synapse in sympathetic ganglia at all but directly innervate the chromaffin cells of the *adrenal medulla* via the splanchnic nerve. These cells release epinephrine, which acts on the heart and blood vessels (see below).

Parasympathetic Efferents Increased baroreceptor activity instructs the NTS to stimulate neurons in the nucleus ambiguus and the dorsal motor nucleus of the vagus (cardioinhibitory area). The target neurons in these two nuclei are preganglionic parasympathetic fibers of the vagus nerve (CN X) that project to the heart. These efferent vagal fibers follow the common carotid arteries, ultimately synapsing in small ganglia in the walls of the atria. There, they release ACh onto the N_2-type nAChRs of the postganglionic parasympathetic neurons. The short postganglionic fibers then innervate the *sinoatrial (SA) node, the atria, and the ventricles,* where they act primarily to slow conduction through the heart (see below).

The principal effectors in the neural control of arterial pressure are the heart, the arteries, the veins, and the adrenal medulla

The cardiovascular system uses several effector organs to control systemic arterial pressure: the heart, arteries, veins, and adrenal medulla (Fig. 23.5).

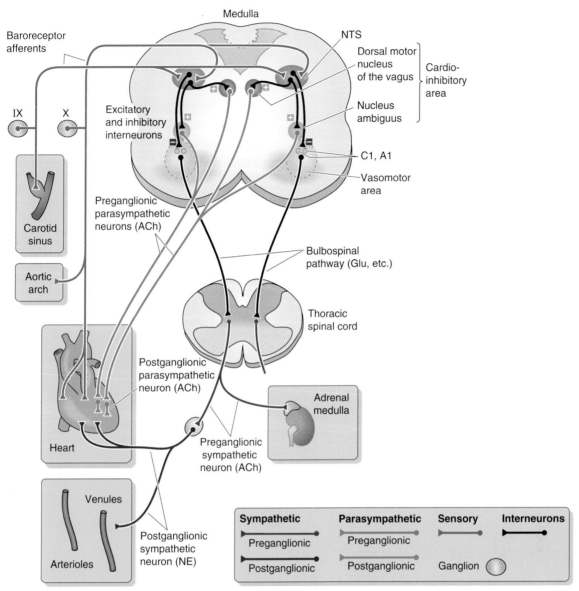

Figure 23.4 Afferent and efferent pathways, as well as medullary control centers for the cardiovascular system. *Glu, etc.,* Glutamate and other neurotransmitters (i.e., norepinephrine and peptides); *NE,* norepinephrine.

Sympathetic Input to the Heart (Cardiac Nerves) ⊙ 23-8 The sympathetic division of the autonomic nervous system influences the heart through the cardiac nerves, which form a plexus near the heart. The postganglionic fibers, which release **norepinephrine,** innervate the SA node, atria, and ventricles. Their effect is to increase both heart rate and contractility. Because it dominates the innervation of the SA node (which is in the right atrium), sympathetic input from the *right* cardiac nerve has more effect on the *heart rate* than does input from the left cardiac nerve. On the other hand, sympathetic input from the *left* cardiac nerve has more effect on *contractility*. In general, the cardiac nerves do not exert a strong tonic cardioacceleratory influence on the heart. At rest, their firing rate is less than that of the vagus nerve.

Parasympathetic Input to the Heart (Vagus Nerve) The vagus normally exerts an intense tonic, parasympathetic activity on the heart through **ACh** released by the postganglionic fibers. Severing of the vagus nerve or administration

of atropine (which blocks the action of ACh) increases heart rate. Vagal stimulation decreases heart rate by its effect on pacemaker activity (see ⊙ 21-6). Just as the actions of the right and left cardiac nerves are somewhat different, the right vagus is a more effective inhibitor of the SA node than the left. The left vagus is a more effective inhibitor of conduction through the atrioventricular (AV) node. Vagal stimulation, to some extent, also reduces cardiac contractility.

Sympathetic Input to Blood Vessels (Vasoconstrictor Response) ⊙ 23-9 The vasoconstrictor sympathetic fibers are disseminated widely throughout the blood vessels of the body. These fibers are most abundant in the kidney and the skin, relatively sparse in the coronary and cerebral vessels, and absent in the placenta. They release norepinephrine, which binds to adrenoceptors on the membrane of VSMCs. In most vascular beds, *vasodilation* is the result of a decrease in the tonic discharge of the vasoconstrictor sympathetic nerves.

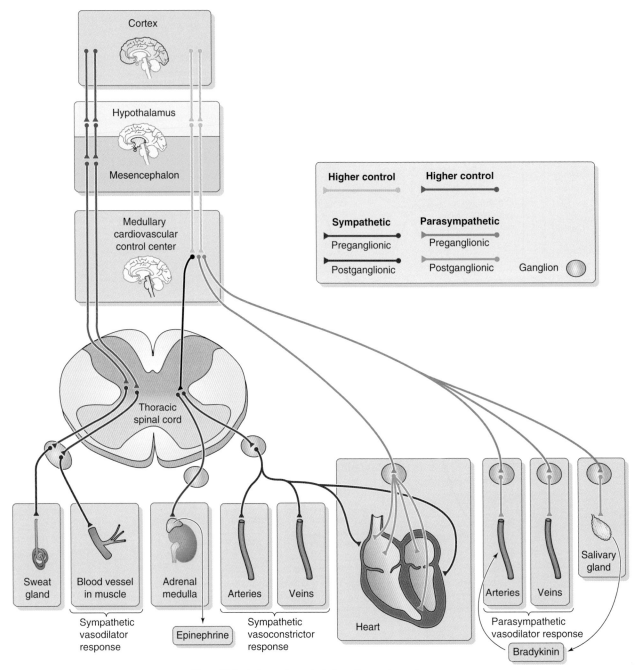

Figure 23.5 Autonomic control of cardiovascular end organs.

Parasympathetic Input to Blood Vessels (Vasodilator Response) Parasympathetic vaso*dilator* fibers are far less common than sympathetic vaso*constrictor* fibers. The parasympathetic vasodilator fibers supply the salivary and some gastrointestinal glands and are also crucial for vasodilation of erectile tissue in the external genitalia. Postganglionic parasympathetic fibers cause vasodilation via release of ACh, nitric oxide (NO; see ⊙ 14-9) and vasoactive intestinal peptide.

Sympathetic Input to Blood Vessels in Skeletal Muscle (Vasodilator Response) ⊙ **23-10** In addition to the more widespread sympathetic vasoconstrictor fibers, skeletal muscle in nonprimates has a special system of sympathetic fibers that produce *vasodilation*. These special fibers innervate the large precapillary vessels in skeletal muscle. While the sympathetic vasodilator pathway receives its instructions from the vasomotor area of the medulla, the sympathetic vasodilator fibers receive their instructions from neurons in the cerebral cortex, which synapse on other neurons in the hypothalamus or in the mesencephalon. The fibers from these second neurons (analogous to the bulbospinal neurons discussed above) transit through the medulla without interruption and reach the spinal cord. There, these fibers synapse on preganglionic sympathetic neurons in the intermediolateral column, just as do other descending neurons. The vasodilatory preganglionic fibers synapse in the sympathetic ganglia on postganglionic neurons that terminate on VSMCs surrounding skeletal muscle blood vessels. These postganglionic vasodilatory fibers release ACh and perhaps other transmitters.

Therefore, blood vessels within skeletal muscle receive both sympathetic adrenergic and sympathetic cholinergic innervation. The cholinergic system, acting directly via muscarinic receptors (see ◉ 14-5), relaxes VSMCs and causes rapid vasodilation. This vasodilation in skeletal muscle occurs in the fight-or-flight response as well as perhaps during the anticipatory response in exercise (see ◉ 14-13). In both cases, mobilization of the sympathetic vasodilator system is accompanied by extensive activation of the sympathetic division, including cardiac effects (i.e., increased heart rate and contractility) and generalized vasoconstriction of all vascular beds *except those in active skeletal muscle.*

Adrenal Medulla Some preganglionic sympathetic fibers in the sympathetic splanchnic nerves also innervate the chromaffin cells in the adrenal medulla, which can be considered equivalent of a sympathetic ganglion. The synaptic terminals of the preganglionic fibers release ACh, which acts on **nAChRs** of the **chromaffin cells** of the adrenal medulla (see ◉ 50-9). Chromaffin cells are thus modified postganglionic neurons that release their transmitters—**epinephrine** and, to a far lesser degree, norepinephrine—into the bloodstream rather than onto a specific end organ. Thus, the adrenal medulla participates as a global effector that through its release of epinephrine causes generalized effects on the circulation as it acts on both the heart and the blood vessels.

The unique combination of agonists and receptors determines the end response in cardiac and vascular effector cells

Adrenergic Receptors in the Heart ◉ 23-11 The *sympathetic* output to the heart affects both heart rate and contractility. Norepinephrine, released by the postganglionic sympathetic neurons, acts on postsynaptic β_1-adrenergic receptors of pacemaker cells in the SA node as well as on similar receptors of myocardial cells in the atria and ventricles. The β_1 adrenoceptor, via the G protein G_s, acts via the cAMP–protein kinase A pathway (see ◉ 3-9) to phosphorylate multiple effector molecules in both pacemaker cells and cardiac myocytes.

In **pacemaker cells,** β_1 agonists stimulate (1) I_f, the diastolic Na^+ current through HCN channels, and (2) I_{Ca}, a Ca^{2+} current through T-type and L-type Ca^{2+} channels. The net effect of these two changes is an increased rate of diastolic depolarization (i.e., phase 4 of the action potential; see Fig. 21.6A) and a negative shift in the threshold for the action potential (see Fig. 21.6C). Because diastole shortens, the *heart rate* increases.

In **myocardial cells,** β_1 agonists exert several parallel **positive inotropic** effects via protein kinase A. In addition, the activated α_s subunit of the G protein can directly activate L-type Ca^{2+} channels. The net effects of these pathways are contractions that are both stronger (see ◉ 21-7) and briefer (see ◉ 22-3).

Cholinergic Receptors in the Heart Parasympathetic output to the heart affects heart rate and, to a much lesser extent, contractility. ACh released by postsynaptic parasympathetic neurons binds to M_2 muscarinic (i.e., G protein–coupled)

receptors on pacemaker cells of the SA node and on ventricular myocytes.

◉ 23-12 In **pacemaker cells,** ACh acts by three mechanisms. (1) ACh triggers a membrane-delimited signaling pathway mediated not by the G-protein α subunits but rather by the $\beta\gamma$ heterodimers (see ◉ 3-7). The newly released $\beta\gamma$ subunits directly open inward-rectifier K^+ channels (GIRK1 or Kir3.1) in pacemaker cells (see ◉ 7-9). The resulting elevation of the K^+ conductance makes the maximum diastolic potential more negative during phase 4 of the action potential. (2) ACh also decreases I_f, thereby reducing the rate of diastolic depolarization. (3) ACh decreases I_{Ca}, thereby both reducing the rate of diastolic depolarization and making the threshold more positive (see Fig. 21.6C). The net effect is a reduction in heart rate.

In **myocardial cells,** ACh has a *minor* **negative inotropic effect,** which could occur by two mechanisms: (1) Activation of the M_2 receptor, via $G\alpha_i$, inhibits adenylyl cyclase, reducing $[cAMP]_i$ and thereby counteracting the effects of adrenergic stimulation. (2) Activation of the M_3 receptor, via $G\alpha_q$, stimulates phospholipase C, raising $[Ca^{2+}]_i$ and thus stimulating nitric oxide synthase (NOS; see ◉ 3-23). The newly formed NO stimulates guanylyl cyclase and increases $[cGMP]_i$, which inhibits L-type Ca^{2+} channels and decreases Ca^{2+} influx.

Adrenergic Receptors in Blood Vessels ◉ 23-13 The sympathetic division of the autonomic nervous system can modulate the tone of vascular smooth muscle in arteries, arterioles, and veins via two distinct routes—postganglionic sympathetic neurons and the adrenal medulla. Whether the net effect of sympathetic stimulation in a particular vessel is vasoconstriction (increased VSMC tone) or vasodilation (decreased VSMC tone) depends on four factors: (1) which agonist is released, (2) which adrenoceptors that agonist binds to, (3) whether receptor occupancy tends to cause vasoconstriction or vasodilation, and (4) which receptor subtypes happen to be present on a particular VSMC.

Which agonist is released is the most straightforward of the factors. Postganglionic sympathetic neurons release norepinephrine, and the adrenal medulla releases primarily epinephrine.

Norepinephrine and epinephrine do not have exclusive affinity for a single type of adrenoceptor. The original α and β designations followed from the observation that norepinephrine appeared to have its greatest activity on α receptors, and epinephrine, on β receptors. However, although norepinephrine binds with a greater affinity to α receptors than to β receptors, it also can activate β receptors. Similarly, although epinephrine binds with a greater affinity to β receptors than to α receptors, it can also activate α receptors. Of course, synthetic agonists may be more specific and potent than either norepinephrine or epinephrine (e.g., the α agonist phenylephrine and β agonist isoproterenol). A finer pharmacological and molecular dissection reveals that both α and β receptors have subgroups (e.g., β_1 and β_2), and even the subgroups have subgroups (see ◉ 14-6). Each of these many adrenoceptor types has a unique pharmacology. Thus, the β_1 receptor has about the same affinity for epinephrine and norepinephrine, but the β_2 receptor has a higher affinity for epinephrine than for norepinephrine.

The *vasoconstriction* elicited by catecholamines is an α_1 effect. Thus, norepinephrine released from nerve terminals acts on the α_1 adrenoceptor, which is coupled to the G protein G_q. The resulting activation of phospholipase C (see ⊙ 3-6) and formation of inositol 1,4,5-trisphosphate (IP_3) lead to a rise in $[Ca^{2+}]_i$ and smooth-muscle contraction. In contrast, *vasodilation,* elicited by epinephrine released from the adrenal medulla, is a β_2 effect. Occupancy of the β_2 adrenoceptor triggers the cAMP–protein kinase A pathway, leading to phosphorylation of myosin light-chain kinase (MLCK; see ⊙ 9-14); this reduces the sensitivity of MLCK to the Ca^{2+}-calmodulin complex, resulting by default in smooth-muscle relaxation.

Many blood vessels are populated with a mixture of α-receptor or β-receptor subtypes, each stimulated to varying degrees by norepinephrine and epinephrine. Therefore, the response of the cell depends on the relative dominance of the subtype of receptor present on the cell surface.

The ultimate outcome in the target tissue (vasoconstriction versus vasodilation) depends on both the heterogeneous mixture of agonists (norepinephrine versus epinephrine) applied and the heterogeneous mixture of VSMC receptors (α_1 and β_2) present in tissues. As an example, consider blood vessels in the skin and heart. Because cutaneous blood vessels have *only* α_1 receptors, they can only vasoconstrict, regardless of whether the agonist is norepinephrine or epinephrine. On the other hand, epinephrine causes coronary blood vessels to dilate because they have a greater number of β_2 receptors than α_1 receptors.

Cholinergic Receptors in or Near Blood Vessels ⊙ **23-14** The addition of ACh to an isolated VSMC causes contraction. In real life, however, ACh dilates blood vessels by binding to muscarinic receptors on neighboring cells and generating *other* messengers that indirectly cause vasodilation. For example, in **skeletal muscle,** ACh may bind to M_2 receptors on the presynaptic membranes of postganglionic sympathetic neurons, decreasing $[cAMP]_i$ and inhibiting the release of norepinephrine. Thus, inhibition of vasoconstriction produces vasodilation.

Nonadrenergic, Noncholinergic Receptors in Blood Vessels Postganglionic parasympathetic nerve terminals may cause vasodilation by co-releasing neurotransmitters other than ACh, such as NO, vasoactive intestinal peptide (VIP), and calcitonin gene–related peptide (CGRP). Postganglionic sympathetic nerve terminals may cause vasoconstriction by co-releasing neuropeptide Y (NPY). NO of neuronal origin acts in the same way as endothelium-derived NO. NPY acts by lowering $[cAMP]_i$; VIP and presumably CGRP act by raising $[cAMP]_i$.

The medullary cardiovascular center tonically maintains blood pressure and is under the control of higher brain centers

The medullary cardiovascular center normally exerts its tonic activity on the sympathetic preganglionic neurons, whose cell bodies lie in the thoracolumbar segments of the spinal cord. However, a variety of somatic and visceral afferents also make connections with this efferent pathway in the spinal cord, and such afferents are responsible for several reflexes that occur at the spinal level. The sympathetic preganglionic neurons are normally so dependent on medullary input that they are not very sensitive to local afferents.

Neurons of the C1 area of the medulla (Fig. 23.4) are responsible for maintaining a normal mean arterial pressure. In general, C1 neurons are tonically active and excite sympathetic preganglionic neurons to produce vasoconstriction (see ⊙ 23-6).

Besides the afferents from the baroreceptors, the medullary cardiovascular center receives afferents from respiratory centers and from higher CNS centers, such as the hypothalamus and cerebral cortex (Fig. 23.5). The **hypothalamus** integrates many cardiovascular responses. The dorsomedial hypothalamic nucleus in the hypothalamus acts on the rostral ventrolateral medulla (see ⊙ 23-4) to mediate vasomotor and cardiac responses (e.g., during exercise and acute stress). The **cerebral cortex** influences the hypothalamic integration areas along both excitatory and inhibitory pathways. Thus, a strong emotion can lead to precipitous hypotension with syncope (i.e., fainting). Conditioned reflexes can also elicit cardiovascular responses.

Secondary neural regulation of arterial blood pressure depends on chemoreceptors

Although baroreceptors are the primary sensors for blood pressure control, a second set of receptors, the peripheral chemoreceptors, also play a role. Whereas input from baroreceptors exerts a *negative* drive on the medullary *vasomotor center,* causing vasodilation, the peripheral chemoreceptors exert a *positive* drive on the vasomotor center, causing vasoconstriction (Fig. 23.6A). As far as the heart is concerned, inputs from *both* the baroreceptors and the peripheral chemoreceptors exert a positive drive on the *cardioinhibitory center;* that is, they both decrease heart rate (compare Figs. 23.1 and 23.6A).

⊙ **23-15** The medullary *respiratory* centers—which include the areas that integrate the input from the peripheral chemoreceptors—strongly influence medullary *cardiovascular* centers. A fall in arterial P_{O_2}, a rise in P_{CO_2}, or a fall in pH stimulates the peripheral chemoreceptors to increase the firing frequency of the afferent nerves to the medulla. In the absence of conflicting input, which we discuss next, the intrinsic response of the medulla to this peripheral chemoreceptor input is to direct efferent pathways to cause *vasoconstriction* and *bradycardia* (Fig. 23.6A). Opposite changes in the P_{O_2}, P_{CO_2}, and pH have the opposite effects.

The **peripheral chemoreceptors**—whose primary role is to regulate ventilation (see ⊙ 32-3)—lie close to the baroreceptors. Just as there are two types of high-pressure baroreceptors (i.e., carotid sinus and aortic arch), there are also two types of peripheral chemoreceptors: the carotid bodies and the aortic bodies (compare the location of the baroreceptor and chemoreceptor systems in Fig. 23.2A and B).

Carotid Bodies The carotid body—or glomus caroticum—is located between the external and internal carotid arteries. Although the human carotid body is small (i.e., ~1 mm^3), it has an extraordinarily high blood flow per unit mass and a minuscule arteriovenous difference for P_{O_2}, P_{CO_2}, and pH—putting it in an excellent position to monitor the composition of the *arterial blood.* The chemosensitive cell in the carotid body is the **glomus cell,** which synapses

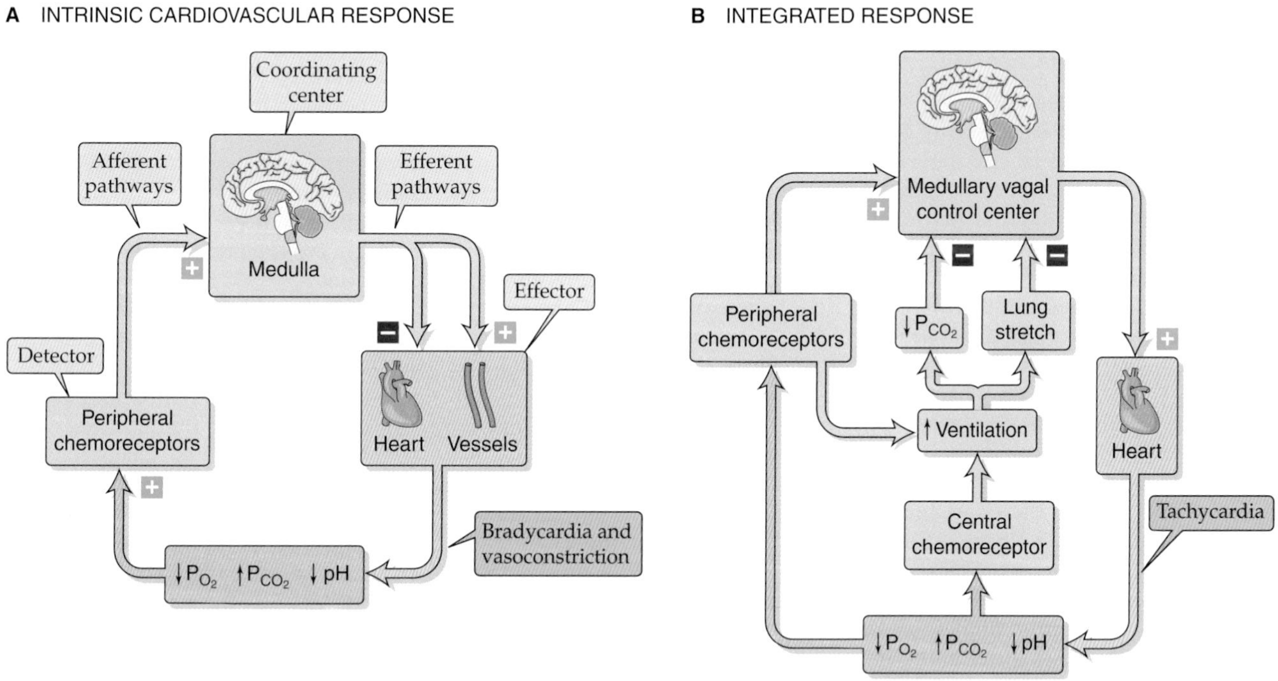

A INTRINSIC CARDIOVASCULAR RESPONSE

B INTEGRATED RESPONSE

Figure 23.6 Chemoreceptor control of the cardiovascular system. In this example, we assume that a decrease in P_{O_2}, an increase in P_{CO_2}, or a decrease in pH is the primary insult *(violet box)*. In (A) the bradycardia occurs only when ventilation is fixed or prevented (e.g., breath-holding). In (B) the effects of breathing overcome the intrinsic cardiovascular response, producing tachycardia.

with nerve fibers that join the glossopharyngeal nerve (CN IX). A fall in arterial P_{O_2}, a rise in arterial P_{CO_2}, or a fall in the pH increases the spike frequency in the sensory fibers of the afferent sinus nerve.

Aortic Bodies The aortic bodies are situated immediately under the concavity of the aortic arch and in the angle between the *right* subclavian and carotid arteries. Aortic bodies may also be present at the angle between the *left* subclavian and common carotid arteries. The aortic glomus cells synapse with nerve fibers that are afferent pathways in the vagus nerve (CN X).

Afferent Fiber Input to the Medulla The most important signal affecting the glomus cells is a low P_{O_2}, which triggers an increase in the firing rate of the sensory fibers. Elsewhere, we discuss ways in which this signal triggers neuronal firing (see 32-3). Like the afferent fibers from the baroreceptors, the afferent fibers from both the carotid body (CN IX) and the aortic bodies (CN X) project to the NTS in the medulla. Indeed, the responses to input from the peripheral chemoreceptors overlap with those to input from the baroreceptors.

Physiological Role of the Peripheral Chemoreceptors in Cardiovascular Control 23-16 The fluctuations in P_{O_2} that normally occur in humans are not large enough to affect the blood pressure or heart rate. For the cardiovascular system, the peripheral chemoreceptors play a role only during severe hypoxia (e.g., hemorrhagic hypotension). As already noted, the *intrinsic* cardiovascular effects of hypoxia on the peripheral chemoreceptors include vasoconstriction and bradycardia (Fig. 23.6A). However, this primary reflex bradycardia is observed only during forced apnea. Under real-life conditions, hypoxia stimulates the peripheral chemoreceptors and thereby increases ventilation (Fig. 23.6B). The resulting

stimulation of pulmonary stretch receptors and decrease in systemic P_{CO_2} indirectly produce tachycardia. Thus, *the physiological response to hypoxia is tachycardia*.

Central Chemoreceptors In addition to peripheral chemoreceptors, *central* chemoreceptors are present in the medulla (see 32-8). However, in contrast to the peripheral chemoreceptors, which primarily sense a low P_{O_2}, the central chemoreceptors mainly sense a low brain pH, which generally reflects a high arterial P_{CO_2}.

Tonic baroreceptor input to the NTS in the medulla stimulates inhibitory interneurons that project onto the vasomotor area. This pathway exerts a considerable restraining influence on sympathetic output, which would otherwise cause vasoconstriction. Thus, cutting of these baroreceptor afferents causes vasoconstriction. The central chemoreceptor also influences the vasomotor area. Indeed, a high arterial P_{CO_2} (i.e., low brain pH), which stimulates the central chemoreceptor, disinhibits the vasomotor area—just as cutting of baroreceptor afferents. Both conditions result in an increase in the sympathetic output and vasoconstriction.

In summary, a low P_{O_2} acting on the peripheral chemoreceptor and a high P_{CO_2} acting on the central chemoreceptor act in concert to enhance vasoconstriction.

REGULATION OF CARDIAC OUTPUT

Cardiac output is the product of the heart rate and stroke volume (see Equation 17.6), and both factors are under the dual control of (1) regulatory mechanisms intrinsic to the heart, and (2) neural and hormonal pathways that are extrinsic to the heart.

Mechanisms intrinsic to the heart modulate both heart rate and stroke volume

Intrinsic Control of Heart Rate As the length of diastole increases, the heart rate necessarily decreases. The diastolic interval is determined by the nature of the action potential fired off by the SA node. Such factors as the maximum diastolic potential, the slope of the diastolic depolarization (phase 4), and the threshold potential all influence the period between one SA node action potential and the next (see Fig. 21.6). Intrinsic modifiers of the SA node pacemaker, such as $[K^+]_o$ and $[Ca^{2+}]_o$, greatly influence the ionic currents responsible for SA node pacemaker activity but are not part of any cardiovascular feedback loops.

Intrinsic Control of Stroke Volume Stroke volume is the difference between end-diastolic volume and end-systolic volume (see Equation 22.2). Various processes intrinsic to the heart affect both of these variables.

The **end**-diastolic **volume (EDV)** depends on the following:

1. **Filling pressure.** Ventricular filling pressure depends to a large degree on *atrial* filling pressure. When increased venous return causes atrial filling pressure to rise, EDV rises as well.
2. **Filling time.** The *longer* the filling time, the greater the EDV. As heart rate rises, diastole shortens to a greater extent than does systole, thereby decreasing EDV.
3. **Ventricular compliance** (reciprocal of the slope of the diastole curve in Fig. 22.11B). As ventricular compliance increases, a given filling pressure will produce a greater increase in ventricular volume, thus resulting in a greater EDV.

The **end**-systolic **volume (ESV)** depends on the following:

1. **Preload** (i.e., end-*diastolic* volume). According to Starling's law of the heart, increase of the EDV increases the stretch on the cardiac muscle and the force of the contraction (see the systole curve in Fig. 22.11B), and thus the stroke volume. Only at a very large EDV does contraction begin to weaken as the muscle fibers are too stretched to generate maximal power (see Fig. 22.11A).
2. **Afterload** (force against which the ventricle ejects its contents). The afterload of the left ventricle is the mean systemic arterial pressure; the afterload of the right ventricle is the mean pulmonary arterial pressure. Increased afterload impedes the heart's ability to empty and thereby increases ESV (see ⊙ **22-5**).
3. **Heart rate.** An increased heart rate leads to greater Ca^{2+} entry into myocardial cells, thereby increasing contractility and reducing ESV (see ⊙ **22-8**).
4. **Contractility.** Positive inotropic agents act by increasing $[Ca^{2+}]_i$ within the myocardial cells (see ⊙ **22-7**), thereby enhancing the force of contraction and decreasing ESV.

Mechanisms extrinsic to the heart also modulate heart rate and stroke volume

The sympathetic and parasympathetic pathways are the efferent limbs of the feedback loops that control mean arterial pressure (Fig. 23.5). These efferent limbs also control cardiac output via heart rate and stroke volume.

Baroreceptor Regulation Baroreceptor responses affect both heart rate and stroke volume, the *product* of which is *cardiac output*. However, baroreceptors do not monitor cardiac output per se but rather arterial pressure. Thus, the baroreceptor response does *not* correct spontaneous alterations in cardiac output unless they happen to change mean arterial pressure. For example, when an increase in the cardiac output matches a commensurate decrease in the peripheral resistance, leaving the mean arterial pressure unchanged, the baroreceptors do not respond.

Chemoreceptor Regulation In Fig. 23.6B, we saw that the integrated response to hypoxia and respiratory acidosis is *tachycardia*. This tachycardia response turns out to be a very helpful feedback mechanism for maintaining cardiac output. For example, a reduced cardiac output lowers arterial P_{O_2}, raises P_{CO_2}, and lowers pH. These changes stimulate the peripheral chemoreceptors, indirectly producing tachycardia and thereby increasing cardiac output. Thus, the chemoreceptor response corrects changes in blood chemistry that are likely to result from reduced cardiac output. Once again, the detector (i.e., the peripheral chemoreceptor) senses changes in the metabolic consequences of altered cardiac output. Changes in cardiac output go unnoticed by the chemoreceptors if they do not affect arterial P_{O_2}, P_{CO_2}, or pH.

The integrated response to high P_{CO_2}—which *indirectly* increases heart rate (Fig. 23.6B)—tends to counteract the *direct* effect of high P_{CO_2} on the heart: a *decrease* in myocardial contractility. High P_{CO_2} leads to intracellular acidosis of the myocardial cells (see ⊙ 28-9). The low pH_i shifts the $[Ca^{2+}]_i$-tension curve of cardiac muscle to higher $[Ca^{2+}]_i$ values, which reflects a lower sensitivity of the cardiac form of troponin C (TNNC1) to $[Ca^{2+}]_i$. Thus, in the absence of reflex tachycardia (Fig. 23.6B), high P_{CO_2} would decrease myocardial force and thereby lower cardiac output.

⊙ 23-17 Low-pressure baroreceptors in the atria respond to increased "fullness" of the vascular system, triggering tachycardia, renal vasodilation, and diuresis

The baroreceptors located at *high*-pressure sites (i.e., the carotid sinus and aortic arch) are not the only stretch receptors involved in feedback regulation of the circulation. Low-pressure baroreceptors—bare ends of myelinated nerve fibers—are located at strategic *low*-pressure sites, including the pulmonary artery, the junction of the atria with their corresponding veins, the atria themselves, and the ventricles (Fig. 23.7A). Distention of these receptors depends largely on venous return to the heart. These low-pressure receptors also help control cardiac output. By regulating both effective circulating volume and cardiac output, these receptors also *indirectly* regulate mean arterial blood pressure.

Atrial Receptors ⊙ **23-18** The most extensively studied low-pressure receptors are the atrial receptors. These are located at the ends of afferent axons—either A or B fibers—that join the vagus nerve (CN X). The A fibers fire in synchrony with atrial systole and therefore monitor heart rate (Fig. 23.7B). The B fibers fire in a burst during ventricular systole (Fig. 23.7B) and gradually increase their firing rate as the atria fill, reaching maximum firing frequency at the

A ANATOMICAL DISTRIBUTION

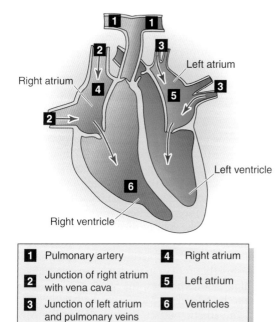

1 Pulmonary artery   **4** Right atrium

2 Junction of right atrium with vena cava   **5** Left atrium

3 Junction of left atrium and pulmonary veins   **6** Ventricles

B RESPONSE OF ATRIAL A– AND B–TYPE RECEPTORS

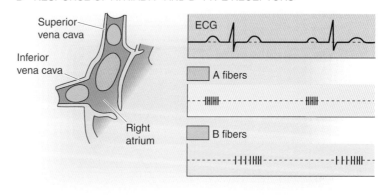

Figure 23.7 Low-pressure receptors. In (B) A-type receptors *(orange)* are located mainly in the body of the right atrium; B-type receptors *(green)* are located mainly in the superior and inferior vena cava. *ECG,* Electrocardiogram.

peak of the *v* wave of the atrial (i.e., jugular) pulse (see Fig. 22.6A). Thus, the B fibers monitor the rising atrial volume. Because the **central venous pressure (CVP)**—the pressure inside large systemic veins leading to the right heart—is the main determinant of right atrial filling, the B fibers also detect changes in CVP. By inference, the atrial B-type stretch receptors primarily monitor effective circulating volume and venous return.

⊙ **23-19** The afferent pathways for the low-pressure receptors are similar to those for high-pressure baroreceptors and peripheral chemoreceptors traveling along the vagus nerve and projecting to the NTS (see ⊙ **23-5**) and other nuclei of the medullary cardiovascular center. To some extent, the efferent pathways and effector organs (i.e., heart and blood vessels) also are similar. However, whereas increased stretch of the high-pressure receptors *lowers* heart rate, increased stretch of the atrial B-type receptors *raises* heart rate—**Bainbridge reflex.** Moreover, whereas increased stretch of the high-pressure receptors causes *generalized* vasodilation, increased stretch of the atrial B-type receptors decreases sympathetic vasoconstrictor output *only to the kidney.* The net effect of increased atrial stretch (i.e., tachycardia and renal vasodilation) is an increase in renal blood flow and an increase in urine output (i.e., diuresis). Decreased atrial stretch has little effect on heart rate but increases sympathetic output to the kidney. Therefore, the high-pressure baroreceptors respond to stretch (i.e., increased blood pressure) by attempting to decrease blood pressure. The low-pressure baroreceptors respond to stretch (i.e., increased fullness) by attempting to eliminate fluid.

⊙ **23-20** The afferent fibers of the atrial receptors that project to the NTS also synapse there with neurons that project to magnocellular neurons in the paraventricular nucleus of the hypothalamus (see Fig. 40.4). These hypothalamic neurons synthesize **arginine vasopressin (AVP)**—also known as antidiuretic hormone (see ⊙ **38-2**)—and then transport it down their axons to the posterior pituitary for release into the blood (see ⊙ **47-3**). Increased atrial stretch lowers AVP secretion, which produces a water diuresis and thus decreases total body water (see ⊙ **40-11**).

⊙ **23-21** In addition to stimulating bare nerve endings, atrial stretch causes a *non*-neural response: When stretched, atrial myocytes release **atrial natriuretic peptide (ANP)** or factor (ANF), a powerful vasodilator. It also causes diuresis (see ⊙ **40-8**) and thus enhances the renal excretion of Na⁺ (i.e., it causes natriuresis), lowering effective circulating volume and blood pressure.

Thus, enhanced atrial filling with consequent stretching of the atrial mechanoreceptors promotes diuresis by: (1) Tachycardia in combination with a reduced sympathetic vasoconstrictor output to the kidney increases renal blood flow. (2) Atrial baroreceptors cause decreased secretion of AVP. (3) The stretch of the atrial myocytes themselves enhances the release of ANP.

Ventricular Receptors Stretching of the ventricular *low-*pressure stretch receptors causes bradycardia and vasodilation, responses similar to those associated with stretching of the arterial *high-*pressure receptors. However, these ventricular receptors do not contribute appreciably to homeostasis of the cardiac output.

Cardiac output is roughly proportional to effective circulating blood volume

⊙ **23-22** The Bainbridge reflex is the name given to the tachycardia caused by an increase in venous return. An increase

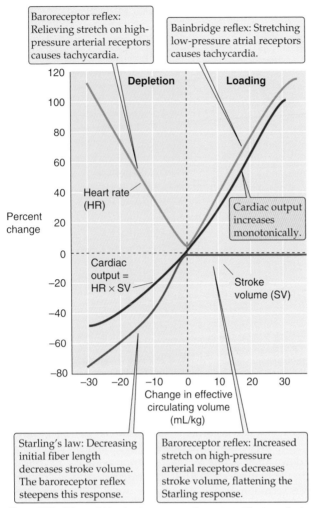

Barorreceptor reflex: Relieving stretch on high-pressure arterial receptors causes tachycardia.

Bainbridge reflex: Stretching low-pressure atrial receptors causes tachycardia.

Starling's law: Decreasing initial fiber length decreases stroke volume. The baroreceptor reflex steepens this response.

Baroreceptor reflex: Increased stretch on high-pressure arterial receptors decreases stroke volume, flattening the Starling response.

Figure 23.8   Effect of blood volume on cardiac output. The investigators changed effective circulating volume (x-axis) by altering blood volume.

in blood volume leads to increased firing of low-pressure B fibers (see Fig. 23.7B) during atrial filling. The efferent limb of this Bainbridge reflex is carried by both parasympathetic and sympathetic pathways to the SA node, which determines heart rate. Effects on cardiac contractility and stroke volume are insignificant. Because the Bainbridge reflex saturates, the increase in heart rate is greatest at low baseline heart rates.

The Bainbridge reflex acts as a counterbalance to the baroreceptor reflex in the control of **heart rate.** The orange curve on the right upper quadrant of Fig. 23.8 illustrates the Bainbridge reflex: increase of the effective circulating volume (i.e., increase of venous return and stimulation of *low-pressure* receptors) increases heart rate. On the other hand, decreased atrial stretch has little effect on heart rate by the Bainbridge reflex. The *orange curve* in the left upper quadrant of Fig. 23.8 illustrates the intervention of the *high-pressure* baroreceptors, whereby a decrease in blood volume does not cause heart rate to fall but rather causes it to rise. Indeed, a significant reduction in blood volume leads to a fall in mean arterial pressure, reduced baroreceptor firing, and—via the cardioinhibitory and cardioaccelleratory areas in the medulla (Fig. 23.4B)—stimulation of the SA node. Therefore, on examination of the full *orange curve* in Fig. 23.8, we see that changes in blood volume or venous return

have a biphasic effect on heart rate. By different mechanisms, volume loading and volume depletion *both* cause a graded increase in heart rate. In general, during volume loading, the Bainbridge reflex prevails, whereas during volume depletion, the high-pressure baroreceptor reflex dominates. *Heart rate is at its minimum when effective circulating volume is normal.*

Stroke volume also shows a peculiar, biphasic dependence on effective circulating volume (*blue curve* in Fig. 23.8) that is the result of two competing effects, Starling's law and the baroreceptor reflex. According to Starling's law, as venous blood volume increases, enhanced ventricular filling increases EDV, thereby improving cardiac performance and thus stroke volume (see ⊙ 22-4). The Starling relationship reflects the *intrinsic* properties of the heart muscle. However, in a real person, the baroreceptor reflex has a major influence on the dependence of stroke volume on blood volume. At low blood volumes, the baroreceptor reflex produces high sympathetic output, increasing contractility and steepening the Starling relationship (blue curve in the left lower quadrant of Fig. 23.8). At high blood volumes, the Starling relationship normally tends to be less steep. Moreover, the baroreceptor reflex reduces sympathetic output, thereby decreasing contractility and further flattening the *blue curve* in the right half of Fig. 23.8.

In contrast to the biphasic response of heart rate and stroke volume to changes in effective circulating volume, **cardiac output** rises monotonically (Fig. 23.8, *red curve*). The reason for this smooth increase is that cardiac output is the product of heart rate *and* stroke volume. The increase in blood volume causes a gradual rise in stroke volume (*blue curve*), offset by a fall in heart rate (*orange curve*), resulting in an overall rise of cardiac output (*red curve*) until blood volume and stroke volume reach normal levels. Further increases in blood volume have no effect on stroke volume (*blue curve*) but increase heart rate (*orange curve*), further increasing cardiac output (*red curve*). Consequently, the dependence of cardiac output on effective circulating volume is the result of the complex interplay among three responses: (1) the Bainbridge reflex, (2) the baroreceptor reflex, and (3) Starling's law.

MATCHING OF VENOUS RETURN AND CARDIAC OUTPUT

Venous return is the blood flow returning to the heart. Most often, the term is used to mean the *systemic* venous return. Because the input of the right heart must equal its output in the steady state, and because the cardiac outputs of the right and left heart are almost exactly the same, the input to the right heart must equal the output of the left heart. Thus, the systemic venous return must match the systemic cardiac output.

Increases in cardiac output cause right atrial pressure to fall

The right atrial pressure (RAP) determines the extent of ventricular filling. In turn, RAP depends on the venous return of blood to the heart.

In a situation such as cardiac arrest, for several seconds, blood continues to flow from the arteries and capillaries into the veins because the arterial pressure continues to exceed the venous pressure. The aortic pressure does not fall to zero during diastole because of the potential energy stored in the elastic recoil of the arterial walls. Similarly, after a cardiac arrest, this potential energy continues to push blood to the venous side until all pressures are equal throughout the vascular tree, and flow stops everywhere.

When blood flow finally ceases after a cardiac arrest, the pressures in the arteries, capillaries, veins, and right atrium are uniform. This pressure is called the **mean systemic filling pressure (MSFP)** and is about +7 mm Hg (point B in Fig. 23.9). MSFP is not zero because MSFP depends on the blood volume and the overall compliance of the entire vascular system.

Cardiovascular physiologists usually work with a **vascular function curve** that treats RAP as the independent variable (plotted on the x-axis in Fig. 23.9) and venous return as the dependent variable (plotted on the y-axis). As RAP becomes less positive, it provides a greater driving pressure (i.e., greater $\Delta P = CVP - RAP$) for the return of blood from the periphery to the right atrium, as it must for cardiac output to increase. Thus, the cardiac output steadily rises as RAP falls. At a normal cardiac output of 5 L/min, RAP is 2 mm Hg (point A in Fig. 23.9). However, as RAP declines and eventually becomes negative, the transmural pressure of the large veins becomes negative, so that the large veins feeding blood to the right atrium collapse. No further increment in venous return can occur, even though the driving pressure, ΔP, is increasing. Therefore, the vascular function curve plateaus at negative values of RAP, around −1 mm Hg.

Changes in blood volume shift the vascular function curve to different RAPs, whereas changes in arteriolar tone alter the slope of the curve

Because the vascular function curve depends on how full the capacitance vessels are, *changing the blood volume* affects the vascular function curve. An increase in blood volume (e.g., a transfusion) shifts the curve to the right. In the example in Fig. 23.10A, the intercept with the x-axis (i.e., MSFP) moves from 7 to 9 mm Hg, as would be expected if more blood were put into a distensible container, whether it is a balloon or the circulatory system. A decrease in blood volume (e.g., hemorrhage) shifts the curve and the x-intercept to the left. Thus, MSFP increases with transfusion and decreases with hemorrhage. However, changes in blood volume do *not* affect the *slope* of the linear portion of the vascular function curve as long as there is no change in either vessel compliance or resistance.

Change in the venomotor tone, by constriction or dilation of *only the veins,* is equivalent to change in the blood volume. Returning to our balloon analogy, even if we hold the

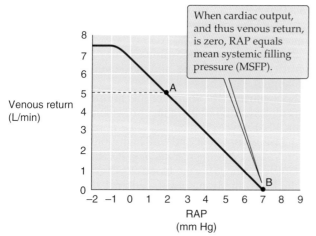

Figure 23.9 Vascular function curve.

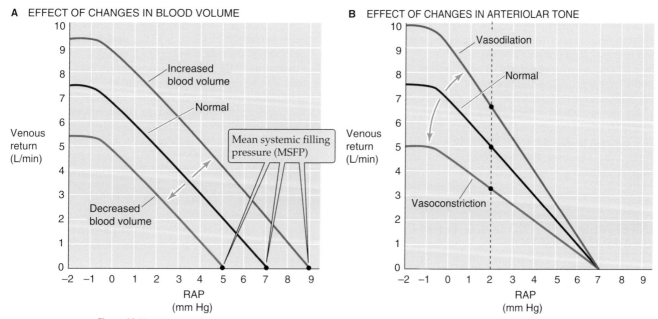

Figure 23.10 Effect of changes in blood volume and vasomotor tone on the vascular function curve. The purple curves are the same as the vascular function curve in Fig. 23.9. In (B) dilation of the arterioles increases CVP and thus raises the driving force (CVP − RAP) for venous return. Constriction of arterioles has the opposite effects.

amount of blood constant, we can increase pressure inside the balloon by increasing the tension in the wall. Because most of the blood volume is in the veins, a pure increase in venomotor tone would be equivalent to a blood transfusion (Fig. 23.10A). Conversely, a pure decrease in venomotor tone would reduce the tension in the wall of the container, shifting the curve to the left, just as in a hemorrhage.

Change in the tone of the arterioles has a very different effect on the vascular function curve. Because the arterioles contain only a minor fraction of the blood volume, changes in the arteriolar tone have little effect on MSFP and thus on the x-intercept. However, changes in the arteriolar tone can have a marked effect on the CVP, which, along with the RAP, determines the driving force for the venous return. Arteriolar constriction flattens the vascular function curve; arteriolar dilation has the opposite effect (Fig. 23.10B). Thus, arteriolar constriction flattens the vascular function curve, whereas arteriolar dilation steepens it.

Because vascular function and cardiac function depend on each other, cardiac output and venous return match at exactly one value of RAP

The classical Starling's law relationship (see Fig. 22.11B), which is valid for both ventricles, is a plot of developed pressure versus EDV. However, we already expressed Starling's law in Fig. 22.11C, plotting stroke work on the y-axis and atrial pressure on the x-axis. Because stroke work—at a fixed arterial pressure and heart rate—is proportional to cardiac output, we can replace stroke work with *cardiac output* on the y-axis of the cardiac performance curve. The result is the red cardiac function curve in Fig. 23.11A.

Cardiac output and venous return depend on RAP, and RAP depends on the cardiac output and venous return. They all depend on each other. There is no absolute dependent or independent variable in this closed circuit because, in the steady state, venous return and cardiac output must be equal.

The only way to produce a *permanent change* in cardiac output, venous return, and RAP is to change at least one of the two function curves. The vascular function curve may be any one of a large family of such curves (Fig. 23.10A and B), depending on the precise blood volume, venomotor tone, and arteriolar tone. Thus, a transfusion of blood shifts the vascular function curve to the right, establishing a new steady-state operating point at a higher RAP (point A → point B in Fig. 23.11B). Similarly, vasodilation would rotate the vascular function curve to a steeper slope, also establishing a new steady-state operating point at a higher RAP.

INTERMEDIATE- AND LONG-TERM CONTROL OF THE CIRCULATION

In addition to the rapidly acting neural mechanisms that control the total peripheral resistance and cardiac output, humoral controls contribute to the homeostasis of the circulation. In most instances, these control systems operate on a time scale of hours or days, far more slowly than the neurotransmitter-mediated reflex control by the CNS.

Two classes of humoral controls influence the circulation:
1. Vasoactive substances released in the blood, or in the proximity of vascular smooth muscle, modulate the vasomotor tone of arteries and veins, affecting blood pressure and the distribution of blood flow.
2. Nonvasoactive substances, which act on targets other than the cardiovascular system, control the effective circulating volume by modulating ECF volume. By determining the filling of the blood vessels, these nonvasoactive agents also modulate the mean arterial pressure and cardiac output.

Endocrine and paracrine vasoactive compounds control the circulatory system on an intermediate- to long-term basis

Vasoactive substances, both endocrine and paracrine, cause blood vessels to contract or to relax (Table 23.1). In many instances, paracrine control dominates over endocrine control. The chemical messengers controlling the blood vessels can be amines, peptides, or proteins; derivatives of arachidonic acid; or gases such as NO.

Biogenic Amines Monoamines may be either vasoconstrictors (epinephrine and serotonin) or vasodilators (histamine).
1. **Epinephrine.** The source of this hormone is the adrenal medulla (see ⊙ 50-8). Epinephrine binds to α_1 **receptors** on VSMCs with less affinity than norepinephrine, causing *vasoconstriction*, and with high affinity to β_2 **receptors** on VSMCs, causing *vasodilation*. Because β_2 receptors are largely confined to the blood vessels of skeletal muscle, the heart, the liver, and the adrenal medulla itself, epinephrine is not a systemic vasodilator. Epinephrine also binds to β_1 receptors in the heart, thereby *increasing the heart rate and contractility* (see ⊙ 23-11).
2. **Serotonin.** Also known as 5-hydroxytryptamine (5-HT; see Fig. 13.6B), this monoamine is synthesized by serotonergic nerves, enterochromaffin cells, and adrenal chromaffin cells. 5-HT is also present in platelets and mast cells. Serotonin binds to **5-HT$_{2A}$ and 5-HT$_{2B}$ receptors** on VSMCs, causing *vasoconstriction*.
3. **Histamine.** Like serotonin, histamine (see Fig. 13.6B) may also be present in nerve terminals. In addition, mast cells release histamine in response to tissue injury and inflammation. Histamine binds to **H$_2$ receptors** on VSMCs, causing *vasodilation*. Although histamine causes vascular smooth muscle to relax, it causes visceral smooth muscle (e.g., bronchial smooth muscle in asthma) to contract.

Peptides Vasoactive peptides may be either vasoconstrictors or vasodilators (Table 23.1).
1. **Angiotensin II (ANG II).** ⊙ 23-23 Part of the renin-angiotensin-aldosterone cascade (see ⊙ 40-2), ANG II, as its name implies, is a powerful *vasoconstrictor*. The liver secretes angiotensinogen into the blood. The enzyme renin, released into the blood by the kidney, then converts angiotensinogen to the decapeptide ANG I. Finally, angiotensin-converting enzyme (ACE), which is present primarily on endothelial cells, particularly those of the lung, cleaves ANG I to the octapeptide ANG II.

ANG II is *normally* not present in plasma concentrations high enough to produce systemic vasoconstriction.

A MATCHING OF A SINGLE CARDIAC FUNCTION CURVE
WITH A SINGLE VASCULAR FUNCTION CURVE

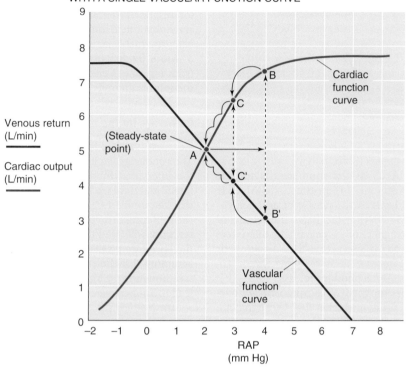

Venous return
(L/min)

Cardiac output
(L/min)

B SHIFT OF VASCULAR FUNCTION CURVE

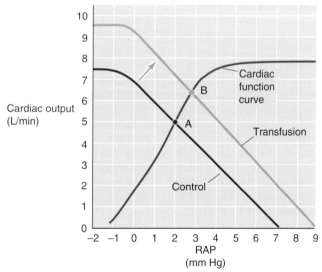

Cardiac output
(L/min)

Figure 23.11 Matching of cardiac output with venous return. The *purple curves* are the same as the vascular function curve in Fig. 23.9. The red cardiac function curves represent Starling's law. In (A), point A is the single RAP at which venous return and cardiac output match. A transient increase in RAP from 2 to 4 mm Hg causes an initial mismatch between cardiac output (point B) and venous return (point B′), which eventually resolves (B′C′A and BCA). In (B), permanently increasing blood volume (transfusion) shifts the vascular function curve to the right (as in Fig. 23.10A), so that a match between the cardiac output and venous return now occurs at a higher RAP (point B).

In contrast, ANG II plays a major role in cardiovascular control during blood loss (see ⊙ 25-7), exercise, and similar circumstances that reduce renal blood flow. Reduced perfusion pressure in the kidney causes the release of renin (see ⊙ 40-2). Plasma ANG II levels rise, leading to an intense vasoconstriction in the splanchnic and renal circulations. The resulting reduced renal blood flow leads to even

more renin release and higher ANG II levels, a dangerous positive-feedback system that can lead to acute renal failure.

ANG II has a range of other effects—besides direct vasoactive effects—that indirectly increase mean arterial pressure: (1) ANG II increases cardiac contractility. (2) It reduces renal plasma flow, thereby enhancing Na^+ reabsorption in the kidney. (3) As discussed in the next

TABLE 23.1 Vasoactive Compounds

VASOCONSTRICTORS	VASODILATORS
Epinephrine (via α_1 receptors)	Epinephrine (via β_2 receptors)
Serotonin	Histamine
ANG II	ANP
AVP	Bradykinins
ET	PGE_2, PGI_2
	NO

section, ANG II and ANG III also stimulate the adrenal cortex to release aldosterone. (4) In the CNS, ANG II stimulates thirst and leads to the release of another vasoconstrictor, AVP. (5) ANG II facilitates the release of norepinephrine by postganglionic sympathetic nerve terminals. (6) Finally, ANG II also acts as a cardiac growth factor.

2. **AVP.** ⊙ **23-24** The posterior pituitary releases AVP. AVP binds to V_{1A} **receptors** on VSMCs, causing *vasoconstriction*, but only at concentrations higher than those that are strongly antidiuretic (see ⊙ **38-2**). Hemorrhagic shock causes enhanced AVP release and a vasoconstriction that contributes to a transient restoration of arterial pressure (see ⊙ **25-5**).

3. **Endothelins (ETs).** Endothelial cells produce ETs (see ⊙ **20-20**) that bind to ET_A **receptors** on VSMCs, causing *vasoconstriction*.

4. **ANP or ANF.** Released from atrial myocytes in response to stretch (see ⊙ **23-21**), this 28–amino-acid peptide binds to **ANP receptor A (NPR1)** on VSMCs, which is membrane-bound guanylyl cyclase, causing *vasodilation*. Because ANP also has powerful diuretic and natriuretic actions, it ultimately reduces plasma volume and therefore blood pressure.

5. **Kinins.** ⊙ **23-25** At least three different kinins exist: (1) the nonapeptide **bradykinin,** which is formed in plasma; (2) the decapeptide **lysyl-bradykinin,** which is liberated from tissues; and (3) **methionyl-lysyl-bradykinin,** which is present in the urine. These kinins are produced by the breakdown of **kininogens,** catalyzed by **kallikreins**—enzymes that are present in plasma and in tissues such as the salivary glands, pancreas, sweat glands, intestine, and kidney. The kinins formed by the action of these kallikreins are eliminated by the **kininases** (kininase I and II). Kininase II is the same as ACE. Thus, the same enzyme (ACE) that generates a vasoconstrictor (ANG II) also disposes of vasodilators (bradykinin). Bradykinin binds to **B2 receptors** on endothelial cells, causing release of NO and prostaglandins and thereby *vasodilation*. Like histamine, the kinins *relax* vascular smooth muscle but *contract* visceral smooth muscle.

Prostaglandins Many tissues synthesize prostaglandins, derivatives of arachidonic acid (see Fig. 3.9). Prostacyclin (prostaglandin I_2 [PGI_2]) binds to prostanoid **IP receptors** on VSMCs, causing strong *vasodilation*. PGE_2 binds to prostanoid EP_2 and EP_4 **receptors** on VSMCs, also causing *vasodilation*. It is doubtful that prostaglandins play a role in systemic vascular control. In veins and also in some arteries, arachidonic acid or

Ca^{2+} ionophores cause endothelium-dependent contractions. Because cyclooxygenase inhibitors prevent this vasoconstrictor response, venous endothelial cells probably metabolize arachidonic acid into a vasoconstrictive cyclooxygenase product, presumably thromboxane A_2.

Nitric Oxide Nitric oxide synthase (NOS) produces NO from arginine in endothelial cells (see ⊙ **20-19**). NO activates the **soluble guanylyl cyclase** in VSMCs, causing *vasodilation*.

Pathways for the renal control of ECF volume are the primary long-term regulators of mean arterial pressure

The *volume of the* ECF includes both the blood plasma and the interstitial fluid. The small solutes in the plasma and interstitial fluid exchange freely across the capillary wall, so that the entire ECF constitutes a single osmotic compartment. Because the plasma volume is a more or less constant fraction (~20%) of the ECF volume, changes in the ECF volume produce proportional changes in plasma volume. Thus, assuming that the compliance of the vasculature is constant (see Equation 19.3), such an increase in plasma volume will lead to an increase in transmural blood pressure.

The *Starling forces* across a capillary (i.e., the hydrostatic and colloid osmotic pressure differences) determine the traffic of fluid between the plasma and the interstitial fluid (see ⊙ **20-16**). Thus, alterations in the Starling forces acting across the capillary wall can affect the plasma volume and therefore blood pressure.

⊙ **23-26** Because of the importance of the ECF volume and Starling forces in determining the plasma volume, one might expect that the body would have specific sensors for ECF volume, interstitial fluid volume, and blood volume. However, the parameter that the body controls in the intermediate- and long-term regulation of the mean arterial pressure is the **effective circulating volume**, the *functional* blood volume that reflects the extent of tissue perfusion, as sensed by the fullness or pressure in the vessels. The control mechanisms that defend effective circulating volume include the two classes of stretch receptors: (1) The high-pressure receptors in the carotid sinus and aorta (see ⊙ **23-1**), which regulate blood pressure in the short term and regulate effective circulating volume in the longer term. (2) The low-pressure receptors (see ⊙ **23-17**), which regulate effective circulating volume by direct and indirect effects on the cardiovascular system. Additional sensors monitoring effective circulating volume (see Table 40.2) are: the baroreceptors in the renal artery, the stretch receptors in the liver, and the atrial myocytes themselves as well as—to some extent—osmoreceptors in the CNS.

These sensors of effective circulating volume send signals to the dominant effector organ—the kidney—to change the rate of Na^+ excretion in the urine. These signals to the kidney follow four parallel effector pathways (see ⊙ **40-1**): (1) the renin–ANG II–aldosterone axis, (2) the autonomic nervous system, (3) the posterior pituitary that releases AVP, and (4) the atrial myocytes that release ANP. Of these four parallel pathways, the most important is the **renin-angiotensin-aldosterone** system. By regulating total body Na^+ content, the kidney determines ECF volume. Therefore, the kidney ultimately governs the blood volume and is thus the principal agent in the long-term control of mean arterial pressure.

CHAPTER 24

SPECIAL CIRCULATIONS

Steven S. Segal

Because each organ in the body has its own unique set of requirements, special circulations within each organ have evolved with their own particular features and regulatory mechanisms. Here, we focus on the circulations of the brain, heart, skeletal muscle, abdominal viscera, and skin.

The blood flow to individual organs must vary to meet the needs of the particular organ, as well as of the whole body

The blood flow to each tissue must meet the nutritional needs of that tissue's parenchymal cells, while at the same time allowing those cells to play their role in the homeostasis of the whole individual. The way in which the circulatory system distributes blood flow must be flexible so that changing demands can be met. Consider the circulatory changes that accompany exercise. Blood flow to active skeletal muscle increases tremendously through both an increase in and a redistribution of cardiac output. Blood flow to the coronary circulation must also rise to meet the demands of exercise. Furthermore, in order to dispose of the heat generated during exercise, the vessels in the skin dilate, thereby promoting heat transfer to the environment. As cardiac output is increasingly directed to active muscle and skin, circulation to the splanchnic and renal circulations decreases, while blood flow to the brain is preserved.

Neural, myogenic, metabolic, and endothelial mechanisms control regional blood flow

The interplay among neural, myogenic, metabolic, and endothelial mechanisms establishes a resting level of vasomotor tone.

Neural Mechanisms The resistance vessels of nearly every organ are invested with fibers of the autonomic nervous system (ANS), particularly those of the sympathetic division (see ◉ 23-13) which modulate local blood flow to meet the needs of particular tissues.

Myogenic Mechanisms The muscular arteries and arterioles that govern vascular resistance are inherently responsive to changes in transmural pressure. Increased pressure and the accompanying stretch of vascular smooth-muscle cells (VSMCs) elicit vasoconstriction (see ◉ 20-18), whereas decreased pressure elicits vasodilation. This myogenic response plays an important role in the autoregulation (see ◉ 20-21) that occurs in the vessels of the brain, heart, skeletal muscle, and kidneys.

Metabolic Mechanisms Throughout the body, the vessels that govern blood flow are sensitive to the local metabolic needs of parenchymal cells. For example, a decrease in P_{O_2} or pH

promotes relaxation of VSMCs, thereby causing vasodilation. In response to activity, excitable cells raise extracellular K^+ concentration ($[K^+]_o$), which also causes vasodilation. Tissues with high energy demands—such as the brain, heart, and skeletal muscle during exercise—rely heavily on such local control mechanisms.

Endothelial Mechanisms Endothelial cells release a variety of vasoactive substances (see Table 20.2). For example, the shear stress exerted by the movement of blood through the vessel lumen stimulates the release of nitric oxide (NO), which relaxes VSMCs and prevents leukocyte adhesion. Endothelial cells and VSMCs also use gap junctions for electrical and chemical signaling between themselves, thereby coordinating their activity during blood flow control. In addition, other factors—which are regulatory in nature—can affect the local circulation. For example, in the heart (see ◉ 24-2) and skeletal muscle, muscle contraction transiently limits blood flow by compressing blood vessels within the tissue.

THE BRAIN

Anastomoses at the circle of Willis and among the branches of distributing arteries protect the blood supply to the brain, which is ~15% of resting cardiac output

The brain accounts for only ~2% of the body's weight, yet it receives ~15% of the resting cardiac output. Of all the organs in the body, the brain is the least tolerant of ischemia. It depends entirely on oxidative sources of energy production. Each day, the human brain oxidizes ~100 g of glucose, which is roughly equivalent to the amount stored as glycogen in the liver. Interruption of cerebral blood flow for just a few seconds causes unconsciousness. If ischemia persists for even a few minutes, irreversible cellular damage is likely.

Arteries Blood reaches the brain through four *source arteries*—the two internal carotid arteries and the two vertebral arteries (Fig. 24.1)—branches of which form the **circle of Willis** at the base of the brain. The internal carotid arteries are the major source of blood to the circle. Three bilateral pairs of *distributing arteries* (anterior, middle, and posterior cerebral arteries) arise from the circle of Willis to envelop the cerebral hemispheres. Each of the four source arteries tends to supply the brain region closest to where the source artery joins the circle of Willis. However, if a stenosis develops in one source artery, other source arteries to the circle of Willis can provide alternative flow.

Veins The veins of the brain are thin-walled structures that have no valves and ultimately drain into the **dural sinuses** (see

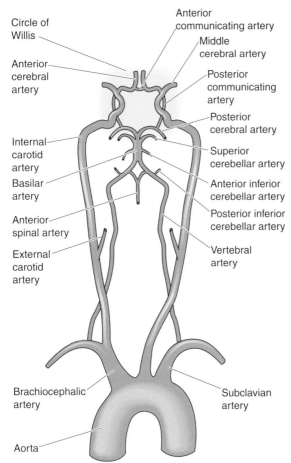

Figure 24.1 Major arterial supply and the circle of Willis.

Circle of Willis

Anterior cerebral artery

Internal carotid artery

Basilar artery

Anterior spinal artery

External carotid artery

Brachiocephalic artery

Aorta

Anterior communicating artery

Middle cerebral artery

Posterior communicating artery

Posterior cerebral artery

Superior cerebellar artery

Anterior inferior cerebellar artery

Posterior inferior cerebellar artery

Vertebral artery

Subclavian artery

Fig. 11.1B). Nearly all of the venous blood from the brain leaves the cranium by way of the **internal jugular vein.**

Capillaries One of the most characteristic features of the brain vasculature is the **blood-brain barrier** (see ⊙ 11-3), which prevents the solutes in the lumen of the capillaries from having direct access to the brain extracellular fluid (BECF). In specialized areas of the brain—the **circumventricular organs** (see ⊙ 11-4)—the capillaries are fenestrated and have permeability characteristics similar to those of capillaries in the intestinal circulation.

Vascular Volume The skull encloses all of the cerebral vasculature, along with the brain and the cerebrospinal fluid compartments. Because the rigid cranium has a fixed total volume, vasodilation and an increase in vascular volume in one region of the brain must be met by reciprocal volume changes elsewhere within the cranium. Precise control of the cerebral blood volume is essential for preventing elevation of the intracranial pressure. With cerebral edema or hemorrhage, or with the growth of a brain tumor, neurological dysfunction can result from the restriction of blood flow due to vascular compression.

Neural, metabolic, and myogenic mechanisms control blood flow to the brain

Cerebral blood flow averages 50 mL/min for each 100 g of brain tissue and, because of autoregulation, is relatively constant. Nevertheless, regional changes in blood distribution occur in response to changing patterns of neuronal activity.

Neural Control *Sympathetic* nerve fibers supplying the brain vasculature originate from postganglionic neurons in the superior cervical ganglia and travel with the internal carotid and vertebral arteries into the skull, branching with the arterial supply. The sympathetic nerve terminals release norepinephrine, which causes contraction of VSMCs. *Parasympathetic* innervation of the cerebral vessels arises from branches of the facial nerve, and elicits modest vasodilation. The cerebral vessels are also supplied with sensory nerves, whose cell bodies are located in the trigeminal ganglia and whose sensory processes can release calcitonin gene–related peptide, a vasodilatory neurotransmitter implicated in migraine.

Metabolic Control Neural activity leads to ATP breakdown and to the local production and release of adenosine, a potent vasodilator. A local increase in brain metabolism also lowers P_{O_2} while raising P_{CO_2} and lowering pH in the nearby BECF. These changes trigger vasodilation and thus a compensatory increase in blood flow. Cerebral VSMCs relax mainly in response to low *extra*cellular pH.

Lowering of *arterial* pH at a constant P_{CO_2} (metabolic acidosis; see ⊙ 28-6) has little effect on cerebral blood flow because arterial H^+ cannot easily penetrate the blood-brain barrier and therefore does not readily reach cerebral VSMCs. On the other hand, lowering of arterial pH by an increase in P_{CO_2} (respiratory acidosis; see ⊙ 28-4) rapidly leads to a fall in the pH around VSMCs because CO_2 readily crosses the blood-brain barrier. This fall in pH of the BECF evokes pronounced dilation of the cerebral vasculature, with an increase in blood flow that occurs within seconds. The fall in arterial P_{CO_2} caused by hyperventilation raises the pH of the BECF, producing cerebral vasoconstriction, decreased blood flow, and dizziness.

A fall in the blood and tissue P_{O_2}—from hypoxemia or impaired cardiac output—may also contribute to cerebral vasodilation, although the effects are less dramatic than those produced by arterial hypercapnia.

Myogenic Control Cerebral resistance vessels are inherently responsive to changes in their transmural pressure. Increases in pressure lead to vasoconstriction, whereas decreases in pressure produce vasodilation.

The neurovascular unit matches blood flow to local brain activity

Neurons, glia, and cerebral blood vessels function as an integrated unit to distribute cerebral blood flow according to local activity within the brain. Synaptic activity generates vasoactive mediators in neurons and astrocytes that can produce vasodilation. Concurrent activation of local interneurons with vascular projections helps to focus the vasomotor response. A reduction in resistance directs increased blood flow to the region of increased neural activity.

Autoregulation maintains a fairly constant cerebral blood flow across a broad range of perfusion pressures

The perfusion pressure to the brain is the difference between the systemic arterial pressure (mean pressure, ~95 mm Hg) and intracranial venous pressure, which is nearly equal to the intracranial pressure (<10 mm Hg). A decrease in cerebral blood flow could thus result from a fall in arterial pressure or a rise in intracranial (or venous) pressure. However, the local control of cerebral blood flow maintains a nearly constant blood flow through perfusion pressures ranging from ~70 to 150 mm Hg. This constancy of blood flow—**autoregulation** (see ⦿ 20-21)—maintains a continuous supply of O_2 and nutrients. Vascular resistance falls with hypotension. This autoregulation of blood flow has both myogenic and metabolic components.

Increases in intracranial pressure compress the brain vasculature and tend to reduce blood flow despite autoregulatory vasodilation. In such cases, the brain regulates its blood flow by inducing reflexive changes in *systemic arterial pressure*. This principle is exemplified by the **Cushing reflex,** an increase in arterial pressure that occurs in response to an increase in intracranial pressure. It appears that intracranial compression causes a local ischemia that stimulates vasomotor centers in the medulla. Increased sympathetic nerve activity in the systemic circulation then triggers a rise in total peripheral resistance.

THE HEART

The coronary circulation receives 5% of the resting cardiac output from the left heart and mostly returns it to the right heart

⦿ **24-1** The heart receives ~5% of the resting cardiac output, although it represents <0.5% of total body weight. The heart normally uses oxidative phosphorylation to generate the ATP required to pump blood. More than 60% of myocardial O_2 consumption in the fasting state is due to the oxidation of fatty acids, with the remainder reflecting oxidation of carbohydrate. The myocardium readily oxidizes ketone bodies (see ⦿ 58-16). When the O_2 supply is adequate, the heart takes up and oxidizes both lactate and pyruvate. When the energetic demand for ATP exceeds the supply of O_2, the heart

can no longer take up lactate, but instead releases lactate by breaking down its own glycogen stores. If hypoxia develops in the myocardium, nociceptive fibers trigger the sensation of referred pain, known as **angina pectoris.** More severe or prolonged insults damage the myocardial tissue, which eventually becomes necrotic: **myocardial infarction.**

The entire blood supply to the myocardium derives from the right and left coronary arteries, which originate at the root of the aorta behind the cusps of the aortic valves (Fig. 24.2). Although the anatomy is subject to individual variation, the **right coronary artery** generally supplies the right ventricle and atrium, and the left coronary artery supplies the left ventricle and atrium. The **left coronary artery** divides near its origin into two principal branches: The **left circumflex artery** sends branches to the left atrium and ventricle, and the **left anterior descending artery** descends to the apex of the heart and branches to supply the interventricular septum and a portion of the right as well as the left ventricle. These arteries course over the heart, branching into segments that penetrate into the tissue and dividing into capillary networks. Capillary density in the human heart exceeds 3000 per square millimeter. The small diameter of cardiac muscle fibers (<20 µm) facilitates O_2 diffusion into the cardiac myocytes, which have a high energetic demand.

Once blood passes through the capillaries, it collects in venules, which drain outward from the myocardium to converge into the epicardial veins. These veins empty into the right atrium via the **coronary sinus.** Other vascular channels drain directly into the cardiac chambers. These include the **thebesian veins,** which drain capillary beds within the ventricular wall. Because the deoxygenated blood carried by the thebesian veins exits predominantly into the ventricles, this blood flow bypasses the pulmonary circulation.

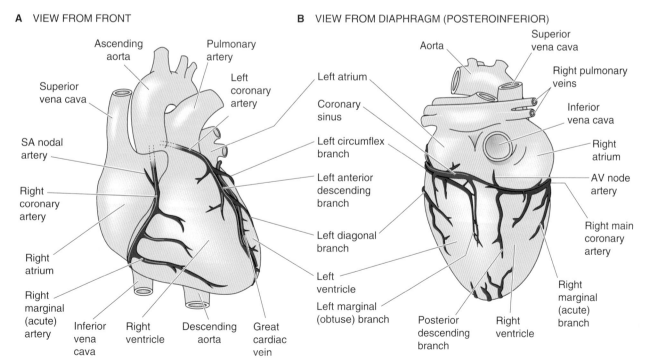

A VIEW FROM FRONT

B VIEW FROM DIAPHRAGM (POSTEROINFERIOR)

Figure 24.2 Heart and coronary circulation. *AV,* Atrioventricular; *SA,* sinoatrial.

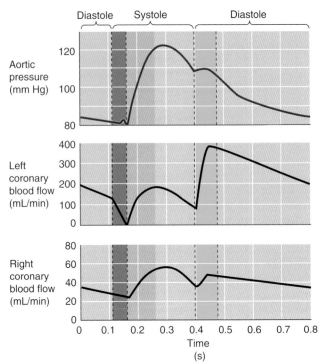

Figure 24.3 Coronary blood flow cycle. Bands at the beginning of systole and diastole reflect isovolumetric contraction and relaxation, respectively.

⊙ 24-2 Extravascular compression impairs coronary blood flow during systole

In other systemic vascular beds, blood flow roughly parallels the pressure profile in the aorta, rising in systole and falling in diastole (see Fig. 22.3). However, in the coronary circulation, flow is somewhat paradoxical: Although the heart is the source of its own perfusion pressure, myocardial contraction effectively compresses the heart's own vascular supply. Therefore, the profile of blood flow through the coronary arteries depends on both the perfusion pressure in the aorta (Fig. 24.3, *top panel*) and the extravascular compression resulting from the contracting ventricles, particularly the left ventricle.

Blood flow in the *left coronary artery* may actually reverse transiently in early systole (Fig. 24.3, *middle panel*) because the force of the left ventricle's isovolumetric contraction compresses the left coronary vessels and the aortic pressure has not yet begun to rise (i.e., aortic valve is still closed). As aortic pressure increases later during systole, coronary blood flow increases, but never reaches peak values. However, early during diastole, when the relaxed ventricles no longer compress the left coronary vessels and aortic pressure is still high, left coronary flow rises rapidly to extremely high levels. All told, ~80% of total left coronary blood flow occurs during diastole.

The profile of flow through the *right coronary artery* (Fig. 24.3, *lower panel*) is very similar to the pressure profile of the aorta. Here, systole contributes a greater proportion of the total flow, and systolic reversal does not occur. The reason for this difference is the lower wall tension developed by the right heart, which pumps against the low resistance of the pulmonary circulation and does not occlude the right coronary vessels during contraction.

During tachycardia, the fraction of the cardiac cycle spent in diastole decreases, minimizing the time available for maximal left coronary perfusion.

Coronary blood flow not only varies in *time* during the cardiac cycle, it also varies with *depth* in the wall of the heart. Blood flows to cardiac myocytes through arteries that penetrate from the epicardium toward the endocardium. During systole, the intramuscular pressure is greatest near the endocardium and least near the epicardium. All things being equal, the perfusion of the endocardium would therefore be less than that of the epicardium. However, total blood flows to the endocardial and epicardial halves are approximately equal because the endocardium has a lower intrinsic vascular resistance, and thus a greater blood flow during *diastole*.

Myocardial blood flow parallels myocardial metabolism

The coronary circulation presents a nearly linear correspondence between myocardial O_2 consumption and myocardial blood flow. This relationship persists in isolated heart preparations, emphasizing that metabolic signals are the principal determinants of O_2 delivery to the myocardium. The heart can meet large increases in O_2 demand only by increasing coronary blood flow, which can exceed 250 mL/min per 100 g with exercise.

Because blood pressure normally varies within fairly narrow limits, the only way to substantially increase blood flow through the coronary circulation during exercise is by vasodilation. The heart relies primarily on metabolic mechanisms to increase the caliber of its coronary vessels. **Adenosine** has received particular emphasis in this regard. An increased metabolic activity of the heart, an insufficient coronary blood flow, or a fall in myocardial P_{O_2} results in adenosine release. Adenosine then diffuses to the VSMCs, activating purinergic receptors to induce vasodilation by lowering $[Ca^{2+}]_i$.

When cardiac work increases, contracting myocytes release K^+, resulting in a transient rise in $[K^+]_o$ that may contribute to the initial increase in coronary perfusion. When the O_2 demand of cardiac myocytes exceeds O_2 supply, a rise in the P_{CO_2} and a fall in the P_{O_2} may also lower coronary vascular resistance and thereby increase local O_2 delivery.

Coronary blood flow is relatively stable between perfusion pressures of ~70 mm Hg and >150 mm Hg. Thus, like that of the brain, the blood flow to the heart exhibits **autoregulation**. In addition to the myogenic response, fluctuations in adenosine and P_{O_2} contribute to coronary autoregulation.

Although sympathetic stimulation directly constricts coronary vessels, accompanying metabolic effects predominate, producing an overall vasodilation

Sympathetic nerves course throughout the heart, following the arterial supply. Stimulation of these nerves causes the heart to beat more frequently and more forcefully. β_1 adrenoceptors on the cardiac myocytes mediate these chronotropic and inotropic responses. The increased metabolic work of the myocardium leads to coronary vasodilation via metabolic pathways. Blocking of β_1 receptors "unmasks" adrenergic vasoconstriction. However, under normal circumstances (i.e., no β blockade), the tendency of the *metabolic* pathways to vasodilate far overwhelms the tendency of the *sympathetic* pathways to vasoconstrict.

Activation of the **vagus nerve** has only a mild vasodilatory effect on the coronary resistance vessels. The release of acetylcholine from the vagus nerve is restricted to the vicinity of the sinoatrial node. Thus, the vagus nerve has a much greater effect on heart rate than on coronary resistance.

Collateral vessel growth can provide blood flow to ischemic regions

When a coronary artery or one of its primary branches becomes abruptly occluded, ischemia can produce necrosis (i.e., a myocardial infarct) in the region deprived of blood flow. However, if a coronary artery narrows *gradually* over time, collateral blood vessels may develop and ameliorate the reduced delivery of O_2 and nutrients to the compromised area, preventing or at least diminishing tissue damage. Collateral vessels originate from existing vessel branches that undergo remodeling with the proliferation of endothelial and smooth-muscle cells.

Vasodilator drugs may compromise myocardial flow through "coronary steal"

A variety of drugs that can promote vasodilation of the coronary arteries are typically prescribed for patients with angina pectoris. Administration of a vasodilator can increase the diameter of blood vessels only in *nonischemic* vascular beds that are parallel to the ischemic ones, which thereby decreases the pressure at the branch point, upstream from the stenosis. The result is **coronary steal.** When vasodilator therapy relieves angina, the favorable result is more likely attributable to the vasodilation of the *noncoronary* systemic vessels, which reduces peripheral resistance, thereby reducing the afterload during systole and thus the work of the heart.

THE SKELETAL MUSCLE

Muscle blood flow at rest is 5 to 10 mL/min for each 100 g of tissue. With maximal aerobic exercise, it may increase 50-fold, reaching 250 mL/min or more for each 100 g of active muscle. The linear correspondence among work rate, O_2 consumption, and muscle blood flow implies a "coupling" between muscle fiber activity and O_2 delivery to capillaries.

A microvascular unit is the capillary bed supplied by a single terminal arteriole

The vascular supply to skeletal muscle begins externally to the tissue in the **feed arteries.** These muscular vessels are the last branches of the arterial supply, located just before entry into the tissue. As much as 30% to 50% of the total resistance to blood flow of skeletal muscle resides in these feed arteries.

The arteriolar network originates from the site at which a feed artery enters the muscle. Within the muscle, arterioles branch through several orders until reaching the **terminal arterioles,** which are the last branches to contain smooth muscle and, therefore, the last branches still able to control blood flow. Thus, the terminal arteriole is the functional equivalent of the precapillary sphincter (see ⊙ 20-2). The group of capillaries supplied by a terminal arteriole represents one **microvascular unit,** which is the smallest functional unit of blood flow control in skeletal muscle. Each unit consists of capillaries that run parallel to the muscle fibers in each direction, for a distance of ≤1 mm, ending in a **collecting venule.**

Because muscle fibers may have lengths of many centimeters, many microvascular units are required to span the distance of each muscle fiber.

⊙ 24-3 Metabolites released by active muscle trigger vasodilation and an increase in blood flow

When skeletal muscle is at rest, its vascular resistance is high, blood flow is low, and the venous O_2 content is only a few milliliters per deciliter lower than the arterial O_2 content. As exercise begins, the terminal arterioles (those closest to the capillaries) dilate first. This vasodilation increases blood flow through capillaries that are already flowing with blood and opens up previously unperfused capillaries, thus increasing the number of perfused capillaries and thereby decreasing the effective intercapillary distance (see ⊙ 20-4). Even before total blood flow increases, the greater demand of active muscle fibers for O_2 produces a large increase in the O_2 extraction ratio (see ⊙ 20-6). As metabolic demand continues to increase, additional O_2 delivery is required.

The vasculature meets increased metabolic demand by progressively dilating the more proximal arteriolar branches and feed arteries. Dilation of the downstream arterioles, without dilation of the proximal arterioles and feed arteries, would result in only a limited ability to increase muscle blood flow because of the high resistance of upstream vessels. Thus, when feed arteries dilate in concert with arterioles, the increase in muscle blood flow is profound.

The primary stimulus triggering vasodilation is the release of vasodilator substances (e.g., adenosine, CO_2, K^+) from active muscle fibers in proportion to the energy expenditure. These metabolites diffuse locally and—acting either directly on VSMCs or indirectly on adjacent endothelial cells—relax the VSMCs of resistance vessels, thereby increasing blood flow in proportion to local demand.

Sympathetic innervation increases the intrinsic tone of resistance vessels

Sympathetic nerve fibers invest the entire resistance network of skeletal muscle, from feed arteries to terminal arterioles. The release of norepinephrine by these nerve terminals activates α-adrenoceptors on VSMCs, leading to vasoconstriction beyond that produced by transmural pressure and myogenic tone. On the other hand, the shear stress of blood flowing past the endothelial cells produces vasodilators, such as NO. The interactions among these vasoconstrictor and vasodilatory mechanisms maintain the intrinsic basal tone of the VSMCs. Venules also constrict in response to sympathetic nerve stimulation but are not directly innervated, and instead respond to norepinephrine that diffuses from the nearby arterioles.

With the onset of exercise, or when high-pressure baroreceptors detect a fall in blood pressure (see ⊙ 23-1), sympathetic firing to skeletal muscle resistance vessels increases to levels that would close the lumens of arterioles in resting skeletal muscle. However, during exercise arterioles remain dilated under the influence of vasodilator metabolites released from surrounding muscle fibers.

During exercise, total blood flow through skeletal muscle increases to as much as 80% of cardiac output. This redistribution of systemic blood flow occurs for two reasons. First, the increase in sympathetic nerve activity constricts the splanchnic circulation, renal circulation (see ⊙ 34-7), and the vessels of *inactive* skeletal muscle. Indeed, only the brain and heart are spared from vasoconstriction. Second, the metabolites released by active skeletal muscle overcome the constriction of arterioles that sympathetic activity would otherwise produce. In addition, substances released during muscle fiber contraction (e.g., NO and adenosine) may inhibit norepinephrine release from sympathetic nerve fibers surrounding the arterioles.

The vasodilatory effects of the metabolites notwithstanding, sympathetic vasoconstrictor activity can limit muscle blood flow, particularly when another large mass of muscle is active simultaneously and requires a substantial portion of cardiac output.

Rhythmic contraction promotes blood flow through the "muscle pump"

During exercise, skeletal muscle undergoes rhythmic changes in length and tension, giving rise to mechanical forces within the tissue analogous to those of the beating heart. The contraction of muscle forces venous blood out of the muscle and impedes arterial inflow. Because valves in the veins prevent backflow of blood, each muscle contraction squeezes and empties the veins, driving blood toward the heart (see ⊙ 22-1). During the subsequent relaxation, the reduction in venous pressure increases the arteriovenous driving force for capillary perfusion. As is true for coronary blood flow, skeletal muscle blood flow is maximal between contractions. This pumping action of skeletal muscle on the vasculature imparts substantial kinetic energy to the blood, thereby reducing the work of the heart. Remarkably, the skeletal muscle pump may generate up to half of the total energy required to circulate blood, an essential contribution for achieving the high blood flows experienced during maximal aerobic exercise.

THE SPLANCHNIC ORGANS

The splanchnic circulation includes the blood flow through the stomach, small intestine, large intestine, pancreas, spleen, and liver. The majority of flow to the liver occurs through the portal vein, which carries the venous blood draining from all of these organs except the liver itself.

The vascular supply to the gut is highly interconnected

The **celiac artery** is the primary blood supply to the stomach, pancreas, and spleen. The **superior and inferior mesenteric arteries** supply the large and small intestines, as well as parts of the stomach and pancreas. The extensive interconnections between its arterial branches provide multiple collateral pathways through which blood can reach each portion of the intestines.

The microvascular network in the small intestine (Fig. 24.4A) is representative of that throughout the gastrointestinal tract. After penetrating the wall of the intestine, small arteries course through the various muscle layers and reach the submucosa, where they branch into arterioles. Some arterioles remain in the submucosa to form a submucosal vascular plexus. Others project toward the intestinal lumen and into the mucosa, including the villi. Venules emerging from the villi and mucosal and muscularis layers converge into veins. These exit the intestinal wall, paralleling the arterial supply.

The arrangement of microvessels within a villus is like a fountain (Fig. 24.4B). The incoming arteriole courses up the center of the villus, branching into many capillaries along the way to the tip of the villus. Capillaries converge into venules and carry blood back to the base of the villus. Capillaries also interconnect the arteriole and the venule all along the villus. These microvessels of villi are highly permeable to solutes of low molecular weight, thereby facilitating the absorption of nutrients.

Because the capillaries in the villi are fenestrated (i.e., they have large pores) and have a large surface area, they are well suited for absorbing nutrients from the intestinal lumen. The

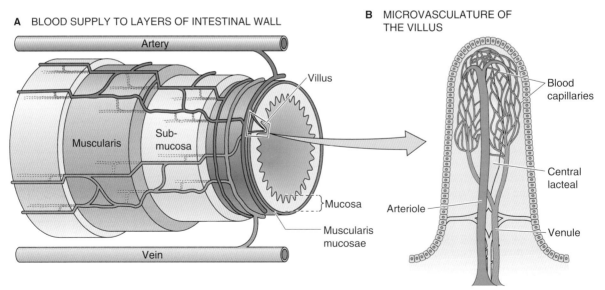

A   BLOOD SUPPLY TO LAYERS OF INTESTINAL WALL

B   MICROVASCULATURE OF THE VILLUS

Artery

Villus

Muscularis

Sub-mucosa

Mucosa

Muscularis mucosae

Vein

Blood capillaries

Central lacteal

Arteriole

Venule

Figure 24.4   Intestinal blood supply.

venous blood carries away the majority of **water-soluble nutrients** absorbed from the gut, eventually delivering them to the portal vein. **Lipophilic nutrients** absorbed from the intestinal lumen enter the central lacteal of the villus, which merges with the intestinal lymphatics. The lymph then delivers these substances into the bloodstream via the thoracic duct.

Blood flow to the gastrointestinal tract increases up to eight-fold after a meal (postprandial hyperemia)

Throughout the gastrointestinal tract, blood flow in each layer of the gut wall closely correlates with the local metabolism. Intestinal blood flow at rest, in the fasting state, is typically 30 mL/min for each 100 g of tissue. However, flow can reach 250 mL/min for each 100 g during peak hyperemia after a meal.

First, the CNS initiates an "anticipatory" response that increases splanchnic blood flow with the mere thought of food—corresponding to the "cephalic phase" of gastric (see ⊚ 42-4) and pancreatic secretion (see ⊚ 43-5).

Second, mucosal metabolic activity during digestion consumes O_2 and produces **vasodilator metabolites** (e.g., adenosine and CO_2) that increases blood flow locally.

Third, the absorption of nutrients generates hyperosmolality in both the blood and the lymphatic vessels of the villus. Hyperosmolality itself stimulates an increase in blood flow.

Fourth, during digestion, the gastrointestinal tract releases several hormones, some of which are vasoactive. Of these, **cholecystokinin** and **neurotensin** (see Table 41.1) may reach high enough concentrations in the local circulation to promote intestinal blood flow. The intestinal epithelium also releases various kinins (e.g., bradykinin and kallidin), which are powerful vasodilators. The magnitude of the postprandial hyperemia further depends on the nature of the luminal content. Bile acids and partially digested fats are particularly effective in promoting hyperemia by acting on chemoreceptors in the intestinal mucosa.

The circulatory system does not distribute the increased splanchnic blood flow equally to all digestive organs, nor does it distribute the flow equally throughout the wall of even one segment of bowel. During and after a meal, as digestion and absorption proceed, blood flow increases sequentially along the gastrointestinal tract, first in the stomach and then in progressively more distal segments of the intestine. In all segments, blood flow through the muscularis layers primarily provides nutrition for the smooth-muscle cells. After a meal, splanchnic blood flow remains elevated for 2 to 4 hours, primarily reflecting the vasodilation in the *mucosal* layer.

Sympathetic activity directly constricts splanchnic blood vessels, whereas parasympathetic activity indirectly dilates them

The gastrointestinal tract is endowed with its own division of the ANS, the **enteric nervous system** (**ENS;** see ⊚ 14-1 and ⊚ 41-1). One of the components of the ENS, the myenteric (or Auerbach's) plexus, releases vasoactive neurotransmitters.

The predominant neural influence is via sympathetic postganglionic fibers, which release norepinephrine that acts on α adrenoceptors on VSMCs and produces vasoconstriction. The vasoconstriction occurs to a similar extent in both the muscularis and mucosal layers, without redistribution of flow between the layers. Vasoconstriction elicited by sympathetic nerve activity can reduce blood flow to <10 mL/min per 100 g of tissue (i.e., ~⅓ of resting values).

Parasympathetic preganglionic fibers travel to the intestine via vagal or pelvic nerves, which contact postganglionic parasympathetic neurons in the intestinal wall. The effect of parasympathetic activity on blood flow is indirect. Parasympathetic activity stimulates intestinal motility and glandular secretion, which in turn increases intestinal metabolism, thereby enhancing blood flow to the gut.

Changes in the splanchnic circulation regulate total peripheral resistance and the distribution of blood volume

The splanchnic circulation serves both as a site of adjustable resistance and as a major reservoir of blood. During exercise, when blood flow increases to active skeletal muscle, sympathetic constriction of the splanchnic resistance vessels decreases the proportion of cardiac output directed to the viscera.

The splanchnic circulation contains ~15% of the total blood volume, with the majority contained in the liver. During increases in sympathetic tone, splanchnic arteriolar constriction reduces perfusion, resulting in the passive collapse of the splanchnic veins. Blood contained in these veins moves into the inferior vena cava, thus increasing the circulating blood volume.

The liver receives its blood flow from both the systemic and the portal circulation

The liver receives nearly one fourth of resting cardiac output. Of this blood flow, ~25% is arterial blood that arrives via the hepatic artery. The remaining 75% of the hepatic blood flow comes from the portal vein, which drains the stomach, intestines, pancreas, and spleen. Because the portal venous blood has already given up much of its O_2 to the gut, the hepatic artery is left to supply ~75% of the O_2 used by the liver. We discuss the anatomy of the hepatic circulation in more detail in Chapter 46 (see ⊚ 46-1).

The mean blood pressure in the portal vein is normally 10 to 12 mm Hg. In contrast, the pressure in the hepatic artery averages 90 mm Hg. These two systems, with very different pressures, feed into the sinusoids (8 to 9 mm Hg). The sinusoids drain into the hepatic veins (~5 mm Hg), and these in turn drain into the vena cava (2 to 5 mm Hg). These remarkable values lead us to three conclusions. First, there must be a very high "precapillary" resistance between the hepatic artery (90 mm Hg) and the sinusoids (8 to 9 mm Hg), causing the arterial pressure to step down to sinusoidal values. Second, because the pressure in the portal vein (10 to 12 mm Hg) is only slightly higher than that in the sinusoids (8 to 9 mm Hg), the precapillary resistance of the portal inflow (75% of the total blood flow entering the liver) must be very low. Third, because the pressure in the sinusoids is only slightly higher than that in the hepatic vein, the resistance of the sinusoids must also be extremely low.

As a result of the unique hemodynamics of the liver, changes in pressure within the hepatic vein have profound effects on fluid exchange across the wall of sinusoids. An elevated vena cava pressure can result in transudation of fluid from the liver into the peritoneal cavity, a condition known as **ascites**.

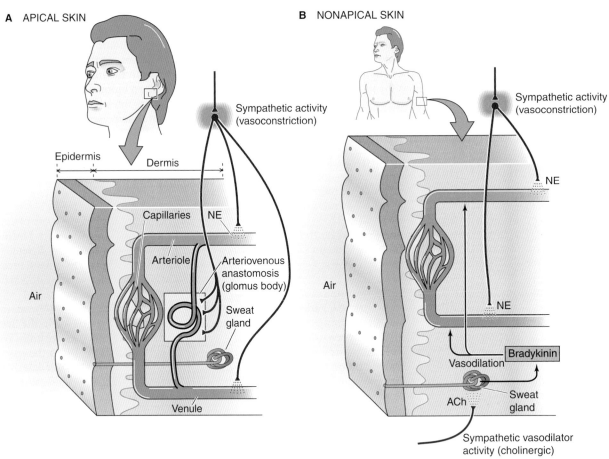

Figure 24.5 Blood flow to the skin. (A) In apical skin, glomus bodies (arteriovenous anastomoses) can reach a density of ~500 per cm² in the nail beds. (B) The nonapical skin lacks glomus bodies. Postganglionic sympathetic fibers release norepinephrine (NE), causing the usual vasoconstriction. Preganglionic sympathetic fibers release acetylcholine (ACh) and cause vasodilation, perhaps mediated by formation of bradykinin.

THE SKIN

The skin is the largest organ of the body

The skin is the major barrier between the internal milieu of the body and the environment of the outside world. The skin is normally overperfused in relation to its nutritional requirements. However, changes in blood flow to the skin also play a central role in the body's temperature regulation (see ⊙ 59-12).

In terms of blood flow, we can divide the skin into "apical" skin (Fig. 24.5A)—which is present on the nose, lips, ears, hands, and feet—and "nonapical" skin (Fig. 24.5B). In skin, capillaries reach only as superficially as the dermis; the epidermis does not have a blood supply. The venules that are part of a plexus of vessels near the dermal-epidermal border (i.e., the most superficial vessels) may contain an appreciable volume of blood. When cutaneous blood flow decreases, this volume of blood also decreases. Local nutritional flow through the precapillary sphincters and capillaries is under the control of local vasodilator metabolites and sensory stimuli (e.g., temperature, touch, pain).

⊙ 24-4 Specialized arteriovenous anastomoses in apical skin help control heat loss

Apical Skin The apical skin at the extremities of the body has a very high surface-to-volume ratio that favors heat loss. Circulation to these apical regions has an unusual feature: *arteriovenous (a-v) anastomoses,* called **glomus bodies.** Glomus bodies of the skin are tiny nodules found in many parts of the body, including the ears, the pads of the fingers and toes, and the nail beds. As the afferent arteriole enters the connective tissue capsule of the glomus body, it becomes a vessel with a small lumen and a thick, muscular wall comprising multiple layers of myoepithelioid cells. These vessels connect with short, thin-walled veins that eventually drain into larger skin veins. The a-v anastomoses, which are involved in heat exchange, are in parallel with the capillaries of the skin, which are involved in nutrient exchange (Fig. 24.5A).

The anastomotic vessels are under neural control and play a critical role in temperature regulation. In these apical regions, blood flow is under the control of sympathetic fibers that release norepinephrine and thereby constrict the arterioles, anastomotic vessels, and venules. The increase in sympathetic tone that occurs in response to decreases in core temperature elicits vasoconstriction in the a-v anastomoses, a fall in blood flow, and a reduction in heat loss. Maximal sympathetic stimulation can completely obliterate the lumen of an anastomotic vessel, thus greatly reducing total blood flow to the skin. On the other hand, when the core temperature rises, the withdrawal of sympathetic tone leads to vasodilation.

Nonapical Skin Vasculature in nonapical skin lacks a-v anastomoses, but possesses two types of sympathetic neurons innervating the vessels of the skin: one releasing *norepinephrine* and another releasing *acetylcholine.*

Vasoconstriction occurs in response to the release of norepinephrine. Blockade of sympathetic innervation to *nonapical* skin in a thermoneutral environment produces little change in skin blood flow, demonstrating that little vasoconstrictor activity is present at rest.

◉ 24-5 Vasodilation in nonapical skin occurs in response to sympathetic neurons that release acetylcholine (see Fig. 25.3). Indeed, blockade of sympathetic innervation to the nonapical skin in a warm environment produces vasoconstriction and a decrease in skin blood flow, demonstrating neurally directed vasodilation before the blockade. The precise mechanism of this vasodilation is obscure.

Mechanical stimuli elicit local vascular responses in the skin

White Reaction If the skin is stroked mildly with a sharp instrument, a blanched line appears in the trailing path of the instrument. The immediate response is attributable to passive expulsion of the blood by the external mechanical force. During the next 15 to 60 seconds, the **white reaction** that ensues is caused by contraction of microvascular VSMCs and pericytes in response to mechanical stimulation. This active response has the effect of emptying the capillary loops, the collecting venules, and the subpapillary venous plexus of blood in a sharply delineated manner.

"Triple Response" If a pointed instrument is drawn across the skin more forcefully, a series of reactions ensues that is collectively known as the **triple response.** Within several seconds, a band of increased redness appears due to a local dilation and increased perfusion of capillaries and venules within the perturbed area. This **red reaction** is independent of innervation and may persist for one to several minutes. The presumed cause is the local release of a vasodilator substance (e.g., histamine) from cells that were disturbed by the mechanical response.

If the stimulus is sufficiently strong or repeated, the reddening of the skin is no longer restricted to the line that was stroked but spreads to the surrounding region. This **flare reaction** is a local nervous response known as the **axon reflex,** and depends on the branching of a single nerve fiber (see Fig. 15.22), so that an action potential travels centrally to the point of fiber branching. From this branch point, the afferent signal travels both orthodromically to the spinal cord and antidromically along the collateral branch.

When the stimulus is even more intense, the skin along the line of injury develops localized swelling known as a **wheal.** This local edema results from an increase in capillary permeability (e.g., in response to histamine) as filtration exceeds absorption. The wheal is preceded by and ultimately replaces the red reaction, appearing within a few minutes from the time of injury, and it is often surrounded by the flare reaction.

CHAPTER 25

INTEGRATED CONTROL OF THE CARDIOVASCULAR SYSTEM

Emile L. Boulpaep

Powerful *systemic* mechanisms operate over both the short term and the long term to control mean arterial pressure and cardiac output. Operating independently of these are *local* mechanisms of control that regulate blood flow at the microcirculatory level. In addition, individual organs have their own unique tools for managing specific circulatory requirements. In this chapter, we will learn how the cardiovascular system integrates the complex systemic, local, and individualized regulatory mechanisms in response to the demands of everyday life.

INTERACTION AMONG THE DIFFERENT CARDIOVASCULAR CONTROL SYSTEMS

The control of the cardiovascular system involves "linear," "branched," and "connected" interactions

We often present physiological responses in a linear sequence or on a **linear chart** (Fig. 25.1A). However, cardiovascular parameters and associated physiological responses are often related by multiple factors, requiring a more complex diagram called a **branching tree** (Fig. 25.1B).

For example, the control of *mean arterial pressure* depends on both *cardiac output* (and all the elements in its branching tree in Fig. 25.1B) and *total peripheral resistance*, which requires a branching tree of its own (Fig. 25.1C). A physiological system with such complex interactions is best represented by a **connected diagram,** which may include feedback loops (Fig. 25.1C, *red arrows*), parameters that appear more than once in the tree (connected by a *red dashed line*), or factors that modulate parameters in two different branches of the tree (connected by *brown arrows*). Several feedback loops may impinge on a single element, and some loops are more dominant than others. The complex interactions among parameters make it difficult to distinguish factors of overriding importance from those of lesser weight. Moreover, when one disturbs a single parameter in a complex physiological system, the initial state of other parameters determines the end state of the system.

Regulation of the entire cardiovascular system depends on the integrated action of multiple subsystem controls as well as noncardiovascular controls

In performing a systems analysis of the entire cardiovascular system, we must consider the interrelationships among its various subsystems. For instance, consider the effects of administering norepinephrine, which has a high affinity for α_1 adrenoceptors, less for β_1 adrenoceptors, and far less for β_2 adrenoceptors. These receptors are present, in varying degrees, in both the blood vessels and the heart. Because α_1 adrenoceptors (high affinity) are present in most vascular beds, we expect widespread vasoconstriction. Because β_2 adrenoceptors (low affinity) are present in only a few vascular beds, we predict little vasodilation. Because β_1 adrenoceptors (intermediate affinity) are present in pacemaker and myocardial cells of the heart, we would anticipate an increase in both heart rate and contractility and therefore an increase in cardiac output.

Although our analysis predicts that the *heart rate* should increase, in most cases the dominant effect of intravenous norepinephrine injection is to slow down the heart. The explanation is that increased peripheral resistance (caused by stimulation of α_1 receptors) and increased cardiac output (caused by stimulation of β_1 receptors) combine to cause a substantial rise in mean arterial pressure. The baroreceptor reflex (*red arrow* on right in Fig. 25.1C) then intervenes to instruct the heart to slow down (see ⊙ 23-1). However, bradycardia may not occur if many vascular beds were dilated before the administration of norepinephrine; in this case, the rise in blood pressure would be modest.

In trying to understand the integrated response of the cardiovascular system to an insult, we must include in our analysis not only all the subsystems of the cardiovascular system but also the pertinent control systems outside the circulation, such as:

1. Autonomic nervous system (ANS).
2. Respiratory system.
3. Hematopoietic organs and liver.
4. Gastrointestinal and urinary systems.
5. Endocrine system.
6. Temperature control system.

We will now consider the integrated cardiovascular responses to four important circulatory "stresses": (1) orthostasis (i.e., standing up), (2) emotional stress, (3) exercise, and (4) hemorrhage.

RESPONSE TO ERECT POSTURE

Because of gravity, standing up (orthostasis) tends to shift blood from the head and heart to veins in the legs

About two thirds of the total blood volume resides in the systemic veins (see ⊙ 19-3). When a recumbent subject assumes an upright position, the blood shifts from the central blood volume reservoirs and other veins to large veins in the dependent limbs. Unless compensatory mechanisms intervene, blood redistribution will lower not only arterial blood pressure but also venous return and thus cardiac output.

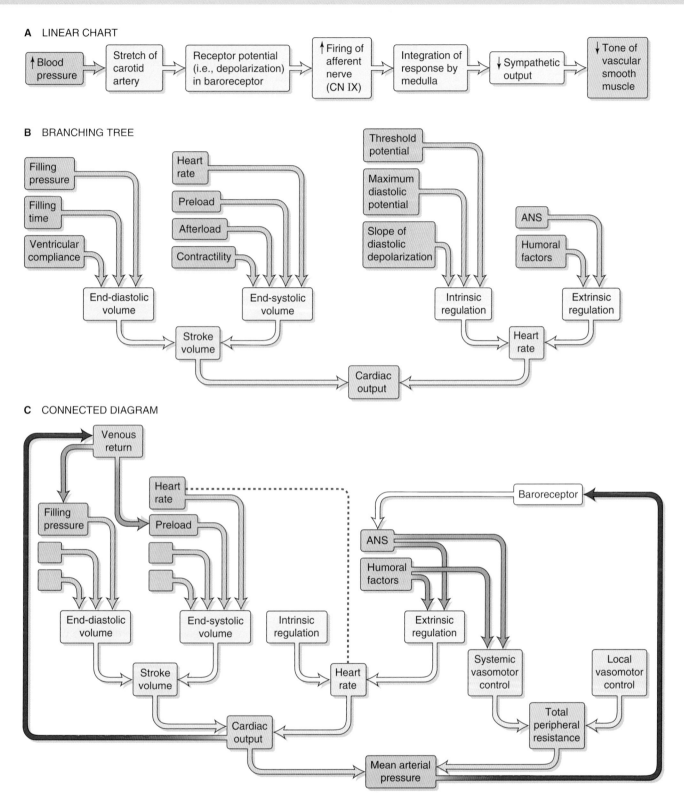

Figure 25.1 Patterns of cardiovascular control. (A) The baroreceptor reflex is depicted as a linear sequence. (B) Cardiac output depends on multiple parameters. (C) A branching tree represents the control of mean arterial pressure. The left limb repeats (B). Superimposed on this simple tree are three more complex interactions: (1) feedback loops *(red arrows),* (2) two occurrences of the same parameter *(connected by the red dashed line),* and (3) examples of parameters exerting effects on two different branches of the tree *(brown arrows). CN,* Cranial nerve.

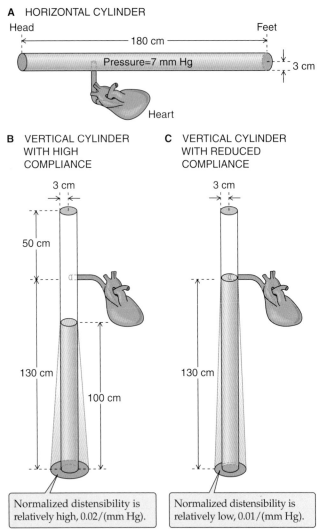

A HORIZONTAL CYLINDER

B VERTICAL CYLINDER WITH HIGH COMPLIANCE

C VERTICAL CYLINDER WITH REDUCED COMPLIANCE

| Normalized distensibility is relatively high, 0.02/(mm Hg). | Normalized distensibility is relatively low, 0.01/(mm Hg). |

Figure 25.2 Model of the orthostatic redistribution of blood. (A) A horizontal tube (3-cm radius, 180 cm long) contains the entire blood volume (5 L). With no blood flow, pressure inside the tube is uniform and corresponds to a mean systemic filling pressure of 7 mm Hg. (B) With the cylinder upright (orthostasis), pressure gradually increases toward the bottom, causing increasingly greater distention of this compliant tube. Because blood volume has shifted to the bottom, the upper level of the blood column is 30 cm below the level of the heart, preventing venous return. (C) Reducing compliance of the tube by half also causes distention to fall by half. With the reduced shift of blood volume, the upper level of the blood column now just reaches the heart.

To illustrate the effect of blood redistribution on venous return, we will represent the entire circulatory system by a horizontal, distensible cylinder 180 cm in length (the height of our person) and 3 cm in radius (Fig. 25.2A). This cylinder holds ~5000 mL of blood (the normal blood volume). If a subject is recumbent and has no heartbeat, and if the cardiovascular system is filled with a normal blood volume of 5000 mL (V_o), the overall compliance of the system will produce a uniform pressure of ~7 mm Hg. If we were to transfuse an additional 100 mL (ΔV) of blood into our cylinder, the mean systemic filling pressure (MSFP) would rise by ~1 mm Hg (ΔP). Thus, for every 2% increase in blood volume, the MSFP of the cylinder increases by 1 mm Hg. In other words, the compliance, expressed as a normalized distensibility, is 0.02/(mm Hg).

If our cylinder is now turned upright, we have a vertical column of blood 180 cm tall, and we must now consider gravity (Fig. 25.2B). The highest pressures will be at the bottom of the cylinder. (Fig. 17.6 shows that orthostasis causes venous pressure at the ankle to rise from 5 to 100 mm Hg.) Therefore, our cylinder will distend maximally at the bottom, and this distention represents a shift in blood volume. The bottom of the cylinder (corresponding to the "dependent areas" of a person) gains volume, whereas the top (i.e., corresponding to the cranial portion of a person) loses blood volume.

The column of blood in our upright, 180-cm-tall cylinder would reach only about 100 cm (Fig. 25.2B). If the heart were 50 cm below the top of the cylinder, then the top of the column would now be ~30 cm below the level of the heart. Therefore, there would be no blood to return to the heart. Moreover, the right arterial pressure (RAP) would be negative (-30 cm H_2O, or about -22 mm Hg). Because the heart cannot create a vacuum this large at its input by "sucking" blood, cardiac output would fall to zero.

The ANS mediates an "orthostatic response" that raises heart rate and peripheral vascular resistance and thus tends to restore mean arterial pressure

Although our model predicts that orthostasis should cause RAP to fall to -22 mm Hg, the body manages to maintain RAP at about $+2$ mm Hg in the upright position. This occurs because pooling of blood in the dependent vessels is much less pronounced during orthostasis than would be predicted by Fig. 25.2B, where ~2.3 L disappeared from the top of the cylinder. The actual amount of pooling in both legs of a real person is only ~500 mL. Four major factors help reduce pooling and maintain RAP.

Nonuniform Initial Distribution of Blood In a recumbent human, most of the blood in large veins is located in the central blood volume (see ⊙ 19-4), that is, the vessels near the heart. If a large fraction of the blood had started off in the head, the orthostatic shift of blood would have been more dramatic, as in Fig. 25.2B. The majority of the 500 mL of blood that pools in the legs during orthostasis comes from the intrathoracic vascular compartments. As one stands, the output from the heart for a number of beats exceeds the venous return into the thoracic pool. This excess blood ends up filling the vessels in the dependent regions of the body. The result is a net transfer of blood—by way of the heart—from the intrathoracic vascular compartments to the dependent vessels.

Nonuniform Distensibility of the Vessels In Fig. 25.2B, we assumed a relative distensibility of 0.02/(mm Hg). If the vessels were *less* distensible, as in Fig. 25.2C, standing would cause a less dramatic shift of blood to the dependent vessels. Assuming a lower distensibility for the leg veins is reasonable because small vessels are far stiffer than larger ones, such as the aorta and vena cava.

Muscle Pumps An important compensation for blood pooling during orthostasis comes from skeletal muscle contraction. When a person stands, the muscles of the legs and abdomen tighten. The presence of valves in the veins, as well as intermittent muscular movement, contributes to the flow of blood upward along the veins (see Fig. 22.6C). Vessels of the abdominal region remain nearly unaffected by orthostasis because the abdominal viscera are contained in a water-filled jacket that is maintained by the tone of the abdominal muscles.

Autonomic Reflexes ◉ 25-1 Because of decreased venous return, cardiac output tends to fall by ~20% soon after one assumes an erect position. However, the fall in cardiac output would be even greater in the absence of autonomic reflexes. The decreased venous return leads to a fall in RAP, which in turn leads to a decrease in stroke volume and thus arterial pressure. High-pressure baroreceptors (see ◉ 23-2) sense this decrease in arterial pressure, which leads to an increased sympathetic output that raises vascular tone throughout the body and increases heart rate and contractility. Together, the constriction of arterioles (which raises total peripheral resistance) and the increased heart rate restore the systemic mean arterial pressure, despite a small decrease in stroke volume. The sympathetic response also increases the tone of the veins, thereby decreasing their diameter and their capacity (compare Fig. 25.2B and C).

In summary, of the four factors that contribute to the stability of RAP during orthostasis, two are anatomical (i.e., nonuniformities of initial blood volume distribution and distensibility) and two are physiological (i.e., muscle pumps and autonomic reflexes). The two physiological mechanisms are both important.

The extent of the **orthostatic response**—how much the heart rate or peripheral vascular resistance increases under the control of the ANS—depends on a variety of factors (Table 25.1), which involve nearly the entire cardiovascular system. Because these factors may differ from person to person or may differ within any one individual according to the circumstances, the orthostatic response is highly variable.

TABLE 25.1 Factors Influencing the Degree of Orthostatic Response[a]

Total blood volume
Distribution of blood volume
Size of vessels in dependent regions of the body
Vascular distensibility
Mean systemic filling pressure (pressure in the absence of cardiac output)
Level at which zero effective pressure is normally located in a particular individual
Degree of tilt
Skeletal muscle tone; strength and rate of intermittent contraction of skeletal muscles
Vascular sufficiency
Abdominal muscle tone
Temperature
Response of low-pressure receptors
Response of high-pressure baroreceptors
Activity of the sympathetic system
Initial heart rate
Initial myocardial contractility
Sensitivity of vascular smooth muscle to sympathetic stimulation

[a]That is, by how much standing up increases heart rate and peripheral vascular resistance.

Postural Hypotension ◉ 25-2 In very sensitive subjects lying on a tilt table, a sudden orthostatic tilt can cause such a large fall in arterial pressure that the individual becomes dizzy or even faints. **Fainting** is caused by a transient fall in arterial pressure that causes cerebral perfusion to become inadequate.

RESPONSES TO ACUTE EMOTIONAL STRESS

The fight-or-flight reaction is a sympathetic response that is centrally controlled in the cortex and hypothalamus

Emotional responses vary greatly among people. A severe emotional reaction can resemble the **fight-or-flight response** in animals (see ◉ 14-10). This defense reaction causes a generalized increase in skeletal muscle tone and increased sensory attention.

Fight-or-flight behavior is an extreme example of an integrated acute stress response that originates entirely within the central nervous system (CNS), without involvement of peripheral sensors or reflexes. The response is due to the activation of sensory centers in the **cortex** (Fig. 25.3), which activate a part of the limbic system called the **amygdala** (see ◉ 10-2). The amygdala in turn activates the **locus coeruleus**, in the pons, as well as hypothalamic nuclei. Noradrenergic neurons in the locus coeruleus project to nearly every part of the CNS (see Fig. 13.5A), including the **hypothalamic paraventricular nucleus (PVN),** which produces both an endocrine and an ANS response. The *endocrine response* of the PVN involves (1) release of arginine vasopressin (AVP) by magnocellular neurons in the PVN (see Fig. 40.4), thereby reducing urine output (see ◉ 38-3), and (2) release of corticotropin-releasing hormone (CRH; see ◉ 50-5) by parvocellular neurons in the PVN, activating the hypothalamic-pituitary-adrenal axis and thereby releasing cortisol, which is important for the metabolic response to stress. The *ANS response* of the PVN involves projections to (1) autonomic nuclei in the brainstem (dorsal motor nucleus of the vagus, rostral ventrolateral medulla, and nucleus tractus solitarii [NTS]) that are part of the **medullary cardiovascular center** (see ◉ 23-4), and (2) direct projections to the **spinal intermediolateral column** (Fig. 25.3).

The overall fight-or-flight response involves the following:
1. **Skeletal muscle blood flow.** Activation of postganglionic sympathetic cholinergic neurons *directly* causes a rapid increase in blood flow to skeletal muscle (see ◉ 23-10). Flow also increases *secondarily* more slowly and less dramatically because the adrenal medulla releases epinephrine, which increase skeletal muscle blood flow.
2. **Cutaneous blood flow.** The **sympathetic** response causes little change in blood flow to skin unless it stimulates sweating. The neural pathway involves sympathetic cholinergic neurons, which release acetylcholine and perhaps vasodilatory neurotransmitters (e.g., calcitonin gene-related peptide, vasoactive intestinal peptide). The acetylcholine causes the secretion of sweat and possibly also the local formation of kinins (see ◉ 23-25). These kinins increase capillary permeability and presumably also dilate arterioles but constrict venules (i.e., increasing the midcapillary pressure). The result would be an increased

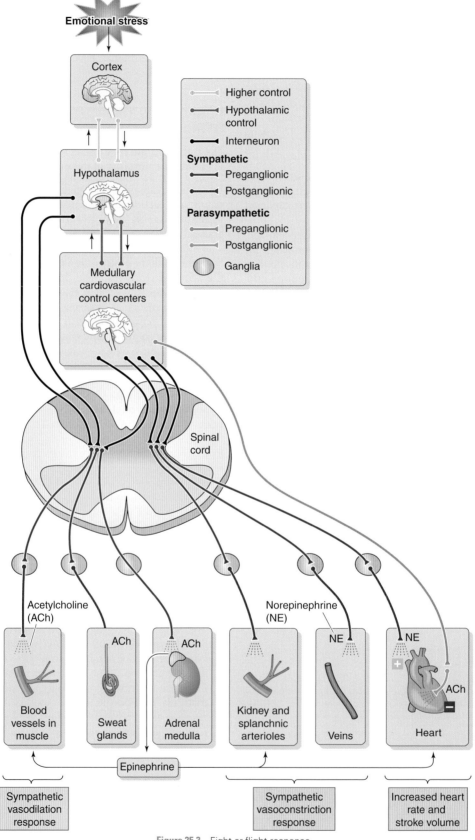

Figure 25.3   Fight-or-flight response.

filtration of fluid from the skin capillaries into the interstitium, causing dermal swelling.

3. **Adrenal medulla.** Preganglionic sympathetic neurons stimulate the release of epinephrine, which causes vasodilation in muscle and vasoconstriction in the kidney and splanchnic beds.
4. **Renal and splanchnic blood flow.** In virtually all vascular beds, increased sympathetic output causes vasoconstriction and thereby decreases blood flow.
5. **Veins.** Most veins constrict in response to sympathetic output.
6. **The heart.** Increased sympathetic output and decreased vagal output cause a rise in heart rate and contractility, so that cardiac output increases.
7. **Blood volume.** High plasma levels of AVP reduce urine output and maintain blood volume.
8. **Mean arterial pressure.** Depending on the balance of vasodilation and vasoconstriction, the overall result of vascular resistance changes may be either a decrease or an increase in total peripheral resistance. Nevertheless, because cardiac output increases, the net result is an increase in arterial pressure.

The common faint reflects mainly a parasympathetic response caused by sudden emotional stress

About one fifth of humans experience one or more episodes of fainting during adolescence. This type of fainting is known as vasodepressor syncope or **vasovagal syncope (VVS)**, which can occur in response to a sudden emotional stress, phlebotomy, the sight of blood, or acute pain. Fainting usually starts when the individual is standing or sitting, rarely when the individual is recumbent. The loss of consciousness is due to a transient fall in perfusion pressure to the brain. The "playing dead" reaction in animals is the equivalent of VVS in humans.

VVS originates with activation of specific areas in the cerebral cortex. Indeed, stimulation of areas in the anterior cingulate gyrus can trigger a faint. Although the exact trigger is not known, VVS has been attributed to activation of the **Bezold-Jarisch reflex.** This reflex causes bradycardia, hypotension, and apnea. In patients, coronary injection of contrast material or of thrombolytic agents can cause VVS, presumably by stimulating ventricular receptors. It is possible that these chemical stimuli activate the same stretch-sensitive arterial baroreceptors (see ⊙ 23-2) that are usually activated by high blood pressure. In humans, triggers clearly distinct from those known to initiate a Bezold-Jarisch reflex can also elicit VVS. Whatever the actual trigger, vagal afferents carry signals to higher CNS centers, which act through autonomic nuclei in the medulla to cause a massive stimulation of the parasympathetic system and abolition of sympathetic tone.

VVS involves changes in several parameters (Fig. 25.4):

1. **Total peripheral resistance.** A massive vasodilation results from the removal of sympathetic tone from the resistance vessels of the skeletal muscle, splanchnic, renal, and cerebral circulations.
2. **Cardiac output.** Intense vagal output to the heart causes bradycardia and decreased stroke volume, resulting in a marked decrease in cardiac output.

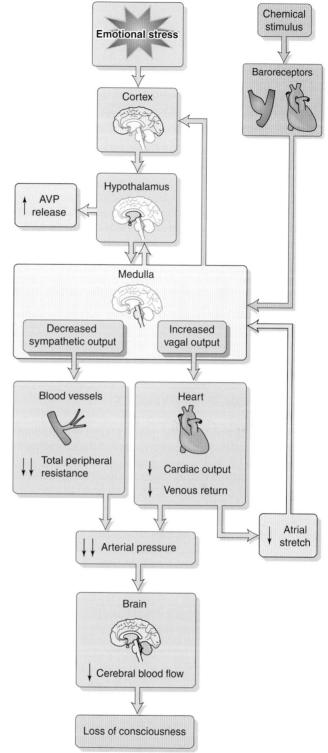

Figure 25.4 Vasovagal syncope.

3. **Arterial pressure.** The combination of a sudden decrease in both total peripheral resistance and cardiac output causes a profound fall in mean arterial pressure.
4. **Cerebral blood flow.** The fall in mean arterial pressure causes global cerebral ischemia. If the decreased cerebral blood flow persists for only a few seconds, the result is

dizziness or faintness. If it lasts for ~10 seconds, the subject loses consciousness.

5. **Other manifestations of altered ANS activity.** Pallor of the skin and sweating (beads of perspiration) are signs that often appear before the loss of consciousness. Intense vagal stimulation of the gastrointestinal tract may cause epigastric pain that is interpreted as nausea. Mydriasis (pupillary dilation) as well as visual blurring can also result from parasympathetic stimulation.

Fainting is more likely to occur in a warm room, after a volume loss (e.g., dehydration or hemorrhage), or after standing up or other maneuvers that tend to lower mean arterial pressure. These stresses might be expected to trigger baroreceptor responses that increase cardiac output and vascular resistance, thereby making fainting less likely. In fact, the integrated pattern of brain activity that orchestrates VVS also appears to suppress the expected baroreceptor reflexes that would otherwise counteract the syncope.

After regaining consciousness, the patient often notices oliguria (reduced urine output), caused by high plasma levels of AVP (also known as antidiuretic hormone; see ⊙ 38-2). Elevated levels of AVP can result in part from the reduced atrial stretch that occurs during periods of decreased venous return (see ⊙ 23-18). The pallor and nausea that persist after fainting may also result from the high levels of circulating AVP.

⊙ 25-3 RESPONSE TO EXERCISE

Adaptation to exercise probably places the greatest demands on circulatory function. The main feature of the cardiovascular response to exercise is an increased cardiac output, up to four or five times the resting cardiac output. The increase in cardiac output during exercise is more the result of increased heart rate (~3 times the control value) than of increased stroke volume (~1.5 times control). The cardiovascular response to exercise has both early and late components and originates from higher centers in the CNS (early), from mechanical and chemical changes triggered by contracting skeletal muscle (delayed), and from various reflexes (delayed).

Early physiologists suggested that muscle contraction triggers an increase in cardiac output

Contracting skeletal muscle produces cardiovascular changes that mimic many of those that occur during exercise. Muscle contraction directly affects the cardiovascular system in two ways (Fig. 25.5)—through a mechanical response that increases venous return and through a chemical response that dilates blood vessels in active muscle.

Mechanical Response: Increased Venous Return The pumping action of contracting skeletal muscle improves venous return (see ⊙ 22-1). As a result, RAP, ventricular end-diastolic pressure, and end-diastolic volume should all increase. According to the Starling mechanism (see ⊙ 22-4), the result should be an increase in stroke volume.

Chemical Response: Local Vasodilation in Active Muscle Enhanced skeletal muscle metabolism produces multiple changes in the chemistry of the interstitial fluid. The P_{O_2} and pH fall, whereas other metabolites (CO_2, lactic acid, K^+, and adenosine) accumulate. Moreover, the accumulation of

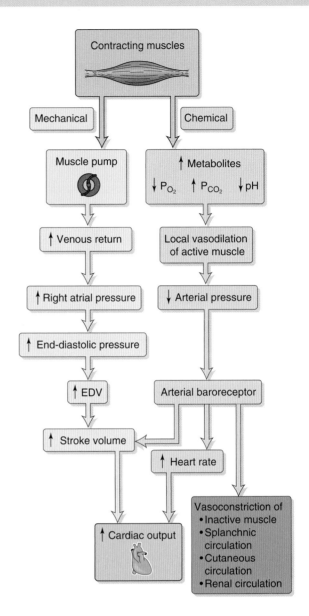

Figure 25.5 Early model of how exercise affects cardiovascular function. *EDV*, End-diastolic volume.

metabolites causes interstitial osmolarity to increase. After a small delay that follows the onset of muscle contraction, the developing chemical changes cause the arterioles to dilate (see ⊙ 20-17), which may lead to an initial fall in arterial pressure. However, this fall is transient because of the intervening baroreceptor response (see ⊙ 23-1), which increases heart rate and stroke volume, both of which enhance cardiac output. At the same time, the baroreceptor reflex vasoconstricts inactive muscle regions as well as the splanchnic, renal, and cutaneous circulations.

Central command organizes an integrated cardiovascular response to exercise

During exercise, a **central command** controls the parallel activation of both the motor cortex (see ⊙ 16-5) and cardiovascular centers. The central command involves such brain areas as the **medial prefrontal cortex** (involved in the mental state of thinking and planning exercise) as well as the insula and anterior cingulate gyrus, which are **cortical parts of the limbic system** (see ⊙ 14-12). Indeed, the medial prefrontal cortex receives multiple limbic inputs. Moreover, both cortical centers modulate stress-related sympathetic outflow, including the sympathetic outflow related to exercise. Stimulation of the H_2 fields of Forel in the ventral thalamus or neurons in the periventricular gray matter of the hypothalamus reproduce all the details of the cardiac response to exercise, even though the muscles are completely quiescent. The central command centers project to the lateral hypothalamus, rostral ventrolateral medulla, and NTS to make autonomic adaptations appropriate for exercise (Fig. 25.6):

1. **Increased cardiac output.** Increased sympathetic output to the heart causes early tachycardia and increased contractility, resulting in a rapid upsurge of cardiac output.

2. **Vasoconstriction.** Sympathetic output from the medulla causes vasoconstriction in inactive muscle regions as well as in the renal, splanchnic, and cutaneous circulations. The net effect is to make more blood available for diversion to the contracting muscles. Except during maximal exercise, the increase in splanchnic and renal resistance does not result in a fall in local blood flow to the abdominal viscera and kidneys. Rather, because the arterial pressure increases along with the renal and splanchnic vascular resistance, the *absolute* blood flow remains close to resting levels in these tissues, even as the flow to the skeletal muscle increases markedly. Cutaneous blood flow eventually rises, which reflects the attempt of the temperature-regulatory system to prevent body temperature from rising too much (see ⊙ 59-11).

3. **Early vasodilation in active muscle.** In dogs—although possibly not in humans—at the initiation of exercise, central command stimulates hypothalamic neurons whose axons bypass the medullary cardiovascular centers and synapse on preganglionic sympathetic neurons in the spinal cord (see ⊙ 23-10). The postganglionic neurons synapse on cholinergic sympathetic vasodilator fibers that innervate the vascular smooth muscle of skeletal muscle and trigger early peripheral vasodilation in active skeletal muscle. As discussed in the next section, the delayed local "chemical" response later reinforces this vasodilation.

Muscle and baroreceptor reflexes, metabolites, venous return, histamine, epinephrine, and increased temperature reinforce the response to exercise

In addition to the events orchestrated by the command center, the integrated cardiovascular response to exercise includes the following delayed responses:

1. **Exercise pressor reflex.** A neural drive called the exercise pressor reflex originates within the exercising muscle itself. Contraction activates stretch receptors that sense muscle tension and may also activate chemoreceptors that sense metabolites. Signals from these receptors travel through small thinly myelinated and unmyelinated sensory fibers from skeletal muscle to the spinal cord and then on to the medullary cardiovascular control centers. This sensory input reinforces the central input to the car-

diovascular control center and thus sustains the sympathetic outflow.

2. **Arterial baroreflexes.** Elevated mean arterial pressure resulting from high cardiac output and vasoconstriction outside active muscle would normally slow the heart. However, during exercise, central command resets the sensitivity of the **arterial baroreflex** so that the heart slows only at much higher arterial pressures. Conversely, if massive vasodilation in exercising skeletal muscle would reduce total peripheral resistance, the baroreceptor reflex maintains mean arterial pressure.

3. **Vasodilation triggered by metabolites in skeletal muscle.** *Metabolites* released locally (Fig. 25.6) dilate the resistance vessels and recruit capillaries that had received no blood flow at rest (see ⊙ 24-3). This vasodilator effect of metabolites thus more than overcomes any vasoconstrictive tendency produced by norepinephrine.

4. **Increased venous return.** The mechanical and the chemical limbs described in Fig. 25.5 further sustain the high cardiac output. Mechanically, the **muscle pump** increases venous return, and stroke volume rises by the **Starling mechanism.**

5. **Histamine release.** As sympathetic tone wanes, cells near the arterioles may release their intracellular stores of histamine, a potent vasodilator, leading to increased extravasation of fluid and enhanced lymph flow.

6. **Epinephrine release.** ⊙ 25-4 The systemic effects of circulating epinephrine on cardiac β_1 adrenoceptors enhance the neural effects on the heart, thus increasing cardiac output. Circulating epinephrine also acts on vascular β_2 adrenoceptors, augmenting vasodilation mainly in skeletal muscle and heart.

7. **Regulation of body core temperature.** As exercise continues, increased metabolism causes body core temperature to rise, activating **temperature-sensitive cells** in the hypothalamus (see ⊙ 59-9). This activation has two effects, both of which promote heat loss through the skin as part of a temperature-regulatory response (see ⊙ 59-10). First, the hypothalamus signals the medulla to inhibit its sympathetic vasoconstrictor outflow to the skin, thereby increasing cutaneous blood flow. Second, the hypothalamus activates sympathetic cholinergic fibers to sweat glands, causing an increase in sweat production as well as an indirect cutaneous vasodilation that may involve kinin formation.

RESPONSE TO HEMORRHAGE

If a person rapidly loses <10% or 20% of total blood volume from a large *vein*, the inadequate intravascular volume causes sequential decreases in central blood volume, venous return, ventricular filling, stroke volume, cardiac output, and thus mean arterial pressure. However, if the blood loss comes from a large peripheral *artery*, the mean arterial pressure in central arteries does not fall until cardiac output falls secondary to decreased venous return.

Large hemorrhages, in which one loses 30% or more of total blood volume, produce **hypovolemic shock.** Shock is a state of peripheral circulatory failure that is characterized

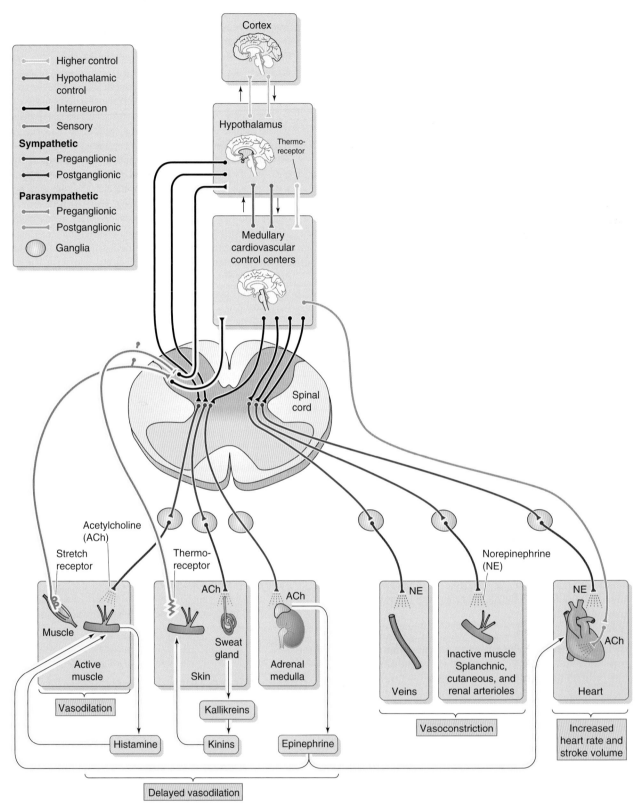

Figure 25.6 Integrated cardiovascular response to exercise. The hypothalamus orchestrates an *early* response, which includes vasodilation of active muscle (the mechanism of which is controversial in humans), vasoconstriction of certain inactive tissues, and increased cardiac output. In addition to those responses shown here, the *delayed* responses *(highlighted in yellow)* include release of histamine, kallikreins, and epinephrine, leading to delayed vasodilation. Delayed local chemical responses from contracting muscles sustain early cardiovascular responses. Cutaneous thermoreceptors trigger delayed vasodilation in the skin.

by inadequate perfusion of the peripheral tissues. During shock, the *systolic* arterial pressure is usually <90 mm Hg, and the *mean* arterial pressure is <70 mm Hg. By the time a significant fall in mean arterial pressure occurs, other signs of shock are evident. The first signs may be narrowing of the pulse pressure and a sensation of faintness when sitting or standing. The subject in hypovolemic shock has cold and moist (i.e., "clammy") skin as well as a rapid and weak pulse. Moreover, urine output drops to <25 mL/hr, even if fluid intake had been normal.

After its abrupt initial fall, arterial pressure tends to return to normal, although blood pressure falls irreversibly in some cases. Under favorable circumstances, the body restores blood pressure toward normal values by mobilizing two lines of defense.

First, circulatory control mechanisms act on the heart and blood vessels to restore cardiac output and to increase peripheral resistance. Second, mechanisms of capillary exchange and fluid conservation restore the intravascular volume.

After hemorrhage, cardiovascular reflexes restore mean arterial pressure

Several cardiovascular reflexes cooperate to compensate for the fall in mean arterial pressure. These reflexes originate from four major groups of receptors (numbered 1 to 4 in Fig. 25.7):

1. **High-pressure baroreceptors.** The fall in arterial pressure leads to a decrease in the firing rate of afferents from

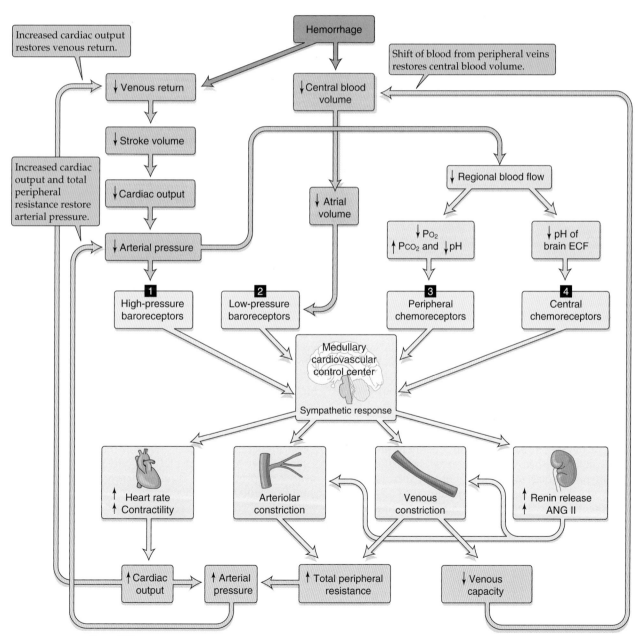

Figure 25.7 Integrated response to hemorrhage. Blood loss triggers four kinds of receptors (numbered 1 to 4) to produce an integrated response orchestrated by the medulla.

the carotid and aortic baroreceptors (see ⊙ 23-1). The resulting enhanced sympathetic output and diminished vagal output increase heart rate and cardiac contractility and also produce venoconstriction and selective arteriolar constriction.

2. **Low-pressure baroreceptors.** ⊙ 25-5 Reduced blood volume directly decreases effective circulating volume, which in turn lessens the activity of low-pressure stretch receptors (see ⊙ 23-17). The resulting increased sympathetic outflow causes vasoconstriction in a number of vascular beds, particularly the kidney, reducing glomerular filtration rate and urine output. The atrial stretch receptors also instruct the hypothalamus to enhance release of AVP, which reduces renal water excretion (see ⊙ 38-3). During shock, the vasoconstrictor effects of AVP appear to be important for maintaining peripheral vascular resistance. Reduced atrial stretch also lowers the level of circulating atrial natriuretic peptide (ANP), thereby reducing salt and water loss by the kidneys (see ⊙ 40-8).

3. **Peripheral chemoreceptors.** As blood pressure drops, perfusion of the carotid and aortic bodies declines, causing local hypoxia near the glomus cells and an increase in the firing rate of the chemoreceptor afferents (see ⊙ 32-5), a response enhanced by increased sympathetic tone to the peripheral chemoreceptor vessels. Increased *chemoreceptor* discharge leads to increased firing of the sympathetic vasoconstrictor fibers and ventilatory changes that indirectly increase heart rate (see ⊙ 23-15).

4. **Central chemoreceptors.** Severe hypotension results in brain ischemia, which leads to a fall in the P_{O_2} of brain ECF as well as a rise in P_{CO_2} and a fall in pH. The acidosis has a profound effect on the central chemoreceptors in the medulla (see ⊙ 32-8) leading to a sympathetic output several-fold more powerful than that caused by baroreceptor reflexes.

⊙ 25-6 These four reflex pathways have in common the activation of a massive sympathetic response that results in the release of norepinephrine from postganglionic sympathetic neurons. In addition, the sympathetic response triggers the **adrenal medulla** to release epinephrine and norepinephrine roughly in proportion to the severity of the hemorrhage. The consequences of the four combined reflex actions are the following responses (Fig. 25.7).

Tachycardia and Increased Contractility Increased sympathetic activity increases heart rate roughly in proportion to the volume of shed blood. Increased sympathetic tone increases myocardial contractility but can increase stroke volume only after venous return also improves.

Arteriolar Constriction Sympathetic constriction of the resistance vessels is most pronounced in the blood vessels of the *extremities, skin, skeletal muscle,* and *abdominal viscera. Renal* blood flow falls rapidly after hemorrhage as a result of the fall in blood pressure but recovers after a few minutes because of autoregulation (see ⊙ 34-5). In hypovolemic shock, renal blood flow falls to a proportionately greater extent than does cardiac output, which explains why severe hemorrhage often results in acute renal failure. Both *coronary blood flow and cerebral blood flow* initially fall after

hemorrhage, but autoregulation can largely restore blood flow to normal.

Venous Constriction. Sympathetic venous constriction decreases both the *capacity* and the compliance of the large veins, thereby tending to restore central venous pressure.

Circulating Vasoactive Agonists. ⊙ 25-7 Sympathetic stimulation of the adrenal medulla causes circulating epinephrine levels to rise. In hemorrhagic shock, ANG II rises to concentrations that are vasoconstrictive. Activation of the sympathetic system also triggers sympathetic cholinergic stimulation of the sweat glands (see ⊙ 24-5), causing the patient's extremities to become clammy.

After hemorrhage, transcapillary refill, fluid conservation, and thirst restore the blood volume

The reflexes discussed in the preceding section compensate for the principal *consequences* of blood loss—decreased blood pressure and reduced cardiac output. The responses discussed here compensate for the *primary disturbance,* the loss of blood volume.

Transcapillary Refill The movement of fluid from the interstitium to the blood plasma is the major defense against reduced blood volume. Starling forces (see ⊙ 20-10) are critically important during hemorrhage and hypovolemic shock. Immediately after hemorrhage, a phase of **hemodilution** develops (i.e., low hematocrit). Within an hour, interstitial fluid replaces ~75% of the shed blood volume. The dilution of **hemoglobin** is more pronounced than the dilution of **plasma proteins** after hemorrhage. Therefore, not only do fluid and electrolytes move from the interstitium to the blood, but proteins also enter the vascular compartment.

Transcapillary refill involves two steps. The first is **fluid movement** from the interstitium to the vasculature. Capillary hydrostatic pressure (P_c) (Fig. 25.8A) depends on arteriolar and venular pressures as well as on the relation of the precapillary to the postcapillary resistance (see ⊙ 19-5) Immediately after the hemorrhage, the upstream arteriolar pressure and the downstream venular pressure both fall, causing P_c to fall (Fig. 25.8B). The Starling forces thus produce a large net movement of fluid and small electrolytes from the interstitium into the capillaries. As compensation occurs, total peripheral resistance increases, in part restoring arteriolar pressure (Fig. 25.8C). However, because precapillary resistance increases more than does postcapillary resistance, P_c remains relatively low, sustaining the net movement of fluid into the capillaries. The entry of protein-free fluid into the capillary gradually modifies the three other Starling forces. First, the interstitial fluid volume decreases, lowering interstitial hydrostatic pressure (P_{if}). Second, the plasma proteins become diluted, so that capillary colloid osmotic pressure (π_c) falls. Finally, the removal of a protein-free solution from the interstitium raises colloid osmotic pressure in the interstitium. The result of these dissipating Starling forces is that transcapillary refill gradually wanes and eventually ceases (see ⊙ 20-16).

The second step in transcapillary refill is the appearance of **plasma proteins** in the blood. These proteins probably

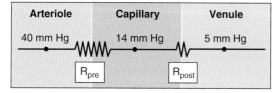

A   NORMAL

Capillary pressure is less than the arithmetic mean between arteriolar and venular pressure because $R_{pre} > R_{post}$.

Arteriole | Capillary | Venule
60 mm Hg | 25 mm Hg | 15 mm Hg
R_{pre} | R_{post} |

B   UNCOMPENSATED HEMORRHAGE

Arteriole | Capillary | Venule
40 mm Hg | 14 mm Hg | 5 mm Hg
R_{pre} | R_{post} |

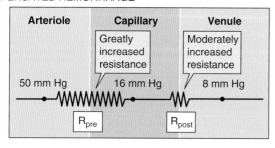

C   COMPENSATED HEMORRHAGE

Arteriole | Capillary | Venule
| Greatly increased resistance | Moderately increased resistance
50 mm Hg | 16 mm Hg | 8 mm Hg
R_{pre} | R_{post} |

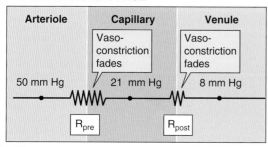

D   DECOMPENSATED HEMORRHAGE

Arteriole | Capillary | Venule
| Vaso-constriction fades | Vaso-constriction fades
50 mm Hg | 21 mm Hg | 8 mm Hg
R_{pre} | R_{post} |

Figure 25.8 Effect of hemorrhage on capillary hydrostatic pressure. (A) In this figure (which is similar to Fig. 19.3A), R_{pre} and R_{post} are the precapillary and postcapillary resistances, respectively. Here, the ratio $R_{post}/R_{pre} = 0.35$. (B) The fall in capillary hydrostatic pressure reverses the Starling forces, causing net movement of fluid from the interstitium to the capillary lumen. (C) Sympathetic stimulation increases total peripheral resistance ($R_{post}/R_{pre} = 0.25$ in this example). (D) Capillary pressure rises ($R_{post}/R_{pre} = 0.45$ in this example).

enter the blood across fenestrae of the mesenteric and hepatic capillaries, two regions in which the interstitium has a very high interstitial colloid osmotic pressure. In addition, hemorrhage rapidly stimulates albumin synthesis by the liver.

Finally, water from the **intracellular** compartments ultimately replaces the lost **interstitial** fluid.

Renal Conservation of Salt and Water Arterial hypotension and lowered renal blood flow reduce the glomerular filtration rate (see ⊙ **34-2**) and therefore diminish the urinary excretion of salt and water. In addition to the direct hemodynamic effects, the reduced effective circulating volume promotes the renal retention of Na^+ by four mechanisms: increased aldosterone (see ⊙ **40-5**) increased sympathetic nerve activity (see ⊙ **40-6**) release of AVP (see ⊙ **40-7**) and inhibition of ANP release (see ⊙ **40-8**). Therefore, the overall response of the kidney to blood loss is to reduce the excretion of water and salt, thereby contributing to the conservation of ECF.

Thirst. The blood hyperosmolality caused by hemorrhage stimulates thirst osmoreceptors (see ⊙ **40-10**). A far more potent stimulus for thirst (see ⊙ **40-12**) is the reduced effective circulating volume and blood pressure caused by severe hemorrhage.

Positive-feedback mechanisms cause irreversible hemorrhagic shock

In some cases, hemorrhagic shock can be irreversible. After an initial fall in arterial pressure and perhaps some recovery, arterial pressure and the perfusion of peripheral tissues may inexorably deteriorate. Moreover, in these cases, the fall in arterial pressure does not reverse even if the physician intervenes at this time and replaces the volume of blood lost as the result of hemorrhage.

Hemorrhagic shock can become irreversible as a result of the failure of multiple response components: (1) the vasoconstrictor response, (2) the capillary refill response, (3) the cardiac response, and (4) the CNS response.

THE RESPIRATORY SYSTEM

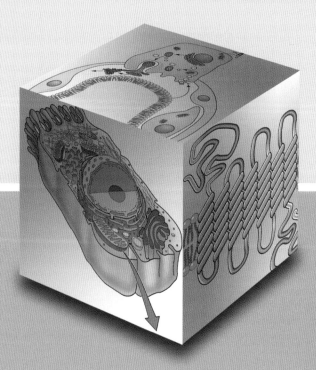

CHAPTER 26

ORGANIZATION OF THE RESPIRATORY SYSTEM

Walter F. Boron

COMPARATIVE PHYSIOLOGY OF RESPIRATION

External respiration is the exchange of O_2 and CO_2 between the atmosphere and the mitochondria

For millennia, people have regarded breathing as being synonymous with life. Life begins and ends with breathing.

By the end of the 18th century, chemists and physiologists appreciated that combustion, putrefaction, and respiration all involve chemical reactions that consume O_2 and produce CO_2. Subsequent advances in the chemistry of gases laid the theoretical foundation for the physiology of O_2 and CO_2.

Later work showed that mitochondrial respiration (i.e., the oxidation of carbon-containing compounds to form CO_2)—also called **internal respiration** or oxidative phosphorylation (see ◉ 58-15)—is responsible for the O_2 consumption and CO_2 production in tissues.

In the chapters on respiratory physiology, we focus on **external respiration,** the dual processes of (1) transporting O_2 from the atmosphere to the mitochondria and (2) transporting CO_2 from the mitochondria to the atmosphere. We will also see that CO_2 is intimately related to acid-base homeostasis.

Diffusion is the major mechanism of external respiration for small aquatic organisms

The most fundamental mechanism of O_2 and CO_2 transport is **diffusion** (see ◉ 5-2). Random movements of molecules such as O_2 and CO_2, whether in a gaseous phase or dissolved in water, result in a net movement of the substance from regions of high concentration to regions of low concentration (Fig. 26.1, *inset*). No expenditure of energy is involved. The driving force for diffusion is the concentration gradient.

Imagine a unicellular organism suspended in a beaker of pond water at 37°C. The water is in equilibrium with an atmosphere that has the usual composition of O_2 and CO_2 (Table 26.1). The partial pressures of O_2 (P_{O_2}) and of CO_2 (P_{CO_2}) in the *dry* air are slightly higher than their corresponding values in the *wet* air immediately above the surface of the water (Box 26.1). It is these partial pressures in wet air that determine the concentrations of dissolved O_2 ($[O_2]_{dis}$) and dissolved CO_2 ($[CO_2]_{dis}$) in the water (Box 26.2 and Fig. 26.2). Thus, the P_{O_2} in the wet air—as well as the water beneath it—will be ~149 mm Hg (or torr), and the P_{CO_2} will be an almost negligible 0.2 mm Hg. These numbers describe

the composition of the **bulk phase** of the pond water, at some distance from the organism. However, because the mitochondria within the organism continuously consume O_2 and produce CO_2, the P_{O_2} at the surface of the mitochondria will be lower than the bulk-phase P_{O_2}, whereas the P_{CO_2} at the mitochondrial surface will be higher than the bulk-phase P_{CO_2} (Fig. 26.1, *right side*). These differences in partial pressure cause O_2 to diffuse from the bulk pond water toward the mitochondria and the CO_2 to diffuse in the opposite direction.

The diffusion of O_2 follows a gradient of decreasing P_{O_2} (Fig. 26.1). The region over which P_{O_2} falls gradually from the bulk pond water toward the outer surface of the plasma membrane is the **extracellular unstirred layer,** so named because no convective mixing occurs in this zone. A similar gradual decline in P_{O_2} drives O_2 diffusion through the **intracellular unstirred layer,** from the inner surface of the plasma membrane to the mitochondria. The abrupt fall in P_{O_2} across the plasma membrane reflects extra resistance to gas flow. The profile for P_{CO_2} is similar, although with the opposite orientation.

The rate at which O_2 or CO_2 moves across the surface of the organism is the **flow** (*units:* moles/s). According to a simplified version of **Fick's law** (see ◉ 5-3), flow is proportional to the concentration difference across this barrier. Because we know from Henry's law that the concentration of a dissolved gas is proportional to its partial pressure in the gas phase, flow is also proportional to the partial-pressure difference (ΔP):

$$\text{Flow} \propto \Delta P \qquad (26.1)$$

Simple diffusion is the mechanism by which O_2 and CO_2 move *short* distances in the respiratory system: between the air and blood in the alveoli, and between the mitochondria and blood of the peripheral circulation.

Convection enhances diffusion by producing steeper gradients across the diffusion barrier

External Convective Systems A purely diffusive system can establish only a relatively small ΔP across the gas exchange barrier of the organism (Fig. 26.1). Yet, for small organisms, even this relatively small ΔP is adequate to meet the demands for O_2 uptake and CO_2 removal. However, when the organism's diameter exceeds ~1 mm, simple diffusion becomes inadequate for gas exchange. One way of ameliorating this problem is to introduce a mechanism for **convection** on

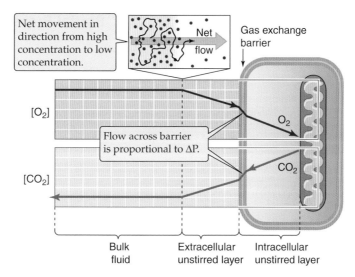

Figure 26.1 Diffusion of O_2 and CO_2 for a single-celled organism. The y-axis of the grids shows the dissolved concentration (or partial pressure) of O_2 and CO_2. The x-axis represents distance (not to scale).

TABLE 26.1 **Composition of Air**

GAS	DRY AIR ATMOSPHERE		WET AIR TRACHEA	
	FRACTION IN AIR (%)	PARTIAL PRESSURE AT SEA LEVEL (mm Hg)	FRACTION IN AIR (%)	PARTIAL PRESSURE AT SEA LEVEL (mm Hg)
Nitrogen	78.09	593.48	73.26	556.78
Oxygen	20.95	159.22	19.65	149.37
Carbon dioxide	0.03	0.23	0.03	0.21
Argon	0.93	7.07	0.87	6.63
Water	0	0	6.18	47
Total	100	760	100	760

the outside surface of the organism. For a paramecium, the beating cilia bring bulk-phase water—having a P_{O_2} of ~154 mm Hg at 25°C and a P_{CO_2} of ~0.2 mm Hg—very near to the cell's surface. This mixing reduces the size of the extracellular unstirred layer, thereby increasing the P_{O_2} and decreasing the P_{CO_2} on the outer surface of the organism. The net effect is that the partial-pressure gradients for both O_2 and CO_2 increase across the gas exchange barrier, leading to a proportionate increase in the flow of both substances.

A filter feeder, such as an oyster or a clam, pumps bulk-phase water past its organ of gas exchange.

In mammals, the bulk phase is the atmosphere and the external convective system is an air pump that includes the chest wall, the respiratory muscles, and the passages through which the air flows (i.e., from the nose up to the alveoli). **Ventilation** is the process of moving air into and out of the lungs. Mammals expand their lungs by developing a negative pressure inside the thorax. Because of the much higher O_2 content of air (about 210 mL O_2/L of air), as opposed to water (~35 mL O_2/L of water), humans need to move far less air than oysters need to move water.

Although we are far more efficient than oysters, the principle of external convective systems is the same: ensure that

the external surface of the gas exchange barrier is in close contact with a fluid whose composition matches—as closely as is practical—that of the bulk phase. In the average adult human, an alveolar ventilation of ~4000 mL/min produces an alveolar P_{O_2} of ~100 mm Hg (versus 149 mm Hg in a wet atmosphere at 37°C), and an alveolar P_{CO_2} of ~40 mm Hg (versus 0.2 mm Hg).

Internal Convective Systems A **circulatory system** is an *internal* convective system that maximizes flow of O_2 and CO_2 across the gas exchange barrier by delivering, to the inner surface of this barrier, blood that has as low a P_{O_2} and as high a P_{CO_2} as is practical. **Perfusion** is the process of delivering blood to the lungs.

Mammals have a sophisticated circulatory system built around a four-chambered heart and separate pulmonary and systemic circulations. The systemic circulatory system carries (by convection) low-P_{O_2} blood from a systemic capillary near the mitochondria to the right ventricle, which pumps the blood to the alveolar wall. At the beginning of a pulmonary capillary, a high alveolar-to-blood P_{O_2} gradient ensures a high O_2 inflow (by diffusion), and blood P_{O_2} rises to match the alveolar (i.e., external) P_{O_2} by the time the blood leaves the pulmonary capillary. The newly oxygenated blood then

BOX 26.1 Wet Gases: Partial Pressures of O_2 and CO_2 in Solutions That Are Equilibrated with Wet Air

Imagine that a beaker of water is equilibrated with a normal atmosphere and that both water and atmosphere have a temperature of 37°C. For dry air (i.e., air containing no water vapor), O_2 makes up ~21% of the total gas by volume (Table 26.1). Thus, if the ambient pressure—or **barometric pressure (PB)**—is 760 mm Hg, the partial pressure of O_2 (P_{O_2}) is 21% of 760 mm Hg, or 159 mm Hg (Fig. 26.2). However, if the air-water interface is reasonably stationary, water vapor will saturate the air immediately adjacent to the liquid. What is the P_{O_2} in this wet air? At 37°C, the partial pressure of water (P_{H_2O}) is 47 mm Hg. Of the total pressure of the wet air, P_{H_2O} makes up 47 mm Hg, and the components of the dry air make up the remaining 760 − 47, or 713 mm Hg. Thus, the partial pressure of O_2 in this wet air is

$$P_{O_2} = \overbrace{F_{O_2}}^{\text{Fraction of dry air that is } O_2} \cdot (P_B - P_{H_2O})$$
$$= (21\%) \cdot (760 \text{ mm Hg} - 47 \text{ mm Hg})$$
$$= 149 \text{ mm Hg}$$

The CO_2 composition of dry air is ~0.03% (Table 26.1). Thus, the partial pressure of CO_2 in wet air is

$$P_{CO_2} = F_{CO_2} \cdot (P_B - P_{H_2O})$$
$$= (0.03\%) \cdot (760 \text{ mm Hg} - 47 \text{ mm Hg})$$
$$= 0.21 \text{ mm Hg}$$

These examples are realistic for respiratory physiology. As we inhale relatively cool and dry air, the nose and other upper respiratory passages rapidly warm and moisturize the passing air so that it assumes the composition of wet air given in Table 26.1.

BOX 26.2 Partial Pressures and Henry's Law

Respiratory physiologists generally express the concentration of a gas, whether it is mixed with another gas (e.g., O_2 mixed with N_2, as is the case for air) or dissolved in an aqueous solution (e.g., O_2 dissolved in water), in terms of partial pressure. **Dalton's law** states that the total pressure (P_{total}) of a mixture of gases is the sum of their individual **partial pressures.** Imagine that we are dealing with an ideal gas (Z) mixed with other gases. Because the ratio of the partial pressure of Z (P_Z) to the total pressure (P_{total}) is its mole fraction (X_Z),

$$P_Z = X_Z \cdot P_{total}$$

Thus, if P_Z in one sample of gas were twice as high as in another, X_Z (i.e., concentration of Z) would also be twice as high.

It may not be immediately obvious why—when Z is dissolved in aqueous solutions—it is still reasonable to express the concentration of Z in terms of P_Z. According to **Henry's law,** when the system is at equilibrium, the concentration of O_2 dissolved in water ($[O_2]_{dis}$) is proportional to P_{O_2} in the gas phase:

$$[O_2]_{dis} = s \cdot P_{O_2}$$

The proportionality constant s is the **solubility;** for O_2, s is ~0.0013 mM/mm Hg at 37°C for a solution mimicking blood plasma. The solubility of CO_2 is ~23-fold higher. Consider a beaker of water at 37°C equilibrated with an atmosphere having a P_{O_2} of 100 mm Hg, the partial pressure in mammalian *arterial* blood plasma:

$$[O_2]_{dis} = \left(0.0013 \frac{mM}{mm \ Hg}\right) \cdot (100 \text{ mm Hg})$$
$$= 0.13 \text{ mM}$$

Now consider a second beaker equilibrated with an atmosphere having a P_{O_2} of 40 mm Hg, the partial pressure of O_2 in *mixed-venous* blood:

$$[O_2]_{dis} = \left(0.0013 \frac{mM}{mm \ Hg}\right) \cdot (40 \text{ mm Hg})$$
$$= 0.05 \text{ mM}$$

If we now place samples of these two solutions on opposite sides of a semipermeable barrier in a closed container, the O_2 gradient across this barrier expressed in terms of concentrations ($\Delta[O_2]$) is 0.13 − 0.05 or 0.08 mM. Expressed in terms of partial pressures (ΔP_{O_2}), this same gradient is 100 − 40 = 60 mm Hg.

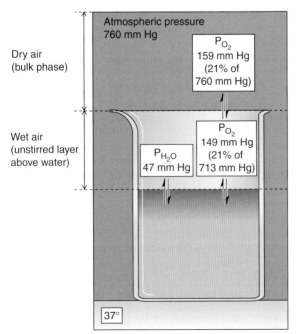

Figure 26.2 Wet versus dry gases. Note that the O_2 partial pressure is less in wet than in dry air.

flows to the left ventricle, which pumps the now-systemic arterial blood (by convection) to the systemic capillaries, where a high blood-to-mitochondria P_{O_2} gradient maximizes the O_2 flux into the mitochondria (by diffusion). The opposite happens with CO_2. Thus, separate pulmonary and systemic circulations ensure maximal gradients for gas diffusion in both the pulmonary and systemic capillaries.

Surface Area Amplification Enhances Diffusion The passive flow of O_2 or CO_2 across a barrier is proportional not only to the concentration gradient, but also to the area of the barrier:

$$\text{Flow} \propto \Delta P \times \text{Area} \qquad \textbf{(26.2)}$$

Indeed, higher animals have increased their ability to exchange O_2 and CO_2 with their environment by increasing the **surface area** across which gas exchange takes place. In an amphibian such as the adult frog, the lungs are simple air sacs with a relatively small surface area. Mammals markedly increase the surface area available for diffusion by developing highly complex lungs with bronchi and a large number of alveoli.

In humans, the lung surface is so large and so thin that O_2 and CO_2 transport across the alveolar wall is ~3-fold faster than necessary—at least when the person is resting at sea level. This redundancy is important, for example, during exercise, when cardiac output can increase markedly. A substantial decrease in surface area, or thickening of the barrier, can be deleterious.

Hemoglobin increases the carrying capacity of the blood for both O_2 and CO_2

In mammals, the external convective system (i.e., ventilatory apparatus), the internal convective system (i.e., circulatory system), and the barrier itself (i.e., alveolar wall) are extraordinarily efficient, but are not sufficient by themselves to ensure the efficient exchange of gases.

Imagine what would happen if the mixed-venous blood flowing along a pulmonary capillary contained only water and salts. The diffusion of O_2 from the alveolar air space into the "blood" is so fast—and the solubility of O_2 in saline is so low—that before the blood could move ~1% of the way down the capillary, the P_{O_2} of the blood would match the P_{O_2} of the alveolar air (i.e., all of the O_2 that *could* move *would* have moved). For the remaining ~99% of the capillary, the P_{O_2} gradient across the barrier would be nil, and no more O_2 would flow into the blood. As a result, at a normal cardiac output, the blood could not carry away enough O_2 from the lungs to the tissues to sustain life. The same would be true in reverse for the elimination of CO_2.

Animals solve this problem with specialized metalloproteins that reversibly bind O_2, greatly increasing the carrying capacity of blood for O_2. The most common—and most efficient—such metalloproteins are the **hemoglobins,** which contain iron. All vertebrates use hemoglobin, which is the chief component of erythrocytes or red blood cells.

The presence of hemoglobin markedly improves the dynamics of O_2 uptake by blood passing through the lungs. Under normal conditions, hemoglobin reversibly binds ~96% of the O_2 that diffuses from the alveolar air spaces to the pulmonary-capillary blood, greatly increasing the carrying capacity of blood for O_2. Hemoglobin also plays a key role in the transport or **carriage** of CO_2 by reversibly binding CO_2 and by acting as a powerful pH buffer.

ORGANIZATION OF THE RESPIRATORY SYSTEM IN HUMANS

Humans optimize each aspect of external respiration

The human respiratory system (Fig. 26.3) has two important characteristics. First, it uses highly efficient convective systems (i.e., ventilatory and circulatory systems) for long-distance transport of O_2 and CO_2. Second, it reserves diffusion exclusively for short-distance movements of O_2 and CO_2. The key components of this respiratory system are the following:

1. **An air pump.** The external convective system consists of the upper respiratory tract and large pulmonary airways,

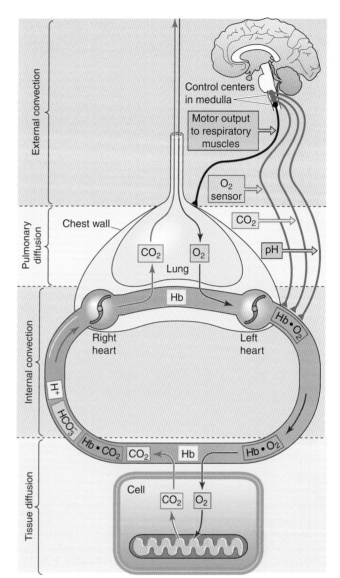

Figure 26.3 Respiratory apparatus in humans.

the thoracic cavity and associated skeletal elements, and the muscles of respiration. These components deliver air to and remove air from the alveolar air spaces—**alveolar ventilation.** Inspiration occurs when muscle contractions increase the volume of the thoracic cavity, thereby lowering intrathoracic pressure; this causes the alveoli to expand passively, which in turn lowers alveolar pressure. Air then flows from the environment to the alveoli, down a pressure gradient. A quiet expiration occurs when the muscles relax. We discuss the mechanics of ventilation in Chapter 27.

2. **Mechanisms for carrying O_2 and CO_2 in the blood.** Red blood cells are highly specialized for transporting O_2 from the lungs to the peripheral tissues and for transporting CO_2 in the opposite direction. They have extremely high levels of hemoglobin and other components that help to rapidly load and unload huge amounts of O_2 and CO_2. Hemoglobin plays a central role in acid-base chemistry, as discussed in Chapter 28, as well as in the carriage of O_2 and CO_2, treated in Chapter 29.

TABLE 26.2 Symbol Conventions in Respiratory Physiology

RESPIRATORY MECHANICS		GAS EXCHANGE	
Main Symbols			
C	Compliance	C	Concentration (or content) in a liquid
		D	Diffusion capacity
f	Respiratory frequency	f	Respiratory frequency
		F	Fraction
P	Pressure	P	Pressure
		Q̇	Flow of blood (perfusion)
R	Resistance	R	Gas exchange ratio
		S	Saturation of hemoglobin
V	Volume of gas	V	Volume of gas
V̇	Flow of gas	V̇	Ventilation
Modifiers (subscripts)			
		a	Systemic arterial
A	Alveolar	A	Alveolar
AW	Airway		
B	Barometric	B	Barometric
		c	Pulmonary capillary
		E	Expired
		I	Inspired
		v	Systemic venous (in any vascular bed)
		v̄	Mixed systemic venous

From Macklem PT: Symbols and abbreviations. In Fishman AP, Fisher AB (eds): Handbook of Physiology, Section 3: The Respiratory System, vol 1, Circulation and Nonrespiratory Functions. Bethesda, MD, American Physiological Society, 1985.

3. **A surface for gas exchange.** The gas exchange barrier in humans consists of the alveoli, which provide a huge but extremely thin surface area for passive diffusion of gases between the alveolar air spaces and the pulmonary capillaries. We discuss the anatomy of the alveoli below in this chapter and explore pulmonary gas exchange in Chapter 30.

4. **A circulatory system.** The internal convective system in humans consists of a four-chambered heart and separate systemic and pulmonary circulations. We discuss the flow of blood to the lungs—**perfusion**—in Chapter 31.

5. **A mechanism for locally regulating the distribution of ventilation and perfusion.** Efficient gas exchange requires that the ratio of ventilation to perfusion be uniform for all alveoli to the extent possible. The lungs attempt to optimize the uniformity of ventilation-perfusion ratios by using sophisticated feedback control mechanisms to regulate local air flow and blood flow, as discussed in Chapter 31.

6. **A mechanism for centrally regulating ventilation.** Unlike the rhythmicity of the heart, that of the respiratory system is not intrinsic to the lungs or the chest wall. Instead, respiratory control centers in the **central nervous system** rhythmically stimulate the muscles of inspiration.

Moreover, these respiratory centers appropriately modify the pattern of ventilation during exercise or other changes in physical or mental activity. Sensors for arterial P_{O_2}, P_{CO_2}, and pH are part of feedback loops that stabilize these three "blood gas" parameters. We discuss these subjects in Chapter 32.

Respiratory physiologists have agreed on a set of symbols to describe parameters that are important for pulmonary physiology and pulmonary function testing (Table 26.2).

Conducting airways deliver fresh air to the alveolar spaces

◉ **26-1** The **parietal pleura,** the wall of the sac that is farthest from the lung, contains blood vessels that are believed to produce an ultrafiltrate of the plasma called **pleural fluid.** About 10 mL of this fluid normally occupies the virtual space between the parietal and the **visceral pleura.** The visceral pleura lies directly on the lung and contains lymphatics that drain the fluid from the pleural space. When the production of pleural fluid exceeds its removal, the volume of pleural fluid increases **(pleural effusion),** limiting the expansion of the lung.

◉ **26-2** We refer to the progressively bifurcating pulmonary airways by their **generation number** (Fig. 26.4): The zeroth generation is the trachea, the first-generation airways are the right and left mainstem bronchi, and so on. Humans have ~23 generations of airways. As generation number increases (i.e., as airways become smaller), the amount of cilia, the number of mucus-secreting cells, the presence of submucosal glands, and the amount of cartilage in the airway walls all gradually decrease. The mucus is important for trapping small foreign particles. The cilia sweep the carpet of mucus—kept moist by secretions from the submucosal glands—up toward the pharynx, where swallowing eventually disposes of the mucus. The cartilage is important for preventing airway collapse, which is especially a problem during expiration (see Chapter 27). Airways maintain some cartilage to about the 10th generation, up to which point they are referred to as **bronchi.**

Beginning at about the 11th generation, the now cartilage-free airways are called **bronchioles.** Up until generation ~16, no alveoli are present, and the air cannot exchange with the pulmonary-capillary blood. The airways from the nose and lips down to the alveoli-free bronchioles are the **conducting airways,** which serve only to move air by convection (i.e., like water moving through a pipe) to those regions of the lung that participate in gas exchange. The most distal conducting airways are the **terminal bronchioles** (generation ~16). The aggregate volume of conducting airways, the **anatomical dead space,** amounts to ~150 mL in healthy young males and >100 mL in females. The anatomical dead space is only a small fraction of the total lung capacity, which averages 5 to 6 L in adults, depending on the size and health of the individual.

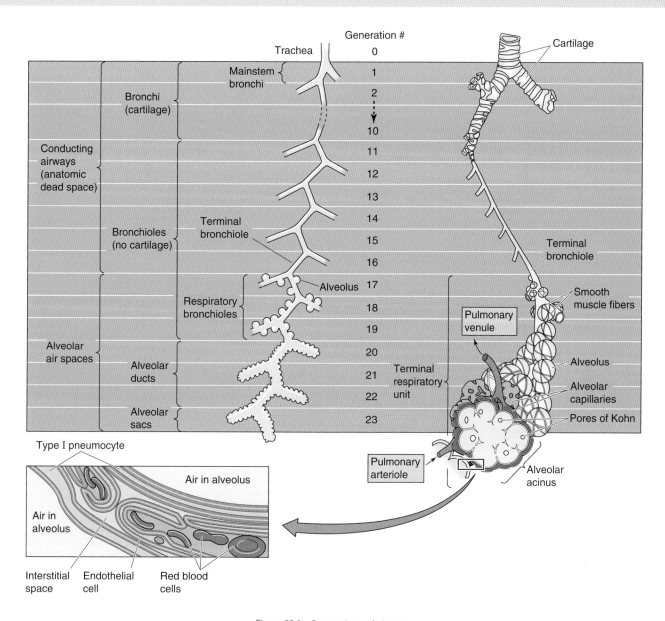

Figure 26.4 Generations of airways.

Alveolar air spaces are the site of gas exchange

Alveoli first appear budding off bronchioles at generation ~17. These **respiratory bronchioles** participate in gas exchange over at least part of their surface. Respiratory bronchioles extend from generation ~17 to generation ~19, the density of alveoli gradually increasing with generation number (Fig. 26.4). Eventually, alveoli completely line the airways. These **alveolar ducts** (generations 20 to 22) finally terminate blindly as **alveolar sacs** (generation 23). The aggregation of all airways arising from a single terminal bronchiole, along with their associated blood and lymphatic vessels, is a **terminal respiratory unit.**

The cross-sectional area of the trachea is ~2.5 cm². Unlike the situation in systemic arteries (see ⊙ 19-1), in which the aggregate cross-sectional area of the branches always exceeds the cross-sectional area of the parent vessel,

the aggregate cross-sectional area falls from the trachea through the first four generations of airways (Fig. 26.5). Thus, the linear velocity of air in the first four generations is higher than that in the trachea, which may be important during coughing (see ⊙ 32-9). In succeeding generations, the aggregate cross-sectional area rises, at first slowly and then very steeply. As a result, the linear velocity falls to very low values.

As air moves into the respiratory bronchioles and further into the terminal respiratory unit, where linear velocity is minuscule, convection becomes less important for the movement of gas molecules, and diffusion dominates. Notice that the long-distance movement of gases from the nose and lips to the end of the generation-16 airways occurs by *convection*. However, the short-distance movement of gases from generation-17 airways to the farthest reaches of the alveolar

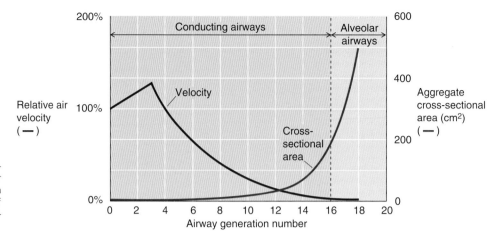

Figure 26.5 Dependence of aggregate cross-sectional area and of linear velocity on generation number. (Data from Bouhuys A: The Physiology of Breathing. New York, Grune & Stratton, 1977.)

ducts occurs by *diffusion,* as does the movement of gases across the gas exchange barrier (~0.6 μm).

The **alveolus** is the fundamental unit of gas exchange. Alveoli are hemispheric structures with diameters that range from 75 to 300 μm. The ~300 million alveoli have an astounding combined surface area of 50 to 100 m² and an aggregate maximal volume of 5 to 6 L in the two lungs. Both the diameter and the surface area depend on the degree of lung inflation.

The alveolar lining consists of two types of epithelial cells, type I and type II alveolar pneumocytes. The cuboidal type II cells exist in clusters and are responsible for elaborating **pulmonary surfactant,** which substantially eases the expansion of the lungs (see ◉ 27-5). The type I cells are much thinner than the type II cells. Thus, even though the two cell types are present in about equal numbers, the type I cells cover 90% to 95% of the alveolar surface and represent the shortest route for gas diffusion. The type II cells appear to serve as repair cells.

The pulmonary capillaries are usually sandwiched between two alveolar air spaces. In fact, the blood forms an almost uninterrupted sheet that flows like a twisted ribbon between abutting alveoli. At the type I cells, the alveolar wall (i.e., pneumocyte plus endothelial cell) is typically 0.15 to 0.30 μm thick.

The lung receives two blood supplies: the pulmonary arteries and the bronchial arteries (Fig. 26.6). The **pulmonary arteries,** by far the major blood supply to the lung, carry the relatively deoxygenated mixed-venous blood. After arising from the right ventricle, they bifurcate as they follow the bronchial tree, and their divisions ultimately form a dense, richly anastomosing array of capillary segments that supply the alveoli. The average erythrocyte spends ~0.75 second in the pulmonary capillaries as it traverses up to three alveoli. After gas exchange in the alveoli, the blood eventually collects in the pulmonary veins.

The **bronchial arteries** are branches of the aorta and carry freshly oxygenated blood to the conducting airways. Because capillaries of the bronchial circulation drain partially into pulmonary veins, there is some **venous admixture** of the partially deoxygenated blood from the bronchial circulation and the newly oxygenated blood (see Fig. 26.6). This mixing represents part of a small physiological **shunt.**

The lungs play important nonrespiratory roles

Although their main function is to exchange O_2 and CO_2 between the atmosphere and the blood, the lungs also play important roles not directly related to external respiration.

Olfaction Ventilation is essential for delivery of odorants to the olfactory epithelium (see Fig. 15.2). Sniffing behavior, especially important for some animals, allows one to sample the chemicals in the air without the risk of bringing potentially noxious agents deep into the lungs.

Processing of Inhaled Air Before It Reaches the Alveoli Strictly speaking, the warming, moisturizing, and filtering of inhaled air in the conducting airways *is* a respiratory function. It is part of the cost of doing the business of ventilation. **Warming** of cool, inhaled air is important because if alveoli and associated blood were substantially cooler than body temperature, the solubility of these alveolar gases in the cool pulmonary-capillary blood would be relatively high. As the blood later warmed, the solubility of these gases would decrease, resulting in air bubbles (i.e., emboli) that could lodge in small systemic vessels and cause infarction. **Moisturizing** is important to prevent the alveoli from becoming desiccated. Finally, **filtering** of particles is important to prevent small airways from being clogged with debris that may also be toxic. Key elements of the filtration process include nasal hairs, a complex anatomy that promotes turbulence and the impaction of particles in the mucus that covers the upper airways, and the sedimentation of tiny particles that become embedded in mucus layers.

Filtering Small Emboli from the Blood ◉ 26-3 The mixed-venous blood contains microscopic emboli, small particles (e.g., blood clots, fat, air bubbles) capable of occluding blood vessels. If these emboli were to reach the systemic circulation and lodge in small vessels that feed tissues with no collateral circulation, the consequences—over time—could be catastrophic. Fortunately, the pulmonary vasculature can trap these emboli before they reach the left heart. If the emboli are sufficiently few and small, the affected alveoli can recover their function. However, if **pulmonary emboli** are sufficiently large or frequent, they can cause serious symptoms or even death.

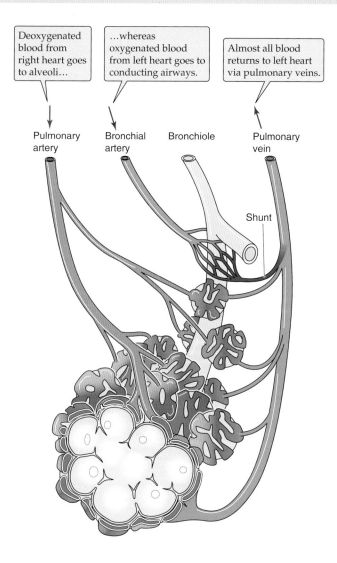

Deoxygenated blood from right heart goes to alveoli…

…whereas oxygenated blood from left heart goes to conducting airways.

Almost all blood returns to left heart via pulmonary veins.

Pulmonary artery

Bronchial artery

Bronchiole

Pulmonary vein

Shunt

Figure 26.6 Blood supply to the airways.

Biochemical Reactions The entire cardiac output passes through the lungs, exposing the blood to the tremendous surface area of the pulmonary-capillary endothelium. Among its many functions, the pulmonary endothelium—representing the vast majority of all endothelial cells in the body—converts angiotensin I (a decapeptide) to angiotensin II (an octapeptide), a reaction catalyzed by angiotensin-converting enzyme (see ⊙ 40-3).

LUNG VOLUMES AND CAPACITIES

The spirometer measures changes in lung volume

The maximal volume of all the airways in an adult—from the nasopharynx to the alveolar sacs—is typically 5 to 6 L. Respiratory physiologists have defined a series of lung "volumes" and "capacities" that, although not corresponding to a particular anatomical locus, are easy to measure with simple laboratory instruments and that can convey important clinical information.

A **spirometer** measures the volume of air inspired and expired and therefore the change in lung volume. Spirometers today are complex computers, some so small that a person can easily hold one in the palm of a hand. The subject blows against a predetermined resistance, and the device performs all the calculations and interpretations. Nevertheless, the principles of spirometric analysis are far easier to conceptualize with an "old-fashioned" spirometer (Fig. 26.7A). This simple spirometer has a movable inverted bell that is partially submerged in water. An air tube extends from the subject's mouth, through the water, and emerges in the bell, just above water level. Thus, when the subject exhales, air enters the bell and lifts it. The change in bell elevation, which we can record on moving paper, reflects the volume of air that the subject exhales.

The amount of air entering and leaving the lungs with each breath is the **tidal volume** (V_T or **TV**). During quiet respirations, the V_T is ~500 mL. The initial portion of the spirograph of Fig. 26.7B illustrates changes in lung volume during quiet breathing. The product of V_T and the frequency of breaths is **total ventilation.**

At the end of a quiet inspiration, the additional volume of air that the subject *could* inhale with a maximal effort is known as the **inspiratory reserve volume (IRV).**

After a quiet expiration, the additional volume of air that one can expire with a maximal effort is the **expiratory reserve volume (ERV).**

⊙ **26-4** Even after a maximal expiratory effort, a considerable amount of air remains inside the lungs—the **residual volume (RV).** Because a spirometer can measure only the air entering or leaving the lungs, we must use other methods to measure RV.

The four primary **volumes** that we have defined—TV, IRV, ERV, and RV—do not overlap (Fig. 26.7B). The lung **capacities** are various combinations of these four primary volumes:

1. **Total lung capacity (TLC)** is the sum of all four volumes.
2. **Functional residual capacity (FRC)** ⊙ **26-5** is the sum of ERV and RV and is the amount of air remaining inside the respiratory system after a quiet expiration. Because FRC includes RV, we cannot measure it using only a spirometer.
3. **Inspiratory capacity (IC)** is the sum of IRV and TV. After a quiet expiration, the IC is the maximal amount of air that one could still inspire.
4. **Vital capacity (VC)** is the sum of IRV, TV, and ERV. In other words, VC is the maximal achievable TV, and depends on several factors, including muscle strength, lung compliance, and skeletal flexibility.

⊙ **26-6** At the end of the spirographic record in Fig. 26.7B, the subject makes a maximal inspiratory effort and then exhales as rapidly and completely as possible. The volume of air exhaled in 1 second under these conditions is the **forced expiratory volume in 1 second (FEV$_1$).** In healthy young adults, FEV$_1$ is ~80% of VC. FEV$_1$ depends on all the factors that affect VC as well as on airway resistance. Thus, VC and FEV$_1$ are valuable for monitoring a variety of pulmonary disorders and the effectiveness of treatment.

The volume of distribution of helium or nitrogen in the lung is an estimate of the RV

Although we cannot use a spirometer to measure RV or any capacity containing RV (i.e., FRC or TLC), we can use approaches based on the **law of conservation of mass.** In

A   SIMPLE SPIROMETER

Expiration makes the bell of the spirometer move upward.

Floating drum

Counter-balance weight

Lungs

Air

Pen

RV
FRC
ERV
TV
IRV
TLC

Water

Recorder

B   SPIROGRAPHIC RECORD

Maximal inspiratory effort.

After maximal inspiration, the subject exhales as much air as fast as possible.

IRV   IC   VC   FEV₁

TV

ERV   TLC

FRC   ←1 s→

RV

Lung volume (L)

Time

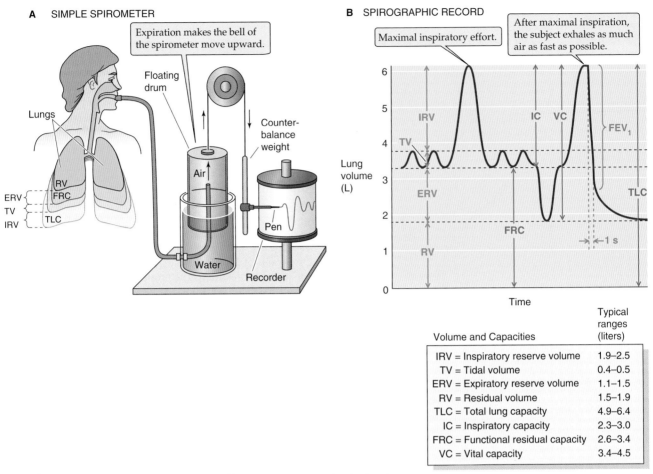

Volume and Capacities	Typical ranges (liters)
IRV = Inspiratory reserve volume	1.9–2.5
TV = Tidal volume	0.4–0.5
ERV = Expiratory reserve volume	1.1–1.5
RV = Residual volume	1.5–1.9
TLC = Total lung capacity	4.9–6.4
IC = Inspiratory capacity	2.3–3.0
FRC = Functional residual capacity	2.6–3.4
VC = Vital capacity	3.4–4.5

Figure 26.7   Workings of a simple spirometer.

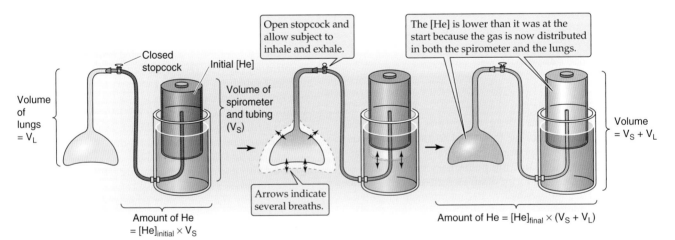

Closed stopcock

Initial [He]

Volume of lungs = V_L

Volume of spirometer and tubing (V_S)

Open stopcock and allow subject to inhale and exhale.

Arrows indicate several breaths.

The [He] is lower than it was at the start because the gas is now distributed in both the spirometer and the lungs.

Volume = $V_S + V_L$

Amount of He = $[He]_{initial} \times V_S$

Amount of He = $[He]_{final} \times (V_S + V_L)$

Figure 26.8   The helium-dilution technique.

a common approach, we compute RV from the **volume of distribution** of an insoluble gas, such as helium (He). The underlying principle is that the concentration of He is the ratio of mass (in moles) to volume (in liters). Thus, if we know the mass and concentration of He, we can calculate the *volume* of the physiological compartment in which the He is distributed. In our case, the subject

breathes air containing He, which cannot escape from the airways.

We begin with a spirometer containing air with 10% He—this is the *initial* He concentration, $[He]_{initial} = 10\%$ (Fig. 26.8). In this example, the initial spirometer volume, $V_{S,initial}$, including all air up to the valve at the subject's mouth, is 2 L. The amount of He in the spirometer system at the outset of our experiment is thus $[He]_{initial} \times V_{S,initial}$, or $(10\%) \times (2\ L)$ = 0.2 L.

We now open the valve at the mouth and allow the subject to breathe spirometer air until the He distributes evenly throughout the spirometer and airways. After equilibration, the *final* He concentration ($[He]_{final}$) is the same in the airways as it is in the spirometer. Because the system does not lose He, the total He content after equilibration must be the same as it was at the outset. In our example, we assume that $[He]_{final}$ is 5%.

If the spirometer and lung volumes at the end of the experiment are the same as those at the beginning,

$$[He]_{initial} \cdot V_S = [He]_{final} \cdot (V_S + V_L) \tag{26.3}$$

Solving for lung volume, we get

$$V_L = V_S \cdot \left(\frac{[He]_{initial}}{[He]_{final}} - 1 \right) \tag{26.4}$$

If we now insert the values from our experiment,

$$V_L = 2L \cdot \left(\frac{10\%}{5\%} - 1 \right) = 2L \tag{26.5}$$

This V_L is the lung volume at the instant we open the valve and allow He to begin equilibrating. If we wish to measure FRC, we open the valve just after the completion of a *quiet* expiration. If we open the valve after a *maximal* expiration, then the computed V_L is RV.

CHAPTER 27

MECHANICS OF VENTILATION

Walter F. Boron

Pulmonary mechanics deals with how the body moves air in and out of the lungs, producing a *change* in lung volume (V_L). When no air is flowing, we are studying **static** properties. When the lungs are changing volume—and air is flowing either in or out—we are studying the more complicated **dynamic** properties.

STATIC PROPERTIES OF THE LUNG

The balance between the outward elastic recoil of the chest wall and the inward elastic recoil of the lungs generates a subatmospheric intrapleural pressure

⊙ **27-1** The interaction between the lungs and the thoracic cage determines V_L. The lungs have a tendency to collapse because of their **elastic recoil,** a *static property*. The chest wall also has an elastic recoil. However, this elastic recoil tends to pull the thoracic cage outward. The stage is thus set for an interaction between the lungs and the chest wall: at equilibrium, the inward elastic recoil of the lungs exactly balances the outward elastic recoil of the chest wall. This interaction between lungs and chest wall does not occur by direct attachment but via the **intrapleural space** between the visceral and parietal pleurae (see ⊙ 26-1). This space is filled with a small amount of pleural fluid and is extremely thin (5 to 35 μm). Because the lungs and chest wall pull away from each other on opposite sides of the intrapleural space, the **intrapleural pressure (P_{IP})** is less than barometric pressure (PB); that is, the intrapleural space is a *relative vacuum.*

Actually, P_{IP} is best thought of as the *intrathoracic pressure*—the pressure everywhere in the thorax *except* in the lumens of blood vessels, lymphatics, and airways. The lumen of the esophagus is at P_{IP} except during peristalsis.

If a subject has finished a quiet expiration—and if PB is 760 mm Hg—P_{IP} is ~756 mm Hg near the mediastinum (Fig. 27.1). Note that P_{IP} is subatmospheric. Because respiratory physiologists historically measured these small pressures with water manometers rather than with less sensitive mercury manometers, it has become customary to express P_{IP} in *centimeters of H_2O* relative to a PB of 0 cm H_2O. Thus, P_{IP} is about −5 cm H_2O at the mediastinum.

Contraction of the diaphragm and selected intercostal muscles increases the volume of the thorax, producing an inspiration

We have seen that the opposing elastic recoils of the lungs and chest wall create a relatively negative P_{IP} that keeps the lungs expanded. Any change in the balance between these elastic recoils will cause V_L to change as well. For example, imagine a healthy person with a functional residual capacity (FRC) of 3 L and a P_{IP} of −5 cm H_2O. If that person now develops **pulmonary fibrosis,** which increases the elastic recoil of the lungs, FRC would decrease because a P_{IP} of −5 cm H_2O would no longer be adequate to keep the resting V_L at 3 L. Moreover, as the lungs shrink, P_{IP} would become more negative, causing chest volume to decrease as well. Under normal circumstances, the key elastic recoil is the one *we* control: the elastic recoil of the chest wall, which we change moment to moment by modulating the tension of the muscles of respiration.

⊙ **27-2** The **muscles of inspiration** expand the chest, increasing the elastic recoil of the chest wall and making P_{IP} more negative. Responding to this enhanced intrathoracic vacuum, the lungs expand passively. The increase in V_L is virtually the same as the increase in thoracic volume. The muscles that produce a quiet inspiration are the **primary muscles of inspiration** and include the diaphragm and many intercostal muscles.

The most important component of the increase in chest volume is the rise in the chest cavity's rostral-caudal diameter, a result of the action of the **diaphragm.** Stimulated by the phrenic nerves, the diaphragm contracts and moves downward into the abdomen ~1 cm during quiet ventilation.

The **external and internal intercostal muscles,** innervated by segmental spinal nerves, span the space between adjacent ribs. The action of each such muscle depends partly on its orientation between ribs but especially—because of the shape of the rib cage—on its position along the rostral-caudal axis and around the dorsal-ventral circumference of the rib cage. Inspiratory neurons preferentially stimulate the most rostral and dorsal *external* intercostals and the parasternal *internal* intercostals, both of which have inspiratory mechanical advantages. The contraction of these muscles has two consequences (Fig. 27.2A). First, the rib cage and the tissues between the ribs stiffen and are therefore better able to withstand the increasingly negative P_{IP}. Second, thoracic volume increases as (a) ribs 2 through 10 rotate upward and outward, increasing the transverse diameter (bucket-handle effect; see Fig. 27.2B), and (b) the upper ribs rotate the sternum upward and outward, increasing the anterior-posterior diameter (water pump–handle effect).

During a **forced** inspiration (e.g., during exercise or before a cough), the **accessory** (or **secondary**) **muscles** of inspiration also come into play:

1. **Scalenes.** These muscles lift the first two ribs.
2. **Sternocleidomastoids.** These muscles lift the sternum outward, contributing to the water pump–handle effect.
3. **Neck and back muscles.** These elevate the pectoral girdle (increasing the cross-sectional area of the thorax) and extend the back (increasing the rostral-caudal length).

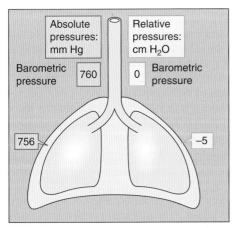

Fig. 27.1 Intrapleural pressures. The values are those after a quiet expiration (i.e., FRC under *static* conditions).

4. **Upper respiratory tract muscles.** The actions of these muscles decrease airway resistance.

Relaxation of the muscles of inspiration produces a quiet expiration

During a *quiet* inspiration, *normal* lungs store enough energy in their elastic recoil to fuel a quiet expiration, just as stretching of a rubber band stores enough energy to fuel the return to initial length. Thus, a quiet expiration is normally passive, accomplished simply by relaxation of the muscles of inspiration. Thus, *there are no primary muscles of expiration.*

During a **forced** expiration (e.g., during exercise or a cough), the **accessory muscles of expiration** help make P_{IP} more positive:

1. **Abdominal muscles** (internal and external oblique, rectoabdominal, and transverse abdominal muscles). Their contraction (Fig. 27.2C) forces the diaphragm upward into the chest cavity, decreasing the rostral-caudal diameter of the thorax.
2. **Intercostals.** A subset of both the *external* and *internal* intercostals has an expiratory mechanical advantage, and reduces both the anterior-posterior and the transverse diameters of the thorax. These actions are particularly important for coughing.
3. **Neck and back muscles.** Lowering of the pectoral girdle reduces the cross-sectional area of the thorax,

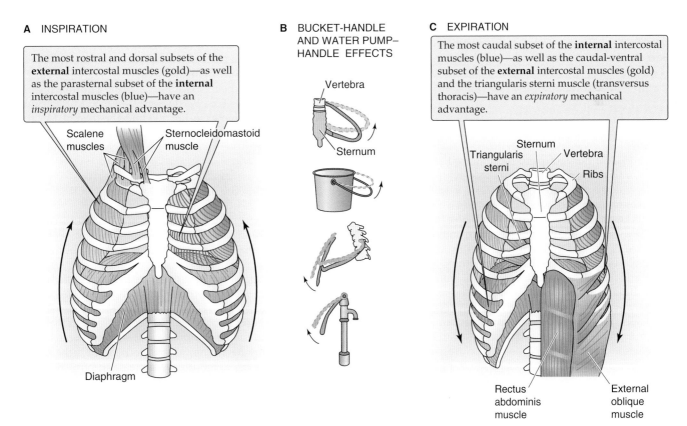

Fig. 27.2 Actions of major respiratory muscles. External intercostal muscles slope obliquely between the ribs, mostly *forward* and *downward*. Internal intercostal muscles also slope obliquely between the ribs, but mostly *backward* and *downward*.

whereas flexion of the trunk reduces the rostral-caudal diameter.

An increase of the static compliance makes it easier to inflate the lungs

Imagine that a person experiences a puncture wound to the chest cavity, so that air enters the thorax from the atmosphere, raising P_{IP} to the same level as PB. This condition is called a **pneumothorax**. With no vacuum to counter their elastic recoil, alveoli tend to collapse—a condition known as **atelectasis**. The upper part of Fig. 27.3A illustrates an extreme hypothetical case in which pressure is atmospheric throughout the thorax. Even so, V_L is not zero because some proximal airways collapse before smaller ones farther downstream, trapping air.

What pressures can we change to re-expand the collapsed lungs? The pressure responsible for maintaining an airway at its present dimensions is the **transmural pressure (P_{TM})**—the *radial* pressure difference across an airway wall at any point along the tracheobronchial tree:

$$P_{TM} = P_{AW} - P_{IP} \qquad \textbf{(27.1)}$$

P_{AW} is the pressure inside the airway, and P_{IP} is the pressure in the interstitial space surrounding the airway. A special case of P_{TM} is the transmural pressure across the *alveolar* wall—**transpulmonary pressure (P_{TP})**:

$$P_{TP} = PA - P_{IP} \qquad \textbf{(27.2)}$$

PA is **alveolar pressure**. When the glottis is open and no air is flowing, the lungs are under **static conditions,** and PA must be 0 cm H_2O:

$$\text{static conditions}: P_{TP} = 0 - P_{IP} = -P_{IP} \qquad \textbf{(27.3)}$$
$$\text{(glottis open)}$$

Thus, with the glottis open under static conditions, the pressure that inflates the alveoli (i.e., P_{TP}) is simply the negative of P_{IP}. We can re-expand the lungs to FRC by any combination of an increase in PA and a decrease in P_{IP}, as long as P_{TP} ends up at 5 cm H_2O (Fig. 27.3A, *lower panels*). Thus, it makes no difference whether we increase PA from 0 to +5 cm H_2O with P_{IP} fixed at zero (the principle behind positive-pressure ventilation in an intensive care unit) or whether we decrease P_{IP} from 0 to −5 cm H_2O with PA fixed at zero (the principle behind physiological ventilation). In both cases, P_{TP}—and thus V_L—increase by the same amount.

A clinician would treat the pneumothorax by inserting a chest tube through the wound into the thoracic cavity and gradually pumping out the intrathoracic air. As we remove air from the thorax, P_{IP} measured under static conditions becomes more negative, P_{TP} becomes correspondingly more positive, and the alveoli eventually re-expand. We can characterize the elastic (or static) properties of the lungs by plotting V_L versus P_{TP} (Fig. 27.3B, *purple curve*). Our approach will be to remove a small amount of air from the thorax, halt (so that we are now under *static conditions*), measure V_L and P_{IP} (i.e., $-P_{TP}$), and then repeat the process until V_L approaches total lung capacity (TLC).

During the reinflation, measured under static conditions, we can divide the effect on V_L into four stages—indicated by the numerals next to the *purple curve* in Fig. 27.3B:

Step 1: **Stable V_L.** Starting from the lowest P_{IP} values, making P_{IP} more negative has little or no effect on V_L because the relatively small P_{TP} is insufficient to overcome surface tension of completely collapsed alveoli and pop them open.

Step 2: **Opening of airways.** Decreasing P_{IP} beyond about −8 cm H_2O produces P_{TP} values that are finally large enough to pop open the most distensible alveoli and gradually recruit others.

Step 3: **Linear expansion of open airways.** After all the alveoli are already open, graded increases in P_{TP} inflates all airways further, causing V_L to increase in a roughly linear fashion.

Step 4: **Limit of airway inflation.** As V_L approaches TLC, decreases in P_{IP} produce ever-smaller increases in V_L, which reflects decreased airway and chest-wall compliance and the limits of muscle strength.

What would happen if, having inflated the lungs to TLC, we allowed P_{IP} to increase to 0 cm H_2O once again? Obviously, the V_L would decrease. However, the lungs follow a different path during deflation (Fig. 27.3B, *red curve*), creating a **P_{IP}-V_L loop.** The difference between the inflation and the deflation paths—**hysteresis**—exists because a greater P_{TP} is required *to pop open* a previously closed airway than *to keep* an open airway from closing. A key player here is pulmonary surfactant; we will discuss surfactant in the next section. During normal ventilation, the lungs exhibit much less hysteresis, and the green P_{IP}-V_L loop in Fig. 27.3B lies close to the red deflation limb of our original loop.

We will borrow a piece of the red curve in Fig. 27.3B and create the middle (i.e., "Normal") curve in Fig. 27.4. Here, P_{TP} is +5 cm H_2O when V_L is at FRC. During a normal inspiration, P_{TP} increases (i.e., P_{IP} decreases) by 2.5 cm H_2O and produces a tidal volume (V_T) of 500 mL. The ratio of ΔV_L to ΔP_{TP} (i.e., the slope of the P_{TP}-V_L curve) is the compliance, a measure of the distensibility of the lungs. In our example,

$$C = \frac{\Delta V_T}{\Delta P_{TP}} = \frac{0.5L}{(7.5-5.0)\,\text{cm H}_2\text{O}} = 0.2\,\frac{1}{\text{cm H}_2\text{O}} \qquad \textbf{(27.4)}$$

◉ **27-3** Because we made this measurement under conditions of zero airflow, C is the **static compliance.** Static compliance, like V_L, is mainly a property of the alveoli. Lungs with a high compliance have a low elastic recoil, and vice versa.

Fig. 27.4 also shows representative P_{TP}-V_L relationships for lungs of patients with pulmonary fibrosis (bottom curve) and emphysema (top curve). In **pulmonary fibrosis,** the disease process causes deposition of fibrous tissue, so that the lung is stiff and difficult to inflate. Patients with **restrictive lung disease,** by definition, have a decreased C. The same ΔP_{TP} that produces a 500-mL V_L increase in normal lungs produces a substantially *smaller* V_L increase in fibrotic lungs.

The situation is reversed in **emphysema,** a common consequence of cigarette smoking that destroys pulmonary tissue and makes the lungs floppy. An important part of the disease process is the destruction of the extracellular matrix by elastase released from macrophages. The same increase in P_{TP} that

A   PNEUMOTHORAX AND LUNG REINFLATION

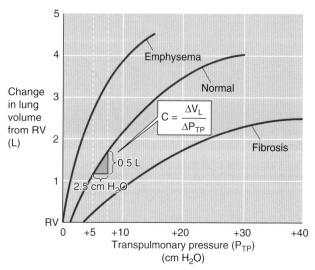

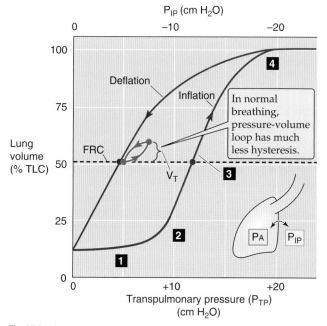

Fig. 27.3 Collapse and reinflation of the lungs. In (A) we assume that P_{IP} rises to PB, so that P_{TP} falls to zero, collapsing the lungs.

produces a 500-mL V_L increase in normal lungs produces a substantially *larger* V_L increase—reflecting an increased C—in lungs with emphysema. In other words, static compliance is much greater (i.e., much less elastic recoil).

Fig. 27.4 Static pressure-volume curves for healthy and diseased lungs.

Because it requires work to inflate the lungs against their elastic recoil, one might think that a little emphysema might be a good thing. Although it is true that patients with emphysema exert less effort to inflate their lungs, the cigarette smoker pays a terrible price for this small advantage. The destruction of pulmonary architecture also makes emphysematous airways more prone to collapse during expiration, which drastically increases airway resistance.

Surface tension at the air-water interface of the airways accounts for most of the elastic recoil of the lungs

What is the basis of the elastic recoil that determines the static compliance of the lungs? The elasticity of pulmonary cells and extracellular matrix—what we might think of as the "anatomical" component of elastic recoil—generally accounts for only a small part. The rest is due to surface tension at the air-water interface of airways, predominantly alveoli. If we eliminate this air-water interface by reinflating the lungs with saline (Fig. 27.5A, *orange curve*) rather than air (*blue curve*), we see that (1) the P_{TP}-V_L relationship exhibits far less hysteresis, and (2) the static compliance is substantially greater (i.e., much less pressure is required to inflate the lungs). These changes occur because the saline-filled lungs lack the air-water interface that generates surface tension. It is this surface tension that is responsible for most of the lung's elastic recoil.

Surface tension is a measure of the force acting to pull a liquid's surface molecules together at an air-liquid interface (Fig. 27.5B). Water molecules in the bulk liquid phase are equally attracted to surrounding water molecules in all directions, so that the net force acting on these "deep" water molecules is zero. However, water molecules at the surface are equally attracted to others in all directions but "up," where no molecules are available to pull surface water molecules toward the air phase. Thus, a net force pulls surface molecules away from the air-water interface toward the bulk water phase.

We can think of the surface water molecules as beads connected by an elastic band. The force that pulls a water

A EFFECT OF SURFACE TENSION ON COMPLIANCE

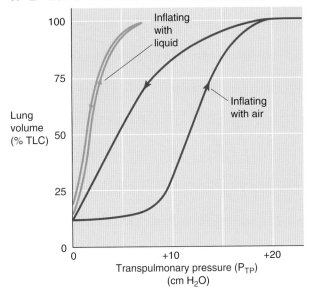

B FLAT AIR-WATER INTERFACE

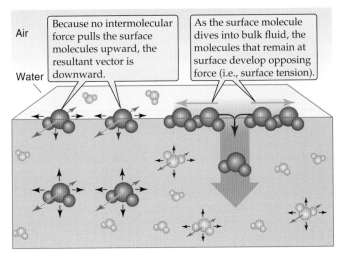

Air

Water

Because no intermolecular force pulls the surface molecules upward, the resultant vector is downward.

As the surface molecule dives into bulk fluid, the molecules that remain at surface develop opposing force (i.e., surface tension).

C DEFINITION OF SURFACE TENSION

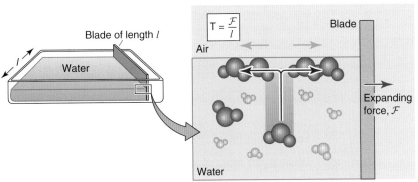

Blade of length *l*

Water

$T = \frac{\mathcal{F}}{l}$

Air

Blade

Expanding force, $\mathcal{F}$

Water

D SPHERICAL AIR-WATER INTERFACE

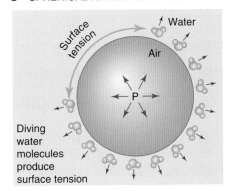

Surface tension

Water

Air

P

Diving water molecules produce surface tension

Fig. 27.5 Effect of surface tension on the lung.

molecule down into the bulk also creates a *tension* between the molecules that remain at the surface, in a direction that is *parallel* to the surface. If we try to overcome this tension and stretch the air-water interface (Fig. 27.5C), thus increasing its area, we must apply force (*F*) to bring water molecules from the bulk liquid (a low-energy state) to the surface (a high-energy state). If the body of water on which we tug has a length of *l*, then the surface tension *(T)* is

$$T = F/l \qquad \textbf{(27.5)}$$

For a simple air-water interface at 37°C, the surface tension is ~70 dynes/cm.

A drop of water falling through the air tends to form into a sphere because this shape has the smallest surface area and thus the lowest energy. Put differently, when the drop is spherical, it is impossible for any additional water molecules to leave the surface.

In the reverse scenario, a spherical air bubble surrounded by water (Fig. 27.5D), unbalanced forces acting on surface water molecules cause them to dive into the bulk, which decreases the surface area and creates tension in the plane

of the air-water interface. This surface tension acts like a belt tightening around one's waist. It tends to decrease the volume of compressible gas inside the bubble and increases its pressure. At equilibrium, the tendency of increased pressure to expand the gas bubble balances the tendency of surface tension to collapse it. The Laplace equation describes this equilibrium:

$$P = \frac{2T}{r} \qquad \textbf{(27.6)}$$

P is the *dependent* variable, the surface tension *T* is a *constant* for a particular interface, and the bubble radius *r* is the *independent* variable. Therefore, the smaller the bubble's radius, the greater the pressure needed to keep the bubble inflated. See ⊙ 19-9 for a description of how Laplace's treatment applies to blood vessels.

Our bubble-in-water analysis is important for the lung because a thin layer of water covers the inner surface of the alveolus. Just as surface tension at the air-water interface of our gas bubble causes the bubble to constrict, it also causes alveoli and other airways to constrict, contributing greatly to elastic recoil.

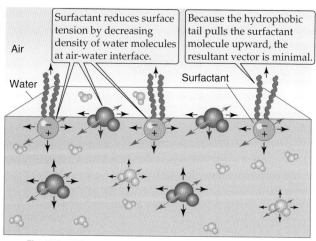

Fig. 27.6 Effect of a surface-active agent on surface tension.

○ 27-4 Pulmonary surfactant is a mixture of lipids—mainly dipalmitoylphosphatidylcholine—and apoproteins

The term **surfactant** means a surface-active agent. Because surfactants have both a hydro*philic* region (strongly attracted to water) and a hydro*phobic* region (strongly repelled by water), they localize to the surface of an air-water interface. An example of a synthetic surfactant is dishwashing detergent.

Detergent molecules orient themselves so that their hydrophilic heads point toward (and interact with) the most superficial water molecules, whereas the hydrophobic tails point toward the air (Fig. 27.6). The hydrophilic surfactant *heads* pull strongly upward on the most superficial water molecules, greatly reducing the net force on these surface water molecules and minimizing their tendency to dive into the bulk water. What prevents surfactant at the air-surfactant interface from diving into the bulk water? The hydrophobic *tails* exert a counterforce, pulling the surfactant upward toward the air. Thus, unlike surface water molecules, which are subjected to a large net force pulling them into the bulk, surfactant experiences a much smaller net force. The greater the surface density of surfactant molecules at the air-water interface (i.e., the smaller the surface occupied by water molecules), the smaller the surface tension.

○ **27-5 Pulmonary surfactant** is a complex mixture of lipids and proteins. Type II alveolar cells, cuboidal epithelial cells that coexist with the much thinner type I cells, synthesize and secrete pulmonary surfactant. Lipids make up ~90% of surfactant and are responsible for the surface-active properties. About half of the lipid is **dipalmitoylphosphatidylcholine (DPPC)**.

Proteins account for the remaining ~10% of pulmonary surfactant. Plasma proteins (mainly albumin) and secretory immunoglobulin A make up about half of the protein, and four **apoproteins** (SP-A, SP-B, SP-C, and SP-D) make up the rest. **SP-A** and **SP-D** contribute to "innate immunity" by acting as opsonins to coat bacteria and viruses, thereby promoting phagocytosis by macrophages resident in the alveoli.

The secretion of pulmonary surfactant occurs by constitutive exocytosis. In the fetus, both synthesis and secretion

are quite low until immediately before birth, when a surge in maternal glucocorticoid levels triggers these processes (see ○ 57-1). Infants born prematurely may thus lack sufficient levels of surfactant and may develop **infant respiratory distress syndrome** (**IRDS**). In postnatal life, several stimuli enhance the surfactant secretion, including hyperinflation of the lungs (e.g., sighing and yawning), exercise, and pharmacological agents (e.g., β-adrenergic agonists, Ca^{2+} ionophores).

Two mechanisms remove components of pulmonary surfactant from the surface of alveoli. Alveolar macrophages degrade some of the surfactant. Type II cells take up the rest, and either recycle or destroy it.

Pulmonary surfactant reduces surface tension and increases compliance

The pulmonary surfactant present at the alveolar air-water interface has three major effects.

First, because surfactant reduces surface tension, it increases compliance, making it far easier to inflate the lungs. If surfactant suddenly disappeared from the lungs, mimicking the situation in IRDS, total elastic recoil would increase (i.e., compliance would *decrease*) twofold or more, causing small airways to collapse partially. The situation would be similar to that described by the fibrosis curve in Fig. 27.4. Because the compliance of the lungs is far lower than normal, an infant with IRDS—compared with a normal infant—must produce far larger changes in P_{TP} (or P_{IP}) to achieve the same increase in V_L. Therefore, infants with low surfactant levels must expend tremendous effort to contract their inspiratory muscles and expand the lungs.

Second, by reducing surface tension, surfactant minimizes fluid accumulation in the alveolus. In the absence of surfactant, the high surface tension of the liquid layer between the air and the alveolar type I cells would cause the "air bubble" to collapse (like the one in Fig. 27.5D), drawing fluid into the alveolar space from the interstitium. The net effect would be to increase the thickness of the liquid layer and thereby impair gas diffusion. With normal levels of surfactant, the surface tension is lower, and the tendency to draw fluid from the interstitium to the alveolar space is balanced by the negative interstitial hydrostatic pressure (i.e., P_{IP}), which favors fluid movement from the alveolar space into the interstitium.

Third, surfactant helps keep alveolar size relatively uniform during the respiratory cycle. This occurs because dynamic changes in the surface density of surfactant tend to put a brake on the expansion of relatively large alveoli during inspiration, and on the collapse of relatively small alveoli during expiration.

DYNAMIC PROPERTIES OF THE LUNG

When air is flowing—that is, under dynamic conditions—one must not only exert the force necessary to maintain the lung and chest wall at a certain volume (i.e., static component of force), but also exert an extra force to overcome the inertia and resistance of the tissues and air molecules (i.e., dynamic component of force).

⦿ 27-6 Airflow is proportional to the difference between alveolar and atmospheric pressure, but inversely proportional to airway resistance

The flow of air through tubes is governed by the same principles governing the flow of blood through blood vessels and the flow of electrical current through wires (see Equation 17.1). Airflow is proportional to driving pressure (ΔP) but inversely proportional to **total airway resistance (R_{AW})**:

$$\dot{V} = \frac{\Delta P}{R_{AW}} = \frac{P_A - P_B}{R_{AW}} \qquad (27.7)$$

$\dot{V}$ (*units:* L/s) is airflow; the dot above the V indicates the time derivative of volume. For the lung, the driving pressure is the difference between alveolar pressure (P_A) and barometric pressure (P_B). Thus, for a fixed resistance, more *airflow* requires a greater ΔP (i.e., more effort). Viewed differently, to achieve a desired airflow, a greater *resistance* requires a greater ΔP.

When airflow is laminar—that is, when air molecules move smoothly in the same direction—we can apply Poiseuille's law, which states that the resistance (R) of a tube is proportional to the viscosity of the gas (η) and length of the tube (*l*) but inversely proportional to the fourth power of the radius:

$$R = \frac{8}{\pi} \cdot \frac{\eta l}{r^4} \qquad (27.8)$$

This equation is the same as Equation 17.11 for laminar blood flow. The key aspect of Equation 27.8 is that airflow is extraordinarily sensitive to changes in airway **radius.** The fourth-power dependence of R on radius means that a 10% decrease in radius causes a 52% increase in R—that is, a 34% *decrease* in airflow.

In principle, it is possible to compute the total airway resistance of the tracheobronchial tree from anatomical measurements, applying Poiseuille's law when the flow is laminar and analogous expressions for airways in which the flow is not laminar. However, because such calculations are not practical for monitoring physiological or pathological changes in R_{AW}, physiologists and physicians must *measure* R_{AW} directly. Rearrangement of Equation 27.7 yields an expression from which we can compute R_{AW}, provided that we know the driving pressure and the airflow that it produces:

$$R_{AW} = \frac{\Delta P}{\dot{V}} = \frac{P_A - P_B}{\dot{V}} \left(units: \frac{cm\ H_2O}{L/s} \right) \qquad (27.9)$$

We can measure airflow directly with a **flowmeter** (pneumotachometer) built into a tube through which the subject breathes, and we can measure P_A during breathing by using a device called a plethysmograph. For example, if the peak V during a quiet inspiration is −0.5 L/s (by convention, a negative value denotes inflow) and P_A at the same instant is −1 cm H_2O, then

$$R_{AW} = \frac{\Delta P}{\dot{V}} = \frac{P_A - P_B}{\dot{V}} = \frac{-1\ cm\ H_2O}{-0.5 L/s} = 2 \frac{cm\ H_2O}{L/s} \qquad (27.10)$$

In normal individuals, R_{AW} is ~1.5 cm H_2O/(L/s) but can range from 0.6 to 2.3. Resistance values are higher in patients with respiratory disease and can exceed 10 cm H_2O/(L/s) in extreme cases.

The resistance that we measure in this way is the *airway resistance*, which represents ~80% of total pulmonary resistance. The remaining 20% represents **tissue resistance**—that is, the friction of pulmonary and thoracic tissues as they slide past one another as the lungs expand or contract.

In the lung, airflow is transitional in most of the tracheobronchial tree

We have seen that Equation 27.7 and Equation 27.9—which are analogous to Ohm's law—describe airflow when it is laminar, as discussed for blood flow (⦿ 17-5). Can we predict whether the airflow is likely to be laminar? If the average velocity of the fluid flowing down the tube passes a critical value, flow becomes **turbulent;** local irregular currents, called vortices, develop randomly, and they greatly increase resistance to flow. Under ideal laboratory conditions, airflow generally is laminar when the dimensionless **Reynolds number** (Re) is <2000:

$$Re = \frac{2r\bar{v}\rho}{\eta} \qquad (27.11)$$

Here *r* is the radius of the tube, $\bar{v}$ is the velocity of the gas averaged over the cross section of the tube, ρ is the density of the gas, and η is its viscosity. When *Re* exceeds ~3000, flow tends to be turbulent. Between *Re* values of 2000 and 3000, flow is unstable and may switch between laminar and turbulent.

Reynolds developed Equation 27.11 to predict turbulence when fluids flow through tubes that are long, straight, smooth, and unbranched. Pulmonary airways, however, are short, curved, bumpy, and bifurcated. The branches are especially problematic, because they set up small eddies. Although these eddies resolve farther along the airways, the air soon encounters yet other bifurcations, which establish new eddies. This sort of airflow is termed **transitional.** Airflow is transitional throughout most of the tracheobronchial tree. Only in the trachea, where the airway radius is large and linear air velocities may be extremely high (e.g., during exercise, coughing), is airflow truly turbulent.

The distinction among laminar, transitional, and turbulent airflow is important because these patterns influence how much energy one must invest to produce airflow. When flow is *laminar* (Equation 27.7), airflow is proportional to ΔP and requires relatively little energy. When flow is *transitional*, one must apply more ΔP to produce the same airflow because producing vortices requires extra energy. Thus, the "effective resistance" increases. When flow is *turbulent*, airflow is proportional not to ΔP but to $\sqrt{\Delta P}$. Thus, we must apply an even greater ΔP to achieve a given flow (i.e., effective resistance is even greater).

The smallest airways contribute only slightly to total airway resistance in healthy lungs

As discussed above, total airway resistance for healthy individuals is ~1.5 cm H_2O/(L/s). The second column of Table 27.1 shows how R_{AW} normally varies with location as air moves from lips to alveoli during a quiet inspiration. A striking feature is that the greatest aggregate resistance is in the pharynx-larynx and large airways (diameter > 2 mm, or before about generation 8). Of the R_{AW} of 1.5 cm H_2O/(L/s)

TABLE 27.1 Airway Resistance[a]

LOCUS	NORMAL	COPD
Pharynx-larynx	0.6	0.6
Airways > 2 mm diameter	0.6	0.9
Airways < 2 mm diameter	0.3	3.5
Total airway resistance	1.5	5.0

[a]Units of resistance are cm H_2O/(L/s).

in a normal subject, 0.6 is in the upper air passages, 0.6 is in the large airways, and only 0.3 is in the small airways.

Because R increases with the fourth power of airway radius (Equation 27.8), it might seem counterintuitive that the small airways have the lowest aggregate resistance. However, although each small airway has a high individual resistance, so many are aligned in parallel that their aggregate resistance is very low. We see this same pattern of resistance in the vascular system, where capillaries make a smaller contribution than arterioles to aggregate resistance.

⊙ **27-7** Table 27.1 also shows how R_{AW} varies for a typical patient with moderately severe **chronic obstructive pulmonary disease (COPD),** a condition in which emphysema or chronic bronchitis increases R_{AW}. COPD is a common and debilitating consequence of cigarette smoking. Notice *where* the disease strikes. Even though COPD increases total airway resistance to 5.0 cm H_2O/(L/s)—3.3-fold greater than in our normal subject—pharynx-larynx resistance does not change at all, and large-airway resistance increases only modestly. Almost all of the increment in R_{AW} is due to a nearly 12-fold increase in the resistance of the smallest airways!

Although small airways normally have a very low aggregate resistance, it is within these small airways that COPD has its greatest and earliest effects. Even a doubling of small-airway resistance from 0.3 to 0.6 cm H_2O/(L/s) in the early stages of COPD would produce such a small increment in R_{AW} that it would be impossible to identify the COPD patient in a screening test based on resistance measurements. In addition to COPD, the other common cause of increased R_{AW} is **asthma.**

Regardless of its cause, increased R_{AW} greatly increases the energy required to move air into and out of the lungs. If the increase in R_{AW} is severe enough, it can markedly limit exercise. In extreme cases, even walking may be more exercise than the patient can manage.

Vagal tone, histamine, and reduced lung volume all increase airway resistance

Several factors can modulate R_{AW}, including the autonomic nervous system (ANS), humoral factors, and changes in the volume of the lungs themselves. The vagus nerve, part of the **parasympathetic** division of the ANS, releases acetylcholine, which acts on an M_3 muscarinic receptor on bronchial smooth muscle (see ⊙ 14-5). The result is bronchoconstriction and therefore an increase in R_{AW}. The muscarinic antagonist atropine blocks this action. Irritants such as cigarette

smoke cause a reflex bronchoconstriction in which the vagus nerve is the efferent limb.

⊙ **27-8** Opposing the action of the vagus nerve is the **sympathetic** division of the ANS, which releases norepinephrine and dilates the bronchi and bronchioles, but reduces glandular secretions. However, these effects are weak because norepinephrine is a poor agonist of the β_2-adrenergic receptors that mediate this effect via cAMP (see ⊙ 14-6).

Humoral factors include **epinephrine,** released by the adrenal medulla. Circulating epinephrine is a far better β_2 agonist than is norepinephrine and therefore a more potent bronchodilator. **Histamine** constricts bronchioles and alveolar ducts and thus increases R_{AW}. Far more potent is the bronchoconstrictor effect of the leukotrienes LTC_4 and LTD_4.

⊙ **27-9** One of the most powerful determinants of R_{AW} is **lung volume** R_{AW} is extremely high at residual volume (RV) but decreases steeply as V_L increases (Fig. 27.7A). One reason for this effect is obvious: all pulmonary airways—including the conducting airways, which account for virtually all of R_{AW}—expand at high V_L, and resistance falls steeply as radius increases (see Equation 27.8). A second reason is the **principle of interdependence**—alveoli tend to hold open their neighbors by exerting **mechanical tethering** (Fig. 27.7B). At high V_L, alveoli dilate more than the adjacent bronchioles, pulling the bronchioles farther open by mechanical tethering. Patients with **obstructive lung disease,** by definition, have an increased R_{AW} at a given V_L (Fig. 27.7A). However, because these patients tend to have a higher-than-normal FRC, they breathe at a higher V_L, where airway resistance is—for them—relatively low.

During inspiration, a sustained negative shift in P_{IP} causes P_A to become transiently more negative

During a quiet respiratory cycle—an inspiration of 500 mL, followed by an expiration—the body first generates negative and then positive values of P_A. The four large gray panels of Fig. 27.8 show the idealized time courses of five key parameters. The uppermost panel is a record of V_L. The next panel is a pair of plots, $-P_{TP}$ and P_{IP}. The third shows the record of P_A. The bottom panel shows a simultaneous record of $\dot{V}$.

On the right side of Fig. 27.8 are the static P_{TP}-V_L curve and the dynamic P_A-V relationship. On the left side is a series of four cartoons that represent snapshots of the key pressures (i.e., P_{IP}, P_{TP}, and P_A) at four points during the respiratory cycle:

a. Before inspiration begins. The lungs are under static conditions at a volume of FRC.
b. Halfway through inspiration. The lungs are under dynamic conditions at a volume of FRC + 250 mL.
c. At the completion of inspiration. The lungs are once again under static conditions but at a volume of FRC + 500 mL.
d. Halfway through expiration. The lungs are under dynamic conditions at a volume of FRC + 250 mL.
e. At the end of expiration/ready for the next inspiration. The lungs are once again under static conditions at a volume of FRC.

The P_{IP} record in the second gray panel of Fig. 27.8 shows that P_{IP} is the same as $-P_{TP}$ whenever the lungs are under

A DEPENDENCE OF TOTAL AIRWAY RESISTANCE ON LUNG VOLUME

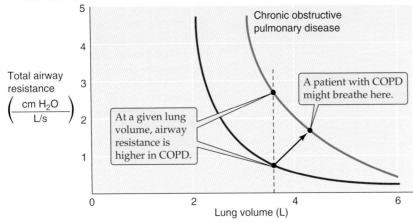

B MECHANICAL TETHERING

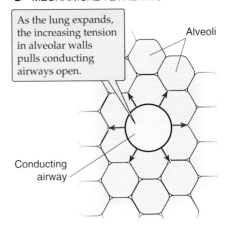

Fig. 27.7 Airway resistance.

static conditions (points *a*, *c*, and *a*). However, during the initial stages of inspiration, P_{IP} rapidly becomes more negative than $-P_{TP}$. This difference between P_{IP} and $-P_{TP}$ is P_A, which must be negative to produce airflow into the lungs. Later during the inspiration, $-P_{TP}$ catches up with P_{IP} so that the difference between them (i.e., P_A) falls to zero and inspiration stops. The relatively negative value of P_{TP} at the end of inspiration reflects the relatively large lung volume. During expiration, P_{IP} is more positive than $-P_{TP}$ to produce expiration.

The P_A record in the third gray panel of Fig. 27.8 shows that P_A is zero under static conditions (points *a*, *c*, and *a*). During inspiration, P_A rapidly becomes negative but then relaxes to zero by the end of inspiration. The opposite is true during expiration.

The bottom gray panel shows that the time course of airflow generally mirrors that of P_A, which drives airflow.

It is important to recognize that our respiratory muscles control P_{IP}, and that P_{IP} plays two very different roles. First, a sudden change in P_{IP} transiently changes P_A and transiently produces airflow—a *dynamic* property. Second, and somewhat more slowly, changes in P_{IP} produce changes in lung volume—a *static* property—that eventually become stable as P_A falls to zero.

Table 27.2 summarizes key aspects of static vs. dynamic properties of the lungs.

Dynamic compliance falls as respiratory frequency rises

In the preceding section, we examined pressure, volume, and flow changes during an idealized respiratory cycle of 5 seconds, which corresponds to a respiratory frequency of 12 breaths/min. The V_L curve in the top gray panel in Fig. 27.8 shows that—at the end of the 2.5 seconds allotted for inspiration or expiration—V_L has already been stable (i.e., the lung has been static) for more than a second. In other words, for a healthy person breathing at a low respiratory frequency, the lungs fully complete their volume changes during inspiration and expiration. Stated differently, the change in P_{TP} is equal to but opposite the change in P_{IP}:

$$C_{static} = \frac{\Delta V_L}{\Delta P_{TP}} = \frac{\Delta V_L}{-\Delta P_{IP}} \quad \text{(27.12)}$$

at very low frequency $\approx$ static conditions

However, at higher frequencies (Fig. 27.9), the shifts in P_{IP} may occur so rapidly that the lungs cannot complete the change in volume. In other words, the ΔV_L (and ΔP_{TP}) is less than we would expect for the ΔP_{IP}, so that the **dynamic compliance** is now less than the static compliance:

$$C_{dynamic} = \frac{\text{smaller } \Delta V_L \ \text{(at high frequency)}}{-\Delta P_{IP}} < C_{static} \quad \text{(27.13)}$$

Even in a healthy person (i.e., normal R_{AW} and normal C_{static}), the $C_{dynamic}$ gradually falls as respiratory frequency rises. However, in patients with increased R_{AW} or increased C_{static}, the lungs may change volume so slowly that $C_{dynamic}$ is substantially less than C_{static}, even at relatively low frequencies.

This analysis greatly oversimplifies what happens in the lungs of real people. Although we have treated the lungs as if there were one value for R_{AW} and one for C_{static}, each conducting airway has its own R_{AW} and each alveolar unit has its own C_{static}, and some alveolar units are slower than others. With disease some respiratory units may become so slow that, at sufficiently high frequencies, very slow airways may drop out of the picture entirely.

Transmural pressure differences cause airways to dilate during inspiration and to compress during expiration

We have noted three factors that modulate airway caliber: (1) the ANS, (2) humoral substances, and (3) V_L (Fig. 27.7). A fourth factor that modulates R_{AW} is the very flow of air through the conducting airway. Airflow alters the pressure difference across the walls of an airway, and this change in transmural pressure (P_{TM}) can cause the airway to dilate or to collapse. Fig. 27.10A through C depicts the pressures along a single hypothetical airway, extending from the level of the alveolus to the lips, under three conditions: during inspiration (Fig. 27.10A), at rest (Fig. 27.10B), and during

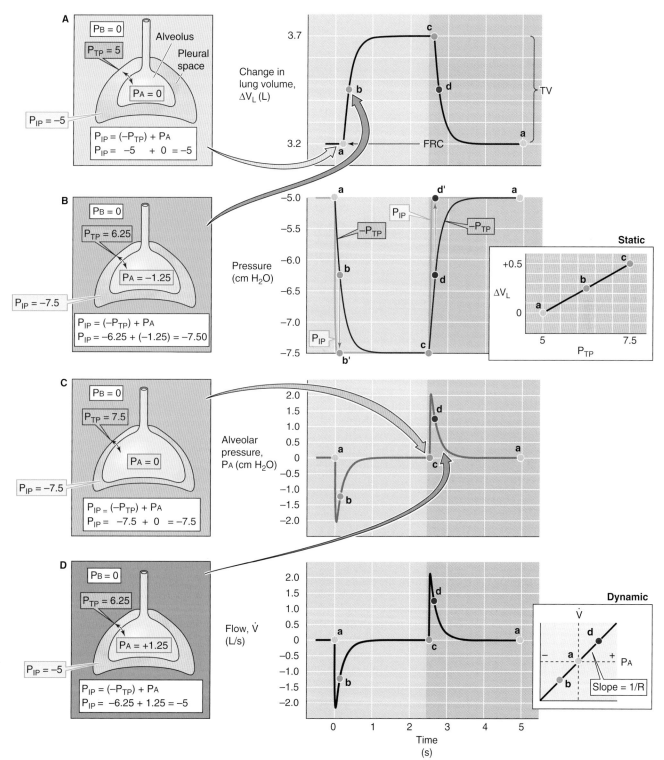

Fig. 27.8 Idealized plots of P_B, P_{IP}, P_{TP}, and P_A during the respiratory cycle. Note that all pressures are in centimeters of H_2O. The *colored points* (labeled *a*, *b*, *c*, and *d*) in each of the central panels correspond to the illustrations on the left with the same-colored backgrounds.

TABLE 27.2 Static Versus Dynamic Properties of the Lungs

	STATIC PROPERTIES	DYNAMIC PROPERTIES
Anatomical correlate	Alveoli and interstitial space	Conducting airways
Key "constant"	Static compliance, C	Airway resistance, R_{AW}
Key pressure	P_{TP} ($P_{TP} = P_A - P_{IP}$)	P_A
What is controlled?	V_L ($C = \Delta V_L / \Delta P_{TP}$)	$\dot{V}$ ($\dot{V} = P_A / R_{AW}$)
Pathology	Restrictive disease (e.g., fibrosis), caused by ↓ C	Obstructive disease (e.g., COPD), caused by ↑R_{AW}

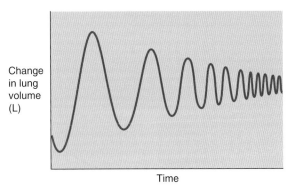

Change in lung volume (L)

Time

Fig. 27.9 Dynamic compliance.

expiration (Fig. 27.10C). In all three cases, the lung is at the same volume, FRC. Because V_L is at FRC, P_{TP} (the P_{TM} for the alveoli) is 5 cm H_2O in all three cases.

Static Conditions First consider static conditions (Fig. 27.10B). In the absence of airflow, the pressures inside all airways must be zero. Considering first the alveoli, P_{TP} is 5 cm H_2O and the P_A is zero, and thus P_{IP} is −5 cm H_2O. The P_{IP} of −5 cm H_2O acts not only on alveoli but also on *all* conducting airways within the thoracic cavity. For these, P_{TM} at any point is the difference between the pressure inside the airway (P_{AW}) and P_{IP} (see Equation 27.1):

$$P_{TM} = P_{AW} - P_{IP} = 0 - (-5 \text{ cm } H_2O) = +5 \text{ cm } H_2O \quad \textbf{(27.14)}$$

In other words, a transmural pressure of +5 cm H_2O acts on *all* thoracic airways, tending to expand them to the extent that their compliance permits.

Inspiration Now consider a vigorous inspiration (Fig. 27.10A). We first exhale to a V_L below FRC and then inhale vigorously, so that the P_A is −15 cm H_2O at the instant that V_L passes through FRC. While the lung is at FRC, P_{TP} must be +5 cm H_2O, and the P_{IP} needed to produce a P_A of −15 cm H_2O is

$$P_{IP} = (-P_{TP}) + P_A$$
$$= -5 \text{ cm } H_2O + (-15 \text{cm } H_2O) \quad \textbf{(27.15)}$$
$$= -20 \text{ cm } H_2O$$

How does this exceptionally negative P_{IP} affect airways upstream from the alveoli? P_{AW} gradually decays from −15 cm H_2O in the alveoli to zero at the lips. The farther we move from the alveoli, the less negative is P_{AW}, and thus the greater is P_{TM}. At a point where P_{AW} is −8 cm H_2O, the transmural pressure opposing the elastic recoil at this point has increased from +5 cm H_2O at rest (Fig. 27.10B) to +12 cm H_2O during

this vigorous inspiration (see Fig. 17.10A). Because P_{TM} has increased, the airway will dilate. The tendency to dilate increases as we move from the alveoli to larger airways. The extent to which an airway *actually* dilates also depends on its compliance. The amount of cartilage supporting the airways gradually increases from none for 11th-generation airways to a substantial amount for the mainstem bronchi. Because the increasing amount of cartilage in the larger airways decreases their compliance, they have an increasing ability to resist changes in caliber produced by a given change in P_{TM}.

Expiration Conducting airways tend to collapse during expiration (Fig. 27.10C). We first inhale to a V_L above FRC and then exhale vigorously, so that P_A is +15 cm H_2O at the instant that V_L passes through FRC. Because the lung is at FRC, P_{TP} must be +5 cm H_2O. The P_{IP} needed to produce a P_A of +15 cm H_2O is

$$P_{IP} = (-P_{TP}) + P_A$$
$$= -5 \text{ cm } H_2O + (+15\text{cm } H_2O) \quad \textbf{(27.16)}$$
$$= +10 \text{ cm } H_2O$$

What is the effect of this very positive P_{IP} on the upstream airways? P_{AW} must decrease gradually from +15 cm H_2O in the alveoli to zero at the lips. The farther we move from the alveolus, the lower the P_{AW} and thus the lower the P_{TM}. At a point where P_{AW} is +8 cm H_2O, the transmural pressure opposing elastic recoil has fallen sharply from +5 cm H_2O at rest (which tends to mildly inflate the airway) to −2 cm H_2O during expiration (which actually tends to squeeze the airway). As we move from the alveoli to larger airways, P_{AW} further decreases. That is, P_{TM} gradually shifts from an inflating force (positive values) to an ever-increasing squeezing force (negative values). Fortunately, these larger airways—with the greatest collapsing tendency—have the most cartilage and thus some resistance to the natural collapsing tendency that develops during expiration. In addition, mechanical tethering (see ⊙ 27-9) helps all conducting airways surrounded by alveoli to resist collapse. Nevertheless, R_{AW} is greater during expiration than it is during inspiration.

The problem of airway compression during expiration is exaggerated in patients with **emphysema,** a condition in which the alveolar walls break down. This process results in fewer and larger air spaces. Although the affected alveoli have an increased compliance and thus a larger diameter at the end of an inspiration, they are flimsy and exert less mechanical tethering on the conducting airways they surround. Thus, patients with emphysema have great difficulty exhaling because their conducting airways are less able to resist the tendency to collapse. One of the strategies that

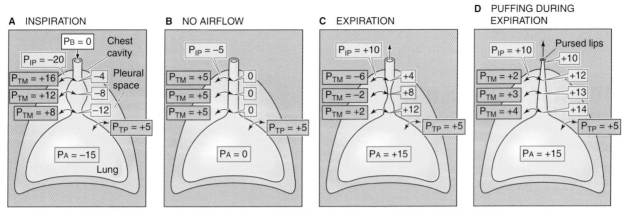

Fig. 27.10 Dilation and collapse of airways with airflow. In all four panels, V_L is FRC. P_{TM} is the transmural pressure across conducting airways. P_{AW} and values in *pale blue balloons* represent pressures inside conducting airways (all in centimeters of H_2O).

these patients spontaneously make is to **exhale through pursed lips.** This maneuver—known as puffing—creates an artificial high resistance at the lips. Because the greatest pressure drop occurs at the location of the greatest resistance, puffing causes a greater share of the P_{AW} drop to occur across the lips than along collapsible, cartilage-free airways. Thus, puffing maintains relatively high P_{AW} values farther along the tracheobronchial tree (Fig. 27.10D) and reduces collapsing tendencies throughout. The greatest collapsing tendencies are reserved for the largest airways that have the most cartilage (see ◉ 26-2). Of course, the patient pays a price for puffing: the high resistance at the lips decreases instantaneous airflow and thus ventilation.

CHAPTER 28

ACID-BASE PHYSIOLOGY

Walter F. Boron

Although present in exceedingly low concentrations in most body fluids, protons nevertheless have a major impact on biochemical reactions and on a variety of physiological processes that are critical for the homeostasis of the entire body and individual cells. Not surprisingly, sophisticated systems evolved to maintain [H⁺] values within narrow and precise ranges in the blood plasma, intracellular fluid, and other compartments.

This chapter provides the introduction to acid-base physiology, including the chemistry of buffers, the CO_2/HCO_3^- buffer system, the competition between the CO_2/HCO_3^- buffer system and other buffers, and the regulation of intracellular pH. In other chapters, we discuss how blood pH—and, by extension, the pH of extracellular fluid—is under the dual control of the respiratory system, which regulates plasma $[CO_2]$ (see Chapter 31), and the kidneys, which regulate plasma $[HCO_3^-]$ (see Chapter 39). In addition, we discuss the control of cerebrospinal fluid pH in Chapter 32.

pH AND BUFFERS

pH values vary enormously among different intracellular and extracellular compartments

An **acid** is any chemical substance (e.g., CH_3COOH, NH_4^+) that can donate an H⁺. A **base**—or **alkali**—is any chemical substance (e.g., CH_3COO^-, NH_3) that can accept an H⁺.

[H⁺] varies over a large range in biological solutions, from >100 mM in gastric secretions to <10 nM in pancreatic secretions. The **pH scale**—an effort to simplify [H⁺] notation—is based on powers of 10:

$$pH \equiv -\log_{10}[H^+] \qquad (28.1)$$

Thus, when [H⁺] is 10^{-7} M, the pH is 7.0. The higher the [H⁺], the lower the pH (Table 28.1). It is worth remembering that a 10-fold change in [H⁺] corresponds to a pH shift of 1, whereas a 2-fold change in [H⁺] corresponds to a pH shift of ~0.3.

Even small changes in pH can have substantial physiological consequences. pH-sensitive molecules include a variety of enzymes, receptors and their ligands, ion channels, transporters, and structural proteins. For most proteins, pH sensitivity is modest. The activity of the Na-K pump, for example, falls by about half when the pH shifts by ~1 pH unit from the optimum pH, which is near the resting pH of the typical cell. However, the activity of phosphofructokinase, a key glycolytic enzyme, falls by ~90% when pH falls by only 0.1.

The overall impact of pH changes on cellular processes can be impressive. For example, cell proliferation in response to mitogenic activation is maximal at the normal, resting intracellular pH but may fall as much as 85% when intracellular pH falls by only 0.4.

Table 28.2 lists the pH values in several body fluids. Because the pH of neutral water at 37°C is 6.81, most major body compartments are alkaline.

Buffers minimize the size of the pH changes produced by adding acid or alkali to a solution

A **buffer** is any substance that reversibly consumes or releases H⁺. Buffers do not *prevent* pH changes, they only help to *minimize* them.

⊙ **28-1** Consider a hypothetical buffer B for which the protonated form $HB^{(n+1)}$, with a valence of $n + 1$, is in equilibrium with its deprotonated form $B^{(n)}$, which has the valence of n:

$$HB^{(n+1)} \rightleftharpoons B^{(n)} + H^+ \qquad (28.2)$$

Here, $HB^{(n+1)}$ is a **weak acid** because it does not fully dissociate; $B^{(n)}$ is its **conjugate weak base**. Conversely, $B^{(n)}$ is a **weak base** and $HB^{(n+1)}$ is its conjugate weak acid. Together, $HB^{(n+1)}$ and $B^{(n)}$ are a **buffer pair**. The **total buffer concentration**, [TB], is the sum of the concentrations of the protonated and unprotonated forms:

$$[TB] = [HB^{(n+1)}] + [B^{(n)}] \qquad (28.3)$$

The valence of the acidic (i.e., protonated) form can be positive, zero, or negative:

$$
\begin{array}{cccc}
\overbrace{NH_4^+}^{\text{Weak acid} \atop (HB^{(n+1)})} & \rightleftharpoons & \overbrace{NH_3}^{\text{Conjugate weak base} \atop (B^{(n)})} & + H^+ \\
H_2CO_3 & \rightleftharpoons & HCO_3^- & + H^+ \\
H_2PO_4^- & \rightleftharpoons & HPO_4^{2-} & + H^+
\end{array}
\qquad (28.4)
$$

In these examples, NH_4^+ (ammonium), H_2CO_3 (carbonic acid), and $H_2PO_4^-$ ("monobasic" inorganic phosphate) are all weak acids, whereas NH_3 (ammonia), HCO_3^- (bicarbonate), and HPO_4^{2-} ("dibasic" inorganic phosphate) are the respective conjugate weak bases. Each buffer reaction is governed by a **dissociation constant,** K:

$$K = \frac{[B^{(n)}][H^+]}{[HB^{(n+1)}]} \qquad (28.5)$$

TABLE 28.1 Relationship Between [H⁺] and pH Values

	[H⁺] (M)	PH	
×10	1×10^{-6}	6.0	1 pH unit
	1×10^{-7}	7.0	
	1×10^{-8}	8.0	
×2	8×10^{-8}	7.1	0.3 pH unit
	4×10^{-8}	7.4	
	2×10^{-8}	7.7	
	1×10^{-8}	8.0	

TABLE 28.2 Approximate pH Values of Various Body Fluids

COMPARTMENT	PH
Gastric secretions (under conditions of maximal acidity)	0.7
Lysosome	5.5
Chromaffin granule	5.5
Neutral H_2O at 37°C	6.81
Cytosol of a typical cell	7.2
Cerebrospinal fluid (CSF)	7.3
Arterial blood plasma	7.4
Mitochondrial inner matrix	7.5
Secreted pancreatic fluid	8.1

If we add to a physiological solution a small amount of HCl—which is a strong acid because it fully dissociates—the buffers in the solution consume almost all added H^+:

$$H^+ + Cl^- + B^{(n)} \rightarrow HB^{(n+1)} + Cl^- \tag{28.6}$$

For each H^+ buffered, one $B^{(n)}$ is *consumed*. The tiny amount of H^+ that is *not buffered* remains free in solution and is responsible for a decrease in pH.

If we instead titrate this same solution with a strong base such as NaOH, H^+ derived from $HB^{(n+1)}$ neutralizes almost all the added OH^-:

$$Na^+ + OH^- + HB^{(n+1)} \rightarrow Na^+ + B^{(n)} + H_2O \tag{28.7}$$

For each OH^- buffered, one $B^{(n)}$ is *formed*. The tiny amount of added OH^- that is not neutralized by the buffer equilibrates with H^+ and H_2O and is responsible for an increase in pH.

A useful measure of the strength of a buffer is its **buffering power (β)**, which is the number of moles of strong base (e.g., NaOH) that one must add to a liter of solution to increase pH by 1 pH unit. This value is equivalent to the amount of strong acid (e.g., HCl) that one must add to decrease the pH by 1 pH unit. Thus, buffering power is

$$\beta \equiv \frac{\overbrace{\Delta[\text{Strong base}]}^{\text{moles/liter}}}{\Delta pH} = -\frac{\overbrace{\Delta[\text{Strong acid}]}^{\text{moles/liter}}}{\Delta pH} \tag{28.8}$$

In the absence of CO_2/HCO_3^-, the buffering power of whole blood (which contains erythrocytes, leukocytes, and platelets) is ~25 mM/pH unit. This value is known as the non-HCO_3^- **buffering power** ($\beta_{\text{non-HCO}_3^-}$). In other words, we would have to add 25 mmol of NaOH to a liter of whole blood to increase the pH by 1 unit, assuming that β is constant over this wide pH range. For blood plasma, which lacks the cellular elements of whole blood, $\beta_{\text{non-HCO}_3^-}$ is only ~5 mM/pH unit, which means that only about one fifth as much strong base would be needed to produce the same pH increase.

According to the Henderson-Hasselbalch equation, pH depends on the ratio $[CO_2]/[HCO_3^-]$

The most important physiological buffer pair is CO_2 and HCO_3^-. The impressive strength of this buffer pair is due to the volatility of CO_2, which allows the lungs to maintain stable CO_2 concentrations in the blood plasma despite ongoing metabolic and buffer reactions that produce or consume CO_2. Imagine that a beaker contains an aqueous solution of 145 mM NaCl (pH = 6.81), but no buffers. We now expose this solution to an atmosphere containing CO_2 (Fig. 28.1). Once the system achieves equilibrium, the concentration of dissolved CO_2 ($[CO_2]_{\text{dis}}$) is governed by **Henry's law** (see Box 26.2):

$$[CO_2]_{\text{Dis}} = s \cdot P_{CO_2} \tag{28.9}$$

At the temperature (37°C) and ionic strength of mammalian blood plasma, the **solubility coefficient, *s*,** is ~0.03 mM/mm Hg. Because the alveolar air with which arterial blood equilibrates has a P_{CO_2} of ~40 mm Hg, or torr, $[CO_2]_{\text{dis}}$ in arterial blood is

$$[CO_2]_a = (0.03 \text{ mM/mm Hg}) \cdot 40 \text{ mm Hg} = 1.2 \text{ mM} \tag{28.10}$$

So far, the entry of CO_2 from the atmosphere into the aqueous solution has had *no effect* on pH. The reason is that we have neither generated nor consumed H^+. CO_2 itself is neither an acid nor a base. If we were considering dissolved N_2 or O_2, our analysis would end here because these gases interact no further with simple aqueous solutions. The aqueous chemistry of CO_2, however, is more complicated, because CO_2 reacts with the solvent (i.e., H_2O) to form carbonic acid:

$$CO_2 + H_2O \xrightarrow{\text{slow}} H_2CO_3 \tag{28.11}$$

⊙ 28-2 This CO_2 **hydration reaction** is very slow. In fact, it is far too slow to meet most physiological needs. The enzyme **carbonic anhydrase,** present in erythrocytes and elsewhere, catalyzes a reaction that effectively bypasses this slow hydration reaction. Carbonic acid is a weak acid that rapidly dissociates into H^+ and HCO_3^-:

$$H_2CO_3 \xrightarrow{\text{fast}} H^+ + HCO_3^- \tag{28.12}$$

This **dissociation reaction** is the first point at which pH falls. Note that the formation of HCO_3^- (the conjugate weak base of H_2CO_3) necessarily accompanies the formation of H^+ in a stoichiometry of 1:1. The observation that pH decreases, even though the above reaction produces the weak base

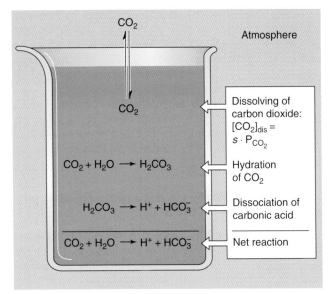

Figure 28.1   Interaction of CO_2 with water.

HCO_3^-, is sometimes confusing. A safe way to reason through such an apparent paradox is to focus always on the fate of the proton: if the reaction forms H^+, pH falls. Thus, even though the dissociation of H_2CO_3 leads to generation of a weak base, pH falls because H^+ forms along with the weak base.

Unlike the hydration of CO_2, the dissociation of H_2CO_3 is extremely fast. Thus, in the absence of carbonic anhydrase, the slow CO_2 hydration reaction limits the speed at which increased $[CO_2]_{dis}$ leads to the production of H^+. HCO_3^- can accept a proton to form its conjugate weak acid (i.e., H_2CO_3) or release a second proton to form its conjugate weak base (i.e., CO_3^{2-}). Because this latter reaction generally is of only minor physiological significance for buffering in mammals, we will not discuss it further.

◉ **28-3** For convenience, we may treat the hydration and dissociation reactions that occur when we expose water to CO_2 as if only one reaction were involved:

$$CO_2 + H_2O \rightleftarrows H_2CO_3 \rightleftarrows H^+ + HCO_3^- \quad \text{(28.13)}$$
$$CO_2 + H_2O \rightleftarrows H^+ + HCO_3^-$$

Moreover, we can define a dissociation constant for this pseudoequilibrium:

$$K = \frac{[H^+][HCO_3^-]}{[CO_2]} \quad \text{(28.14)}$$

In logarithmic form, this equation becomes

$$pH = pK + \log \frac{[HCO_3^-]}{[CO_2]} \quad \text{(28.15)}$$

Finally, we may express $[CO_2]$ in terms of P_{CO_2}, recalling from Henry's law that $[CO_2] = s \cdot P_{CO_2}$:

$$pH = pK + \log \frac{[HCO_3^-]}{s \cdot P_{CO_2}} \quad \text{(28.16)}$$

This is the **Henderson-Hasselbalch** equation, a logarithmic restatement of the CO_2/HCO_3^- equilibrium in Equation 28.14. Its central message is that pH depends not on $[HCO_3^-]$ or P_{CO_2}

per se, but on their *ratio*. Human arterial blood has a P_{CO_2} of ~40 mm Hg and an $[HCO_3^-]$ of ~24 mM. If we assume that the pK governing the CO_2/HCO_3^- equilibrium is 6.1 at 37°C, then

$$pH = 6.1 + \log \frac{24 \text{ mM}}{(0.03 \text{ mM/mm Hg} \times 40 \text{ mm Hg})} = 7.40 \quad \text{(28.17)}$$

Thus, the Henderson-Hasselbalch equation correctly predicts the normal pH of arterial blood.

Because it is the kidney that controls $[HCO_3^-]$ in the blood plasma (see ◉ 39-3), and because it is the lung that controls P_{CO_2} (see Fig. 31.2), the pH of blood plasma is under the dual control of both organ systems, a concept embodied by a whimsical variant of the Henderson-Hasselbalch equation:

$$pH = \text{Constent} + \frac{\text{Kidney}}{\text{Lungs}} \quad \text{(28.18)}$$

ACID-BASE CHEMISTRY IN THE PRESENCE OF BOTH CO_2/HCO_3^- AND NON-HCO_3^- BUFFERS—THE DAVENPORT DIAGRAM

Real biological systems are mixtures of CO_2/HCO_3^- and many non-HCO_3^- buffers. Thus, to understand the effects of acid-base disturbances in a biological system, we must consider multiple competing equilibria—one for CO_2/HCO_3^- (described by Equation 28.16) and one for each of the non-HCO_3^- buffers (each described by its version of Equation 28.5). Obtaining a precise solution to such clinically relevant problems is impossible. One approach is to use a computer to make increasingly more precise approximations of the correct answer. Another, more intuitive approach is to use a graphical method to estimate the final pH. The Davenport diagram is the best such tool.

The Davenport diagram is a graphical tool for interpreting acid-base disturbances in blood

◉ **28-4** What happens to the pH of blood—a complex mixture that includes many HCO_3^- buffers—when P_{CO_2} doubles? This is an example of **respiratory acidosis**—"acidosis" because pH falls, and "respiratory" because pulmonary problems (Table 28.3) are the most common causes of an increase in the P_{CO_2} of arterial blood.

In analyzing respiratory acidosis, we simplify matters by lumping together the actions of all non-HCO_3^- buffers, so that $H^+ + B^{(n)} \rightleftarrows HB^{(n+1)}$ represents the reactions of *all* non-HCO_3^- buffers, regardless of their pK values and concentrations. When we raise P_{CO_2}, almost all of the newly formed H^+ reacts with $B^{(n)}$ to form $HB^{(n+1)}$ so that the free $[H^+]$ rises only slightly.

$$CO_2 + H_2O \rightarrow HCO_3^- + H^+ \quad \begin{array}{l} \text{Non-}HCO_3^- \text{ buffers} \\ \text{consume almost all the} \\ H^+ \text{ produced by } CO_2. \\ \rightarrow B^{(n)} \end{array}$$
$$\downarrow$$
$$HB^{(n+1)}$$

$$\text{(28.19)}$$

TABLE 28.3 The Four Major Acid-Base Disorders

DISORDER	PROXIMATE CAUSE(S)	CLINICAL CAUSES	CHANGES IN ARTERIAL ACID-BASE PARAMETERS
Respiratory acidosis	↑ P_{CO_2}	↓ Alveolar ventilation (e.g., drug overdose) ↓ Lung-diffusing capacity (e.g., pulmonary edema) Ventilation-perfusion mismatch	pH: ↓ [HCO_3^-]: ↑ P_{CO_2}: ↑

Respiratory alkalosis	↓ P_{CO_2}	↑ Alveolar ventilation caused by:
		   Hypoxia (e.g., acclimatization to high altitude)
		   Anxiety
		   Aspirin intoxication
			pH: ↑ [HCO_3^-]: ↓
			 P_{CO_2}: ↓

Metabolic acidosis	Addition of acids other than CO_2 or H_2CO_3 Removal of alkali (fixed P_{CO_2})	↓ Urinary secretion of H^+ (e.g., renal failure) Ketoacidosis (e.g., diabetes mellitus) Lactic acidosis (e.g., shock) HCO_3^- loss (e.g., severe diarrhea)	pH: ↓ [HCO_3^-]: ↓ P_{CO_2}: No change
Metabolic alkalosis	Addition of alkali Removal of acids other than CO_2 or H_2CO_3 (fixed P_{CO_2})	HCO_3^- load (e.g., $NaHCO_3$ therapy) Loss of H^+ (e.g., severe vomiting)	pH: ↑ HCO_3^-: ↑ P_{CO_2}: No change

In this simplified approach, the final pH depends on two competing buffer reactions—one involving CO_2/HCO_3^- and the other involving $HB^{(n+1)}/B^{(n)}$. Computing the final pH requires using a graphical approach for solving two simultaneous equations, one for each buffer reaction, which we will consider in the next two sections.

The CO_2/HCO_3^- Buffer The first of the two equations that we must solve simultaneously is a rearrangement of the Henderson-Hasselbalch equation (see Equation 28.16):

$$[HCO_3^-] = s \cdot P_{CO_2} \cdot 10^{\left(pH - pK_{CO_2}\right)} \qquad (28.20)$$

◉ 28-5 For a P_{CO_2} of 40 mm Hg, the equation requires that [HCO_3^-] be 24 mM when pH is 7.40—as in normal arterial blood plasma. If pH decreases by 0.3 at this same P_{CO_2}, Equation 28.20 states that [HCO_3^-] must fall by half to 12 mM. Conversely, if pH increases by 0.3, [HCO_3^-] must double to 48 mM. The blue column of Table 28.4 lists the [HCO_3^-] values that Equation 28.20 predicts for various pH values when P_{CO_2} is 40 mm Hg. Plotting these [HCO_3^-] values against pH yields the blue curve labeled "P_{CO_2} = 40 mm Hg" in Fig. 28.2. This curve, which is known as a CO_2 isobar, or **isopleth,** represents all possible combinations of [HCO_3^-] and pH at a P_{CO_2} of 40 mm Hg. Table 28.4 also summarizes [HCO_3^-] values prevailing at P_{CO_2} values of 20 and 80 mm Hg. Note that at a P_{CO_2} of 20 (orange column), representing **respiratory alkalosis** (Table 28.3)—"respiratory" because, clinically, it results from hyperventilation and "alkalosis" because the pH rises—[HCO_3^-] values are half those for a P_{CO_2} of 40 at the same pH. At a P_{CO_2} of 80 (green column), representing respiratory acidosis, [HCO_3^-] values are twice those at a P_{CO_2} of 40. Each of the isopleths in Fig. 28.2 rises exponentially with pH. The slope of each isopleth also rises exponentially with pH and represents the open-system buffering power (β_{open}) for CO_2/HCO_3^-. The system is *open* because CO_2 can freely exchange with the environment to keep P_{CO_2} constant. In a beaker (Fig. 28.1), the stability of P_{CO_2} is the result of the exchange of CO_2 dissolved in water with the CO_2 gas in the overlying atmosphere. In the body, the stability of P_{CO_2} is the result of changes in alveolar ventilation, as we will see in Chapter 31. At a particular pH, an isopleth representing a higher P_{CO_2} (i.e., a higher [HCO_3^-]) has a steeper slope, which represents the buffering power of the CO_2/HCO_3^- buffer pair.

Non-HCO_3^- Buffers The second of the two equations that we must solve simultaneously describes the titration curve created by the lumped reactions of all of the non-HCO_3^- buffers. In Fig. 28.2, we summarize these reactions by the red line, the slope of which represents the non-HCO_3^- buffering power ($\beta_{non-HCO_3^-}$).

Solving the Problem Fig. 28.2 is a Davenport diagram, a combination of the three CO_2 isopleths we discussed and the red line that represents the non-HCO_3^- titration curve ($\beta_{non-HCO_3^-}$ for whole blood = 25 mM/pH unit). The intersection of this red line with the CO_2 isopleth for a P_{CO_2} of 40—at the point labeled "Start"—represents the initial conditions for arterial blood, where both CO_2/HCO_3^- and non-HCO_3^- buffers are simultaneously in equilibrium.

We are now in a position to answer the question raised at the beginning of this section: What will be the final pH when we increase the P_{CO_2} of whole blood from 40 to 80 mm Hg? The final equilibrium conditions for this case of *respiratory acidosis* must be described by a point that lies simultaneously on the red non-HCO_3^- titration line and the green isopleth for 80 mm Hg. Obtaining the answer using the Davenport diagram requires a three-step process:

Step 1: Identify the point at the intersection of the initial P_{CO_2} isopleth and the initial non-HCO_3^- titration line (Fig. 28.2, "Start").
Step 2: Identify the isopleth describing the *final* P_{CO_2} (80 mm Hg in this case).
Step 3: Follow the non-HCO_3^- titration line to its intersection with the final P_{CO_2} isopleth. In Fig. 28.2, this intersection occurs at point A, which corresponds to a pH of 7.19 and an [HCO_3^-] of 29.25 mM.

TABLE 28.4 **Relationship Between [HCO₃⁻] and pH at Three Fixed Levels of P_CO₂**

	[HCO₃⁻] (mM)		
pH	P_CO₂ = 20 mm Hg	= 40 mm Hg	= 80 mm Hg
7.1	6 mM	12 mM	24 mM
7.2	8	15	30
7.3	10	19	38
7.4	12	24	48
7.5	15	30	60 P_CO₂
7.6	19	38	76
7.7	24	48	96

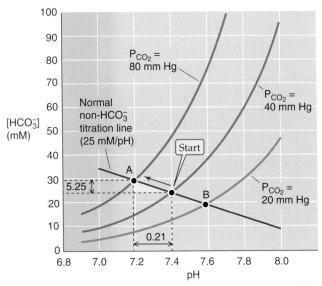

Figure 28.2 Davenport diagram. The *red arrow* represents the transition from a normal acid-base status for blood ("Start") to respiratory acidosis *(point A),* produced by raising P_CO₂ from 40 to 80 mm Hg. *Point B* represents respiratory alkalosis produced by lowering P_CO₂ to 20 mm Hg.

In the *absence* of non-HCO₃⁻ buffers, this same doubling of P_CO₂ causes a larger pH decrease, from 7.4 to 7.1.

By following three similar steps, we can use the Davenport diagram to predict the final pH and [HCO₃⁻] under conditions of a *respiratory alkalosis.* For example, what would be the effect of decreasing P_CO₂ by half, from 40 to 20 mm Hg? In Fig. 28.2 follow the red non-HCO₃⁻ titration line from "Start" to its intersection with the orange isopleth for a P_CO₂ of 20 mm Hg (point B), which corresponds to a pH of 7.60 and an [HCO₃⁻] of 19 mM. If the solution had *not* contained non-HCO₃⁻ buffers, halving the P_CO₂ would have caused a larger pH increase, from 7.4 to 7.7.

Adding or removing an acid or base—at a constant P_CO₂—produces a "metabolic" acid-base disturbance

◉ **28-6** The effect of adding HCl to blood plasma is rather complex because this solution contains both CO₂/HCO₃⁻ and non-HCO₃⁻ buffers (Fig. 28.3, *stage 1*). This disturbance is

called **metabolic acidosis,** "metabolic" because it can arise because of metabolic derangements (Table 28.3), and "acidosis" because pH falls. When we add 10 mmol of HCl to 1 L of solution in a beaker, the open-system CO₂/HCO₃⁻ buffer pair neutralizes most of the added H⁺, non-HCO₃⁻ buffers handle some, and a minute amount of added H⁺ remains free and lowers pH (Fig. 28.3, *stage 2A*). Because the system is open, the CO₂ formed during buffering of the added H⁺ escapes to the atmosphere. If this buffering reaction were occurring within the body, the newly formed CO₂ would enter the blood and escape first into the alveolar air, and then into the atmosphere.

How much of the added H⁺ (Δ[strong acid] = 10 mM) follows each of the three pathways in this example of *metabolic acidosis*? Answering this question requires dealing with two competing equilibria, the CO₂/HCO₃⁻ and the non-HCO₃⁻ buffering reactions. As for respiratory acid-base disturbances, we cannot precisely solve the equations governing metabolic acid-base disturbances. However, we can use the Davenport diagram on the left of Fig. 28.3 to obtain a graphical estimate of the final pH and [HCO₃⁻] through a four-step process:

Step 1: Identify the point describing the initial conditions (Fig. 28.3, "Start" in graph on left).
Step 2: Following the *black arrow* labeled "2," move downward (in the direction of decreased [HCO₃⁻]) by 10 mM—the concentration of added H⁺—to the point labeled with an asterisk.
Step 3: Through the asterisk, draw a line (Fig. 28.3, *black line* in left graph) that is parallel to the non-HCO₃⁻ titration line.
Step 4: Following the *black arrow* labeled "4," move to the intersection of the new *black line* and the original P_CO₂ isopleth. This intersection occurs at *point C,* which corresponds to a pH of 7.26 and an [HCO₃⁻] of 17.4 mM.

As a shortcut, we could bypass the two *black arrows* and simply follow the *red arrow* along the CO₂ isopleth from "Start" to *point C.*

We now can return to the question of how much of the added H⁺ follows each of the three pathways in Fig. 28.3, *stage 2A.* Because [HCO₃⁻] decreased by 24 − 17.4 = 6.6 mM, the amount of H⁺ buffered by CO₂/HCO₃⁻ must have been 6.6 mmol in each liter. Almost all of the remaining H⁺ that we added, nearly 3.4 mmol, must have been buffered by non-HCO₃⁻ buffers. A tiny amount of the added H⁺, ~0.000,015 mmol, must have remained unbuffered and was responsible for decreasing pH from 7.40 to 7.26 (Fig. 28.3, *stage 3A*).

Fig. 28.3 also shows what would happen if we added 10 mmol of a strong base such as NaOH to our 1-L solution. This disturbance is called **metabolic alkalosis,** "metabolic" because it can arise because of metabolic derangements (Table 28.3), and "alkalosis" because pH rises. The open-system CO₂/HCO₃⁻ buffer pair neutralizes most of the added OH⁻, non-HCO₃⁻ buffers handle some, and a minute amount of added OH⁻ remains unbuffered, thus raising pH (Fig. 28.3, *stage 2B*). The Davenport diagram on the right of Fig. 28.3 shows how much of the added OH⁻ follows each of the three pathways in this example of *metabolic alkalosis.* The approach is similar to the one we used above for metabolic acidosis, except that in this case, we generate a new black line

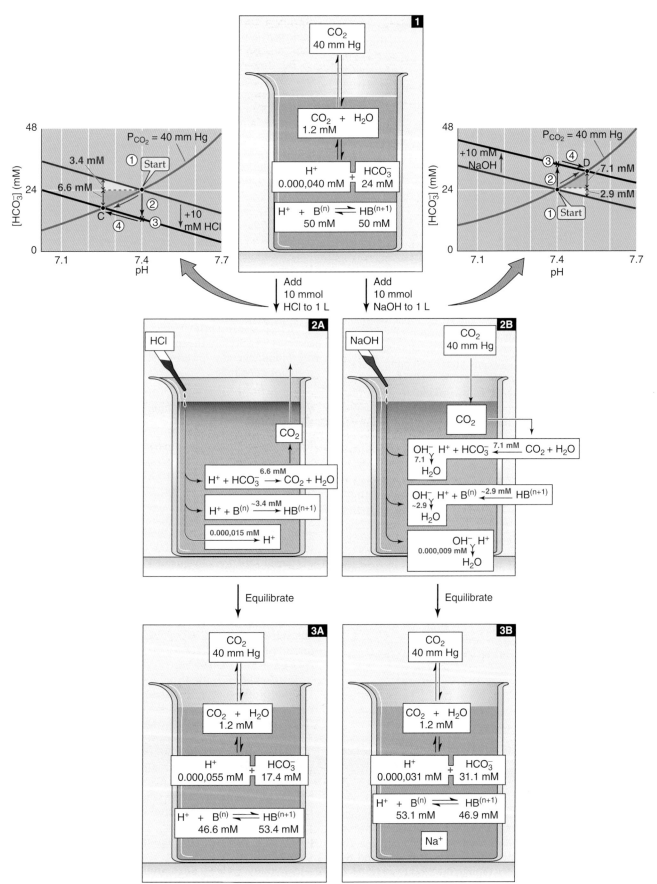

Figure 28.3 Metabolic acidosis and alkalosis in the presence of both CO_2/HCO_3^- and non-HCO_3^- buffers. The *red arrows* in the Davenport diagrams represent the transition to metabolic acidosis *(point C)* and metabolic alkalosis *(point D)*.

that is displaced 10 mM *above* the non-HCO_3^- titration line. We follow the P_{CO_2} isopleth to its intersection with this *black line* at *point D*, which corresponds to a final pH of 7.51 and an $[HCO_3^-]$ of 31.1 mM. Thus, $[HCO_3^-]$ rose by 31.1 − 24.0 = 7.1 mM. This is the amount of added OH^- that CO_2/HCO_3^- buffered. Non-HCO_3^- buffers must have buffered almost all of the remaining OH^- that we added, ~2.9 mmol in each liter. The unbuffered OH^-, which was responsible for the pH increase, must have been in the nanomolar range (Fig. 28.3, *stage 3B*).

A metabolic change can compensate for a respiratory disturbance

Thus far, we have considered what happens during *primary* respiratory and metabolic acid-base disturbances. When challenged by such acid or alkaline loads in the blood plasma, the body **compensates** by altering $[HCO_3^-]$ or P_{CO_2}, returning pH toward its initial value and minimizing the magnitude of the overall pH change.

◉ **28-7** In Fig. 28.4A we revisit an example, originally introduced in Fig. 28.2, in which we produced a primary respiratory acidosis by increasing P_{CO_2} from 40 to 80 mm Hg (*red arrow* in Fig. 28.4A between "Start" and *point A* at pH 7.19). If the high P_{CO_2} persists, the only way we can restore pH toward its initial value of 7.40 is to add an alkali (e.g., HCO_3^- or OH^-) or remove an acid (e.g., H^+), all of which are equivalent. Adding 10 mmol of OH^- to 1 L, for example, superimposes a metabolic *alkalosis* on the primary respiratory *acidosis*—a **metabolic compensation to respiratory acidosis.**

The Davenport diagram predicts the consequences of adding 10 mmol of OH^- to 1 L. We start by generating a black line that is parallel to the red non-HCO_3^- titration line, but displaced upward by 10 mM. Point A_1, the intersection of the black line and the P_{CO_2} isopleth for 80 mm Hg, represents a final pH of 7.29, still lower than the normal 7.40, but much higher than the 7.19 prevailing before compensation.

◉ **28-8** If we add an additional 14 mmol OH^-, for a total addition of 24 mmol OH^- to 1 L, pH returns to exactly its initial value of 7.40 (*point A_2* in Fig. 28.4A). In other words, we can perfectly compensate for doubling P_{CO_2} from 40 ("Start") to 80 mm Hg (*point A*) by adding an amount of OH^- equivalent to the amount of HCO_3^- that was present (i.e., 24 mM) at "Start." *Perfect* compensation of respiratory acidosis is an example of **isohydric hypercapnia** (i.e., *same* pH at a *higher* P_{CO_2}):

$$pH = 6.1 + \log \frac{\overbrace{48 \text{ mM}}^{\text{Doubled}[HCO_3^-]}}{(0.03 \text{ mM/mm Hg}) \times \underbrace{80 \text{ mm Hg}}_{\text{Doubled } P_{CO_2}}} \quad \textbf{(28.21)}$$

$$= 7.4$$

The kidneys are responsible for the metabolic compensation to a primary respiratory acidosis. They acutely sense high P_{CO_2} and may also sense chronically low blood pH. The response is to increase both the secretion of acid into the urine and the transport of HCO_3^- into the blood (see ◉ **39-4**), thereby raising plasma pH—a compensatory metabolic

alkalosis. The renal compensation to a substantial respiratory acidosis is not perfect, so that pH remains below the normal value of 7.40.

The kidneys can also perform a **metabolic compensation to a respiratory alkalosis.** In Fig. 28.4B we revisit a second example, originally introduced in Fig. 28.2, in which we produced a primary respiratory alkalosis by decreasing P_{CO_2} from 40 to 20 mm Hg (*red arrow* in Fig. 28.4B between "Start" and *point B* at pH 7.60). We can compensate for most of this respiratory alkalosis by adding 10 mmol of H^+ to each liter of solution or by removing 10 mmol $NaHCO_3$ or $NaOH$, all of which produce the same effect. We generate a *black line* that is parallel to the red non-HCO_3^- titration line but is displaced downward by 10 mM. *Point B_1* (pH 7.44), at the intersection of the *black line* and the P_{CO_2} isopleth for 20 mm Hg, represents a partial compensation.

If we add an additional 2 mmol H^+, for a total addition of 12 mmol of H^+ to each liter, pH returns to exactly its initial value of 7.40 (*point B_2* in Fig. 28.4B). When we halve P_{CO_2}, we need only add an amount of H^+ equivalent to halve the amount of HCO_3^- that was present (24/2 = 12 mM) at "Start."

In response to a primary respiratory alkalosis, the kidneys secrete less acid into the urine and transport less HCO_3^- into the blood, thereby lowering plasma pH—a compensatory metabolic acidosis.

A respiratory change can compensate for a metabolic disturbance

Just as metabolic changes can compensate for respiratory disturbances, respiratory changes can compensate for metabolic ones. In Fig. 28.5A we return to an example originally introduced on the left side of Fig. 28.3, in which we produced a primary metabolic acidosis by adding 10 mmol of HCl to 1 L of arterial blood (*red arrow* in Fig. 28.5A between "Start" and *point C* at pH 7.26). Other than removing the H^+ (or adding OH^- to neutralize the H^+), the only way we can restore pH toward the initial value of 7.40 is to lower P_{CO_2}. That is, we can superimpose a respiratory *alkalosis* on the primary metabolic *acidosis*—a **respiratory compensation to a metabolic acidosis.** For example, we can compensate for most of the metabolic acidosis by reducing P_{CO_2} from 40 to 30 mm Hg. Starting at C, follow the *black line* from the P_{CO_2} isopleth for 40 mm Hg to the new isopleth for 30 mm Hg at *point C_1* (pH 7.34). This maneuver represents a *partial* compensation.

If we reduce P_{CO_2} by an additional 6.6 mm Hg to 23.4 mm Hg, we produce a perfect compensation, which we represent in Fig. 28.5A by following the *black line* from C until we reach pH 7.40 at *point C_2*, which is on the P_{CO_2} isopleth for 23.4 mm Hg.

Not surprisingly, the respiratory system is responsible for the respiratory compensation to a primary metabolic acidosis. The low plasma pH or $[HCO_3^-]$ stimulates the peripheral chemoreceptors (see ◉ **32-4**) and, if sufficiently long-standing, also the central chemoreceptors (see ◉ **32-7**). The result is an increase in alveolar ventilation, which lowers P_{CO_2} (see Fig. 31.2) and thus provides the respiratory compensation.

The body achieves a **respiratory compensation to a primary metabolic alkalosis** in just the opposite manner. In Fig. 28.5B, we revisit an example originally presented on the right

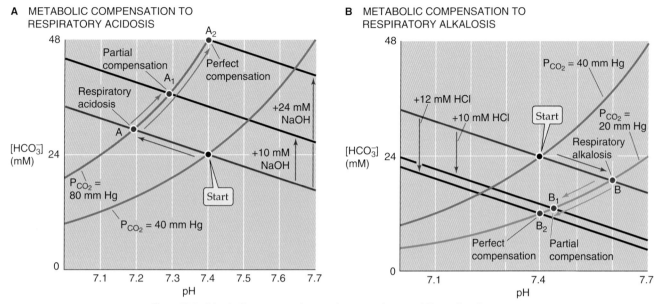

Figure 28.4 Metabolic compensation to primary respiratory acid-base disturbances.

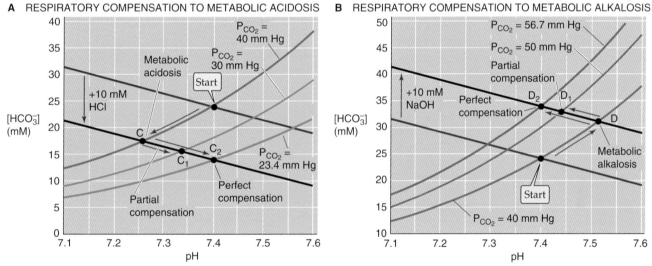

Figure 28.5 Respiratory compensation to primary metabolic acid-base disturbances.

side of Fig. 28.3, in which we produce a primary metabolic alkalosis by adding 10 mmol of NaOH to 1 L (*red arrow* in Fig. 28.5B between "Start" and *point D* at pH 7.51). If we now increase P_{CO_2} from 40 to 50 mm Hg, we partially compensate for the metabolic alkalosis by moving from D to D_1 (pH 7.44). If we raise P_{CO_2} by an additional 6.7 mm Hg to ~56.7 mm Hg, the compensation is perfect, and pH returns to 7.40 (D_2).

In response to a primary metabolic alkalosis, the respiratory system decreases alveolar ventilation and thereby raises P_{CO_2}. The compensatory respiratory acidosis is the least "perfect" of the four types of compensation we have discussed. The reason is that one can decrease alveolar ventilation—and thus oxygenation—only so far before compromising one's very existence.

In a real person, each of the four primary acid-base disturbances—points A, B, C, and D in Fig. 28.4 and

28.5—occurs in the extracellular fluid. In each case, the body's first and almost instantaneous response is to use extracellular buffers to neutralize part of the acid or alkaline load. In addition, cells rapidly take up some of the acid or alkaline load and thus participate in the buffering, as discussed below. Furthermore, renal tubule cells may respond to a *metabolic* acidosis of extrarenal origin (e.g., diabetic ketoacidosis) by increasing acid secretion into the urine, or to a metabolic alkalosis (e.g., $NaHCO_3$ therapy) by decreasing acid secretion—examples of *metabolic* compensation to a *metabolic* disturbance. *Points C and D* in Fig. 28.5 include the effects of the actual acid or alkaline load, extracellular and intracellular buffering, and any renal (i.e., "metabolic") response. Fig. 28.6A and B summarize the four primary acid-base disturbances and the partial compensation of each.

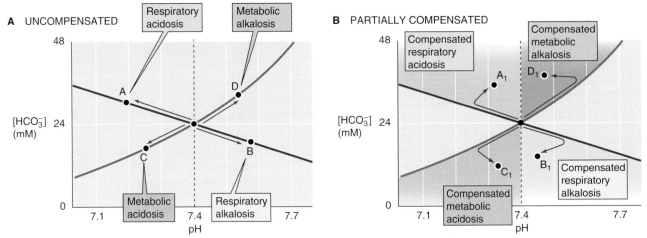

A UNCOMPENSATED

Respiratory acidosis

Metabolic alkalosis

B PARTIALLY COMPENSATED

Compensated respiratory acidosis

Compensated metabolic alkalosis

[HCO$_3^-$] (mM)

Metabolic acidosis

Respiratory alkalosis

Compensated metabolic acidosis

Compensated respiratory alkalosis

Figure 28.6 Acid-base states represented by position on a Davenport diagram.

pH REGULATION OF INTRACELLULAR FLUID

Clinicians focus on the acid-base status of blood plasma, the fluid compartment whose acid-base status is easiest to assess. However, far more biochemical reactions and other processes occur *inside* than *outside* cells. Thus, the most important biological fluid for pH regulation is the cytosol, and it is possible to monitor intracellular pH (pH$_i$) in the laboratory. The pH of cells both influences, and is influenced by, extracellular pH.

Ion transporters at the plasma membrane closely regulate the pH inside of cells

Fig. 28.7A shows a hypothetical cell with three acid-base transporters: an electroneutral Na/HCO$_3$ cotransporter (NBCn1) a Na-H exchanger (NHE1), and a Cl-HCO$_3$ or anion exchanger (AE2). NBCn1 and NHE1 are prototypic **acid extruders,** transporters that tend to *raise* intracellular pH (pH$_i$). Both use the energy of the Na$^+$ gradient to either import HCO$_3^-$ or export H$^+$ from the cytosol. The Cl-HCO$_3$ exchanger AE2 is a prototypic **acid loader,** a transporter that tends to *lower* pH$_i$. AE2, driven by the steep out-to-in Cl$^-$ gradient, moves HCO$_3^-$ out of the cell. In our example, the chronic acid extrusion via NBCn1 and NHE1 balances the chronic acid loading via AE2, producing a steady state. Several other acid extruders and acid loaders may contribute to pH$_i$ regulation, and each cell type has a characteristic complement of such transporters.

Imagine that we use a micropipette to inject HCl into the cell in Fig. 28.7A. This injection of an **acute acid load**—a one-time-only introduction of a fixed quantity of acid—causes an immediate fall in pH$_i$ (Fig. 28.7B, *black curve*), an example of **intracellular metabolic acidosis.** If we add HCl to a beaker, the pH remains low indefinitely. However, when we acutely acid-load a cell, pH$_i$ spontaneously recovers to the initial value. This pH$_i$ recovery cannot be due to passive H$^+$ efflux out of the cell, inasmuch as the electrochemical gradient for H$^+$ usually favors H$^+$ influx. Hence, the pH$_i$ recovery reflects the active transport of acid from the cell—a *metabolic compensation to a metabolic acid load*. Studies of pH$_i$ regulation show that, during an acute load, acid extruders

tend to accelerate, whereas acid loaders tend to decelerate. Hence, pH$_i$ increases until it reaches its initial value, where the rates of acid extrusion and acid loading once more come into balance.

One of the most powerful modulators of these transporters are changes in extracellular pH (pH$_o$). In general, a low pH$_o$ slows the rate of pH$_i$ recovery from acute acid loads and reduces the final steady-state pH$_i$ (Fig. 28.7B, *red curve*), whereas a high pH$_o$ does the opposite (*blue curve*).

Cells also spontaneously recover from acute alkaline loads. If we inject a cell with potassium hydroxide (KOH) (Fig. 28.7C), pH$_i$ rapidly increases but then slowly recovers to its initial value (Fig. 28.7D, *black curve*), which reflects stimulation of acid loading and inhibition of acid extrusion. pH$_i$ continues to decrease until it reaches its initial value, where the rates of acid extrusion and acid loading once more come into balance. The injection of OH$^-$ represents a metabolic alkalosis, whereas increased Cl-HCO$_3$ exchange represents a metabolic compensation.

⊙ 28-9 Changes in intracellular pH are often a sign of changes in extracellular pH, and vice versa

In the steady state, the rates of acid extrusion (e.g., Na/HCO$_3$ cotransport) and acid loading (e.g., Cl-HCO$_3$ exchange) exactly balance. Any disturbance in this balance will shift pH$_i$. For example, extracellular *metabolic* acidosis inhibits acid extrusion and stimulates acid loading, thus lowering steady-state pH$_i$. Conversely, extracellular metabolic alkalosis leads to a slow increase in steady-state pH$_i$. Generally, a change in pH$_o$ causes pH$_i$ to shift in the same direction, but by a smaller amount.

⊙ **28-10** Extracellular *respiratory* acidosis (Fig. 28.8, top two panels) generally affects pH$_i$ in three phases. First, the increase in extracellular [CO$_2$]$_{dis}$ creates an inwardly directed gradient for CO$_2$. This dissolved gas rapidly enters the cell and produces HCO$_3^-$ and H$^+$. This **intracellular respiratory acidosis** manifests itself as a rapid fall in pH$_i$ (Fig. 28.8, *phase A in lower panel*).

The cell recovers from this acid load, but only feebly (Fig. 28.8, *phase B in lower panel*) because the decrease in pH$_o$ inhibits acid extrusion and stimulates acid loading.

A RESPONSE TO INTRACELLULAR METABOLIC ACIDOSIS

B RECORD OF INTRACELLULAR pH

C RESPONSE TO INTRACELLULAR METABOLIC ALKALOSIS

D RECORD OF INTRACELLULAR pH

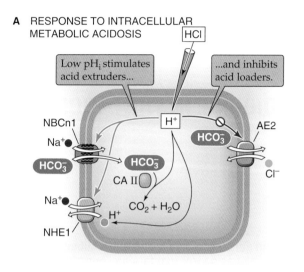

Figure 28.7 Recovery of a cell from intracellular acid and alkali loads. *CA II,* Carbonic anhydrase II.

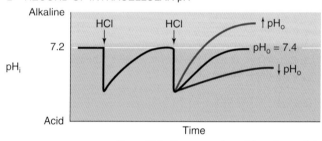

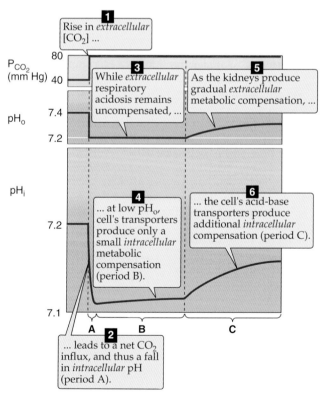

Figure 28.8 Response of cell to extracellular respiratory acidosis.

Finally, the extracellular respiratory acidosis stimulates the kidneys to upregulate acid-base transporters and thus stimulate urinary acid secretion (see ⊚ 39-4). The net effect, over a period of hours or days, is an extracellular metabolic compensation that causes pH_o to increase gradually (Fig. 28.8, *phase C in upper panel*). As pH_o rises, it gradually relieves the inhibition of NBCn1 and NHE1 and other acid extruders and relieves the stimulation of Cl-HCO_3 exchange and other acid loaders. Thus, *intra*cellular pH recovers in parallel with *extra*cellular pH, albeit by a smaller amount (Fig. 28.8, *phase C in lower panel*). The pH_i recovery represents an **intracellular metabolic compensation** to the intracellular respiratory acidosis.

Although different cell types may use different complements of acid-base transporters, the example in Fig. 28.8 illustrates that the fate of pH_i is closely intertwined with that of interstitial fluid, and thus blood plasma. During respiratory acid-base disturbances, the lungs generate the insult, and virtually every other cell in the body must defend itself against it. In the case of metabolic acid-base disturbances, however, some cells may generate the insult, whereas the others attempt to defend themselves against it. From a teleological perspective, one can imagine that the primary reason that the body regulates the pH of the blood plasma and extracellular fluids is to allow the cells to regulate their pH_i properly. The primary reason why the clinical assessment of blood acid-base parameters can be useful is that these parameters tend to parallel cellular acid-base status.

CHAPTER 29

TRANSPORT OF OXYGEN AND CARBON DIOXIDE IN THE BLOOD

Walter F. Boron

CARRIAGE OF O_2

The amount of O_2 dissolved in blood is far too small to meet the metabolic demands of the body

Blood carries oxygen in two forms. More than 98% of the O_2 normally binds to hemoglobin within the **erythrocytes,** also known as red blood cells or RBCs (see Chapter 18). A tiny fraction physically dissolves in the aqueous phases of both blood plasma and the cytoplasm of blood cells (predominantly RBCs). What is the significance of the O_2 that is bound to hemoglobin?

Imagine that we expose a liter of blood plasma, initially free of O_2, to an atmosphere having the same P_{O_2} as alveolar air—100 mm Hg. Oxygen will move from the atmosphere to the plasma until an equilibrium is established, at which time the concentration of **dissolved O_2 ($[O_2]_{dis}$)** in the blood obeys **Henry's law** (see Box 26.2):

$$[O_2]_{dis} = k_{O_2} \cdot P_{O_2} \tag{29.1}$$

If we express P_{O_2} in units of mm Hg at 37°C and $[O_2]_{dis}$ in units of (mL of O_2 gas)/(dL of blood), then the solubility k_{O_2} is ~0.003 mL O_2/(dL of blood · mm Hg). For arterial blood,

$$[O_2]_{dis} = \frac{0.003 \text{ mL } O_2}{100 \text{ mL blood} \cdot \text{mm Hg}} \cdot 100 \text{ mm Hg} \tag{29.2}$$

$$= 0.3 \text{ mL } O_2/100 \text{ mL blood}$$

Is such an O_2-carrying capacity adequate for supplying O_2 to the systemic tissues? If these tissues could extract all the O_2 dissolved in arterial blood so that no O_2 remained in venous blood, and if cardiac output were 5000 mL/min, then—according to the Fick principle (see ◉ 20-7)—the delivery of dissolved O_2 to the tissues would be

$$\underbrace{\dot{V}_{O_2}}_{\substack{O_2 \\ \text{delivery}}} = \underbrace{\frac{5000 \text{ mL blood}}{\text{min}}}_{\text{Blood flow}} \cdot \underbrace{\frac{0.3 \text{ mL } O_2}{100 \text{ mL blood}}}_{\substack{O_2 \text{ concentration} \\ \text{in plasma}}} \tag{29.3}$$

$$= 15 \text{ mL } O_2/\text{min}$$

However, the average 70-kg human at rest consumes O_2 at the rate of ~250 mL/min. Dissolved O_2 could supply the body's metabolic demands only if cardiac output increased by a factor of 250/15, or nearly 17-fold! Thus, the body cannot rely on dissolved O_2 as a mechanism for O_2 carriage.

Hemoglobin consists of two α and two β subunits, each of which has an iron-containing "heme" and a polypeptide "globin"

◉ 29-1 Normal adult **hemoglobin (Hb)** is a tetramer, each monomer consisting of a heme and a globin (Fig. 29.1A). Each heme coordinates a single iron atom. The **globin** is a polypeptide, either an α chain (141 amino acids) or a highly homologous β chain (146 amino acids). The α and β chains have similar conformations, a series of seven helices enveloping a single heme. Thus, the complete Hb molecule has the stoichiometry $[\alpha(\text{heme})]_2[\beta(\text{heme})]_2$ and can bind as many as four O_2 molecules, one for each iron atom.

Heme is a general term for a metal ion chelated to a porphyrin ring (Fig. 29.1B). For Hb, the metal is iron in the Fe^{2+} or ferrous state. The interaction among O_2, Fe^{2+}, and porphyrin causes the complex to have a red color when fully saturated with O_2 (e.g., arterial blood) and a purple color when devoid of O_2 (e.g., venous blood).

Hb can bind O_2 only when the iron is in the Fe^{2+} state. The Fe^{2+} in Hb can become oxidized to ferric iron (Fe^{3+}), either spontaneously or under the influence of compounds such as nitrites or sulfonamides. The result of such an oxidation is **methemoglobin (metHb),** which is incapable of binding O_2. Inside the RBC, heme-containing enzymes called **methemoglobin reductases** reduce metHb back to Hb, so that only about 1.5% of total Hb is usually in the metHb state. In the rare case in which a genetic defect results in a deficiency of this enzyme, metHb may represent 25% or more of the total Hb. Such a deficiency results in a decreased O_2-carrying capacity, leading to tissue hypoxia.

The globin portion of Hb provides an environment that is crucial for the O_2-heme interaction. To be useful, this interaction must be fully reversible under physiological conditions, allowing repetitive capture and release of O_2. About 20 amino acids in the globin cradle the heme so that O_2 loosely and *reversibly* binds to Fe^{2+}. A crucial histidine residue interacts with the Fe^{2+} and helps transmit to the rest of the Hb tetramer the information that an O_2 molecule is or is not bound to the Fe^{2+}. When all four hemes are devoid of O_2, each of the four histidines pulls its Fe^{2+} above the *plane of its porphyrin ring* (the blue conformation in Fig. 29.1C), distorting the porphyrin ring. The various components of the Hb tetramer are so tightly interlinked, as if by a snugly fitting system of levers and joints, that no one subunit can leave this **tensed (T) state** unless they all leave it

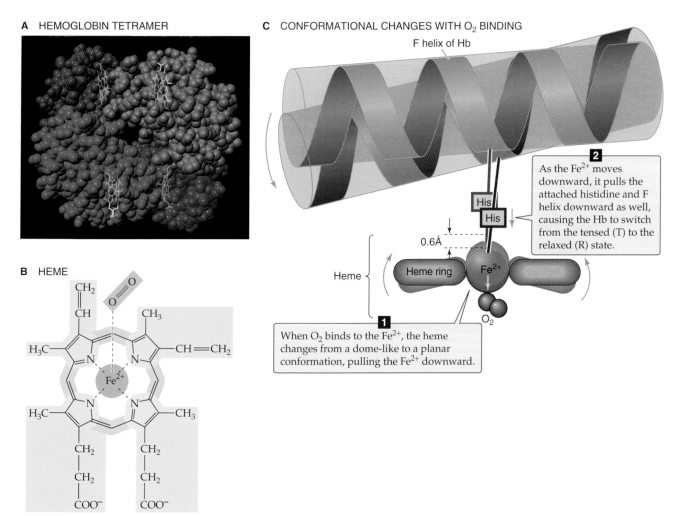

Figure 29.1 Structure of hemoglobin.

together. Because the shape of the heme in the T state sterically inhibits the approach of O_2, empty Hb has a very low affinity for O_2.

When one O_2 binds to one of the Fe^{2+} atoms, the Fe^{2+} tends to move down into the plane of the porphyrin ring. If the Fe^{2+} actually *could* move, it would flatten the ring. When enough O_2 molecules bind, enough energy builds up and all four subunits of the Hb simultaneously snap—cooperatively—into the **relaxed (R) state,** whether or not they are bound to O_2. In this R state, with its flattened heme, the Hb molecule has an O_2 affinity that is ~150-fold greater than that in the T state. Thus, when P_{O_2} is zero, all Hb molecules are in the T state and have a low O_2 affinity. When P_{O_2} is very high, all Hb molecules are in the R state and have a high O_2 affinity. At intermediate P_{O_2} values, an equilibrium exists between Hb molecules in the T and R states.

⊙ **29-2 Myoglobin (Mb)** is another heme-containing, O_2-binding protein that is specific for muscle. Mb functions as a *monomer,* homologous to either an α or a β chain of Hb. Mb has a much higher O_2 affinity than Hb. In the capillaries, Hb can thus hand off O_2 to an Mb inside a muscle cell; this Mb then transfers its O_2 to the next Mb, and so on, which speeds diffusion of O_2 through the muscle cell.

The Hb-O_2 dissociation curve has a sigmoidal shape because of cooperativity among the four subunits of the Hb molecule

Imagine that we expose whole blood (see ⊙ 18-1) to a gas phase with a P_{O_2} that we can set at any one of several values. For example, we could incubate the blood with a P_{O_2} of 40 mm Hg, typical of mixed-venous blood, and centrifuge a sample to separate plasma from erythrocytes, as one would for determining hematocrit (see ⊙ 18-1). Next, we could individually determine the O_2 content of the plasma (i.e., dissolved O_2) and packed RBCs. If we know how much water is inside the RBCs, we can subtract the amount of O_2 dissolved in this water from the total O_2, arriving at the amount of O_2 bound to Hb.

Repeating this exercise over a range of P_{O_2} values, we obtain the red curve in Fig. 29.2. The right-hand y-axis gives the O_2 bound to Hb in the units (mL O_2)/(dL blood). The left-hand y-axis gives the same data in terms of **percent O_2 saturation** of Hb (S_{O_2} or "Sat"). The percent saturation of Hb is

$$\% \text{ Saturation of Hb} = \frac{O_2 \text{ actually bound to Hb}}{O_2 \text{ capacity of Hb}} \cdot 100 \quad \textbf{(29.5)}$$

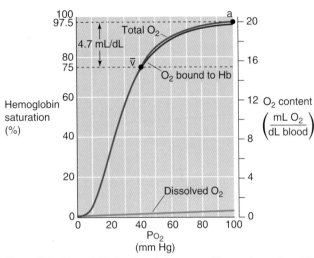

Figure 29.2 Normal Hb-O_2 dissociation curve. The y-axis on the *right* shows O_2 content. For the *red curve* (O_2 content of Hb), we assume 15 g Hb/dL of blood and an O_2 capacity of 1.35 mL O_2/g Hb. The *brown curve* is the sum of the *red* and *purple curves*. The y-axis on the left, which pertains only to the *red curve*, gives the percentage of Hb saturation or S_{O_2}.

$$\underbrace{\dot{V}_{O_2}}_{\substack{O_2 \\ \text{consumption} \\ \text{by tissues}}} = \underbrace{\frac{5000\,\text{mL blood}}{\text{min}}}_{\text{Blood flow}} \cdot \underbrace{\frac{4.7\,\text{mL } O_2}{100\,\text{mL blood}}}_{\substack{\text{a-}\bar{\text{v}} \\ \text{difference} \\ \text{for total} \\ O_2 \text{ content}}} \qquad (29.7)$$

$$= \sim\!235\,\text{mL } O_2/\text{min}$$

By either increasing cardiac output by ~6% or decreasing the P_{O_2} of mixed-venous blood, the body could meet a demand of 250 mL O_2/min. We spend our lives moving endlessly from point *a* in Fig. 29.2 to point $\bar{v}$ (as we deliver O_2 to the tissues) and then back to point *a* (as we take up more O_2 from alveolar air).

Because the plot of $[O_2]_{\text{dis}}$ versus P_{O_2} is linear (Fig. 29.2, *green curve*), the amount of O_2 that can dissolve in blood plasma has no theoretical maximum. Thus, breathing 100% O_2 would raise arterial P_{O_2} by ~6-fold, so that ~1.8 mL of O_2 would be dissolved in each deciliter of arterial blood. Even so, Hb would still carry the vast majority of O_2. Hence, a decrease in the Hb content of the blood—known as **anemia**—can markedly reduce O_2 carriage. The body can compensate for decreased Hb content in the same two ways that, in the above example, we increased the $\dot{V}_{O_2}$ from 235 to 250 mL O_2/min. First, it can increase cardiac output. Second, it can increase O_2 extraction, thereby reducing mixed-venous O_2 content. Anemia leads to pallor of the mucous membranes and skin, reflecting the decrease in the red Hb pigment. Impaired O_2 delivery may cause lethargy and fatigue. The accompanying increase in cardiac output may manifest itself as palpitations and a systolic murmur. Shortness of breath may also be a part of the syndrome.

◉ **29-4** Might increasing Hb content increase maximal O_2 content and thus provide a competitive advantage for athletes? Even in normal individuals, [Hb] in RBC cytoplasm is already extremely high (see ◉ 18-6). Hypoxia (e.g., adaptation to high altitude) leads to the increased production of erythropoietin (see ◉ 18-5), a hormone that somewhat increases the amount of Hb per erythrocyte, but especially increases their number. Indeed, a few instances have been highly publicized in the international press, in which elite athletes have infused themselves with erythrocytes or injected themselves with recombinant erythropoietin. However, an excessive increase in hematocrit—**polycythemia**—has the adverse effect of increasing blood viscosity and thus vascular resistance (see Fig. 18.6). The consequences include increased blood pressure in both the systemic and pulmonary circulations, and a mismatch of ventilation to perfusion within the lung. Such a ventilation-perfusion mismatch leads to hypoxia (see ◉ 31-9), and thus *desaturation* of arterial Hb.

The different colors of arterial and venous blood reflect difference in light absorbance between oxygenated and deoxygenated Hb. Clinicians now routinely use the **pulse oximeter**, which exploits these differences to obtain simple, noninvasive measurements of the arterial O_2 saturation (Sa_{O_2}) of Hb in patients.

The purplish color of desaturated Hb produces the physical sign known as **cyanosis**, a purplish coloration of the skin and mucous membranes. Cyanosis results not from the

Notice that the curve in Fig. 29.2 is sigmoidal or S-shaped, owing to the **cooperativity** among the four O_2-binding sites on the Hb molecule. The P_{O_2} at which the Hb is half saturated is known as the **P_{50}**. The difference in Hb saturation—and the accompanying change in color—at relatively low versus high P_{O_2} values is the basis for an important clinical tool, the pulse oximeter.

◉ **29-3** At the P_{O_2} prevailing in normal arterial blood (Pa_{O_2})—approximately 100 mm Hg—the Hb saturation (Sa_{O_2}) is ~97.5% or 19.7 mL O_2/dL bound to Hb. The dissolved O_2 (*green curve* in Fig. 29.2) would add an additional 0.3 mL O_2/dL for a **total O_2 content** of 20.0 mL O_2/dL (point *a* on the *brown curve* in Fig. 29.2). In mixed-venous blood, in which P_{O_2} ($P\bar{v}_{O_2}$) is ~40 mm Hg, the Hb saturation ($S\bar{v}_{O_2}$) is ~75% or 15.2 mL O_2/dL bound to Hb. The dissolved O_2 would add 0.1 mL O_2/dL for a total of 15.3 mL O_2/dL (point $\bar{v}$ in Fig. 29.3). The difference in total O_2 content between points *a* and $\bar{v}$, the a-$\bar{v}$ difference, is the amount of O_2 that the lungs add to the blood in the pulmonary capillaries, which is the same amount that all the tissues extract from the blood in the systemic capillaries:

$$\underbrace{\Delta C(a-\bar{v})_{O_2}}_{\substack{\text{a-}\bar{\text{v}} \\ \text{difference for total} \\ O_2 \text{ content}}} = \underbrace{\frac{20.0\,\text{mL } O_2}{\text{dL blood}}}_{\substack{O_2 \text{ content of} \\ \text{arterial} \\ \text{blood}}} - \underbrace{\frac{15.3\,\text{mL } O_2}{\text{dL blood}}}_{\substack{O_2 \text{ content of} \\ \text{mixed-venous} \\ \text{blood}}} \qquad (29.6)$$

$$= \frac{4.7\,\text{mL } O_2}{\text{dL blood}}$$

Of the total a-$\bar{v}$ difference of 4.7 mL O_2/dL, Hb provides 4.5 mL O_2/dL or nearly 96% of the O_2 that the lungs add and the systemic tissues extract from blood. Is this a-$\bar{v}$ difference in O_2 content enough to satisfy the metabolic demands of the body (i.e., ~250 mL O_2/min)? Using the Fick principle, as we did in Equation 29.3, we see that the combination of a cardiac output of 5 L/min and an a-$\bar{v}$ difference of 4.7 mL/dL would be nearly adequate:

absence of saturated or oxygenated Hb, but from the *presence* of desaturated Hb. Thus, an anemic patient with poorly saturated Hb might have too little unsaturated Hb for it to manifest as cyanosis. The clinician's ability to detect cyanosis also depends on other factors, such as the subject's skin pigmentation and the lighting conditions for the physical examination.

Increases in temperature, [CO₂], and [H⁺], all of which are characteristic of metabolically active tissues, cause Hb to dump O₂

Metabolically active tissues not only have a high demand for O_2, they also are warm, produce large amounts of CO_2, and are acidic. Indeed, high temperature, high P_{CO_2}, and low pH of metabolically active tissues all decrease the O_2 affinity of Hb by acting at nonheme sites to shift the equilibrium between the T and R states of Hb more toward the low-affinity T state. The net effect is that metabolically active tissues can signal Hb in the *systemic* capillaries to release more O_2 than usual, whereas less active tissues can signal Hb to release less. In the *pulmonary* capillaries—where temperature is lower than in active tissues, P_{CO_2} is relatively low and pH is high—these same properties promote O_2 uptake by Hb.

Temperature Increasing the temperature causes the Hb-O_2 dissociation curve to *shift to the right*, whereas decreasing the temperature has the opposite effect (Fig. 29.3). Comparing the three Hb-O_2 dissociation curves in Fig. 29.3 at the P_{O_2} of mixed-venous blood (40 mm Hg), we see that the amount of O_2 bound to Hb becomes progressively less at higher temperatures. In other words, high temperature decreases the O_2 affinity of Hb and leads to release of O_2.

Acid Respiratory acidosis (see ⊙ 28-4) shifts the Hb-O_2 dissociation curve to the right (Fig. 29.4A). This decrease in O_2 affinity is known as the **Bohr effect**. A mild respiratory acidosis occurs physiologically as erythrocytes enter the systemic capillaries. There, the increase in extracellular P_{CO_2} causes CO_2 to enter erythrocytes, which leads to a fall in intracellular pH (see ⊙ 28-10). Other acidic metabolites may also lower extracellular and, therefore, intracellular pH. Thus, this intracellular respiratory acidosis has two components—a decrease in pH and an increase in P_{CO_2}. *Both* contribute to the rightward shift of the Hb-O_2 dissociation curve.

The effect of acidosis per se on the Hb-O_2 dissociation curve (Fig. 29.4B)—the **pH-Bohr effect**—accounts for most of the overall Bohr effect. Hb is an outstanding H⁺ buffer, and thus decreases in pH lead to the protonation of Hb, which in turn reduces the affinity of Hb for O_2, and thereby shifts the dissociation curve to the right.

Carbon Dioxide ⊙ 29-5 The isolated effect of hypercapnia per se on the Hb-O_2 dissociation curve (Fig. 29.4C) represents a small portion—the **CO₂-Bohr effect**—of the overall Bohr effect. As P_{CO_2} increases, CO_2 combines with unprotonated amino groups on Hb (Hb-NH_2) to form **carbamino groups** (Hb-NH-COO⁻), predominantly at the four amino termini of the globin chains, the β chains more so than the α chains. The result is that the reaction with CO_2 reduces the affinity of Hb for O_2, and thereby shifts the dissociation curve to the right.

In conclusion, the Hb-O_2 dissociation curve shifts to the right under conditions prevailing in the capillaries of metabolically active systemic tissues—increased temperature (Fig.

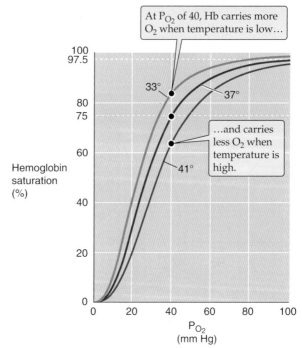

Figure 29.3 Effect of temperature changes on the Hb-O_2 dissociation curve.

29.3), decreased pH (Fig. 29.4B), and increased P_{CO_2} (Fig. 29.4C). These right shifts are synonymous with decreased O_2 affinity. Thus, high metabolic rates promote the unloading of O_2 from Hb.

⊙ 29-6 2,3-Diphosphoglycerate reduces the affinity of adult, but not of fetal, Hb

The affinity of Hb for O_2 is very sensitive to the presence of the glycolytic metabolite 2,3-diphosphoglycerate (2,3-DPG) and, to a lesser extent, organic phosphates such as ATP. The concentration of **2,3-DPG** in the cytosol is about the same as that of Hb (i.e., ~5.5 mM). Indeed, 2,3-DPG binds to Hb in a 1:1 stoichiometry, interacting with a central cavity formed by the two β chains.

The result is to reduce the affinity of Hb for O_2, and thereby shift the dissociation curve to the right (Fig. 29.5). This effect is important both in the adaptation to hypoxia and in the physiology of fetal Hb.

Decreasing the P_{O_2} of RBCs stimulates glycolysis, which leads to increased levels of 2,3-DPG. Indeed, chronic hypoxia, anemia, and acclimation to high altitude are all associated with an increase in 2,3-DPG levels and thus lower the O_2 affinity of Hb. Reducing the affinity is a two-edged sword. At the relatively high P_{O_2} in alveoli, where the Hb-O_2 dissociation curve is fairly flat, this decrease in O_2 affinity reduces O_2 *uptake*—but only slightly. At the low P_{O_2} in systemic tissues, where the Hb-O_2 dissociation curve is steep, this decrease in O_2 affinity markedly increases the O_2 *release*. The net effect is enhanced O_2 unloading to metabolizing tissues, which is more important than P_{O_2} per se.

The **fetal hemoglobin (HbF)** in fetal erythrocytes has a much higher O_2 affinity than the predominant Hb inside adult RBCs (HbA). This difference is crucial for the fetus,

A RESPIRATORY ACID-BASE DISTURBANCES

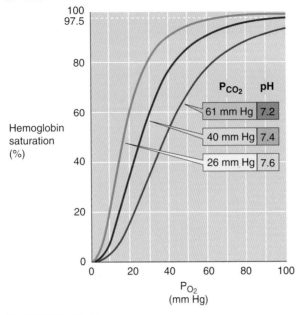

B EFFECT OF pH

C EFFECT OF CO_2

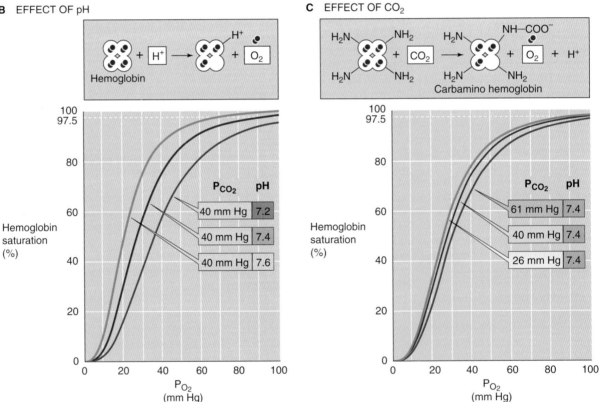

Figure 29.4 Effect of acidosis and hypercapnia on the Hb-O_2 dissociation curve (Bohr effect).

whose blood must extract O_2 from maternal blood in the placenta (see ◉ 56-1). The explanation for this difference is that two γ chains in HbF replace the two β chains of HbA, and the γ chains of HbF bind 2,3-DPG less avidly than do the β chains of HbA. With less 2,3-DPG bound, HbF has a higher O_2 affinity, and thus a *left*-shifted dissociation curve.

◉ **29-7** O_2 is not the only gas that can bind to the Fe^{2+} of Hb; carbon monoxide (CO), nitric oxide (NO), and H_2S can also bind to Hb and snap it into the R state, and

CO binds to Hb with an affinity that is ~200-fold greater than that of O_2. Thus, the maximal O_2 capacity falls to the extent that CO binds to Hb. However, the major problem in **carbon monoxide poisoning** is that, as CO snaps Hb into the R state, it greatly increases the O_2 affinity of Hb and shifts the Hb-O_2 dissociation curve far to the left. When Hb reaches the systemic capillaries in CO poisoning, its tenacity for O_2 is so high that the bright red blood cannot release sufficient O_2 to the tissues. Thus, a victim

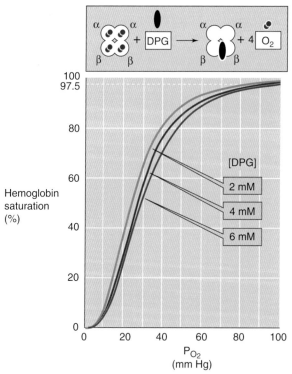

Figure 29.5 Effect of 2,3-DPG on O_2 affinity of Hb. After lowlanders spent about 2 days at an altitude of ~4500 m, their cytosolic [2,3-DPG] increased by ~50%, shifting the Hb-O_2 dissociation curve to the right.

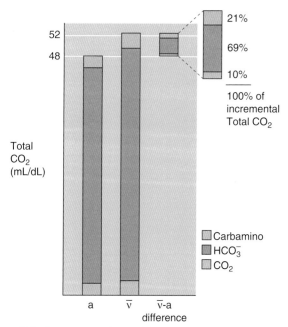

Figure 29.6 Constituents of "total CO_2 in blood." The left bar (a) represents arterial blood; the middle bar ($\bar{v}$), mixed-venous blood; and the right bar, the incremental CO_2 that the blood picks up in the systemic capillaries.

with an average of one CO and three O_2 bound to each Hb can die of asphyxia.

CARRIAGE OF CO_2

Blood carries "total CO_2" mainly as HCO_3^-

The blood carries CO_2 and in three major forms:

1. **Dissolved carbon dioxide.** $[CO_2]_{dis}$ follows Henry's law (see Box 26.2), and it is in the millimolar range in both blood plasma and blood cells. It makes up only ~5% of the total CO_2 of arterial blood (gold portion of leftmost bar in Fig. 29.6).

2. **Bicarbonate.** ⊙ 29-8 In arterial blood, HCO_3^- is ~24 mM, so that HCO_3^- represents ~90% of total CO_2 (purple portion of leftmost bar in Fig. 29.6).

3. **Carbamino compounds.** By far the most important carbamino compound is carbamino hemoglobin (Hb-NH-COO^-), which forms rapidly and reversibly as CO_2 reacts with free amino groups on Hb (see ⊙ 29-5). In arterial blood, carbamino compounds account for ~5% of total CO_2 (blue portion of leftmost bar in Fig. 29.6).

The reason we group together these three CO_2-related compounds under the term total CO_2 is that the methods used for assaying blood HCO_3^- in modern clinical laboratories does not distinguish among them.

CO_2 uptake by RBCs depends critically on channels, carbonic anhydrase, the Cl-HCO_3 exchanger, and Hb

⊙ **29-9** The total CO_2 concentration of arterial blood is ~26 mM, or ~48 mL of CO_2 gas/dL (measured at STP). HCO_3^- constitutes ~90% of this 48 mL/dL, with CO_2 and carbamino compounds contributing ~5% each (bar a in Fig. 29.6). As

blood courses through the systemic capillary beds, it picks up ~4 mL/dL of CO_2, so that the total CO_2 of mixed-venous blood is ~52 mL/dL (bar $\bar{v}$ in Fig. 29.6). In what forms does blood carry this *incremental* 4 mL/dL of CO_2 to the lungs? About 10% of the incremental CO_2 moves as dissolved CO_2, ~69% as HCO_3^-, and ~21% as carbamino compounds (rightmost two bars in Fig. 29.6). Therefore, dissolved CO_2 and carbamino CO_2 are far more important for carrying *incremental* CO_2 to the lungs than we might have surmised, given their contribution to *total* CO_2 in arterial blood.

Fig. 29.7 summarizes the events that occur as incremental CO_2 enters systemic capillaries. As fast as biological oxidations in the mitochondria produce CO_2, this gas diffuses out of cells, through the extracellular space, across the capillary endothelium, and into the blood plasma. Some of the incremental CO_2 (~11%) remains in blood plasma—either as CO_2 per se or HCO_3^-—throughout its journey to the lungs.

However, the remaining ~89% of incremental CO_2 enters the RBCs, predominantly through two "gas channels," **aquaporin 1 (AQP1)** and the **Rh complex**. In the RBC cytosol, a tiny fraction of the CO_2 can remain CO_2; most undergoes conversion to or carbamino compounds (mainly carbamino-Hb) or HCO_3^-. Favoring the formation of HCO_3^- is an extremely high activity of **carbonic anhydrases** (see ⊙ 28-2) and the export of HCO_3^- via the **Cl-HCO_3 exchanger AE1**. Favoring the formation of carbamino compounds and HCO_3^- is the powerful buffering of H^+ by Hb. Note that as O_2 dissociates from HbO_2 (for diffusion, ultimately, into the surrounding mitochondria), the Hb becomes better at forming carbamino-Hb, and Hb becomes a better buffer for H^+. Conversely, the interaction of CO_2 and H^+ with HbO_2 promotes the dissociation of O_2. These processes conspire to make RBCs extraordinarily effective at picking up CO_2 and releasing O_2 in the systemic capillaries. In the pulmonary capillaries, these same processes promote the highly efficient release of CO_2 and uptake of O_2.

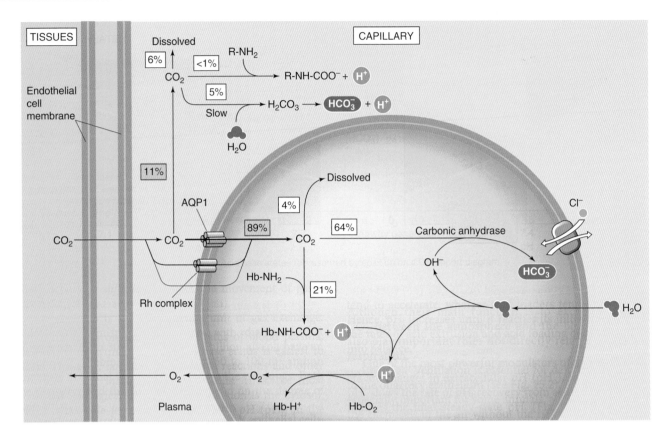

Figure 29.7 Carriage of CO_2 from systemic capillaries to the lungs.

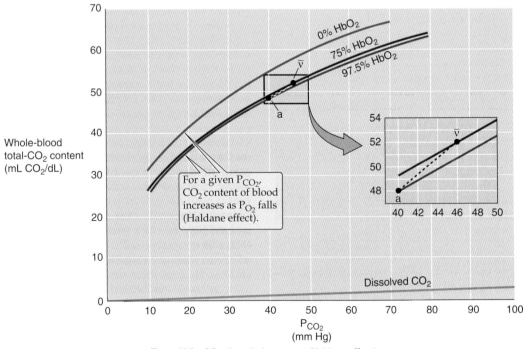

Figure 29.8 CO_2 dissociation curves (Haldane effect).

The high Po$_2$ in the lungs causes the blood to dump CO$_2$

The carriage of total CO$_2$ in the blood depends on the three blood-gas parameters—P$_{CO_2}$, plasma pH, and P$_{O_2}$. The three plots in the main portion of Fig. 29.8 are **CO$_2$ dissociation curves**—analogous to O$_2$ dissociation curves (Fig. 29.2). Each plot in Fig. 29.8 shows how changes in P$_{CO_2}$ affect the total-CO$_2$ content of blood. Although pH per se does not appear in this diagram, pH decreases as P$_{CO_2}$ increases along the x-axis (i.e., respiratory acidosis; see ⊙ 28-4). The blue plot is the CO$_2$ dissociation curve when P$_{O_2}$ is zero (S$_{O_2}$ ≅ 0% Hb). The next two plots are CO$_2$ dissociation curves for P$_{O_2}$ values of 40 mm Hg (S$_{O_2}$ ≅ 75%; purple curve) and 100 mm Hg (S$_{O_2}$ ≅ 97.5%; red curve). The green line at the bottom shows that *dissolved* CO$_2$ rises only slightly with increases in P$_{CO_2}$.

Fig. 29.8 shows that, at any **P$_{CO_2}$**, total CO$_2$ content rises as **P$_{O_2}$** (or Hb saturation) falls—the **Haldane effect.** Thus, as blood enters systemic capillaries and releases O$_2$, the CO$_2$-carrying capacity rises so that blood picks up extra CO$_2$. Conversely, as blood enters the pulmonary capillaries and binds O$_2$, the CO$_2$-carrying capacity falls so that blood dumps extra CO$_2$. The Haldane effect is the flip side of the coin from the pH-Bohr and CO$_2$-Bohr effects. First, just as H$^+$ binding lowers the O$_2$ affinity of Hb, O$_2$ binding destabilizes protonated hemoglobin (Hb-H$^+$), promoting H$^+$ release. By mass action, this H$^+$ reduces CO$_2$-carrying capacity by favoring the formation of CO$_2$ from both carbamino Hb and HCO$_3^-$ (Fig. 29.7). Second, just as carbamino formation lowers the O$_2$ affinity of Hb, O$_2$ binding destabilizes carbamino Hb (Hb-NH-COO$^-$), promoting CO$_2$ release.

In the inset to Fig. 29.8, point *a* on the red curve represents arterial blood, with a P$_{CO_2}$ of 40 mm Hg and a P$_{O_2}$ of 100 mm Hg (S$_{O_2}$ ≅ 97.5%). Point $\bar{v}$ on the purple curve represents mixed-venous blood, with a P$_{CO_2}$ of 46 mm Hg but a P$_{O_2}$ of only 40 mm Hg (S$_{O_2}$ ≅ 75%). The difference between the total CO$_2$ contents represented by the two points (i.e., 52 versus 48 mL/dL) represents the 4 mL/dL of CO$_2$ the blood takes up as it passes through systemic capillaries. If it were not for the Haldane effect, the P$_{CO_2}$ mixed-venous P$_{CO_2}$ would have to increase to ~49 mm Hg—and pH would have to correspondingly decrease—for blood to carry 4 mL/dL of CO$_2$.

CHAPTER 30

GAS EXCHANGE IN THE LUNGS

Walter F. Boron

The complex anatomy of the pulmonary tree, the mechanics of the ventilatory system, and the carriage for O_2 and CO_2 combine to serve two essential purposes: the ready diffusion of O_2 from the alveolar air to the pulmonary-capillary blood, and the movement of CO_2 in the opposite direction. In this chapter, we consider principles that govern these diffusive events and factors that, in certain diseases, can limit gas exchange.

DIFFUSION OF GASES

⊙ 30-1 Gas flow across a barrier is proportional to diffusing capacity and concentration gradient (Fick's law)

The movements of both O_2 and CO_2 across the alveolar blood-gas barrier occur by simple **diffusion** (see ⊙ 5-2). Random motion alone causes a net movement of molecules from areas of high concentration to areas of low concentration. Of course, the body must do work—in the form of ventilation and circulation—to create the concentration gradients down which O_2 and CO_2 diffuse.

Suppose that a barrier that is permeable to O_2 separates two air-filled compartments (Fig. 30.1A). The partial pressures (see Box 26.2) of O_2 on the two sides are P_1 and P_2.

The **net movement** of O_2 from side 1 to side 2 is proportional to the *difference* between the two partial pressures:

$$\text{Flow}_{net} \propto (P_1 - P_2) \tag{30.1}$$

Thus, when P_1 is 100 mm Hg (or torr) and P_2 is 95 mm Hg, the net flow is 5-fold greater than when P_1 is 100 mm Hg and P_2 is 99 mm Hg.

The term **flow** describes the number of O_2 molecules moving across the entire area of the barrier per unit time (*units:* moles/s). Respiratory physiologists usually measure the flow of a gas such as O_2 as the volume of gas moving per unit time. V refers to the volume, and $\dot{V}$ is its time derivative (volume of gas moving per unit time), or flow.

The proportionality constant in Equation 30.1 is the **diffusing capacity** for the lung, D_L (*units:* mL/[min · mm Hg]). Thus, the flow of gas becomes

$$\dot{V}_{net} = D_L \cdot (P_1 - P_2) \tag{30.2}$$

This equation is a simplified version of **Fick's law** (see ⊙ 5-3), which states that net flow is proportional to the concentration gradient, expressed here as the partial-pressure gradient.

Applying Fick's law to the diffusion of gas across the alveolar wall is a bit more complicated. Rather than a simple barrier separating two compartments filled with dry gas, a wet barrier covered with a film of water on one side will separate a volume filled with moist air from a volume of blood plasma at 37°C (Fig. 30.1B). Now we can examine how the physical characteristics of the gas and the barrier contribute to D_L.

⊙ 30-2 Two *properties of the gas*—molecular weight (MW) and solubility in water—contribute to D_L. First, **Graham's law** states that diffusion is inversely proportional to the square root of molecular weight. Second, Fick's law states that the flow of the gas across the wet barrier is proportional to the *concentration* gradient of the gas dissolved in water. According to **Henry's law** (see Box 26.2), these concentrations are proportional to the respective partial pressures, and the proportionality constant is the solubility of the gas (*s*). Therefore, poorly soluble gases (e.g., N_2, He) diffuse poorly across the alveolar wall.

Two *properties of the barrier*—area and thickness—contribute to D_L. First, the net flow of O_2 is proportional to the **area (A)** of the barrier, describing the odds that an O_2 molecule will collide with the barrier. Second, the net flow is inversely proportional to the **thickness (a)** of the barrier, including the water layer. The thicker the barrier, the more gently P_{O_2} falls through the barrier (i.e., the smaller O_2 partial pressure gradient). An analogy is the slope of the trail that a skier takes from a mountain peak to the base. Whether the skier takes a steep "expert" trail or a shallow "beginner's" trail, the end points of the journey are the same. However, the trip is much faster along the steeper trail!

Finally, a combined property of both the barrier and the gas also contributes to D_L, a proportionality constant k that describes the interaction of the gas with the barrier.

Replacing D_L in Equation 30.2 with an area, solubility, thickness, molecular weight, and the proportionality constant yields

$$\dot{V}_{net} = \underbrace{\left[k \frac{A \cdot s}{a\sqrt{MW}} \right]}_{D_L} (P_1 - P_2) \tag{30.3}$$

A DRY, HOMOGENEOUS BARRIER

B ALVEOLAR WALL

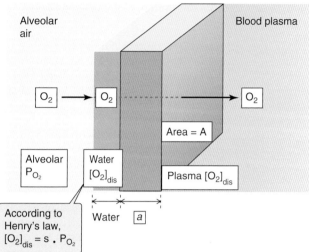

Fig. 30.1 Diffusion of a gas across a barrier.

The total flux of a gas between alveolar air and blood is the summation of multiple diffusion events along each pulmonary capillary during the respiratory cycle

If we assume that the alveolar air, the blood-gas barrier, and pulmonary-capillary blood are uniform in space and time, then we can modify Equation 30.3 to describe the net diffusion of O_2 ($\dot{V}_{O_2}$) from alveolar air to pulmonary-capillary blood:

$$\dot{V}_{O_2} = \underbrace{\left[k \frac{A \cdot s}{a \sqrt{MW}} \right]}_{DL_{O_2}} (P_{A_{O_2}} - P_{c_{O_2}}) \quad \textbf{(30.4)}$$

Here, DL_{O_2} is the diffusing capacity for O_2, $P_{A_{O_2}}$ is the O_2 partial pressure in the alveolar air, and $P_{c_{O_2}}$ is the comparable parameter in pulmonary-capillary blood. However, Equation 30.4—as sophisticated as it may seem—is not valid for understanding O_2 uptake into the lungs as a whole, during a single breath. The reason is that DL_{O_2}, $P_{A_{O_2}}$, and $P_{c_{O_2}}$ all vary in space or time. (1) DL_{O_2} increases during inspiration as the alveolar area increases and thickness decreases, and then does the opposite during expiration. (2) $P_{A_{O_2}}$ rises during the initial phase of inspiration as O_2-rich air enters the alveoli, and then falls off during the rest of the respiratory cycle as O_2 diffuses into the pulmonary capillaries. (3) $P_{c_{O_2}}$ —as we shall see below—gradually rises as the blood travels the pulmonary capillary. In addition, all three parameters vary—at rest and during the respiratory cycle—among alveolar units throughout the lungs. The complications that we have raised for O_2 diffusion apply as well to CO_2 diffusion.

Although we cannot insert a single set of fixed values for DL_{O_2}, $P_{A_{O_2}}$, and $P_{c_{O_2}}$ into Equation 30.4 and hope to describe the overall flow of O_2 between all alveoli and their pulmonary capillaries throughout the entire respiratory cycle, we can use a similar version of Fick's law to describe gas flow between air and blood for a *single piece of alveolar wall* (and its apposed capillary wall) at a *single time* during the respiratory cycle.

The *total amount* of O_2 flowing from all alveoli to all pulmonary capillaries throughout the entire respiratory cycle is simply the sum of all individual diffusion events, added up over all pieces of alveolar wall (and their apposed pieces of capillary wall) and over all times in the respiratory cycle:

$$\text{Overall } \dot{V}_{O_2} = \overset{\substack{\text{All pieces} \\ \text{of alveolar} \\ \text{wall}}}{\sum} \overset{\substack{\text{All times} \\ \text{in respiratory} \\ \text{cycle}}}{\sum} \left(DL_{O_2}(P_{A_{O_2}} - P_{c_{O_2}}) \right) \quad \textbf{(30.5)}$$

Here, DL_{O_2}, $P_{A_{O_2}}$, and $P_{c_{O_2}}$ are the "microscopic" values for one piece of alveolar wall, at one instant in time.

Even though the version of Fick's law in Equation 30.5 does indeed describe O_2 diffusion from alveolar air to pulmonary-capillary blood, it is not of much practical value for *predicting* O_2 uptake. However, we can easily compute the uptake of O_2 *that has already taken place* by use of the **Fick principle** (see ⊙ 20-7). The rate of O_2 uptake by the lungs is the difference between the rate at which O_2 leaves the lungs via the pulmonary veins and the rate at which O_2 enters the lungs via the pulmonary arteries. The rate of O_2 *departure from* the lungs is the product of blood flow (i.e., cardiac output, $\dot{Q}$) and the O_2 content of pulmonary venous blood, which is virtually the same as that of systemic arterial blood (Ca_{O_2}). Remember that "content" (see ⊙ 29-3) is the sum of dissolved O_2 and O_2 bound to hemoglobin (Hb). Similarly, the rate of O_2 *delivery to* the lungs is the product of $\dot{Q}$ and the O_2 content of pulmonary arterial blood, which is the same as that of the mixed-venous blood ($C\bar{v}_{O_2}$). Thus, the difference between the rates of O_2 departure and O_2 delivery is

$$\underbrace{\text{Overall } \dot{V}_{O_2}}_{\substack{\text{Rate of} \\ O_2 \text{ uptake} \\ \text{by lungs}}} = \underbrace{\dot{Q} \cdot Ca_{O_2}}_{\substack{\text{Rate of} \\ O_2 \text{ departure} \\ \text{from lungs}}} - \underbrace{\dot{Q} \cdot C\bar{v}_{O_2}}_{\substack{\text{Rate of} \\ O_2 \text{ delivery} \\ \text{to lungs}}} \quad \textbf{(30.6)}$$

$$= \dot{Q} \cdot (Ca_{O_2} - C\bar{v}_{O_2})$$

For a cardiac output of 5 L/min, a Ca_{O_2} of 20 mL O_2/dL blood, and a $C\bar{v}_{O_2}$ of 15 mL O_2/dL blood, the rate of O_2 uptake by the pulmonary-capillary blood is

$$\underbrace{\text{Overall } \dot{V}_{O_2}}_{\substack{\text{Rate of} \\ O_2 \text{ uptake} \\ \text{by lungs}}} = \underbrace{\frac{5000 \text{ mL of blood}}{\text{min}}}_{\text{Cardiac output}} \times \underbrace{(20-15)\frac{\text{mL } O_2}{100 \text{ mL blood}}}_{\substack{a-\bar{v} \text{ difference of} \\ O_2 \text{ content}}}$$

$$= 250 \text{ mL } O_2/\text{min} \quad \textbf{(30.7)}$$

The flow of O_2, CO, and CO_2 between alveolar air and blood depends on the interaction of these gases with red blood cells

We have been treating O_2 transport as if it involved only the diffusion of the gas across a homogeneous barrier. In fact, the barrier is a three-ply structure comprising an alveolar epithelial cell, a capillary endothelial cell, and the intervening interstitial space containing extracellular matrix. The barrier is remarkable not only for its impressive surface area (50 to 100 m^2) and thinness (~0.6 µm) but also for its strength, which derives mainly from type IV collagen in the lamina densa of the basement membrane (often <50 nm) within the extracellular matrix.

One could imagine that, as O_2 diffuses from the alveolar air to the Hb inside an erythrocyte (red blood cell, or RBC), the O_2 must cross a series of discrete mini-barriers, with a unique mini-diffusing capacity governing each step and contributing to a so-called **membrane diffusing capacity (D_M)** because it primarily describes how O_2 diffuses through various membranes.

For most of the O_2 entering the blood, the final step is binding to Hb (see ◉ **29-1**), which occurs at a finite rate:

$$\text{Rate of } O_2 \text{ uptake by hemoglobin} = (\theta \cdot V_c) P_{O_2} \quad \textbf{(30.8)}$$

θ is a rate constant that describes how many milliliters of O_2 gas bind to the Hb in 1 mL of blood each minute, and for each millimeter of mercury (mm Hg) of partial pressure. V_c is the volume of blood in the pulmonary *capillaries*. The product $\theta \cdot V_c$ has the same dimensions as D_M (*units:* mL/[min · mm Hg]), and both contribute to the overall diffusing capacity:

$$\frac{1}{D_L} = \frac{1}{D_M} + \frac{1}{\theta \cdot V_c} \quad \textbf{(30.9)}$$

Because O_2 binds to Hb so rapidly, its "Hb" term $1/(\theta \cdot V_c)$ is probably only ~5% as large as its "membrane" term $1/D_M$.

For carbon monoxide (CO), which binds to Hb even more tightly than does O_2 (see ◉ **29-7**)—but far more slowly—$\theta \cdot V_c$ is quantitatively far more important. The overall uptake of CO, which pulmonary specialists use to compute D_L (see ◉ **30-3**), depends about equally on the D_M and $\theta \cdot V_c$ terms.

In summary, although we will generally refer to "diffusing capacity" as if it represented only the diffusion across a homogeneous barrier (i.e., the D_M term), one must keep in mind its more complex nature.

DIFFUSION AND PERFUSION LIMITATIONS ON GAS TRANSPORT

The diffusing capacity normally limits the uptake of CO from alveolar air to blood

Imagine that a subject breathes air containing 0.1% CO for a brief period of time. If we assume that barometric pressure (P_B) is 760 mm Hg and that P_{H_2O} is 47 mm Hg at 37°C, then we can compute the P_{CO} of the wet inspired air entering the alveoli (see Box 26.1):

$$P_{CO} = \overbrace{F_{I_{CO}}}^{\substack{\text{Fraction of inspired} \\ \text{dry air that is CO}}} \cdot (P_B - P_{H_2O}) \quad \textbf{(30.10)}$$
$$= 0.1\% \cdot (760 - 47) \text{ mm Hg}$$
$$= \sim 0.7 \text{ mm Hg}$$

If the subject does not smoke cigarettes or live in a polluted environment, the initial P_{CO} of the mixed-venous blood entering the pulmonary capillaries will be ~0 mm Hg. Thus, a small gradient (~0.7 mm Hg) drives CO diffusion from alveolar air into blood plasma (Fig. 30.2A). As CO enters the blood plasma, it diffuses into the cytoplasm of RBCs, where it binds tightly to Hb. The flow of CO from alveolus to RBC is so slow, and the affinity and capacity of Hb to bind CO is so great, that Hb binds almost all incoming CO. Because only a small fraction of the total CO in the pulmonary-capillary blood remains free in solution, P_{CO} in the capillary (Pc_{CO})—which is proportional to *free* [CO] in the capillary—rises only slightly above 0 mm Hg as the blood courses down the capillary (Fig. 30.2B). Thus, by the time the blood reaches the end of the capillary (~0.75 second later), Pc_{CO} is still far below alveolar P_{CO} (PA_{CO}). In other words, CO fails to reach **diffusion equilibrium** between the alveolus and the blood.

What factors influence how much CO the blood takes up as it flows down the capillary? The principles that we develop here apply equally well to O_2 and CO_2. We use the Fick principle (see Equation 30.6) to quantitate, after the fact, how much CO has entered the blood:

$$\text{Overall } \dot{V}_{CO} = \dot{Q} \cdot \left(Cc'_{CO} - C\bar{v}_{CO}\right) \quad \textbf{(30.11)}$$

Overall $\dot{V}_{CO}$ is the total flow of CO along the entire length of all capillaries throughout the lungs; $\dot{Q}$ is cardiac output, Cc'_{CO} is the CO content of blood at the *end* of the pulmonary capillary (dissolved and bound to Hb), indicated by the prime; and $C\bar{v}_{CO}$ is the CO content of mixed-venous blood at the *beginning* of the capillary. If we assume that $C\bar{v}_{CO}$ is zero, then Equation 30.11 simplifies to

$$\text{Overall } \dot{V}_{CO} = \dot{Q} \cdot Cc'_{CO} \quad \textbf{(30.12)}$$

How does CO uptake depend on $D_{L_{CO}}$ and $\dot{Q}$? For basal conditions, we assume that $D_{L_{CO}}$ and $\dot{Q}$ each have relative values of 1 and that the curve in Fig. 30.2B describes the trajectory of Pc_{CO}. Cc'_{N_2O} will also have a relative value of 1. According to the Fick principle, the total amount of CO moving into the blood along the capillary is

$$\text{Overall } \dot{V}_{CO} = \dot{Q} \cdot Cc'_{CO} \quad \textbf{(30.13)}$$
$$= 1 \cdot 1$$
$$= 1$$

What would happen if we kept $\dot{Q}$ constant, but doubled $D_{L_{CO}}$? Fick's law predicts that the flow of CO into the blood for each diffusion event along the capillary would double. Thus, along the entire capillary, Pc_{CO} would rise twice as steeply as in Fig. 30.2B. As a result, Cc'_{N_2O} and thus $\dot{V}_{CO}$ would also double.

Reducing $D_{L_{CO}}$ by half would have the opposite effect: Cc'_{N_2O} and thus $\dot{V}_{CO}$ would also halve. Therefore, CO uptake is proportional to $D_{L_{CO}}$ over a wide range of $D_{L_{CO}}$

A CO DIFFUSION

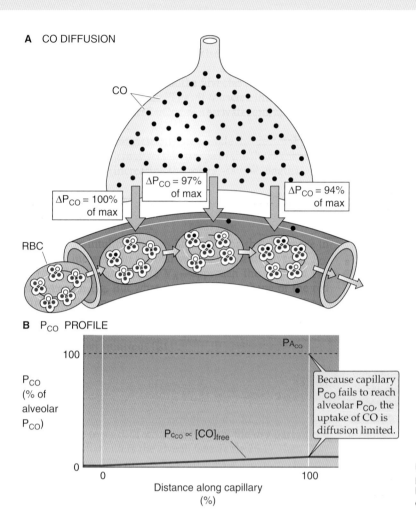

B P_{CO} PROFILE

Because capillary P_{CO} fails to reach alveolar P_{CO}, the uptake of CO is diffusion limited.

$P_{Cco} \propto [CO]_{free}$

P_{CO} (% of alveolar P_{CO})

Distance along capillary (%)

Fig. 30.2 Diffusion of CO. In (A) ΔP_{CO} is the CO partial-pressure gradient from alveolar air to pulmonary-capillary blood. As the RBC enters the capillary, O_2 occupies three of the four sites on Hb. In (B) $P_{A_{CO}}$ is alveolar P_{CO}.

TABLE 30.1 Alveolar Transport of CO

	$D_{L_{CO}}$	$\dot{Q}$	×	Cc'_{CO}	=	$\dot{V}_{CO}$
Vary D_L ($\dot{Q}$ constant)	2	1		2		2
	1	1		1		1
	½	1		½		½
Vary $\dot{Q}$ (D_L constant)	1	½		2		1
	1	1		1		1
	1	2		½		1

The values in the table are all relative to "control" values of unity.
Cc'_{CO}, CO content of the blood at the end of the capillary; D_L, diffusing capacity; DL_{CO}, diffusing capacity of the lungs for CO; $\dot{Q}$, cardiac output; $\dot{V}_{CO}$, overall rate of CO uptake by the pulmonary-capillary blood.

values (Table 30.1, *upper half*). Of course, if it were possible to make DL_{CO} extremely high, then capillary P_{CO} would rise so fast that CO would equilibrate with the Hb before the end of the capillary, and capillary P_{CO} would reach alveolar P_{CO}. However, for realistic values of DL_{CO}—as well as low alveolar P_{CO} levels and normal Hb concentrations—CO would fail to reach equilibrium by the end of the capillary.

How would alteration of blood flow affect $\dot{V}_{CO}$? If $\dot{Q}$ were halved and the dimensions of the capillary remained constant, then the contact time of the blood with the alveolar capillary would double. Thus, at any distance down the capillary, twice as much cumulative time would be available for CO diffusion. The trajectory of capillary P_{CO} versus distance would be twice as steep as in Fig. 30.2B, and Cc'_{N_2O} would also be twice as great. However, because we achieved this increase in Cc'_{N_2O} by cutting $\dot{Q}$ in half, the product $\dot{Q} \cdot Cc'_{N_2O} = \dot{V}_{CO}$ would be the same as that in the basal state (Table 30.1, *lower half*).

Doubling $\dot{Q}$ would cause capillary P_{CO} to rise only half as steeply as in Fig. 30.2B, but still would have no effect on $\dot{V}_{CO}$. Thus, for the range of D_L and $\dot{Q}$ values in this example, *CO uptake is unaffected by changes in blood flow.*

The uptake of CO is more or less proportional to the D_L for CO, and rather insensitive to perfusion. Therefore, we say that the uptake of CO is **diffusion limited** because it is the diffusing capacity that predominantly limits CO transport. We can judge whether the transport of a gas is predominantly diffusion limited by comparing the partial pressure of the gas at the end of the pulmonary capillary with the alveolar partial pressure. *If the gas does not reach diffusion equilibrium (i.e., if the end-capillary partial pressure fails to reach the alveolar partial pressure), then transport is predominantly diffusion limited.* However, if the gas does reach diffusion

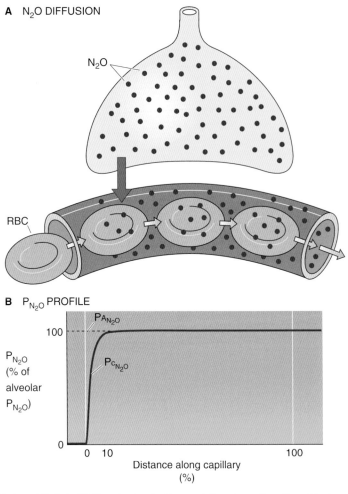

A   N₂O DIFFUSION

N₂O

RBC

B   P$_{N_2O}$ PROFILE

P$_{A_{N_2O}}$

100

P$_{N_2O}$
(% of
alveolar
P$_{N_2O}$)

Pc$_{N_2O}$

0

0   10   100

Distance along capillary
(%)

Fig. 30.3   Diffusion of N₂O. In (B) P$_{A_{N_2O}}$ is alveolar P$_{N_2O}$ and Pc$_{N_2O}$ is capillary P$_{N_2O}$. The key difference between the handling of N₂O and CO is that Hb does not buffer N₂O.

equilibrium, then its transport is perfusion limited, as discussed next.

Perfusion normally limits the uptake of N₂O from alveolar air to blood

Unlike CO, nitrous oxide ("laughing gas," N₂O) does not bind to Hb. Therefore, when a subject inhales N₂O, the gas distributes into the blood plasma and the RBC cytoplasm, but Hb does not buffer the N₂O (Fig. 30.3A). Consequently, as blood courses down the pulmonary capillary, the free [N₂O]—and thus capillary P$_{N_2O}$ (Pc$_{N_2O}$)—rises very rapidly (Fig. 30.3B). By the time the blood is ~10% of the way along the capillary, Pc$_{N_2O}$ has reached alveolar P$_{N_2O}$ (P$_{A_{N_2O}}$), and N₂O is thus in diffusion equilibrium between alveolus and blood. In other words, no net transfer of N₂O from alveoli to blood occurs in the distal 90% of the capillary! The reason N₂O reaches diffusion equilibrium—whereas CO does not—is not that D$_{L_{N_2O}}$ is particularly high, or that we chose a high inspired P$_{N_2O}$. The key difference is that, because N₂O does not bind to Hb, relatively little N₂O need enter the blood before Pc$_{N_2O}$ rises to match P$_{A_{N_2O}}$.

How does N₂O uptake by the lungs depend on D$_{L_{N_2O}}$ and $\dot{Q}$? If the N₂O content of the mixed-venous blood entering the pulmonary capillary (C$\bar{v}_{N_2O}$) is zero, then

$$\text{Overall } \dot{V}_{N_2O} = \dot{Q} \cdot Cc'_{N_2O} \qquad \textbf{(30.14)}$$

Cc'$_{N_2O}$ is the N₂O content of the blood at the end of the pulmonary capillary and consists represents entirely of N₂O physically dissolved in blood.

We can approach the uptake of N₂O in the same way we did the uptake of CO. We begin, under basal conditions, with relative values of 1 for D$_{L_{N_2O}}$, $\dot{Q}$, and end-capillary N₂O content (Cc'$_{N_2O}$). Thus, the initial $\dot{V}_{N_2O}$ is $\dot{Q} \cdot$ Cc'$_{N_2O}$ = 1.

Doubling D$_{L_{N_2O}}$ doubles the flow of N₂O into the blood for each diffusion event, causing Pc$_{N_2O}$ to rise twice as steeply as in Fig. 30.3B. However, even though N₂O comes into diffusion equilibrium twice as fast as before, Cc'$_{N_2O}$ and $\dot{V}_{N_2O}$ remain unaffected. Cutting D$_{L_{N_2O}}$ in half also would have no effect on $\dot{V}_{N_2O}$. Thus, N₂O uptake is insensitive to these changes in D$_{L_{N_2O}}$ (Table 30.2, *upper half*). In other words, the *uptake* of N₂O is *not diffusion* limited.

What would be the effect of reducing $\dot{Q}$ by half while holding D$_{L_{N_2O}}$ constant? If capillary dimensions remain constant, the halving of $\dot{Q}$ would double the contact time of blood with the alveolus and make the Pc$_{N_2O}$ trajectory along the capillary twice as steep as in Fig. 30.3B. Thus, Cc'_{N_2O} remains unchanged at 1. However, because we reduced $\dot{Q}$ by half, $\dot{V}_{N_2O}$ also falls by half. Conversely, doubling $\dot{Q}$ causes $\dot{V}_{N_2O}$ to double. Thus, N_2O uptake is more or less proportional to blood flow (i.e., perfusion) over a wide range of $\dot{Q}$ values (Table 30.2, *lower half*). For this reason, we say that N_2O transport is predominantly **perfusion limited.** *The transport of a gas is predominantly perfusion limited if the gas in the capillary comes into equilibrium with the gas in the alveolar air by the end of the capillary.*

The uptake of CO provides an estimate of D_L

As one would intuit from Equation 30.4, **pulmonary diffusing capacity** may decrease in diseases that cause the thickness of the blood-gas barrier to increase (e.g., interstitial pulmonary fibrosis), or the surface area for gas exchange to decrease (e.g., emphysema). Thus, being able to measure D_L would be valuable, both as a diagnostic tool and as a means to follow the progression of such diseases.

TABLE 30.2 Alveolar Transport of N_2O

	$D_{L_{N_2O}}$	$\dot{Q}$	×	Cc'_{N_2O}	=	$\dot{V}_{N_2O}$
Vary D_L ($\dot{Q}$ constant)	2	1		1		1
	1	1		1		1
	½	1		1		1
Vary $\dot{Q}$ (D_L constant)	1	½		1		½
	1	1		1		1
	1	2		1		2

Which gas could we use to estimate D_L? We certainly do *not* want to use N_2O, whose uptake is *perfusion* limited. After all, $\dot{V}_{N_2O}$ is more or less proportional to changes in $\dot{Q}$, but virtually insensitive to changes in D_L (Table 30.2). However, CO is an excellent choice because its uptake is *diffusion* limited, so that changes in the parameter of interest (i.e., D_L) have nearly a proportionate effect on $\dot{V}_{CO}$ (Table 30.1). As we have seen in Equation 30.5, Fick's law applies to individual diffusion events in different pieces of alveolar blood-gas barrier, and at different times in the respiratory cycle. Here, we will use a version of Fick's law that applies to the overall $\dot{V}_{CO}$, as well as the *average* values for $D_{L_{CO}}$, alveolar P_{CO}, and pulmonary-capillary P_{CO} that reflect properties of all alveoli throughout both lungs at all times in the respiratory cycle:

$$\text{Overall } \dot{V}_{CO} = D_{L_{CO}} \cdot (\overline{P}_{A_{CO}} - \overline{P}_{c_{CO}}) \tag{30.15}$$

Solving for $D_{L_{CO}}$:

$$D_{L_{CO}} = \frac{\dot{V}_{CO}}{(\overline{P}_{A_{CO}} - \overline{P}_{c_{CO}})} \tag{30.16}$$

◉ **30-3** The most commonly used approach for measuring D_L is the **single-breath technique** (Fig. 30.4). The subject makes a maximal expiratory effort to residual volume (see ◉ 26-4) and then makes a maximal inspiration of air containing CO and a tracer gas like helium, and holds the breath for 10 seconds. We use the helium—which has a low water solubility and thus a negligible transport across the blood-gas barrier—to compute the extent to which the CO/He mixture is diluted in the alveoli. As the subject exhales, we obtain a sample of alveolar air and analyze for $P_{A_{CO}}$ and $P_{A_{He}}$. This approach provides enough information to

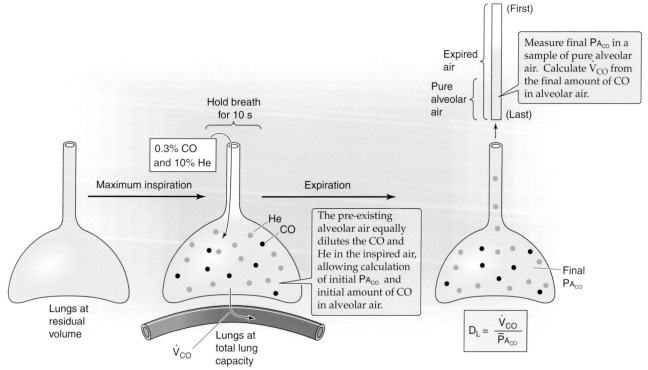

Expired air

Pure alveolar air

(First)

Measure final $P_{A_{CO}}$ in a sample of pure alveolar air. Calculate $\dot{V}_{CO}$ from the final amount of CO in alveolar air.

(Last)

Hold breath for 10 s

0.3% CO and 10% He

Maximum inspiration

Expiration

He CO

The pre-existing alveolar air equally dilutes the CO and He in the inspired air, allowing calculation of initial $P_{A_{CO}}$ and initial amount of CO in alveolar air.

Lungs at residual volume

$\dot{V}_{CO}$

Lungs at total lung capacity

Final $P_{A_{CO}}$

$$D_L = \frac{\dot{V}_{CO}}{\overline{P}_{A_{CO}}}$$

Fig. 30.4 Single-breath method for estimating $D_{L_{CO}}$.

calculate PA_{CO} and $\dot{V}_{CO}$, and thus to compute DL_{CO} during the 10-second breath-holding period.

A normal value for DL_{CO} is ~25 mL CO taken up per minute for each millimeter of mercury of partial pressure driving CO diffusion and for each milliliter of blood having a normal Hb content. The value of DL_{CO} determined in the pulmonary function laboratory depends about equally on D_M (i.e., the "membrane" component of D_L) in Equation 30.9 and $\theta \cdot V_c$.

Because V_c is proportional to the Hb content of the blood, a patient with **anemia**—a condition with decreased Hb content—can have a reduced DL_{CO} even though the diffusion pathways in the lung (i.e., D_M) are perfectly normal.

⊙ 30-4 For both O_2 and CO_2, transport is normally perfusion limited

Uptake of O_2 Blood enters the pulmonary capillaries (Fig. 30.5A) with the P_{O_2} of mixed-venous blood, typically 40 mm Hg. Capillary P_{O_2} reaches the alveolar P_{O_2} of ~100 mm Hg about one third of the way along the capillary (Fig. 30.5B, *black curve*). This P_{O_2} profile along the pulmonary capillary is intermediate between that of CO in Fig. 30.2B (where CO fails to reach diffusion equilibrium) and N_2O in Fig. 30.3B (where N_2O reaches diffusion equilibrium ~10% of the way along the capillary). The transport of O_2 is similar to that of CO in that both molecules bind to Hb. Why, then, does O_2 reach **diffusion equilibrium,** whereas CO does not?

The uptake of O_2 differs from that of CO in three important respects. First, the Hb that enters the pulmonary capillary is already heavily preloaded with O_2, with a ~75% saturation (see ⊙ 29-3)—versus ~0% for CO. Thus, the available O_2-binding capacity of Hb is relatively low. Second, the alveolar P_{O_2} is extremely high, compared to PA_{CO} (i.e., ~100 mm Hg versus <1 mm Hg), so that the initial rate of O_2 diffusion from the alveolus into pulmonary-capillary blood is immense. Third, D_L for O_2 is higher than that for CO, owing to a greater $\theta \cdot V_c$. As a result of these three factors, Hb in pulmonary-capillary blood rapidly approaches its equilibrium carrying capacity for O_2 along the first third of the capillary. Because capillary P_{O_2} reaches alveolar P_{O_2}, O_2 transport is **perfusion limited,** as is the case for N_2O.

Because O_2 normally reaches diffusion equilibrium so soon along the capillary, the lung has a tremendous **D_L reserve** for O_2 uptake. This reserve is extremely important during **exercise,** when cardiac output can increase substantially, thereby decreasing the contact time of the blood with the pulmonary capillaries. Nevertheless, even with vigorous exercise, P_{O_2} reaches virtual equilibrium with the alveolar air by the end of the capillary (Fig. 30.5C, *green curve*)—except in some elite athletes. Thus, because the uptake of O_2 usually remains perfusion limited, the increase in $\dot{Q}$ during exercise leads to a corresponding increase in $\dot{V}_{O_2}$, which carries obvious survival benefits.

Like exercise, **high altitude** stretches out the P_{O_2} profile along the capillary (Fig. 30.5D, *red curve*). The reasons are two, both of which stem from the low barometric pressure at altitude, which leads to a proportional decrease in ambient P_{O_2} (see ⊙ 61-1) and thus to a fall in alveolar P_{O_2}. First, the low PA_{O_2} causes the alveolar-capillary P_{O_2} gradient at the beginning of the capillary to fall, reducing the absolute

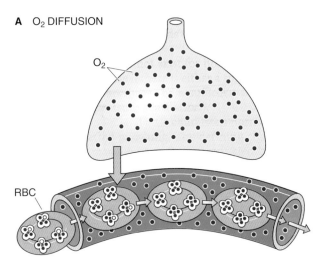

A O_2 DIFFUSION

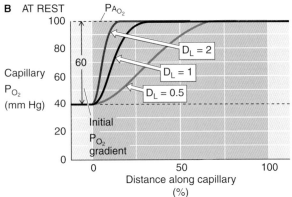

B AT REST

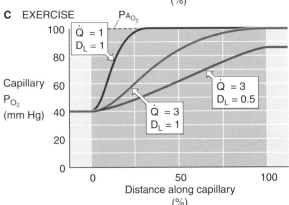

C EXERCISE

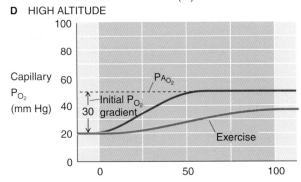

D HIGH ALTITUDE

Fig. 30.5 Diffusion of O_2. In (A), as the RBC enters the capillary, O_2 occupies three of the four sites on Hb. In (B) through (D), PA_{O_2} is alveolar P_{O_2}. In (B) and (D), $\dot{Q}$ is constant.

A CO₂ DIFFUSION

B P_CO₂ PROFILE

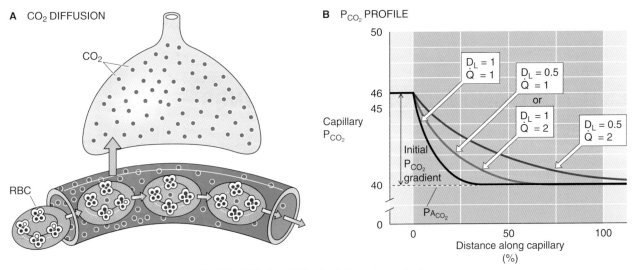

Fig. 30.6 Diffusion of CO_2. In (B), P_{ACO_2} is alveolar P_{CO_2}.

O_2 transport rate. Second, because at altitude $P\bar{v}_{O_2}$ is lower, we now operate on a steeper part of the Hb-O_2 dissociation curve (see Fig. 29.2). Thus, a given increment in the O_2 content of the pulmonary-capillary blood occurs with a smaller increase in P_{O_2}.

The combination of exercise and high altitude can cause O_2 transport to become diffusion limited even in healthy individuals (Fig. 30.5D, *green curve*). If the subject also has a pathological condition that lowers $D_{L_{O_2}}$, then transport may become diffusion limited even more readily at altitude. Obviously, any combination of exercise, high altitude, and reduced $D_{L_{O_2}}$ compounds the problems for O_2 transport.

Escape of CO₂ Mixed-venous blood entering the pulmonary capillary has a P_{CO_2} of ~46 mm Hg, whereas the alveolar P_{CO_2} is ~40 mm Hg (Fig. 30.6A). Thus, CO_2 diffuses in the opposite direction of O_2—from blood to alveolus—and P_{CO_2} falls along the pulmonary capillary (Fig. 30.6B, *black curve*), eventually reaching **diffusion equilibrium.** Thus, *CO_2 excretion is perfusion limited.* The decrease in D_L that occurs in certain lung diseases (see next section) or heavy exercise (Fig. 30.6B, *red* and *blue curves*) may cause the transport of CO_2 to become diffusion limited.

Pathological changes that reduce D_L do not necessarily produce hypoxia

The measured pulmonary diffusing capacity for CO falls in disease states accompanied by a thickening of the alveolar blood-gas barrier, a reduction in the surface area (i.e., capillaries) available for diffusion, or a decrease in the amount of Hb in the pulmonary capillaries. Examples of pathological processes accompanied by a decrease in D_L include the following:

Diffuse interstitial pulmonary fibrosis, a fibrotic process causing a thickening of the interstitium, thickening of alveolar walls, and destruction of capillaries.

Chronic obstructive pulmonary disease (COPD; see ⊙ **27-7)** can lead to a destruction of pulmonary capillaries and thus a reduction in both (1) surface area available for diffusion, and (2) total pulmonary-capillary Hb content.

Loss of functional lung tissue, as caused by surgical removal of lung tissue. D_L falls because of a decrease in both (1) surface area, and (2) total pulmonary-capillary Hb content.

Anemia, in which the fall in total Hb content decreases the $\theta \cdot V_c$ component of $D_{L_{CO}}$.

Although pulmonary diseases can cause both a decrease in D_L and hypoxemia (i.e., a decrease in arterial P_{O_2}), it is not necessarily true that the decrease in D_L is the sole or even the major cause of the hypoxemia. The same diseases that lower D_L also upset the distribution of ventilation and perfusion throughout the lung. As discussed in Chapter 31, mismatching of ventilation to perfusion among various regions of the lungs can be a powerful influence leading to hypoxemia. Furthermore, because the lung has a sizeable D_L reserve for O_2 (and perhaps for CO_2 as well), D_L would have to decrease to about one third of its normal value for O_2 transport to become diffusion limited.

CHAPTER 31

VENTILATION AND PERFUSION OF THE LUNGS

Walter F. Boron

Although diffusion is at the very heart of gas exchange (see Chapter 30), two other parameters are vital. Ventilation and perfusion—convective processes that require energy—establish the gradients along which O_2 and CO_2 diffuse. **Ventilation** is the convective movement of air that exchanges gases between the atmosphere and the alveoli. In the first part of the present chapter, we consider the importance of ventilation for determining alveolar P_{O_2} and P_{CO_2}, and also see that ventilation varies from one group of alveoli to the next. **Perfusion** is the convective movement of blood that carries the dissolved gases to and from the lung. In the second part, we examine the special properties of the pulmonary circulation and see that, like ventilation, perfusion varies in different regions of the lung. Finally, in the third part, we see that the matching of ventilation to perfusion and vice versa—and the distribution of ventilation-perfusion ratios among alveolar units—is critical for gas exchange and thus for the composition of the arterial blood gases: P_{O_2}, P_{CO_2}, and pH.

VENTILATION

About 30% of total ventilation in a respiratory cycle is wasted ventilating anatomical dead space (i.e., conducting airways)

Total ventilation ($\dot{V}_T$) is the volume of air moved out of the lungs per unit of time:

$$\dot{V}_T = \frac{V}{t} \tag{31.1}$$

Here V is the volume of air exiting the lungs during a *series of breaths*. Note that we are using $\dot{V}$ differently than in Chapter 27, where $\dot{V}$ represented flow through an airway at a particular *instant* in time. A practical definition is that $\dot{V}_T$ is the product of tidal volume (TV or V_T) and the respiratory frequency (f). Thus, for someone with a tidal volume of 0.5 L, breathing 12 breaths/min,

$$\dot{V}_T = V_T \cdot f$$
$$= (0.5\,L) \cdot (12/min) \tag{31.2}$$
$$= 6\,L/min$$

Because total ventilation usually is reported in L/min, it is sometimes called **minute ventilation.**

Before an inspiration, the conducting airways are filled with "stale" air having the same composition as alveolar air (Fig. 31.1, *step 1*); we will see why shortly. During inspiration, ~500 mL of "fresh" atmospheric air (high P_{O_2}/low P_{CO_2}) enters the body (*step 2*). However, only the first 350 mL reaches the alveoli; the final 150 mL remains in the conducting airways (i.e., nose, pharynx, larynx, trachea, and other airways without alveoli)—the **anatomical dead space V_D.** These figures are typical for a 70-kg person; V_T and V_D are roughly proportional to body size. During inspiration, ~500 mL of air also enters the alveoli. However, the first 150 mL is stale air previously in the conducting airways; only the final 350 mL is fresh air. By the end of inspiration, the 500 mL of air that entered the alveoli (150 mL of stale air plus 350 mL of fresh air) has mixed by diffusion with the pre-existing alveolar air (Fig. 31.1, *step 3*). During expiration (*step 4*), the first 150 mL of air emerging from the body is the fresh air left in the conducting airways from the previous inspiration. As the expiration continues, 350 mL of stale alveolar air sequentially moves into the conducting airways and then exits the body—for a total of 500 mL of air leaving the body. Simultaneously, 500 mL of air leaves the alveoli. The first 350 mL is the same 350 mL that exited the body. The final 150 mL of stale air to exit the alveoli remains in the conducting airways, as we are ready to begin the next inspiration.

Thus, with each 500-mL inspiration, only the *initial* 350 mL of fresh air entering the body reaches the alveoli. With each 500-mL expiration, only the *final* 350 mL of air exiting the body comes from the alveoli. One 150-mL bolus of *fresh air* shuttles back and forth between the atmosphere and conducting airways. Another 150-mL bolus of *stale air* shuttles back and forth between the conducting airways and alveoli. **Dead-space ventilation** ($\dot{V}_D$) is the volume of the stale air so shuttled per minute. **Alveolar ventilation** ($\dot{V}_A$) is the volume of fresh air per minute that actually reaches the alveoli, or the volume of stale alveolar air that reaches the atmosphere. Thus, total ventilation—a reflection of the work invested in breathing—is the sum of the wasted dead-space ventilation and the useful alveolar ventilation. In our example,

			liters / breath	breaths / minute	liters / minute	
$\dot{V}_D =$	$V_D \cdot f$	$= 0.150$	$\cdot$	12	$= 1.8$	(31.3)
$\dot{V}_A = (V_T - V_D) \cdot f$	$= 0.350$	$\cdot$	12	$= 4.2$	
$\dot{V}_T =$	$V_T \cdot f$	$= 0.500$	$\cdot$	12	$= 6.0$	

so that the dead-space ventilation is 30% of the total ventilation.

The dead space that we have been discussing is, more precisely, the **anatomical dead space**—the volume of the conducting airways. It specifically omits the volume of the alveolar airways. We can also define the **physiological dead space**—the volume of the ventilatory system that does *not* engage in gas exchange with the pulmonary capillary blood. In a healthy person, the anatomical and physiological dead

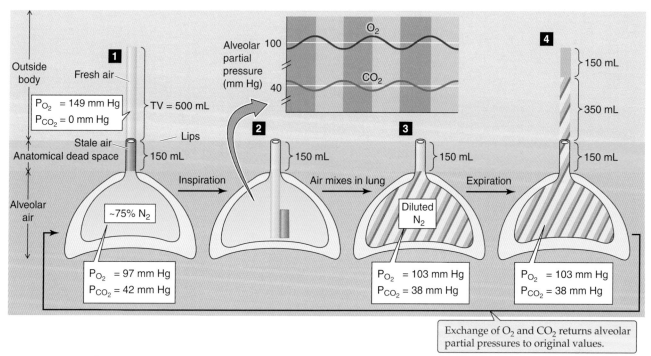

Fig. 31.1 Ventilation of dead space and alveolar space during a respiratory cycle. *Inset* shows how the alveolar P_{O_2} and P_{O_2} oscillate with each breath, as inspiration delivers fresh air (high P_{O_2}, low P_{CO_2}) to the alveoli, and then pulmonary capillary blood flow pulls away O_2 but delivers CO_2.

spaces are virtually identical—the volume of the conducting airways. However, if some alveoli are ventilated but not perfused by pulmonary-capillary blood, these unperfused alveoli, like conducting airways, do not engage in gas exchange. The air in such unperfused alveoli, known as **alveolar dead space,** contributes to the physiological dead space:

$$\frac{\text{Physiological}}{\text{dead space}} = \frac{\text{Anatomical}}{\text{dead space}} + \frac{\text{Alveolar}}{\text{dead space}} \quad \textbf{(31.4)}$$

The anatomical and physiological dead spaces could be very different in a patient with a **pulmonary embolism,** a condition in which a mass such as a blood clot wedges into and obstructs part or all of the pulmonary circulation. Alveoli downstream from the embolus are ventilated but not perfused; that is, they are alveolar dead space. Thus, although the anatomical dead space might be normal, the physiological dead space would be increased.

In a pulmonary function laboratory, we would measure physiological dead space as the volume that does not contain CO_2. Recall that appreciable levels of CO_2 can come only from the blood perfusing the alveoli.

Alveolar ventilation is the ratio of CO_2 production rate to CO_2 mole fraction in alveolar air

In addition to the approach in Equation 31.3, we can calculate $\dot{V}_A$ from alveolar P_{CO_2}. The body produces CO_2 via oxidative metabolism at a rate of ~200 mL/min. *In the*

steady state, this rate of CO_2 production $(\dot{V}_{CO_2})$ must equal the rate at which the CO_2 enters the alveoli, and the rate at which we exhale the CO_2. Of course, this 200 mL/min of exhaled CO_2 is part of the ~4200 mL of total alveolar air that we exhale each minute. Therefore, the exhaled 200 mL of CO_2 is ~5% of the exhaled 4200 mL of alveolar air:

$$\frac{\begin{array}{c}\text{Volume of } CO_2 \\ \text{leaving alveoli} \\ \text{in 1 min} \end{array}}{\begin{array}{c}\text{Volume of air} \\ \text{leaving alveoli} \\ \text{in 1 min} \end{array}} = \begin{pmatrix}\text{Volume} \\ \text{fraction} \\ \text{of } CO_2 \text{ in} \\ \text{alveolar air}\end{pmatrix} = (CO_2 \text{ mole fraction})_A$$

$$\frac{\dot{V}_{CO_2}}{\dot{V}_A} = \frac{200 \text{ mL}}{4200 \text{ mL}} = 5\% \quad \textbf{(31.5)}$$

Rearranging the foregoing equation and solving for $\dot{V}_A$ yields

$$\dot{V}_A = \underbrace{\frac{\dot{V}_{CO_2}}{(CO_2 \text{ mole fraction})_A}} = k\frac{\dot{V}_{CO_2}}{P_{A_{CO_2}}} \quad \textbf{(31.6)}$$

By historical accident, we measure the two volume terms under different conditions:
1. Body temperature and pressure, saturated with water vapor (BTPS) for $\dot{V}_A$.
2. Standard temperature and pressure/dry (STPD) for $\dot{V}_{CO_2}$. The factor 0.863 accounts for these differences:

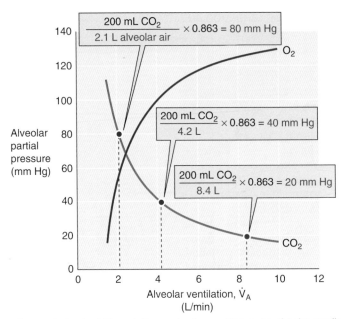

Fig. 31.2 Dependence of alveolar CO_2 and O_2 on alveolar ventilation. As alveolar ventilation increases, alveolar P_{O_2} and P_{O_2} approach their values in inspired air.

$$\dot{V}_A = 0.863 \cdot \frac{\overset{(mL/min, STPD)}{\dot{V}_{CO_2}}}{\underset{(mm\,Hg \cdot L/mL)}{P_{A_{CO_2}}}}$$

$$(L/min, BTPS) \quad (mm\,Hg \cdot L/mL) \quad (mm\,Hg\ at\ 37°C) \quad \textbf{(31.7)}$$

This is the **alveolar ventilation equation**. We determine $\dot{V}_{CO_2}$ by collecting a known volume of expired air over a fixed time period and analyzing its CO_2 content. For a 70-kg human, $\dot{V}_{CO_2}$ is ~200 mL/min. We can determine P_{CO_2} by sampling the expired air at the end of an expiration—an alveolar gas sample (Fig. 31.1, *step 4*). This **end-tidal** $P_{A_{CO_2}}$ is ~40 mm Hg. In practice, clinicians generally measure *arterial* P_{CO_2} ($P_{A_{CO_2}}$), and assume that alveolar and arterial P_{CO_2} are identical because CO_2 is perfusion limited (see Fig. 30.6). Inserting these values into the alveolar ventilation equation, we have

$$\dot{V}_A = 0.863 \cdot \frac{\dot{V}_{CO_2}}{P_{A_{CO_2}}} = 0.863 \cdot \frac{200\ mL/min}{40\ mm\,Hg} = 4.315\ L/min$$

$$\textbf{(31.8)}$$

For the sake of simplicity—and consistency with our example in Equation 31.3—we round this figure to 4.2 L/min.

Alveolar and arterial P_{CO_2} are inversely proportional to alveolar ventilation

Viewing Equation 31.7 from a different perspective illustrates one of the most important concepts in respiratory physiology: Other things being equal, alveolar P_{CO_2} is inversely proportional to alveolar ventilation. Rearranging Equation 31.7 yields

$$P_{A_{CO_2}} = 0.863 \cdot \frac{\dot{V}_{CO_2}}{\dot{V}_A} \qquad \textbf{(31.9)}$$

In other words, if CO_2 production is fixed, then doubling $\dot{V}_A$ causes $P_{A_{CO_2}}$ to fall to half of its initial value. Conversely, halving $\dot{V}_A$ causes $P_{A_{CO_2}}$ to double. Because, *arterial* P_{CO_2} is virtually the same as *alveolar* P_{CO_2} (see Fig. 30.6), changes in $\dot{V}_A$ affect both $P_{A_{CO_2}}$ and $P_{a_{CO_2}}$.

The *blue curve* in Fig. 31.2 illustrates the principle. Imagine that your tissues are producing 200 mL/min of CO_2. *In a steady state*, your lungs must blow off 200 mL of CO_2 each minute. If your lungs are exhaling 4200 mL/min of alveolar air, then the 200 mL of expired CO_2 must dissolve in the 4200 mL of exhaled alveolar air (*center red point* in Fig. 31.2), and $P_{A_{CO_2}}$ must be ~40 mm Hg.

◉ 31-1 What would happen if your alveolar ventilation doubled, to 8400 mL/min? This is an example of **hyperventilation.** Eventually, you would reach a new steady state in which the rate at which you blow off CO_2 would exactly match the rate at which you produce CO_2 (i.e., 200 mL/min). But what would be the $P_{A_{CO_2}}$? Because each minute you now are blowing off 8400 mL of alveolar air (i.e., twice normal) but still only 200 mL of CO_2 (*right red point* in Fig. 31.2), your $P_{A_{CO_2}}$ must be half normal, or ~20 mm Hg. Not only does the hyperventilation cause *alveolar* P_{CO_2} to fall by half, it also causes *arterial* P_{CO_2} to fall by half. Thus, hyperventilation leads to **respiratory alkalosis** (see ◉ 28-5).

What would happen if, instead of doubling alveolar ventilation, you halved it from 4200 to 2100 mL/min? This is an example of **hypoventilation.** What would $P_{A_{CO_2}}$ be in the new steady state? Because each minute you must exhale 200 mL of CO_2, but this can be diluted in only 2100 mL—half the usual amount of alveolar air (*left red point* in Fig. 31.2)—the alveolar [CO_2] must double from ~40 to 80 mm Hg. Of course, this doubling of *alveolar* P_{CO_2} is paralleled by a doubling of *arterial* P_{CO_2}, leading to a **respiratory acidosis** (see ◉ 28-4).

Therefore, the steady-state alveolar and arterial P_{CO2} values are inversely proportional to alveolar ventilation. The higher the $\dot{V}_A$ the lower the $P_{A_{CO_2}}$. If $\dot{V}_A$ were infinitely high, then $P_{A_{CO_2}}$ would theoretically fall nearly to zero, the P_{CO_2} of inspired air.

Fig. 34.1 illustrates another example of this principle: blood [creatinine] is inversely proportional to glomerular filtration rate.

◉ 31-2 Alveolar and arterial P_{O_2} rise with increased alveolar ventilation

It should be intuitive that, as illustrated by the red curve in Fig. 31.2, increases in alveolar ventilation cause alveolar P_{O_2} to rise and—at an infinite $\dot{V}_A$—approach the inspired P_{O_2} of ~149 mm Hg. But what determines the shape of the red curve? Answering this question requires knowing the ratio of CO_2 production to O_2 consumption, which depends on the *kind of fuel* the tissues burn (see Table 58.3), and is termed the **respiratory quotient (RQ):**

$$RQ = \frac{\dot{V}_{CO_2}}{\dot{V}_{O_2}} \qquad \textbf{(31.10)}$$

If the tissues are burning carbohydrate, RQ is 1, which is a good place to start. If we consider only the *dry* part of the inspired air that enters the alveoli (see Table 26.1), then PI_{N2} is $713 \times 0.78 = 557$, PI_{O2} is $713 \times 0.2095 = 149$ mm Hg, and PI_{CO2} is ~0. As pulmonary-capillary blood takes up incoming O_2, in the steady state it replaces the O_2 with an equal number of CO_2 molecules (RQ = 1). Because the exchange of O_2 for CO_2 is precisely 1 for 1, alveolar P_{O_2} is what is left of the inspired P_{O_2} after metabolism replaces some alveolar O_2 with CO_2. If the *blue curve* in Fig. 31.2 tells us that $P_{A_{CO_2}}$ is 40 mm Hg, then

$$P_{A_{O_2}} = P_{I_{O_2}} - P_{A_{CO_2}} = 149 - 40 = 109 \text{ mm Hg} \qquad \textbf{(31.11)}$$

A typical fat-containing Western-pattern diet produces an RQ of ~0.8, so that 8 molecules of CO_2 replace 10 molecules of O_2 in the alveolar air. This 8-for-10 replacement has two consequences. First, the volume of alveolar air falls slightly during gas exchange. Because the non-H_2O pressure remains at 713 mm Hg, this volume contraction concentrates the N_2 and dilutes the O_2. Second, the volume of *expired* alveolar air is slightly less than the volume of *inspired* air.

The **alveolar gas equation** describes how alveolar P_{O_2} depends on RQ:

$$RQ = 1: P_{A_{O_2}} = P_{I_{O_2}} - P_{A_{CO_2}} \qquad \textbf{(31.12)}$$

General case: $$P_{A_{O_2}} = P_{I_{O_2}} - P_{A_{CO_2}} \cdot \left(F_{I_{O_2}} + \frac{1 + F_{I_{O_2}}}{RQ} \right) \quad \textbf{(31.13)}$$

FI_{O2} is the fraction of inspired *dry* air that is O_2, which is ~0.21 for room air (see Table 26.1). Imagine that we first found that $P_{A_{CO_2}}$ is 40 mm Hg and that we know that RQ is 0.8. What is $P_{A_{O_2}}$?

$$P_{A_{O_2}} = P_{I_{O_2}} - P_{A_{CO_2}} \cdot \left(F_{I_{O_2}} + \frac{1 - F_{I_{O_2}}}{RQ} \right)$$

$$P_{A_{O_2}} = 149 - 40 \cdot \underbrace{\left(0.21 + \frac{1 - 0.21}{0.8} \right)}_{1.2} \qquad \textbf{(31.14)}$$

$$= 149 - 48$$

$$= 101 \text{ mm Hg}$$

Because of the action of gravity on the lung, regional ventilation in an upright subject is normally greater at the base than the apex

Not all alveoli are ventilated to the same extent. Imagine that a subject who is standing up breathes air containing ^{133}Xe. Because Xe—like He and N_2—has a very low water solubility, it has a very low diffusing capacity (see ◉ 30-1) and—over a short period—remains almost entirely within the alveoli. Imaging the ^{133}Xe radioactivity can provide a map of alveolar ventilation (Fig. 31.3A).

This sort of analysis shows that alveolar ventilation in a standing person gradually falls from the base to the apex of the lung (Fig. 31.3B). Why? The answer is **gravity,** which causes alveoli to be less inflated in *dependent* regions—that is, regions closer to the center of the earth or, in the case of a standing person, the base of the lung. A person reclining on the right side would ventilate the dependent lung tissue on the right side better than the elevated lung tissue on the left.

Restrictive and obstructive pulmonary diseases can exacerbate the nonuniformity of ventilation

Even in microgravity, where we would expect no regional differences in ventilation, ventilation would still be nonuniform at the *microscopic* or *local* level because of seemingly random differences in local static compliance (C_{static}) and airway resistance (R_{AW}) that occur in healthy individuals. In fact, such local differences in the ventilation of alveolar units are probably more impressive than gravity-dependent regional differences. Moreover, pathological changes in compliance and resistance can substantially increase the local differences and thus the nonuniformity of ventilation.

Restrictive Pulmonary Disease Restrictive pulmonary diseases include disorders that decrease the static compliance of alveoli (e.g., fibrosis) as well as disorders that limit the expansion of the lung (e.g., pulmonary effusion). These diseases—and the decreases in C_{static}—affect some regions of the lungs more than others. In affected regions with lower C_{static} values, usual changes in intrapleural pressure (P_{IP}) produce smaller volume changes and thus reduced local ventilation. The result is increased *nonuniformity* of ventilation.

Obstructive Pulmonary Disease Obstructive pulmonary diseases include disorders (e.g., asthma, chronic obstructive pulmonary disease [COPD]) that increase the resistance of conducting airways. These diseases affect some regions of the lungs more than others. Because flowing air follows the pathway of least resistance, a local increase in R_{AW} can reduce the ventilation to downstream alveoli, and increase *nonuniformity* of ventilation.

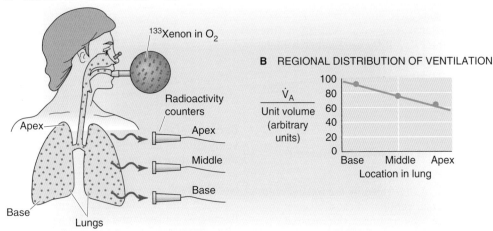

A DETECTION OF INSPIRED ^{133}Xe

^{133}Xenon in O_2

Radioactivity counters

Apex

Apex

Middle

Base

Base

Lungs

B REGIONAL DISTRIBUTION OF VENTILATION

$\dfrac{\dot{V}_A}{\text{Unit volume (arbitrary units)}}$

Location in lung: Base — Middle — Apex

Fig. 31.3 Distribution of ventilation. Data from West JB: Respiratory Physiology—The Essentials, 4th ed. Baltimore, Williams & Wilkins, 1990.

PERFUSION OF THE LUNG

The pulmonary circulation has low pressure and resistance but high compliance

◉ **31-3** The pulmonary circulatory system handles the same cardiac output as the systemic circulation. However, the systemic circulation is a *high-pressure* system. This high pressure is necessary to pump blood to the top of the brain in a standing position. The systemic circulation also needs to be a high-pressure system because it is a high-*resistance* system. It uses this high resistance to control the distribution of blood flow. Thus, at rest, a substantial fraction of the systemic capillaries are closed, which gives the system the flexibility to redistribute large amounts of blood (e.g., to muscle during exercise). The mean pressure of the aorta is ~95 mm Hg. At the opposite end of the circuit is the right atrium, which has a mean pressure of ~2 mm Hg. Thus, the driving pressure for blood flow through the systemic circulation is ~93 mm Hg. Given a cardiac output ($\dot{Q}$) of 5 L/min or 83 mL/s, we can compute the resistance of the systemic system using an equation like Ohm's law:

$$R_{systemic} = \frac{\Delta P}{\dot{Q}} = \frac{93 \text{ mm Hg}}{83 \text{ mL blood/s}} = 1.1 \text{ PRU} \qquad \text{(31.15)}$$

◉ **31-4** In contrast, the pulmonary circulation is a *low-pressure* system. It can afford to be a low-pressure system because it needs to pump blood only to the top of the lung. Moreover, it *must* be a low-pressure system to avoid the consequences of Starling forces (see ◉ **20-10**) that would otherwise flood the lung with edema fluid. The mean pressure in the pulmonary artery is only ~15 mm Hg. Because the mean pressure of the left atrium, at the other end of the circuit, is ~8 mm Hg, and because the cardiac output of the right heart is the same as for the left, we have:

$$R_{pulmonary} = \frac{\Delta P}{\dot{Q}} = \frac{7 \text{ mm Hg}}{83 \text{ mL blood/s}} = 0.08 \text{ PRU} \qquad \text{(31.16)}$$

Thus, the total resistance of the pulmonary circulation is less than one tenth that of the systemic system, which explains how the pulmonary circulation accomplishes its mission at such low pressures. Unlike in the systemic circulation, where most of the pressure drop occurs in the arterioles, in the pulmonary circulation almost the entire pressure drop occurs rather uniformly between the pulmonary artery and the end of the capillaries. In particular, the arterioles make a much smaller contribution to resistance in the pulmonary circulation than in the systemic circulation.

◉ **31-5** What properties of the pulmonary vasculature give it such a low resistance? Together, the two lungs have ~300 *million* alveoli. However, they may have as many as 280 *billion* highly anastomosing capillary segments, or nearly 1000 such capillary segments per alveolus—creating a surface for gas exchange of ~100 m². It is easy to imagine why some have described the pulmonary capillary bed as a nearly continuous flowing sheet of blood surrounding the alveoli—and low capillary resistance.

Pulmonary blood vessels are generally shorter and wider than their systemic counterparts. Arterioles are also present in much higher numbers in the pulmonary circulation. Although the pulmonary arterioles contain smooth muscle and can constrict, these vessels are far less muscular than their systemic counterparts, and their resting tone is low. These properties combine to produce a vascular system with an unusually **low resistance.**

The walls of pulmonary vessels have another key property: thinness, like the walls of veins elsewhere in the body. The thin walls and paucity of smooth muscle give the pulmonary vessels a **high compliance,** which allows the vessels to dilate in response to modest increases in pulmonary arterial pressure.

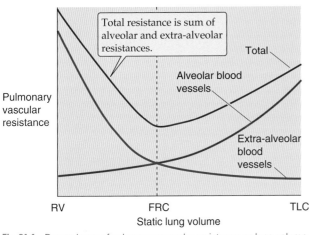

Fig. 31.4 Dependence of pulmonary vascular resistance on lung volume. Data from Murray JF: The Normal Lung, 2nd ed. Philadelphia, WB Saunders, 1986.

TABLE 31.1 Changes or Agents That Affect Pulmonary Vascular Resistance

DILATORS	CONSTRICTORS
↑ PA_{O_2}	↓ PA_{O_2}
↓ PA_{CO_2}	↑ PA_{CO_2}
↑ pH	↓ pH
Histamine, H_2 agonists	Histamine, H_1 agonists
PGI_2 (prostacyclin), PGE_1	Thromboxane A_2, $PGF_{2\alpha}$, PGE_2
β-adrenergic agonists (e.g., isoproterenol)	α-adrenergic agonists
Bradykinin	Serotonin
Theophylline	Angiotensin II
Acetylcholine	
NO	

PG, Prostaglandin.

Overall pulmonary vascular resistance is minimal at functional residual capacity

Because pulmonary blood vessels are so compliant, they are especially susceptible to deformation by external forces.

Alveolar Vessels Alveolar vessels include the capillaries, as well as slightly larger vessels that are also surrounded on all sides by alveoli. The resistance of these alveolar vessels is minimal at residual volume, but gradually increases with increases in lung volume (V_L), as the expanding alveoli crush the vessels (Fig. 31.4).

Extra-alveolar Vessels The resistance of extra-alveolar vessels has the opposite dependence on V_L, compared to intra-alveolar vessels. Because they are not surrounded by alveoli, extra-alveolar vessels are extremely sensitive to P_{IP}. The resistance of extra-alveolar vessels is maximal at residual volume—when P_{IP} is most positive—crushing the vessels. However, the resistance gradually decreases with increases in V_L, as the increasingly negative P_{IP} pulls the vessels open (Fig. 31.4).

In summary, the net effect of the *opposite* resistance profiles of the intra- and extra-alveolar vessels is to produce a biphasic dependence of resistance on V_L, with a minimal pulmonary vascular resistance at about functional residual capacity (FRC).

Increases in pulmonary arterial pressure reduce pulmonary vascular resistance by recruiting and distending pulmonary capillaries

Although the pulmonary circulation is a low-resistance system under resting conditions, it has a remarkable ability to lower its resistance even further. During exercise, 2-fold to 3-fold increases in cardiac output may elicit only a minor increase in mean pulmonary arterial pressure. In other words, a slight increase in pulmonary arterial pressure is somehow able to markedly *decrease* resistance and thus markedly *increase* flow.

Under "resting" conditions (i.e., at relatively low values of pulmonary arterial pressure), some pulmonary capillaries are open and conducting blood, others are open but not conducting substantial amounts of blood, and still others are

closed. Why should some capillaries be **open** but have no flow? In a highly anastomosing capillary network, tiny differences in driving pressure and resistance allow pathways with relatively low resistances to steal flow from neighbors with slightly higher resistances, leaving some "open" pathways heavily underutilized. A familiar example is a garden hose with hundreds of tiny holes, only some of which—at low pressure—conduct water.

Why should some parallel vessels be **closed**? Popping open a previously closed vessel requires that the perfusion pressure overcome the tone of the vascular smooth muscle and reach that vessel's **critical closing pressure**, which varies from vessel to vessel.

Recruitment Imagine that the pressure inside a pulmonary arteriole starts out at a fairly low level. As pressure increases, some vessels that were completely *closed* may now open. Similarly, capillaries that previously had been *open but not conducting* now begin to conduct blood. The greater the increase in perfusion pressure, the greater the number of open and conducting vessels. This recruitment of additional parallel capillary pathways reduces overall vascular resistance.

Distention Once a vessel is open and conducting, further pressure increases cause the vessel to dilate. The net effect is a reduction in overall pulmonary resistance.

⊙ 31-6 Hypoxia is a strong vasoconstrictor, opposite to its effect in the systemic circulation

In addition to lung volume and perfusion pressure, several other factors can modulate pulmonary vascular resistance.

Oxygen The effects of changes in P_{O_2}, P_{CO_2}, and pH on pulmonary vascular resistance (Table 31.1) are opposite to those in the systemic circulation. Hypoxia causes pulmonary vasoconstriction. What appears to be critical is the P_{O_2} in the *alveolar air* adjacent to the vessel.

⊙ 31-7 **Hypoxic vasoconstriction** occurs in isolated lung tissue and thus does not rely on either the nervous system or systemic hormones. Rather, the low P_{O_2} is generally believed to act directly on the pulmonary vascular smooth-muscle cells.

How this occurs is unknown, but hypothesized mechanisms include all those proposed for the sensing of hypoxia by the peripheral chemoreceptor, which we discuss below (see ⊙ 32-6).

Hormones and Other Humoral Agents The pulmonary blood vessels are relatively *unresponsive* to hormones and—aside from P_{O_2}—other signaling molecules. Table 31.1 summarizes the actions of some factors that modify pulmonary vascular resistance.

Because of gravity, regional perfusion in an upright subject is far greater near the base than the apex of the lung

When it comes to perfusion—as with ventilation—not all alveoli are created equal. First, *microscopic* differences in pulmonary vascular resistance lead to corresponding local differences in perfusion. Second, pathological processes can exacerbate these differences. Third, gravity causes large *regional* differences in perfusion that we can assess by using ^{133}Xe imaging. In Fig. 31.5A, we equilibrate a saline solution with gas containing ^{133}Xe and then inject the solution intravenously as the patient holds his or her breath. When it reaches the lungs, the poorly soluble ^{133}Xe rapidly enters the alveolar air. A lung scan reveals the distribution of radioactivity, which here reflects the regional uniformity of *perfusion.*

When the patient is upright, perfusion ($\dot{Q}$) is greatest near the base of the lungs and falls toward low levels near the apex (Fig. 31.5B). Note that although regional $\dot{Q}$ is highest *near* the base of the lung, $\dot{Q}$ falls off somewhat from this peak as we approach the extreme base. With exercise, perfusion increases in all regions of the lung, but more so near the apex, so that the nonuniformity of perfusion is less.

Why should $\dot{Q}$ have this peculiar height dependence? The basic answer is the same as for the similar question we raised about the regional nonuniformity of *ventilation:* **gravity.** Thus, standing on your head will reverse the flow-height relationship.

⊙ 31-8 Fig. 31.5C shows how we can divide the upright lung into four zones based on the relationships among various pressures. We define the first three zones based on how *alveolar* blood vessels are affected by the relative values of three pressures: alveolar pressure (P_A), the pressure inside pulmonary arterioles (P_{PA}), and the pressure inside pulmonary venules (P_{PV}). In the fourth zone, we instead focus on how extra-alveolar vessels are affected by intrapleural pressure (P_{IP}).

Zone 1: $P_A > P_{PA} > P_{PV}$ At the level of the left atrium, (1) the *mean* P_{PA} is ~15 mm Hg, which corresponds to ~20 cm H_2O (Fig. 31.5C, *lower illustration for zone 3*) and (2) the mean P_{PV} is ~8 mm Hg, or ~10 cm H_2O.

As we move upward closer to the apex of an upright lung, the actual pressures in the pulmonary arterioles and venules fall by 1 cm H_2O for each 1 cm of vertical ascent. For alveoli 20 cm above the level of the left atrium, the mean P_{PA} would be 0 cm H_2O (Fig. 31.5C, *zone 1*), and P_{PV} would be about −10 cm H_2O. The pressure inside the pulmonary capillary (Pc) would be intermediate. Blood would still flow through this capillary (driving pressure ≅ 10 cm H_2O) were it not for the pressure inside the surrounding alveoli,

which is 0 cm H_2O between breaths. Therefore, because P_A is much higher than Pc, the negative transmural pressure gradient (P_{TM}; see ⊙ 17-2) tends to crush the capillary and reduce blood flow.

Zone 1 conditions do not exist for normal people at rest. However, they can arise if there is either a sufficient decrease in P_{PA} (e.g., in hemorrhage) or a sufficient increase in P_A (e.g., in **positive-pressure ventilation**).

Zone 2: $P_{PA} > P_A > P_{PV}$ These conditions normally prevail from the apex to the mid-lung. The defining characteristic of zone 2 is that mean P_{PA} and P_{PV} are sufficiently high that they sandwich P_A (Fig. 31.5C, *zone 2*). Thus, at the arteriolar end, the positive P_{TM} causes the alveolar vessel to dilate. Further down the capillary, Pc gradually falls below P_A, so that the negative P_{TM} squeezes the vessel. Downward in zone 2, the crushing force decreases because the hydrostatic pressures in the arteriole, capillary, and venule all rise in parallel (Fig. 31.5C, *upper → lower illustrations for zone 2*). Simultaneously, resistance decreases. The conversion of a closed vessel (or one that is open but not conducting) to a conducting one by increased P_{PA} and P_{PV} is an example of **recruitment.**

Zone 3: $P_{PA} > P_{PV} > P_A$ These conditions prevail in the middle to lower lung. The defining characteristic of zone 3 is that mean P_{PA} and P_{PV} are so high that they both exceed P_A (Fig. 31.5C, *zone 3*). Thus, P_{TM} is positive along the entire length of the alveolar vessel, tending to dilate it. Downward in zone 3, the hydrostatic pressures in the arteriole, capillary, and venule all continue to rise, causing the vessel to dilate more and more—an example of **distention** (Fig. 31.5C, *upper → lower illustrations for zone 3*). This distention causes a gradual decrease in resistance of the capillaries as we move downward in zone 3. Hence, although the driving force ($P_{PA} − P_{PV}$) remains constant, perfusion increases toward the base of the lung.

Zone 4: $P_{PA} > P_{PV} > P_A$ These conditions prevail at the extreme base of the lungs. In zone 4, the *intra-alveolar vessels* behave as in zone 3; they dilate more as we descend toward the base of the lung. However, the *extra-alveolar vessels* behave differently. At the base of the lung, P_{IP} is least negative. Thus, as we approach the extreme base of the lung, the distending forces acting on the extra-alveolar blood vessels fade, and the resistance of these extra-alveolar vessels increases (Fig. 31.5C, *zone 4*). Thus, $\dot{Q}$ begins to fall from its peak as we approach the extreme base of the lungs (Fig. 31.5B).

MATCHING VENTILATION AND PERFUSION

The greater the ventilation-perfusion ratio, the higher the P_{O_2} and the lower the P_{CO_2} in the alveolar air

⊙ 31-9 In Fig. 31.2 we saw that, all other factors being equal, alveolar ventilation determines alveolar $P_{A_{O_2}}$ and $P_{A_{CO_2}}$. The greater the ventilation, the more closely $P_{A_{O_2}}$ and $P_{A_{CO_2}}$ approach their respective values in inspired air. However, in Fig. 31.2 we were focusing on *total* alveolar ventilation and how this influences the *average* $P_{A_{O_2}}$ and $P_{A_{CO_2}}$.

We have already learned that both ventilation and perfusion each vary among alveoli. The greater the local ventilation, the more closely the composition of local alveolar air approaches that of the inspired air. Similarly, because blood

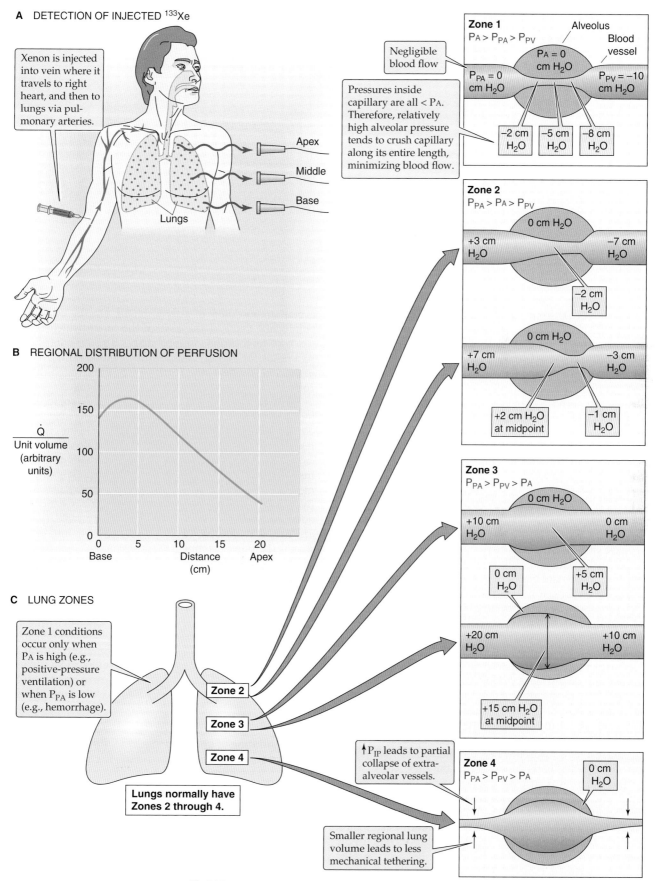

A DETECTION OF INJECTED ^{133}Xe

Xenon is injected into vein where it travels to right heart, and then to lungs via pulmonary arteries.

Apex

Middle

Base

Lungs

Zone 1
$P_A > P_{PA} > P_{PV}$

Alveolus

Blood vessel

Negligible blood flow

$P_A = 0$ cm H_2O

$P_{PA} = 0$ cm H_2O

$P_{PV} = -10$ cm H_2O

Pressures inside capillary are all < P_A. Therefore, relatively high alveolar pressure tends to crush capillary along its entire length, minimizing blood flow.

−2 cm H_2O −5 cm H_2O −8 cm H_2O

Zone 2
$P_{PA} > P_A > P_{PV}$

0 cm H_2O

+3 cm H_2O

−7 cm H_2O

−2 cm H_2O

0 cm H_2O

+7 cm H_2O

−3 cm H_2O

+2 cm H_2O at midpoint   −1 cm H_2O

B REGIONAL DISTRIBUTION OF PERFUSION

$\dfrac{\dot{Q}}{\text{Unit volume}}$ (arbitrary units)

200

150

100

50

0

0   5   10   15   20
Base   Distance   Apex
              (cm)

Zone 3
$P_{PA} > P_{PV} > P_A$

0 cm H_2O

+10 cm H_2O

0 cm H_2O

0 cm H_2O +5 cm H_2O

+20 cm H_2O

+10 cm H_2O

+15 cm H_2O at midpoint

C LUNG ZONES

Zone 1 conditions occur only when P_A is high (e.g., positive-pressure ventilation) or when P_{PA} is low (e.g., hemorrhage).

Zone 2

Zone 3

Zone 4

Lungs normally have Zones 2 through 4.

↑P_{IP} leads to partial collapse of extra-alveolar vessels.

Smaller regional lung volume leads to less mechanical tethering.

Zone 4
$P_{PA} > P_{PV} > P_A$

0 cm H_2O

Fig. 31.5 Physiological nonuniformity of pulmonary perfusion.

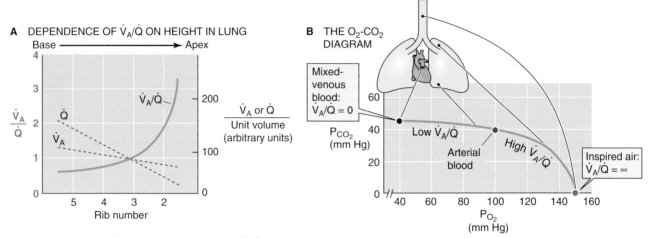

Fig. 31.6 Regional differences in $\dot{V}_A/\dot{Q}$ ratio and alveolar gas composition. Data from West JB: Ventilation/Blood Flow and Gas Exchange. Oxford, UK, Blackwell, 1985.

flow removes O_2 from the alveolar air and adds CO_2, the greater the perfusion, the more closely the composition of local alveolar air approaches that of mixed-venous blood. Thus, the local **ventilation-perfusion ratio** ($\dot{V}_A/\dot{Q}$) determines the local $P_{A_{O_2}}$ and $P_{A_{CO_2}}$.

You might view the alveoli as a sports venue where ventilation and perfusion are engaged in a continuous struggle over control of the composition of alveolar air. To the extent that ventilation gains the upper hand, $P_{A_{O_2}}$ rises and $P_{A_{CO_2}}$ falls. To the extent that perfusion holds sway, these parameters change in the opposite direction.

Because of gravity, the regional $\dot{V}_A/\dot{Q}$ ratio in an upright subject is greater at the apex of the lung than at the base

We have already seen that when a subject is upright in a gravitational field, ventilation falls from the base to the apex of the lung (Fig. 31.3B) and that perfusion also falls, but more steeply (Fig. 31.5B). Thus, it is not surprising that the ratio $\dot{V}_A/\dot{Q}$ itself varies with height in the lung (Fig. 31.6A). $\dot{V}_A/\dot{Q}$ is lowest near the base, where $\dot{Q}$ exceeds $\dot{V}_A$, and increases toward the apex, where falls more precipitously than $\dot{V}_A$.

Table 31.2 shows how differences in $\dot{V}_A/\dot{Q}$ at the apex and base of the lungs influence the regional composition of alveolar air. At the apex, where $\dot{V}_A/\dot{Q}$ is highest, alveolar P_{O_2} and P_{CO_2} most closely approach their values in inspired air. Because both O_2 and CO_2 transport across the blood-gas barrier are **perfusion limited** (see ⊙ 30-4), blood leaving the apex has the same high P_{O_2} and low P_{CO_2} as the alveolar air. Of course, the relatively low P_{CO_2} produces a *respiratory alkalosis* (see ⊙ 28-5) in the blood leaving the apex.

The situation is just the opposite near the base of the lung, where $\dot{V}_A/\dot{Q}$ is lowest. What impact do these different regions of the lung, each with its own $\dot{V}_A/\dot{Q}$ ratio, have on the composition of systemic arterial blood? Each region makes a contribution that is proportional to its blood flow (see the rightmost column in Table 31.2). Because the apex is poorly perfused, it makes only a small contribution to the

overall composition of arterial blood. On the other hand, pulmonary tissue at the base of the lungs, which receives ~26% of total cardiac output, makes a major contribution. As a result, the average composition of blood exiting the lung more closely reflects the composition of the blood that had equilibrated with the air in the base of the lung.

⊙ **31-10** The **O_2-CO_2 diagram** is a helpful tool for depicting how different $\dot{V}_A/\dot{Q}$ ratios throughout the lung produce different blood-gas compositions. The curve in Fig. 31.6B represents all possible combinations of P_{O_2} and P_{CO_2} in the alveolar air or end-pulmonary-capillary blood. The H_2O-saturated **inspired air** (P_{O_2} = 149, P_{CO_2} = ~0 mm Hg) represents the rightmost extreme of the diagram (*blue point on curve*, Fig. 31.6B). By definition, the $\dot{V}_A/\dot{Q}$ ratio of inspired air is ∞, because it does not come into contact with pulmonary-capillary blood. The **mixed-venous blood** (P_{O2} = 40, P_{CO_2} = 46 mm Hg) represents the other extreme (*dark magenta point on curve*, Fig 31.6B). By definition, the $\dot{V}_A/\dot{Q}$ ratio of mixed-venous blood is zero, because it has not yet come into contact with alveolar air. With the end points of the diagram established, we can now predict—with the help of the alveolar gas equation (see Equation 31.3), as well as the Bohr and Haldane effects (see Chapter 29)—all possible combinations of P_{O_2} and P_{CO_2} in the alveoli and end-pulmonary-capillary blood throughout the lung. As shown in Fig. 31.6B, the base, midportion, and apex of the lungs—as well as arterial blood—correspond to points along the O_2-CO_2 diagram between mixed-venous blood at one extreme and inspired air at the other.

The ventilation of unperfused alveoli (local $\dot{V}_A/\dot{Q}$ = ∞) triggers compensatory bronchoconstriction and a fall in surfactant production

The effects of gravity on ventilation and perfusion cause regional $\dot{V}_A/\dot{Q}$ to vary widely. Microscopic or local physiological and pathological variations in ventilation and perfusion can cause even greater mismatches of $\dot{V}_A/\dot{Q}$, the extremes of which are alveolar dead-space ventilation (this section) and shunt (next section).

TABLE 31.2 Effect of Regional Differences in $\dot{V}_A/\dot{Q}$ on the Composition of Alveolar Air and Pulmonary-Capillary Blood

LOCATION	FRACTION OF TOTAL LUNG VOLUME	$\dot{V}_A/\dot{Q}$	P_{O_2} (mm Hg)	P_{CO_2} (mm Hg)	pH	$\dot{Q}$ (L/min)
Apex	7%	3.3	132	28	7.55	0.07
Base	13%	0.6	89	42	7.38	1.3
Overall	100%	0.84[a]	100	40	7.40	5.0

[a]Because the transport of both O_2 and CO_2 is perfusion limited, we assume that end-capillary values of P_{O_2} and P_{O_2} are the same as their respective alveolar values. If the overall alveolar ventilation for the two lungs is 4.2 L/min, and if the cardiac output (i.e., perfusion) is 5 L/min, then the overall $\dot{V}_A/\dot{Q}$ ratio for the two lungs is (4.2 L/min)/(5 L/min) = 0.84.
Modified from West JB: Ventilation/Blood Flow and Gas Exchange. Oxford, UK, Blackwell, 1989.

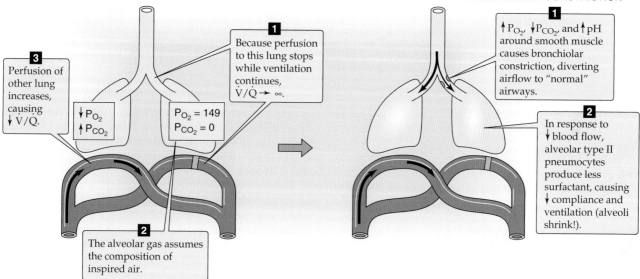

A ALVEOLAR DEAD-SPACE VENTILATION WITHOUT COMPENSATION **B** COMPENSATION: BRONCHIOLAR CONSTRICTION

1 Because perfusion to this lung stops while ventilation continues, $\dot{V}/\dot{Q} \rightarrow \infty$.

3 Perfusion of other lung increases, causing $\downarrow\dot{V}/\dot{Q}$.

$\downarrow P_{O_2}$ $\uparrow P_{CO_2}$

$P_{O_2} = 149$ $P_{CO_2} = 0$

2 The alveolar gas assumes the composition of inspired air.

1 $\uparrow P_{O_2}$, $\downarrow P_{CO_2}$, and $\uparrow$pH around smooth muscle causes bronchiolar constriction, diverting airflow to "normal" airways.

2 In response to $\downarrow$ blood flow, alveolar type II pneumocytes produce less surfactant, causing $\downarrow$ compliance and ventilation (alveoli shrink!).

Fig. 31.7 Extreme $\dot{V}_A/\dot{Q}$ mismatch and compensatory response—alveolar dead-space ventilation.

Alveolar Dead-Space Ventilation At one end of the spectrum of $\dot{V}_A/\dot{Q}$ mismatches is the elimination of blood flow to a group of alveoli. If we ligated the pulmonary artery feeding one lung, the affected alveoli receives no perfusion even though ventilation would initially continue normally (Fig. 31.7A). The ventilation of the unperfused alveoli is called *alveolar dead-space ventilation* because it does not contribute to gas exchange.

A natural cause of alveolar dead-space ventilation is a pulmonary embolism, which obstructs blood flow to a group of alveoli. Because one task of the lung is to filter small emboli from the blood (see ⊚ 26-3), the lung must deal with small regions of alveolar dead-space ventilation on a recurring basis. At the instant the blood flow ceases, the alveoli supplied by the affected vessel(s) contain normal alveolar air. However, each cycle of inspiration and expiration replaces some stale alveolar air with fresh air, the alveolar gas gradually achieves the composition of moist inspired air, with alveolar P_{O_2} rising to ~149 mm Hg and P_{CO_2} falling to ~0 mm Hg (Fig. 31.7A, *step 2*). By definition, alveolar dead space has a V_A/Q ratio of ∞, as described by the "Inspired air" blue point on the x-axis of an O_2-CO_2 diagram (Fig. 31.6B).

Redirection of Blood Flow Blocking blood flow to one group of alveoli diverts blood to other "normal" alveoli, which

then become somewhat hyperperfused. Thus, the blockage not only increases $\dot{V}_A/\dot{Q}$ in alveoli downstream from the blockage, but also decreases $\dot{V}_A/\dot{Q}$ in other regions. Redirection of blood flow thus accentuates the nonuniformity of ventilation.

Regulation of Local Ventilation Because alveolar dead-space ventilation causes alveolar P_{CO_2} to fall to ~0 mm Hg in downstream alveoli, it leads to a respiratory alkalosis (see ⊚ 28-5) in the surrounding interstitial fluid. These local changes trigger a compensatory **bronchiolar constriction** in the adjacent tissues (Fig. 31.7B), so that over a period of seconds to minutes, airflow partially diverts away from the unperfused alveoli and toward normal alveoli, to which blood flow is also being diverted. This compensation makes teleological sense, because it tends to correct the $\dot{V}_A/\dot{Q}$ shift in both the unperfused and normal alveoli. The precise mechanism of bronchiolar constriction is unknown, although bronchiolar smooth muscle may contract—at least in part—in response to a high extracellular pH.

The elimination of perfusion has a second consequence. Downstream from the blockage, alveolar type II pneumocytes become starved for nutrients, including the lipids they need to make surfactant. As a result, **surfactant**

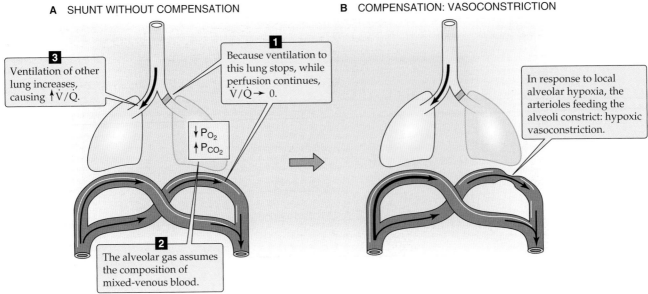

A SHUNT WITHOUT COMPENSATION

3
Ventilation of other lung increases, causing ↑V/Q.

1
Because ventilation to this lung stops, while perfusion continues, $\dot{V}/\dot{Q} \rightarrow 0$.

↓P_{O_2}
↑P_{CO_2}

2
The alveolar gas assumes the composition of mixed-venous blood.

B COMPENSATION: VASOCONSTRICTION

In response to local alveolar hypoxia, the arterioles feeding the alveoli constrict: hypoxic vasoconstriction.

Fig. 31.8 Extreme $\dot{V}_A/\dot{Q}$ mismatch and compensatory response—shunt.

production *falls* over a period of hours to days. The result is a local decrease in compliance, further reducing local ventilation.

These compensatory responses—which tend to normalize $\dot{V}_A/\dot{Q}$ distribution—work well only if the alveolar dead space is relatively small, so that an ample volume of healthy tissue remains into which the airflow can divert.

The perfusion of unventilated alveoli (local $\dot{V}_A/\dot{Q} = 0$) triggers a compensatory hypoxic vasoconstriction

Shunt Alveolar dead-space ventilation is at one end of the spectrum of $\dot{V}_A/\dot{Q}$ mismatches. At the opposite end is shunt—the flow of blood past unventilated alveoli. If we ligate a mainstem bronchus, then inspired air cannot refresh alveoli distal to the obstruction (Fig. 31.8A). As a result, mixed-venous blood perfusing the unventilated alveoli "shunts" from the right heart to the left heart, without benefit of ventilation. When the low-O_2 shunted blood mixes with high-O_2 unshunted blood (which *is* ventilated), the result is that the mixture has a lower-than-normal P_{O_2}, causing hypoxia in the systemic arteries. It is possible to calculate the extent of the shunt from the degree of hypoxia.

Natural causes of airway obstruction include aspiration of a **foreign body** or the presence of a **tumor** in the lumen of a conducting airway. The collapse of alveoli (**atelectasis**) also produces a right-to-left shunt, a pathological example of which is pneumothorax. Atelectasis also occurs naturally in dependent regions of the lungs, where surfactant levels gradually decline. Sighing or yawning stimulates surfactant release and can reverse physiological atelectasis.

Imagine that a child aspirates a peanut. Initially, the air trapped distal to the obstruction has the composition of normal alveolar air. However, pulmonary-capillary blood gradually extracts O_2 from the trapped air and adds CO_2. Eventually, the P_{O_2} and P_{CO_2} of the trapped air drift to their values in **mixed-venous blood.** If the shunt is small, so that

it does not materially affect the P_{O_2} or P_{CO_2} of the systemic arterial blood, then the alveoli will have a P_{O_2} of 40 mm Hg and a P_{CO_2} of 46 mm Hg. By definition, shunted alveoli have a $\dot{V}_A/\dot{Q}$ of zero and are represented by the "Mixed-venous blood" magenta point on an O_2-CO_2 diagram (Fig. 31.6B).

Redirection of Airflow Blocking airflow to one group of alveoli simultaneously diverts air to normal parts of the lung, which then become somewhat hyperventilated. Thus, shunt not only decreases $\dot{V}_A/\dot{Q}$ in unventilated alveoli, but also increases $\dot{V}_A/\dot{Q}$ in other regions. The net effect is a widening of the nonuniformity of $\dot{V}_A/\dot{Q}$ ratios.

Asthma Although less dramatic than complete airway obstruction, an incomplete occlusion also decreases $\dot{V}_A/\dot{Q}$. An example is asthma, in which hyperreactivity of airway smooth muscle increases local airway resistance and decreases ventilation of alveoli distal to the pathology.

Normal Anatomical Shunts The **thebesian veins** drain some of the blood from the heart. Other veins drain about half the blood that the **bronchial arteries** supply to the *conducting* airways. The drainage from both sets of veins mix with oxygenated blood and thus represents part of the anatomical right-to-left shunt.

Pathological Shunts In Chapter 57, we discuss examples of right-to-left shunts. For example, generalized hypoxemia in the newborn can constrict the pulmonary vasculature, as we will see in the next paragraph, leading to pulmonary hypertension and the shunting of blood via the foramen ovale or a patent ductus arteriosus.

Regulation of Local Perfusion The alveoli that derive from a single terminal bronchiole surround the pulmonary arteriole that supplies these alveoli. Thus, the vascular smooth-muscle cells of this pulmonary arteriole are bathed in an interstitial fluid whose composition reflects that of the local alveolar gas. In the case of shunt, the vascular smooth-muscle cells sense a decrease in P_{O_2}, an increase in P_{CO_2}, and a fall in pH. The decrease in local alveolar P_{O_2} triggers a compensatory **hypoxic pulmonary vasoconstriction** (see ⊙ 31-7), which the accompanying respiratory acidosis augments (Fig. 31.8B). Note that this response is just the opposite of that of *systemic* arterioles, which *dilate* in response to hypoxia (see ⊙ 20-17). Hypoxic pulmonary vasoconstriction makes teleological sense because it diverts blood flow away from unventilated alveoli toward normal alveoli, to which airflow is also being diverted. This compensation tends to correct the $\dot{V}_A / \dot{Q}$ shift in both the unventilated and normal alveoli.

Even if whole-lung $\dot{V}_A$ and $\dot{Q}$ are normal, exaggerated local $\dot{V}_A/\dot{Q}$ mismatches produce hypoxia and respiratory acidosis

Even a normal person has lung regions with $\dot{V}_A / \dot{Q}$ values ranging from ~0.6 to 3.3 (Table 31.2). Even a normal person has local variations in $\dot{V}_A / \dot{Q}$ due to alveolar dead-space ventilation as well as physiological and anatomical shunts. These physiological $\dot{V}_A / \dot{Q}$ mismatches produces an arterial P_{CO_2} (i.e., ~40 mm Hg) that we regard as "normal" and an arterial P_{O_2} (i.e., ~100 mm Hg) that we also regard as "normal."

If pathological processes exaggerate the normal $\dot{V}_A / \dot{Q}$ *distribution*, the result is respiratory acidosis and hypoxia. Pathological $\dot{V}_A / \dot{Q}$ mismatches cause the range of $\dot{V}_A / \dot{Q}$ ratios to broaden beyond the physiological range (Table 31.2). Some alveoli may be true alveolar dead space (i.e., perfusion absent, $\dot{V}_A / \dot{Q} = \infty$), but others may be more modestly underperfused. Some alveoli may be totally shunted (i.e., ventilation absent, $\dot{V}_A / \dot{Q} = 0$), but others may be more modestly underventilated. Thus, the left ventricle receives a mixture of blood from alveoli with $\dot{V}_A / \dot{Q}$ ratios from ∞ to zero, corresponding to all of the points along the O_2-CO_2 diagram in Fig. 31.6B. What is the composition of this mixed blood? Even if total $\dot{V}_A$ and total $\dot{Q}$ remain normal, pathologically high $\dot{V}_A / \dot{Q}$ ratios in some alveoli cannot make up for pathologically low ratios in others, and vice versa. The result of uncompensated pathological $\dot{V}_A / \dot{Q}$ mismatching is always respiratory acidosis and hypoxia. The sophisticated compensatory responses to alveolar dead-space ventilation and shunt—discussed above—are important because they help to minimize these mismatches and the respiratory acidosis and hypoxia.

CHAPTER 32

CONTROL OF VENTILATION

George B. Richerson and Walter F. Boron

OVERVIEW OF THE RESPIRATORY CONTROL SYSTEM

Breathing is one of those things in life that you almost never think about until something goes wrong with it. However, those with pulmonary disease become intensely aware of breathing, as do people who overexert themselves, especially at high altitude. Dyspnea (i.e., feeling of being short of breath) is one of the most unpleasant sensations in life. Swimmers and SCUBA divers, musicians who sing or play wind instruments, Lamaze practitioners, and anyone with a bed partner who snores also focus intensely on breathing. It is common for respiratory output to be the last brain function to be lost in comatose patients, in which case its cessation marks the onset of brain death. Thus, despite our common tendency to ignore breathing, control of ventilation is one of the most important of all brain functions.

The ventilatory-control mechanism must accomplish two tasks. First, it must establish the *automatic rhythm* for contraction of respiratory muscles. Second, it must adjust this rhythm to accommodate changing *metabolic* demands (as reflected by changes in blood P_{O_2}, P_{CO_2}, and pH), varying *mechanical* conditions (e.g., changing posture), and a range of episodic *nonventilatory* behaviors (e.g., speaking, sniffing, eating).

Automatic centers in the brainstem activate the respiratory muscles rhythmically and subconsciously

The rhythmic output of the central nervous system (CNS) to muscles of ventilation normally occurs automatically, without any conscious effort. This output depends upon a vast array of interconnected neurons—located primarily in the medulla oblongata, but also in the pons and other brainstem regions. These neurons are called **respiratory-related neurons (RRNs)** because they fire more action potentials during specific parts of the respiratory cycle. For example, some neurons have peak activity during inspiration, and others, during expiration. Some RRNs are **interneurons** (i.e., they make local connections), others are **premotor neurons** (i.e., they innervate motor neurons), and still others are **motor neurons** (i.e., they innervate muscles of respiration). A subset of these neurons, thought to be in the medulla oblongata, are able to independently generate a respiratory rhythm—and are known as the **central pattern generator (CPG;** see ⊙ **16-2**). Together the neurons

of the respiratory network distribute signals appropriately to various pools of cranial and spinal motor neurons, which directly innervate the respiratory muscles (Fig. 32.1).

The most important respiratory motor neurons are those that send axons via the phrenic nerve to innervate the diaphragm, one of the *primary muscles of inspiration* (see ⊙ **27-2**). When respiratory output increases (e.g., during exercise), activity also appears in motor neurons that innervate a wide variety of *accessory* muscles of inspiration and expiration.

Each of these muscles is active at different times within the respiratory cycle, and the brain can alter this timing depending on prevailing conditions. It is the job of the premotor neurons to orchestrate the appropriate patterns of activity among the different pools of motor neurons. The pattern of alternating inspiratory and expiratory activity that occurs under normal conditions during non–rapid eye movement (NREM) sleep, at rest, and during mild exercise is called **eupnea**. During eupnea, neural output to respiratory muscles is highly regular, with rhythmic bursts of activity during inspiration only to the diaphragm and certain intercostal muscles. Expiration occurs purely as a result of cessation of inspiration and passive elastic recoil (see ⊙ **27-1**) of the chest wall and lungs. During more intense exercise, the amplitude and frequency of phrenic nerve activity increase, and additional activity appears in nerves that supply accessory muscles of inspiration. With this increased effort, the accessory muscles of expiration also become active, thereby producing more rapid exhalation and permitting the next inspiration to begin sooner (i.e., increasing respiratory frequency).

Peripheral and central chemoreceptors—which sense P_{O_2}, P_{CO_2}, and pH—drive the CPG

The CPG for breathing is the clock that times the automatic cycling of inspiration and expiration. In some cases, the CPG stops "ticking" in the absence of **tonic drive** inputs, which results in the absence of ventilation, or **apnea**. Although this tonic drive comes from many sources, the most important are the central and peripheral chemoreceptors, which monitor the **arterial blood gas** parameters—O_2, CO_2, and pH levels. Unlike the frequency of a clock, that of the respiratory CPG changes with the strength of the drive from the chemoreceptors, resulting in changes in both depth and frequency of ventilation.

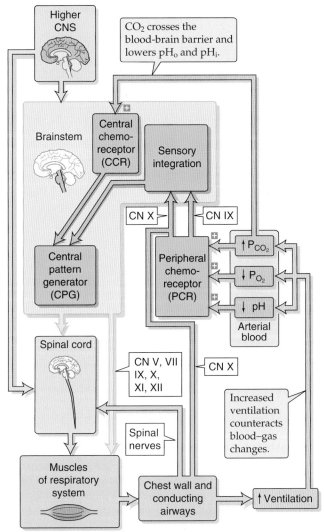

Fig. 32.1 Control of ventilation.

The **peripheral chemoreceptors,** located in the carotid bodies in the neck and aortic bodies in the thorax, are primarily sensitive to decreases in arterial P_{O_2}, although high P_{CO_2} and low pH also stimulate them and enhance their sensitivity to hypoxia. They convey their sensory information to the medulla via the glossopharyngeal nerve (cranial nerve [CN] IX) and vagus nerve (CN X). The **central chemoreceptors,** located on the brain side of the blood-brain barrier (see ◉ 11-3), sense increases in arterial P_{CO_2} and—much more slowly—decreases in arterial pH, but not arterial P_{O_2}. All three signals trigger an increase in alveolar ventilation that tends to return these arterial blood-gas parameters to normal. Thus, the chemoreceptors, in addition to supplying tonic drive to the CPG, form the critical sensory end of a **negative-feedback system** that uses respiratory output to stabilize arterial P_{O_2}, P_{CO_2}, and pH (Fig. 32.1).

Other receptors as well as higher brain centers also modulate ventilation

Left alone, the respiratory CPG would tick regularly for an indefinite period. However, many inputs to the CPG cause the clock to speed up or slow down. For example, respiratory output is often highly irregular during many behaviors that use the respiratory muscles (e.g., eating, talking, and yawning). During NREM sleep or quiet wakefulness, and with anesthesia, the CPG is unperturbed and *does* run regularly.

A variety of receptors in the lungs and airways provide sensory feedback that the medulla integrates and uses to alter respiratory output. The mechanoreceptors and chemoreceptors in the lungs and lower (i.e., distal) airways send their sensory information to the respiratory neurons of the medulla via CN X, and those in the upper airways send information via CN IX.

Nonrespiratory brainstem nuclei and higher centers in the CNS also interact with respiratory control centers, which allows the ventilatory system to accommodate such activities as speaking, playing a musical instrument, swallowing, and vomiting. These interconnections also allow respiratory control to be highly integrated with the autonomic nervous system, the sleep-wake cycle, emotions, and other aspects of brain function.

NEURONS THAT CONTROL VENTILATION

The neurons that generate the respiratory rhythm are located in the medulla

A classical method for determining which parts of the CNS are responsible for controlling respiratory output is to transect the neuraxis at different levels and to observe changes in breathing.

A century ago, Lumsden found that transection of the CNS between the medulla and spinal cord causes ventilation to cease as a result of loss of the descending input to phrenic and intercostal motor neurons in the spinal cord. However, even after a spinomedullary transection, respiratory activity continues in muscles innervated by motor neurons whose cell bodies reside in the brainstem. During the period that would have been an inspiration, the nostrils continue to flare, and the muscles of the tongue, pharynx, and larynx continue to maximize airway caliber—although this respiratory activity cannot sustain life. Thus, spinomedullary transection blocks ventilation by interrupting output to the diaphragm, not by eliminating the respiratory rhythm. Thus, the neural machinery driving ventilation lies above the spinal cord.

The dorsal and ventral respiratory groups contain many neurons that fire in phase with respiratory motor output

In the 1930s, Gesell and colleagues used extracellular microelectrode recordings to monitor single neurons, finding that many neurons within the medulla increase their firing rate during one of the phases of the respiratory cycle. Some of these neurons fire more frequently during inspiration—**inspiratory neurons**—whereas others fire more often during expiration—**expiratory neurons.**

Such mapping has proved very useful in defining neurons that are candidates for *controlling* ventilation. On each side of the medulla, two large concentrations of RRNs—the dorsal and ventral respiratory groups—are grossly organized into sausage-shaped columns, oriented along the long axis of the medulla (Fig. 32.2). Many neurons of these two regions tend to fire exclusively during either inspiration or expiration.

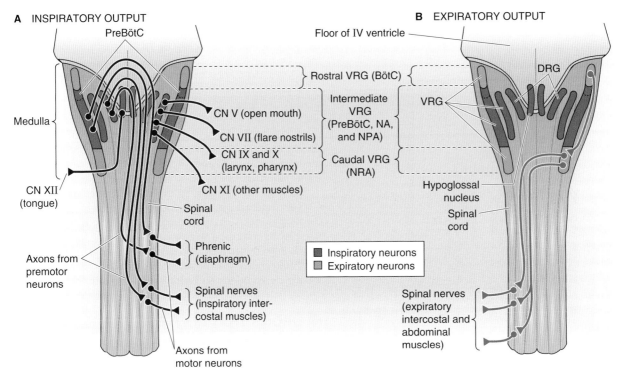

A INSPIRATORY OUTPUT
PreBötC
Medulla
CN V (open mouth)
CN VII (flare nostrils)
CN IX and X (larynx, pharynx)
CN XI (other muscles)
CN XII (tongue)
Spinal cord
Axons from premotor neurons
Phrenic (diaphragm)
Spinal nerves (inspiratory intercostal muscles)
Axons from motor neurons
Rostral VRG (BötC)
Intermediate VRG (PreBötC, NA, and NPA)
Caudal VRG (NRA)

Inspiratory neurons
Expiratory neurons

B EXPIRATORY OUTPUT
Floor of IV ventricle
DRG
VRG
Hypoglossal nucleus
Spinal cord
Spinal nerves (expiratory intercostal and abdominal muscles)

Fig. 32.2 Dorsal and ventral respiratory groups and their motor output. These are dorsal views of the brainstem and spinal cord, with the cerebellum removed. The color coding indicates whether the neurons are primarily inspiratory *(red)* or primarily expiratory *(green)*.

The dorsal respiratory group processes sensory input and contains primarily inspiratory neurons

⊙ **32-1** The **dorsal respiratory group (DRG)** primarily contains inspiratory neurons. It extends for about one third of the length of the medulla and is located bilaterally in and around the **nucleus tractus solitarii (NTS),** which receives *sensory* input from all viscera of the thorax and abdomen and plays an important role in control of the autonomic nervous system (see ⊙ 14-11). The NTS is viscerotopically organized, with the respiratory portion of the NTS ventrolateral to the **tractus solitarius,** just beneath the floor of the caudal end of the fourth ventricle (Fig. 32.2). These NTS neurons, as well as some immediately adjacent neurons in the dorsal medulla, make up the DRG.

As might be surmised from the sensory role of the NTS, one of the major functions of the DRG is the *integration* of sensory information from the respiratory system. Indeed, some of the DRG neurons receive sensory input—via the glossopharyngeal (CN IX) and vagus (CN X) nerves—from peripheral chemoreceptors, as well as from receptors in the lungs and airways (see above). Some of the RRNs in the DRG are local *interneurons.* Others are *premotor neurons,* projecting directly to various pools of motor neurons—primarily inspiratory—in the spinal cord and ventral respiratory group (Fig. 32.2).

The ventral respiratory group is primarily motor and contains both inspiratory and expiratory neurons

The **ventral respiratory group (VRG)** contains both inspiratory and expiratory neurons. The VRG lies within and around a series of nuclei that form a column of neurons extending from the pons nearly to the spinal cord and is thus considerably longer than the DRG (Fig. 32.2). Like the DRG, the VRG contains local *interneurons* and *premotor* neurons. In contrast to the DRG, the VRG also contains *motor* neurons that innervate muscles of the pharynx and larynx, as well as viscera of the thorax and abdomen. Sensory information related to pulmonary function comes indirectly via the DRG. Thus, the VRG plays more of an efferent role, whereas the DRG primarily plays an afferent role.

The VRG consists of three regions that perform specific functions: (1) The **rostral VRG** or **Bötzinger complex (BötC)** contains *interneurons* that drive the expiratory activity of the caudal region. (2) The **intermediate VRG** contains somatic *motor* neurons whose axons leave the medulla via CN IX and CN X. These fibers supply the pharynx, larynx, and other structures, thus maximizing the caliber of the upper airways during inspiration. The intermediate VRG also contains *premotor* neurons that project to inspiratory motor neurons in the spinal cord and medulla. Within the rostral pole of the intermediate VRG is a group of inspiratory neurons defined as the **pre-Bötzinger complex (preBötC),** which, as we will see below, may be part of the respiratory CPG, contributing to generation of the respiratory rhythm. (3) The **caudal VRG** contains expiratory *premotor* neurons that travel down the spinal cord to synapse on motor neurons that innervate accessory muscles of expiration, such as abdominal and certain intercostal muscles.

The respiratory CPG for eupnea could reside in a single site or in multiple sites, or could emerge from a complex network

Restricted-Site Model A small region in the rostral VRG—the preBötC (Fig. 32.2)—generates rhythmic motor output in the phrenic nerve and hypoglossal nerve (CN XII, which innervates the tongue, an accessory muscle of inspiration). Destroying the preBötC in the isolated brainstem causes respiratory output to cease. These and other experiments led to the hypothesis that the preBötC is the site of the respiratory CPG.

Distributed Oscillator Models A different theory is that there is more than one CPG, any one of which could take over the job of generating the respiratory rhythm, depending on the conditions.

Emergent Property Model The most common early explanation for generation of the respiratory rhythm is that no individual region of the DRG or VRG is sufficient to generate the rhythm but that many of them are necessary. A normal rhythm would require the component neurons in multiple brainstem regions to be "wired up" in a specific way.

Although none of the models we have discussed is universally accepted, some of their elements are not mutually exclusive.

⊙ 32-2 CHEMICAL CONTROL OF VENTILATION

In fulfilling its mission to exchange O_2 and CO_2 between the atmosphere and the capillaries of the systemic circulation, the respiratory system attempts to regulate the blood-gas parameters, that is, the arterial levels of O_2, CO_2, and pH. These are overwhelmingly the most important influences on breathing. The body senses these parameters via two sets of chemoreceptors—the peripheral chemoreceptors and the central chemoreceptors. Hypoxia, hypercapnia, and acidosis all cause an increase in ventilation, which tends to raise P_{O_2}, to lower P_{CO_2}, and to raise pH, thereby correcting deviations in the three blood-gas parameters. Although small variations in arterial P_{CO_2} and P_{O_2} occur with activities such as sleep, exercise, talking, and panting, the control of arterial blood gases is so tight in normal individuals that it is rare for arterial P_{CO_2} to change from the normal 40 mm Hg by more than a few mm Hg. Thus, the peripheral and central chemoreceptors form the vital sensory arm of a negative-feedback mechanism that stabilizes arterial P_{O_2}, P_{CO_2}, and pH.

PERIPHERAL CHEMORECEPTORS

⊙ 32-3 Peripheral chemoreceptors (carotid and aortic bodies) respond to hypoxia, hypercapnia, and acidosis

A decrease in arterial P_{O_2} is the primary stimulus for the peripheral chemoreceptors. Increases in P_{CO_2} and decreases in pH also stimulate these receptors and make them more responsive to hypoxia.

Sensitivity to Decreased Arterial P_{O_2} Perfusion of the carotid body with blood having a low P_{O_2}—but a normal P_{CO_2} and pH—causes a prompt and reversible increase in the firing rate of axons in the carotid sinus nerve. Fig. 32.3A

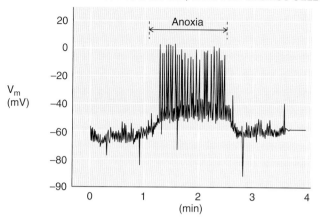

A EFFECT OF ANOXIA ON SINGLE, ISOLATED GLOMUS CELL

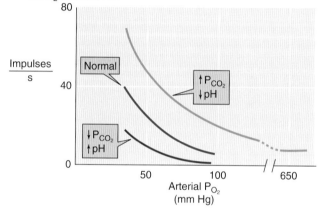

B EFFECT OF RESPIRATORY ACID-BASE DISTURBANCES ON O_2 SENSITIVITY

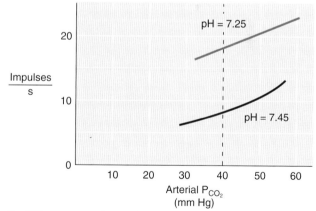

C EFFECT OF pH CHANGES ON CO_2 SENSITIVITY

Fig. 32.3 Chemosensitivity of the carotid body. In (B) and (C), the y-axis represents the frequency of action potentials in single sensory fibers from the carotid body. V_m, Membrane potential. (A, Data from Buckler KJ, Vaughan-Jones RD: Effects of hypoxia on membrane potential and intracellular calcium in rat neonatal carotid body type I cells. J Physiol 476:423–428, 1994; B, data from Cunningham DJC, Robbins PA, Wolff CB: Integration of respiratory responses to changes in alveolar partial pressures of CO_2 and O_2 and in arterial pH. In Cherniack NS, Widdicombe J [eds]: Handbook of Physiology, Section 3: The Respiratory System, vol 2. Bethesda, MD, American Physiological Society, 1986, pp 475–528; C, data from Biscoe TJ, Purves MJ, Sampson SR: The frequency of nerve impulse in single carotid body chemoreceptor afferent fibers recorded in vivo with intact circulation. J Physiol 208:121–131, 1970.)

shows an illustrative experiment on an isolated chemoreceptor cell of the carotid body. Under normal acid-base conditions, increasing P_{O_2} above the normal value of ~100 mm Hg has only trivial effects on the firing rate of the nerve. However, at normal values of P_{CO_2} and pH (Fig. 32.3B, *blue curve*), decreasing P_{O_2} to values <100 mm Hg causes a progressive increase in the firing rate.

Sensitivity to Increased Arterial P_{CO_2} The carotid body can sense hypercapnia in the absence of hypoxia or acidosis. During in vitro experiments, it is possible to maintain a constant extracellular pH (pH_o) while increasing P_{CO_2} by keeping the ratio $[HCO_3^-]/P_{CO_2}$ constant (see ◉ 28-8). The *purple curve* in Fig. 32.3C shows the results of experiments in which graded increases in P_{CO_2}—at a fixed blood pH of 7.45 and a fixed P_{O_2} of 80 mm Hg—produced graded increases in the firing rate of the carotid sinus nerve.

Sensitivity to Decreased Arterial pH ◉ **32-4** The carotid body also can sense acidosis in the absence of hypoxia or hypercapnia. The *green curve* in Fig. 32.3C shows the results of experiments that are the same as those represented by the *purple curve*, except that blood pH was fixed at 7.25 rather than at 7.45. Over the entire range of P_{CO_2} values, the firing rate of the carotid sinus nerve is greater at a pH of 7.25 than at 7.45. Thus, metabolic acidosis (see ◉ 28-6) stimulates the carotid body.

In summary, besides being sensitive to hypoxia, the carotid body is sensitive to *both* components of respiratory acidosis—high P_{CO_2} and low pH. In fact, respiratory acidosis makes the carotid body more sensitive to hypoxia (Fig. 32.3B, *orange curve*), whereas respiratory alkalosis has the opposite effect (Fig. 32.3B, *red curve*).

◉ 32-5 The glomus cell is the chemosensor in the carotid and aortic bodies

The body has two sets of peripheral chemoreceptors: the **carotid bodies,** one located at the bifurcation of each of the common carotid arteries, and the **aortic bodies,** scattered along the underside of the arch of the aorta (Fig. 32.4A). The carotid *bodies* should not be confused with the carotid *sinus*, which is the bulbous initial portion of the internal carotid artery that serves as a *baroreceptor*. Similarly, the aortic *bodies* should not be confused with baroreceptors of the aortic arch.

The major function of the carotid and aortic bodies is to sense hypoxia in the arterial blood and signal cells in the medulla to increase ventilation. This signaling occurs via afferents of the glossopharyngeal nerve (CN IX) for the carotid bodies and of the vagus nerve (CN X) for the aortic bodies.

Aside from their chemosensitivity, three features characterize the carotid bodies. First, they are extremely small: each weighs only ~2 mg. Second, for their size, they receive an extraordinarily high blood flow—the greatest of any tissue in the body. Their blood flow, normalized for weight, is ~40-fold higher than that of the brain. Third, they have a very high metabolic rate, 2- to 3-fold greater than that of the brain. Thus, even though the metabolic rate is high, the blood flow is so much higher that the composition of blood (e.g., P_{O_2}, P_{CO_2}, and pH) in carotid body capillaries approaches that of systemic arteries.

The chemosensitive cells of the carotid body are the type I or **glomus cells.** They are ~10 μm in diameter, are roughly

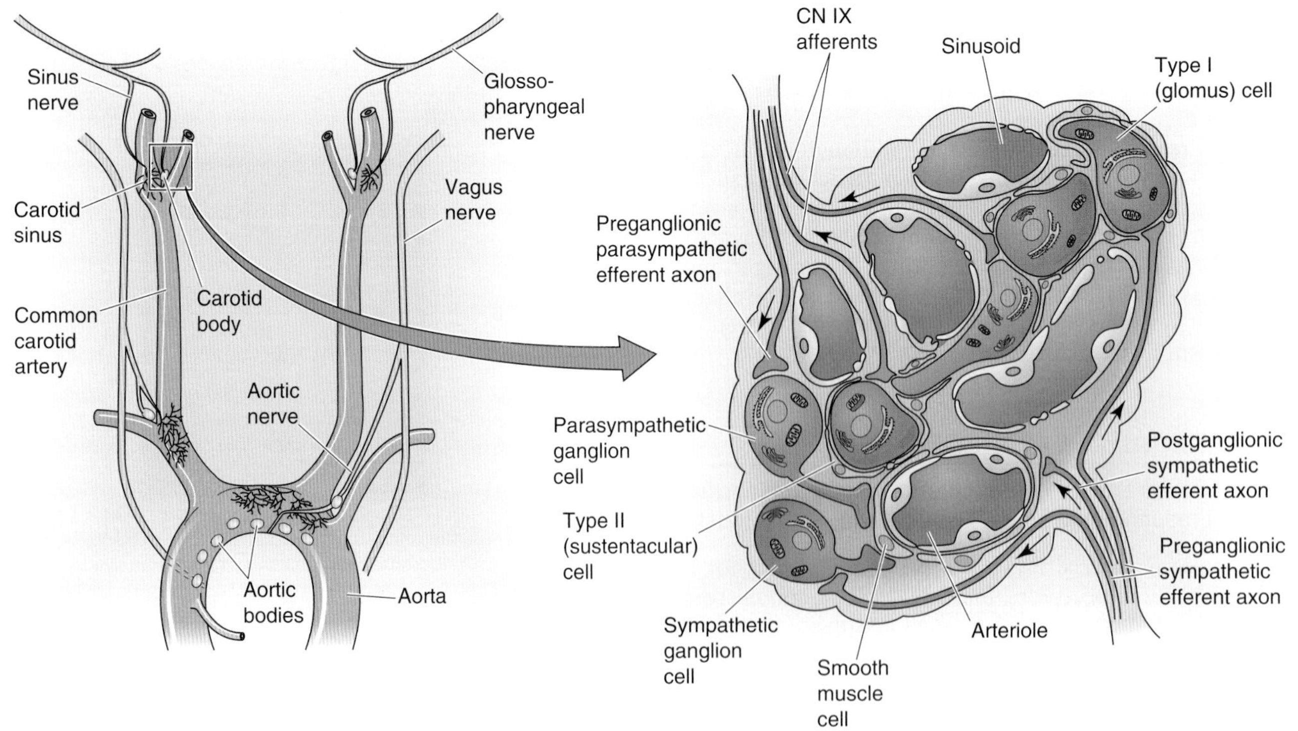

A LOCATION OF CAROTID AND AORTIC BODIES

B MICROSCOPIC ANATOMY OF CAROTID BODY

Fig. 32.4 Anatomy of the peripheral chemoreceptors. (B, Data from Williams PL, Warwick R [eds]: Splanchnology. In Gray's Anatomy. Philadelphia, WB Saunders, 1980.)

spherical, and occur in clusters (Fig. 32.4B). Adjacent glomus cells may communicate with each other via gap junctions. Glomus cells are neuroectodermal in origin and share many characteristics with neurons of the peripheral nervous system as well as with adrenal chromaffin cells (see ◉ 50-8).

Sensory endings of the carotid sinus nerve (a branch of CN IX) impinge on carotid body glomus cells. Neurotransmitter release from the glomus cells triggers action potentials in the carotid sinus nerve, which makes its first synapse on neurons of the NTS (part of the DRG) and thereby signals the medulla that the systemic arterial blood has a low P_{O_2}, a high P_{CO_2}, or a low pH.

Surrounding individual clusters of glomus cells are the type II or **sustentacular cells** (Fig. 32.4B), which are supporting cells similar to glia. Also close to the glomus cells is a dense network of **fenestrated capillaries.** This vascular anatomy as well as the exceptionally high blood flow puts the glomus cells in an ideal position to monitor the arterial blood gases with fidelity.

Hypoxia, hypercapnia, and acidosis inhibit K⁺ channels, raise glomus cell [Ca²⁺]ᵢ, and release neurotransmitters

The sensitivity of the glomus cell to hypoxia, hypercapnia, and acidosis is a special case of chemoreception that we discussed in connection with sensory transduction. It is interesting that one cell type—the glomus cell—is able to sense all three blood-gas parameters. The final common pathway for the response to all three stimuli (Fig. 32.5) is an inhibition of K⁺ channels, depolarization of the glomus cell, possible firing of action potentials, opening of voltage-gated Ca²⁺ channels, an increase in [Ca²⁺]ᵢ, secretion of neurotransmitters, and stimulation of the afferent nerve fiber. What differs among the three pathways is how the stimulus inhibits K⁺ channels.

Hypoxia ◉ **32-6** Investigators have proposed three mechanisms by which low P_{O_2} might inhibit K⁺ channels. First, some evidence suggests that a heme-containing protein responds to a decrease in P_{O_2} by lowering the open probability of closely associated K⁺ channels. Second, in rabbit glomus cells, hypoxia raises [cAMP]ᵢ, which inhibits a cAMP-sensitive K⁺ current. Third, small decreases in P_{O_2} inhibit reduced nicotinamide adenine dinucleotide phosphate oxidase (NADPH oxidase) in mitochondria, thus increasing the ratio of reduced glutathione (GSH) to oxidized glutathione (GSSG; see ◉ 46-5), which directly inhibits certain K⁺ channels. Regardless of how hypoxia inhibits which K⁺ channels, the resulting depolarization activates voltage-gated Ca²⁺ channels.

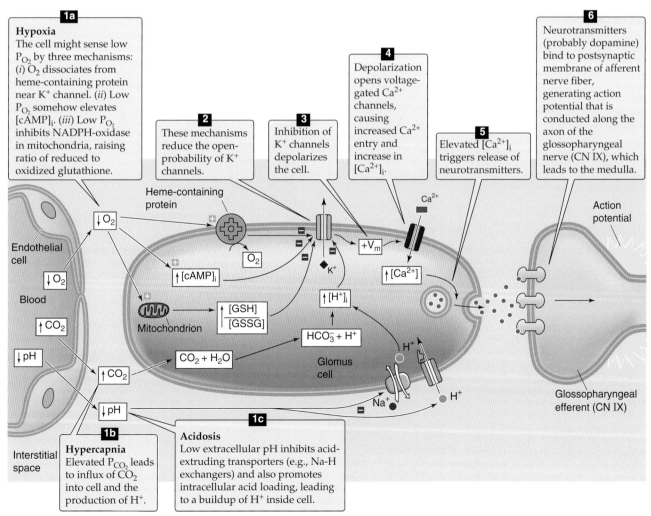

Fig. 32.5 Response of glomus cell to hypoxia, hypercapnia, and acidosis. V_m, Membrane potential.

Hypercapnia An increase in P_{CO_2} causes CO_2 to move into the glomus cell, thereby generating H^+ and leading to a virtually instantaneous fall of intracellular pH (pH_i). As pH_i decreases, the protons appear to inhibit high-conductance K^+ channels. The result is a depolarization, a rise in $[Ca^{2+}]_i$, and the release of neurotransmitter.

Extracellular Acidosis A decrease in pH_o inhibits acid-base transporters that elevate pH_i and stimulates acid-base transporters that lower pH_i, thereby leading to a slow fall in pH_i. Thus, even at a constant P_{CO_2}, extracellular acidosis (i.e., metabolic acidosis) triggers the same cascade of events as was outlined above for hypercapnia, albeit more slowly.

◉ 32-7 CENTRAL CHEMORECEPTORS

When the blood-gas parameters are nearly normal, the central chemoreceptors are the primary source of feedback for assessing the effectiveness of ventilation and also the major source of tonic drive for breathing. Just as the peripheral chemoreceptors are primarily sensitive to arterial hypoxia, the neurons that act as central chemoreceptors are primarily sensitive to arterial *hypercapnia*, which generally presents itself as respiratory acidosis (i.e., a decrease in pH_o brought

about by a rise in P_{CO_2}; see ◉ 28-4). However, the actual parameter sensed appears to be a low pH in or around the chemoreceptor neurons.

The blood-brain barrier separates the central chemoreceptors in the medulla from arterial blood

The primary stimulus driving respiration during respiratory acidosis is not actually an increase in arterial P_{CO_2} but probably the ensuing pH decrease within brain tissue. Most evidence indicates that the central chemoreceptors are at a site within the brain parenchyma that responds to changes both in arterial P_{CO_2} and cerebrospinal fluid (CSF) pH.

If P_{CO_2} increases suddenly, the increase in ventilation begins rapidly, augmenting first the *depth* and later the *frequency* of inspirations. However, the response may take as long as 10 minutes to develop fully (Fig. 32.6A). If, instead, the acid-base disturbance in arterial blood is a *metabolic* acidosis of comparable magnitude (i.e., a decrease in pH_o and $[HCO_3^-]_o$ at a fixed P_{CO_2}; see ◉ 28-6), ventilation increases much more slowly and the steady-state increase is substantially less.

The reason for these observations is that the central chemoreceptors are located within the brain parenchyma (Fig. 32.6B) and are bathed in **brain extracellular fluid (BECF)**,

A EFFECT OF BREATHING CO_2 ON VENTILATION

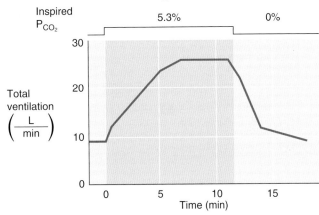

B LOCATION OF CENTRAL CHEMORECEPTOR NEURONS

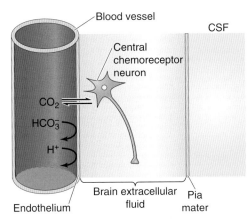

C DEPENDENCE OF CSF pH ON BLOOD pH

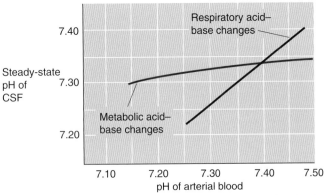

D DEPENDENCE OF VENTILATION ON CSF pH

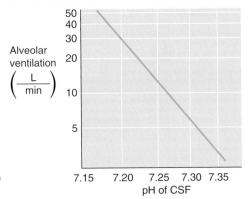

Fig. 32.6 Effect of arterial hypercapnia on brain pH and ventilation. (A, Data from Padget P: The respiratory response to carbon dioxide. Am J Physiol 83:384–389, 1928; B, data from Fencl V: Acid-base balance in cerebral fluids. In Cherniack NS, Widdicombe J [eds]: Handbook of Physiology, Section 3: The Respiratory System, vol 2, part 1. Bethesda, MD, American Physiological Society, 1986, pp 115–140; C, data from Fencl V, Miller TB, Pappenheimer JR: Studies on the respiratory response to disturbances of acid-base balance, with deductions concerning the ionic composition of cerebral interstitial fluid. Am J Physiol 210:459–472, 1966.)

which is separated from arterial blood by the **blood-brain barrier (BBB)**. The BBB has a high permeability to O_2 and CO_2 but a low permeability to ions such as Na^+, Cl^-, H^+, and $[HCO_3^-]_o$ (see ◉ 11-6). An increase in arterial P_{CO_2} rapidly leads to a P_{CO_2} increase of similar magnitude in the BECF, in the CSF, and inside brain cells. The result is an acidosis in each of these compartments.

Although raising arterial P_{CO_2} causes the pH of the BECF and CSF to fall rapidly, the choroid plexus (see ◉ 11-2) and perhaps the BBB partially restore the pH of these compartments by actively transporting HCO_3^- from the blood into the CSF. Thus, after many hours or days of respiratory acidosis in the arterial blood, the low-pH signal in the BECF and CSF gradually wanes. Even so, respiratory acid-base disturbances lead to substantial changes in the steady-state pH of the BECF and CSF (Fig. 32.6C, *purple curve*).

In contrast to its high CO_2 permeability, the BBB's permeability to ions such as H^+ and HCO_3^- is low. For this reason, and because the BBB actively regulates the pH of the BECF and CSF, *metabolic* acid-base disturbances alter steady-state brain pH only 10% to 35% as much as identical blood pH changes during *respiratory* acid-base disturbances (Fig. 32.6C, *red curve*). Therefore, ventilation is much less sensitive to changes in arterial pH and $[HCO_3^-]$ at constant arterial P_{CO_2}. Ventilation correlates uniquely with the pH of the BECF (Fig. 32.6D), regardless of whether respiratory or metabolic acid-base disturbances produce the pH changes.

◉ 32-8 Central chemoreceptors are located in the ventrolateral medulla and other brainstem regions

Early work on central chemoreceptors by Hans Loeschcke, Marianne Schläfke, and Robert Mitchell identified candidate regions near the surface of the **ventrolateral medulla (VLM;** Fig. 32.7). The application of acidic solutions to the rostral or caudal VLM leads to a prompt increase in ventilation. This and other work led to the conclusion that *the* central chemoreceptors are located near the surface of the VLM.

More recent work with brain slices and cultured cells show that acidosis stimulates neurons in many brainstem nuclei, including the medullary raphé (Fig. 32.7, inset) and the NTS—both in the medulla—as well as the locus coeruleus and hypothalamus. Multiple sensors may be another example of redundancy in a critical system. Alternatively,

some may come into play only under special circumstances, such as during severe acid-base disturbances or during sleep, when airway obstruction leads to arousal.

Some neurons of the medullary raphé and VLM are unusually pH sensitive

Certain medullary raphé neurons are unusually pH sensitive. In brain slices and in tissue culture, small decreases in extracellular pH raise the firing rate of one subset of medullary raphé neurons (Fig. 32.7) and lower the firing rate of another. In both types of chemosensitive neurons, metabolic and respiratory disturbances have similar effects on firing, which indicates that the primary stimulus is a decrease in either extracellular or intracellular pH, rather than an increase in P_{CO_2}.

Serotonergic neurons of the raphé and VLM have many properties that would be expected of central respiratory chemoreceptors. Many infants who have died of **sudden infant death syndrome (SIDS)** have a deficit of serotonergic neurons, which is consistent with a prevailing theory that a subset of SIDS infants have a defect in central respiratory chemoreception.

INTEGRATED RESPONSES TO HYPOXIA, HYPERCAPNIA, AND ACIDOSIS

In real life, it is rare for arterial P_{O_2} to fall without accompanying changes in P_{CO_2} and pH. In addition, changes in individual blood-gas parameters may independently affect both the peripheral and the central chemoreceptors. How does the respiratory system as a whole respond to changes in multiple blood-gas parameters?

Hypoxia accentuates the acute response to respiratory acidosis

Respiratory Acidosis When the blood-gas parameters are nearly normal, respiratory acidosis (increased P_{CO_2}/decreased pH) stimulates ventilation more than does hypoxia. If an animal breathes an air mixture containing CO_2, the resultant respiratory acidosis causes ventilation to increase rapidly. Because both peripheral and central chemoreceptors respond to respiratory acidosis, both could contribute to the

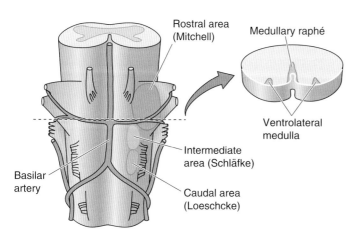

Fig. 32.7 Chemosensitive neurons in the VLM and raphé. The figure shows a ventral view of a cat medulla showing chemosensitive areas named after the three physiologists who first described them. The slice to the *right* shows the location of serotonergic neurons in the VLM and medullary raphé nuclei. (Data from Dermietzel R: Central chemosensitivity, morphological studies. In Loeschke HL [ed]: Acid-base Homeostasis of the Brain Extracellular Fluid and the Respiratory Control System. Stuttgart, Germany, Thieme Edition/Publishing Sciences Group, 1976, pp 52–66.)

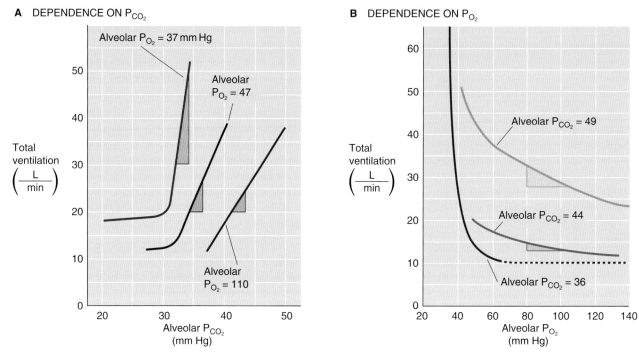

Fig. 32.8 Integrated ventilatory response to changes in P_{CO_2} (A) and P_{O_2} (B). The *shaded triangles* indicate the slopes. (A, Data from Nielsen M, Smith H: Studies on the regulation of respiration in acute hypoxia. Acta Physiol Scand 24:293–313, 1952; B, data from Loeschcke HH, Gertz KH: Einfluss des O_2-Druckes in der Ein-atmungsluft auf die Atemtätigkeit der Menschen, geprüft unter Konstanthaltung des alveolaren CO_2-Druckes. Pflugers Arch Ges Physiol 267:460–477, 1958.)

response. It appears that the central chemoreceptors account for 65% to 80% of the integrated response to respiratory acidosis under normoxic conditions. However, the response of the peripheral chemoreceptors is considerably more rapid than that of the central chemoreceptors, which require several minutes to develop a maximal response.

At an alveolar P_{O_2} that is somewhat higher than normal, raising the alveolar P_{CO_2} causes a linear increase in steady-state ventilation (Fig. 32.8A, *red curve*). Lowering the alveolar P_{O_2} has two effects (Fig. 32.8A, *other two curves*). First, at a given P_{CO_2}, hypoxia increases ventilation, which reflects the response of the peripheral chemoreceptors to hypoxia. Second, hypoxia increases the *sensitivity* of the integrated response to respiratory acidosis. That is, the slopes of the curves increase.

Metabolic Acidosis Severe metabolic acidosis (e.g., diabetic ketoacidosis) leads to profound hyperventilation, known as **Kussmaul breathing.** This hyperventilation can drive arterial P_{CO_2} down to low levels in an attempt to compensate for the metabolic acidosis. Acutely, the main stimulus for hyperventilation comes from peripheral chemoreceptors. Because a severe decrease in arterial pH does produce a small fall in CSF pH, central chemoreceptors also participate in this response. If the insult persists for many hours, CSF pH falls even farther, and central chemoreceptor drive becomes more prominent.

Respiratory acidosis accentuates the acute response to hypoxia

At an arterial P_{CO_2} that is slightly lower than normal, lowering alveolar P_{O_2} has very little effect on ventilation until P_{O_2} falls below 50 mm Hg (Fig. 32.8B, *red curve*).

The eventual response at very low P_{O_2} values indicates that the peripheral chemoreceptors play a vital, fail-safe role in responding to extreme hypoxia, as at high altitudes. Raising the arterial P_{CO_2} (i.e., respiratory acidosis) has two effects (Fig. 32.8B, *other two curves*). First, at a given P_{O_2}, respiratory acidosis increases ventilation, which reflects the dual contributions of the peripheral and central chemoreceptors to hypercapnia and acidosis. Second, respiratory acidosis increases the *sensitivity* of the integrated response to hypoxia. That is, the curves become steeper.

MODULATION OF VENTILATORY CONTROL

The major parameters that feedback on the respiratory control system are the arterial blood-gas parameters—P_{O_2}, P_{CO_2}, and pH. In addition, the respiratory system receives input from two other major sources: (1) a variety of stretch and chemical/irritant receptors that monitor the size of the airways and the presence of noxious agents, and (2) higher CNS centers that modulate respiration during nonrespiratory activities.

Stretch and chemical/irritant receptors in the airways and lung parenchyma provide feedback about lung volume and the presence of irritants

Sensors within the lungs and upper airways detect foreign bodies, chemical irritants, or immunological challenges and help protect the lungs—one of the few organs that have direct access to the outside world. Sensors also detect changes in lung volume as part of a feedback mechanism that helps control output to respiratory muscles. Respiratory afferent fibers from sensors in the thorax travel with CN X, and those from sensors in the upper airways travel with CN IX. Both synapse within the DRG in the medulla (see ⊙ 32-1).

Higher brain centers coordinate ventilation with other behaviors and can override the brainstem's control of breathing

The role of the CNS in controlling ventilation is far more complex than generating a regular pattern of inspirations and expirations, and then modifying this pattern in response to input from mechanical and chemical sensors (Box 32.1). The CNS also must balance the need to control P_{O_2}, P_{CO_2}, and pH with the need to control ventilation for nonrespiratory purposes, such as speaking and sniffing. In addition, the CNS must coordinate breathing with behaviors that require the *absence* of airflow, such as chewing, swallowing, and vomiting.

Coordination with Voluntary Behaviors That Use Respiratory Muscles Numerous voluntary actions initiated in the cerebral cortex involve a change in airflow—voluntarily hyperventilating, breath holding, speaking, singing, whistling, and playing musical wind instruments. Although voluntary control over muscles of respiration can be exquisitely precise, this control is not absolute. For example, voluntary breath holding can last only so long before being overwhelmed by ventilatory drive from chemoreceptors. The cerebral cortex controls the respiratory system by at least two major mechanisms. First, some cortical neurons send axons to respiratory centers in the medulla. Second, some cortical premotor neurons send axons to motor neurons that control muscles of respiration. One consequence of this dual control mechanism is that lesions in specific areas of the cerebral cortex can abolish voluntary breath holding, a condition known as **respiratory apraxia.**

Coordination with Complex Nonventilatory Behaviors One of the jobs of the brain is to coordinate complex behaviors such as yawning, chewing, swallowing, sucking, defecating, grunting, and vomiting. During yawning and vomiting, for example, groups of neurons orchestrate an array of simultaneous actions, only some involving the respiratory system. The premotor neurons that project from medullary respiratory centers to respiratory motor neurons are probably distinct from descending pathways involved in these complex nonventilatory behaviors.

Modification by Affective States Fear, horror, rage, and passion can be associated with major and highly characteristic changes in the respiratory pattern. For example, if a child runs in front of the car you are driving, the sudden application of the brakes is almost always accompanied by an equally sudden and rapid inspiration, with mouth open widely, increasing lung volume to nearly total lung capacity. The tendency of prevarications to be associated with changes in the breathing pattern is the basis for one part of the polygraph test used as a **lie detector.** Descending pathways from the limbic system (see ⊙ 14-12) of the forebrain may mediate these emotional effects on breathing.

BOX 32.1 Sighs, Yawns, Coughs, and Sneezes

The respiratory apparatus engages in a variety of motor behaviors that help maintain normal lung function and gas exchange by protecting the alveoli from collapse or preventing obstruction of the upper airways.

Sigh or "Augmented Breath"
A sigh is a slow and deep inspiration, held for just a moment, followed by a longer-than-normal expiratory period. A normal person sighs ~6 times per hour. Local collapse of alveoli (atelectasis) may initiate a sigh, which is an important mechanism for stimulating release of surfactant (see ⊙ 27-5) and thus reopening these alveoli. Hypoxia and respiratory acidosis increase sigh frequency, consistent with the idea that sighs counteract decreased alveolar ventilation.

Yawn
An exaggerated sigh, a yawn takes lung volume to total lung capacity for several seconds. The mouth is fully open. In the extreme case, the arms are stretched upward, the neck is extended to elevate the pectoral girdle, and the back is extended—maneuvers that maximize lung volume (see ⊙ 26-5). Yawning is even more effective than sighing in opening up the most resistant atelectatic alveoli. Yawns may (1) minimize atelectasis as one prepares for sleep, and (2) reverse—on arousal—the atelectasis that has accumulated during sleep.

Cough Reflex ⊙ 32-9
Coughing is important for ridding the tracheobronchial tree of inhaled foreign substances. There is probably no single class of "cough receptors." The tickling sensation that is relieved by a cough is analogous to the cutaneous itch and is probably mediated by C-fiber receptors. *Thus, a cough is a respiratory scratch.*

When *lower airway* receptors trigger a cough, it begins with a small inspiration that increases the coughing force. Mechanosensitive and irritant receptors in the *larynx* can trigger either coughing or apnea. When they trigger a cough, the inspiration is absent, which minimizes the chances that the offending foreign body will be pulled deeper into the lungs. In either case, a forced expiratory effort against a closed glottis raises intrathoracic and intra-abdominal pressures to very high levels. The glottis then opens suddenly, and the pressure inside the larynx falls almost instantaneously to near-atmospheric levels. This sudden drop in luminal pressure produces dramatic increases in the *axial* (alveolus to trachea) pressure gradient that drives air flow (see ⊙ 27-6).

Sneeze
Sensors in the nose detect irritants and can evoke a sneeze. A sneeze differs from a cough in that a sneeze is almost always preceded by a deep inspiration. Like a cough, a sneeze involves an initial buildup of intrathoracic pressure behind a closed glottis. Unlike a cough, a sneeze involves pharyngeal constriction during the buildup phase and an explosive forced expiration through the nose as well as the mouth. This expiration is accompanied by contraction of facial and nasal muscles, so that the effect is to dislodge foreign bodies from the nasal mucosa.

THE URINARY SYSTEM

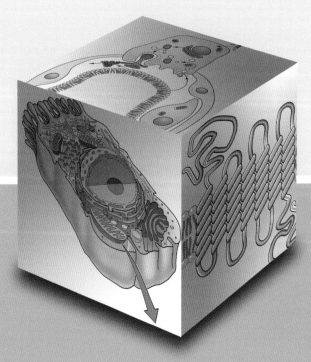

CHAPTER 33

ORGANIZATION OF THE URINARY SYSTEM

Gerhard Giebisch[†] and Peter S. Aronson

The kidneys serve three essential functions. First, they act as filters, removing metabolic products and toxins from the blood and excreting them through the urine. Second, they regulate the body's fluid status, electrolyte balance, and acid-base balance. Third, the kidneys produce or activate hormones that are involved in erythrogenesis, Ca^{2+} metabolism, and the regulation of blood pressure and blood flow.

FUNCTIONAL ANATOMY OF THE KIDNEY

We begin this discussion with a macroscopic view and progress to the microscopic level as we describe the **nephron,** the functional unit of the kidney that is repeated approximately 1 million times within each kidney.

The kidneys are paired, retroperitoneal organs with vascular and epithelial elements

The human kidneys are paired, bean-shaped structures that lie behind the peritoneum on each side of the vertebral column (Fig. 33.1A). They extend from the twelfth thoracic vertebra to the third lumbar vertebra. In men, each kidney weighs 125 to 170 g, whereas in women, each kidney weighs 115 to 155 g.

A fibrous, almost nondistensible capsule covers each kidney (Fig. 33.1B). In the middle of the concave surface, a slit in the capsule—the **hilus**—serves as the port of entry for the renal artery and nerves and as the site of exit for the renal vein, the lymphatics, and the ureter. The hilus opens into a shallow space called the **renal sinus,** which includes the urine-filled spaces: the **renal pelvis** proper and its extensions, the **major** and the **minor calyces.** Blood vessels and nerves also pass through the sinus.

A section of the kidney (Fig. 33.1B) reveals two basic layers, the cortex (granular outer region) and the medulla (darker inner region). The granularity of the **cortex** results from the presence of glomeruli, microscopic tufts of capillaries, and a large number of highly convoluted epithelial structures in the form of tubules. The **medulla** lacks glomeruli and consists of a parallel arrangement of tubules and small blood vessels.

The medulla is subdivided into 8 to 18 conical **renal pyramids,** whose bases face the cortical-medullary border; the tip of each pyramid terminates in the renal pelvis. At the

tip of each pyramid are perforations, almost invisible to the naked eye, through which urine flows into the minor calyces of the renal sinus.

The kidneys have a very high blood flow and glomerular capillaries flanked by afferent and efferent arterioles

The kidneys receive ~20% of the cardiac output. The renal circulation has a unique sequence of vascular elements: a high-resistance arteriole (the afferent arteriole), followed by a high-pressure glomerular capillary network for filtration, followed by a second high-resistance arteriole (the efferent arteriole), followed by a low-pressure capillary network that surrounds the renal tubules (peritubular capillaries).

The main features of the renal vascular system are illustrated in Fig. 33.1B and C. For nephrons in the *superficial* portion of the cortex, the efferent arterioles are the origin of a dense peritubular capillary network that supplies oxygen and nutrients to the tubules in the cortex.

The efferent arterioles of *juxtamedullary* glomeruli descend into the renal papillae to form hairpin-shaped vessels called the **vasa recta,** which provide capillary networks for tubules in the medulla. Some 90% of the blood entering the kidney perfuses superficial glomeruli and cortex; only ~10% perfuses juxtamedullary glomeruli and medulla.

The functional unit of the kidney is the nephron

Each kidney consists of 800,000 to 1,200,000 nephrons, each an independent entity until the point at which its initial collecting tubule merges with another tubule (Fig. 33.2).

A nephron consists of a glomerulus and a tubule. The **glomerulus** is a cluster of blood vessels from which the plasma filtrate originates. The **tubule** is an epithelial structure consisting of many subdivisions, designed to convert the filtrate into urine. **Bowman's capsule** or the **glomerular capsule** surrounds the glomerulus and contains **Bowman's space,** which is contiguous with the lumen of the tubule. It is here that filtrate passes from the vascular system into the tubule system.

The remainder of the nephron consists of subdivisions of the tubule (Fig. 33.2). The epithelial elements of the nephron include Bowman's capsule, the proximal tubule, thin descending and thin ascending limbs of the loop of Henle, thick ascending limb of the loop of Henle, distal convoluted tubule, and connecting tubule. The connecting tubule leads

---

[†]Deceased.

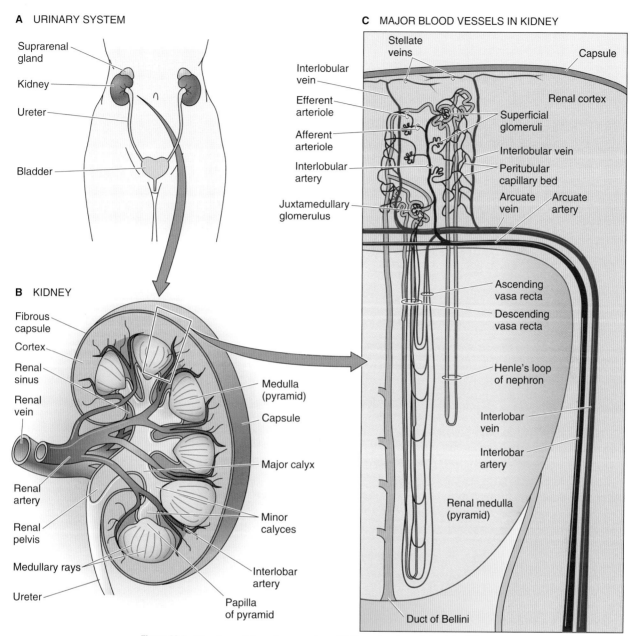

A URINARY SYSTEM

Suprarenal gland
Kidney
Ureter
Bladder

B KIDNEY

Fibrous capsule
Cortex
Renal sinus
Renal vein
Renal artery
Renal pelvis
Medullary rays
Ureter
Medulla (pyramid)
Capsule
Major calyx
Minor calyces
Interlobar artery
Papilla of pyramid

C MAJOR BLOOD VESSELS IN KIDNEY

Stellate veins
Interlobular vein
Efferent arteriole
Afferent arteriole
Interlobular artery
Juxtamedullary glomerulus
Capsule
Renal cortex
Superficial glomeruli
Interlobular vein
Peritubular capillary bed
Arcuate vein
Arcuate artery
Ascending vasa recta
Descending vasa recta
Henle's loop of nephron
Interlobar vein
Interlobar artery
Renal medulla (pyramid)
Duct of Bellini

Figure 33.1 Structure of the urinary system. (B) Posterior view of the right kidney.

further into the initial collecting tubule, the cortical collecting tubule, and medullary collecting ducts.

Within the renal cortex, one can distinguish two populations of nephrons (Fig. 33.2). **Superficial nephrons** have short loops extending to the boundary between outer and inner medulla. **Juxtamedullary nephrons,** which play a special role in the production of a concentrated urine, have long loops that extend as far as the tip of the medulla.

The renal corpuscle has three components: vascular elements, the mesangium, and Bowman's capsule and space

The **renal corpuscle,** the site of formation of the glomerular filtrate, comprises a glomerulus, Bowman's space, and Bowman's capsule (Fig. 33.3A).

In the kidney, foot processes of the podocytes (Fig. 33.3A) cover the glomerular capillaries. Glomerular filtrate drains into Bowman's space and flows into the proximal tubule at the urinary pole of the renal corpuscle.

The **glomerular filtration barrier** between the glomerular capillary lumen and Bowman's space comprises four elements with different functional properties (Fig. 33.3B): (1) a glycocalyx covering the luminal surface of endothelial cells, (2) the endothelial cells, (3) the glomerular basement membrane, and (4) epithelial podocytes.

The **glycocalyx** consists of negatively charged glycosaminoglycans that may play a role in preventing leakage of large negatively charged macromolecules.

The endothelial cells of the glomerular capillaries are almost completely surrounded by the glomerular basement membrane and a layer of **podocyte foot processes**

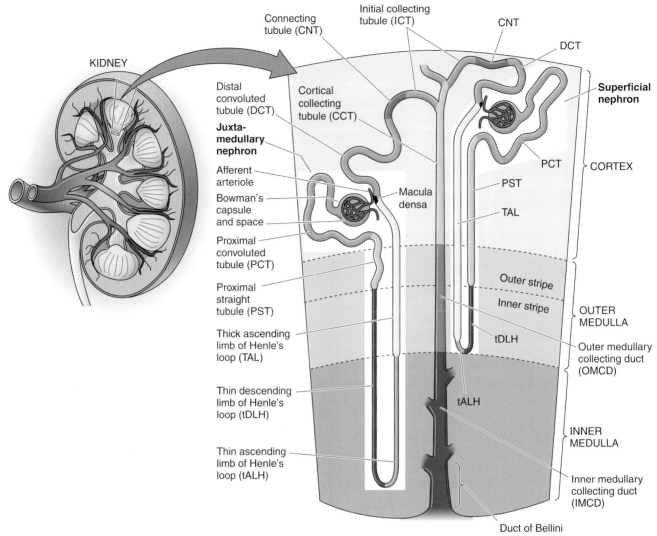

Figure 33.2 Structure of the nephron.

(Fig. 33.4). Filtration occurs at the peripheral portion of the capillary wall, which is covered with basement membrane and podocytes. The **endothelial cells** contain large **fenestrations,** 70-nm holes that provide no restriction to the movement of water and small solutes—including proteins or other large molecules—out of the lumen of the capillary.

The **basement membrane,** located between endothelial cells and podocyte foot processes (Fig. 33.3B), separates the endothelial layer from the epithelial layer in all parts of the glomerular tuft. The basement membrane makes an important contribution to the permeability characteristics of the filtration barrier by restricting intermediate-sized to large solutes (molecular weight > 1 kDa). Because the basement membrane contains **heparan sulfate proteoglycans (HSPGs),** it especially restricts large, negatively charged solutes (see Fig. 34.3).

Podocytes have interdigitating foot processes that cover the basement membrane (Fig. 33.4). Between these interdigitations (the nose-like structures in Fig. 33.3B) are **filtration slits** (Fig. 33.3C); the interdigitations are connected by thin diaphragmatic structures—the **slit diaphragms**—with pores ranging in size from 4 to 14 nm. Glycoproteins with negative charges cover the podocyte bodies, the interdigitations,

and the slit diaphragms. These negative charges contribute to the restriction of filtration of large anions (see Fig. 34.3). The extracellular domains of the integral membrane proteins **nephrin** and **NEPH1** from adjacent podocytes appear to zip together to help form the slit diaphragm. **Podocin** and other proteins also contribute to the slit diaphragm (Fig. 33.3D).

◉ **33-1** Supporting the glomerular capillary loops is a network of contractile **mesangial cells,** which secrete the extracellular matrix. This network is continuous with the smooth-muscle cells of the afferent and efferent arterioles. The matrix extends to the "extraglomerular" mesangial cells (Fig. 33.3A). The **juxtaglomerular apparatus (JGA)** includes the extraglomerular mesangial cells, the macula densa, and the granular cells. The **macula densa** (from the Latin *macula* [spot] + *densa* [dense]) is a patch of specialized tubule epithelial cells—at the transition between the TAL and the distal tubule—that contacts its own glomerulus (Fig. 33.3A). The **granular cells** in the wall of afferent arterioles, also called juxtaglomerular cells, are specialized smooth-muscle cells that produce, store, and release the enzyme renin (see ◉ **40-3**). The JGA is part of a complex feedback mechanism that regulates renal blood flow and filtration rate,

A GLOMERULUS AND BOWMAN'S CAPSULE

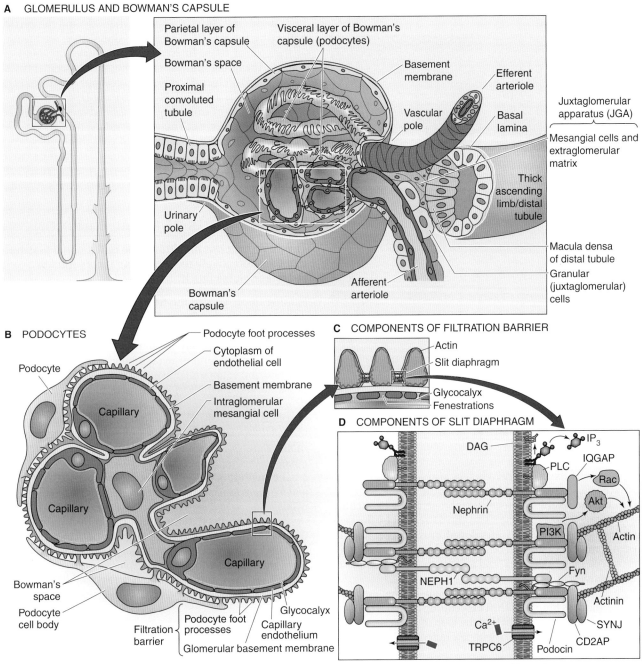

Figure 33.3 Glomerulus and Bowman's capsule, with podocytes and slit diaphragm. *Akt,* Protein kinase B; *CD2AP,* CD2-associated protein; *DAG,* diacylglycerol; *Fyn,* a Src kinase; *IP₃,* inositol 1,4,5-trisphosphate; *IQ-GAP,* IQ motif containing GTPase activating protein; *NEPH1,* member 1 of the NEPH protein family, interacts with nephrin; *PI3K,* phosphatidylinositol 3-kinase; *PLC,* phospholipase C; *Rac,* a GTPase; *SYNJ,* synaptojanin; *TRPC6,* transient receptor potential cation channel, subfamily C, member 6. (C and D, modified from Zenker M, Machuca E, Antignac C: Genetics of nephrotic syndrome: New insights into molecules acting at the glomerular filtration barrier. *J Mol Med* 87:849–857, 2009.)

and it also indirectly modulates Na⁺ balance and systemic blood pressure.

The tubule components of the nephron include the proximal tubule, loop of Henle, distal tubule, and collecting duct

Fig. 33.5 illustrates the ultrastructure of the cells of the different tubule segments. Table 33.1 lists these segments and

their abbreviations. The proximal tubule can be subdivided into three segments: S1, S2, and S3. The S1 segment starts at the glomerulus and includes the first portion of the PCT. The S2 segment starts in the second half of the PCT and continues into the first half of the PST. Finally, the S3 segment includes the distal half of the PST that extends into the medulla.

Both the apical (luminal) and basolateral (peritubular) membranes of proximal-tubule cells are extensively amplified

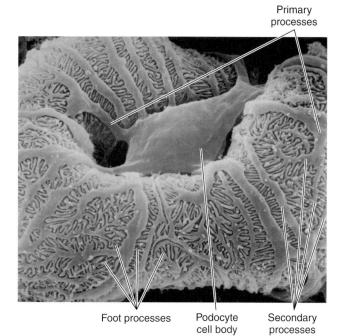

Primary processes

Foot processes   Podocyte cell body   Secondary processes

Figure 33.4 Glomerular capillary covered by the foot processes of podocytes. This scanning electron micrograph shows a view of glomerular capillary from the vantage point of Bowman's space.

(Fig. 33.5A and B). The apical membrane has infoldings in the form of a well-developed *brush border.*

The *basolateral membranes* of proximal-tubule cells form numerous interdigitations, bringing abundant mitochondria in close contact with the plasma membrane. The interdigitations of the lateral membranes also form an extensive extracellular compartment bounded by the tight junctions at one end and by the basement membrane of the epithelium at the other end. From the S1 to the S3 segments, the cells exhibit a progressively less developed brush border, diminished complexity of lateral cell interdigitations, a lower basolateral cell membrane area, and a decrease in the number of mitochondria.

In comparison with the S3 segment of the proximal tubule, the cells lining the **thin descending limb (tDLH)** and **thin ascending limb (tALH)** of the loop of Henle are far less complex (Fig. 33.5C and D), with few mitochondria and little cell membrane amplification.

Epithelial cells lining the **thick ascending limb** of the loop of Henle (TAL), which terminates at the macula densa, are characterized by tall interdigitations and numerous mitochondria within extensively invaginated basolateral membranes (Fig. 33.5E).

We subdivide the distal tubule into three segments: the distal convoluted tubule (starting at the macula densa), the connecting tubule, and the initial collecting tubule.

The **distal convoluted tubule (DCT)** begins at the macula densa and ends at the transition to the connecting tubule (Fig. 33.5F). The cells of the DCT are similar in structure to those of the thick ascending limb.

The **connecting tubule (CNT),** which ends at the transition to the initial collecting tubule, consists of two cell types: CNT cells and intercalated cells (Fig. 33.5G).

The two segments following the CNT, the **initial collecting tubule (ICT,** up to the first confluence) and the **cortical collecting tubule (CCT,** after the confluence), are identical at the cellular level. **Intercalated cells** make up about one third of the lining of these collecting-tubule segments (Fig. 33.5H and I). **Principal cells** make up about two thirds of the cells of the ICT and CCT (Fig. 33.5H and I).

The **medullary collecting duct** is lined mostly by one cell type that increases in cell height toward the papilla (Fig. 33.5J and K). The number of intercalated cells diminishes beginning at the outer medullary collecting duct. At the extreme end of the medullary collecting duct (i.e., the "papillary" collecting duct or duct of Bellini), the cells are extremely tall.

MAIN ELEMENTS OF RENAL FUNCTION

The nephron forms an ultrafiltrate of the blood plasma and then selectively reabsorbs the tubule fluid or secretes solutes into it

Starling forces govern the flow of fluid across the capillary walls in the **glomerulus** and result in net filtration. In glomerular capillaries, the filtrate flows into Bowman's space, which is contiguous with the lumen of the proximal tubule.

The main function of renal tubules is to recover most of the fluid and solutes filtered at the glomerulus. The retrieval of the largest fraction of glomerular filtrate occurs in the **proximal tubule,** which *reabsorbs* NaCl, NaHCO$_3$, filtered nutrients (e.g., glucose and amino acids), divalent ions (e.g., Ca^{2+}, HPO$_4^{2-}$, and SO$_4^{2-}$), and water. Finally, the proximal tubule *secretes* NH$_4^+$ and a variety of endogenous and exogenous solutes into the lumen.

The main function of the **loop of Henle**—tDLH, tALH, and TAL—is to participate in forming concentrated or dilute urine.

The classic **distal tubule** and the **collecting-duct system** perform the fine control of salt and water excretion. Although only small fractions of the glomerular filtrate reach these most distally located nephron sites, these tubule segments are where several hormones (e.g., aldosterone, arginine vasopressin) exert their main effects on electrolyte and water excretion.

The JGA is a region where each thick ascending limb contacts its glomerulus

Elements of the JGA play two important regulatory roles. First, if the amount of fluid and NaCl reaching a nephron's **macula densa** (Fig. 33.3F) increases, the glomerular filtration rate of *that nephron* falls. We discuss this phenomenon of **tubuloglomerular feedback** in Chapter 34 (see ⦿ 34-6).

The second regulatory mechanism comes into play during a decrease in the pressure of the renal artery feeding the various afferent arterioles. When the baroreceptor in the afferent arteriole senses decreased stretch in the arteriole wall, it directs neighboring granular cells to increase their release of **renin** into the general circulation. The renin-angiotensin-aldosterone axis is important in the long-term control of **systemic arterial blood pressure** (see ⦿ 40-2).

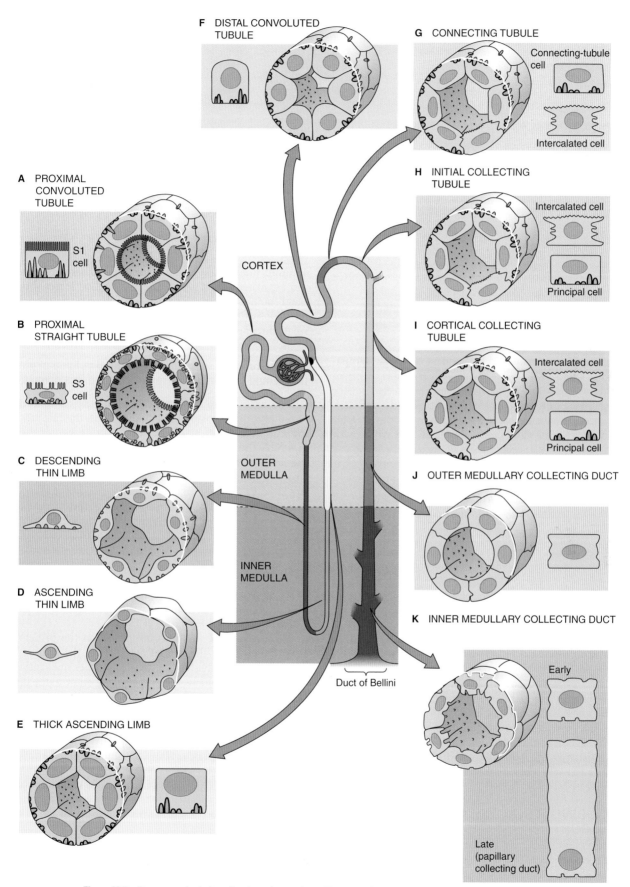

Figure 33.5 Structure of tubule cells along the nephron. Because of the wide range of tubule diameters along the nephron, the scaling factors for tubule cross sections differ for panels (A) to (K). However, the individual cells next to the tubule cross sections are drawn to the same scale.

TABLE 33.1 Tubule Segments of the Nephron

TUBULE SEGMENT	ABBREVIATION
Proximal convoluted tubule	PCT
Proximal straight tubule	PST
Thin descending limb of loop of Henle	tDLH
Thin ascending limb of loop of Henle	tALH
Thick ascending limb of loop of Henle	TAL
Distal convoluted tubule	DCT
Connecting tubule	CNT
Initial collecting tubule	ICT
Cortical collecting tubule	CCT
Outer medullary collecting duct	OMCD
Inner medullary collecting duct	IMCD

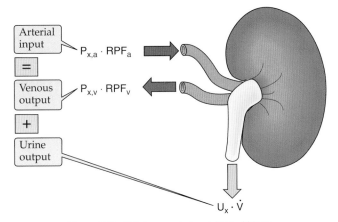

Figure 33.6   Solute mass balance in the kidney.

Sympathetic nerve fibers to the kidney regulate renal blood flow, glomerular filtration, and tubule reabsorption

The autonomic innervation to the kidneys is entirely **sympathetic;** the kidneys lack parasympathetic nerve fibers. Sympathetic stimulation to the kidneys has three major effects. First, the catecholamines cause vasoconstriction. Second, the catecholamines strongly enhance Na^+ reabsorption by proximal-tubule cells. Third, as a result of the dense accumulation of sympathetic fibers near the granular cells of the JGA, increased sympathetic nerve activity dramatically stimulates renin secretion.

The kidneys, as endocrine organs, produce renin, 1,25-dihydroxyvitamin D, erythropoietin, prostaglandins, and bradykinin

Besides **renin** production by the JGA granular cells, the kidneys play several other endocrine roles. Proximal-tubule cells convert circulating 25-hydroxyvitamin D to the active metabolite, **1,25-dihydroxyvitamin D.** This hormone controls Ca^{2+} and phosphorus metabolism and is important for developing and maintaining bone structure.

Fibroblast-like cells in the cortex and outer medulla secrete **erythropoietin (EPO)** in response to a fall in the local tissue P_{O_2}. EPO stimulates the development of red blood cells by action on hematopoietic stem cells in bone marrow. In chronic renal failure, the deficiency of EPO leads to severe anemia that can be treated with recombinant EPO.

The kidney releases **prostaglandins** and several **kinins,** paracrine agents that control circulation within the kidney. These substances are generally vasodilators and may play a protective role when renal blood flow is compromised.

MEASURING RENAL CLEARANCE AND TRANSPORT

This subchapter focuses on clearance measurements, which compare the rate at which the glomeruli filter a substance (water or a solute) with the rate at which the kidneys excrete it into the urine. By measuring the difference between the amounts filtered and excreted for a particular substance, we can estimate the net amount reabsorbed or secreted by the renal tubules and can thus gain insight into the three basic functions of the kidney: glomerular **filtration,** tubule **reabsorption,** and tubule **secretion.**

The clearance of a solute is the virtual volume of plasma that would be totally cleared of a solute in a given time

All solutes excreted into the urine ultimately come from the blood plasma perfusing the kidneys. Thus, the rate at which the kidney excretes a solute into the urine equals the rate at which the solute disappears from the plasma, provided the kidney does not produce, consume, or store the solute. Imagine that, in 1 minute, 700 mL of plasma flow through the kidneys. This plasma contains 0.7 L × 142 mM or ~100 mmol of Na^+. Of this Na^+, the kidneys remove and excrete into the urine only a tiny amount, ~0.14 mmol. In principle, these 0.14 mmol of Na^+ could have come from only 1 mL of plasma, had all Na^+ ions been removed (i.e., cleared) from this volume. The **clearance** of a solute is the virtual volume of blood plasma (per unit time) needed to supply the amount of solute that appears in the urine. Thus, in our example, Na^+ clearance was 1 mL/min, even though 700 mL of plasma flowed through the kidneys.

Renal clearance methods are based on the principle of mass balance and the special anatomy of the kidney (Fig. 33.6). For any solute (X) that the kidney does not synthesize, degrade, or accumulate, the only route of entry to the kidney is the renal artery, and the only two routes of exit are the renal vein and the ureter. Because the input of X equals the output of X, $P_{X,a}$ and $P_{X,v}$ are plasma concentrations of X in the renal artery and renal vein, respectively. RPF_a and RPF_v are rates of **renal plasma flow (RPF)** in the renal artery and vein, respectively. U_X is the concentration of X in urine. $\dot{V}$ is urine flow (the overdot represents the time derivative of volume). The product $U_X \cdot \dot{V}$ is the **urinary excretion rate,** the amount of X excreted in urine per unit time.

$$\underbrace{\underset{\frac{mmole}{mL}}{P_{X,a}} \cdot \underset{\frac{mL}{min}}{RPF_a}}_{\text{Arterial input of X}} = \underbrace{\left(\underset{\frac{mmole}{mL}}{P_{X,v}} \cdot \underset{\frac{mL}{min}}{RPF_v} \right)}_{\text{Venous output of X}} + \underbrace{\left(\underset{\frac{mmole}{mL}}{U_X} \cdot \underset{\frac{mL}{min}}{\dot{V}} \right)}_{\text{Urine output of X}} \quad \textbf{(33.1)}$$

In developing the concept of renal clearance, we transform Equation 33.1 in two ways, both based on the assumption that the kidneys clear all X from an incoming volume of arterial plasma. First, we replace RPF_a with the inflow of the virtual volume—the clearance of X (C_X)—that provides just that amount of X that appears in the urine. Second, we assign the virtual venous output a value of zero. Thus, Equation 33.1 becomes

$$\overbrace{P_{X,a} \cdot C_X}^{\substack{\text{Virtual} \\ \text{arterial input}}} = \overbrace{0}^{\substack{\text{Virtual} \\ \text{venous output}}} + \overbrace{(U_X \cdot \dot{V})}^{\substack{\text{Actual} \\ \text{urine output}}} \qquad \textbf{(33.2)}$$

Solving for clearance yields

$$C_X = \frac{U_X \cdot \dot{V}}{P_X} \qquad \textbf{(33.3)}$$

This is the classic **clearance equation** that describes the virtual volume of plasma that would be *totally cleared* of a solute in a given time. We need to know only three parameters to compute the clearance of a solute X:
1. The concentration of X in the urine (U_X)
2. The volume of urine formed in a given time ($\dot{V}$)
3. The concentration of X in systemic blood plasma (P_X), which is the same as $P_{X,a}$ in Equation 33.1

⊙ **33-2** Together, the three basic functions of the kidney—glomerular filtration, tubule reabsorption, and tubule secretion—determine the renal clearance of a solute. In the special case in which the kidneys completely clear X from plasma during a *single passage* through the kidneys ($P_{X,v} = 0$ in Equation 33.1), the renal clearance of X equals RPF_a in Equation 33.1. Because **para-aminohippurate (PAH)** is just such a special solute, its clearance is a good estimate of RPF_a, which we simplify to RPF.

For all solutes that *do not* behave like PAH, the renal venous plasma still contains some X. Thus, the virtual volume cleared of X in a given time is less than the total RPF. For most solutes, then, clearance describes a virtual volume of plasma that would be *totally cleared* of a solute, whereas in reality a much larger volume of plasma is *partially cleared* of the solute.

We can use a clearance approach to estimate another important renal parameter: **glomerular filtration rate (GFR),** which is the volume of fluid filtered into Bowman's capsule per unit time. Imagine a solute X that fulfills two criteria. First, X is freely filtered (i.e., concentration of X in Bowman's space is the same as that in blood plasma). Second, the tubules do not absorb, secrete, synthesize, degrade, or accumulate X. Thus, the amount of X that appears in the urine per unit time ($U_X \cdot \dot{V}$) is the same as the amount of X that the glomerulus filters per unit time ($P_X \cdot GFR$):

$$\overbrace{P_X \cdot GFR}^{\substack{\text{Input to} \\ \text{Bowman's space}}} = \overbrace{U_X \cdot \dot{V}}^{\substack{\text{Output into} \\ \text{urine}}} \qquad \textbf{(33.4)}$$

The input to Bowman's space is also known as the **filtered solute load** and is generally given in mmol/min (or mg/min). Rearranging Equation 33.4, we have

$$GFR = \frac{U_X \cdot \dot{V}}{P_X} \qquad \textbf{(33.5)}$$

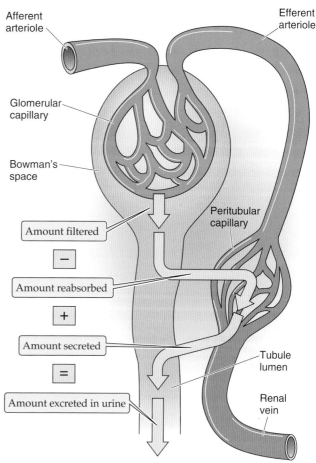

Figure 33.7 Factors contributing to the net urinary excretion of a substance.

Equation 33.5 is in exactly the same form as the classic clearance equation (Equation 33.3). In other words, GFR is C_X if X has the required properties.

A solute's urinary excretion is the algebraic sum of its filtered load, reabsorption by tubules, and secretion by tubules

The homeostasis of body fluids critically depends on the ability of the kidneys to determine the amount of a given solute that they excrete into the urine. Renal excretion rate (E_X) depends on three factors (Fig. 33.7):
1. The rate of filtration of X (F_X), known as the **filtered load** ($F_X = GFR \cdot P_X$)
2. The rate of reabsorption of X (R_X) by the tubules
3. The rate of secretion of X (S_X) by the tubules
This interrelationship is expressed quantitatively by

$$\overbrace{E_x}^{\substack{\text{Amount} \\ \text{excreted} \\ \text{per unit} \\ \text{time}}} = \overbrace{F_x}^{\substack{\text{Amount} \\ \text{filtered} \\ \text{per unit} \\ \text{time}}} - \overbrace{R_x}^{\substack{\text{Amount} \\ \text{reabsorbed} \\ \text{per unit} \\ \text{time}}} + \overbrace{S_x}^{\substack{\text{Amount} \\ \text{secreted} \\ \text{per unit} \\ \text{time}}} \qquad \textbf{(33.6)}$$

For some substances (e.g., inulin), no reabsorption or secretion occurs. For most substances, *either* reabsorption *or* secretion determines the amount present in the final urine. However, for some substances, *both* reabsorption *and* secretion determine excretion.

A   URETERS AND BLADDER
B   SMOOTH-MUSCLE ACTION POTENTIAL

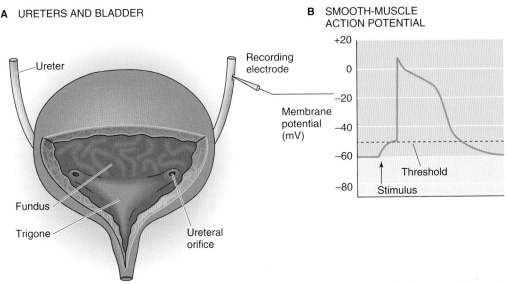

Figure 33.8 (A) Anatomy of the ureters and bladder. (B) Ureteral smooth-muscle cell action potential.

A useful parameter for gauging how the kidney handles a freely filtered solute is the **fractional excretion (FE)**, which is the ratio of the amount excreted in the urine ($U_X \cdot \dot{V}$) to the filtered load ($P_X \cdot GFR$):

$$FE_X = \frac{U_X \cdot \dot{V}}{P_X \cdot GFR} \qquad (33.7)$$

THE URETERS AND BLADDER

By the time the fluid leaves the most distal portion of the collecting duct, the fluid has the composition of final urine. Thus, the renal pelvis, ureters, bladder, and urethra do not substantially modify the urine volume or composition.

The ureters propel urine from the renal pelvis to the bladder by peristaltic waves conducted along a syncytium of smooth-muscle cells

The **ureters** serve as conduits for the passage of urine from the renal pelvis into the urinary bladder (Fig. 33.1A). Each ureter loops over the top of the common iliac artery and vein on the same side of the body and courses through the pelvis. The ureters enter the lower posterior portion of the bladder (**ureterovesical junction**), pass obliquely through its muscular wall, and open into the bladder lumen 1 to 2 cm above, and lateral to, the orifice of the urethra (Fig. 33.8A). The two ureteral orifices, connected by a ridge of tissue, and the urethral orifice form the corners of a triangle (**bladder trigone**). A flap-like valve of mucous membrane covers each ureteral orifice. This anatomical valve, in conjunction with the physiological valve-like effect created by the ureter's oblique pathway through the bladder wall, prevents reflux of urine back into the ureters during contraction of the bladder.

The lumen of each ureter is lined by **transitional epithelium,** which is above a submucosal layer of connective tissue, as well as an inner longitudinal and an outer circular layer of smooth muscle. Ureteral **smooth muscle** functions as a syncytium and is thus an example of unitary smooth muscle. Gap junctions conduct electrical activity from cell to cell. Chemical or mechanical stimuli (e.g., stretch) or a supra-threshold membrane depolarization may trigger an **action potential** (Fig. 33.8B) of the plateau type (see Fig. 9.13A).

Contraction of ureteral smooth muscle is similar to that of other smooth muscle in which Ca^{2+}-calmodulin activates myosin light-chain kinase (MLCK).

Ureteral **peristaltic waves** originate from electrical **pacemakers** in the proximal portion of the renal pelvis. These waves propel urine along the ureters and into the bladder. Blockade of ureteral outflow to the bladder, as by a kidney stone, causes the ureter to dilate and increases the baseline hydrostatic pressure over a period of 1 to 3 hours. This pressure is transmitted in retrograde fashion to the nephrons, creating a stopped-flow condition in which glomerular filtration nearly comes to a halt. **Hydronephrosis,** dilation of the pelvis and calyces of the kidney, can evolve over hours to days. Patients complain of severe pain (renal colic) resulting from distention of involved structures. If not cleared, the obstruction can cause marked renal dysfunction and even acute renal failure.

Although ureteral peristalsis can occur without innervation, the autonomic nervous system can modulate peristalsis. As in other syncytial smooth muscle, autonomic control of the ureters occurs by diffuse transmitter release from multiple varicosities formed as the postganglionic axon courses over the smooth-muscle cell. *Sympathetic* input modulates ureteral contractility as norepinephrine acts by excitatory α-adrenergic receptors and inhibitory β-adrenergic receptors. *Parasympathetic* input enhances ureteral contractility via acetylcholine, either by directly stimulating muscarinic cholinergic receptors or by causing postganglionic sympathetic fibers to release norepinephrine, which then can stimulate α adrenoceptors.

Sympathetic, parasympathetic, and somatic fibers innervate the urinary bladder and its sphincters

The urinary bladder consists of a main portion (body) that collects urine and a funnel-shaped extension (neck) that connects with the urethra (Fig. 33.8A). A transitional

TABLE 33.2 Urethral Sphincters

	INTERNAL SPHINCTER	EXTERNAL SPHINCTER
Type of muscle	Smooth	Skeletal
Nerve reaching the structure	Hypogastric	Pudendal
Nature of innervation	Autonomic	Somatic

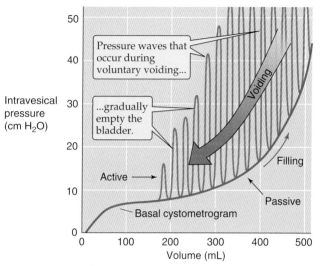

Figure 33.9 A cystometrogram.

epithelium lines the bladder lumen. Three poorly defined layers of smooth muscle make up the bulk of the bladder wall, the so-called **detrusor muscle.** At the lower tip of the trigone, the bladder lumen opens into the posterior urethra (i.e., distal part of bladder neck). The wall of the posterior urethra contains *smooth*-muscle fibers of the detrusor muscle interspersed with elastic tissue, together forming the **internal sphincter** (Table 33.2). Immediately adjacent is the **external sphincter,** made up of voluntary, mainly slow-twitch *striated*-muscle fibers.

◉ **33-3** The bladder and sphincters receive sympathetic and parasympathetic (autonomic) as well as somatic (voluntary) innervation.

Bladder filling activates stretch receptors, initiating the micturition reflex, a spinal reflex under control of higher central nervous system centers

Bladder **tone** is defined by the relationship between bladder volume and internal (intravesical) pressure. The record of the relationship between volume and pressure is a **cystometrogram** (Fig. 33.9, *blue curve*). Increasing bladder volume from 0 to ~50 mL produces a moderately steep increase in pressure. Additional volume increases up to ~300 mL produce almost no pressure increase; this high compliance reflects relaxation of bladder smooth muscle. At volumes >400 mL, additional increases in volume produce steep increments in passive pressure. Bladder tone, up to the point of triggering the micturition reflex, is independent of extrinsic bladder innervation.

During the **storage phase,** stretch receptors in the bladder send afferent signals to the brain via the pelvic splanchnic nerves. One first senses the urge for voluntary bladder emptying at a volume of ~150 mL and senses fullness at 400 to 500 mL. Nevertheless, until a socially acceptable opportunity to void presents itself, efferent impulses from the brain, in a learned reflex, inhibit presynaptic parasympathetic neurons

that would otherwise stimulate the detrusor muscle. Voluntary contraction of the external urinary sphincter probably also contributes to storage.

The **voiding phase** begins with a voluntary relaxation of the external urinary sphincter, followed by relaxation of the internal sphincter. When a small amount of urine reaches the proximal (posterior) urethra, afferents signal the cortex that voiding is imminent. The micturition reflex now continues as the pons no longer inhibits the parasympathetic preganglionic neurons that innervate the detrusor muscle. As a result, the bladder contracts, expelling urine. Once this micturition reflex has started, the initial bladder contractions lead to further trains of sensory impulses from stretch receptors, thus establishing a self-regenerating process (Fig. 33.9, *red spikes* moving to the left). At the same time, the cortical centers inhibit the external sphincter muscles. Voluntary urination also involves the voluntary contraction of abdominal muscles, which further raises bladder pressure and thus contributes to voiding and complete bladder emptying.

The basic bladder reflex may be either facilitated or inhibited by higher centers in the central nervous system that set the level at which the threshold for voiding occurs.

Because of the continuous flow of urine from the kidneys to the bladder, the function of the various sphincters, and the nearly complete emptying of the bladder during micturition, the entire urinary system is normally sterile.

CHAPTER 34

GLOMERULAR FILTRATION AND RENAL BLOOD FLOW

Gerhard Giebisch[†] and Peter S. Aronson

GLOMERULAR FILTRATION

A high glomerular filtration rate is essential for maintaining stable and optimal extracellular levels of solutes and water

⊙ **34-1** Glomerular ultrafiltration results in the formation of a fluid—the **glomerular filtrate**—with solute concentrations that are similar to those in plasma water. However, proteins, other high-molecular-weight compounds, and protein-bound solutes are present at reduced concentration. The glomerular filtrate, like filtrates formed across other body capillaries, is free of formed blood elements, such as red and white blood cells.

⊙ **34-2** Compared with other organs, the kidneys receive an extraordinarily large amount of blood flow—normalized to the mass of the organ—and filter an unusually high fraction of this blood flow. Under normal conditions, the **glomerular filtration rate (GFR)** of the two kidneys is 125 mL/min, or 180 L/day. Such a high rate of filtrate formation ensures that the entire extracellular fluid (ECF) is filtered by the kidneys >10 times a day. A high blood flow and a high GFR allow the kidneys to eliminate harmful materials rapidly by filtration.

Population studies show that GFR is proportional to body surface area. Because the surface area of an average 70-kg man is 1.73 m², the normal GFR in men is often reported as 125 mL/min per 1.73 m² of body surface area. In women, this figure is 110 mL/min per 1.73 m².

The clearance of inulin is a measure of glomerular filtration rate

The ideal **glomerular marker** for measuring GFR would be a substance X that has the same concentration in the glomerular filtrate as in plasma and that also is not reabsorbed, secreted, synthesized, broken down, or accumulated by the tubules (Table 34.1). In Equation 33.4, we saw that

$$
\underbrace{\overbrace{P_X \cdot GFR}^{\text{Input into Bowman's space}}}_{\frac{mg}{mL} \cdot \frac{mL}{min}} = \underbrace{\overbrace{U_X \cdot \dot{V}}^{\text{Output into urine}}}_{\frac{mg}{mL} \cdot \frac{mL}{min}}
\tag{34.1}
$$

P_X is the concentration of the solute in plasma, GFR is the sum of volume flow of filtrate from the plasma into all

Bowman's spaces, U_X is the urine concentration of the solute, and $\dot{V}$ is the urine flow. Rearranging this equation, we have

$$
GFR = \frac{U_X \times \dot{V}}{P_X}
$$
$$
\frac{mL}{min} = \frac{(mg/mL) \times (mL/min)}{(mg/mL)}
\tag{34.2}
$$

Note that Equation 34.2 has the same form as the clearance equation (see Equation 33.3) and is identical to Equation 33.5. Thus, the plasma clearance of a glomerular marker is the GFR.

Inulin is an exogenous starch-like fructose polymer that has a molecular weight of 5000 Da. Inulin is freely filtered at the glomerulus, but neither reabsorbed nor secreted by the renal tubules. Inulin also fulfills the additional requirements listed in Table 34.1 for an ideal glomerular marker.

Although the inulin clearance is the most reliable method for measuring GFR, it is not practical for clinical use. One must administer inulin intravenously to achieve reasonably constant plasma inulin levels. Another deterrent is that the chemical analysis for determining inulin levels in plasma and urine is sufficiently demanding to render inulin unsuitable for routine use in a clinical laboratory.

The clearance of creatinine is a useful clinical index of glomerular filtration rate

We can avoid the problems of intravenous infusion of a GFR marker such as inulin by using an *endogenous* substance with inulin-like properties. **Creatinine** is such a substance, and **creatinine clearance (C_{Cr})** is commonly used to estimate GFR in humans. In clinical practice, determining C_{Cr} is an easy and reliable means of assessing the GFR, and such determination avoids the need to inject anything into the patient. One merely obtains samples of venous blood and urine, analyzes them for creatinine concentration, and makes a simple calculation (see Equation 34.3 below).

The source of plasma creatinine is the normal metabolism of **creatine phosphate** in muscle. In men, this metabolism generates creatinine at the rate of 20 to 25 mg/kg body weight per day (i.e., ~1.5 g/day in a 70-kg man). In women, the value is 15 to 20 mg/kg body weight per day (i.e., ~1.2 g/day in a 70-kg woman), owing to a lower muscle mass. In the steady state, the rate of urinary creatinine excretion equals this rate of metabolic production. Because metabolic production of

---

[†] Deceased.

TABLE 34.1 Criteria for Use of a Substance to Measure GFR

1. Substance must be freely filterable in the glomeruli.
2. Substance must be neither reabsorbed nor secreted by the renal tubules.
3. Substance must not be synthesized, broken down, or accumulated by the kidney.
4. Substance must be physiologically inert (not toxic and without effect on renal function).

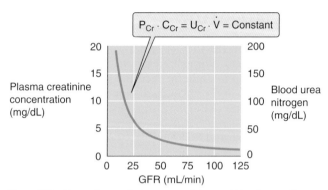

$$P_{Cr} \cdot C_{Cr} = U_{Cr} \cdot \dot{V} = Constant$$

Plasma creatinine concentration (mg/dL)

Blood urea nitrogen (mg/dL)

GFR (mL/min)

Figure 34.1 Dependence of plasma creatinine and blood urea nitrogen on the GFR.

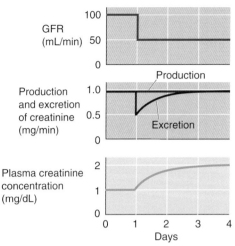

Figure 34.2 Effect of suddenly decreasing the GFR on plasma creatinine concentration.

creatinine largely depends on muscle mass, the daily excretion of creatinine depends strongly not only on gender but also on age, because elderly patients tend to have lower muscle mass.

Frequently, clinicians make a further simplification, using the **endogenous plasma concentration of creatinine (P_{Cr})**, normally 1 mg/dL, as an instant index of GFR. This use rests on the inverse relationship between P_{Cr} and C_{Cr}: in the steady state, when metabolic production in muscle equals the urinary excretion rate ($U_{Cr} \cdot \dot{V}$) of creatinine, and both remain fairly constant, this equation predicts that a plot of P_{Cr} versus C_{Cr} (i.e., P_{Cr} versus GFR) is a rectangular hyperbola (Fig. 34.1). For example, in a healthy person whose GFR is 100 mL/min, plasma creatinine concentration is ~1 mg/dL. The product of GFR (100 mL/min) and P_{Cr} (1 mg/dL) is thus 1 mg/min, which is the rate both of creatinine production and of creatinine excretion. If GFR suddenly drops to 50 mL/min (Fig. 34.2, *top*), the kidneys will initially filter and excrete less creatinine (Fig. 34.2, *middle*), although the production rate is unchanged. As a result, the plasma creatinine level will rise to a new steady state, which is reached at a P_{Cr} of 2 mg/dL (Fig. 34.2, *bottom*). At this point, the product of the reduced GFR (50 mL/min) and the elevated P_{Cr} (2 mg/dL) will again equal 1 mg/min, the rate of endogenous production of creatinine. Similarly, if GFR were to fall to one fourth of normal, P_{Cr} would rise to 4 mg/dL. This concept is reflected in the right-rectangular hyperbola of Fig. 34.1.

$$C_{Cr} = \frac{U_{Cr} \cdot \dot{V}}{P_{Cr}} \approx GFR \qquad \textbf{(34.3)}$$

Molecular size and electrical charge determine the filterability of solutes across the glomerular filtration barrier

The glomerular filtration barrier consists of four elements (see Fig. 33.3B and C): (1) the glycocalyx overlying the endothelial cells, (2) endothelial cells, (3) the glomerular basement membrane, and (4) epithelial podocytes. Layers 1, 3, and 4 are covered with negative charges from anionic proteoglycans.

The permselectivity of the glomerular barrier for different solutes is estimated by the ratio of solute concentration in the ultrafiltrate versus the plasma (UF_X/P_X). The ratio UF_X/P_X, also known as the **sieving coefficient** for the solute X, depends on molecular weight and effective molecular radius. Substances of low **molecular weight** (<5500 Da) and small **effective molecular radius** (e.g., water, urea, glucose, and inulin) appear in the filtrate in the same concentration as in plasma ($UF_X/P_X \approx 1$). In these instances, no sieving of the contents of the fluid moving through the glomerular "pores" occurs, so that the water moving through the filtration slits by convection carries the solutes with it. As a result, the concentration of the solute in the filtrate is the same as that in bulk plasma. The situation is different for substances with a molecular weight that is greater than ~14 kDa, such as lysozyme. Larger and larger macromolecules are increasingly restricted from passage.

◉ **34-3** In addition to molecular weight and radius, **electrical charge** also makes a major contribution to the permselectivity of the glomerular barrier. Fig. 34.3 is a plot of the clearance ratio for uncharged, positively charged, and negatively charged dextran molecules of varying molecular size. Two conclusions can be drawn from these data. First, *neutral* dextrans with an effective molecular radius of <2 nm pass readily across the glomerular barrier. For dextrans with a larger radius, the clearance ratio decreases with an increase in molecular size, so that passage ceases when the radius exceeds 4.2 nm. Second, *anionic* dextrans (e.g., dextran sulfates) are restricted from filtration, whereas for the same molecular radius, *cationic* dextrans (e.g., diethylaminoethyl dextrans) pass more readily into the filtrate. For negatively charged dextrans, the relationship between charge and filterability is characterized by a left shift of the curve relating molecular size to clearance ratio, whereas the opposite is true for positively charged dextrans.

Because albumin is highly negatively charged, its clearance ratio is nearly zero, similar to that of anionic dextrans (Fig. 34.3, *green curve*). Glomerular diseases causing loss of negative charge in the glomerular barrier lead to the development of albuminuria.

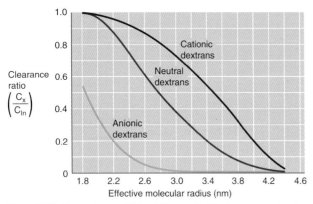

Figure 34.3 Dependence of filterability on electrical charge and molecular size. (Data from Bohrer MP, Baylis C, Humes HD, et al: Permselectivity of the glomerular capillary wall: Facilitated filtration of circulating polycations. J Clin Invest 61:72–78, 1978.)

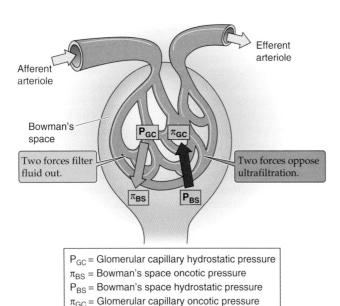

P_{GC} = Glomerular capillary hydrostatic pressure
π_{BS} = Bowman's space oncotic pressure
P_{BS} = Bowman's space hydrostatic pressure
π_{GC} = Glomerular capillary oncotic pressure

Figure 34.4 Forces affecting glomerular ultrafiltration.

Hydrostatic pressure in glomerular capillaries favors glomerular ultrafiltration, whereas oncotic pressure in capillaries and hydrostatic pressure in Bowman's space oppose it

As is the case for filtration in other capillary beds, glomerular ultrafiltration depends on the product of the ultrafiltration coefficient (K_f) and net Starling forces. (see ◉ 20-2)

$$GFR = K_f \cdot \underbrace{[(P_{GC} - P_{BS}) - (\pi_{GC} - \pi_{BS})]}_{P_{UF}} \qquad \textbf{(34.4)}$$

Fig. 34.4 provides a schematic overview of the driving forces affecting ultrafiltration. **Hydrostatic pressure in the glomerular capillary (P_{GC})** favors ultrafiltration. **Hydrostatic pressure in Bowman's space (P_{BS})** opposes ultrafiltration. **Oncotic pressure in the glomerular capillary (π_{GC})** opposes ultrafiltration. **Oncotic pressure of the filtrate in Bowman's space (π_{BS})** favors ultrafiltration. Thus, two forces

favor filtration (P_{GC} and π_{BS}), and two oppose it (P_{BS} and π_{GC}).

The **net driving force favoring ultrafiltration (P_{UF})** at any point along the glomerular capillaries is the difference between the hydrostatic pressure difference and the oncotic pressure difference between the capillary and Bowman's space. Thus, GFR is proportional to the **net hydrostatic force ($P_{GC} - P_{BS}$)** minus the **net oncotic force ($\pi_{GC} - \pi_{BS}$)**.

RENAL BLOOD FLOW

Renal blood flow (RBF) is ~1 L/min out of the total cardiac output of 5 L/min. Normalized for weight, this blood flow amounts to ~350 mL/min for each 100 g of tissue, which is 7-fold higher than the normalized blood flow to the brain. **Renal** plasma **flow (RPF)** is

$$RPF = (1 - Hct) \cdot RBF \qquad \textbf{(34.5)}$$

Given a hematocrit (Hct) of 0.40, the "normal" RPF is ~600 mL/min.

◉ 34-4 Increased glomerular plasma flow leads to an increase in glomerular filtration rate

GFR increases with glomerular plasma flow (Fig. 34.5A). However, this increase is not linear. Compared with the normal situation, the GFR increases only moderately with *increasing* RPF, but decreases greatly with *decreasing* RPF. Indeed, clinical conditions causing an acute fall in renal perfusion result in an abrupt decline in GFR.

The relationship between GFR and RPF defines a parameter known as the **filtration fraction (FF),** which is the volume of filtrate that forms from a given volume of plasma entering the glomeruli:

$$FF = \frac{GFR}{RPF} \qquad \textbf{(34.6)}$$

Because the normal GFR is ~125 mL/min and the normal RPF is ~600 mL/min, the normal FF is ~0.2. Because GFR saturates at high values of RPF, FF is greater at low plasma flows than it is at high plasma flows (Fig. 34.5B).

Afferent and efferent arteriolar resistances control both glomerular plasma flow and glomerular filtration rate

The renal microvasculature has two unique features. First, this vascular bed has two major sites of resistance control, the afferent and the efferent arterioles. Second, it has two capillary beds in series, the glomerular and the peritubular capillaries. As a consequence of this unique architecture, significant pressure drops occur along both arterioles (Fig. 34.6), glomerular capillary pressure is relatively high throughout, and peritubular capillary pressure is relatively low. Selective constriction or relaxation of the afferent and efferent arterioles allows for highly sensitive control of the hydrostatic pressure in the intervening glomerular capillary, and thus of glomerular filtration.

A   GFR VERSUS PLASMA FLOW

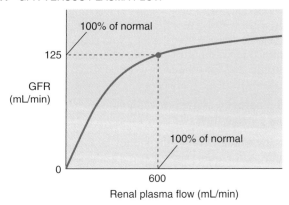

B   FF VERSUS PLASMA FLOW

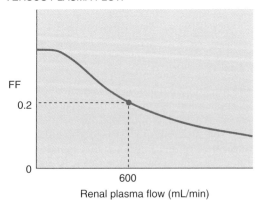

Figure 34.5   Dependence of the GFR and filtration fraction on renal plasma flow.

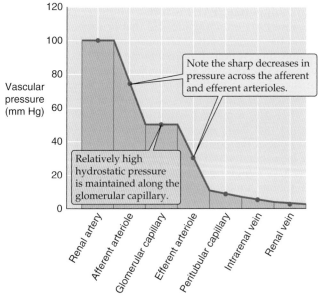

Figure 34.6   Pressure profile along the renal vasculature.

Fig. 34.7A provides an idealized example in which we reciprocally change afferent and efferent arteriolar resistance while keeping total arteriolar resistance—and thus glomerular plasma flow—constant. Compared with an

initial condition in which the afferent and efferent arteriolar resistances are the same (Fig. 34.7A, *top panel*), constricting the *afferent* arteriole while relaxing the efferent arteriole lowers P_{GC} (Fig. 34.7A, *middle panel*). Conversely, constricting the *efferent* arteriole while relaxing the afferent arteriole raises P_{GC} (Fig. 34.7A, *lower panel*). From these idealized P_{GC} responses, one might predict that an increase in afferent arteriolar resistance would decrease the GFR and that an increase in efferent arteriolar resistance should have the opposite effect. However, physiological changes in the afferent and efferent arteriolar resistance usually do not keep overall arteriolar resistance constant. Thus, changes in arteriolar resistance generally lead to changes in glomerular plasma flow, which, as discussed above, can influence GFR independent of glomerular capillary pressure.

Fig. 34.7B and C show somewhat more realistic effects on RPF and GFR as we change the resistance of a *single* arteriole. With a selective increase of *afferent* arteriolar resistance (Fig. 34.7B), both capillary pressure and RPF decrease, which leads to a monotonic decline in the GFR. In contrast, a selective increase of *efferent* arteriolar resistance (Fig. 34.7C) causes a steep increase in glomerular capillary pressure but a decrease in RPF. As a result, over the lower range of resistances, GFR increases with efferent resistance as an increasing P_{GC} dominates. On the other hand, at higher resistances, GFR begins to fall as the effect of a declining RPF dominates. These opposing effects on glomerular capillary pressure and RPF account for the biphasic dependence of GFR on efferent resistance.

The examples in Fig. 34.7B and C, in which only afferent or efferent resistance is increased, are still somewhat artificial. During sympathetic stimulation, or in response to ANG II, both afferent *and* efferent resistances increase. Thus, RPF decreases. The generally opposing effects on GFR of increasing both afferent resistance (Fig. 34.7B) and efferent resistance (Fig. 34.7C) explain why the combination of both keeps GFR fairly constant despite a decline in RPF.

Peritubular capillaries provide tubules with nutrients and retrieve reabsorbed fluid

Peritubular capillaries originate from the efferent arterioles of the superficial and juxtamedullary glomeruli (see Fig. 33.1C). The capillaries from the superficial glomeruli form a dense network in the cortex, and those from the juxtamedullary glomeruli follow the tubules down into the medulla, where the capillaries are known as the vasa recta. The peritubular capillaries have two main functions. First, these vessels deliver oxygen and nutrients to the epithelial cells. Second, they are responsible for taking up from the interstitial space the fluid and solutes that the renal tubules reabsorb.

Lymphatic capillaries are mainly found in the cortex, in association with blood vessels. They provide an important route for removing protein from the interstitial fluid. Proteins leak continuously from the peritubular capillaries into the interstitial fluid. Total renal lymph flow is small and amounts to <1% of RPF.

Blood flow in the renal cortex exceeds that in the renal medulla

Measurements of regional blood flow in the kidney show that ~90% of the blood leaving the glomeruli in efferent arterioles

A   RECIPROCAL CHANGES IN AFFERENT AND EFFERENT ARTERIOLAR RESISTANCE

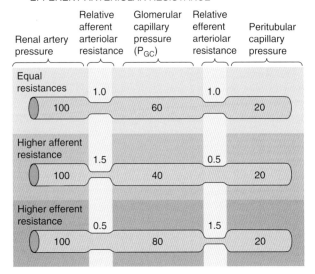

B   CONSTRICTION OF ONLY *AFFERENT* ARTERIOLE

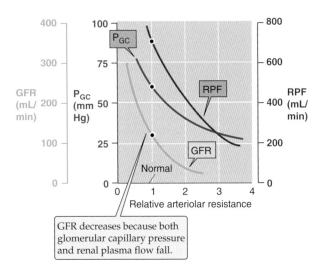

GFR decreases because both glomerular capillary pressure and renal plasma flow fall.

C   CONSTRICTION OF ONLY *EFFERENT* ARTERIOLE

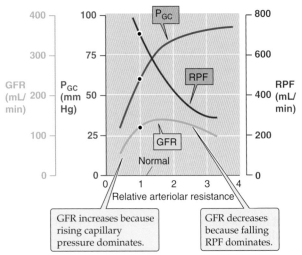

GFR increases because rising capillary pressure dominates.

GFR decreases because falling RPF dominates.

Figure 34.7   Role of afferent and efferent arteriolar resistance on pressure and flows. In (A) the sum of afferent and efferent arteriolar resistances is always 2, whereas in (B) and (C) the total resistance changes.

perfuses cortical tissue. The remaining 10% perfuses the renal medulla, with only 1% to 2% reaching the papilla. The relatively low blood flow through the medulla, a consequence of the high resistance of the long vasa recta, is important for minimizing washout of the hypertonic medullary interstitium and thus for producing a concentrated urine.

The clearance of para-aminohippurate is a measure of renal plasma flow

For any solute (X) that the kidney neither metabolizes nor produces, the only route of entry to the kidney is the renal artery, and the only two routes of exit are the renal vein and the ureter (see Fig. 33.6):

$$\overbrace{P_{X,a} \cdot RPF_a}^{\substack{\text{Arterial input} \\ \text{of X}}} = (\overbrace{P_{X,v} \cdot RPF_v}^{\substack{\text{Venous output} \\ \text{of X}}}) + (\overbrace{U_X \cdot \dot{V}}^{\substack{\text{Urine output} \\ \text{of X}}}) \quad (34.7)$$

$$\underbrace{\frac{mmol}{mL}}_{} \quad \underbrace{\frac{mL}{min}}_{} \qquad \underbrace{\frac{mmol}{mL}}_{} \quad \underbrace{\frac{mL}{min}}_{} \qquad \underbrace{\frac{mmol}{mL}}_{} \quad \underbrace{\frac{mL}{min}}_{}$$

The foregoing equation (a restatement of Equation 33.1) is an application of the Fick principle used for measurements of regional blood flow. To estimate arterial RPF (RPF_a)—or, more simply, RPF—we could in principle use the clearance of *any substance* that the kidney measurably excretes into the urine, as long as it is practical to obtain samples of systemic arterial plasma, renal venous plasma, and urine. The problem, of course, is sampling blood from the renal vein.

However, we can avoid the need for sampling the renal vein if we choose a substance that the kidneys clear so efficiently that they leave almost *none* in the renal vein. **Para-aminohippurate (PAH)** is such a substance (see ⊙ 33-2). Because PAH is an organic acid that is not normally present in the human body, PAH must be administered by continuous intravenous infusion. Some PAH binds to plasma proteins, but a significant amount remains freely dissolved in the plasma and therefore filters into Bowman's space. However, the kidney filters only ~20% of the RPF (i.e., FF = ~0.2), and a major portion of the PAH remains in the plasma that flows out of the efferent arterioles. PAH diffuses out of the peritubular capillary network and reaches the basolateral surface of the proximal-tubule cells. These cells have a high capacity to secrete PAH from blood into the tubule lumen against large concentration gradients. This PAH-secretory system is so efficient that—as long as we do not overwhelm it by infusing too much PAH—almost no PAH (~10%) remains in the renal venous blood. We can therefore assume that all the PAH presented to the kidney appears in the urine:

$$\text{PAH excreted} = \frac{\text{PAH filtered}}{\text{in glomerulus}} + \frac{\text{PAH secreted in urine}}{\text{by tubules}}$$

$$(34.8)$$

In the example of Fig. 34.8, the concentration of filterable PAH in the arterial blood plasma (P_{PAH}) is 10 mg/dL or 0.1 mg/mL. If RPF is 600 mL/min, then the arterial load of PAH to the kidney is 60 mg/min. Of this amount, 12 mg/min appears in the glomerular filtrate. If the tubules secrete

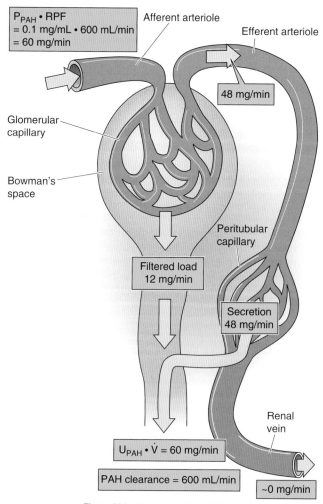

$P_{PAH} \cdot RPF$
= 0.1 mg/mL • 600 mL/min
= 60 mg/min

Afferent arteriole

Efferent arteriole

48 mg/min

Glomerular capillary

Bowman's space

Peritubular capillary

Filtered load 12 mg/min

Secretion 48 mg/min

Renal vein

$U_{PAH} \cdot \dot{V}$ = 60 mg/min

PAH clearance = 600 mL/min

~0 mg/min

Figure 34.8   Renal handling of PAH.

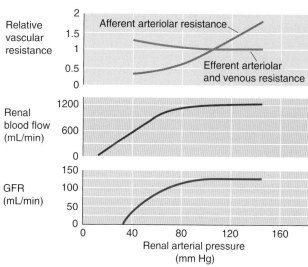

Figure 34.9   Autoregulation of RBF and GFR. (Data on RBF from Arend-shorst WJ, Finn WF, Gottschalk CW: Autoregulation of renal blood flow in the rat kidney. Am J Physiol 228:127–133, 1975.)

the remaining 48 mg/min, then the entire 60 mg/min of PAH presented to the kidney appears in the urine. That is, in the idealized example of Fig. 34.8, during a single passage of blood the kidneys clear 100% of PAH presented to them. In practice, the kidneys excrete only ~90% of the arterial load of PAH, provided P_{PAH} does not exceed 12 mg/dL. The excretion of 90% rather than 100% of the arterial load of PAH reflects the 10% of the RBF that perfuses the medulla, where the tubules do not secrete PAH.

As long as we do not infuse too much PAH—that is, as long as virtually no PAH remains in the renal venous blood—Equation 34.7 reduces to the equation for the clearance of PAH:

$$C_{PAH} = RPF = \frac{U_{PAH} \cdot \dot{V}}{P_{PAH}} \qquad \textbf{(34.9)}$$

If we apply this equation to the example in Fig. 34.8,

$$C_{PAH} = RPF = \frac{60\,mg/min}{10\,mg/dL} = \frac{60\,mg/min}{0.1\,mg/mL} = 600\,mL/min$$

$$\textbf{(34.10)}$$

To compute RPF, we need to collect a urine sample to obtain ($U_{PAH} \cdot \dot{V}$) and a blood sample to obtain P_{PAH}.

However, the blood sample need not be arterial. For example, one can obtain venous blood from the arm, inasmuch as skeletal muscle extracts negligible amounts of PAH.

CONTROL OF RENAL BLOOD FLOW AND GLOMERULAR FILTRATION

Autoregulation keeps renal blood flow and glomerular filtration rate relatively constant

◉ 34-5 An important feature of the renal circulation is its remarkable ability to maintain RBF and GFR within narrow limits, although mean arterial pressure may vary between ~80 and 170 mm Hg (Fig. 34.9, *middle and bottom panels*). Stability of blood flow—known as **autoregulation** (see Fig. 20.9)—is also a property of the vascular beds serving two other vital organs, the brain and the heart. Perfusion to all three of these organs must be preserved in emergency situations, such as hypotensive shock. Autoregulation of the renal blood supply is independent of the influence of renal nerves and circulating hormones, and persists even when one perfuses isolated kidneys with erythrocyte-free solutions. Autoregulation of RBF—and, consequently, autoregulation of GFR, which depends on RBF (Fig. 34.5A)—stabilizes the filtered load of solutes that reaches the tubules over a wide range of arterial pressures. Autoregulation of RBF also protects the fragile glomerular capillaries against increases in perfusion pressure that could lead to structural damage.

The kidney autoregulates RBF by responding to a rise in renal arterial pressure with a proportional increase in the resistance of the afferent arterioles. Autoregulation comes into play during alterations in arterial pressure that occur, for example, during changes in posture, light to moderate exercise, and sleep. It is the *afferent arteriole* where the autoregulatory response occurs, and where the resistance to flow rises with increasing perfusion pressure (Fig. 34.9, *top panel*). In contrast, *efferent* arteriolar resistance, glomerular and peritubular capillary resistances, as well as venous resistance all change very little over the range of normal to high renal arterial pressures. However, in the range of *low renal* perfusion pressures—as in congestive heart failure—efferent arteriolar resistance increases, and thereby minimizes decreases in GFR.

Two basic mechanisms—equally important—underlie renal autoregulation: a myogenic response of the smooth muscle of the afferent arterioles and a tubuloglomerular feedback mechanism.

Myogenic Response The afferent arterioles have the inherent ability to respond to changes in vessel circumference by contracting or relaxing—a myogenic response (see ◉ 20-22). The mechanism of contraction is the opening of stretch-activated nonselective cation channels in vascular smooth muscle. The resultant depolarizing leads to an influx of Ca^{2+} that stimulates contraction.

Tubuloglomerular Feedback ◉ **34-6** The juxtaglomerular apparatus (JGA; see ◉ 33-1) mediates tubuloglomerular feedback (TGF). The macula densa cells in the thick ascending limb sense an increase in GFR and, in classic feedback fashion, translate this to a contraction of the afferent arteriole, a fall in P_{GC} and RPF, and hence a decrease in GFR.

The mechanism of TGF is thought to be the following:

1. An increase in arterial pressure leads to increases in glomerular capillary pressure, RPF, and GFR.
2. Increased GFR leads to an increased delivery of Na^+, Cl^-, and fluid into the proximal tubule and, ultimately, to the macula densa cells of the JGA.
3. Macula densa cells do not sense flow per se, but the higher luminal $[Na^+]$ or $[Cl^-]$ resulting from high flow. Increases in luminal $[Na^+]$ and $[Cl^-]$—via the apical Na/K/Cl cotransporter of the macula densa cell—translate to parallel increases in *intracellular* $[Na^+]$ and $[Cl^-]$. Indeed, blocking the Na/K/Cl cotransporter with furosemide not only blocks the uptake of Na^+ and Cl^- into the macula densa cells, but also interrupts TGF.
4. The rise in $[Cl^-]_i$, in conjunction with a basolateral Cl^- channel, leads to a depolarization.
5. The depolarization activates a basolateral nonselective cation channel, which allows Ca^{2+} to enter the macula densa cell.
6. Increased $[Ca^{2+}]_i$ causes the macula densa cell to release paracrine agents, particularly adenosine and ATP, which breaks down to adenosine.
7. Adenosine, binding to A_1 adenosine receptors on the smooth-muscle cells, triggers contraction of nearby vascular smooth-muscle cells.
8. Increased afferent arteriolar resistance decreases GFR, counteracting the initial increase in GFR.

Volume expansion and a high-protein diet increase glomerular filtration rate by reducing tubuloglomerular feedback

Both the intrinsic sensitivity of the macula densa mechanism and the initial set-point for changes in flow are sensitive to changes in the ECF volume. Expansion of the ECF decreases the sensitivity of the overall feedback loop. Conversely, volume contraction increases the sensitivity of TGF, thus helping preserve fluid by reducing GFR. Many of these effects may be mediated by ANG II, which is a required cofactor for TGF responses.

Of clinical importance is the observation that a **high-protein diet** increases GFR and RPF by indirectly lowering the sensitivity of the TGF mechanism. A high-protein diet somehow enhances NaCl reabsorption proximal to the macula densa, so that luminal [NaCl] at the macula densa falls. As a consequence, the flow in the loop of Henle (and thus GFR) must be higher to raise [NaCl] to a given level at the macula densa. A high-protein diet may thereby decrease TGF, increasing glomerular capillary pressure. This sequence of events may lead, particularly in the presence of intrinsic renal disease, to progressive glomerular damage.

Four factors that modulate renal blood flow and glomerular filtration rate play key roles in regulating effective circulating volume

Changes in effective circulating volume (see ◉ 23-26) trigger responses in four parallel effector pathways that ultimately modulate either renal hemodynamics or renal Na^+ reabsorption. The four effector pathways (see Fig. 40.1) are (1) the renin-angiotensin-aldosterone axis, (2) the sympathetic nervous system, (3) arginine vasopressin (AVP), and (4) atrial natriuretic peptide (ANP).

Renin-Angiotensin-Aldosterone Axis In terms of renal hemodynamic effects, the most important part of the renin-angiotensin-aldosterone axis is its middle member, the peptide hormone ANG II. ANG II has multiple actions on renal hemodynamics. The net effect of ANG II on blood flow and GFR depends on multiple factors. Under normal conditions, the effect of ANG II is primarily to mediate *efferent* arteriolar constriction, an effect that tends to maintain GFR when renal perfusion is reduced. The reason is that prostaglandins counteract any tendency of ANG II to constrict the *afferent* arteriole. Indeed, inhibition of prostaglandin production by NSAIDs unmasks the constriction of the afferent arteriole, resulting in a decline in GFR.

Sympathetic Nerves ◉ **34-7** Sympathetic tone to the kidney may increase either as part of a general response—as occurs with pain, stress, trauma, hemorrhage, or exercise—or as part of a more selective renal response to a decrease in effective circulating volume (see ◉ 23-19). In either case, sympathetic nerve terminals release **norepinephrine** into the interstitial space. At relatively high levels of nerve stimulation, both afferent and efferent arteriolar resistances rise, thus generally decreasing RBF and GFR. The observation that the RBF may fall more than the GFR is consistent with a preferential *efferent* arteriolar constriction. With maximal nerve stimulation, however, afferent vasoconstriction predominates and leads to drastic reductions in both RBF and GFR.

In addition, sympathetic stimulation triggers granular cells to increase their release of renin, raising levels of ANG II, which acts as described above. Finally, sympathetic activation—even at levels too low to reduce RBF and GFR—causes increased reabsorption of Na^+ by proximal tubules.

Arginine Vasopressin In response to increases in the osmotic pressure of the ECF, the posterior pituitary releases AVP—also known as antidiuretic hormone. Although the principal effect of this small polypeptide is to increase water absorption in the collecting duct, AVP also increases vascular resistance. Despite physiological fluctuations of circulating AVP levels, total RBF and GFR remain nearly constant. Nevertheless, AVP may decrease blood flow to the renal *medulla*, thereby minimizing the washout of the hypertonic medulla; this hypertonicity is essential for forming a concentrated urine.

In humans, severe decreases in effective circulating volume (e.g., shock) cause a massive release of AVP (see ◉ 23-20). Only under these conditions does AVP produce a systemic vasoconstriction and thus contribute to maintaining systemic blood pressure.

Atrial Natriuretic Peptide Atrial myocytes release ANP in response to increased atrial pressure and thus effective circulating volume (see ◉ 23-21). ANP markedly vasodilates afferent and efferent arterioles, thereby increasing cortical and medullary blood flow, and lowers the sensitivity of the TGF mechanism. The net effect is an increase in RPF and GFR. ANP also affects renal hemodynamics indirectly by inhibiting secretion of renin (thus lowering ANG II levels).

Even without affecting GFR, low levels of ANP can be natriuretic by inhibiting Na^+ reabsorption by tubules. First, ANP inhibits aldosterone secretion by the adrenal gland (and thereby reduces Na^+ reabsorption). Second, ANP acts *directly* to inhibit Na^+ reabsorption by the inner medullary collecting duct. At higher levels, ANP decreases systemic arterial pressure and increases capillary permeability. ANP plays a role in the diuretic response to the redistribution of ECF and plasma volume into the thorax that occurs during space flight and water immersion.

CHAPTER 35

TRANSPORT OF SODIUM AND CHLORIDE

Gerhard Giebisch[†] and Peter S. Aronson

The kidneys help to maintain the body's **extracellular fluid (ECF)** volume by regulating the amount of Na^+ in the urine. Sodium salts (predominantly NaCl) are the most important contributor to the osmolality of the ECF; hence, where Na^+ goes, water follows. This chapter focuses on how the kidneys maintain the ECF volume by regulating excretion of Na^+ and its most prevalent anion, Cl^-.

The normal daily urinary excretion of Na^+ is only a tiny fraction of the total Na^+ filtered by the kidneys (Fig. 35.1). The filtered load of Na^+ is the product of the glomerular filtration rate (GFR, ~180 L/day) and the plasma Na^+ concentration of ~142 mM, or ~25,500 mmol/day. For individuals on a typical Western diet containing ~120 mmol of Na^+, the kidneys reabsorb ~99.6% of the filtered Na^+ by the time the tubule fluid reaches the renal pelvis. Therefore, even minute variations in the fractional reabsorptive rate can lead to changes in total-body Na^+ that markedly alter ECF volume and, hence, body weight and blood pressure.

Na^+ AND Cl^- TRANSPORT BY DIFFERENT SEGMENTS OF THE NEPHRON

Na^+ and Cl^- reabsorption decreases from proximal tubules to Henle's loops to classic distal tubules to collecting tubules and ducts

Fig. 35.2 summarizes the segmental distribution of Na^+ reabsorption along the nephron. The **proximal tubule** reabsorbs the largest fraction of filtered Na^+ (~67%). Because [Na^+] in *tubule fluid* (or TF_{Na}) remains almost the same as that in *plasma* (i.e., $TF_{Na}/P_{Na} = 1.0$) throughout the length of the proximal tubule, it follows that the [Na^+] in the *reabsorbate* is virtually the same as that in plasma. Because Na^+ salts are the dominant osmotically active solutes in the filtrate, reabsorption must be a nearly isosmotic process (i.e., water is reabsorbed along with Na^+).

The **loop of Henle** reabsorbs a smaller but significant fraction of filtered Na^+ (~25%). Because of the low water permeability of the **thick ascending limb (TAL)**, this nephron segment reabsorbs Na^+ faster than it reabsorbs water, so that [Na^+] in the tubule fluid entering the distal convoluted tubule has decreased substantially ($TF_{Na}/P_{Na} \cong 0.45$).

The segments between the **distal convoluted tubule (DCT)** and the **cortical collecting tubule (CCT)**, inclusive, reabsorb ~5% of the filtered Na^+ load under normal conditions. Finally, the medullary collecting duct reabsorbs ~3% of the filtered Na^+ load.

[†]Deceased.

The tubule reabsorbs Na^+ via both the transcellular and paracellular pathways

The tubule can reabsorb Na^+ and Cl^- via both transcellular and paracellular pathways (Fig. 35.3A). In the **transcellular pathway,** Na^+ and Cl^- sequentially traverse the apical and basolateral membranes before entering the blood. In the **paracellular pathway,** these ions move entirely by an extracellular route, through the tight junctions between cells.

Transcellular Na^+ Reabsorption The basic mechanism of transcellular Na^+ reabsorption is similar in all nephron segments. The *first step* is the passive entry of Na^+ into the cell across the **apical membrane.** Because the intracellular Na^+ concentration ([Na^+]$_i$) is low and the cell voltage is negative with respect to the lumen, the electrochemical gradient is

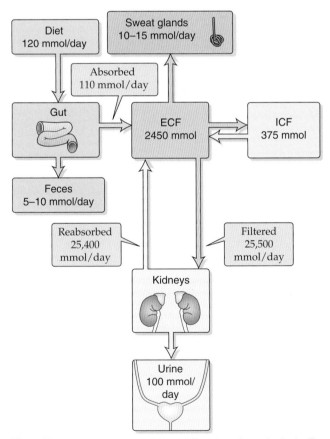

Figure 35.1 Distribution and balance of Na^+ throughout the body. The values in the *boxes* are approximations. *ICF*, Intracellular fluid.

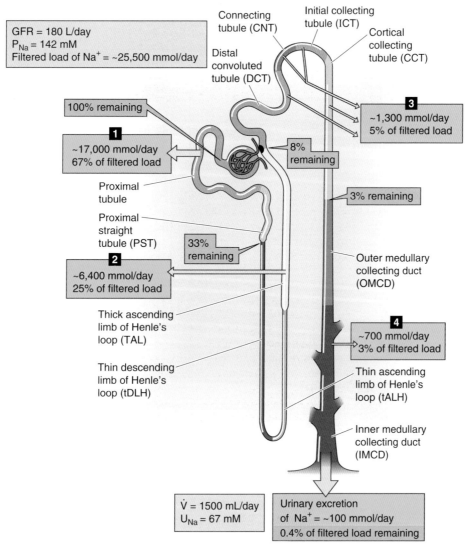

GFR = 180 L/day
P_Na = 142 mM
Filtered load of Na⁺ = ~25,500 mmol/day

Connecting tubule (CNT)

Initial collecting tubule (ICT)

Cortical collecting tubule (CCT)

Distal convoluted tubule (DCT)

100% remaining

1
~17,000 mmol/day
67% of filtered load

3
~1,300 mmol/day
5% of filtered load

8% remaining

Proximal tubule

3% remaining

Proximal straight tubule (PST)

33% remaining

Outer medullary collecting duct (OMCD)

2
~6,400 mmol/day
25% of filtered load

Thick ascending limb of Henle's loop (TAL)

4
~700 mmol/day
3% of filtered load

Thin descending limb of Henle's loop (tDLH)

Thin ascending limb of Henle's loop (tALH)

Inner medullary collecting duct (IMCD)

V̇ = 1500 mL/day
U_Na = 67 mM

Urinary excretion of Na⁺ = ~100 mmol/day
0.4% of filtered load remaining

Figure 35.2 Estimates of renal handling of Na⁺ along the nephron. The *numbered yellow boxes* indicate the absolute amount of Na⁺—as well as the fraction of the filtered load—that various nephron segments reabsorb. The *green boxes* indicate the fraction of the filtered load that remains in the lumen at these sites. The values in the boxes are approximations. P_{Na}, Plasma sodium concentration; U_{Na}, urine sodium concentration; $\dot{V}$, urine flow.

favorable for passive Na⁺ entry across the apical membrane (Fig. 35.3B).

The *second step* of transcellular Na⁺ reabsorption is the active extrusion of Na⁺ out of the cell across the **basolateral membrane** (Fig. 35.3B). This Na⁺ extrusion is mediated by the Na-K pump, which keeps $[Na^+]_i$ low (~15 mM) and $[K^+]_i$ high (~120 mM).

Paracellular Na⁺ Reabsorption The basic mechanism of paracellular Na⁺ transport is similar among nephron segments: the transepithelial electrochemical gradient for Na⁺ drives transport. However, both the **transepithelial voltage** (V_{te}) and luminal $[Na^+]$ vary along the nephron (Table 35.1). As a result, the net driving force for Na⁺ is positive—favoring passive Na⁺ reabsorption—only in the S2 and S3 segments of the proximal tubule and in the TAL. In the other segments, the net driving force is negative—favoring passive Na⁺ diffusion from blood to lumen ("backleak").

In addition, Na⁺ can move uphill from lumen to blood via **solvent drag** across the tight junctions. In this case, the movement of H_2O from the lumen to the lateral intercellular space—energized by the active transport of Na⁺ into the lateral intercellular space—also sweeps Na⁺ and Cl⁻ in the same direction.

Nephron segments also vary in their **leakiness** to Na⁺ ions. This leakiness is largely a function of the varying ionic conductance of the paracellular pathway between cells across the tight junction, due to the expression of different claudins.

The leakiness of an epithelium has serious repercussions for the steepness of the ion gradients that the epithelium can develop and maintain. For both Na⁺ and Cl⁻, the ability of specific nephron segments to establish large concentration gradients correlates with the degree of tightness, which limits the backflux of ions between cells.

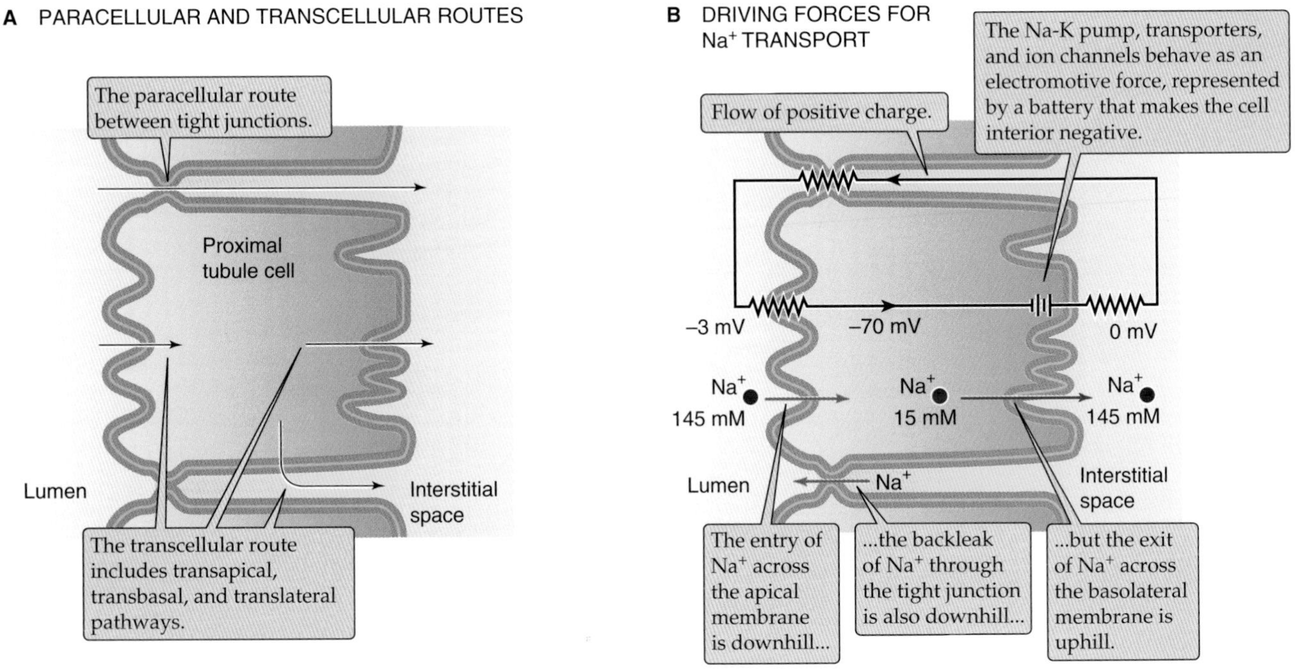

A PARACELLULAR AND TRANSCELLULAR ROUTES

The paracellular route between tight junctions.

Proximal tubule cell

Lumen

Interstitial space

The transcellular route includes transapical, transbasal, and translateral pathways.

B DRIVING FORCES FOR Na⁺ TRANSPORT

The Na-K pump, transporters, and ion channels behave as an electromotive force, represented by a battery that makes the cell interior negative.

Flow of positive charge.

−3 mV   −70 mV   0 mV

Na^+ 145 mM Na^+ 15 mM Na^+ 145 mM

Lumen Na^+ Interstitial space

The entry of Na^+ across the apical membrane is downhill...

...the backleak of Na^+ through the tight junction is also downhill...

...but the exit of Na^+ across the basolateral membrane is uphill.

Figure 35.3 Transcellular and paracellular mechanisms of Na^+ and Cl^- reabsorption.

TABLE 35.1 Transepithelial Driving Forces for Na⁺

	LUMINAL [Na⁺]	TRANSEPITHELIAL CHEMICAL DRIVING FORCE[a,b]	TRANSEPITHELIAL VOLTAGE (ELECTRICAL DRIVING FORCE)[b,c]	TRANSEPITHELIAL ELECTROCHEMICAL DRIVING FORCE[b]
Proximal tubule, S1	142 mM	0 mV	−3 mV	−3 mV
Proximal tubule, S3	142 mM	0 mV	+3 mV	+3 mV
TAL	100 mM	−9 mV	+15 mV	+6 mV
DCT	70 mM	−19 mV	−5 to +5 mV	−24 to −14 mV
CCT	40 mM	−34 mV	−40 mV	−74 mV

[a]The chemical driving force is calculated assuming a plasma [Na⁺] of 142 mM and is given in mV.
[b]A negative value promotes passive Na⁺ movement from blood to lumen (i.e., backleak or secretion), whereas a positive value promotes passive Na⁺ movement from lumen to blood (i.e., reabsorption).
[c]A negative value indicates that the lumen is negative with respect to the blood.

Na⁺ AND Cl⁻, AND WATER TRANSPORT AT THE CELLULAR AND MOLECULAR LEVEL

Na⁺ reabsorption involves apical transporters or epithelial Na⁺ channels and a basolateral Na-K pump

Proximal Tubule Along the first half of the tubule (Fig. 35.4A), a variety of cotransporters in the *apical membrane* couples the downhill uptake of Na⁺ to the uphill uptake of solutes such as glucose, amino acids, phosphate, sulfate, lactate, and citrate. Many of these **Na⁺-driven cotransporters** are electrogenic, carrying net positive charge into the cell. Thus, both the low [Na⁺]ᵢ and the negative apical membrane voltage fuel the secondary active uptake of these other solutes. In addition to being coupled to the cotransporters, Na⁺ entry is also coupled to the extrusion of H⁺ through the electroneutral **Na-H exchanger 3 (NHE3)**.

Both cotransporters and exchangers exploit the downhill Na⁺ gradient across the apical cell membrane that is

established by the **Na-K pump** in the *basolateral membrane*. The Na-K pump—and, to a lesser extent, the **electrogenic Na/HCO₃ cotransporter 1 (NBCe1)**—are also responsible for the second step in Na⁺ reabsorption, moving Na⁺ from cell to blood. K⁺ channels establish the negative voltage across the basolateral membrane and permit the recycling of K⁺ that had been transported into the cell by the Na-K pump.

Thin Limbs of Henle's Loop Na⁺ transport by the thin descending and thin ascending limbs of Henle's loop is almost entirely passive and paracellular.

Thick Ascending Limb ⊙ 35-1 Two major pathways contribute to Na⁺ reabsorption in the TAL: transcellular and paracellular (Fig. 35.4B). The *transcellular pathway* includes two major mechanisms for the uptake of Na⁺ across the apical membrane. **Na/K/Cl cotransporter 2 (NKCC2)** couples the inward movement of 1 Na⁺, 1 K⁺, and 2 Cl⁻ ions in an electroneutral process driven by the downhill concentration gradients of Na⁺ and Cl⁻. The second entry pathway for Na⁺

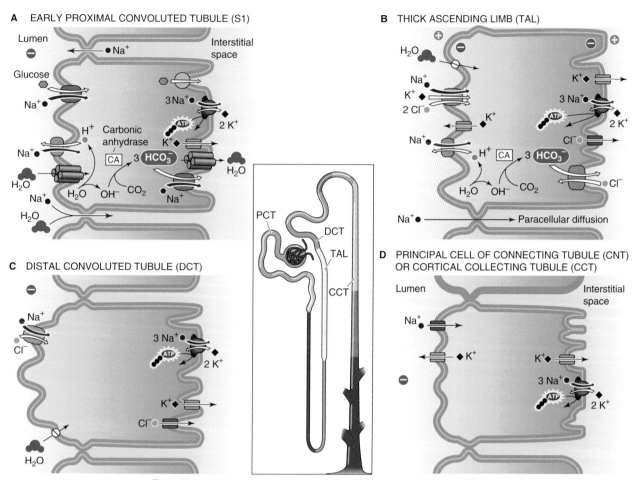

Figure 35.4 Cell models of Na⁺ reabsorption. *PCT,* Proximal convoluted tube.

is an **NHE3.** As in the proximal tubule, the basolateral Na-K pump keeps $[Na^+]_i$ low and moves Na^+ to the blood.

Two features of the apical step of Na^+ reabsorption in the TAL are noteworthy. First, the **loop diuretics** (e.g., furosemide and bumetanide) inhibit Na/K/Cl cotransport. Second, a large fraction of the K^+ that NKCC2 brings into the cell recycles to the lumen via apical K^+ channels. These channels are essential for replenishing luminal K^+ and thus for maintaining adequate Na/K/Cl cotransport.

A key aspect of the *paracellular pathway* for Na^+ reabsorption in the TAL is a **lumen-positive V_{te}** (Fig. 35.4B). Nearly all other epithelia have a lumen-negative V_{te} because the apical membrane voltage is less negative than the basolateral membrane voltage. The TAL is just the opposite. Its lumen-positive V_{te} develops because the apical membrane potential is more negative than the basolateral membrane potential, hence the V_{te} is lumen positive. Because the TAL has a low water permeability, removing luminal NaCl leaves the remaining tubule fluid *hypo-osmotic.* Hence, the TAL is sometimes referred to as the **diluting segment.**

The lumen-positive V_{te} provides the driving force for the diffusion of Na^+ across the tight junctions, accounting for approximately half of the Na^+ reabsorption by the TAL. The lumen-positive V_{te} also drives the passive reabsorption of K^+, Ca^{2+}, and Mg^{2+} via the paracellular pathway.

Distal Convoluted Tubule Na^+ reabsorption in the DCT occurs almost exclusively by the transcellular route (Fig. 35.4C). The *apical step* of Na^+ uptake is mediated by an electroneutral **Na/Cl cotransporter** (**NCC**) that is highly sensitive to **thiazide diuretics.** Although the thiazides produce less diuresis than do the loop diuretics, the thiazides are nevertheless effective in removing excess Na^+ from the body. The *basolateral step* of Na^+ reabsorption, as in other cells, is mediated by the Na-K pump. Because the DCT, like the TAL, has a low water permeability, removing luminal NaCl leaves the remaining tubule fluid even more hypo-osmotic. Hence, the DCT is also part of the "diluting segment."

Initial and Cortical Collecting Tubules ◉ 35-2 Na^+ reabsorption in the connecting tubule, **initial collecting tubule (ICT),** and cortical collecting tubule (CCT) is transcellular and mediated by the **principal cell** (Fig. 35.4D). Na^+ crosses the *apical membrane* of the principal cell via the **epithelial Na^+ channel (ENaC).** This channel is unique in that low levels of the diuretic drug **amiloride** specifically block it. Amiloride is a relatively mild diuretic because Na^+ reabsorption along the collecting duct is modest. The *basolateral step* of Na^+ reabsorption is again mediated by the Na-K pump, which also provides the electrochemical driving force for the apical entry of Na^+.

Medullary Collecting Duct The inner and outer medullary collecting ducts reabsorb only a minute amount of Na^+, ~3% of the filtered load (Fig. 35.2). It is likely that ENaC mediates the apical entry of Na^+ in these segments and that the Na-K pump extrudes Na^+ from the cell across the basolateral membrane (Fig. 35.4D).

Cl^- reabsorption involves both paracellular and transcellular pathways

Proximal Tubule The proximal tubule reabsorbs Cl^- by both the transcellular and the paracellular routes, with the *paracellular* believed to be the dominant one in the early proximal tubule (Fig. 35.5A). The *transcellular pathway* is more appreciable in the late proximal tubule (Fig. 35.5B), where the energetically uphill influx of Cl^- across the apical membrane occurs via an exchange of luminal Cl^- for cellular anions (e.g., formate, oxalate, HCO_3^- and OH^-), mediated at least in part by the anion exchanger SLC26A6. Cl-base exchange is an example of *tertiary* active transport: the apical NHE3, itself a *secondary* active transporter, provides the H^+ that neutralizes base in the lumen, thereby sustaining the gradient for Cl-anion exchange. The basolateral exit step for transcellular Cl^- movement may occur in part via a **Cl^- channel** and the **K/Cl cotransporters.**

Passive Cl^- reabsorption via the *paracellular pathway* is driven by different electrochemical Cl^- gradients in the early versus the late proximal tubule (Fig. 35.5A versus B).

Thick Ascending Limb Cl^- reabsorption in the TAL takes place largely by Na/K/Cl cotransport across the apical membrane (Fig. 35.5C), as we already noted in our discussion of Na^+ reabsorption (Fig. 35.4B). The exit of Cl^- across the basolateral cell membrane via Cl^- channels.

Distal Convoluted Tubule Cl^- reabsorption by the DCT (Fig. 35.5D) occurs by a mechanism that is somewhat similar to that in the TAL, except the apical step occurs via NCC, as discussed above in connection with Na^+ reabsorption by the DCT (Fig. 35.4C). Cl^- channels that are probably similar to those in the TAL mediate the basolateral Cl^- exit step.

Collecting Ducts The ICT and the CCT reabsorb Cl^- by two mechanisms. First, the principal cell generates a V_{te} (~40 mV, lumen negative) that is favorable for *paracellular* diffusion of Cl^- (Fig. 35.5E). Second, the β-type intercalated cells reabsorb Cl^- via a *transcellular* process in which **pendrin** mediates Cl^- uptake across the apical membrane in exchange for HCO_3^-, and Cl^- exits via channels in the basolateral membrane (Fig. 35.5F). Moreover, two cycles of Cl-HCO_3 exchange via pendrin may operate in parallel with one cycle of Na-dependent Cl-HCO_3 exchange via NDCBE to produce net electroneutral NaCl entry across the apical membrane of β-intercalated cells (Fig. 35.5F). Neither the α-type intercalated cells nor the principal cells participates in transcellular Cl^- reabsorption.

Water reabsorption is passive and secondary to solute transport

Proximal Tubule ⊙ **35-3** The pathway for water movement across the proximal-tubule epithelium appears to be a combination of transcellular and paracellular transit, with the transcellular route dominating. The reabsorbate is

isosmotic. The reason for the high rate of water movement through the proximal-tubule cell is the presence of a high density of aquaporin 1 (AQP1) **water channels** in both the apical and basolateral membranes.

Loop of Henle and Distal Nephron Two features distinguish water and Na^+ transport in the distal nephron. First, the TAL and all downstream segments have a relatively low water permeability in the absence of AVP (or antidiuretic hormone). Second, the combination of NaCl reabsorption and low water permeability allows these nephron segments to generate a low luminal [Na^+] and osmolality with respect to the surrounding interstitial fluid. Given this large osmotic gradient across the epithelium, the distal nephron is poised to reabsorb water passively from a hypo-osmotic luminal fluid into the isosmotic blood when AVP increases the water permeability.

The kidney's high O_2 consumption reflects a high level of active Na^+ transport

Because virtually all Na^+ transport ultimately depends on the activity of the ATP-driven Na-K pump and, therefore, on the generation of ATP by oxidative metabolism, it is not surprising that renal O_2 consumption is extraordinarily large. Despite their low weight (<0.5% of body weight), the kidneys are responsible for 7% to 10% of total O_2 consumption.

⊙ 35-4 REGULATION OF Na^+ AND Cl^- TRANSPORT

The body regulates "effective circulating volume" by regulating Na^+ excretion.

Three factors that respond to decreases in effective circulating volume—the renin-angiotensin-aldosterone axis, renal sympathetic nerve activity, and AVP (see ⊙ 23-26)—do so in part by increasing Na^+ reabsorption in various nephron segments. Likewise, several factors that respond to increases in effective circulating volume—including atrial natriuretic peptide and dopamine—do so in part by reducing Na^+ reabsorption in various segments of the nephron. That is, they produce a **natriuresis.**

Glomerulotubular balance stabilizes fractional Na^+ reabsorption by the proximal tubule in the face of changes in the filtered Na^+ load

When hemodynamic changes (e.g., caused by a high-protein diet, intense exercise, severe pain, or anesthesia) alter GFR and thus the Na^+ load presented to the nephron, *proximal tubules respond by reabsorbing a relatively constant fraction of the Na^+ load*. This constancy of fractional Na^+ reabsorption along the proximal tubule—**glomerulotubular (GT) balance**—is independent of external neural and hormonal control, and prevents spontaneous fluctuations in GFR from causing marked changes in Na^+ excretion.

The distal nephron also increases Na^+ reabsorption in response to an increased Na^+ load

The tubules of the distal nephron, like their proximal counterparts, also increase their absolute magnitude of Na^+

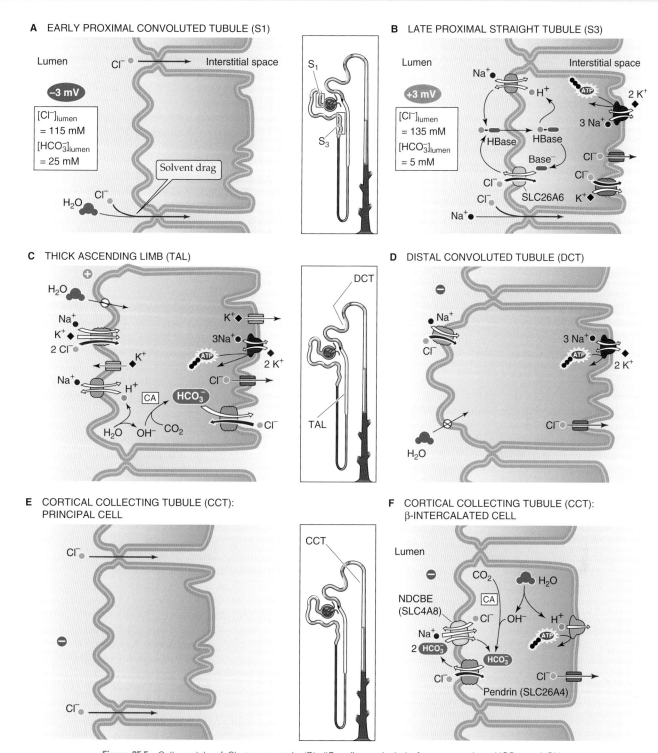

A EARLY PROXIMAL CONVOLUTED TUBULE (S1)

Lumen

Cl⁻

Interstitial space

−3 mV

$[Cl^-]_{lumen}$ = 115 mM
$[HCO_3^-]_{lumen}$ = 25 mM

Solvent drag

H_2O Cl⁻

S_1

S_3

B LATE PROXIMAL STRAIGHT TUBULE (S3)

Lumen

Na⁺

Interstitial space

+3 mV

$[Cl^-]_{lumen}$ = 135 mM
$[HCO_3^-]_{lumen}$ = 5 mM

H⁺

ATP

2 K⁺

3 Na⁺

HBase HBase

Base⁻

Cl⁻

Cl⁻ Cl⁻

Cl⁻ SLC26A6 K⁺

Na⁺

C THICK ASCENDING LIMB (TAL)

H_2O

Na⁺
K⁺
2 Cl⁻

K⁺

Na⁺ H⁺

CA

H_2O OH⁻ CO_2

K⁺

3Na⁺

ATP 2 K⁺

Cl⁻

HCO_3^-

Cl⁻

DCT

TAL

D DISTAL CONVOLUTED TUBULE (DCT)

Na⁺

Cl⁻

3 Na⁺

ATP 2 K⁺

H_2O

Cl⁻

E CORTICAL COLLECTING TUBULE (CCT): PRINCIPAL CELL

Cl⁻

Cl⁻

CCT

F CORTICAL COLLECTING TUBULE (CCT): β-INTERCALATED CELL

Lumen

CO_2 H_2O

CA

NDCBE (SLC4A8)

Cl⁻ OH⁻ H⁺

Na⁺

ATP

2 HCO_3^-

HCO_3^-

Cl⁻ Cl⁻

Pendrin (SLC26A4)

Figure 35.5 Cell models of Cl⁻ transport. In (B), "Base" may include formate, oxalate, HCO_3^-, and OH⁻. "HBase" represents the conjugate weak acid (e.g., formic acid). *CA,* Carbonic anhydrase.

reabsorption in response to increased flow and Na⁺ delivery. The principle is that the fall of luminal [Na⁺] along the length of the tubule is less steep when flow increases. Because the transport mechanisms responsible for Na⁺ reabsorption by the distal nephron are more effective at higher luminal [Na⁺] values, reabsorption at any site increases with flow.

Four parallel pathways that regulate effective circulating volume all modulate Na⁺ reabsorption

Renin-Angiotensin-Aldosterone Axis ⊙ 35-5 **ANG II**— the second element in the renin-angiotensin-aldosterone axis—binds to AT₁ receptors at the apical and basolateral membranes of proximal-tubule cells and, predominantly via protein kinase C, stimulates NHE3. ANG II also upregulates expression of NHE3 and NKCC2 in the TAL. Moreover, ANG II upregulates NCC activity in the DCT and stimulates apical Na^+ channels in the ICT. These effects promote Na^+ reabsorption.

⊙ **35-6 Aldosterone**—the final element in the renin-angiotensin-aldosterone axis—stimulates Na^+ reabsorption by NCC in the DCT and by the ENaC in the late DCT, connecting tubule, and collecting ducts. Normally, <10% of the filtered Na^+ load is under humoral control by aldosterone. Nevertheless, the sustained loss of even a small fraction of the filtered Na^+ load would exceed the daily Na^+ intake significantly. Accordingly, the lack of aldosterone that occurs in adrenal insufficiency (Addison disease) can lead to severe Na^+ depletion, contraction of the ECF volume, low plasma volume, and hypotension.

⊙ **35-7** Aldosterone acts on its target tissues by binding to cytoplasmic **mineralocorticoid receptors (MRs)** that then translocate to the nucleus and upregulate transcription. Thus, the effects of aldosterone require a few hours to manifest themselves because they depend on the increased production of aldosterone-induced proteins. The ultimate cellular actions of aldosterone include upregulation of apical ENaCs, apical K^+ channels, the basolateral Na-K pump, and mitochondrial metabolism.

⊙ **35-8** Because MRs distinguish poorly between glucocorticoids and mineralocorticoids, and because plasma concentrations of glucocorticoids greatly exceed those of aldosterone, one would expect glucocorticoids to exert a mineralocorticoid effect and cause Na^+ retention. Under normal conditions, this does not happen because of the enzyme **11β-hydroxysteroid dehydrogenase 2 (11β-HSD2).** This enzyme irreversibly converts cortisol into cortisone, an inactive metabolite with low affinity for MRs. In sharp contrast, the enzyme does *not* metabolize aldosterone. Thus, 11β-HSD2 enhances the apparent specificity of MRs by protecting them from illicit occupancy by cortisol. As may be expected, an 11β-HSD2 deficiency may cause **apparent mineralocorticoid excess (AME),** with abnormal Na^+ retention, hypokalemia, and hypertension. Carbenoxolone, a specific inhibitor of 11β-HSD2, prevents metabolism of cortisol in target cells, thus permitting abnormal activation of MRs by this glucocorticoid. Another inhibitor of 11β-HSD2 is glycyrrhetinic acid, a component of "natural" **licorice.** Thus, natural licorice can also cause the symptoms of AME.

Sympathetic Division of the Autonomic Nervous System Sympathetic nerve terminals in the kidney release norepinephrine, which has two major *direct* effects on Na^+ reabsorption. First, high levels of sympathetic stimulation markedly reduce renal blood flow and, therefore, GFR. A decreased filtered load of Na^+ will tend to cause Na^+ excretion to fall. Second, even low levels of sympathetic stimulation activate

α-**adrenergic receptors** in proximal tubules. This activation stimulates both the apical NHE3 and basolateral Na-K pump (Fig. 35.4A), thereby increasing Na^+ reabsorption, independent of any hemodynamic effects. Conversely, surgical denervation of the kidneys can reduce blood pressure in patients with resistant hypertension.

Arginine Vasopressin (Antidiuretic Hormone) ⊙ **35-9** Released by the posterior pituitary, AVP binds to a **V_2 receptor** at the basolateral membrane of target cells. Acting via G_s, the AVP increases $[cAMP]_i$. The overall renal effect of AVP in humans is to produce urine with a high osmolality and thereby retain water (see ⊙ 38-3). However, AVP also stimulates Na^+ reabsorption by increasing the number of open Na^+ channels in the apical membrane.

Atrial Natriuretic Peptide ⊙ **35-10** Of the four parallel effectors that control effective circulating volume, ANP is the only one that promotes natriuresis. A polypeptide released by atrial myocytes, ANP stimulates a receptor guanylyl cyclase to generate cGMP. The major effects of ANP are hemodynamic. It causes renal vasodilation by increasing blood flow to both the cortex and the medulla. Increased blood flow to the *cortex* raises GFR and increases the Na^+ load to the proximal tubule and to the TAL. Increased blood flow to the *medulla* washes out the medullary interstitium, thus decreasing osmolality and ultimately reducing passive Na^+ reabsorption in the thin ascending limb. The combined effect of increasing cortical and medullary blood flow is to increase the Na^+ load to the distal nephron and thus to increase urinary Na^+ excretion. In addition to having hemodynamic effects, ANP directly inhibits Na^+ transport in the inner medullary collecting duct, perhaps by decreasing the activity of nonselective cation channels in the apical membrane.

Dopamine decreases Na⁺ reabsorption

In addition to ANP (see previous section), dopamine has significant natriuretic action, in part due to inhibition of Na^+ reabsorption at the level of the tubule cell.

From circulating L-dopa, proximal-tubule cells use L-amino acid decarboxylase (see Fig. 13.6C) to form dopamine, which they then secrete into the tubule lumen. Na^+ loading increases the synthesis and urinary excretion rate of dopamine, whereas a low Na^+ diet has the opposite effect. Dopamine causes renal vasodilation, which increases Na^+ excretion. Dopamine also directly inhibits Na^+ reabsorption at the level of tubule cells. Indeed, D1 dopamine receptors are present in the renal cortex, where they lead to an increase in $[cAMP]_i$. The result is an inhibition of apical NHE3 in the proximal tubule and inhibition of the basolateral Na-K pump in multiple tubule segments. In humans, administering low doses of dopamine leads to natriuresis.

CHAPTER 36

TRANSPORT OF UREA, GLUCOSE, OTHER ORGANIC SOLUTES, PHOSPHATE, CALCIUM, AND MAGNESIUM

Gerhard Giebisch[†] and Peter S. Aronson

The kidney plays a central role in controlling the plasma levels of a wide range of solutes that are present at low concentrations in the body. The renal excretion of a solute depends on three processes—filtration, reabsorption, and secretion. The kidney filters and then totally reabsorbs some of the substances we discuss in this chapter (e.g., glucose). Others it filters and also secretes (e.g., the organic anion para-aminohippurate [PAH]). Still others, the kidney filters, reabsorbs, and secretes (e.g., urea).

UREA

⊙ 36-1 The kidney filters, reabsorbs, and secretes urea

The liver generates urea from NH_4^+, the primary nitrogenous end product of amino-acid catabolism (see Fig. 46.10). The primary route for urea excretion is the urine. The normal plasma concentration of urea is 2.5 to 6 mM. Clinical laboratories report plasma urea levels as **blood urea nitrogen (BUN)** in the units (mg of elemental nitrogen)/(dL plasma); normal values are 7 to 18 mg/dL. For a 70-kg human ingesting a typical Western diet and producing 1.5 to 2 L/day of urine, the urinary excretion of urea is ~450 mmol/day.

The kidney freely filters urea at the glomerulus, and then it both reabsorbs and secretes it. Because the tubules reabsorb more urea than they secrete, the amount of urea excreted in the urine is less than the quantity filtered. In the example shown in Fig. 36.1A (i.e., average urine flow), the kidneys excrete ~40% of the filtered urea. The primary sites for urea reabsorption are the proximal tubule and the medullary collecting duct, whereas the primary sites for secretion are the thin limbs of the loop of Henle.

In the very early **proximal tubule** (Fig. 36.1B), [urea] in the lumen is the same as in blood plasma. However, water reabsorption tends to increase [urea] in the lumen, thereby generating a favorable transepithelial gradient that drives urea reabsorption by **diffusion** via the transcellular or paracellular pathway. In addition, some urea may be reabsorbed by **solvent drag** (see ⊙ 20-8) across the tight junctions. The greater the fluid reabsorption along the proximal tubule, the greater the reabsorption of urea via both diffusion and solvent drag.

In more distal urea-permeable nephron segments, urea moves via facilitated diffusion through the **urea transporters (UTs).**

In *juxtamedullary* nephrons, as the tubule fluid in the **thin descending limb (tDLH)** approaches the tip of the loop of Henle, [urea] is higher in the medullary interstitium than in the lumen (see ⊙ 38-1). Thus, the deepest portion of the tDLH *secretes* urea via facilitated diffusion (Fig. 36.1C) mediated by the urea transporter **UT-A2.** As the fluid turns the corner to flow up the **thin ascending limb (tALH),** the tubule cells continue to secrete urea into the lumen, probably also by facilitated diffusion (Fig. 36.1D).

The tDLH of *superficial* nephrons is located in the inner stripe of the outer medulla. Here, the interstitial [urea] is higher than the luminal [urea] because the vasa recta carry urea from the inner medulla. Because the tDLH cells of these superficial nephrons appear to have UT-A2 along their entire length, these cells *secrete* urea. Thus, both superficial and probably also juxtamedullary nephrons contribute to urea secretion, raising urea delivery to ~110% of the filtered load at the level of the cortical collecting ducts.

⊙ 36-2 Finally, the **inner medullary collecting duct (IMCD)** *reabsorbs* urea via a transcellular route involving apical and basolateral steps of facilitated diffusion (Fig. 36.1E). The **UT-A1** urea transporter moves urea across the apical membrane of the IMCD cell, whereas **UT-A3** probably mediates urea movement across the basolateral membrane. Arginine vasopressin (AVP)—which is also known as antidiuretic hormone (ADH)—stimulates UT-A1 and UT-A3.

Urea excretion rises with increasing urinary flow

Because urea transport depends primarily on urea concentration differences across the tubule epithelium, changes in urine flow unavoidably affect renal urea handling (Fig. 36.2). At low urine flow, when the tubule reabsorbs considerable water and, therefore, much urea, the kidneys excrete only ~15% of filtered urea (see Fig. 38.4). However, the kidneys may excrete as much as 70% of filtered urea at high urine flow, when the tubules reabsorb relatively less water and urea. During the progression of renal disease, the decline of glomerular filtration rate (GFR) leads to a low urine flow and urea retention, and thus an increase in BUN.

[†]Deceased.

A HANDLING OF UREA ALONG NEPHRON

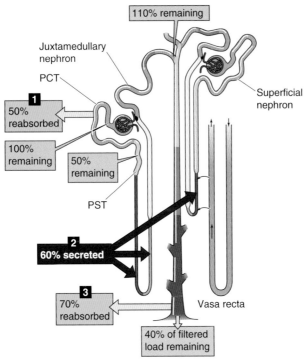

B PROXIMAL TUBULE

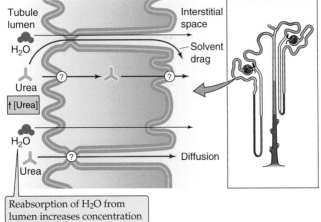

Reabsorption of H₂O from lumen increases concentration of urea in the lumen.

C THIN DESCENDING LIMB (tDLH)

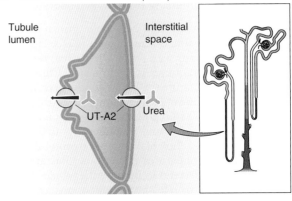

D THIN ASCENDING LIMB (tALH)

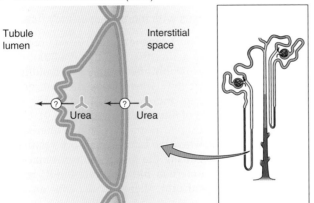

E INNER MEDULLARY COLLECTING DUCT (IMCD)

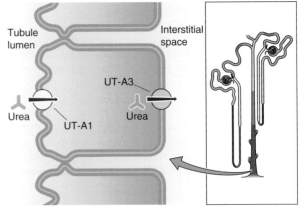

Figure 36.1 Urea handling by the kidney. In (A) we assume a normal urine flow and thus a urea excretion of 40% of the filtered load. The *numbered yellow boxes* indicate the fraction of the filtered load that various nephron segments *reabsorb*. The *red box* indicates the fraction of the filtered load jointly *secreted* by both superficial and juxtamedullary nephrons. The *green boxes* indicate the fraction of the filtered load that remains in the lumen at various sites. The values in the boxes are approximations.

GLUCOSE

The proximal tubule reabsorbs glucose via apical, electrogenic Na/glucose cotransport and basolateral facilitated diffusion

The fasting plasma glucose concentration is normally 4 to 5 mM (70 to 100 mg/dL). The kidneys freely filter glucose at the glomerulus and then reabsorb it, so that only trace amounts normally appear in the urine (Fig. 36.3A). The

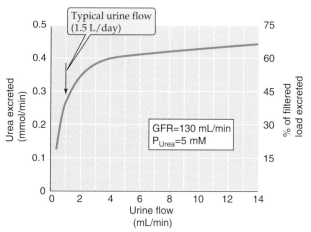

Figure 36.2 Urea excretion versus urine flow. P_{Urea}, Plasma concentration of urea. (Data from Austin JH, Stillman E, Van Slyke DD: Factors governing the excretion rate of urea. J Biol Chem 46:91–112, 1921.)

proximal tubule reabsorbs nearly all the filtered load of glucose, mostly along the first third of this segment. More distal segments reabsorb almost all of the remainder. In the proximal tubule, luminal [glucose] is initially equal to plasma [glucose]. As the early proximal tubule reabsorbs glucose, luminal [glucose] drops sharply, falling to levels far lower than those in the interstitium. Accordingly, glucose reabsorption occurs against a concentration gradient and must, therefore, be active.

Glucose reabsorption is transcellular; glucose moves from the lumen to the proximal tubule cell via Na/glucose cotransport, and from cytoplasm to blood via facilitated diffusion (Fig. 36.3B and C). At the apical membrane, **Na/glucose cotransporters** (**SGLT1, SGLT2**) couple the movements of D-glucose (but not L-glucose) and Na^+. The electrochemical gradient of Na^+ drives the uphill transport of glucose into the cell (i.e., secondary active transport), thereby concentrating glucose in the cytoplasm.

In the early part of the proximal tubule (S1 segment), a high-capacity, low-affinity transporter called **SGLT2** mediates apical glucose uptake (Fig. 36.3B). This cotransporter has an Na^+-to-glucose stoichiometry of 1:1 and is responsible for 90% of the glucose reabsorption. Indeed, SGLT2 inhibitors have recently become available to treat patients with hyperglycemia due to diabetes mellitus. In the later part of the proximal tubule (S3 segment), a high-affinity, low-capacity cotransporter called **SGLT1** is responsible for apical glucose uptake (Fig. 36.3C). Because this cotransporter has an Na^+-to-glucose stoichiometry of 2:1

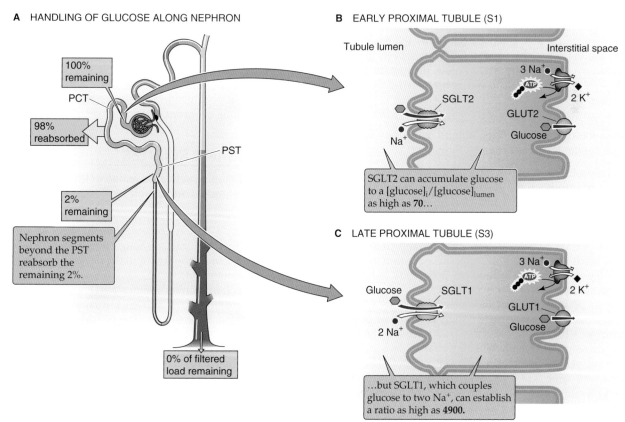

Figure 36.3 Glucose handling by the kidney. The *yellow box* indicates the fraction of the filtered load that the proximal tubule reabsorbs. The *green boxes* indicate the fraction of the filtered load that remains in the lumen at various sites. The values in the boxes are approximations. *PCT,* Proximal convoluted tubule; *PST,* proximal straight tubule.

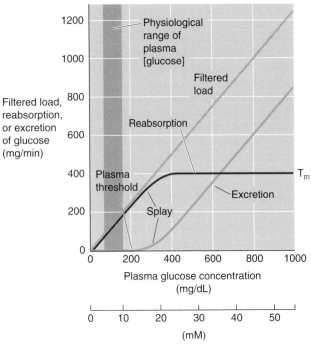

Figure 36.4 Glucose titration curve. T_m is the transport maximum for reabsorption. The darker vertical band represents the physiological range of plasma [glucose], which spans from a fasting [glucose] to the peak value after a meal.

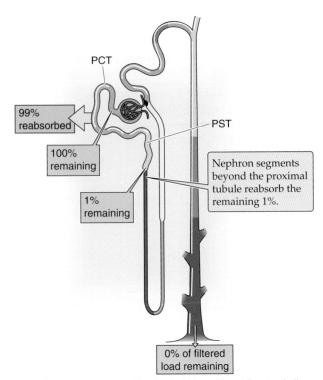

Figure 36.5 Amino-acid handling by the kidney. The *yellow box* indicates the fraction of the filtered load that the proximal tubule reabsorbs. The *green boxes* indicate the fraction of the filtered load that remains in the lumen at various sites. The values in the boxes are approximations. *PCT*, Proximal convoluted tubule; *PST*, proximal straight tubule.

(i.e., far more electrochemical energy per glucose molecule), it can generate a far larger glucose gradient across the apical membrane.

Once inside the cell, glucose exits across the basolateral membrane via a member of the **GLUT** family of glucose transporters. These transporters—quite distinct from the SGLTs—are Na$^+$-*independent* and move glucose by facilitated diffusion.

Glucose excretion in the urine occurs only when the plasma concentration exceeds a threshold

The relationship between plasma [glucose] and the rate of glucose reabsorption is the **glucose titration curve.** Fig. 36.4 shows how rates of glucose filtration (*orange curve*), excretion (*green curve*), and reabsorption (*red curve*) vary when plasma [glucose] is increased by infusing intravenous glucose. As plasma [glucose] rises—at constant GFR—from control levels to ~200 mg/dL, glucose excretion remains zero. It is only above a **threshold** of ~200 mg/dL (~11 mM) that glucose appears in the urine. Glucose excretion rises linearly as plasma [glucose] increases further. Because the threshold is considerably higher than the normal plasma [glucose] of ~100 mg/dL (~5.5 mM), and because the body effectively regulates plasma [glucose], healthy people do not excrete any glucose in the urine, even after a meal. Likewise, patients with *diabetes mellitus,* who have chronically elevated plasma glucose concentrations, do not experience glucosuria until the blood sugar level exceeds this threshold value.

The glucose titration curve shows a second property, **saturation.** The rate of glucose reabsorption reaches a plateau—the **transport maximum (T_m)**—at ~400 mg/min. The

reason for the T_m value is that the SGLTs now become fully saturated. Therefore, these transporters cannot respond to further increases in filtered glucose.

Fig. 36.4A also shows that the rate of glucose reabsorption reaches the T_m gradually, not abruptly. This **splay** in the titration curve probably reflects both anatomical and kinetic differences among nephrons.

OTHER ORGANIC SOLUTES

The proximal tubule reabsorbs amino acids using a wide variety of apical and basolateral transporters

The total concentration of amino acids in the blood is ~2.4 mM. These L-amino acids are largely those absorbed by the gastrointestinal tract, although they also may be the products of protein catabolism or of the de novo synthesis of nonessential amino acids.

The glomeruli freely filter amino acids (Fig. 36.5). Because amino acids are important nutrients, it is advantageous to retrieve them from the filtrate. The proximal tubule reabsorbs >98% of these amino acids via a transcellular route, using a wide variety of amino-acid transporters. At the *apical* membrane, amino acids enter the cell via Na$^+$-driven or H$^+$-driven transporters as well as amino-acid exchangers. At the *basolateral* membrane, amino acids exit the cell via amino-acid exchangers—some of which are Na$^+$ dependent—and also by facilitated diffusion.

With a few exceptions, the kinetics of amino-acid reabsorption resembles that of glucose: the titration curves show

A HANDLING OF OLIGOPEPTIDES
ALONG NEPHRON

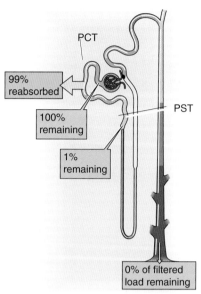

B PROXIMAL TUBULE: OLIGOPEPTIDES

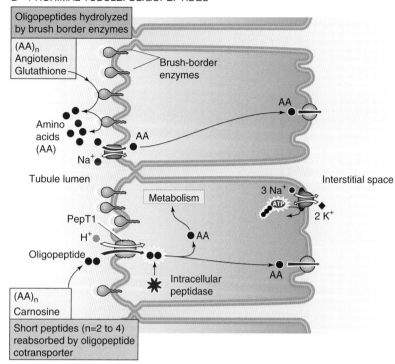

Figure. 36.6 Oligopeptide handling by the kidney. The *yellow box* indicates the fraction of the filtered load that the proximal tubule reabsorbs. The *green boxes* indicate the fraction of the filtered load that remains in the lumen at various sites. The values in the boxes are approximations. *PCT,* Proximal convoluted tubule; *PST,* proximal straight tubule.

saturation and transport maxima (T_m). In contrast to the case of glucose, in which the T_m is relatively high, the T_m values for amino acids are generally low. As a consequence, when plasma levels of amino acids increase, the kidneys excrete the amino acids in the urine, thus limiting the maximal plasma levels.

An H⁺-driven cotransporter takes up oligopeptides across the apical membrane, whereas endocytosis takes up proteins and other large organic molecules

Oligopeptides The proximal tubules reabsorb ~99% of filtered oligopeptides (Fig. 36.6A). Segments beyond the proximal tubule contribute little to peptide transport.

Several peptidases are present at the outer surface of the brush-border membrane of proximal-tubule cells (Fig. 36.6B), just as they are in the small intestine (see ◉ 45-1) These brush-border enzymes (e.g., γ-glutamyltransferase, aminopeptidases, endopeptidases, and dipeptidases) hydrolyze many peptides, including angiotensin II, thereby releasing into the tubule lumen the free constituent amino acids and oligopeptides. Tubule cells reabsorb the resulting free amino acids as described in the previous section. The cell also absorbs the resulting oligopeptides (two to five residues)—as well as other peptides (e.g., carnosine) that are resistant to brush-border enzymes—using the apical H/oligopeptide cotransporters **PepT1** and **PepT2**. PepT1 is a low-affinity, high-capacity system in the early proximal tubule, whereas PepT2 is a high-affinity, low-capacity transporter in the late proximal segments—analogous in their properties to SGLT2 and SGLT.

Once inside the cell, the oligopeptides undergo hydrolysis by cytosolic peptidases.

Proteins Although the glomerular filtration barrier generally prevents the filtration of large amounts of protein, this restriction is incomplete. For example, the albumin concentration in the filtrate is very low (4 to 20 mg/L), only 0.01% to 0.05% of the plasma albumin concentration. Nevertheless, given a GFR of 180 L/day, the filtered albumin amounts to 0.7 to 3.6 g/day. In contrast, albumin excretion in the urine normally is only ~30 mg/day. Thus, the tubules reabsorb some 96% to 99% of filtered albumin (Fig. 36.7A). In addition to albumin, the tubules extensively reabsorb low-molecular-weight proteins that are relatively freely filtered (e.g., lysozyme, light chains of immunoglobulins, and β₂-microglobulin), SH-containing peptides (e.g., insulin), and other polypeptide hormones (e.g., parathyroid hormone [PTH], atrial natriuretic peptide [ANP], and glucagon). It is therefore not surprising that tubule injury can give rise to proteinuria even in the absence of glomerular injury.

Proximal-tubule cells use **receptor-mediated endocytosis** to reabsorb proteins and polypeptides (Fig. 36.7B). The first step is binding to receptors at the apical membrane, followed by internalization into clathrin-coated endocytic vesicles. The vesicles target to lysosomes, where acid-dependent proteases largely digest the contents over a period that is on the order of minutes for peptide hormones and many hours or even days for other proteins. The cells ultimately release the low-molecular-weight end products of digestion, largely amino acids, across the basolateral membrane into

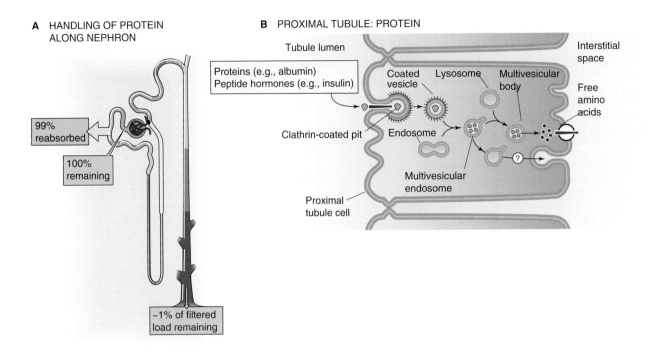

A HANDLING OF PROTEIN ALONG NEPHRON

99% reabsorbed

100% remaining

~1% of filtered load remaining

B PROXIMAL TUBULE: PROTEIN

Tubule lumen

Proteins (e.g., albumin)
Peptide hormones (e.g., insulin)

Clathrin-coated pit

Coated vesicle

Lysosome

Endosome

Multivesicular endosome

Multivesicular body

Interstitial space

Free amino acids

Proximal tubule cell

Figure 36.7 Protein handling by the kidney. The *yellow box* indicates the fraction of the filtered load that the proximal tubule reabsorbs. The *green boxes* indicate the fraction of the filtered load that remains in the lumen at various sites. The values in the boxes are approximations.

TABLE 36.1 Components of Total Plasma Phosphate

	mg/dL	mM	% OF TOTAL
Ionized HPO_4^{2-} and $H_2PO_4^-$	2.1	0.7	50
Diffusible phosphate complexes	1.5	0.5	40
Nondiffusible (protein-bound) phosphate	0.6	0.2	10
Total phosphate	4.2	1.4	100

the peritubular circulation. A small subset of proteins avoid the lysosomes and moves by transcytosis for release at the basolateral membrane.

The kidney plays a major role in the metabolism of small proteins and peptide hormones. Renal extraction rates may account for as much as 80% of the total metabolic clearance.

PHOSPHATE

The metabolism of **inorganic phosphate (P_i)** depends on bone, the gastrointestinal tract, and the kidneys (see Fig. 52.2). About half of total plasma phosphate (Table 36.1) is in an ionized form, and the rest is either complexed to small solutes (~40%) or bound to protein (10% to 15%). The plasma concentration of total P_i varies rather widely, between 0.8 and 1.5 mM (2.5 to 4.5 mg/dL of elemental phosphorus). Thus, the filterable phosphate (i.e., both the ionized and complexed) varies between ~0.7 and 1.3 mM. At a normal blood pH of 7.4, 80% of the ionized plasma phosphate is **HPO_4^{2-}** and the rest

is **$H_2PO_4^-$**. Assuming that the total plasma phosphate concentration is 4.2 mg/dL, that only the free and complexed phosphate is filterable, and that the GFR is 180 L/day, each day the kidneys filter ~7000 mg of phosphate. Because this amount is more than an order of magnitude greater than the total extracellular pool of phosphate (see Fig. 52.2) it is clear that the kidney must reabsorb most of the phosphate filtered in the glomerulus.

⊙ 36-3 The proximal tubule reabsorbs phosphate via apical Na/phosphate cotransporters

The proximal tubule reabsorbs 80% to 95% of the filtered phosphate (Fig. 36.8A). More distal nephron segments reabsorb a negligible fraction of the filtered phosphate. Thus, the kidneys excrete 5% to 20% of the filtered load of phosphate in the urine under normal conditions.

The proximal tubule reabsorbs most of the filtered phosphate by the transcellular route (Fig. 36.8B). Phosphate ions enter the cell across the *apical* membrane by secondary active transport, energized by the apical electrochemical Na^+ gradient. At least three separate **Na/phosphate cotransporters** contribute: NaPi-IIa, NaPi-IIc, and PiT-2. The passive exit of phosphate across the *basolateral* membrane occurs by mechanisms that are still unknown (Fig. 36.8B).

Phosphate excretion in the urine already occurs at physiological plasma concentrations

Phosphate handling by the kidney shares some of the properties of renal glucose handling, including threshold, saturation with T_m kinetics, and splay (Fig. 36.9). However, important differences

A HANDLING OF PHOSPHATE ALONG NEPHRON

PCT

80% to 95% reabsorbed

100% remaining

PST

5% to 20% remaining

For individuals on a low-P_i diet, P_i excretion is minimal.

5% to 20% of filtered load remaining on a normal diet.

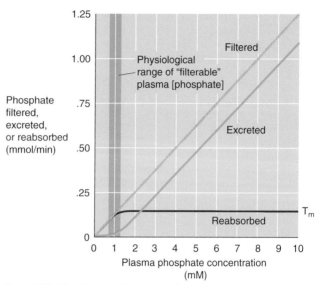

Phosphate filtered, excreted, or reabsorbed (mmol/min)

Physiological range of "filterable" plasma [phosphate]

Filtered

Excreted

Reabsorbed

T_m

Plasma phosphate concentration (mM)

Figure. 36.9 Phosphate titration curves. The plasma phosphate concentration is the filterable phosphate (i.e., ionized plus complexed to small solutes). The dark vertical band is the approximate range of normal filterable values.

B PROXIMAL TUBULE

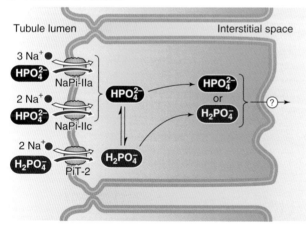

Tubule lumen

Interstitial space

3 Na$^+$

HPO_4^{2-}

NaPi-IIa

HPO_4^{2-}

2 Na$^+$

HPO_4^{2-}

NaPi-IIc

HPO_4^{2-} or $H_2PO_4^-$

?

2 Na$^+$

$H_2PO_4^-$

PiT-2

$H_2PO_4^-$

Figure. 36.8 Phosphate handling by the kidney. The numbered *yellow boxes* indicate the fraction of the filtered load that various nephron segments reabsorb. The *green boxes* indicate the fraction of the filtered load that remains in the lumen at various sites. The values in the boxes are approximations. *PCT,* Proximal convoluted tubule; *PST,* proximal straight tubule.

exist. First, some phosphate excretion (*green curve*) occurs even at normal levels of plasma [phosphate]. Thus, a small increment in the plasma [phosphate] results in significant acceleration of phosphate excretion (i.e., to higher values along the *green curve*). Second, the kidney reaches the T_m for phosphate (*red curve*) at the high end of normal plasma [phosphate] values.

⊙ 36-4 Parathyroid hormone inhibits apical Na/phosphate uptake, promoting phosphate excretion

The most important hormonal regulator of phosphate handling by the kidney is **PTH,** which inhibits phosphate reabsorption

and thus promotes phosphate excretion. PTH binds to **PTH 1 receptors (PTH1Rs),** which appear to couple to *two* heterotrimeric G proteins. The first ($G\alpha_s$) activates adenylyl cyclase and, via cAMP, stimulates protein kinase A (PKA). The second ($G\alpha_q$), particularly at low PTH levels, activates phospholipase C (PLC), and then protein kinase C (PKC). Once activated, PKA and PKC promote endocytotic removal of NaPi from the apical membrane with targeting for degradation in lysosomes, which reduces phosphate reabsorption.

⊙ 36-5 Fibroblast growth factor 23 and other phosphatonins also inhibit apical Na/phosphate uptake, promoting phosphate excretion

Phosphatonins are the circulating factors that cause renal phosphate wasting in diseases such as oncogenic osteomalacia, autosomal dominant hypophosphatemic rickets, and X-linked hypophosphatemic rickets. In these diseases, phosphatonins—including fibroblast growth factor 23 (**FGF23**)—cause the kidneys to excrete more phosphate.

In response to *hyper*phosphatemia, osteocytes release FGF23, which acts via the **receptor tyrosine kinase FGFR1** and the coreceptor **Klotho** to reduce the expression of Na/phosphate cotransporters and thereby augment renal phosphate excretion.

CALCIUM

Binding to plasma proteins and formation of Ca^{2+}-anion complexes influence the filtration and reabsorption of Ca^{2+}

The *total* calcium concentration in plasma is normally 2.2 to 2.6 mM (8.8 to 10.6 mg/dL). Table 36.2 summarizes the forms of calcium in the plasma. Some 40% binds to plasma proteins, mainly albumin, and constitutes the nonfilterable fraction. The **filterable** portion, ~60% of total plasma calcium, consists of two moieties. The first, ~15% of the total, complexes with small anions such as carbonate, citrate, phosphate, and sulfate. The second, ~45% of total calcium, is the ionized calcium (Ca^{2+}) that one may measure with Ca^{2+}-sensitive electrodes or dyes. It is the concentration of this

free, ionized calcium that the body tightly regulates; plasma [Ca^{2+}] normally is 1.0 to 1.3 mM (4.0 to 5.2 mg/dL).

TABLE 36.2 Components of Total Plasma Calcium

	mg/dL	mM	% OF TOTAL
Ionized Ca^{2+}	4.7	1.2	~45%
Filterable calcium complexes	1.4	0.3	~15%
Non-filterable (protein-bound) calcium	3.9	1.0	~40%
Total calcium	10.0	2.5	100%

The proximal tubule reabsorbs two thirds of filtered Ca^{2+}, with more distal segments reabsorbing nearly all of the remainder

The kidney reabsorbs ~99% of the filtered load of calcium, principally at the proximal tubule, the thick ascending limb (TAL), and the distal convoluted tubule (DCT) (Fig. 36.10A).

Proximal Tubule The proximal tubule reabsorbs ~65% of the filtered calcium, a process that is *not* subject to hormonal control. Virtually all proximal-tubule Ca^{2+} reabsorption occurs via the paracellular route (Fig. 36.10B). The passive paracellular reabsorption of calcium is very dependent on luminal [Ca^{2+}]. Water reabsorption tends to increase luminal [Ca^{2+}], generating a favorable transepithelial gradient that drives passive Ca^{2+} reabsorption by diffusion via the

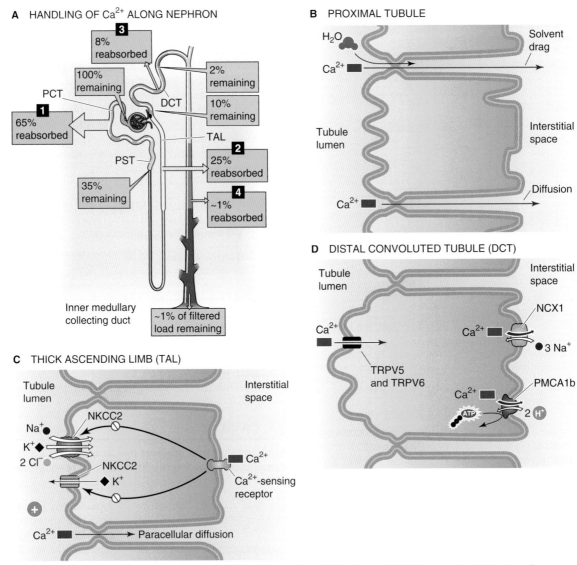

Figure. 36.10 Calcium handling by the kidney. The numbered *yellow boxes* indicate the approximate fraction of the filtered load that various nephron segments *reabsorb*. The *green boxes* indicate the fraction of the filtered load that remains in the lumen at various sites. The values in the boxes are approximations.

paracellular pathway. In addition, some calcium reabsorption may occur via solvent drag across the tight junctions.

Thick Ascending Limb The TAL reabsorbs ~25% of the filtered calcium (Fig. 36.10C). Most of the Ca^{2+} reabsorption in the TAL occurs passively via a paracellular route, driven by the lumen-positive voltage. Thus, it is not surprising that loop diuretics, which block the generation of the lumen-positive transepithelial voltage, acutely inhibit Ca^{2+} reabsorption.

Distal Convoluted Tubule The DCT reabsorbs ~8% of the filtered Ca^{2+} load (Fig. 36.10D). Despite the relatively small amount of Ca^{2+} delivered, the DCT is a major regulatory site for Ca^{2+} excretion. In contrast to the proximal tubule and TAL, the DCT reabsorbs Ca^{2+} predominantly via an active, transcellular route (see next section).

The quantitative contribution of the collecting ducts and tubules to Ca^{2+} reabsorption is quite small (~1% of the filtered load).

Transcellular Ca^{2+} movement is a two-step process, involving passive Ca^{2+} entry through apical channels and basolateral extrusion by electrogenic Na/Ca exchange and a Ca pump

Apical Ca^{2+} entry in the DCT is passive (Fig. 36.10D), mediated by the epithelial Ca^{2+} channels **TRPV5** and **TRPV6** (ECaC1 and ECaC2).

Both primary and secondary active transporters participate in basolateral Ca^{2+} extrusion against a steep electrochemical gradient. The primary active transporter is an ATP-driven plasma-membrane Ca^{2+} ATPase or pump (**PMCA1b**). The Na-Ca exchanger **NCX1** also extrudes Ca^{2+} across the basolateral membrane of tubule cells.

Parathyroid hormone and vitamin D stimulate—whereas high plasma Ca^{2+} inhibits—Ca^{2+} reabsorption

Parathyroid Hormone ◉ **36-6** The most important regulator of renal Ca^{2+} reabsorption is **PTH,** which stimulates Ca^{2+} reabsorption in the DCT and the connecting tubule. Regarding TRPV5, PTH increases transcription and open probability, and inhibits endocytosis, thereby stimulating Ca^{2+} reabsorption. In addition to its effects to stimulate apical Ca^{2+} entry, PTH also upregulates expression of calbindin and NCX1.

As we saw in our discussion of phosphate handling, PTH acts by binding to the PTH1R receptor, which ultimately activates two kinases, PKA, and PKC, both of which are essential for the action of PTH on apical Ca^{2+} entry.

Vitamin D ◉ **36-7** Acting on gene transcription, vitamin D increases Ca^{2+} reabsorption in the distal nephron; this renal reabsorption complements the major Ca^{2+}-retaining action of vitamin D, Ca^{2+} absorption in the gastrointestinal tract (see ◉ **52-9**). In renal tubule cells, vitamin D upregulates TRPV5 and Ca^{2+}-binding proteins, which contribute to enhanced Ca^{2+} reabsorption by keeping $[Ca^{2+}]_i$ low during increased Ca^{2+} traffic through the cell.

Plasma Ca^{2+} Levels Extracellular Ca^{2+} binds to a basolateral **Ca^{2+}-sensing receptor (CaSR)** in the TAL (Fig. 36.10C), which leads to a reduction in the lumen-positive transepithelial potential. CaSR activation also leads to a reduction

in paracellular Ca^{2+} permeability in this nephron segment. Because Ca^{2+} reabsorption in the TAL is predominantly passive and paracellular, these CaSR-mediated decreases in driving force and permeability lead to reduced Ca^{2+} reabsorption and thus increased Ca^{2+} excretion, tending to compensate for hypercalcemia.

MAGNESIUM

Most Mg^{2+} reabsorption takes place along the thick ascending limb

Approximately 99% of the total body stores of magnesium reside either within bone (~54%) or within the intracellular compartment (~45%), mostly muscle. Renal magnesium excretion plays an important role in maintaining physiological plasma magnesium levels. The body maintains the total magnesium concentration in blood plasma within narrow limits, 0.8 to 1.0 mM (1.8 to 2.2 mg/dL). Of this total, ~30% is protein bound (Table 36.3). The remaining ~70% of total magnesium, which is **filterable**, is made up of two components. Less than 10% is complexed to anions such as phosphate, citrate, and oxalate, thus leaving ~60% of the total as free, ionized magnesium (Mg^{2+}).

Disturbances of Mg^{2+} metabolism usually involve abnormal *losses*, and these occur most frequently during gastrointestinal malabsorption and diarrhea, in the course of renal disease, and following the administration of diuretics.

Normally, 5% or less of the filtered magnesium load appears in the urine (Fig. 36.11A). In contrast to the predominantly "proximal" reabsorption pattern of the major components of the glomerular filtrate, Mg^{2+} reabsorption occurs mainly along the TAL.

Normally, the **proximal tubule** reabsorbs only ~15% of the filtered magnesium load (Fig. 36.11B). Water reabsorption along the proximal tubule causes luminal $[Mg^{2+}]$ to double compared with the value in Bowman's space, thereby establishing a favorable Mg^{2+} electrochemical gradient for passive, paracellular Mg^{2+} reabsorption. Solvent drag may also contribute to the paracellular reabsorption of Mg^{2+}.

The **TAL** absorbs ~70% of the filtered magnesium load (Fig. 36.11C). The driving force for paracellular Mg^{2+} reabsorption is the lumen-positive voltage of the TAL. The tight-junction proteins **claudin 16** and **claudin 19** (see ◉ **2-17**) account for the high paracellular cation permeability.

Mg^{2+} reabsorption along the **DCT**, which is predominantly transcellular (Fig. 36.11D), accounts for only ~10% of

TABLE 36.3 Components of Total Plasma Magnesium

	mg/dL	mM	% OF TOTAL
Ionized Mg^{2+}	1.3	0.56	62
Filterable magnesium complexes	0.1	0.06	7
Non-filterable (protein-bound) magnesium	0.6	0.28	31
Total magnesium	2.0	0.90	100

A HANDLING OF Mg²⁺ ALONG NEPHRON

C THICK ASCENDING LIMB (TAL)

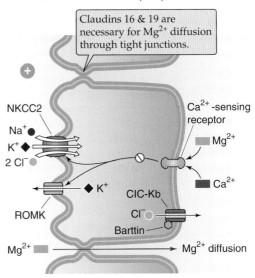

B PROXIMAL TUBULE

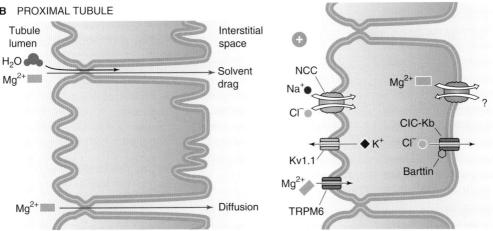

D DISTAL CONVOLUTED TUBULE (DCT)

Figure. 36.11 Magnesium handling by the kidney. The numbered *yellow boxes* indicate the fraction of the filtered load that various nephron segments reabsorb. The *green boxes* indicate the fraction of the filtered load that remains in the lumen at various sites. The values in the boxes are approximations. *CCT,* Cortical collecting tubule; *ICT,* initial collecting tubule; *OMCD,* outer medullary collecting duct; *PCT,* proximal convoluted tubule; *PST,* proximal straight tubule.

the filtered load. Mg²⁺ entry across the apical membrane may take place via the **TRPM6** cation channel. Because both luminal and intracellular Mg²⁺ are in the millimolar range, the key driving force is the inside-negative membrane potential. The efflux of K⁺ through apical Kv1.1 K⁺ channels neutralizes the entry of positive charge via Mg²⁺ uptake. The mechanism of Mg²⁺ extrusion across the basolateral membrane may be secondary active transport by Na-Mg exchange.

Mg²⁺ reabsorption increases with depletion of Mg²⁺ or Ca²⁺, or with elevated parathyroid hormone levels

Mg²⁺ Depletion In response to low plasma [Mg²⁺], the kidney reduces fractional excretion of Mg²⁺ to very low levels (<2%). This adaptive response is due to upregulation of Mg²⁺ reabsorption in the TAL and DCT.

Hormones PTH is the most important hormone for Mg²⁺ regulation, increasing distal Mg²⁺ reabsorption. AVP, glucagon, and calcitonin all stimulate Mg²⁺ reabsorption in the TAL, acting via cAMP and PKA. Many of these hormones probably act by modulating passive Mg²⁺ movement through the paracellular pathway, either by changing NaCl transport and transepithelial voltage or by increasing paracellular permeability.

CHAPTER 37

TRANSPORT OF POTASSIUM

Gerhard Giebisch[†] and Peter S. Aronson

POTASSIUM BALANCE AND THE OVERALL RENAL HANDLING OF POTASSIUM

Changes in K+ concentrations can have major effects on cell and organ function

The distribution of K+ in the body differs strikingly from that of Na+. Whereas Na+ is largely extracellular, K+ is the most abundant intracellular cation. Some 98% of the total-body K+ content (~50 mmol/kg body weight) is inside cells; only 2% is in the extracellular fluid (ECF). The body tightly maintains the plasma [K+] at 3.5 to 5.0 mM.

A *high* [K+] inside cells and a relatively *low* extracellular [K+] is necessary for maintaining the steep K+ gradient across cell membranes that is largely responsible for the membrane potential of excitable and nonexcitable cells. Therefore, changes in extracellular [K+] can cause severe disturbances in excitation and contraction.

K+ homeostasis involves external K+ balance between environment and body, and internal K+ balance between intracellular and extracellular compartments

Fig. 37.1 illustrates processes that govern K+ balance and the distribution of K+ in the body: (1) gastrointestinal (GI) intake, (2) renal and extrarenal excretion, and (3) the internal distribution of K+ between the intracellular and extracellular fluid compartments. The first two processes accomplish external K+ balance (i.e., body versus environment), whereas the last achieves internal K+ balance (i.e., intracellular versus extracellular fluids).

External K+ Balance The relationship between dietary K+ intake and K+ excretion determines external K+ balance. The *dietary intake* of K+ is approximately equal to that of Na+, 60 to 80 mmol/day. This K+ intake is approximately equal to the entire K+ content of the ECF, which is only about 65 to 75 mmol. For the plasma K+ content to remain constant, the body must excrete K+ via renal and extrarenal mechanisms at the same rate as K+ ingestion. Moreover, because dietary K+ intake can vary over a wide range, it is important that these K+-excretory mechanisms be able to adjust appropriately to variable K+ intake. The kidney is largely responsible for K+ excretion, although the GI tract plays a minor role. The kidneys excrete 90% to 95% of the daily K+ intake; the colon excretes 5% to 10%.

Internal K+ Balance Maintaining normal intracellular and extracellular [K+] requires not only the *external* K+ balance just described, but also the appropriate distribution of K+ within the body. Most of the K+ is inside cells—particularly muscle cells, which represent a high fraction of body mass (Fig. 37.1). Of the total intracellular K+ content of ~3000 mmol, shuttling as little as 1% to or from the ECF would cause a 50% change in extracellular [K+], with severe consequences for neuromuscular function.

Ingested K+ moves transiently into cells for storage before excretion by the kidney

By far, the most common source of a K+ load is dietary K+. When one ingests K+ salts, both the small intestine (see ⊚ 44-1) and the colon (see ⊚ 44-2) absorb the K+. A release of K+ from damaged tissue can lead to a severe, even lethal, increase in plasma [K+] (i.e., **hyperkalemia**). However, even a large meal presents the body with a K+ load that could produce hyperkalemia if it were not for mechanisms that buffer and ultimately excrete this K+.

Some four fifths of an ingested K+ load temporarily moves into cells, so that plasma [K+] rises only modestly, as shown in the upper panel of Fig. 37.2. Were it not for this translocation, plasma [K+] could reach dangerous levels. The transfer of excess K+ into cells is rapid and almost complete after an hour (lower panel of Fig. 37.2, gold curve). With a delay, the kidneys begin to excrete the surfeit of K+ (lower panel of Fig. 37.2, brown curve), removing from the cells the excess K+ that they had temporarily stored.

⊙ **37-1** What processes mediate the temporary uptake of K+ into cells during K+ loading? As shown in Fig. 37.3, the hormones insulin, epinephrine (a β-adrenergic agonist), and aldosterone all promote the transfer of K+ from extracellular to intracellular fluid via the ubiquitous Na-K pump.

Acid-base disturbances also affect internal K+ distribution. As a rule, *acidemia* leads to hyperkalemia as tissues release K+. *Extracellular* acidosis inhibits Na-H exchange and Na/HCO_3 cotransport (Fig. 37.4), both raising $[H^+]_i$ (i.e., lowering pH_i) and lowering $[Na^+]_i$. The *intracellular* acidosis compromises both the Na-K pump and the Na/K/Cl cotransporter NKCC2, both of which move K+ into cells. In addition, low pH_i lessens the binding of K+ to nondiffusible intracellular anions, promoting K+ efflux. In parallel, the low $[Na^+]_i$ reduces the supply of intracellular Na+ to be extruded by the Na-K pump and thus inhibits K+ uptake by the Na-K pump. These mechanisms all promote hyperkalemia.

Conversely, *alkalemia* causes cells to take up K+ and thus leads to **hypokalemia**.

[†]Deceased.

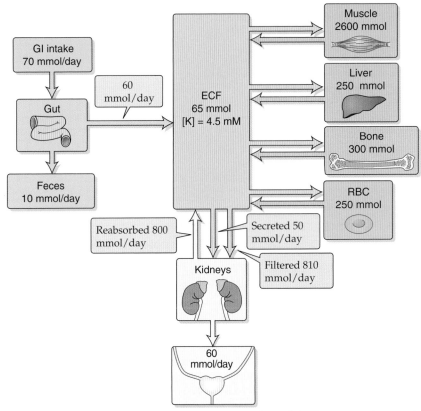

Figure 37.1 Distribution and balance of K⁺ throughout the body. Intracellular K⁺ concentrations are similar in all tissues in the four *purple boxes*. The values in the boxes are approximations. *RBC,* Red blood cell.

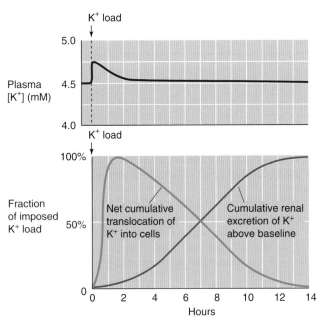

Figure 37.2 K⁺ handling following an acute K⁺ load. (Data from Cogan MG: Fluid and Electrolytes: Physiology and Pathophysiology. Norwalk, CT, Appleton & Lange, 1991.)

The kidney excretes K⁺ by a combination of filtration, reabsorption, and secretion

At a normal glomerular filtration rate and at physiological levels of plasma [K⁺], the kidney filters ~800 mmol/day of K⁺, far more than the usual dietary intake of 60 to 80 mmol/day. Therefore, to

achieve K⁺ balance, the kidneys normally need to excrete 10% to 15% of the filtered K⁺. Under conditions of low dietary K⁺ intake, the kidneys excrete 1% to 3% of filtered K⁺, so that—with a normal- or low-K⁺ diet—the kidneys could, in principle, achieve K⁺ balance by *filtration* and *reabsorption* alone. However, with a chronic high intake of dietary K⁺, when the kidneys must rid the body of excess K⁺, urinary K⁺ excretion may exceed 150% of the total amount of filtered K⁺. Therefore, even if the tubules reabsorb none of the filtered K⁺, they must be capable of secreting an amount equivalent to at least 50% of the filtered K⁺ load.

POTASSIUM TRANSPORT BY DIFFERENT SEGMENTS OF THE NEPHRON

The proximal tubule reabsorbs most of the filtered K⁺, whereas the distal nephron reabsorbs or secretes K⁺, depending on K⁺ intake

Fig. 37.5 summarizes the pattern of K⁺ transport along the nephron under conditions of low or normal/high K⁺ intake. In either case, the kidney filters K⁺ in the glomerulus and then extensively reabsorbs it along the proximal tubule (~80%) and the loop of Henle (~10%), so that only ~10% of the filtered K⁺ enters the distal convoluted tubule (DCT). Moreover, in either case, the **medullary collecting duct (MCD)** reabsorbs K⁺. The K⁺ handling depends critically on dietary K⁺ in five nephron segments: the DCT, the connecting tubule (CNT), the initial collecting tubule (ICT), the cortical collecting tubule (CCT), and the MCD.

Low Dietary K⁺ When the body is trying to conserve K⁺, the "classic distal tubule" (i.e., DCT, CNT, and ICT) and CCT all reabsorb K⁺, so that only a small fraction of the filtered load (1% to 3%) appears in the urine (Fig. 37.5A).

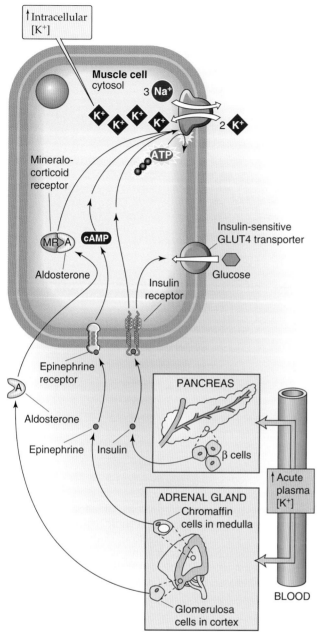

Figure 37.3   K+ uptake into cells in response to high plasma [K+].

reabsorption of K^+ is very dependent on the luminal [K^+] and transepithelial voltage (V_{te}). Water reabsorption tends to increase [K^+] in the lumen, generating a favorable transepithelial gradient that drives passive absorption by diffusion across the paracellular pathway from lumen to blood.

In addition, some K^+ may be reabsorbed by solvent drag (see ◉ 20-8) across tight junctions. The greater the fluid reabsorption along the proximal tubule, the greater the reabsorption of K^+ via both electrodiffusion and solvent drag.

Although the proximal tubule reabsorbs K^+ via paracellular pathways, the proximal tubule has several cellular pathways for K^+ movement that do not directly participate in K^+ reabsorption (Fig. 37.6A): (1) a basolateral Na-K pump, a feature common to all tubule cells; (2) apical and basolateral K^+ channels; and (3) a basolateral K/Cl cotransporter (KCC).

K^+ reabsorption along the TAL occurs predominantly via a transcellular route that exploits secondary active Na/K/Cl cotransport

The TAL of the loop of Henle reabsorbs K^+ predominantly by a transcellular mechanism (Fig. 37.6B), using the apical NKCC2, a typical example of a secondary active transporter (see ◉ 5-12). A characteristic feature of NKCC2 is its sensitivity to a class of diuretics that have their main site of action in the TAL. Therefore, administering so-called **loop diuretics** such as furosemide or bumetanide blocks net reabsorption of Na^+, Cl^-, and K^+.

The apical K^+ conductance—which mainly reflects ROMK and BK_{Ca} channels—is also important for the function of NKCC2 (Fig. 37.6B). The major function of the apical K^+ channel is to provide a mechanism for recycling much of the K^+ from cell to lumen, so that luminal [K^+] does not fall so low as to jeopardize Na/K/Cl cotransport (see ◉ 35-1).

K^+ secretion by principal and intercalated cells of the ICT and CCT involves active K^+ uptake across the basolateral membrane

The *early* portion of the classic distal tubule (i.e., DCT) secretes K^+ but at a relatively low rate. However, a high rate of K^+ secretion into the tubule fluid is one of the distinguishing features of *late* portions of the classic distal tubule (i.e., CNT and ICT) and of the CCT. Of the two cell types in the ICT and CCT, it is the **principal cell** that is mainly responsible for secretion of K^+, and it does so by a transcellular process (Fig. 37.6C). The three key elements of the principal cell are (1) an Na-K pump for active K^+ uptake at the basolateral membrane, (2) a relatively high apical K^+ permeability due to the ROMK channel, and (3) a favorable electrochemical driving force for K^+ exit across the apical membrane. In addition, K^+ may move from cell to lumen via an apical KCC (see Fig. 5.7I).

◉ 37-2 K^+ reabsorption by intercalated cells involves apical uptake via an H-K pump

Ultrastructurally, the ICT and CCT are nearly identical (see Fig. 33.5H and I); they are made up of ~70% principal cells (which secrete K^+) and ~30% intercalated cells (some of which reabsorb K^+).

POTASSIUM TRANSPORT AT THE CELLULAR AND MOLECULAR LEVELS

Passive K^+ reabsorption along the proximal tubule follows Na^+ and fluid movements

The proximal tubule reabsorbs most of the filtered K^+, a process occurring via two paracellular mechanisms (Fig. 37.6A): electrodiffusion and solvent drag. The passive paracellular

Normal or High Dietary K^+   When external K^+ balance demands that the kidneys excrete K^+, the ICT, CCT, and the more proximal portion of the MCD *secrete* K^+ into the tubule lumen (Fig. 37.5B). Together, these segments, known as the **distal K^+ secretory system,** account for most of the urinary excretion of K^+.

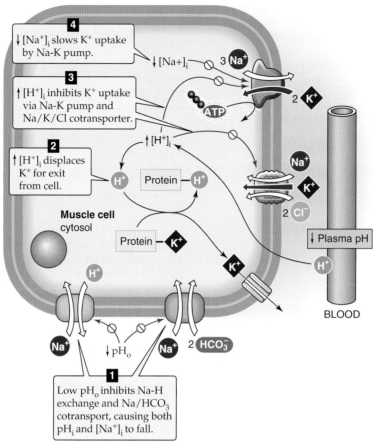

4
↓[Na$^+$]$_i$ slows K$^+$ uptake by Na-K pump.

3
↑[H$^+$]$_i$ inhibits K$^+$ uptake via Na-K pump and Na/K/Cl cotransporter.

2
↑[H$^+$]$_i$ displaces K$^+$ for exit from cell.

↓[Na+]$_i$ 3 Na$^+$

ATP   2 K$^+$

↑[H$^+$]$_i$

H$^+$ Protein — H$^+$

Muscle cell
cytosol

Na$^+$

K$^+$

Cl$^-$ 2

Protein — K$^+$

↓ Plasma pH

K$^+$

H$^+$

BLOOD

H$^+$

Na$^+$ ↓pH$_o$ Na$^+$ 2 HCO$_3^-$

1
Low pH$_o$ inhibits Na-H exchange and Na/HCO$_3$ cotransport, causing both pH$_i$ and [Na$^+$]$_i$ to fall.

Figure 37.4   Effect of acidosis on K$^+$ uptake into cells.

As discussed above, the ICT, CCT, and MCD reabsorb K$^+$ in response to K$^+$ depletion (Fig. 37.5A). This K$^+$ reabsorption is transcellular (Fig. 37.6D), mediated by both α- and β-intercalated cells in two steps: (1) an *active step* mediated by an apical ATP-driven H-K pump (see ⊙ 5-9), and (2) a *passive step* mediated by a basolateral K$^+$ channel.

K$^+$ reabsorption along the medullary collecting duct is both passive and active

The capacity for K$^+$ *secretion* diminishes from the cortical CT to the MCD. Indeed, the MCD is responsible for K$^+$ *reabsorption*. This K$^+$ removal from the MCD lumen can occur by passive movement via the paracellular pathway—which has a significant K$^+$ permeability—driven by a favorable K$^+$ concentration gradient.

REGULATION OF RENAL POTASSIUM EXCRETION

Increased luminal flow increases K$^+$ secretion

One of the most potent stimuli of K$^+$ secretion is the rate of fluid flow along the distal K$^+$-secretory system (i.e., ICT and CCT). Under almost all circumstances, an increase in luminal flow increases K$^+$ secretion (Fig. 37.7) and a similar relationship holds between final urine flow and K$^+$ excretion. Accordingly, the increased urine flow that occurs with extracellular volume expansion, osmotic diuresis, or administration of several diuretic agents (e.g., acetazolamide, furosemide, thiazides) leads to enhanced K$^+$ excretion—**kaliuresis.**

When luminal flow increases and sweeps newly secreted K$^+$ downstream, the resulting fall in luminal [K$^+$] steepens the K$^+$ gradient across the apical membrane and consequently increases passive K$^+$ flux from cell to lumen.

An increased lumen-negative transepithelial potential increases K$^+$ secretion

The apical step of K$^+$ secretion in the ICT and CCT occurs by diffusion of K$^+$ from the principal cell to the lumen, a process that depends on the apical electrochemical K$^+$ gradient (Fig. 37.6C). Increases in luminal [Na$^+$]—enhancing apical Na$^+$ entry through **epithelial Na$^+$ channels (ENaCs;** see ⊙ 35-2) depolarize the apical membrane, favoring the exit of K$^+$ from cell to lumen (i.e., K$^+$ secretion).

The diuretic amiloride has the same effect on K$^+$ secretion as decreasing luminal [Na$^+$]. By blocking apical ENaCs, amiloride hyperpolarizes the apical membrane and reduces the electrochemical gradient for K$^+$ secretion. Thus, amiloride is a K$^+$-sparing diuretic.

Low luminal [Cl$^-$] enhances K$^+$ secretion

Lowering luminal Cl—replacing it with an anion (e.g., SO$_4^{2-}$ or HCO$_3^-$) that the tubule reabsorbs poorly—promotes K$^+$

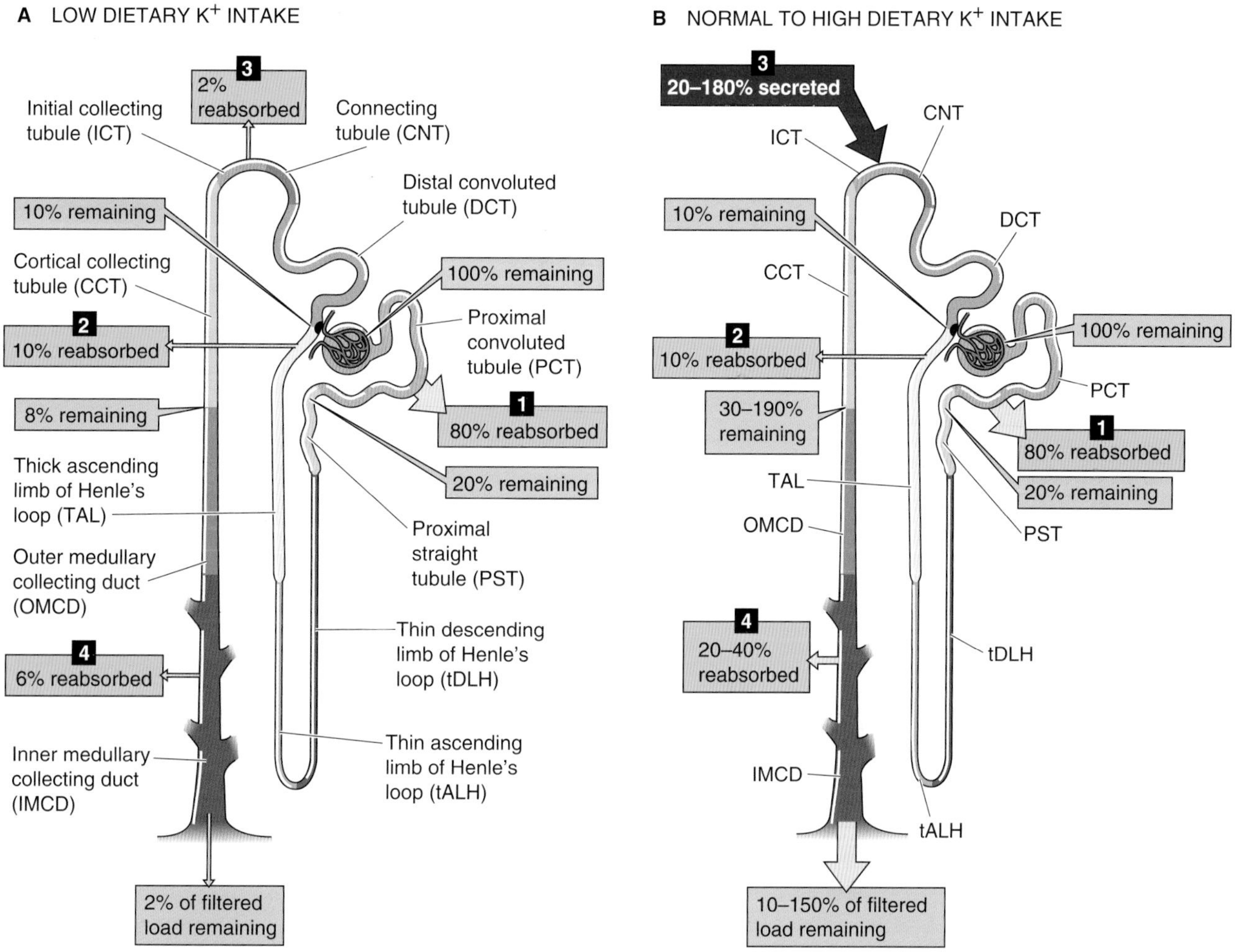

A   LOW DIETARY K⁺ INTAKE

B   NORMAL TO HIGH DIETARY K⁺ INTAKE

Figure 37.5   K⁺ handling along the nephron. The numbered *yellow boxes* indicate the fraction of the filtered load that various nephron segments reabsorb. The *red box* in (B) indicates the fraction of the filtered load secreted by the ICT and CCT. The *green boxes* indicate the fraction of the filtered load that remains in the lumen at these sites. The values in the boxes are approximations that reflect the joint contributions of both juxtamedullary and superficial nephrons.

loss into the urine, independent of changes in the lumen-negative V_{te}. Underlying this effect may be a KCC in the apical membrane of the principal cell of the ICT and CCT (Fig. 37.6C). Lowering luminal [Cl⁻] increases the cell-to-lumen Cl⁻ gradient, which presumably stimulates K/Cl cotransport, and thus K⁺ secretion.

Aldosterone increases K⁺ secretion

Both mineralocorticoids and glucocorticoids cause kaliuresis.

Mineralocorticoids   Aldosterone, the main native mineralocorticoid, induces K⁺ secretion in the ICT and CCT, particularly when its effects are prolonged. Aldosterone increases the transcription of genes that enhance Na⁺ reabsorption and, secondarily, K⁺ secretion in the *principal cells* of the ICT and CCT (Fig. 37.6C). Three factors act in concert to promote K⁺ secretion. First, over a period of a few hours, aldosterone increases the basolateral K⁺ uptake by stimulating the Na-K pump. Over a few days, elevated aldosterone levels also lead to a marked amplification of the area of the basolateral membrane of principal cells, as well as to a

corresponding increase in the number of Na-K pump molecules. Second, mineralocorticoids stimulate apical ENaCs, thus depolarizing the apical membrane and increasing the driving force for K⁺ diffusion from cell to lumen. Third, aldosterone increases the K⁺ conductance of the apical membrane.

Glucocorticoids   Under physiological conditions, glucocorticoids enhance K⁺ excretion, largely by increasing flow along the distal K⁺-secretory system (i.e., ICT and CCT). The flow increases because glucocorticoids increase the glomerular filtration rate and, probably, lower the water permeability of the distal K⁺-secretory system.

High K⁺ intake promotes renal K⁺ secretion

Dietary K⁺ Loading   An increase in dietary K⁺ intake causes, after some delay, an increase in urinary K⁺ excretion (Fig. 37.5B). If the period of high-K⁺ intake is prolonged, a condition of tolerance (**K⁺ adaptation**) develops in which the kidneys become able to excrete large doses of K⁺—even previously lethal doses—with only a small rise in plasma [K⁺].

A PROXIMAL TUBULE

B THICK ASCENDING LIMB (TAL)

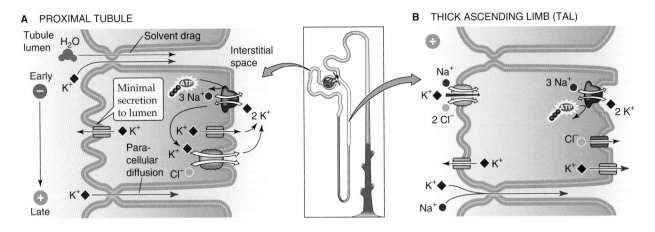

C CORTICAL COLLECTING TUBULE (CCT):
PRINCIPAL CELL

D CORTICAL COLLECTING TUBULE (CCT):
α-INTERCALATED CELL

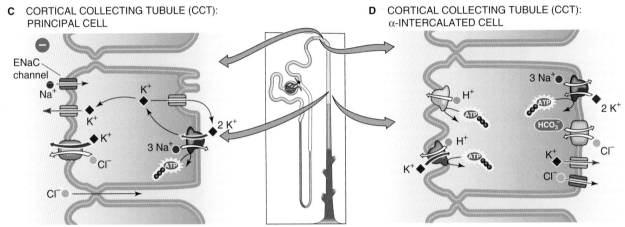

Figure 37.6 Cellular models of K⁺ transport along the nephron.

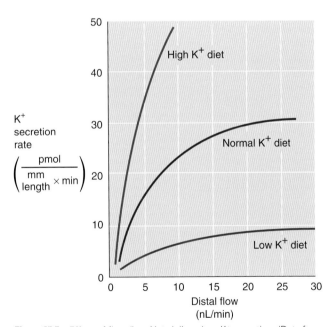

Figure 37.7 Effect of flow (i.e., Na⁺ delivery) on K⁺ excretion. (Data from Stanton BA, Giebisch G: Renal potassium transport. In Windhager EE [ed]: Handbook of Physiology, Section 8: Renal Physiology. New York, Oxford University Press, 1992, pp 813–874.)

Dietary K⁺ Deprivation In response to K⁺ restriction, the kidneys retain K⁺ (Fig. 37.5A). The rate of urinary K⁺ excretion may fall to 1% to 3% of the filtered load.

Acidosis decreases K⁺ secretion

Acid-base disturbances (see Table 28.3) have marked effects on renal K⁺ transport. In general, either metabolic alkalosis or respiratory alkalosis leads to increased K⁺ excretion. Conversely, acidosis reduces K⁺ excretion, although this response is more variable than that to alkalosis. Changes in systemic acid-base parameters affect K⁺ transport mainly by acting on the distal K⁺-secretory system.

The cellular events underlying the renal response to acid-base disturbances most likely involve effects of pH_i on both the basolateral Na-K pump and the apical K⁺ channels of the principal cells in the ICT and CCT.

Epinephrine reduces K⁺ excretion

By both extrarenal and renal mechanisms, **epinephrine** lowers K⁺ excretion. First, epinephrine enhances K⁺ uptake by extrarenal tissues (see ◉ 37-1) thereby lowering plasma [K⁺] and reducing the filtered K⁺ load. Second, catecholamines directly inhibit K⁺ secretion in nephron segments downstream of the ICT.

CHAPTER 38

URINE CONCENTRATION AND DILUTION

Gerhard Giebisch[†] and Peter S. Aronson

WATER BALANCE AND THE OVERALL RENAL HANDLING OF WATER

The kidney can generate urine as dilute as 40 mOsm (one seventh of plasma osmolality) or as concentrated as 1200 mOsm (four times plasma osmolality)

In the steady state, water intake and output must be equal (Table 38.1). The body's three major sources of water are (1) ingested water, (2) water contained in the foods eaten, and (3) water produced by aerobic metabolism as mitochondria convert foodstuffs and O_2 to CO_2 and H_2O.

The major route of water loss is usually through the kidneys, the organs that play the central role in regulating water balance. The values summarized in Table 38.1 will obviously vary, depending on diet, physical activity, and the environment (e.g., temperature and humidity).

The kidney adjusts its water output to compensate for either abnormally high or abnormally low water intake, or for abnormally high water losses via other routes. The kidney excretes a variable amount of solute, depending especially on salt intake. However, with consumption of a normal diet, the excreted solute is ~600 milliosmoles/day. For average conditions of water and solute intake and output, these 600 milliosmoles are dissolved in a daily urine output of 1500 mL. A key principle is that, regardless of the volume of water they excrete, the kidneys must excrete ~600 milliosmoles/day. Stated somewhat differently, the product of urine osmolality and urine output is approximately constant:

$$\text{Osmoles excreted/day} = \underbrace{U_{Osm}}_{\substack{\text{Urine} \\ \text{osmolality}}} \times \underbrace{\dot{V}}_{\substack{\text{Urine} \\ \text{output/day}}} \quad \textbf{(38.1)}$$

Therefore, to excrete a wide range of water volumes, the human kidney must produce urine having a wide range of osmolalities. For example, when the kidney excretes the 600 milliosmoles dissolved in 1500 mL of urine each day, urine osmolality must be 400 milliosmolar (i.e., 400 mOsm):

$$U_{Osm} = \frac{\text{osmoles excreated/day}}{\dot{V}}$$
$$= \frac{600 \text{ milliosmoles/day}}{15 \text{ L/day}} = 400 \text{ mOsm} \quad \textbf{(38.2)}$$

When the intake of water is especially high, the human kidney can generate urine having an osmolality as low as ~40 mOsm. Because the kidneys must still excrete 600

milliosmoles of solutes, the urine volume in an extreme **water diuresis** would be as high as ~15 L/day.

$$\dot{V} = \frac{\text{osmoles excreated/day}}{U_{Osm}}$$
$$= \frac{600 \text{ milliosmoles/day}}{40 \text{ mOsm}} = 15 \text{ L/day} \quad \textbf{(38.3)}$$

However, when it is necessary to conserve water (e.g., with restricted water intake or excessive loss by sweat or stool), the kidney is capable of generating urine with an osmolality as high as ~1200 mOsm. Therefore, with an average solute load, the minimal urine volume can be as low as ~0.5 L/day:

$$\dot{V} = \frac{\text{osmoles excreated/day}}{U_{Osm}}$$
$$= \frac{600 \text{ milliosmoles/day}}{1200 \text{ mOsm}} = 0.5 \text{ L/day} \quad \textbf{(38.4)}$$

Therefore, the kidney is capable of diluting the urine ~7-fold with respect to blood plasma, but it is capable of concentrating the urine only ~4-fold. Renal failure reduces both the concentrating and diluting ability.

WATER TRANSPORT BY DIFFERENT SEGMENTS OF THE NEPHRON

The kidney concentrates urine by driving water via osmosis from the tubule lumen into a hyperosmotic interstitium

The kidney generates *dilute* urine by pumping salts out of the lumen of tubule segments that are relatively impermeable to water. What is left behind is tubule fluid that is hypo-osmotic (dilute) with respect to the blood.

How does the kidney generate *concentrated* urine? The kidney uses osmosis as the driving force to concentrate the contents of the tubule lumen. The kidney generates the osmotic gradient by creating a hyperosmotic interstitial fluid in a confined compartment, the renal medulla. The final step for making a hyperosmotic urine—controlled by regulated water permeability—is allowing the lumen of the medullary collecting duct (MCD) to equilibrate with the hyperosmotic interstitium, resulting in a concentrated urine.

Although net absorption of H_2O occurs to a variable degree all along the nephron, not all segments alter the osmolality of the tubule fluid. The proximal tubule, *regardless of the final osmolality of the urine,* reabsorbs two thirds of the filtered

---

[†] Deceased.

TABLE 38.1 Input and Output of Water

INPUT	
SOURCE	AMOUNT (mL)
Ingested fluids	1200
Ingested food	1000
Metabolism	300
Total	2500

OUTPUT	
ROUTE	AMOUNT (mL)
Urine	1500
Feces	100
Skin/sweat	550
Exhaled air	350
Total	2500

(Modified from Valtin H: Renal Dysfunction: Mechanisms Involved in Fluid and Solute Imbalance. Boston, Little, Brown, 1979, p 21.)

fluid isosmotically (i.e., the fluid reabsorbed has nearly the same osmolality as plasma). The loop of Henle and the distal convoluted tubule (DCT) reabsorb salt in excess of water, so that the tubule fluid leaving the DCT is hypo-osmotic. *Whether the final urine is dilute or concentrated* depends on whether water reabsorption occurs in more distal segments: the initial and cortical collecting tubules (ICT and CCT) and the outer and inner medullary collecting ducts (OMCD and IMCD). **Arginine vasopressin (AVP)**—also called **antidiuretic hormone (ADH)**—regulates the variable fraction of water reabsorption in these four nephron segments.

Tubule fluid is isosmotic in the proximal tubule, becomes dilute in the loop of Henle, and then either remains dilute or becomes concentrated by the end of the collecting duct

Fig. 38.1 shows two examples of how tubule-fluid osmolality (expressed as the ratio TF_{Osm}/P_{Osm}) changes along the nephron. The first is a case of water restriction, in which the kidneys maximally concentrate the urine and excrete a minimal volume of water **(antidiuresis).** The second is a case of ingestion of excess water, in which the kidneys produce a large volume of dilute urine **(water diuresis).** In both cases, the tubule fluid does not change in osmolality along the proximal tubule, and it becomes hypotonic to plasma by the end of the thick ascending limb of the loop of Henle (TAL), also known as the diluting segment (see ◉ 35-1). The fluid exiting the DCT is hypo-osmotic with respect to plasma, regardless of the final urine osmolality (Fig. 38.1).

Under conditions of restricted water intake or **hydropenia,** elevated levels of AVP increase the water permeability of the nephron from the ICT to the end of the IMCD. As a result, the osmolality of the tubule fluid increases along the ICT (Fig. 38.1, *red curve*), achieving the osmolality of the cortical interstitium—which is the same as the osmolality of plasma (~290 mOsm)—by the end of this nephron segment (also the end of the classic distal tubule in Fig. 38.1). No additional increase in osmolality occurs along the CCT, because the tubule fluid is already in osmotic equilibrium with the surrounding cortical interstitium. However, in the MCDs, the luminal osmolality rises sharply as

the tubule fluid equilibrates with the surrounding medullary interstitium, which becomes increasingly more hyperosmotic from the corticomedullary junction to the papillary tip. Eventually the tubule fluid reaches osmolalities that are as much as four times higher than the plasma. Thus, the MCDs are responsible for concentrating the final urine.

In summary, the two key elements in producing a concentrated urine are (1) the hyperosmotic medullary interstitium that provides the osmotic gradient, and (2) the AVP that raises the water permeability of the distal nephron.

Under conditions of **water loading,** depressed AVP levels cause the water permeability of the distal nephron to remain low. However, the continued reabsorption of NaCl along the distal nephron effectively separates salt from water and leaves a relatively hypo-osmotic fluid behind in the tubule lumen. Thus, the tubule fluid becomes increasingly hypo-osmotic from the DCT throughout the remainder of the nephron (Fig. 38.1, *blue curve*).

GENERATION OF A HYPEROSMOTIC MEDULLA AND URINE

The renal medulla is hyperosmotic to blood plasma during both antidiuresis (low urine flow) and water diuresis

The loop of Henle plays a key role in both the dilution and the concentration of the urine. The main functions of the loop are to remove NaCl—more so than water—from the lumen and deposit this NaCl in the interstitium of the renal medulla. By separating tubule NaCl from tubule water, the loop of Henle participates *directly* in forming dilute urine. Conversely, because the TAL deposits this NaCl into the medullary interstitium, thus making it hyperosmotic, the loop of Henle is *indirectly* responsible for elaborating concentrated urine. As discussed below, urea also contributes to the hyperosmolality of the medulla.

Fig. 38.2A shows approximate values of osmolality in the tubule fluid and interstitium during an *antidiuresis* produced, for example, by water restriction. Fig. 38.2B illustrates the comparable information during a *water diuresis* produced, for example, by high water intake. In *both* conditions, interstitial osmolality progressively rises from the cortex to the tip of the medulla (corticomedullary osmolality gradient). The difference between the two conditions is that the maximal interstitial osmolality during antidiuresis, ~1200 mOsm (Fig. 38.2A), is more than twice that achieved during water diuresis, ~500 mOsm (Fig. 38.2B).

Because of the NaCl pumped out of the rather water-impermeable TAL, the tubule fluid at the end of this segment is hypo-osmotic to the cortical interstitium during both antidiuresis and water diuresis. However, beyond the TAL, luminal osmolalities differ considerably between antidiuresis and diuresis. In *antidiuresis,* the fluid becomes progressively more concentrated from the ICT to the end of the nephron (Fig. 38.2A). In contrast, during *water diuresis,* the hypo-osmolality of the tubule fluid is further accentuated as the fluid passes along segments from the DCT to the end of the nephron segments that are relatively water impermeable and continue to pump NaCl out of the lumen (Fig. 38.2B). During *antidiuresis,* the tubule fluid in the ICT, CCT, OMCD, and IMCD more or less equilibrates with the interstitium, but it fails to do so during *water diuresis.* This marked difference in osmotic equilibration reflects the action of AVP, which increases water permeability in each of the previously mentioned four segments.

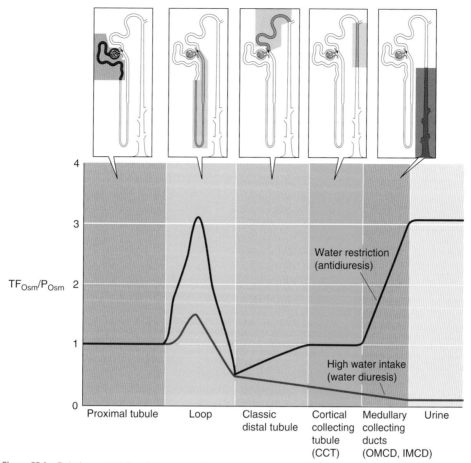

Figure 38.1 Relative osmolality of the tubule fluid along the nephron. Plotted on the y-axis is the ratio of the osmolality of the tubule fluid (TF_{Osm}) to the osmolality of the plasma (P_{Osm}); plotted on the x-axis is a representation of distance along the nephron. The *red record* is the profile of relative osmolality (i.e., TF_{Osm}/P_{Osm}) for water restriction, whereas the *blue record* is the profile for high water intake. (Data from Gottschalk CW: Micropuncture studies of tubular function in the mammalian kidney. Physiologist 4:33–55, 1961.)

In the interstitium, [Na⁺], [Cl⁻], and [urea] all rise along the axis from the cortex to the papillary tip of the renal medulla (Fig. 38.3). In the *outer* medulla, a steep rise in interstitial [Na⁺] and [Cl⁻]—owing to the pumping of NaCl out of the TAL—is largely responsible for producing the hyperosmolality. Although urea makes only a minor contribution in the outermost portion of the outer medulla, [urea] rises steeply from the middle of the outer medulla to the papilla. At the tip of the papilla, urea and NaCl each contribute half of the interstitial osmolality. This steep interstitial [urea] profile in the inner medulla (Fig. 38.3) is the result of the unique water and urea permeabilities of the collecting tubules and ducts (Fig. 38.2A).

⊙ 38-1 The IMCD reabsorbs urea, producing high levels of urea in the interstitium of the inner medulla

Because urea comes from protein breakdown, urea delivery to the kidney—and, therefore, the contribution of urea to the medullary hyperosmolality—is larger with consumption of protein-rich diets. Indeed, investigators have long known that the higher the dietary protein content, the greater the concentrating ability.

Urea Handling The kidney filters urea in the glomerulus and reabsorbs about half in the proximal tubule (Fig. 38.4, *step 1*). In juxtamedullary nephrons, the tDLH and the tALH secrete urea into the tubule lumen (Fig. 38.4, *step 2*). Some

urea reabsorption occurs along the TAL up through the CCT (Fig. 38.4, *step 3*). Finally, the IMCD reabsorbs urea (Fig. 38.4, *step 4*). The net effect is that the kidney excretes less urea into the urine than it filters. In Fig. 38.4 we consider an example in which maximal AVP produces minimal urine flow (i.e., antidiuresis), a condition already illustrated in Fig. 38.2A.

As the tubule fluid enters the TAL, the [urea] is several-fold higher than it is in the plasma because ~100% of the filtered load of urea remains, as earlier nephron segments have reabsorbed water. All nephron segments from the TAL to the OMCD, inclusive, have low permeabilities to urea. In the presence of AVP, however, all segments from the ICT to the end of the nephron have high water permeabilities and continuously reabsorb fluid. As a result, luminal [urea] gradually rises, beginning at the ICT and reaching a concentration as much as 8-fold to 10-fold higher than that in blood plasma by the time the tubule fluid reaches the end of the OMCD.

The **IMCD** differs in an important way from the three upstream segments: Although AVP increases *only water permeability* in the ICT, CCT, and OMCD, AVP increases water *and urea permeability* in the IMCD. In the IMCD, the high luminal [urea] and the high urea permeabilities of the apical membrane (via the urea transporter **UT-A1**; see ⊙ 36-2) and basolateral membrane (via **UT-A3**) promote the outward facilitated diffusion of urea from the IMCD lumen, through the IMCD cells, and into the medullary interstitium (Fig. 38.4, *step 4*). As a result,

A WATER RESTRICTION (ANTIDIURESIS)

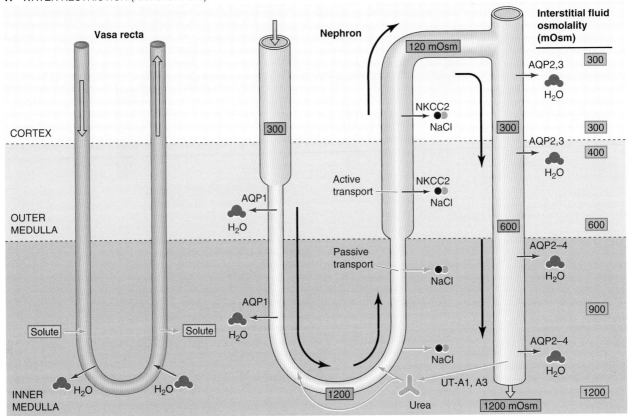

B HIGH WATER INTAKE (WATER DIURESIS)

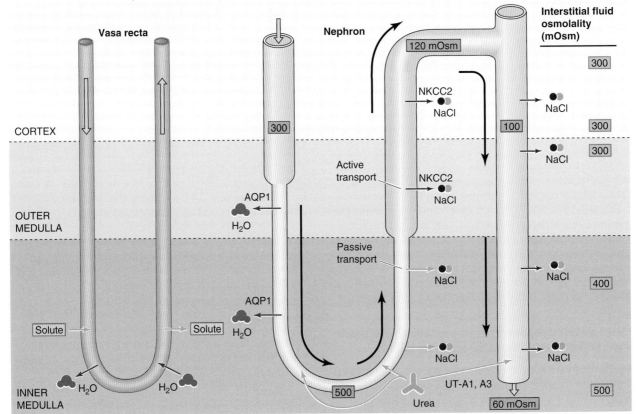

Figure 38.2 Nephron and interstitial osmolalities. (A) Water restriction (antidiuresis). (B) High water intake (water diuresis). The numbers in the boxes are osmolalities (in mOsm) along the lumen of the nephron and along the corticomedullary axis of the interstitium. In (A) the interstitial osmolality values in the *green boxes* come from Fig. 38.7. The outflow of blood from the vasa recta is greater than the inflow, which reflects the uptake of water reabsorbed from the collecting ducts. *Blue arrows* indicate passive water movements. *Green arrows* indicate passive solute movements. *Red arrows* indicate active solute movements. *NKCC2,* Na/K/Cl cotransporter 2.

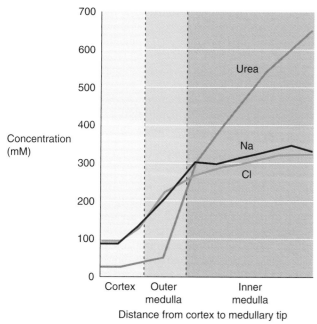

Figure 38.3 Concentration profiles of Na⁺, Cl⁻, and urea along the corticomedullary axis. The data are from hydropenic dogs. (Data from Ullrich KJ, Kramer K, Boylan JW: Present knowledge of the counter-current system in the mammalian kidney. Progr Cardiovasc Dis 3:395–431, 1961.)

urea accumulates in the interstitium and contributes about half of the total osmolality in the deepest portion of the inner medulla. In addition, in the outer portion of the inner medulla, active urea reabsorption occurs via an Na/urea cotransporter in the apical membrane of the early IMCD.

Because of the accumulation of urea in the inner medullary interstitium, [urea] is higher in the interstitium than it is in the lumen of the **tDLH** and **tALH** of juxtamedullary (i.e., long-loop) nephrons. This concentration gradient drives urea into the tDLH via **UT-A2** and into the tALH via an unidentified transporter (Fig. 38.4, *step 2*). The secretion of urea into the tDLH and tALH accounts for two important observations: First, more urea (i.e., a greater fraction of the filtered load) emerges from the tALH than entered the tDLH. Second, as noted above, [urea] in the TAL is considerably higher than that in blood plasma.

Urea Recycling The processes that we have just described—(1) absorption of urea from IMCD into the interstitium (Fig. 38.4 *step 4*), (2) secretion of urea from the interstitium into the thin limbs (see Fig. 38.4, *step 2*), and (3) delivery of urea up into the cortex and back down via nephron segments from the TAL to the IMCD—are the three elements of a loop. This **urea recycling** is responsible for the buildup of a high [urea] in the inner medulla. A small fraction

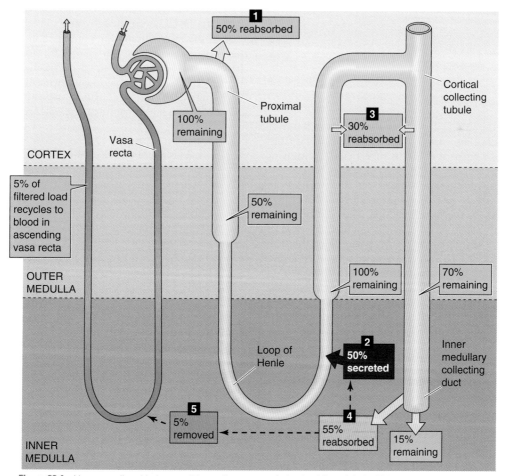

Figure 38.4 Urea recycling. Under conditions of water restriction (antidiuresis), the kidneys excrete ~15% of the filtered urea. The *numbered yellow boxes* indicate the fraction of the filtered load that various nephron segments *reabsorb*. The *red box* indicates the fraction of the filtered load *secreted* by the tALH, and the *brown box* indicates the fraction of the filtered load *carried away* by the vasa recta. The *green boxes* indicate the fraction of the filtered load that remains in the lumen at various sites. The values in the boxes are approximations.

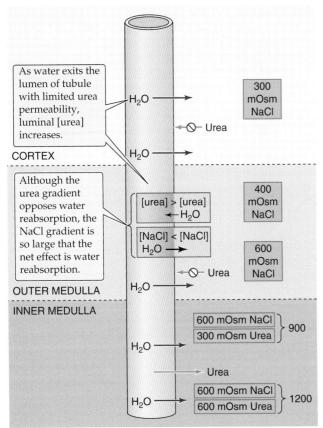

As water exits the lumen of tubule with limited urea permeability, luminal [urea] increases.

CORTEX

Although the urea gradient opposes water reabsorption, the NaCl gradient is so large that the net effect is water reabsorption.

OUTER MEDULLA

INNER MEDULLA

H₂O

Urea

300 mOsm NaCl

H₂O

400 mOsm NaCl

[urea] > [urea] ← H₂O

[NaCl] < [NaCl] H₂O →

600 mOsm NaCl

Urea

H₂O

600 mOsm NaCl
300 mOsm Urea } 900

H₂O

Urea

600 mOsm NaCl
600 mOsm Urea } 1200

H₂O

Figure 38.5 Opposing effects of NaCl and urea gradients on urine concentrating ability along the collecting duct during antidiuresis. The numbers in the *green boxes* indicate the osmolalities (in mOsm) of the interstitial fluid.

osmolality from the cortex to the tip of the papilla (Fig. 38.5). Thus, along the entire length of the tubule, the osmotic gradient across the collecting-duct epithelium favors the reabsorption of water from lumen to interstitium.

A complicating factor is that two solutes—NaCl and urea—contribute to the osmotic gradient across the tubule wall. As fluid in the collecting-duct lumen moves from the corticomedullary junction to the papillary tip, the [NaCl] gradient across the tubule wall always favors the osmotic reabsorption of water (Fig. 38.5). For urea, the situation is just the opposite. However, because the ICT, CCT, and OMCD are all relatively impermeable to urea, water reabsorption predominates in the presence of AVP and gradually causes luminal [urea] to increase in these segments. Because the interstitial [urea] is low in the cortex, a rising luminal [urea] in the ICT and CCT *opposes* water reabsorption in these segments. Even when the tubule crosses the corticomedullary junction, courses toward the papilla, and is surrounded by interstitial fluid with an ever-increasing [urea], the transepithelial urea gradient still favors water movement into the lumen, which is a handicap for the osmotic concentration of the tubule fluid.

The IMCD partially compensates for this problem by acquiring, in response to AVP, a high permeability to urea (Fig. 38.5). The result is a relatively low reflection coefficient for urea (σ_{urea}; see ⊙ 20-11), which converts any transepithelial difference in [urea] into a smaller difference in effective osmotic pressure (see ⊙ 5-15). Thus, water reabsorption continues from the IMCD even though [urea] in tubule fluid exceeds that in the interstitium. The combination of a high interstitial [NaCl] and high σ_{NaCl} ($\sigma_{NaCl} = 1.0$), along with a low σ_{urea} ($\sigma_{urea} = 0.74$), promotes NaCl-driven water *reabsorption*. The high AVP-induced urea permeability has the additional effect of raising interstitial [urea], which further reduces the adverse effect of the high luminal [urea] on water reabsorption.

of the urea that the IMCD deposits in the interstitium moves into the vasa recta (Fig. 38.4, *step 5*), which removes it from the medulla and returns it either to superficial nephrons or to the general circulation.

The preceding discussion focused on the situation in *antidiuresis,* in which AVP levels are high and the kidney concentrates urea in the inner medulla. The converse situation pertains in *water diuresis,* when circulating levels of AVP are low. The kidney reabsorbs *less* water along the ICT, CCT, OMCD, and IMCD. Furthermore, with low AVP levels, the IMCD has *lower* permeability to both urea and water. In addition, urea may be actively secreted by an apical Na-urea exchanger located in the apical membrane of the most distal portions of the IMCD. Therefore, during water diuresis, the interstitial [urea] is lower, and more urea appears in the urine.

The MCD produces a concentrated urine by osmosis, driven by the osmotic gradient between the medullary interstitium and the lumen

The wall of the MCD has three important permeability properties: (1) in the absence of AVP, it is relatively impermeable to water, urea, and NaCl along its entire length; (2) AVP increases its water permeability along its entire length; and (3) AVP increases its urea permeability along just the terminal portion of the tube (IMCD). The collecting duct traverses a medullary interstitium that has a stratified, ever-increasing

REGULATION BY ARGININE VASOPRESSIN

⊙ **38-2** Large-bodied neurons in the paraventricular and supraoptic nuclei of the hypothalamus synthesize AVP, a nonapeptide also known as ADH. These neurons package the AVP and transport it along their axons to the posterior pituitary, where they release AVP through a breech in the blood-brain barrier into the systemic circulation (see ⊙ 40-9) AVP has synergistic effects on two target organs. First, at rather high circulating levels, such as those seen in hypovolemic shock, AVP acts on vascular smooth muscle to cause *vasoconstriction* (see ⊙ 23-24) and thus to increase blood pressure. Second, and more importantly, AVP acts on the kidney, where it is the major regulator of water excretion. AVP increases water reabsorption by increasing (1) the water permeabilities of the collecting tubules and ducts, (2) NaCl reabsorption in the TAL, and (3) urea reabsorption by the IMCD.

⊙ 38-3 AVP increases water permeability in all nephron segments beyond the DCT

Of the water remaining in the DCT, the kidney reabsorbs a variable fraction in the segments from the ICT to the end of the nephron. Absorption of this final fraction of water is under the control of circulating AVP.

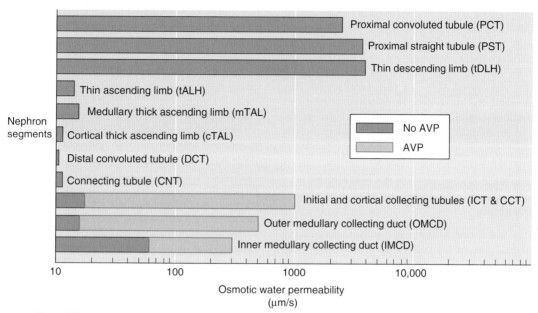

Figure 38.6 Water permeability in different nephron segments. Note that the x-axis scale is logarithmic. (Modified from Knepper MA, Rector FC: Urine concentration and dilution. In Brenner BM [ed]: *The Kidney.* Philadelphia, WB Saunders, 1996, pp 532–570.)

Fig. 38.6 summarizes the water permeability of various nephron segments. The water permeability is highest in the proximal tubule and tDLH. The constitutively high water permeability in these segments reflects the abundant presence of **AQP1** water channels in the apical and basolateral cell membranes.

In the absence of AVP, the next tubule segments, the ICT and CCT, have rather low water permeabilities, whereas the MCDs are virtually impermeable to water. However, AVP dramatically increases the water permeabilities of the collecting tubules (ICT and CCT) and ducts (OMCD and IMCD) by causing **AQP2** water channels to insert into the apical membrane (see below). A third type of water channel, **AQP3**, is present in the basolateral cell membranes of MCDs. Like AQP1, AQP3 is *insensitive* to AVP.

Given the favorable osmotic gradients discussed in the preceding subchapter, high levels of AVP cause substantial water reabsorption to occur in AVP-sensitive nephron segments. In contrast, when circulating levels of AVP are low, for instance after ingestion of large amounts of water, the water permeability of these nephron segments remains low. Therefore, the fluid leaving the DCT remains hypo-osmotic as it flows down more distal nephron segments. In fact, in the absence of AVP, continued NaCl absorption makes the tubule fluid even more hypo-osmotic, which results in a large volume of dilute urine (Fig. 38.1).

⦿ 38-4 AVP, via cAMP, causes vesicles containing AQP2 to fuse with apical membranes of principal cells of collecting tubules and ducts

AVP binds to **V₂ receptors** in the basolateral membrane of the principal cells from the ICT to the end of the nephron (Fig. 38.7). Receptor binding activates the G_s heterotrimeric

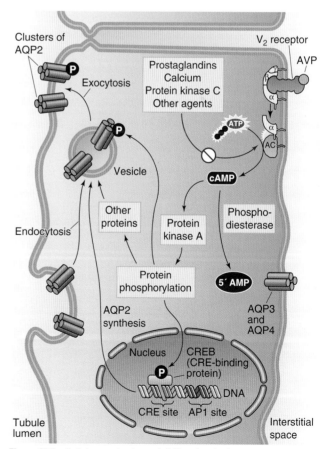

Figure 38.7 Cellular mechanism of AVP action in the collecting tubules and ducts. *AC,* Adenylyl cyclase; *AP1,* activator protein 1; *CRE,* cAMP response element.

G protein, stimulating adenylyl cyclase to generate cAMP. The latter activates protein kinase A, which phosphorylates AQP2 and additional proteins that play a role in the trafficking of intracellular vesicles containing AQP2 and the fusion of these vesicles with the apical membrane. The result is an increase in the *density* of AQP2 in the apical membrane. When AVP levels in the blood decline, endocytosis retrieves the water channel–containing aggregates from the apical membrane and shuttles them back to the cytoplasmic vesicle pool.

AVP increases NaCl reabsorption in the outer medulla and urea reabsorption in the IMCD, enhancing urinary concentrating ability

AVP promotes water reabsorption not only by increasing the water permeability of the collecting tubules and ducts, but also by enhancing the osmotic gradients across the walls of the IMCD and perhaps the OMCD. In the *outer* medulla, AVP acts through the cAMP pathway to increase NaCl reabsorption by the TAL. AVP acts by stimulating the apical Na/K/Cl cotransporter **NKCC2** and K$^+$ recycling across the apical membrane. The net effect is to increase the osmolality of the outer medullary interstitium and thus enhance the osmotic gradient favoring water reabsorption by the OMCD.

In the *inner* medulla, AVP enhances the urea permeability of the terminal two thirds of the IMCD (see ◉ 38-1). The AVP-dependent increase in [cAMP]$_i$ that triggers the apical insertion of AQP2-containing vesicles also leads to a phosphorylation of apical **UT-A1** and basolateral **UT-A3** urea transporters, increasing their activity. The result is a substantial increase in urea reabsorption and thus the high interstitial [urea] that is indirectly responsible for generating the osmotic gradient that drives water reabsorption in the inner medulla.

CHAPTER 39

TRANSPORT OF ACIDS AND BASES

Gerhard Giebisch[†] and Peter S. Aronson

The lungs and the kidneys are largely responsible for regulating the acid-base balance of the blood. They do so by independently controlling the two major components of the body's major buffering system: CO_2 and HCO_3^- (Fig. 39.1).

ACID-BASE BALANCE AND THE OVERALL RENAL HANDLING OF ACID

Whereas the lungs excrete the large amount of CO_2 formed by metabolism, the kidneys are crucial for excreting nonvolatile acids

The kidneys play a critical role in helping the body rid itself of excess acid that accompanies the intake of food or that forms in certain metabolic reactions. By far, the largest potential source of acid is CO_2 production, which occurs during oxidation of carbohydrates, fats, and most amino acids. An adult ingesting a typical Western diet produces ~15,000 mmol/day of CO_2 (Fig. 39.1). This CO_2 would act as an acid if it went on to form H^+ and HCO_3^- (see ⊙ 28-2). Fortunately, the lungs excrete this prodigious amount of CO_2, preventing the CO_2 from forming H^+.

However, metabolism also generates **nonvolatile acids**—such as sulfuric acid, phosphoric acid, and various organic acids—that the lungs cannot handle. In addition, metabolism generates **nonvolatile bases,** which end up as HCO_3^-. Subtracting the metabolically generated base from the metabolically generated acid leaves a net endogenous H^+ production of ~40 mmol/day for a person weighing 70 kg. The strong acids contained in a typical Western acid-ash diet (20 mmol/day of H^+ gained) and the obligatory loss of bases in stool (10 mmol/day of OH^- lost) represent an additional acid load to the body of 30 mmol/day. Thus, the body is faced with a total load of nonvolatile acids (i.e., not CO_2) of ~70 mmol/day—or ~1 mmol/kg body weight—derived from metabolism, diet, and intestinal losses.

Were it not for the tightly controlled excretion of H^+ by the kidney, the daily load of ~70 mmol of nonvolatile acids would progressively lower plasma pH and, in the process, exhaust the body's stores of bases, especially HCO_3^-. The result would be death by relentless acidification. Indeed, one of the characteristic symptoms of renal failure is severe acidosis caused by acid retention. The kidneys continuously monitor the acid-base parameters of the extracellular fluid (ECF) and adjust their rate of acid secretion to maintain the pH of ECF within narrow limits.

In summary, although the lungs excrete an extremely large amount of a *potential* acid in the form of CO_2, the kidneys play an equally essential role in the defense of the normal acid-base equilibrium, because they are the sole effective route for neutralizing *nonvolatile* acids.

To maintain acid-base balance, the kidney must not only reabsorb virtually all filtered HCO_3^- but also secrete generated nonvolatile acids

In terms of acid-base balance, the major task of the kidney is to secrete acid into the urine and thus to neutralize the nonvolatile acids that metabolism produces. However, before the kidney can begin to achieve this goal, it must deal with a related and even more serious problem: retrieving from the tubule fluid virtually all HCO_3^- filtered by the glomeruli.

Each day, the glomeruli filter 180 L of blood plasma, each liter containing 24 mmol of HCO_3^-, so that the daily filtered load of HCO_3^- is 180 L × 24 mM = 4320 mmol. If this filtered HCO_3^- were all left behind in the urine, the result would be equivalent to an acid load in the blood of 4320 mmol, or a catastrophic metabolic acidosis (see ⊙ 28-6). The kidneys avoid this problem by reclaiming virtually all the filtered HCO_3^- through secretion of H^+ into the tubule lumen and titration of the 4320 mmol/day of filtered HCO_3^- to CO_2 and H_2O (Fig 39.1).

After the kidney reclaims virtually all the filtered HCO_3^- (i.e., 4320 mmol/day), how does it deal with the acid load of 70 mmol/day produced by metabolism, diet, and intestinal losses?

The kidney does not simply eliminate the 70 mmol/day of nonvolatile acids by filtering and then excreting them in the urine. Rather, the body deals with the 70-mmol/day **acid challenge** in three steps:

Step 1: Extracellular HCO_3^- neutralizes *most* of the H^+ load:

$$HCO_3^- + \underbrace{H^+}_{\text{Acid load}} \rightarrow CO_2 + H_2O \tag{39.1}$$

Thus, HCO_3^- decreases by an amount that is equal to the H^+ it consumes, and an equal amount of CO_2 is produced in the process. Non-HCO_3^- buffers in the blood neutralize most of the remaining H^+ load:

$$B^- + \underbrace{H^+}_{\text{Acid load}} \rightarrow BH \tag{39.2}$$

[†] Deceased.

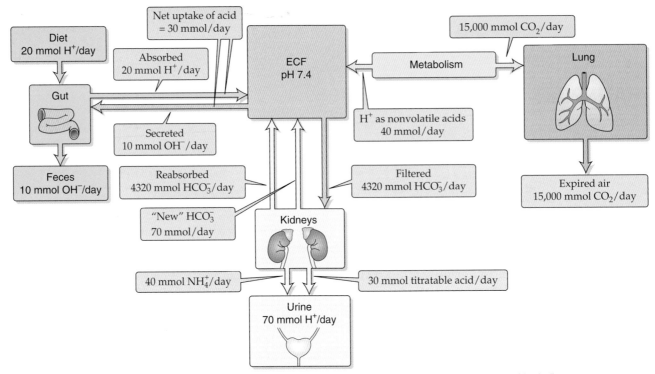

Figure 39.1   Acid-base balance. All values are for a 70-kg human consuming a typical Western acid-ash diet. The values in the boxes are approximations.

TABLE 39.1 Components of Net Urinary Acid Excretion

	1	2	3
Net urinary acid excretion	= Excreted H⁺ bound to phosphate (as $H_2PO_4^-$), creatinine, and uric acid	+ Excreted H⁺ bound to NH_3 (as NH_4^+)	− Excretion of filtered HCO_3^-

Thus, B⁻, too, decreases by an amount that is equal to the H⁺ it consumes.

Step 2: The lungs excrete the CO_2 formed by the process in Equation 39.1. The body does not excrete the BH generated by the process in Equation 39.2, but rather converts it back into B⁻, as discussed below.

Step 3: The kidneys regenerate the HCO_3^- and B⁻ in the ECF by creating new HCO_3^- at a rate that is equal to the rate of H⁺ production (i.e., ~70 mmol/day). Most of this new HCO_3^- replenishes the HCO_3^- consumed by the neutralization of nonvolatile acids, so that extracellular $[HCO_3^-]$ is maintained at ~24 mM. The remainder of this new HCO_3^- regenerates B⁻:

$$HCO_3^- + BH \rightarrow \underset{\substack{\text{Regenerated} \\ \text{base}}}{B^-} + CO_2 + H_2O \qquad (39.3)$$

Again, the lungs excrete the CO_2 formed as indicated in Equation 39.3, just as they excrete the CO_2 formed by the process in Equation 39.1. Thus, by generating new HCO_3^-, the kidneys maintain constant levels of both HCO_3^- and the deprotonated forms of non-HCO_3^- buffers (B⁻) in the ECF.

⊙ **39-1** Table 39.1 lists the three components of net urinary acid excretion. Historically, component 1 is referred to as **titratable acid,** the amount of base one must add

to a sample of urine to bring its pH back up to the pH of blood plasma. The titratable acid does *not* include the H⁺ the kidneys excrete as NH_4^+, which is component 2. Because the pK of the NH_3 / NH_4^+ equilibrium exceeds 9, almost all of the total ammonium buffer in the urine is in the form of NH_4^+, and titrating urine from an acid pH to a pH of 7.4 will not appreciably convert NH_4^+ to NH_3. If no filtered HCO_3^- were lost in component 3, the generation of new HCO_3^- by the kidneys would be the sum of components 1 and 2. To the extent that filtered HCO_3^- is lost in the urine, the new HCO_3^- must exceed the sum of components 1 and 2.

Secreted H⁺ titrates HCO_3^- to CO_2 (HCO_3^- reabsorption) and also titrates filtered non-HCO_3^- buffers and endogenously produced NH_3

As we have seen, the kidney can reabsorb nearly all of the filtered HCO_3^- and excrete additional acid into the urine as both titratable acid and NH_4^+. The common theme of these three processes is **H⁺ secretion** from the blood into the lumen. Thus, the secreted H⁺ can have three fates. It can titrate (1) filtered HCO_3^-, (2) filtered phosphate (or other filtered buffers that contribute to the "titratable acid"), and (3) NH_3, both secreted and, to a lesser extent, filtered.

A HCO₃⁻ REABSORPTION

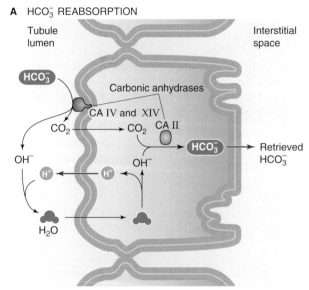

B FORMATION OF TITRATABLE ACID

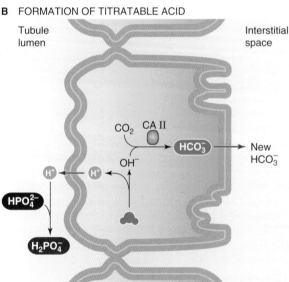

C AMMONIUM EXCRETION

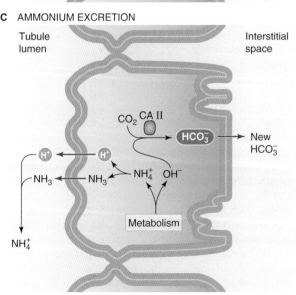

Figure 39.2 Titration of luminal buffers by secreted H⁺. (A and B) Generic models of H⁺ secretion at various sites along the nephron. The *red arrows* represent diverse transport mechanisms. (C) Ammonium handling by the proximal tubule.

Titration of Filtered HCO₃⁻ (HCO₃⁻ Reabsorption) Extensive reabsorption reclaims almost all of the filtered HCO₃⁻ (>99.9%). The kidney reabsorbs HCO₃⁻ at specialized sites along the nephron. However, regardless of the site, the basic mechanism of HCO₃⁻ reabsorption is the same (Fig. 39.2A): H⁺ transported into the lumen by the tubule cell titrates filtered HCO₃⁻ to CO_2 plus H_2O. One way that this titration can occur is by H⁺ interacting with HCO₃⁻ to form H_2CO_3, which in turn dissociates to yield H_2O and CO_2. However, the reaction $H_2CO_3 \rightarrow H_2O + CO_2$ is far too slow to convert the entire filtered load of HCO₃⁻ to CO_2 plus H_2O. The enzyme carbonic anhydrase (CA)—which is present in many tubule segments—bypasses this slow reaction by splitting HCO₃⁻ into CO_2 and OH⁻. The secreted H⁺ neutralizes this OH⁻ so that the net effect is to accelerate the production of H_2O and CO_2.

The apical membranes of these H⁺-secreting tubules are highly permeable to CO_2, so that the CO_2 produced in the lumen, as well as the H_2O, diffuses into the tubule cell. Inside the tubule cell, the CO_2 and H_2O regenerate intracellular H⁺ and HCO₃⁻ with the aid of CA. Finally, the cell exports these two products, thereby moving the H⁺ out across the apical membrane into the tubule lumen and the HCO₃⁻ out across the basolateral membrane into the blood. Thus, for each H⁺ secreted into the lumen, one HCO₃⁻ disappears from the lumen, and one HCO₃⁻ appears in the blood.

Titration of Filtered Non-HCO₃⁻ Buffers (Titratable-Acid Formation) The H⁺ secreted into the tubules can interact with buffers other than HCO₃⁻ and NH_3. The titration of the non-NH_3, non-HCO₃⁻ buffers (B⁻)—mainly HPO_4^{2-}, creatinine, and urate—to their conjugate weak acids (HB) constitutes the titratable acid (see ⊙ 39-1).

$$H^+ + B^- \rightarrow \underbrace{BH}_{\text{Titratable acid}} \qquad \text{(39.4)}$$

The major proton acceptor in this category of buffers excreted in the urine is HPO_4^{2-}. Fig. 39.2B shows the fate of H⁺ as it protonates phosphate from its divalent form (HPO_4^{2-}) to its monovalent form ($H_2PO_4^-$). Because low luminal pH inhibits the apical Na/phosphate cotransporter (NaPi) in the proximal tubule, and NaPi carries $H_2PO_4^-$ less effectively than HPO_4^{2-} (see Fig. 36.8B) the kidneys tend to excrete H⁺-bound phosphate in the urine. For each H⁺ it transfers to the lumen to titrate HPO_4^{2-}, the tubule cell generates one new HCO₃⁻ and transfers it to the blood (Fig. 39.2B).

Titration of Filtered and Secreted NH₃ (Ammonium Excretion) The third class of acceptors of luminal H⁺ is NH_3. Glomerular filtration contributes only a negligible quantity of NH_3 because plasma $[NH_3]$ concentration is exceedingly low. Instead, urinary NH_3 derives mainly from diffusion into the lumen from the proximal-tubule cell (Fig. 39.2C). In the case of the proximal tubule, the conversion of glutamine to α-ketoglutarate (α-KG) generates two NH_4^+ ions, which form two NH_3 and two H⁺ ions. In addition, the metabolism of α-KG generates two OH⁻ ions, which CA converts to HCO₃⁻ ions. This new HCO₃⁻ then enters the blood.

In summary, when renal-tubule cells secrete H⁺ into the lumen, this H⁺ simultaneously titrates three kinds of buffers: (1) HCO₃⁻, (2) HPO_4^{2-} and other buffers that become the "titratable acid," and (3) NH_3. Each of these three buffers competes with the other two for available H^+.

ACID-BASE TRANSPORT BY DIFFERENT SEGMENTS OF THE NEPHRON

Most nephron segments secrete H^+ to varying degrees.

The nephron reclaims virtually all the filtered HCO_3^- in the proximal tubule (~80%), thick ascending limb (~10%), and distal nephron (~10%)

The kidney reabsorbs the largest fraction of filtered HCO_3^- (~80%) along the proximal tubule (Fig. 39.3A). By the end of the proximal tubule, luminal pH falls to ~6.8, which represents only a modest transepithelial H^+ gradient compared with the plasma pH of 7.4. Thus, the proximal tubule is a high-capacity, low-gradient system for H^+ secretion. The thick ascending limb of the loop of Henle (TAL) reabsorbs an additional 10% of filtered HCO_3^-, so that by the time the tubule fluid reaches the distal convoluted tubule (DCT), the kidney has reclaimed ~90% of the filtered HCO_3^-. The rest of the distal nephron—from the DCT to the inner medullary collecting duct (IMCD)—reabsorbs almost all the remaining ~10% of the filtered HCO_3^-, lowering luminal pH to ~4.4. Thus, the collecting tubules and ducts are a low-capacity, high-gradient system for H^+ transport.

The nephron generates new HCO_3^-, mostly in the proximal tubule

The kidney generates new HCO_3^- in two ways (Fig. 39.3B). It titrates filtered buffers such as HPO_4^{2-} to produce "titratable acid," and it titrates secreted NH_3 to NH_4^+. In healthy people, NH_4^+ excretion is the more important of the two and contributes ~60% of *net* acid excretion or new HCO_3^-.

Formation of Titratable Acid The extent to which a particular buffer contributes to titratable acid (Fig. 39.2B) depends on the amount of buffer in the lumen and luminal pH. The titratable acid due to *phosphate* is already substantial at the end of the proximal tubule. Beyond the proximal tubule, the titratable acid due to phosphate rises only slightly because acid secretion slightly exceeds phosphate reabsorption.

NH_4^+ Excretion Of the new HCO_3^- that the nephron generates, ~60% (~40 mmol/day) is the product of net NH_4^+ excretion (Fig. 39.3B), which is the result of five processes: (1) the proximal tubule actually secretes slightly more than ~40 mmol/day of NH_4^+, (2) the TAL reabsorbs some NH_4^+ and deposits it in the interstitium, (3) some of this interstitial NH_4^+ recycles back to the proximal tubule and thin descending limb (tDLH), (4) some of the interstitial NH_4^+ enters the lumen of the collecting duct, and, finally, (5) some of the interstitial NH_4^+ enters the vasa recta and leaves the kidney.

ACID-BASE TRANSPORT AT THE CELLULAR AND MOLECULAR LEVELS

The secretion of acid from the blood to the lumen—whether for reabsorption of filtered HCO_3^-, formation of titratable acid, or NH_4^+ excretion—shares three steps: (1) transport of H^+ (derived from H_2O) from tubule cell to lumen, which leaves behind intracellular OH^-; (2) conversion of intracellular OH^- to HCO_3^-, catalyzed by CA; and (3) transport of newly formed HCO_3^- from tubule cell to blood. In addition, because the buffering power of filtered non-HCO_3^- buffers is not high enough for these buffers to accept sufficient luminal H^+, the adequate formation of new HCO_3^- requires that the kidney generate buffer de novo. This buffer is NH_3.

H^+ moves across the apical membrane from tubule cell to lumen by Na-H exchange, electrogenic H pumping, and K-H pumping

Although the kidney could, in principle, acidify the tubule fluid either by secreting H^+ or by reabsorbing OH^- or HCO_3^-, the secretion of H^+ appears to be solely responsible for acidifying tubule fluid. At least three mechanisms can extrude H^+ across the apical membrane; not all of these are present in any one cell.

Na-H Exchanger NHE3 moves more H^+ from tubule cell to lumen than any other transporter. NHE3 is present not only throughout the proximal tubule (Fig. 39.4A and B) but also in the TAL (Fig. 39.4C) and DCT.

Because apical NHE3 secretes H^+ in exchange for luminal Na^+, apical H^+ secretion ultimately depends on the activity of the basolateral Na-K pump.

Electrogenic H Pump A second mechanism for apical H^+ secretion by tubule cells is the electrogenic H pump, a vacuolar-type ATPase. The ATP-driven H pump can establish steep transepithelial H^+ concentration gradients, thus lowering the urine pH to ~4.0 to 5.0.

The apical electrogenic H pumps are located mainly in a subpopulation of intercalated cells (α cells) of the CNT, ICT, and cortical collecting tubule (CCT) and in cells of the IMCD and outer medullary collecting duct (OMCD; Fig. 39.4D). However, H pumps are also present in the apical membrane of the proximal tubule (Fig. 39.4A and B), the TAL (Fig. 39.4C), and the DCT.

H-K Exchange Pump A third type of H^+-secretory mechanism is present in the α cells of the ICT and CCT, and the cells of the OMCD (Fig. 39.4D): an electroneutral H-K pump.

CAs in the lumen and cytosol stimulate H^+ secretion by accelerating the interconversion of CO_2 and HCO_3^-

The CAs play an important role in renal acidification by catalyzing the interconversion of CO_2 to HCO_3^-. Inhibition of CAs by sulfonamides, such as acetazolamide, profoundly slows acid secretion. CAs may act at three distinct sites of acid-secreting tubule cells (Fig. 39.4): the extracellular face of the apical membrane, the cytoplasm, and the extracellular face of the basolateral membrane.

Apical CA (CA IV) By promoting the conversion of luminal HCO_3^- to CO_2 plus OH^-, apical CA prevents the lumen from becoming overly acidic and thus substantially promotes HCO_3^- reabsorption. Thus, CA promotes high rates of HCO_3^- reabsorption along the early proximal tubule (Fig. 39.4A).

Cytoplasmic CA (CA II) Cytoplasmic CA accelerates the conversion of intracellular CO_2 and OH^- to

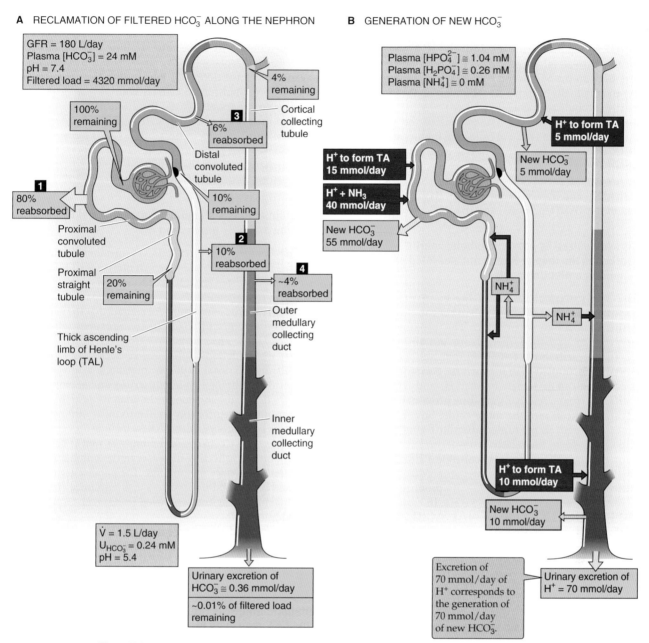

A RECLAMATION OF FILTERED HCO$_3^-$ ALONG THE NEPHRON

GFR = 180 L/day
Plasma [HCO$_3^-$] = 24 mM
pH = 7.4
Filtered load = 4320 mmol/day

100% remaining

1 80% reabsorbed

Proximal convoluted tubule

Proximal straight tubule   20% remaining

Thick ascending limb of Henle's loop (TAL)

4% remaining

3 6% reabsorbed

Cortical collecting tubule

Distal convoluted tubule

10% remaining

2 10% reabsorbed

~4% reabsorbed **4**

Outer medullary collecting duct

Inner medullary collecting duct

V̇ = 1.5 L/day
U$_{HCO_3^-}$ = 0.24 mM
pH = 5.4

Urinary excretion of HCO$_3^-$ ≅ 0.36 mmol/day

~0.01% of filtered load remaining

B GENERATION OF NEW HCO$_3^-$

Plasma [HPO$_4^{2-}$] ≅ 1.04 mM
Plasma [H$_2$PO$_4^-$] ≅ 0.26 mM
Plasma [NH$_4^+$] ≅ 0 mM

H$^+$ to form TA 5 mmol/day

New HCO$_3^-$ 5 mmol/day

H$^+$ to form TA 15 mmol/day

H$^+$ + NH$_3$ 40 mmol/day

New HCO$_3^-$ 55 mmol/day

NH$_4^+$

NH$_4^+$

H$^+$ to form TA 10 mmol/day

New HCO$_3^-$ 10 mmol/day

Excretion of 70 mmol/day of H$^+$ corresponds to the generation of 70 mmol/day of new HCO$_3^-$.

Urinary excretion of H$^+$ = 70 mmol/day

Figure 39.3   Acid-base handling along the nephron. In (A) the *numbered yellow boxes* indicate the fraction of the filtered load reabsorbed by various nephron segments. The *green boxes* indicate the fraction of the filtered load that remains in the lumen at various sites. In (B) *the red boxes* indicate the moieties of acid secretion associated with either the formation of titratable acid (TA) or the secretion of NH$_4^+$. The *yellow boxes* indicate the formation of new HCO$_3^-$ or NH$_4^+$ reabsorption by the TAL. The values in the boxes are approximations.

HCO$_3^-$ (Fig. 39.4). As a result, CA II increases the supply of H$^+$ for apical H$^+$ extrusion and the supply of HCO$_3^-$ for the basolateral HCO$_3^-$ exit step. In the CNT, ICT, and CCT, the intercalated cells (which engage in acid-base transport) contain CA II, whereas the principal cells do not.

Basolateral CA (CA IV and CA XII)   The role played by basolateral CA IV and CA XII (an integral membrane protein with an extracellular catalytic domain) is not yet understood.

Inhibition of CA   The administration of drugs that block CAs, such as acetazolamide, strongly inhibits

HCO$_3^-$ reabsorption along the nephron, leading to the excretion of an alkaline urine. Because acetazolamide reduces the reabsorption of Na$^+$, HCO$_3^-$, and water, this drug is also a **diuretic** (i.e., it promotes urine output).

HCO$_3^-$ efflux across the basolateral membrane takes place by electrogenic Na/HCO$_3$ cotransport and Cl-HCO$_3$ exchange

Two mechanisms are responsible for HCO$_3^-$ transport from the cell into the peritubular fluid: electrogenic Na/HCO$_3$ cotransport and Cl-HCO$_3$ exchange.

Electrogenic Na/HCO₃ Cotransport In proximal-tubule cells, the electrogenic Na/HCO₃ cotransporter NBCe1 (see Fig. 5.7D) is responsible for much of the HCO_3^- transport across the basolateral membrane. NBCe1 is expressed at highest levels in the S1 portion of the proximal tubule (Fig. 39.4A) and gradually becomes less abundant in the more distal proximal-tubule segments (Fig. 39.4B).

Cl-HCO₃ Exchange In the S3 segment of the proximal tubule, as well as in the TAL and collecting tubules and ducts, Cl-HCO₃ exchangers participate in transepithelial acid-base transport. The AE1 anion exchanger (see Fig. 5.8D) is found in the basolateral membranes of α-intercalated cells of the CNT, the ICT, and the CCT (Fig. 39.4D). Basolateral AE2 is present in the TAL (Fig. 39.4C) and the DCT.

NH₄⁺ is synthesized by proximal tubules, partly reabsorbed in the loop of Henle, and secreted passively into papillary collecting ducts

⦿ **39-2** The **proximal tubule** is the main site of renal NH_4^+ synthesis, although almost all other tubule segments have the capacity to form NH_4^+. The proximal tubule forms NH_4^+ in cytosol largely from glutamine, which enters tubule cells both from luminal and peritubular fluid via Na^+-coupled cotransporters. Ammonium is a weak acid that can dissociate to form H^+ and NH_3. When NH_3 diffuses from a relatively alkaline proximal-tubule or collecting-duct cell into the more acidic lumen, the NH_3 becomes "trapped" in the lumen after buffering the newly secreted H^+ to form the relatively impermeant NH_4^+. This titration of luminal NH_3 to NH_4^+ continues along the TAL and collecting ducts.

⦿ 39-3 REGULATION OF RENAL ACID SECRETION

The kidney appropriately modulates H^+ secretion and NH_3 synthesis in response to a variety of physiological and pathophysiological challenges.

⦿ 39-4 Respiratory acidosis stimulates renal H⁺ secretion

The four fundamental pH disturbances are respiratory acidosis and alkalosis, and metabolic acidosis and alkalosis (see Fig. 28.6A). In each case, the initial and almost instantaneous line of defense is the action of buffers—both in the extracellular and intracellular compartments—to *minimize* the magnitude of the pH changes. However, *restoring* the pH to a value as close to "normal" as possible requires slower compensatory responses from the lungs or kidneys.

In respiratory acidosis, in which the primary disturbance is an increase in arterial P_{CO_2}, the compensatory response is an increase in renal H^+ secretion, which translates to increased production of new HCO_3^- via excretion of titratable acid and NH_4^+. The opposite occurs in respiratory alkalosis. These changes in H^+ secretion tend to correct the distorted $[HCO_3^-]/[CO_2]$ ratios that occur in primary respiratory acid-base derangements.

Respiratory acidosis stimulates H^+ secretion in at least three ways. First, an *acute* elevated P_{CO_2} directly stimulates proximal-tubule cells to secrete H^+. Proximal-tubule cells directly sense basolateral CO_2. In part, the mechanism is the exocytotic insertion of H pumps into the apical membranes of proximal-tubule cells. Second, acute respiratory acidosis also causes exocytotic insertion of H pumps into the apical membranes of intercalated cells in distal nephron segments. Third, *chronic* respiratory acidosis leads to adaptive responses that upregulate acid-base transporters. These adaptive changes allow the kidney to produce a metabolic compensation to the respiratory acidosis (see ⦿ 28-7).

Metabolic acidosis stimulates both proximal H⁺ secretion and NH₃ production

The first compensatory response to metabolic acidosis is increased alveolar ventilation, which blows off CO_2 and thus corrects the distorted $[HCO_3^-]/[CO_2]$ ratio in a primary metabolic acidosis. The kidneys can also participate in the compensatory response—assuming, of course, that the acidosis is not the consequence of renal disease. Proximal-tubule cells can directly sense an *acute* fall in basolateral $[HCO_3^-]$, which results in a stimulation of proximal H^+ secretion. In intercalated cells in the distal nephron, metabolic acidosis stimulates apical membrane H pump insertion and activity.

In *chronic* metabolic acidosis, the adaptive responses of the proximal tubule are probably similar to those outlined above for chronic respiratory acidosis. These include upregulation of apical NHE3 and electrogenic H pumps, as well as basolateral NBCe1, perhaps reflecting increases in the number of transporters on the surface membranes. The parallel activation of apical and basolateral transporters may minimize changes in pH_i, while increasing transepithelial HCO_3^- reabsorption.

In addition to increased H^+ secretion, the other adjustable parameter needed to produce new HCO_3^- is enhanced NH_3 secretion. Together, the two increase NH_4^+ excretion. Indeed, the excretion of NH_4^+ into the urine increases markedly as a result of the adaptive response to chronic metabolic acidosis.

Metabolic alkalosis reduces proximal H⁺ secretion and, in the CCT, may even provoke HCO₃⁻ secretion

When $[HCO_3^-]$ in the peritubular blood is higher than normal (e.g., during metabolic alkalosis) luminal H^+ secretion falls. As a result, HCO_3^- reabsorption, the excretion of both titratable acid and NH_4^+—the appropriate homeostatic response.

Extracellular volume contraction—via ANG II, aldosterone, and sympathetic activity—stimulates renal H⁺ secretion

A decrease in *effective circulating volume* stimulates Na^+ reabsorption by four parallel pathways (see ⦿ 40-1), including activation of the renin-angiotensin-aldosterone axis (and thus an increase in ANG II levels) and stimulation of renal sympathetic nerves (and thus the release of norepinephrine). Both ANG II and norepinephrine stimulate Na-H exchange in the proximal tubule. Because the proximal tubule couples Na^+ and H^+ transport, volume contraction increases not only

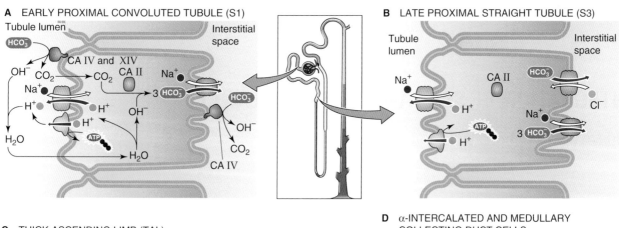

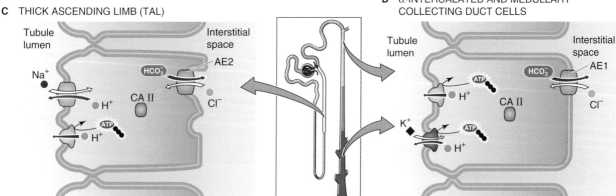

Figure 39.4 Cell models of H⁺ secretion.

Na⁺ reabsorption but also H⁺ secretion, producing a **contraction alkalosis.** Similarly, ANG II stimulates acid secretion by α-intercalated cells in the distal nephron. **Volume expansion** has the opposite effect. On a longer time scale, volume depletion also increases aldosterone levels, thereby enhancing H⁺ secretion in cortical and medullary collecting ducts (see below). Thus, the regulation of effective circulating volume takes precedence over the regulation of plasma pH.

Hypokalemia increases renal H⁺ secretion

Acid-base disturbances can cause changes in K⁺ homeostasis. The opposite is also true. Because a side effect of K⁺ depletion is increased renal H⁺ secretion, K⁺ depletion is frequently associated with metabolic alkalosis. In the proximal tubule, hypokalemia leads to a marked increase in apical Na-H exchange and basolateral Na/HCO₃ cotransport. As in other cells, in tubule cells the pH falls during K⁺ depletion. The resulting chronic cell acidification may lead to adaptive responses that activate Na-H exchange and electrogenic Na/HCO₃ cotransport. In the proximal tubule, K⁺ depletion also

markedly increases NH₃ secretion and NH₄⁺ excretion, thus increasing urinary H⁺ excretion as NH₄⁺. Finally, K⁺ depletion stimulates apical K-H exchange in α-intercalated cells of the ICT and CCT (see ⦿ 37-2) and enhances H⁺ secretion as a side effect of K⁺ retention.

Both glucocorticoids and mineralocorticoids stimulate acid secretion

Chronic adrenal insufficiency leads to acid retention and, potentially, to life-threatening metabolic acidosis. Both glucocorticoids and mineralocorticoids stimulate H⁺ secretion, but at different sites along the nephron.

Glucocorticoids (e.g., cortisol) enhance Na-H exchange in the proximal tubule and thus stimulate H⁺ secretion.

Mineralocorticoids (e.g., aldosterone) stimulate H⁺ secretion, in part by directly stimulating H⁺ secretion in the collecting tubules and ducts by increasing the activity of the apical electrogenic H pump and basolateral Cl-HCO₃ exchanger (Fig. 39.4D).

CHAPTER 40

INTEGRATION OF SALT AND WATER BALANCE

Gerhard Giebisch[†] and Peter S. Aronson

Two separate but closely interrelated control systems regulate the volume and osmolality of the extracellular fluid (ECF). It is important to regulate the **ECF volume** to maintain blood pressure, which is essential for adequate tissue perfusion and function. The body regulates ECF volume by adjusting the total-body content of NaCl. It is important to regulate the **extracellular osmolality** because hypotonic or hypertonic osmolalities cause changes in cell volume that seriously compromise cell function, especially in the central nervous system (CNS). The body regulates extracellular osmolality by adjusting total-body water content. These two homeostatic mechanisms—for ECF volume and osmolality—use different sensors, different hormonal transducers, and different effectors (Table 40.1). However, they have one thing in common: some of their effectors, although different, are located in the kidney. In the case of the ECF volume, the control system modulates the urinary excretion of Na^+. In the case of osmolality, the control system modulates the urinary excretion of solute-free water or simply free water.

Sodium Balance The maintenance of the ECF volume, or Na^+ balance, depends on signals that reflect the adequacy of the circulation—the so-called effective circulating volume, discussed below. Low- and high-pressure baroreceptors send afferent signals to the brain (see ◉ 23-3), which translates this "volume signal" into several responses that can affect ECF volume or blood pressure over either the short or the long term. The short-term effects (over a period of seconds to minutes) occur as the autonomic nervous system and humoral mechanisms modulate the activity of the heart and blood vessels to control blood pressure. The long-term effects (over a period of hours to days) consist of nervous, humoral, and hemodynamic mechanisms that modulate renal Na^+ excretion (see ◉ 35-4). In the first part of this chapter, we discuss the entire feedback loop, of which Na^+ excretion is the effector.

Water Balance The maintenance of osmolality, or water balance, depends on receptors in the hypothalamus that detect changes in the plasma osmolality. These receptors send signals to areas of the brain that (1) control thirst and thus regulate free-water intake, and (2) control the production of arginine vasopressin (AVP)—also known as antidiuretic hormone (ADH)—and thus regulate free-water excretion by the kidneys. In the second part of this chapter, we discuss the entire feedback loop, of which water excretion is merely the end point.

[†] Deceased.

CONTROL OF EXTRACELLULAR FLUID VOLUME

In the steady state, Na⁺ intake via the gastrointestinal tract equals Na⁺ output from renal and extrarenal pathways

The two principal solutes in the ECF are Na^+ and Cl^-. **Sodium** is one of the most abundant ions in the body, totaling ~58 mmol/kg body weight. **Chloride** totals ~33 mmol/kg body weight.

By definition, in the steady state, the total-body content of water and electrolytes is constant. For Na^+, this concept can be expressed as

$$\text{Oral } Na^+ \text{ intake} = \text{Renal } Na^+ \text{ output} + \text{Extrarenal } Na^+ \text{ output} \quad (40.1)$$

Under normal circumstances, extrarenal Na^+ output is negligible. However, large fluid losses from the gastrointestinal tract (e.g., vomiting, diarrhea) or skin (e.g., excessive sweating, extensive burns) can represent substantial extrarenal Na^+ losses. The kidney responds to such deficits by reducing renal Na^+ excretion. Conversely, in conditions of excessive Na^+ intake, the kidneys excrete the surfeit of Na^+.

The kidneys increase Na⁺ excretion in response to an increase in ECF volume, not to an increase in extracellular Na⁺ concentration

In contrast to many other renal mechanisms of electrolyte excretion, the renal excretion of Na^+ depends on the *amount* of Na^+ in the body and not on the Na^+ *concentration* in ECF. Because the amount of Na^+ is the product of ECF volume and the extracellular Na^+ concentration, and because the osmoregulatory system keeps plasma osmolality constant within very narrow limits, it is actually the *volume* of ECF that acts as the signal for Na^+ homeostasis.

It is not the ECF volume as a whole, but the effective circulating volume, that regulates Na⁺ excretion

Although we have referred to the overall expansion of the ECF volume as the signal for increased urinary Na^+ excretion, this is an oversimplification. Only certain regions of the ECF compartment are important for this signaling. For an expansion in ECF volume to stimulate Na^+ excretion—either acutely or chronically—the expansion must make itself evident in parts of the ECF compartment where the ECF volume sensors are

TABLE 40.1 **Comparison of the Systems Controlling ECF Volume and Osmolality**

	REGULATION OF ECF VOLUME AND BLOOD PRESSURE	REGULATION OF OSMOLALITY	
What is sensed?	Effective circulating volume	Plasma osmolality	
Sensors	Carotid sinus, aortic arch, renal afferent arteriole, atria	Hypothalamic osmoreceptors	
Efferent pathways	Renin-angiotensin-aldosterone axis, sympathetic nervous system, AVP, ANP	AVP	Thirst
Effector	*Short term:* Heart, blood vessels *Long term:* Kidney	Kidney	Brain: drinking behavior
What is affected?	*Short term:* Blood pressure *Long term:* Na$^+$ excretion	Renal water excretion	Water intake

located, namely, in blood-filled compartments. *ECF volume* per se is not the critical factor in regulating renal Na$^+$ excretion.

The critical parameter that the body recognizes is the **effective circulating volume** (see ⊙ 23-26)—not something that we can identify anatomically. Rather, effective circulating volume is a *functional* blood volume that reflects the extent of tissue perfusion in specific regions, as evidenced by the fullness or pressure within their blood vessels. Normally, changes in effective circulating volume parallel those in total ECF volume. However, in certain diseases (e.g., congestive heart failure) *total* ECF volume is grossly expanded even though *effective* circulating volume is low.

⊙ 40-1 Decreases in effective circulating volume trigger four parallel effector pathways to decrease renal Na$^+$ excretion

Fig. 40.1 shows the elements of the feedback loop that controls the effective circulating volume. As summarized in Table 40.2, sensors that monitor changes in effective circulating volume are **baroreceptors** located in both high-pressure (see ⊙ 23-1) and low-pressure (see ⊙ 23-17) areas of the circulation. Although most are located within the vascular tree of the thorax, additional baroreceptors are present in the kidney—particularly in the afferent arterioles—as well as in the CNS and liver. Of the pressures at these sites, it is renal perfusion pressure that is most important for long-term regulation of Na$^+$ excretion, and thus blood pressure. The sensors shown in Fig. 40.1 generate four distinct hormonal or neural signals (pathways 1 to 4 in the figure).

In the first pathway, the kidney itself senses a reduced effective circulating volume and directly stimulates a hormonal effector pathway, the **renin-angiotensin-aldosterone system** (see ⊙ 40-2). In addition, increased renal perfusion pressure itself can increase Na$^+$ excretion independent of the renin-angiotensin-aldosterone system.

The second and third effector pathways are neural. Baroreceptors detect decreases in effective circulating volume and communicate these via afferent neurons to the medulla of the brainstem. Emerging from the medulla are two types of efferent signals that ultimately act on the kidney. In one, increased activity of the **sympathetic division** of the autonomic nervous system reduces renal blood flow and directly stimulates Na$^+$ reabsorption, thereby reducing Na$^+$ excretion

(see ⊙ 40-6). In the other effector pathway, the **posterior pituitary** increases its secretion of AVP, which leads to conservation of water. This AVP mechanism becomes active only after large declines in effective circulating volume.

The final pathway is hormonal. Reduced effective circulating volume decreases the release of **atrial natriuretic peptide (ANP),** thus reducing Na$^+$ excretion (see ⊙ 40-8).

All four parallel effector pathways correct the primary change in effective circulating blood volume. An increase in effective circulating volume promotes Na$^+$ excretion (thus reducing ECF volume), whereas a decrease in effective circulating volume inhibits Na$^+$ excretion (thus raising ECF volume).

⊙ 40-2 Increased activity of the renin-angiotensin-aldosterone axis is the first of four parallel pathways that correct a low effective circulating volume

The **renin-angiotensin-aldosterone** axis (Fig. 40.2) promotes Na$^+$ retention via the actions of both ANG II and aldosterone.

⊙ **40-3** **Angiotensinogen** is synthesized by the liver and released into the systemic circulation. Another protein, **renin,** is produced and stored in the **granular cells** of the renal **juxtaglomerular apparatus** (JGA; see ⊙ 33-1). Decreases in effective circulating volume stimulate these cells to release renin, which is a protease that cleaves angiotensinogen, releasing the decapeptide **angiotensin I (ANG I).** **Angiotensin-converting enzyme (ACE)** rapidly removes the two C-terminal amino acids from the physiologically inactive ANG I to form the physiologically active octapeptide **ANG II.** ACE is present on the luminal surface of vascular endothelia throughout the body and is abundantly present in the endothelium-rich lungs. ACE in the kidney—particularly in the endothelial cells of the afferent and efferent arterioles, and also in the proximal tubule—can produce enough ANG II to exert *local* vascular effects.

⊙ **40-4** The principal factor controlling plasma ANG II levels is renin release from JGA granular cells. A decrease in effective circulating volume manifests itself to the JGA—and thus stimulates renin release—in three ways (Fig. 40.1):

1. **Decreased systemic blood pressure (sympathetic effect on JGA).** A low effective circulating volume, sensed by baroreceptors located in the central arterial

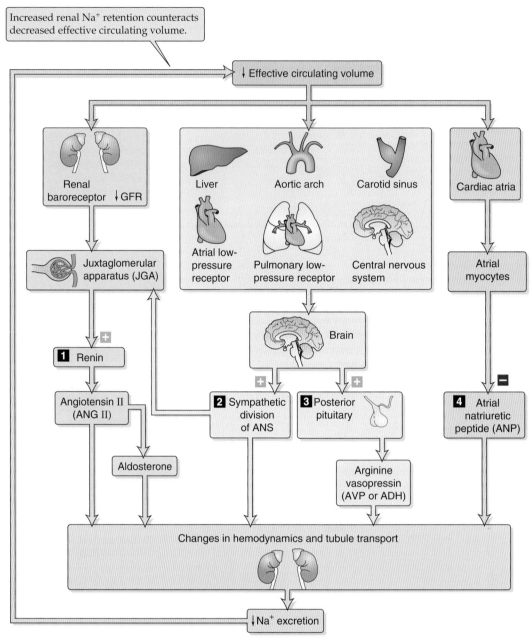

Figure 40.1   Feedback control of effective circulating volume. A low effective circulating volume triggers four parallel effector pathways (numbered *1* to *4*) that act on the kidney, either by changing the hemodynamics or by changing Na+ transport by the renal-tubule cells. *ANS,* Autonomic nervous system.

TABLE 40.2 ECF Volume Receptors

"Central" vascular sensors
High pressure
JGA (renal afferent arteriole)
Carotid sinus
Aortic arch
Low pressure
Cardiac atria
Pulmonary vasculature
Sensors in the CNS (less important)
Sensors in the liver (less important)

circulation, signals medullary control centers to increase sympathetic outflow to the JGA, which in turn increases renin release.

2. **Decreased NaCl concentration at the macula densa (NaCl sensor).** Decreased effective circulating volume tends to increase filtration fraction, thereby increasing Na+ and fluid reabsorption by the proximal tubule and reducing the flow of tubule fluid through the loop of Henle. Na+ reabsorption in the thick ascending limb (TAL) then decreases luminal [Na+] more than if tubular flow were higher. The resulting decrease in luminal [NaCl] at the macula densa stimulates renin release.

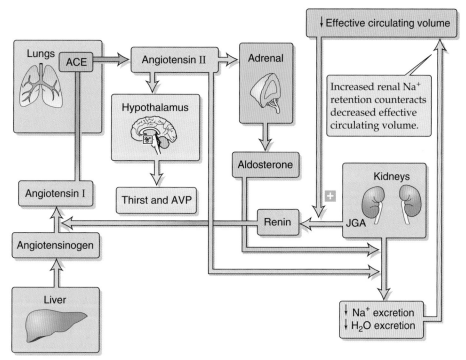

Figure 40.2 Renin-angiotensin-aldosterone axis.

3. **Decreased renal perfusion pressure (renal baroreceptor).** ⊙ **40-5** Stretch receptors in the granular cells of the *afferent* arterioles sense the decreased distention, resulting in increased renin release.

The ANG II formed by the sequential action of renin and ACE has several important actions as follows:

1. **Stimulation of aldosterone release from glomerulosa cells in the adrenal cortex.** In turn, aldosterone promotes Na$^+$ reabsorption in the distal tubule and collecting tubules and ducts (see ⊙ **35-6**).
2. **Vasoconstriction of renal and other systemic vessels.** ANG II increases Na$^+$ reabsorption by altering renal hemodynamics. One mechanism is that, at high concentrations, ANG II constricts the efferent more than the afferent arterioles. The result is increased filtration fraction and reduced *hydrostatic pressure* in the downstream peritubular capillaries and hence enhanced reabsorption of Na$^+$ and fluid by the proximal tubule.
3. **Enhanced tubuloglomerular feedback.** ANG II raises the sensitivity and lowers the set-point of the tubuloglomerular feedback mechanism (see ⊙ **34-6**), so that an increase in Na$^+$ and fluid delivery to the macula densa elicits a more pronounced fall in the glomerular filtration rate (GFR).
4. **Enhanced Na-H exchange.** ANG II promotes Na$^+$ reabsorption in the proximal tubule, TAL, and initial collecting tubule.
5. **Renal hypertrophy.** Over a prolonged time, ANG II induces hypertrophy of renal-tubule cells.
6. **Stimulated thirst and AVP release.** ANG II acts on specific centers in the brain (see ⊙ **40-10**) and the hypothalamus, where it increases the sensation of thirst and stimulates secretion of AVP from the posterior pituitary, both of which increase total-body free water.

This ANG II effect represents an intersection between the systems for regulating effective circulating volume and osmolality.

Increased sympathetic nerve activity, increased AVP, and decreased ANP are the other three parallel pathways that correct a low effective circulating volume

Renal Sympathetic Nerve Activity ⊙ **40-6** The second of the four parallel effector pathways for the control of effective circulating volume is the sympathetic nervous system. Enhanced activity of the renal sympathetic nerves has two *direct* effects on Na$^+$ reabsorption: (1) increased renal vascular resistance and (2) increased Na$^+$ reabsorption by tubule cells. In addition, increased sympathetic tone has an *indirect* effect—enhancing renin release from granular cells (see previous section). These multiple actions of sympathetic traffic to the kidney reduce GFR and enhance Na$^+$ reabsorption, thereby increasing Na$^+$ retention and increasing effective circulating volume.

Arginine Vasopressin (Antidiuretic Hormone) ⊙ **40-7** The posterior pituitary releases AVP primarily in response to increases in extracellular *osmolality*. Indeed, AVP mainly increases distal-nephron water permeability, promoting water retention (see ⊙ **38-3**). However, the posterior pituitary also releases AVP in response to large reductions in effective circulating volume (e.g., hemorrhage), and secondary actions of AVP—vasoconstriction (see ⊙ **23-24**) and promotion of renal Na$^+$ retention (see ⊙ **35-9**)—are appropriate for this stimulus.

Atrial Natriuretic Peptide ⊙ **40-8** Of the four parallel effectors that correct a low effective circulating volume (Fig. 40.1), ANP is the only one that does so by *decreasing* its activity. As its name implies, ANP promotes **natriuresis** (i.e., Na$^+$ excretion) (see ⊙ **35-10**). Atrial myocytes synthesize and store

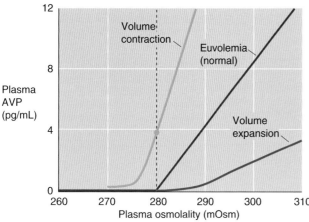

Figure 40.3 Dependence of AVP release on plasma osmolality. Data from Robertson GL, Aycinena P, Zerbe RL: Neurogenic disorders of osmoregulation. Am J Med 72:339–353, 1982.

ANP and release ANP in response to stretch (a low-pressure volume sensor; see ⊙ **23-21**). Thus, reduced effective circulating volume inhibits ANP release and reduces Na⁺ excretion.

CONTROL OF WATER CONTENT (EXTRACELLULAR OSMOLALITY)

Two elements control water content and thus whole-body osmolality: (1) the kidneys, which control water excretion, and (2) thirst mechanisms, which control the oral intake of water. These two effector mechanisms are part of negative-feedback loops that begin within the hypothalamus. An increase in osmolality stimulates separate osmoreceptors to secrete AVP (which reduces renal excretion of free water) and to trigger thirst (which, if fulfilled, increases intake of free water). As a result, the two complementary feedback loops stabilize osmolality and thus [Na⁺].

Increased plasma osmolality stimulates hypothalamic osmoreceptors that trigger the release of AVP, inhibiting water excretion

An increase in the osmolality of the ECF is the primary signal for the secretion of AVP from the posterior pituitary gland. Ingesting large volumes of water causes plasma osmolality to fall, thus leading to reduced AVP secretion.

In healthy individuals, plasma osmolality is ~290 mOsm. The **threshold** for AVP release is somewhat lower, ~280 mOsm (Fig. 40.3, *red curve*). Increasing the osmolality by only 1% higher than this level is sufficient to produce a detectable increase in plasma [AVP], which rises steeply with further increases in osmolality. Thus, hyperosmolality leads to increased levels of AVP, which completes the feedback loop by causing the kidneys to retain free water.

Hypothalamic neurons synthesize AVP and transport it along their axons to the posterior pituitary, where they store it in nerve terminals prior to release

⊙ **40-9** Osmoreceptors of the CNS appear to be located in two areas that breech the blood-brain barrier: the organum

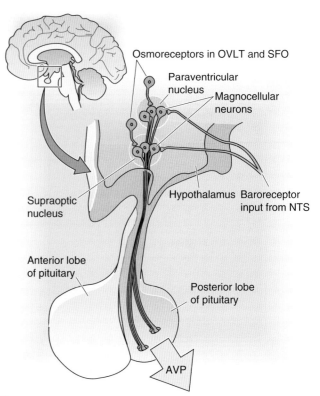

Figure 40.4 Control of AVP synthesis and release by osmoreceptors. Signals from atrial low-pressure baroreceptors travel with the vagus nerve to the nucleus tractus solitarii (NTS); a second neuron carries the signal to the hypothalamus.

vasculosum of the lamina terminalis (OVLT) and the subfornical organ (SFO), two of the circumventricular organs (see Fig. 11.3). Specific neurons in these regions (Fig. 40.4) are able to sense changes in *plasma* osmolality. Elevated osmolality increases the activity of mechanosensitive cation channels located in the neuronal membrane, which results in depolarization and thus an increased frequency of action potentials. Hypo-osmolality causes a striking decrease of frequency. The osmosensitive neurons project to large-diameter neurons in the supraoptic and paraventricular nuclei of the anterior hypothalamus (Fig. 40.4). These neurons synthesize AVP, package it into granules, and transport the granules along their axons to nerve terminals in the posterior lobe of the pituitary, which is part of the brain. When stimulated by the osmosensitive neurons, these **magnocellular neurons** release the stored AVP into the posterior pituitary—an area that also lacks a blood-brain barrier—and AVP enters the general circulation. The half-life of AVP in the circulation is 18 minutes.

⊙ 40-10 Increased osmolality stimulates a second group of osmoreceptors that trigger thirst, which promotes water intake

The second efferent pathway of the osmoregulatory system is **thirst,** which regulates the oral intake of water. Like the osmoreceptors that trigger AVP release, the osmoreceptors that trigger thirst are located in two circumventricular organs, the OVLT and the SFO. Also like the

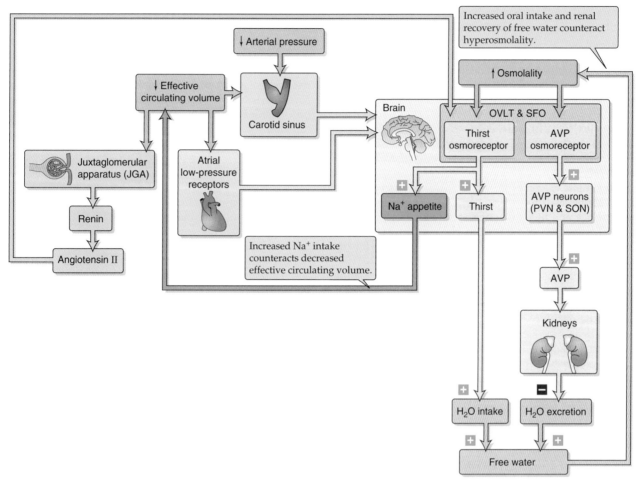

Figure 40.5 Feedback systems involved in the control of osmolality. *PVN,* Paraventricular nucleus; *SON,* supraoptic nucleus of the hypothalamus.

osmoreceptors that trigger AVP release, those that trigger thirst respond to the cell shrinkage that is caused by hyperosmolar solutions.

Hyperosmolality triggers two parallel feedback-control mechanisms that have a common end point (Fig. 40.5): an increase in whole-body free water. In response to hyperosmolality, the AVP osmoreceptors in the hypothalamus trigger other neurons to release AVP. The result is the insertion of aquaporin 2 (AQP2) water channels in the collecting duct of the kidney, an increase in the reabsorption of water, and, therefore, a reduced *excretion* of free water. In response to hyperosmolality, the thirst osmoreceptors stimulate an appetite for water that leads to the increased *intake* of free water. The net effect is an increase in whole-body free water and, therefore, a reduction in osmolality.

⊙ 40-11 Several nonosmotic stimuli also enhance AVP secretion

Although an increase in plasma osmolality is the primary trigger for AVP release, several other stimuli increase AVP release, including a decrease in **effective circulating volume** or arterial pressure and pregnancy (Fig. 40.5). Conversely, volume expansion diminishes AVP release.

Reduced Effective Circulating Volume As noted above a mere 1% rise in plasma *osmolality* stimulates AVP release by a detectable amount. However, fairly large reductions in *effective circulating volume* (5% to 10%) are required to stimulate AVP release of similar amounts. Nevertheless, once the rather high threshold for nonosmotic release of AVP is exceeded, AVP release rises steeply with further volume depletion. The interaction between osmotic and volume stimuli on AVP release is illustrated in Fig. 40.3, which shows that the effective circulating volume modifies the **slope** of the relationship between plasma AVP levels and osmolality, as well as the osmotic **threshold** for AVP release. At a fixed osmolality, volume contraction (Fig. 40.3, *green curve*) increases the rate of AVP release. Therefore, during volume depletion, a low plasma osmolality (e.g., 280 mOsm) that would normally suppress AVP release allows AVP secretion to continue (Fig. 40.3, *green dot*). This leftward shift of the osmolality threshold for AVP release is accompanied by an increased slope, reflecting an increased sensitivity of the osmoreceptors to changes in osmolality.

Fig. 40.5 summarizes the three pathways by which decreased effective circulating volume and low arterial pressure enhance AVP release: (1) A reduction in left atrial pressure—produced by volume depletion—via low-pressure receptors in the left atrium decreases the firing rate of vagal afferents (see ⊙ 23-20). These afferents signal brainstem neurons in the nucleus tractus solitarii, causing magnocellular neurons in the hypothalamus to release AVP (Fig. 40.4). Indeed, at constant osmolality, AVP secretion varies inversely with left atrial pressure. (2) Low effective circulating volume triggers granular cells in the JGA to release renin. This leads to the formation of ANG II, which acts on receptors in the OVLT and the SFO to stimulate AVP release. (3) A fall in the arterial pressure similarly causes high-pressure carotid sinus baroreceptors to stimulate AVP release (see ⊙ 23-1).

Two clinical examples in which reduced effective circulating volume leads to increases in AVP are severe **hemorrhagic shock** and **hypovolemic shock** (e.g., shock resulting from excessive loss of ECF, as in cholera). In both cases, the water retention caused by AVP release accounts for the accompanying hyponatremia.

A clinical example in which reduced effective circulating volume can lead to an *inappropriate* increase in AVP levels is **congestive heart failure.** In this situation, the water retention may be so severe that the patient develops **hyponatremia** (i.e., hypo-osmolality).

Volume Expansion In contrast to volume contraction, chronic volume *expansion* reduces AVP secretion, as a consequence of the rightward shift of the threshold to higher osmolalities and of a decline in the slope (Fig. 40.3, *blue curve*). In other words, volume expansion decreases the sensitivity of the central osmoreceptors to changes in plasma osmolality. A clinical example is **hyperaldosteronism.** With normal thirst and water excretion, the chronic Na^+ retention resulting from the hyperaldosteronism would expand the ECF volume isotonically, thus leaving plasma $[Na^+]$ unchanged. However, because chronic volume expansion downregulates AVP release, the kidneys do not retain adequate water, which results in slight **hypernatremia** (i.e., elevated plasma $[Na^+]$) and very modest hyperosmolality.

Pregnancy Leftward shifts in the threshold for AVP release and thirst often occur during pregnancy. Pregnancy is therefore often associated with a decrease of 8 to 10 mOsm in plasma osmolality. A similar but smaller change may also occur in the late phase of the menstrual cycle.

Other Factors Pain, nausea, and several drugs (e.g., morphine, nicotine, and high doses of barbiturates) *stimulate* AVP secretion. In contrast, alcohol and drugs that block the effect of morphine (opiate antagonists) *inhibit* AVP secretion and thus promote diuresis. Some malignant tumors secrete large amounts of AVP. Such secretion of inappropriate amounts of "antidiuretic hormone" leads to pathological retention of water with dilution of the plasma electrolytes, particularly Na^+. If progressive and uncorrected, this condition may lead to life-threatening deterioration of cerebral function.

⊙ 40-12 Decreased effective circulating volume and low arterial pressure also trigger thirst

Large decreases in effective circulating volume and blood pressure not only stimulate the release of AVP but also profoundly stimulate the sensation of thirst. In fact, hemorrhage is one of the most powerful stimuli of hypovolemic thirst: "Thirst among the wounded on the battlefield is legendary" (Fitzsimons JT: Angiotensin, thirst and sodium appetite. *Physiol Rev* 78:583–686, 1998). Therefore, three distinct stimuli—hyperosmolality, profound volume contraction, and large decreases in blood pressure—lead to the sensation of thirst. Low effective circulating volume and low blood pressure stimulate thirst centers in the hypothalamus via the same pathways by which they stimulate AVP release (Fig. 40.5).

Defense of the effective circulating volume usually has priority over defense of osmolality

Under physiological conditions, the body regulates plasma *volume* and plasma *osmolality* independently. This clear separation of defense mechanisms against volume and osmotic challenges breaks down when more dramatic derangements of fluid or salt metabolism occur. In general, the body defends volume at the expense of osmolality. Examples include severe reductions in absolute blood volume (e.g., hemorrhage) and decreases in effective circulating volume even when absolute ECF volume may be expanded (e.g., congestive heart failure, nephrotic syndrome, and liver cirrhosis). All are conditions that strongly stimulate both Na^+- *and* water-retaining mechanisms. However, hyponatremia can be the consequence.

THE GASTROINTESTINAL SYSTEM

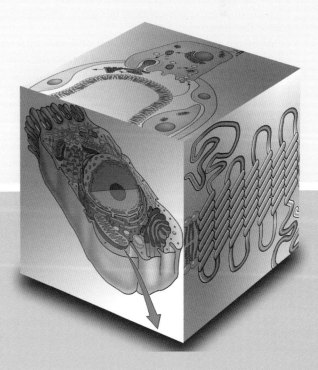

CHAPTER 41

ORGANIZATION OF THE GASTROINTESTINAL SYSTEM

Henry J. Binder

The gastrointestinal tract is a tube that is specialized along its length for the sequential processing of food

The gastrointestinal (GI) tract consists of both the series of hollow organs stretching from the mouth to the anus and the several accessory glands and organs that add secretions to these hollow organs (Fig. 41.1). Each of these hollow organs, which are separated from each other at key locations by sphincters, has evolved to serve a specialized function. The mouth and oropharynx are responsible for chopping food into small pieces, lubricating it, initiating carbohydrate and fat digestion, and propelling the food into the esophagus. The esophagus acts as a conduit to the stomach. The stomach (see Chapter 42) temporarily stores food and also initiates digestion by churning and by secreting proteases and acid. The small intestine (see Chapters 44 and 45) continues the work of digestion and is the primary site for the absorption of nutrients. The large intestine (see Chapters 44 and 45) reabsorbs fluids and electrolytes and also stores the fecal matter before expulsion from the body. The accessory glands and organs include the salivary glands, pancreas, and liver. The pancreas (see Chapter 43) secretes digestive enzymes into the duodenum, in addition to secreting HCO_3^- to neutralize gastric acid. The liver secretes bile (see Chapter 46), which the gallbladder stores for future delivery to the duodenum during a meal. Bile contains bile acids, which play a key role in the digestion of fats.

Although the anatomy of the wall of the GI tract varies along its length, certain organizational themes are common to all segments. Fig. 41.2, a cross section through a generic piece of stomach or intestine, shows the characteristic layered structure of mucosa, submucosa, muscle, and serosa.

The **mucosa** consists of the epithelial layer, as well as an underlying layer of loose connective tissue known as the **lamina propria,** which contains capillaries, enteric neurons, and immune cells (e.g., mast cells), as well as a thin layer of smooth muscle known as the *lamina muscularis mucosae* (literally, the muscle layer of the mucosa). The surface area of the epithelial layer is amplified by several mechanisms. Most cells have microvilli on their apical surfaces. In addition, the layer of epithelial cells can be evaginated to form **villi** or invaginated to form **crypts** (or glands). Finally, on a larger scale, the mucosa is organized into large folds.

The **submucosa** consists of loose connective tissue and larger blood vessels. The submucosa may also contain glands that secrete material into the GI lumen.

The **muscle layer,** the *muscularis externa,* includes two layers of smooth muscle. The inner layer is circular, whereas the outer layer is longitudinal. Enteric neurons are present between these two muscle layers.

The **serosa** is an enveloping layer of connective tissue that is covered with squamous epithelial cells.

Assimilation of dietary food substances requires digestion as well as absorption

The sedentary human body requires ~30 kcal/kg body weight each day. This nutrient requirement is normally acquired by the oral intake of multiple food substances that the GI tract then assimilates. Both the small and large intestines absorb water and electrolytes, but only the small intestine absorbs lipids, carbohydrates, and amino acids.

To facilitate absorption, the GI tract digests the food by both mechanical and chemical processes.

Mechanical disruption of ingested food begins in the mouth with chewing (mastication). The mechanical processes that alter food composition to facilitate absorption continue in the stomach, both to initiate protein and lipid enzymatic digestion and to allow passage of gastric contents through the pylorus into the duodenum. This change in the size and consistency of gastric contents is necessary because solids that are >2 mm in diameter do not pass through the pylorus.

Digestion requires enzymes secreted in the mouth, stomach, pancreas, and small intestine

Digestion involves the conversion of dietary food nutrients to a form that the small intestine can absorb. For carbohydrates and lipids, these digestive processes are initiated in the mouth by salivary and lingual enzymes: amylase for carbohydrates and lipase for lipids. Protein digestion is initiated in the stomach by gastric proteases (i.e., pepsins), whereas additional lipid digestion in the stomach occurs primarily as a result of the lingual lipase that is swallowed, although some gastric lipase is also secreted. Carbohydrate digestion does not involve any secreted gastric enzymes.

Digestion is completed in the small intestine by the action of both pancreatic enzymes and enzymes at the brush border of the small intestine. Pancreatic enzymes, which include lipase, chymotrypsin, and amylase, are critical for the digestion of lipids, protein, and carbohydrates, respectively. The enzymes on the luminal surface of the small intestine (e.g., brush-border disaccharidases and dipeptidases) complete the digestion of carbohydrates and proteins.

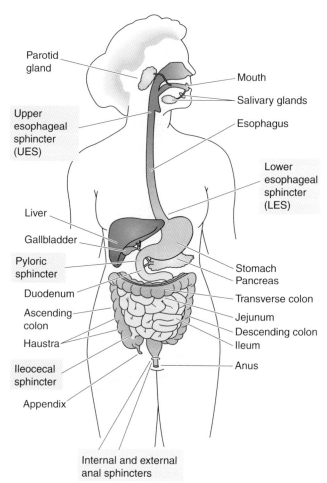

Figure 41.1 Major components of the human digestive system.

Ingestion of food initiates multiple endocrine, neural, and paracrine responses

Digestion of food involves multiple secretory, enzymatic, and motor processes that are closely coordinated with one another. The necessary control is achieved by neural and hormonal processes that are initiated by dietary food substances; the result is a coordinated series of motor and secretory responses.

Endocrine, neural, and paracrine mechanisms all contribute to digestion. All three include sensor and transmitter processes. An **endocrine** mechanism involves the release of a transmitter (e.g., peptide) into the blood.

A **neural** mechanism involves the activation of nerves and neurotransmitters that influence either secretory or motor activity.

The third mechanism of neurohumoral control is **paracrine.** In this mechanism, a transmitter is released from a sensor cell, and it affects adjacent cells without either entering the blood or activating neurons.

In addition to the primary response that leads to the release of one or more digestive enzymes, other signals terminate these secretory responses. Enteric neurons are important throughout the initiation and termination of the responses.

In addition to its function in nutrition, the GI tract plays important roles in excretion, fluid and electrolyte balance, and immunity

Although its primary roles are digesting and absorbing nutrients, the GI tract also excretes **waste material.** Fecal material includes nondigested/nonabsorbed dietary food products, colonic bacteria and their metabolic products, and several excretory products.

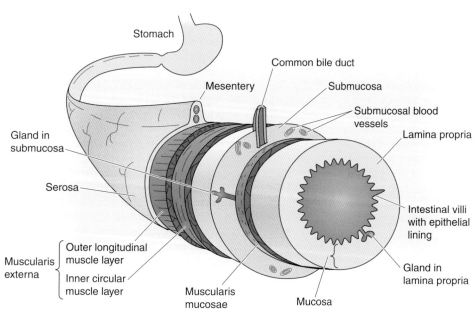

Figure 41.2 Wall of the GI tract, as exemplified by the wall of a segment of the duodenum.

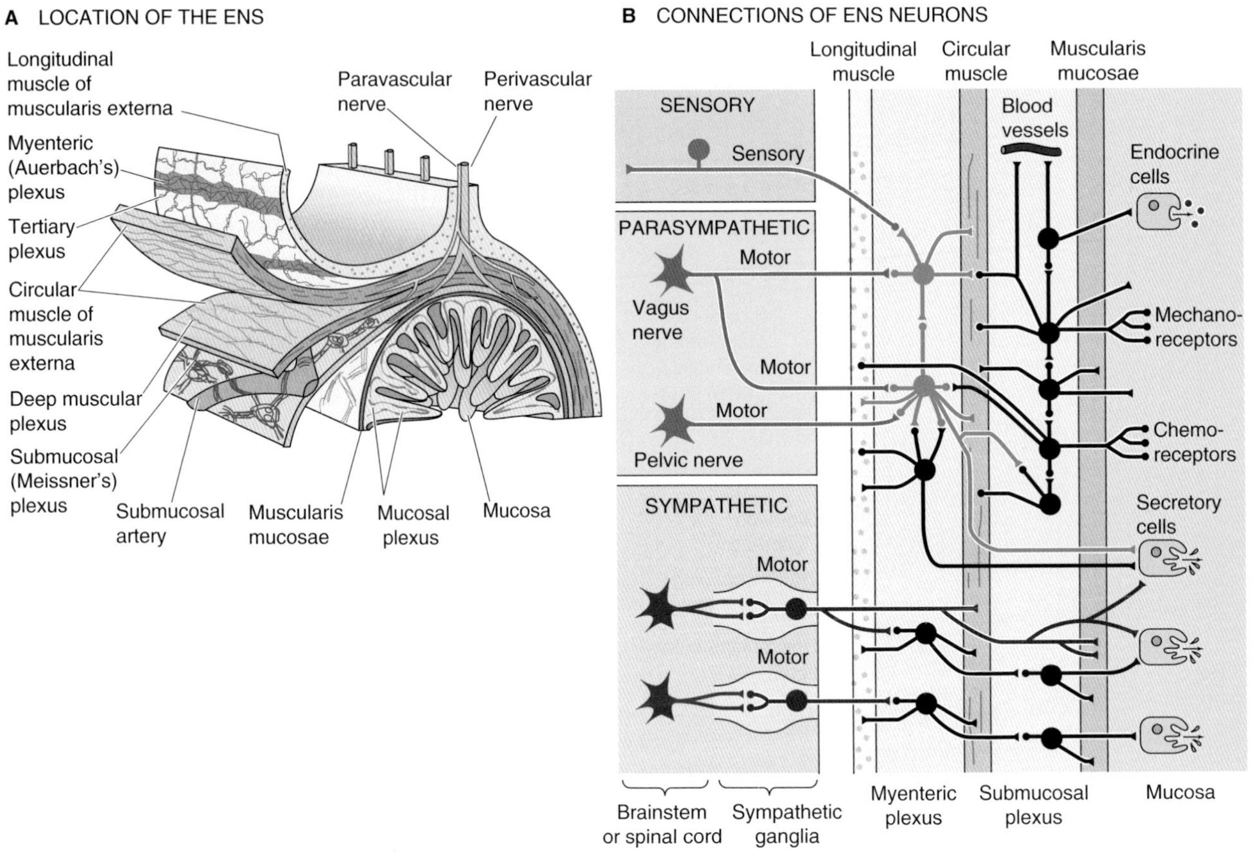

A LOCATION OF THE ENS

B CONNECTIONS OF ENS NEURONS

Figure 41.3 Schematic representation of the typical circuitry of the ENS.

The small intestine is presented with 8 to 9 L/day of fluid, an amount that includes ~1 L/day that the intestine itself secretes. Almost all this water is reabsorbed in the small and large intestine; therefore, stool has relatively small amounts of water (~0.1 L/day).

The GI tract also contributes to **immune function.** The mucosal immune system, or **gut-associated lymphoid tissue (GALT),** consists of both organized aggregates of lymphoid tissue and diffuse populations of immune cells. These immune cells include lymphocytes that reside between the epithelial cells lining the gut, as well as lymphocytes and mast cells in the lamina propria. GALT has two primary functions: (1) to protect against potential microbial pathogens, including bacteria, protozoans, and viruses; and (2) to permit immunological *tolerance* to both the potentially immunogenic dietary substances and the bacteria that normally reside primarily in the lumen of the large intestine.

The mucosal immune system is important because the GI tract has the largest area of the body in potential direct contact with infectious, toxic, and immunogenic material. Approximately 80% of the immunoglobulin-producing cells are found in the small intestine.

REGULATION OF GASTROINTESTINAL FUNCTION

The ENS is a "minibrain" with sensory neurons, interneurons, and motor neurons

⊙ **41-1** The **enteric nervous system (ENS)** is the primary neural mechanism that controls GI function and is one of

the three divisions of the autonomic nervous system (ANS), along with the sympathetic and parasympathetic divisions. One indication of the importance of the ENS is the number of neurons consigned to it. The ENS consists of >100 million neurons, roughly the number in the spinal cord or in the rest of the entire ANS. The ENS is located solely within GI tissue, but it can be modified by input from the brain. Neurons of the ENS are primarily, but not exclusively, clustered in one of two collections of neurons (Fig. 41.3A): the submucosal plexus and the myenteric plexus. The **submucosal (or Meissner's) plexus** is found in the submucosa only in the small and large intestine. The **myenteric (or Auerbach's) plexus** is located between the circular and longitudinal muscle layers throughout the GI tract from the proximal end of the esophagus to the rectum.

The ENS is a complete reflex circuit and can operate totally within the GI tract, without the participation of either the spinal cord or the cephalic brain. As with other neurons, the activity of the ENS is the result of the generation of action potentials by single neurons and the release of chemical neurotransmitters that affect either other neurons or effector cells (i.e., epithelial or muscle cells). The ENS consists of sensory circuits, interneuronal connections, and secretomotor neurons (Fig. 41.3B). Sensory (or **afferent**) neurons monitor changes in luminal activity, including distention (i.e., smooth-muscle tension), chemistry (e.g., pH, osmolality, levels of specific nutrients), and mechanical stimulation. These sensory neurons activate **interneurons,** which relay signals that activate **efferent** secretomotor neurons that in turn stimulate or inhibit a wide range of effector cells:

smooth-muscle cells, epithelial cells that secrete or absorb fluid and electrolytes, submucosal blood vessels, and enteric endocrine cells.

The largely independent function of the ENS has given rise to the concept of a GI "minibrain." Because the efferent responses to several different stimuli are often quite similar, a generalized concept has developed that the ENS possesses multiple preprogrammed responses. Efferent responses controlled by the ENS may also be modified by input from autonomic ganglia, which are in turn under the influence of the spinal cord and brain. In addition, the ENS receives input directly from the brain via parasympathetic nerves (i.e., the vagus nerve).

Acetylcholine, peptides, and bioactive amines are the ENS neurotransmitters that regulate epithelial and motor function

Acetylcholine (ACh) is the primary preganglionic and postganglionic neurotransmitter regulating both secretory function and smooth-muscle activity in the GI tract. In addition, many other neurotransmitters are present in enteric neurons. Among the peptides, **vasoactive intestinal peptide (VIP)** has an important role in both inhibition of intestinal smooth muscle and stimulation of intestinal fluid and electrolyte secretion. Also playing an important role in GI regulation are other peptides (e.g., enkephalins, somatostatin, and substance P), amines (e.g., serotonin), and nitric oxide (NO).

The brain-gut axis is a bidirectional system that controls GI function via the ANS, GI hormones, and the immune system

Neural control of the GI tract is a function of not only intrinsic nerves (i.e., the ENS) but also nerves that are extrinsic to the GI tract. These extrinsic pathways are composed of elements of both the parasympathetic and, to a lesser extent, the sympathetic nervous system and are under the control of autonomic centers in the brainstem.

Parasympathetic innervation of the GI tract from the pharynx to the distal colon is through the vagus nerve; the distal third of the colon receives its parasympathetic innervation from the pelvic nerves. The preganglionic fibers of the parasympathetic nerves use ACh as their neurotransmitter and synapse on some neurons of the ENS (Fig. 41.3B). These ENS neurons are thus postganglionic parasympathetic fibers, and their cell bodies are, in a sense, the parasympathetic ganglion. These postganglionic parasympathetic fibers use mainly ACh as their neurotransmitter. Parasympathetic stimulation increases secretion and motility. The parasympathetic nerves also contain afferent fibers that carry information to autonomic centers in the medulla from chemoreceptors, osmoreceptors, and mechanoreceptors in the mucosa. The loop that is initiated by these afferents, and completed by the aforementioned parasympathetic efferents, is known as a **vagovagal reflex.**

The postganglionic **sympathetic** fibers either synapse in the ENS or directly innervate effector cells (Fig. 41.3B).

Table 41.1 summarizes peptide hormones made by the GI tract as well as their major actions.

In addition to the "hard-wired" communications involved in sensory input and motor output, communication via the gut-brain axis also requires significant participation of the **immune system.** Neuroimmune regulation of both epithelial and motor function in the small and large intestine primarily involves **mast cells** in the lamina propria of the intestine. Chemical mediators released by mast cells (e.g., histamine) directly affect both intestinal smooth-muscle cells and epithelial cells.

In conclusion, three parallel components of the gut-brain axis—the ENS, GI hormones, and the immune system—control GI function, an arrangement that provides substantial redundancy. Such redundancy permits fine-tuning of the regulation of digestive processes and provides "backup" or "fail-safe" mechanisms that ensure the integrity of GI function, especially at times of impaired function (i.e., during disease).

GASTROINTESTINAL MOTILITY

Tonic and rhythmic contractions of smooth muscle are responsible for churning, peristalsis, and reservoir action

The motor activity of the GI tract performs three primary functions. First, it produces segmental contractions that are associated with nonpropulsive movement of the luminal contents. The result is the increased mixing—or **churning**—that enhances the digestion and absorption of dietary nutrients. Second, GI motor activity produces **peristalsis**, a progressive wave of relaxation followed by contraction. The result is **propulsion,** or the propagated movement of food and its digestive products in a caudal direction. Third, motor activity allows some hollow organs—particularly the stomach and large intestine—to hold the luminal content, exerting a **reservoir function.** This reservoir function is made possible by **sphincters** that separate the organs of the GI tract. All these functions are primarily accomplished by the coordinated activity of **smooth muscle.**

The electrical and mechanical properties of intestinal smooth muscle needed for these functions include both tonic (i.e., sustained) contractions and rhythmic contractions (i.e., alternating contraction and relaxation) of individual muscle cells. The intrinsic rhythmic contractility is a function of the membrane voltage (V_m) of the smooth-muscle cell. V_m can either oscillate in a subthreshold range at a low frequency (several cycles per minute), referred to as **slow-wave activity,** or reach a threshold for initiating a true **action potential.** The integrated effect of the slow waves and action potentials determines the smooth-muscle activity of the GI tract.

These activities are regulated, in large part, by both neural and hormonal stimuli. Both excitatory and inhibitory neurotransmitters can modulate smooth-muscle contractility. In general, ACh is the predominant neurotransmitter of *excitatory* motor neurons, whereas VIP and NO are the neurotransmitters of *inhibitory* motor neurons.

An additional, unique factor in the aforementioned regulatory control is that luminal food and digestive products activate mucosal chemoreceptors and mechanoreceptors, thus inducing hormone release or stimulating the ENS and controlling smooth-muscle function.

TABLE 41.1 GI Peptide Hormones

HORMONE	SOURCE	TARGET	ACTION
Cholecystokinin	I cells in duodenum and jejunum and neurons in ileum and colon	Pancreas	↑ Enzyme secretion
		Gall bladder	↑ Contraction
Gastric inhibitory peptide	K cells in duodenum and jejunum	Pancreas	Exocrine: ↓ fluid absorption Endocrine: ↑ insulin release
Gastrin	G cells, antrum of stomach	Parietal cells in body of stomach	↑ H⁺ secretion
Gastrin-releasing peptide	Vagal nerve endings	G cells in antrum of stomach	↑ Gastrin release
Guanylin	Ileum and colon	Small and large intestine	↑ Fluid absorption
Motilin	Endocrine cells in upper GI tract	Esophageal sphincter Stomach Duodenum	↑ Smooth-muscle contraction
Neurotensin	Endocrine cells, widespread in GI tract	Intestinal smooth muscle	Vasoactive stimulation of histamine release
Peptide YY	Endocrine cells in ileum and colon	Stomach	↓ Vagally mediated acid secretion
		Pancreas	↓ Enzyme and fluid secretion
Secretin	S cells in small intestine	Pancreas	↑ HCO_3^- and fluid secretion by pancreatic ducts
		Stomach	↓ Gastric acid secretion
Somatostatin	D cells of stomach and duodenum, δ cells of pancreatic islets	Stomach	↓ Gastrin release
		Intestine	↑ Fluid absorption/↓ secretion ↑ Smooth-muscle contraction
		Pancreas	↓ Endocrine/exocrine secretions
		Liver	↓ Bile flow
Substance P	Enteric neurons	Enteric neurons	Neurotransmitter
VIP	ENS neurons	Small intestine	↑ Smooth-muscle relaxation ↑ Secretion by small intestine
		Pancreas	↑ Secretion by pancreas

Segments of the GI tract have both longitudinal and circular arrays of muscles and are separated by sphincters that consist of specialized circular muscles

The muscle layers of the GI tract consist almost entirely of smooth muscle. Exceptions are the striated muscle of (1) the upper esophageal sphincter (UES), which separates the hypopharynx from the esophagus; (2) the upper third of the esophagus; and (3) the external anal sphincter. As shown above in Fig. 41.2, the two smooth-muscle layers are arranged as an inner circular layer and an outer longitudinal layer. The myenteric ganglia of the ENS are located between the two muscle layers.

The segments of the GI tract through which food products pass are hollow, low-pressure organs that are separated by specialized circular muscles or **sphincters.** These sphincters function as barriers to flow by maintaining a positive **resting pressure** that serves to separate the two adjacent organs, in which lower pressures prevail. Sphincters thus regulate both antegrade (forward) and retrograde (reverse) movement. As a general rule, stimuli proximal to a sphincter cause sphincteric relaxation, whereas stimuli distal to a sphincter induce sphincteric contraction. Changes in sphincter pressure are

coordinated with the smooth-muscle contractions in the organs on either side. This coordination depends on both the intrinsic properties of sphincteric smooth muscle and neurohumoral stimuli.

Location of a sphincter determines its function

Six sphincters are present in the GI tract (Fig. 41.1), each with a different resting pressure and different response to various stimuli. An additional sphincter, the sphincter of Oddi, regulates movement of the contents of the common bile duct and pancreatic duct into the duodenum.

Upper Esophageal Sphincter Separating the pharynx and the upper part of the esophagus is the **UES**, which consists of striated muscle and has the highest resting pressure of all the GI sphincters. The swallowing mechanism (i.e., deglutition), which involves the oropharynx and the UES, is largely under the control of the **swallowing center** in the medulla. Respiration and deglutition are closely integrated.

The UES is closed during inspiration, thereby diverting atmospheric air to the glottis and away from the esophagus. During swallowing, the situation reverses, with closure of the

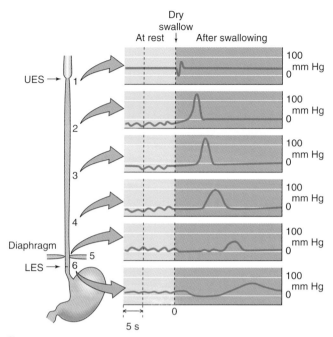

Dry
swallow
At rest ↓ After swallowing

UES → 1

2

3

4

Diaphragm
5
LES → 6

5 s

0

Figure 41.4 Esophageal intraluminal pressures at different points along the esophagus during swallowing. (Data from Conklin JL, Christensen J: Motor functions of the pharynx and esophagus. In Johnson LR [ed]: Physiology of the Gastrointestinal Tract, 3rd ed. New York, Lippincott-Raven, 1994, pp 903–928.)

glottis and inhibition of respiration, but with relaxation of the UES (Fig. 41.4). These changes permit the entry of food contents into the esophagus and not into the airways of the respiratory tract.

Lower Esophageal Sphincter The esophagus is separated from the stomach by the lower esophageal sphincter (**LES**). The primary functions of the LES are (1) to permit coordinated movement of ingested food into the stomach from the esophagus after swallowing or deglutition, and (2) to prevent reflux of gastric contents into the esophagus.

Swallowing and the function of the UES and LES are closely integrated into the function of the esophagus. Under normal circumstances, esophageal muscle contractions are almost exclusively peristaltic and are initiated by swallowing. Deglutition initiates relaxation of the UES and propagated contractions, first of the UES and then of the muscles along the esophagus (Fig. 41.4). In the meantime, the LES has already relaxed. The result of the advancing peristaltic wave is the caudad propulsion of a bolus toward the stomach.

Distention of the esophagus (in the absence of swallowing) also initiates propulsive esophageal contractions distal to the site of distention, as well as relaxation of the LES. Reflux of gastric contents into the lower part of the esophagus also produces such a local distention, without a swallow, and elicits the same response: peristaltic contractions that clear the esophagus of refluxed gastric material. Peristalsis that is initiated by swallowing is called **primary peristalsis,** whereas that elicited by distention of the esophagus is referred to as **secondary peristalsis.**

Pyloric Sphincter The pylorus is the sphincter that separates the stomach from the duodenum. The pressure of the pyloric sphincter regulates, in part, gastric emptying and prevents duodenal-gastric reflux. However, although a specific pyloric sphincter is present, it is quite short and is a relatively

poor barrier (i.e., it can resist only a small pressure gradient).

Ileocecal Sphincter The valve-like structure that separates the ileum and cecum is called the **ileocecal sphincter.** Similar to other GI sphincters, the ileocecal sphincter maintains a positive resting pressure and is under the control of the vagus nerve, sympathetic nerves, and the ENS. Distention of the ileum results in relaxation of the sphincter, whereas distention of the proximal (ascending) colon causes contraction of the ileocecal sphincter. As a consequence, ileal flow into the colon is regulated by luminal contents and pressure, both proximal and distal to the ileocecal sphincter.

Internal and External Anal Sphincters The "anal sphincter" actually consists of both an internal and an external sphincter. The **internal anal sphincter** has both circular and longitudinal smooth muscle and is under involuntary control. The **external anal sphincter,** which encircles the rectum, contains only striated muscle but is controlled by both voluntary and involuntary mechanisms. The high resting pressure of the overall anal sphincter predominantly reflects the resting tone of the *internal* anal sphincter. Distention of the rectum by colonic contents (i.e., stool), initiates the **rectosphincteric reflex** by relaxing the internal sphincter. If defecation is not desired, continence is maintained by an involuntary reflex that contracts the external anal sphincter. If defecation is desired, a series of both voluntary and involuntary events occurs that includes relaxation of the external anal sphincter, contraction of abdominal wall muscles, and relaxation of pelvic wall muscles. In contrast, if a delay in defecation is needed or desired, voluntary contraction of the external anal sphincter is usually sufficient to override the series of reflexes initiated by rectal distention.

Motility of the small intestine achieves both churning and propulsive movement

The two classes of small-intestinal motor activity are churning (or mixing) and propulsion of the bolus of luminal contents. **Churning**—which is accomplished by segmental, nonpropulsive contractions—mixes the luminal contents with pancreatic, biliary, and small-intestinal secretions, thus enhancing the digestion of dietary nutrients in the lumen. Churning or mixing movements are the result of contractions of *circular* muscle in segments flanked at either end by receiving segments that relax. Churning does not advance the luminal contents along the small intestine. In contrast, **propulsion**—which is accomplished by propagated, peristaltic contractions—results in caudad movement of the intestinal luminal contents. Peristaltic propulsion occurs as a result of contraction of the *circular* muscle and relaxation of the *longitudinal* muscle in the propulsive or upstream segment, together with relaxation of the *circular* muscle and contraction of the *longitudinal* muscle in the downstream receiving segment. Thus, circular smooth muscle in the small intestine participates in both churning and propulsion.

In the **fasting state,** the small intestine is relatively quiescent but exhibits synchronized, rhythmic changes in both electrical and motor activity (Fig. 41.5). The interdigestive myoelectric or **migrating motor complex (MMC)** is the term used to describe these rhythmic contractions of the small intestine that are observed in the fasting state. MMCs in humans occur at intervals of 90 to 120 minutes and consist of four distinct phases: (1) a prolonged quiescent period,

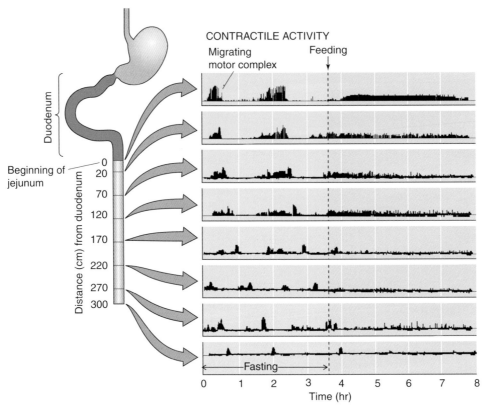

Figure 41.5   Records of intraluminal pressure along the intestine in the fasting and fed states. (Data from Itoh Z, Sekiguchi T: Interdigestive motor activity in health and disease. Scand J Gastroenterol Suppl 82:121–134, 1983.)

(2) a period of increasing action potential frequency and contractility, (3) a period of peak electrical and mechanical activity that lasts a few minutes, and (4) a period of declining activity that merges into the next quiescent period. The slow propulsive contractions that characterize phases 2 to 4 of the MMCs clear the small intestine of its residual content, including undigested food, bacteria, desquamated cells, and intestinal and pancreatic biliary secretions. MMCs usually originate in the stomach and often travel to the distal end of the ileum, but ~25% are initiated in the duodenum and proximal part of the jejunum.

Feeding terminates MMCs and initiates the appearance of the fed motor pattern (Fig. 41.5).

A major determinant of the MMC pattern is the hormone **motilin,** a 22–amino-acid peptide that is synthesized in the duodenal mucosa and released just before the initiation of phase 3 of the MMC cycle.

Motility of the large intestine achieves both propulsive movement and a reservoir function

The human large intestine has four primary functions. First, the colon absorbs large quantities of fluid and electrolytes and converts the liquid content of ileocecal material to solid or semisolid stool. Second, the colon avidly absorbs the short-chain fatty acids (SCFAs) formed by the catabolism (or fermentation) of dietary carbohydrates that are not absorbed in the small intestine. The abundant colonic microflora accomplish this fermentation. Third, the storage of colonic content represents a reservoir function of the large intestine. Fourth, the colon eliminates its contents in a regulated and controlled fashion, largely under voluntary

control. To accomplish these important activities, the large intestine functionally acts as two distinct organs. The proximal (or ascending and transverse) part of the colon is the site where most of the fluid and electrolyte absorption occurs and where bacterial fermentation takes place. The distal (or descending and rectosigmoid) portion of the colon provides final desiccation, as well as reservoir function, and serves as a storage organ for colonic material before defecation.

Similarly to small-intestinal motor activity, colonic contractions are regulated by myogenic, neurogenic, and hormonal factors.

The **proximal colon** has two types of motor activity, nonpropulsive segmentation and mass peristalsis. **Nonpropulsive "segmentation"** is generated by slow-wave activity that produces circular-muscle contractions that churn the colonic contents and move them in an orad direction (i.e., toward the cecum). The segmental contractions that produce the churning give the colon its typical appearance of segments or haustra (Fig. 41.1). One to three times a day, a so-called **mass peristalsis** occurs in which a portion of the colonic contents is propelled distally 20 cm or more. Such mass peristaltic contractions are the primary form of propulsive motility in the colon and may be initiated by eating.

In the **distal colon,** the primary motor activity is nonpropulsive segmentation that is produced by annular or segmental contractions. It is also here that these contents are stored before an occasional mass peristalsis that propels them into the rectum. The **rectum** itself is kept nearly empty by nonpropulsive segmentation until it is filled by mass peristalsis of the distal end of the colon. Filling of the rectum triggers a series of reflexes in the internal and external anal sphincters that lead to defecation.

CHAPTER 42

GASTRIC FUNCTION

Henry J. Binder

The stomach plays several important roles in human nutrition and has secretory, motor, and humoral functions. These activities are not separate and distinct, but rather represent integrated functions that are required to initiate the normal digestive process.

The stomach has several specific **secretory** products. In addition to acid, these products include pepsinogen, mucus, bicarbonate, intrinsic factor, and water. The stomach also has several important **motor** functions that regulate the intake of food, its mixing with gastric secretions and reduction in particle size, and the exit of partially digested material into the duodenum. Moreover, the stomach produces important **humoral agents**—gastrin, histamine, and somatostatin—that have both endocrine and paracrine actions. These agents are primarily important in the regulation of gastric secretion.

FUNCTIONAL ANATOMY OF THE STOMACH

The mucosa is composed of surface epithelial cells and glands

The wall of the stomach consists of both mucosal and muscle layers. The stomach can be divided, based on its gross anatomy, into three major segments (Fig. 42.1): (1) A specialized portion of the stomach called the **cardia** is located just distal to the gastroesophageal junction and is devoid of the acid-secreting parietal cells. (2) The body or corpus is the largest portion of the stomach; its most proximal region is called the fundus. (3) The distal portion of the stomach is called the antrum. The surface area of the gastric mucosa is substantially increased by the presence of gastric glands, which consist of a pit, a neck, and a base. These glands contain several cell types, including mucous, parietal, chief, and endocrine cells. The surface epithelial cells, which have their own distinct structure and function, secrete HCO_3^- and mucus.

Marked cellular heterogeneity exists not only *within* segments (e.g., glands versus surface epithelial cells) but also *between* segments of the stomach.

The proximal portion of the stomach secretes acid, pepsinogens, intrinsic factor, bicarbonate, and mucus, whereas the distal part releases gastrin and somatostatin

Corpus The primary secretory products of the proximal part of the stomach—acid (protons), pepsinogens, and intrinsic factor—are made by distinct cells in glands of the corpus. The two primary cell types in the gastric glands of the body of the stomach are parietal cells and chief cells.

Parietal cells (or oxyntic cells) secrete both acid and intrinsic factor, a glycoprotein that is required for cobalamin (vitamin B_{12}) absorption in the ileum.

Chief cells (or peptic cells) secrete pepsinogens, but not acid.

Glands from the corpus of the stomach also contain **mucus-secreting cells,** which are confined to the neck of the gland (Fig. 42.1), and five or six **endocrine cells.** Among these endocrine cells are **enterochromaffin-like (ECL) cells,** which release histamine.

Antrum The glands in the antrum of the stomach do not contain parietal cells. Therefore, the antrum does not secrete either acid or intrinsic factor. Glands in the antral mucosa contain **chief cells** and **endocrine cells;** the endocrine cells include the so-called **G cells** and **D cells,** which secrete gastrin and somatostatin, respectively (see Table 41.1).

The stomach accommodates food, mixes it with gastric secretions, grinds it, and empties the chyme into the duodenum

In addition to its secretory properties, the stomach also has multiple motor functions. These functions are the result of gastric smooth-muscle activity, which is integrated by both neural and hormonal signals. Gastric motor functions include both propulsive and retrograde movement of food and liquid, as well as a nonpropulsive movement that increases intragastric pressure.

At least four events can be identified in the overall process of gastric filling and emptying: (1) receiving and providing temporary storage of dietary food and liquids; (2) mixing food and water with gastric secretory products, including pepsin and acid; (3) grinding food so that particle size is reduced to enhance digestion and to permit passage through the pylorus; and (4) regulating the exit of retained material from the stomach into the duodenum (i.e., gastric emptying of chyme) in response to various stimuli.

The mechanisms by which the stomach receives and empties liquids and solids are significantly different. Emptying of *liquids* is primarily a function of the smooth muscle of the *proximal* part of the stomach, whereas emptying of *solids* is regulated by *antral* smooth muscle.

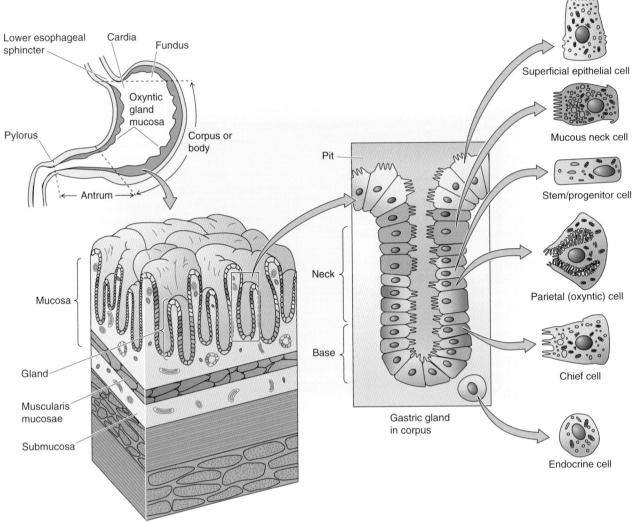

Figure 42.1 Anatomy of the stomach.

ACID SECRETION

The parietal cell has a specialized tubulovesicular structure that increases apical membrane area when the cell is stimulated to secrete acid

In the basal state, the rate of acid secretion is low. Tubulovesicular membranes are present in the apical portion of the resting, nonstimulated parietal cell and contain the H-K pump (or H,K-ATPase) that is responsible for acid secretion. Upon stimulation, cytoskeletal rearrangement causes the tubulovesicular membranes that contain the H-K pump to fuse into the canalicular membrane (Fig. 42.2). The result is a substantial increase (50- to 100-fold) in the surface area of the apical membrane of the parietal cell, as well as the appearance of microvilli. This fusion is accompanied by insertion of the H-K pumps, as well as K^+ and Cl^- channels, into the canalicular membrane.

An H-K pump is responsible for gastric acid secretion by parietal cells

The parietal-cell H-K pump is a member of the gene family of P-type ATPases (see ◉ 5-9).

A RESTING   **B** STIMULATED

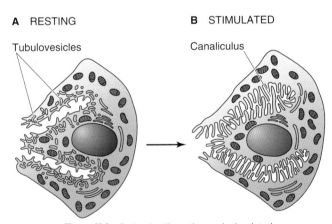

Figure 42.2 Parietal cell: resting and stimulated.

Omeprazole is a potent inhibitor of parietal-cell H-K pump activity and is an extremely effective drug in the control of gastric acid secretion in both normal subjects and patients with hypersecretory states.

The key step in gastric acid secretion is extrusion of H^+ into the lumen of the gastric gland in exchange for K^+

(Fig. 42.3). The K^+ taken up into the parietal cells is recycled to the lumen through K^+ channels. The final component of the process is passive movement of Cl^- into the gland lumen. The net result is the secretion of HCl. Secretion of acid across the apical membrane by the H-K pump results in a rise in parietal-cell pH. The adaptive response to this rise in pH includes passive uptake of CO_2 and H_2O, which the enzyme **carbonic anhydrase (CA)** converts to HCO_3^- and H^+. The H^+ is the substrate of the H-K pump. The HCO_3^- exits across the basolateral membrane via a Cl-HCO_3 exchanger (AE2), which also provides some of the Cl^- required for net HCl movement across the apical/canalicular membrane.

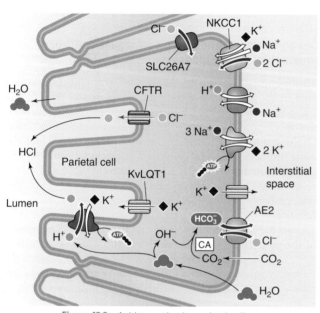

Figure 42.3   Acid secretion by parietal cells.

Three secretagogues (acetylcholine, gastrin, and histamine) directly and indirectly induce acid secretion by parietal cells

The action of secretagogues on gastric acid secretion occurs via at least two parallel and perhaps redundant mechanisms (Fig. 42.4). In the first, acetylcholine (ACh), gastrin, and histamine bind **directly** to their respective receptors on the parietal-cell membrane and synergistically stimulate acid secretion. ACh (see Fig. 14.5) is released from endings of the vagus nerve (cranial nerve X), and gastrin is released from G cells. Histamine (see Fig. 13.6B) is synthesized from histidine in ECL cells of the lamina propria. In the second mechanism, ACh and gastrin **indirectly** induce acid secretion as a result of their stimulation of histamine release from ECL cells.

The three acid secretagogues act through either Ca^{2+}/diacylglycerol or cAMP

Stimulation of acid secretion by ACh, gastrin, and histamine is mediated by a series of intracellular signal-transduction processes similar to those responsible for the action of other agonists in other cell systems. All three secretagogues bind to specific G protein–coupled receptors on the parietal-cell membrane (Fig. 42.5).

Antral and duodenal G cells release gastrin, whereas ECL cells in the corpus release histamine

○ **42-1** Gastrin has three major effects on GI cells: (1) stimulation of acid secretion by parietal cells (Fig. 42.4), (2) release of histamine by ECL cells, and (3) regulation of mucosal growth in the corpus of the stomach, as well as in the small and large intestine.

Gastrin exists in several different forms, but the two major forms are G-17, or "little gastrin," a 17–amino-acid linear peptide, and G-34, or "big gastrin," a 34–amino-acid

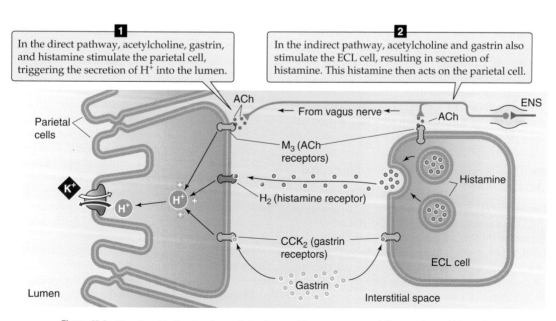

1 In the direct pathway, acetylcholine, gastrin, and histamine stimulate the parietal cell, triggering the secretion of H^+ into the lumen.

2 In the indirect pathway, acetylcholine and gastrin also stimulate the ECL cell, resulting in secretion of histamine. This histamine then acts on the parietal cell.

Figure 42.4   Direct and indirect actions of the three acid secretagogues: ACh, gastrin, and histamine.

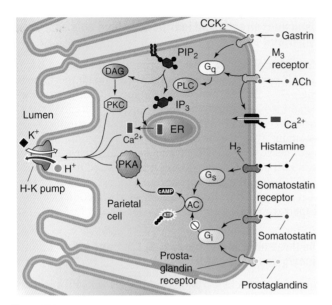

Figure 42.5 Receptors and signal-transduction pathways in the parietal cell. *AC,* Adenylyl cyclase; *DAG,* diacylglycerol; *ER,* endoplasmic reticulum; *PIP₂,* phosphatidylinositol 4,5-bisphosphate; *PKA,* protein kinase A; *PKC,* protein kinase C; *PLC,* phospholipase C.

peptide. Gastrin and **cholecystokinin (CCK),** a related hormone, have identical C-terminal tetrapeptide sequences that possess all the biological activities of both gastrin and CCK.

Specialized endocrine cells in both the antrum and duodenum make each of the two gastrins. **Antral G cells** are the primary source of G-17, whereas **duodenal G cells** are the primary source of G-34. Antral G cells have microvilli on their apical membrane surface and are referred to as an *open-type* endocrine cell. These G cells release gastrin in response to luminal peptides and amino acids, as well as in response to **gastrin-releasing peptide (GRP),** a 27–amino-acid peptide that is released by vagal nerve endings. As discussed below, gastrin release is inhibited by somatostatin, which is released from adjacent D cells.

ECL cells in the **corpus** of the stomach synthesize histamine. The central role of histamine and ECL cells is consistent with the observation that H₂ receptor antagonists (i.e., H₂ blockers), such as cimetidine and ranitidine, not only block the direct action of histamine on parietal cells but also substantially inhibit the acid secretion stimulated by ACh and gastrin (which activate ECL cells). The effectiveness of H₂ blockers in controlling acid secretion after stimulation by most agonists is well established in humans.

⊙ 42-2 Gastric D cells release somatostatin, the central inhibitor of acid secretion

Gastric acid secretion is under close control of not only the stimulatory pathways discussed above but also the inhibitory pathways. The major inhibitory pathway involves the release of **somatostatin,** a polypeptide hormone made by D cells in the antrum and corpus of the stomach. Somatostatin is also made by the δ cells of the pancreatic islets (see ⊙ 51-13) and by neurons in the hypothalamus (see ⊙ 48-6).

Somatostatin inhibits gastric acid secretion by both direct and indirect mechanisms (Fig. 42.6). In the **direct pathway,**

somatostatin binds to a receptor on the basolateral membrane of the parietal cell and antagonizes the stimulatory effect of histamine and thus inhibits gastric acid secretion by parietal cells. The source of this somatostatin can be either *paracrine* (i.e., D cells present in the corpus of the stomach, near the parietal cells) or *endocrine* (i.e., D cells in the antrum).

Somatostatin also acts via two **indirect pathways.** In the corpus of the stomach, D cells release somatostatin, which inhibits the release of *histamine* from ECL cells (Fig. 42.6). Because histamine is an acid secretagogue, somatostatin thus reduces gastric acid secretion. In the antrum of the stomach, D cells release somatostatin, which inhibits the release of *gastrin* from G cells. Because gastrin is another acid secretagogue, somatostatin also reduces gastric acid secretion by this route. The gastrin released by the G cell feeds back on itself by stimulating D cells to release the inhibitory somatostatin.

Several enteric hormones ("enterogastrone") and prostaglandins inhibit gastric acid secretion

Multiple processes in the duodenum and jejunum participate in the negative-feedback mechanisms that inhibit gastric acid secretion. Fat, acid, and hyperosmolar solutions in the duodenum are potent inhibitors of gastric acid secretion. Of these inhibitors, lipids are the most potent, but acid is also quite important. Several candidate hormones have been suggested as mediators of this acid inhibition (Table 42.1).

Prostaglandin E₂ (PGE₂) inhibits parietal-cell acid secretion, probably by inhibiting histamine's activation of parietal-cell function at a site that is distal to the histamine receptor. PGE₂ appears to bind to an EP₃ receptor on the basolateral membrane of the parietal cell (see Fig. 42.5) and stimulates G^{αi} which, in turn, inhibits adenylyl cyclase. In addition, prostaglandins also indirectly inhibit gastric acid secretion by reducing histamine release from ECL cells and gastrin release from antral G cells.

⊙ 42-3 A meal triggers three phases of acid secretion

Basal State The rate of acid secretion between meals (i.e., during the interdigestive phase) is low. This interdigestive period, however, follows a circadian rhythm; acid secretion is lowest in the morning before awakening and is highest in the evening. Acid secretion is a direct function of the number of parietal cells, which is also influenced, at least in part, by body weight. Thus, men have higher rates of basal acid secretion than do women. Considerable variability in basal acid secretion is also seen among normal individuals, and the resting intragastric pH can range from 3 to 7.

Acid secretion is enhanced several-fold by eating (Fig. 42.7). However, the time course of intragastric pH after a meal can vary considerably despite stimulation of acid secretion. The reason is that intragastric pH depends not only on gastric acid secretion but also on the buffering power of food and the rate of gastric emptying of both acid and partially digested material into the duodenum.

Regulation of acid secretion during a meal can be best characterized as including three separate but interrelated phases: the *cephalic,* the *gastric,* and the *intestinal* phases.

Cephalic Phase ⊙ 42-4 The smell, sight, taste, thought, and swallowing of food initiate the cephalic phase, which is primarily mediated by the vagus nerve (Fig. 42.6). Stimulation

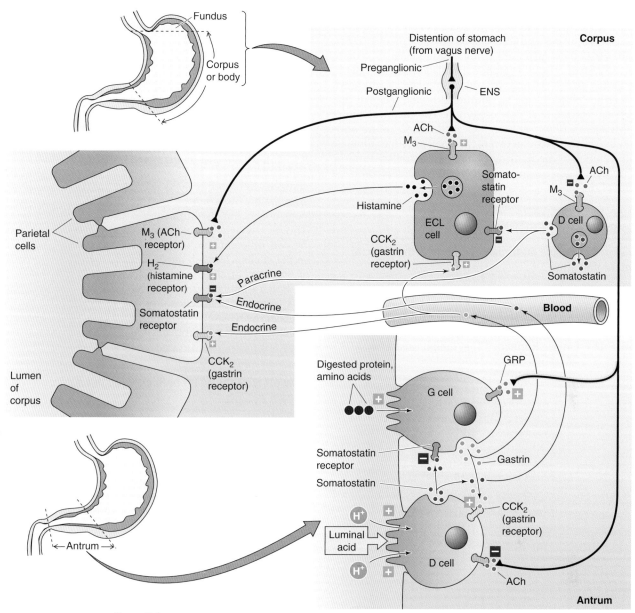

Figure 42.6 Regulation of gastric acid secretion in the corpus and the antrum of the stomach.

of the vagus nerve results in four distinct physiological events that together result in enhanced gastric acid secretion. First, in the body of the stomach, vagal postganglionic nerves release ACh, which stimulates parietal-cell H^+ secretion directly. Second, in the lamina propria of the body of the stomach, the ACh released from vagal endings triggers histamine release from ECL cells, which stimulates acid secretion. Third, in the antrum, *peptidergic* postganglionic parasympathetic vagal neurons, as well as other enteric nervous system (ENS) neurons, release GRP, which induces gastrin release from antral G cells. This gastrin stimulates gastric acid secretion both directly by acting on parietal cells and indirectly by promoting histamine release from ECL cells. Fourth, in both the antrum and the corpus, the vagus nerve inhibits D cells, thereby reducing their release of somatostatin and reducing the background inhibition of gastrin release. Thus, the cephalic phase stimulates acid

secretion directly and indirectly by acting on the parietal cell. The cephalic phase accounts for *~30% of total acid secretion* and occurs before the entry of any food into the stomach.

Gastric Phase Entry of food into the stomach initiates the two primary stimuli for the gastric phase of acid secretion (Fig. 42.8). First, the food distends the gastric mucosa, which activates a vagovagal reflex as well as local ENS reflexes. Second, partially digested proteins (peptones) stimulate antral G cells.

In addition to the two stimulatory pathways acting during the gastric phase, a third pathway *inhibits* gastric acid secretion (Fig. 42.6). Low intragastric pH stimulates antral D cells to release somatostatin. Because somatostatin inhibits the release of gastrin by G cells, the net effect is a reduction in gastric acid secretion.

The gastric phase of acid secretion, which occurs primarily as a result of gastrin release, accounts for *50% to 60% of total gastric acid secretion.*

Intestinal Phase The presence of amino acids and partially digested peptides in the proximal portion of the small intestine stimulates acid secretion by three mechanisms (Fig. 42.9). First, these peptones stimulate duodenal G cells to secrete gastrin, just as peptones stimulate antral G cells in the gastric phase. Second, peptones stimulate an unknown endocrine cell to release an additional humoral signal that has been referred to as entero-oxyntin. The chemical nature of this agent has not yet been identified. Third, amino acids absorbed by the proximal part of the small intestine stimulate acid secretion by mechanisms that require further definition.

Approximately *5% to 10% of total gastric acid secretion* is a result of the intestinal phase.

PEPSINOGEN SECRETION

Chief cells secrete multiple pepsinogens that initiate protein digestion

The chief cells in gastric glands, as well as mucous cells, secrete **pepsinogens,** a group of proteolytic proenzymes (i.e., zymogens or inactive enzyme precursors). They are

TABLE 42.1 **Enteric Hormones That Inhibit Gastric H+ Secretion**

HORMONE	SOURCE
CCK	I cells of duodenum and jejunum and neurons in ileum and colon
Secretin	S cells in small intestine
VIP	ENS neurons
GIP	K cells in duodenum and jejunum
Neurotensin	Endocrine cells in ileum
Peptide YY	Endocrine cells in ileum and colon
Somatostatin	D cells of stomach and duodenum, δ cells of pancreatic islets

activated to pepsins by cleavage of an N-terminal peptide. **Pepsins** are endopeptidases that initiate the hydrolysis of ingested protein in the stomach. Pepsinogen secretion in the basal state is ~20% of its maximal secretion after stimulation.

Two groups of agonists stimulate chief cells to secrete pepsinogen. Chief cells have receptors for **secretin, VIP (vasoactive intestinal peptide),** β_2 **adrenergic** receptors, and **EP$_2$** receptors for **PGE$_2$** (see Fig. 3.9). Chief cells also have M$_3$ muscarinic receptors for **ACh,** as well as receptors for the **gastrin/CCK** family of peptides.

Of the agonists just listed, the most important for pepsinogen secretion is ACh released in response to vagal stimulation. ACh not only stimulates chief cells to release pepsinogen, but also stimulates parietal cells to secrete acid. This gastric acid produces additional pepsinogen secretion by two different mechanisms. First, in the stomach, a fall in pH elicits a local cholinergic reflex that results in further stimulation of chief cells to release pepsinogen. Thus, the ACh that stimulates chief cells can come both from the vagus and from the local reflex. Second, in the duodenum, acid triggers the release of secretin from S cells. By an endocrine effect, this secretin stimulates the chief cells to release more pepsinogen.

Low pH is required for both pepsinogen activation and pepsin activity

As mentioned above, pepsinogen is inactive and requires activation to pepsin to initiate protein digestion. This activation occurs by spontaneous cleavage of a small N-terminal peptide fragment (the activation peptide), but only at a pH that is <5.0 (Fig. 42.10).

Once pepsins are formed, their *activities* are also pH dependent. They have optimal activity at a pH between 1.8 and 3.5. Pepsin action results in the release of small peptides and amino acids (peptones) that stimulate the release of gastrin from antral G cells.

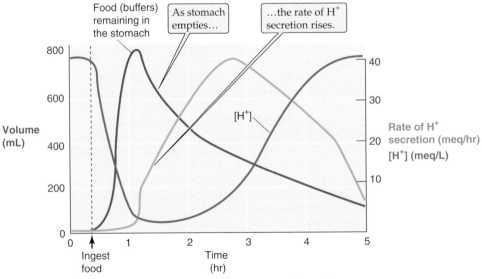

Figure 42.7   Effect of eating on acid secretion.

PROTECTION OF THE GASTRIC SURFACE EPITHELIUM AND NEUTRALIZATION OF ACID IN THE DUODENUM

At maximal rates of H$^+$ secretion, the parietal cell can drive the intraluminal pH of the stomach to 1 or less (i.e., [H$^+$] > 100 mM) for long periods. How is it that the epithelial cells are not destroyed by this acidity? Moreover, why do pepsins in the gastric lumen not digest the epithelial cells? The answer to both questions is the so-called **gastric diffusion barrier.**

The diffusion barrier, which is both physiological and anatomical, is characterized by at least two components:

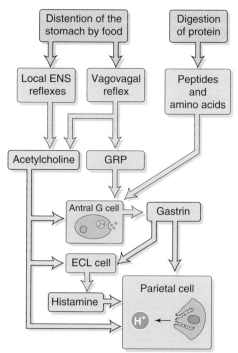

Figure 42.8 Gastric phase of gastric acid secretion.

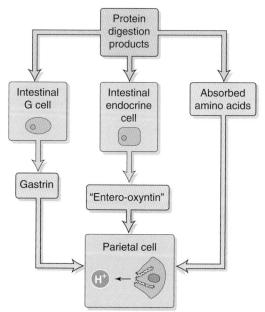

Figure 42.9 Intestinal phase of gastric acid secretion.

(1) a mucous gel layer varying in thickness between 50 and 200 μm overlying the surface epithelial cells, and (2) an HCO$_3^-$-containing microclimate adjacent to the surface epithelial cells that maintains a relatively high local pH.

Vagal stimulation and irritation stimulate gastric mucous cells to secrete mucins

⊙ **42-5** The **mucous gel layer** is largely composed of mucins, phospholipids, electrolytes, and water. Gastric **mucins** are high-molecular-weight glycoproteins that form a protective layer over the gastric mucosa.

Mucus is secreted by three different mucous cells: surface mucous cells (i.e., on the surface of the stomach), mucous neck cells (i.e., at the point where a gastric pit joins a gastric gland), and glandular mucous cells (i.e., in the gastric glands in the antrum). This mucous gel layer provides protection against injury from noxious luminal substances, including acid, pepsins, bile acids, and ethanol. Mucin also lubricates the gastric mucosa to minimize the abrasive effects of intraluminal food.

The two primary stimuli for inducing mucus secretion are vagal stimulation and physical and chemical irritation of the gastric mucosa by ingested food.

Gastric surface cells secrete HCO$_3^-$, stimulated by acetylcholine, acids, and prostaglandins

Surface epithelial cells both in the corpus and in the antrum of the stomach secrete HCO$_3^-$, which is an extremely important part of the gastric mucosal protective mechanism. The mucous gel layer provides an unstirred layer under which the secreted HCO$_3^-$ remains trapped and maintains a local pH of ~7.0 versus an intraluminal pH in the bulk phase of 1 to 3 (Fig. 42.11).

Mucus protects the gastric surface epithelium by trapping an HCO$_3^-$-rich fluid near the apical border of these cells

The paradox of how HCl secreted by the parietal cells emerges from the gland and into the gastric lumen may be explained by a process known as **viscous fingering.** Because the liquid emerging from the gastric gland is both extremely acidic and presumably under pressure, it tunnels through the mucous layer covering the opening of the gastric gland

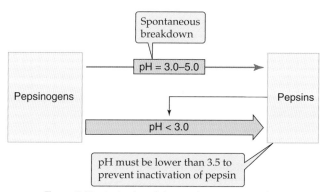

Figure 42.10 Activation of the pepsinogens to pepsins.

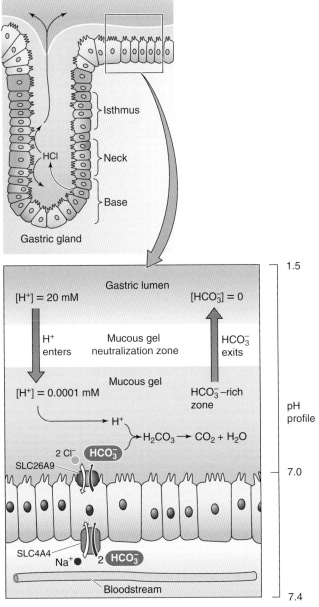

Figure 42.11 Diffusion barrier in the surface of the gastric mucosa.

from **S cells** in the duodenum. Secretin stimulates the secretion of fluid and HCO_3^- by the pancreas (see ⊙ 43-3), thus leading to intraduodenal neutralization of the acid load from the stomach. Maximal HCO_3^- secretion is a function of the amount of acid entering the duodenum, as well as the length of duodenum exposed to acid. Thus, high rates of gastric acid secretion trigger the release of large amounts of secretin, which greatly stimulates pancreatic HCO_3^- secretion, which in turn neutralizes the increased duodenal acid load.

In addition to *pancreatic* HCO_3^- secretion, the duodenal acid load resulting from gastric acid secretion is partially neutralized by *duodenal* HCO_3^- secretion. This duodenal HCO_3^- secretion occurs in the proximal—but not the distal—part of the duodenum under the influence of prostaglandins.

FILLING AND EMPTYING OF THE STOMACH

Gastric motor activity plays a role in filling, churning, and emptying

Gastric motor activity has three functions. First, relaxing of gastric smooth muscle allows the stomach to serve as a **reservoir** for ingested material. This response occurs primarily in the proximal portion of the stomach. Second, **churning** of the ingested material alters it to a form that can rapidly empty from the stomach through the pylorus. And third, the pyloric antrum, pylorus, and proximal part of the duodenum function as a single unit for **emptying** into the duodenum the modified gastric contents (chyme).

The proximal and distal regions of the stomach differ in the motor function responsible for storing, processing, and emptying liquids and solids. The proximal part of the stomach is the primary location for storage of both liquids and solids. The distal portion of the stomach is primarily responsible for churning the solids and generating smaller liquid-like material, which then exits the stomach in a manner similar to that of ingested liquids. Thus, the gastric emptying of liquids and of solids is closely integrated.

Filling of the stomach is facilitated by both receptive relaxation and gastric accommodation

Even a dry swallow relaxes both the lower esophageal sphincter and the proximal part of the stomach. Of course, the same happens when we swallow food. These relaxations facilitate the entry of food into the stomach. Relaxation in the fundus is primarily regulated by a vagovagal reflex and has been called **receptive relaxation**. In a **vagovagal reflex**, afferent fibers running with the vagus nerve carry information to the central nervous system (CNS), and efferent vagal fibers carry the signal from the CNS to the stomach and cause relaxation by a mechanism that is neither cholinergic nor adrenergic. The result is that intragastric volume increases without an increase in intragastric pressure. If vagal innervation to the stomach is interrupted, gastric pressure rises much more rapidly.

Quite apart from the receptive relaxation, the stomach can also relax in response to gastric filling per se (Fig. 42.12A). This phenomenon is the result of *active* dilation of the fundus, called **gastric accommodation**. Vagotomy abolishes a major portion of gastric accommodation. However,

onto the surface of the stomach. However, this stream of acid apparently does not spread laterally, but rather rises to the surface as a "finger" and thus does not neutralize the HCO_3^- in the microenvironment between the surface epithelial cells and the mucus.

The mucus/HCO_3^- layer plays an important role in preventing autodigestion of the gastric mucosa.

Acid entry into the duodenum induces S cells to release secretin, triggering the pancreas and duodenum to secrete HCO_3^-

Low pH in the duodenum serves as a signal for the secretion of alkali to neutralize gastric acid in the duodenum. The key factor in this neutralization process is **secretin**. A low duodenal pH, with a threshold of 4.5, triggers the release of secretin

A GASTRIC ACCOMMODATION

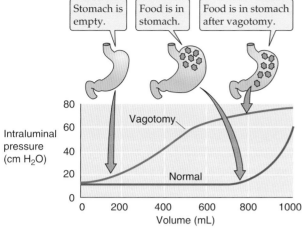

B GASTRIC EMPTYING

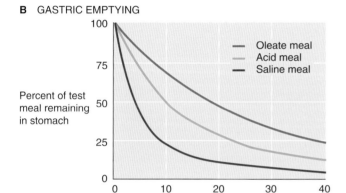

Figure 42.12 Gastric filling and emptying. (B, Data from Dooley CP, Reznick JB, Valenzuela JE: Variations in gastric and duodenal motility during gastric emptying of liquid meals in humans. Gastroenterology 87:1114–1119, 1984.)

A PROPULSION

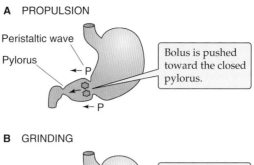

B GRINDING

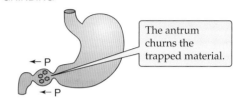

C RETROPULSION

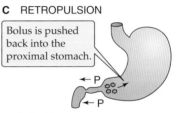

Figure 42.13 Mechanical actions of the stomach on its contents.

the role of the vagus nerve in gastric accommodation is one of modulation. It is generally believed that the **ENS** (see ⊙ 41-1) is the primary regulator permitting the storage of substantial amounts of solids and liquids in the proximal part of the stomach without major increases in intragastric pressure.

The stomach churns its contents until the particles are small enough to be gradually emptied into the duodenum

The substance most rapidly emptied by the stomach is isotonic saline or water. Emptying of these liquids occurs without delay and is faster the greater the volume of fluid. Acidic and caloric fluids leave the stomach more slowly, whereas fatty materials exit even more slowly (Fig. 42.12B).

Solids must first be reduced in size (i.e., trituration) to <2 mm before they are emptied into the duodenum by mechanisms similar to those for liquids. Movement of solid particles toward the antrum is accomplished by the interaction of propulsive gastric contractions and occlusion of the pylorus, a process termed **propulsion** (Fig. 42.13A). Gastric

contractions are initiated by the gastric pacemaker, which is located on the greater curvature, approximately at the junction of the proximal and middle portions of the stomach. These contractions propel the luminal contents toward the pylorus, which is partially closed by contraction of the pyloric musculature before delivery of the bolus. This increase in pyloric resistance represents the coordinated response of antral, pyloric, and duodenal motor activity. Once a bolus of material is trapped near the antrum, it is churned to help reduce the size of the particles, a process termed **grinding** (Fig. 42.13B). Only a small portion of gastric material—that containing particles <2 mm—is propelled through the pylorus to the duodenum. Thus, most gastric contents are returned to the body of the stomach for pulverization and shearing of solid particles, a process known as **retropulsion** (Fig. 42.13C). These processes of propulsion, grinding, and retropulsion repeat multiple times until the gastric contents are emptied.

Modification of gastric contents is associated with the activation of multiple feedback mechanisms. This feedback usually arises from the duodenum (and beyond) and almost always results in a delay in gastric emptying. Thus, as small squirts of gastric fluid leave the stomach, chemoreceptors and mechanoreceptors—primarily in the proximal but also in the distal portion of the small intestine—sense low pH, high caloric content, lipid, certain amino acids (i.e., tryptophan), or changes in osmolarity. These signals all decrease the rate of gastric emptying by a combination of neural and hormonal signals, including the vagus nerve, secretin, CCK, and gastric inhibitory peptide (GIP) released from duodenal mucosa.

CHAPTER 43

PANCREATIC AND SALIVARY GLANDS

Fred S. Gorelick and Christopher R. Marino

OVERVIEW OF EXOCRINE GLAND PHYSIOLOGY

The pancreas and major salivary glands are compound exocrine glands

The exocrine pancreas and major salivary glands are compound exocrine glands—specialized secretory organs that contain a branching ductular system through which they release their secretory products. The principal function of these exocrine glands is to aid in the digestion of food. The saliva produced by the salivary glands lubricates ingested food and initiates the digestion of starch. Pancreatic juice, rich in HCO_3^- and digestive enzymes, neutralizes the acidic gastric contents that enter the small intestine and also completes the intraluminal digestion of ingested carbohydrate, protein, and fat. Each of these exocrine glands is under the control of neural and humoral signals that generate a sequential and coordinated secretory response to an ingested meal.

Morphologically, the pancreas and salivary glands are divided into small but visible **lobules,** each of which is drained by a single **intralobular duct** (Fig. 43.1A). Groups of lobules separated by connective tissue septa are drained by larger **interlobular ducts.** These interlobular ducts empty into a **main duct** that connects the entire gland to the lumen of the gastrointestinal tract.

Within the lobules reside the functional **secretory unit** composed of an acinus and a small intercalated duct. The acinus is a cluster of 15 to 100 acinar cells that secrete proteins into the lumen of the acinus. Acinar cells from both the pancreas and salivary glands also secrete an isotonic, plasma-like fluid that accompanies the secretory proteins. The final acinar secretion is a protein-rich product known as the primary secretion.

The lumen of each acinus is connected to an **intercalated duct.** The intercalated ducts fuse to form progressively larger ducts that ultimately coalesce to form the intralobular duct that drains the lobule. The epithelial cells lining the ducts play an important role in modifying the fluid and electrolyte composition of the primary secretion. Thus, the final exocrine gland secretion represents the combined product of two distinct epithelial-cell populations, the acinar cell and the duct cell.

In addition to acini and ducts, exocrine glands contain a rich supply of nerves and blood vessels. Postganglionic **parasympathetic** and **sympathetic** fibers contribute to the autonomic regulation of secretion through the release of cholinergic, adrenergic, and peptide neurotransmitters that bind to receptors on the acinar and duct cells. These *efferent* fibers also regulate blood flow. Both central and reflex pathways contribute to the neural regulation of exocrine secretion.

Acinar cells are specialized protein-synthesizing cells

Acinar cells of the pancreas (Fig. 43.1B) and salivary glands (Fig. 43.7, *below*) are polarized epithelial cells specialized for the production and export of large quantities of protein. Thus, the acinar cell is equipped with extensive rough endoplasmic reticulum. However, the most characteristic feature of the acinar cell is the abundance of electron-dense secretory granules at the apical pole of the cell. These granules are storage pools of secretory proteins, and they are poised to release their contents after stimulation of the cell by neurohumoral agents. The secretory granules of pancreatic acinar cells contain the mixture of zymogens (inactive enzyme precursors) and enzymes required for digestion. The secretory granules of salivary acinar cells contain either α-amylase (in the parotid glands) or mucins (in the sublingual glands).

The pancreatic acinar cell has served as an important model for elucidating protein synthesis and export via the **secretory pathway.**

Exocytosis, the process by which secretory granules release their contents, is a complex series of events that involves the movement of the granules to the apical membrane, fusion of these granules with the membrane, and release of their contents into the acinar lumen. Secretion is triggered by stimulation of cell-surface receptors by either hormones or neurotransmitters (neurohumoral stimulation).

Duct cells are epithelial cells specialized for fluid and electrolyte transport

Pancreatic and salivary duct cells are polarized epithelial cells specialized for the transport of electrolytes across distinct apical and basolateral membrane domains. Duct epithelial cells contain specific membrane transporters and an abundance of mitochondria to provide energy for active transport, and they exhibit varying degrees of basolateral membrane infolding that increases the membrane surface area of pancreatic duct cells (Fig. 43.1C) and salivary duct cells (Fig. 43.7C, *below*).

A ORGANIZATION OF THE PANCREAS

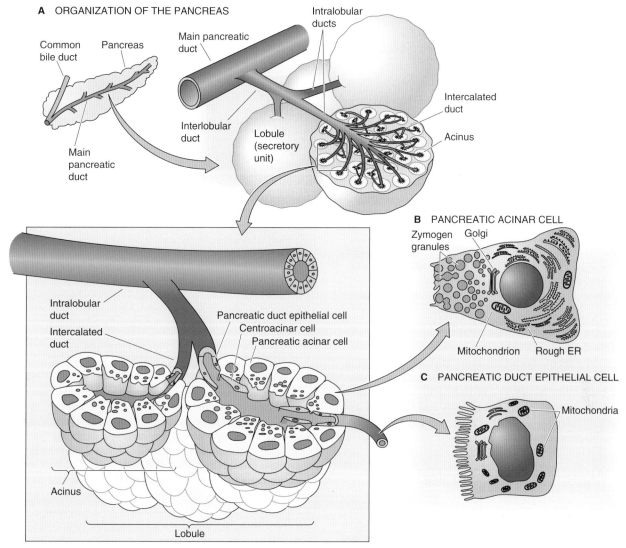

Fig. 43.1 Pancreatic acinus and duct morphology.

Ion transport in duct cells is regulated by neurohumoral stimuli that act through specific receptors located on the basolateral membrane.

Goblet cells contribute to mucin production in exocrine glands

In addition to acinar and duct cells, exocrine glands contain varying numbers of goblet cells. These cells secrete high-molecular-weight glycoproteins known as **mucins** (see ◉ 42-5). When hydrated, mucins form **mucus.** Mucus has several important functions, including lubrication, hydration, and mechanical protection of surface epithelial cells.

PANCREATIC ACINAR CELL

◉ 43-1 The acinar cell secretes digestive proteins in response to stimulation

When the acinar cells are in an unstimulated state, they secrete low levels of digestive proteins via a **constitutive secretory pathway.** Acinar cells stimulated by neurohumoral agents secrete proteins via a **regulated pathway.**

The acinar cell exhibits two distinct patterns of regulated secretion: monophasic and biphasic (Fig. 43.2). Increasing levels of an agonist that generates a *monophasic* dose-response relationship (e.g., gastrin-releasing peptide [GRP]) causes secretion to reach a maximal level that does not fall with higher concentrations of the agent. In contrast, increasing levels of a secretagogue that elicits a *biphasic* dose-response relationship (e.g., cholecystokinin and carbachol) causes secretion to reach a maximal level that decreases at still higher concentrations.

Acetylcholine and cholecystokinin mediate the regulated secretion of proteins by pancreatic acinar cells

Although at least a dozen different receptors are present on the plasma membrane of the pancreatic acinar cell, the most important in regulating protein secretion are the **M₃ muscarinic acetylcholine (ACh) receptor** and the **cholecystokinin (CCK)** receptor.

M₃ and CCK receptors have many similarities: both are basolateral, both are linked to the $G\alpha_q$ heterotrimeric G protein, both use the phospholipase C (PLC)/Ca^{2+} signal-transduction pathway (see ◉ 3-13), and both lead

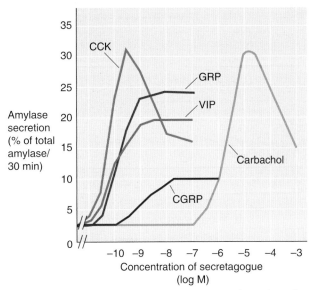

Fig. 43.2 Effects of pancreatic secretagogues on amylase release from isolated pancreatic acini. (Data from Jensen RT: Receptors on pancreatic acinar cells. In Johnson LR [ed]: Physiology of the Gastrointestinal Tract. New York, Raven Press, 1994, pp 1377–1446.)

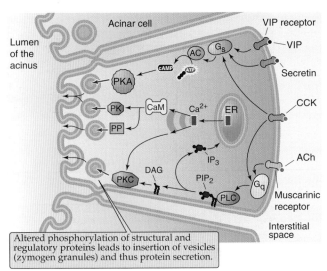

Fig. 43.3 Stimulation of protein secretion from the pancreatic acinar cell. The pancreatic acinar cell has at least two pathways for stimulating the insertion of zymogen granules and thus releasing digestive enzymes. *AC*, Adenylyl cyclase; *CaM*, calmodulin; *CGRP*, calcitonin gene–related peptide; *PIP₂*, phosphatidylinositol 4,5-bisphosphate; *PK*, protein kinases other than PKA and PKC; *PP*, phosphoprotein phosphatases.

to increased enzyme secretion from the acinar cell (Fig. 43.2).

Numerous other receptors—including those for secretin (see ◉ **43-3**), somatostatin (see ◉ **48-6** and ◉ **51-13**) and vasoactive intestinal peptide (VIP; see Table 41.1)—are also found on the pancreatic acinar cell.

Ca²⁺ is the major second messenger for the secretion of proteins by pancreatic acinar cells

Ca²⁺ Generation of a cytosolic Ca^{2+} signal is a complex summation of cellular events (see ◉ **3-14**). Even when the acinar cell is in the resting state, the cytosolic free Ca^{2+} level ($[Ca^{2+}]_i$) oscillates slowly. Maximal stimulatory (i.e., physiological) concentrations of CCK or ACh increase the frequency of the oscillations but have less effect on the amplitude.

cAMP Secretin, VIP, and CCK increase cAMP production and thus activate protein kinase A (PKA) in pancreatic acinar cells (Fig. 43.3).

In addition to proteins, the pancreatic acinar cell secretes a plasma-like fluid

Besides secreting proteins, acinar cells in the pancreas secrete an isotonic, plasma-like fluid (Fig. 43.4). This NaCl-rich fluid hydrates the dense, protein-rich material that the acinar cells secrete. The fundamental transport event is the secretion of Cl⁻ across the apical membrane. For transcellular (plasma-to-lumen) movement of Cl⁻ to occur, Cl⁻ must move into the cell across the basolateral membrane. In the acinar cell basolateral Cl⁻ uptake occurs via an Na/K/Cl cotransporter. The Na-K pump generates the Na⁺ gradient that energizes the Na/K/Cl cotransporter. The K⁺ entering through the Na-K pump and via the Na/K/Cl cotransporter exits through K⁺ channels that are also located on the basolateral membrane. Thus, a pump, a cotransporter, and a channel are necessary to sustain the basolateral uptake of Cl⁻ into the acinar cell.

The rise in $[Ca^{2+}]_i$ produced by basolateral Cl⁻ uptake drives the secretion of Cl⁻ down its electrochemical gradient through channels in the apical membrane. As the transepithelial voltage becomes more lumen negative, Na⁺ moves through the cation-selective paracellular pathway (i.e., tight junctions) to join the Cl⁻ secreted into the lumen. Water also moves through this paracellular pathway, as well as via aquaporin water channels on the apical and basolateral membranes. Therefore, the net effect of these acinar cell transport processes is the production of an isotonic, NaCl-rich fluid that accounts for ~25% of total pancreatic fluid secretion.

PANCREATIC DUCT CELL

◉ 43-2 The pancreatic duct cell secretes isotonic NaHCO₃

The principal physiological function of the pancreatic duct cell is to secrete an HCO₃⁻-rich fluid that alkalinizes and hydrates the protein-rich primary secretions of the acinar cell. The apical step of transepithelial HCO₃⁻ secretion (Fig. 43.5) is mediated in part by a **Cl-HCO₃ exchanger** that secretes intracellular HCO₃⁻ into the duct lumen. Luminal Cl⁻ must be available for this exchange process to occur. Although some luminal Cl⁻ is present in the primary secretions of the acinar cell, anion channels on the apical membrane of the duct cell provide additional Cl⁻ to the lumen in a process called *Cl⁻ recycling*. The most important of these anion channels is the **cystic fibrosis transmembrane conductance regulator (CFTR),** a cAMP-activated Cl⁻ channel that is present on the apical membrane of pancreatic duct cells.

The intracellular HCO₃⁻ that exits the duct cell across the apical membrane arises from two pathways. The first is direct uptake of HCO₃⁻ via an electrogenic Na/HCO₃ cotransporter. The second mechanism is the generation of intracellular HCO₃⁻ from CO₂ and OH⁻, catalyzed by carbonic

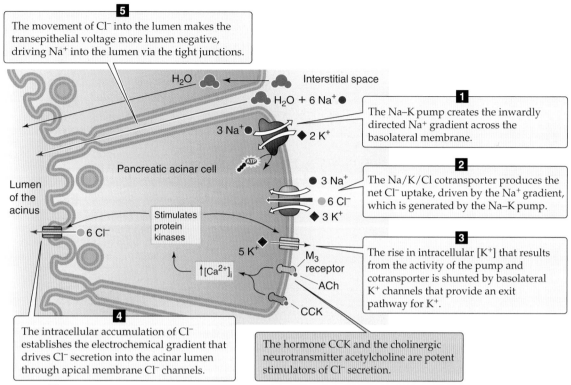

Fig. 43.4 Stimulation of isotonic NaCl secretion by the pancreatic acinar cell. Both ACh and CCK stimulate NaCl secretion, probably through phosphorylation of basolateral and apical ion channels.

anhydrase (see ⊙ 28-2). The pancreatic duct cell accounts for ~75% of total pancreatic fluid secretion.

⊙ 43-3 Secretin (via cAMP) and ACh (via Ca²⁺) stimulate HCO₃⁻ secretion by pancreatic ducts

Secretin is the most important humoral regulator of ductal HCO_3^- secretion. Activation of the **secretin receptor** on the duct cell stimulates adenylyl cyclase, which raises $[cAMP]_i$ and thereby activates PKA. Secretin acts by stimulating the apical CFTR Cl⁻ channel and the basolateral Na/HCO₃ cotransporter.

HCO_3^- secretion is also regulated by the parasympathetic division of the autonomic nervous system. The postganglionic parasympathetic neurotransmitter **ACh,** acts through **muscarinic receptors** on the duct cell.

COMPOSITION, FUNCTION, AND CONTROL OF PANCREATIC SECRETION

Pancreatic juice is a protein- and HCO₃⁻-rich, alkaline secretion

Humans produce ~1.5 L of pancreatic fluid each day. The pancreas has the highest rates of protein synthesis and secretion of any organ in the body. Each day the pancreas delivers between 15 and 100 g of protein into the small intestine.

The human pancreas secretes >20 proteins, some of which are listed in Table 43.1. Most of these proteins are either inactive digestive enzyme precursors—**zymogens**—or active digestive enzymes. The secretory proteins responsible for digestion can be classified according to their substrates: **proteases** hydrolyze proteins, **amylases** digest carbohydrates, **lipases** and phospholipases break down lipids, and **nucleases** digest nucleic acids.

Bicarbonate secreted by duct cells neutralizes the acidic gastric secretions that enter the duodenum and allows digestive enzymes to function properly; HCO_3^- also facilitates the micellar solubilization of lipids and mucosal cell function.

⊙ 43-4 CCK from duodenal I cells stimulates acinar enzyme secretion, and secretin from S cells stimulates HCO₃⁻ and fluid secretion by ducts

CCK plays a central role in regulating pancreatic secretion. CCK is released from neuroendocrine cells (**I cells;** see Table 41.1) present in the duodenal mucosa (Fig. 43.3). In response to a meal, plasma CCK levels increase 5- to 10-fold within 10 to 30 minutes.

The most potent stimulator of CCK release from I cells is **lipid** in the duodenal lumen. Protein digestive products (i.e., peptones, amino acids) also increase CCK release, but carbohydrate and acid have little effect.

Secretin is the most potent humoral stimulator of fluid and HCO_3^- secretion by the pancreas (Fig. 43.5). Secretin is released from neuroendocrine cells (S cells) in the mucosa of the small intestine in response to duodenal acidification and, to a lesser extent, bile acids and lipids. To stimulate secretin secretion, duodenal pH must fall to <4.5. Like CCK levels, secretin levels increase after the ingestion of a meal. However, when these levels are reached experimentally by administration of exogenous secretin, pancreatic HCO_3^- secretion is less than that generated by a meal. These findings suggest that secretin is acting in concert with CCK, ACh, and other agents to stimulate HCO_3^- secretion.

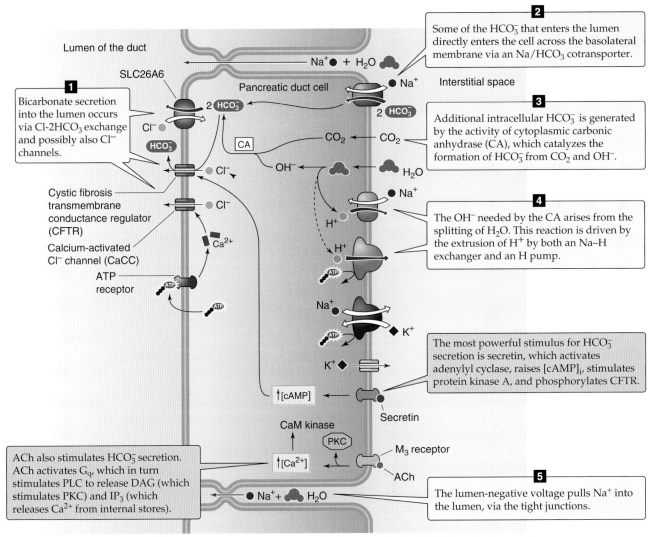

Lumen of the duct

2 Some of the HCO_3^- that enters the lumen directly enters the cell across the basolateral membrane via an Na/HCO_3 cotransporter.

SLC26A6

Pancreatic duct cell

Interstitial space

1 Bicarbonate secretion into the lumen occurs via Cl-$2HCO_3$ exchange and possibly also Cl^- channels.

3 Additional intracellular HCO_3^- is generated by the activity of cytoplasmic carbonic anhydrase (CA), which catalyzes the formation of HCO_3^- from CO_2 and OH^-.

Cystic fibrosis transmembrane conductance regulator (CFTR)

Calcium-activated Cl^- channel (CaCC)

ATP receptor

4 The OH^- needed by the CA arises from the splitting of H_2O. This reaction is driven by the extrusion of H^+ by both an Na–H exchanger and an H pump.

The most powerful stimulus for HCO_3^- secretion is secretin, which activates adenylyl cyclase, raises $[cAMP]_i$, stimulates protein kinase A, and phosphorylates CFTR.

Secretin

CaM kinase

PKC

M_3 receptor

ACh

ACh also stimulates HCO_3^- secretion. ACh activates G_q, which in turn stimulates PLC to release DAG (which stimulates PKC) and IP_3 (which releases Ca^{2+} from internal stores).

5 The lumen-negative voltage pulls Na^+ into the lumen, via the tight junctions.

Fig. 43.5 HCO_3^- secretion by the cells of the pancreatic duct. Secretin, via cAMP, phosphorylates and opens CFTR Cl^- channels. Exit of Cl^- through apical Cl^- channels depolarizes the basolateral membrane, generating the electrical gradient favoring electrogenic Na/HCO_3 cotransport. *CaM,* Calmodulin.

A meal triggers cephalic, gastric, and intestinal phases of pancreatic secretion

The digestive period has been divided into three phases (Table 43.2) based on the site at which food acts to stimulate pancreatic secretion, just as for gastric secretion (see ◉ 42-3). These three phases (cephalic, gastric, and intestinal) are sequential and follow the progression of a meal from its initial smell and taste to its movement through the gastrointestinal tract (Fig. 43.6). These phases act in a coordinated fashion to maximize efficiency of the digestive process.

Cephalic Phase ◉ **43-5** During the cephalic phase, the sight, taste, and smell of food usually generates only a modest increase in fluid and electrolyte secretion (Fig. 43.6A). However, these factors have prominent effects on enzyme secretion. In humans, the cephalic phase is short-lived and dissipates rapidly when food is removed. The cephalic phase is mediated by neural pathways. The efferent signal travels along vagal pathways to stimulate pancreatic secretion via ACh, an effect blocked by atropine. The cephalic phase does not depend on gastrin or CCK release, but it is probably mediated by the stimulation of muscarinic receptors on the *acinar* cell.

Gastric Phase During the gastric phase (Fig. 43.6A), the presence of food in the stomach modulates pancreatic secretion by (1) affecting the release of hormones, (2) stimulating neural pathways, and (3) modifying the pH and availability of nutrients in the proximal part of the small intestine. The presence of specific peptides or amino acids (peptones) stimulates gastrin release from G cells in the antrum of the stomach and, to a much lesser extent, G cells in the proximal part of the duodenum. The gastrin/CCK_2 receptor and the CCK_1 receptor are closely related (see ◉ 42-1). Gastric distention stimulates low levels of pancreatic secretion, probably through a vagovagal gastropancreatic reflex. Although the presence of food in the stomach affects pancreatic secretion, the most important role for chyme in controlling pancreatic secretion occurs after the gastric contents enter the small intestine.

Intestinal Phase During the intestinal phase, chyme entering the proximal region of the small intestine stimulates a major pancreatic secretory response by three major mechanisms (Fig. 43.6B). First, gastric acid entering the duodenum stimulates duodenal **S cells** to release secretin, which, in turn, stimulates duct cells to secrete HCO_3^- and fluid. A threshold duodenal pH of <4.5 is needed to activate S-cell secretion. Second, lipids and, to a lesser degree, peptones stimulate duodenal I cells to release CCK, which stimulates acinar cells to release digestive enzymes. Finally, the same stimuli that trigger I cells also activate a vagovagal enteropancreatic reflex that predominantly stimulates acinar cells.

The pattern of enzyme secretion—mediated by the CCK and vagovagal pathways—depends on the contents of the meal. For example, a *liquid meal* elicits a response that is only ~60% of maximal. In contrast, a *solid meal*, which contains larger particles and is slowly released from the stomach, elicits a prolonged response. Meals rich in *calories* cause the greatest response.

The pancreas has large reserves of digestive enzymes for carbohydrates and proteins, but not for lipids

The exocrine pancreas stores more enzymes than are required for digesting a meal. The greatest pancreatic reserves are those required for carbohydrate and protein digestion. The reserves of enzymes required for lipid digestion—particularly for triglyceride hydrolysis—are more limited. These observations have important clinical implications because they indicate that individuals can tolerate large pancreatic resections for tumors without fear of developing maldigestion or diabetes postoperatively. When fat maldigestion or diabetes does develop because of pancreatic disease, the gland must have undergone extensive destruction.

Fat in the distal part of the small intestine inhibits pancreatic secretion

Once maximally stimulated, pancreatic secretion begins to decrease after several hours. Nevertheless, the levels of secretion remain adequate for digestion. Regulatory systems only gradually return secretion to its basal (interdigestive) state. The regulatory mechanisms responsible for this feedback inhibition are less well characterized than those responsible for stimulating pancreatic secretion. The presence of fat in the distal end of the small intestine reduces pancreatic secretion in most animals, including humans. This inhibition may be mediated by **peptide YY (PYY),** which is present in neuroendocrine cells in the ileum and colon.

Several mechanisms protect the pancreas from autodigestion

Premature activation of pancreatic enzymes within acinar cells may lead to autodigestion and could play a role in initiating pancreatitis. To avoid such injury, the acinar cell has mechanisms for preventing enzymatic activity (Table 43.3).

SALIVARY ACINAR CELL

Different salivary acinar cells secrete different proteins

The organizational structure of the salivary glands (Fig. 43.7A) is similar to that of the pancreas (Fig. 43.1A), with secretory acinar units draining into progressively larger ducts. The **acinar cells** of the parotid glands secrete a serous (i.e., watery) product that contains an abundance of α-**amylase.** Many acinar cells of the sublingual glands secrete a mucinous product that is composed primarily of **mucin glycoproteins.** Fig. 43.7B shows an acinar cell that contains both serous and mucous granules.

Cholinergic and adrenergic neural pathways are the most important physiological activators of regulated secretion by salivary acinar cells

Salivary glands are predominately controlled by the autonomic nervous system (see Chapter 14). The major agonists

TABLE 43.1 Major Digestive Proteins of the Pancreatic Acinar Cell

Zymogens

Trypsinogens

Chymotrypsinogen

Proelastase

Proprotease E

Procarboxypeptidase A

Procarboxypeptidase B

Active Enzymes

α-Amylase

Carboxyl ester lipase

Lipase

RNAase

DNAase

Colipase

TABLE 43.2 Three Phases of Pancreatic Secretion

PHASE	STIMULANT	REGULATORY PATHWAY	% OF MAXIMUM ENZYME SECRETION
Cephalic	Sight Smell Taste Mastication	Vagal pathways	25
Gastric	Distention Gastrin?	Vagal-cholinergic	10–20
Intestinal	Amino acids Fatty acids H+	CCK Secretin Enteropancreatic reflexes	50–80

A CEPHALIC AND GASTRIC PHASES

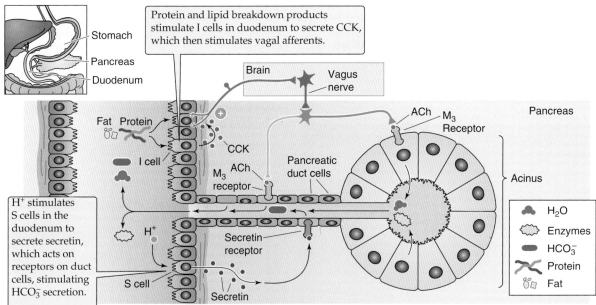

B INTESTINAL PHASE

Protein and lipid breakdown products stimulate I cells in duodenum to secrete CCK, which then stimulates vagal afferents.

H⁺ stimulates S cells in the duodenum to secrete secretin, which acts on receptors on duct cells, stimulating HCO_3^- secretion.

Fig. 43.6 Three phases of pancreatic secretion.

of salivary acinar secretion are ACh and norepinephrine, which are released from postganglionic parasympathetic and sympathetic nerve terminals, respectively (see Fig. 14.5 and Table 43.4). The cholinergic receptor on the salivary acinar cell is the muscarinic M_3 glandular subtype. The adrenergic receptors identified on these cells include both the α and β subtypes. Both cholinergic and adrenergic neurotransmitters can stimulate exocytosis by salivary acinar cells.

Both cAMP and Ca²⁺ mediate salivary acinar secretion

Protein secretion by the salivary acinar cell, as by the pancreatic acinar cell, is associated with increases in both $[cAMP]_i$ and $[Ca^{2+}]_i$. Activation of cAMP via the β-adrenergic receptor is the most potent stimulator of amylase secretion in the rat parotid gland. Activation of Ca^{2+} signaling pathways via the α-adrenergic, muscarinic, and substance P receptors also stimulates amylase secretion by the parotid gland, but in general, these Ca^{2+} signaling pathways have a greater effect on fluid secretion.

Fluid and electrolyte secretion is the second major function of salivary acinar cells, accounting for ~90% of total salivary volume output under stimulatory conditions. The mechanisms in salivary acinar cells are similar to those in pancreatic acinar cells (Fig. 43.4). The primary secretion of the salivary acinar cell is isotonic and results largely from the basolateral uptake of Cl^- through Na/K/Cl cotransporters, working in conjunction with Na-K pumps and basolateral K^+ channels. Secretion of Cl^- and water into the lumen is mediated by apical Cl^- and aquaporin water channels. Na^+ and some water reach the lumen via paracellular routes.

SALIVARY DUCT CELL

Salivary duct cells produce a hypotonic fluid that is poor in NaCl and rich in KHCO₃

In the salivary glands, as in the pancreas, the ducts modify the composition of the isotonic, plasma-like primary secretion of the acinar cells. As the fluid exits the salivary acinus, it passes through an intercalated duct (Fig. 43.7A), with typical **intercalated duct cells** (Fig. 43.7C). Later, abundant mitochondria and infoldings of the basolateral membrane give the basal portion of the duct cells a characteristic striated appearance—hence the term striated **duct cell** (Fig. 43.7B).

TABLE 43.3 **Mechanisms That Protect the Acinar Cell From Autodigestion**

PROTECTIVE FACTOR	MECHANISM
Packaging of many digestive proteins as zymogens	Precursor proteins lack enzymatic activity
Selective sorting of secretory proteins and storage in zymogen granules	Restricts the interaction of secretory proteins with other cellular compartments
Protease inhibitors in the zymogen granule	Block the action of prematurely activated enzymes
Condensation of secretory proteins at low pH	Limits the activity of active enzymes
Nondigestive proteases	Degrade active enzymes

A ORGANIZATION OF THE SALIVARY GLANDS

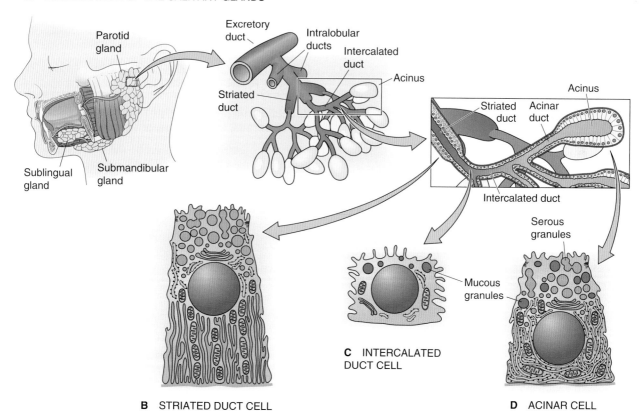

Fig. 43.7 Salivary gland distribution and cellular morphology. (A) Humans have three main bilateral salivary glands. The parotid glands are located in front of each ear, the submandibular glands are located laterally beneath each jaw bone, and the sublingual glands are located in the floor of the mouth, underneath both sides of the tongue.

TABLE 43.4 **Autonomic Control of Salivary Secretion**

AUTONOMIC PATHWAY	NEUROTRANSMITTER	RECEPTOR	SIGNALING PATHWAY	CELLULAR RESPONSE
Parasympathetic	ACh	Muscarinic (M_3)	Ca^{2+}	Fluid > protein secretion
	Substance P	Tachykinin (NK_1)	Ca^{2+}	Fluid > protein secretion
Sympathetic	Norepinephrine	α-adrenergic	Ca^{2+}	Fluid > protein secretion
	Norepinephrine	β-adrenergic	cAMP	Protein ≫ fluid secretion

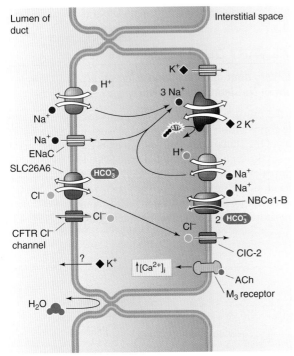

Fig. 43.8 Salivary duct transporters.

In general, salivary duct cells absorb Na^+ and Cl^- and, to a lesser extent, secrete K^+ and HCO_3^-.

Reabsorption of Na^+ by salivary duct cells is a two-step transcellular process (Fig. 43.8). First, Na^+ enters the cell from the lumen through apical epithelial Na^+ channels (ENaCs). Second, the basolateral Na-K pump extrudes this Na^+.

Reabsorption of Cl^- is also a two-step transcellular process (Fig. 43.8). Entry of Cl^- across the apical membrane occurs via a Cl-HCO_3 exchanger and CFTR. To a certain extent, apical CFTR also recycles Cl^- absorbed by the Cl-HCO_3 exchanger. Thus, CFTR may facilitate both HCO_3^- secretion and Cl^- reabsorption through bidirectional Cl^- movement across the apical membrane. Exit of Cl^- across the basolateral membrane of duct cells occurs via Cl^- channels.

Secretion of HCO_3^- occurs via pathways (Fig. 43.8) similar to those in pancreatic ducts and involves apical Cl-HCO_3 exchangers and CFTR, as well as basolateral Na/HCO_3 cotransporters (see Fig. 5.7).

Secretion of K^+ occurs through the basolateral uptake of K^+ via the Na-K pump (Fig. 43.8). The mechanism of K^+ exit across the apical membrane is not well established.

Parasympathetic stimulation decreases Na^+ absorption, whereas aldosterone increases Na^+ absorption by duct cells

Regulation of duct cell transport processes is less well understood in the salivary glands than in the pancreas. In the intact salivary gland (i.e., acini and ducts), secretion is stimulated primarily by *parasympathetic* input via ACh. In the duct cell, cholinergic agonists, acting through muscarinic receptors (mostly M_3).

Activation of the β-adrenergic receptor increases $[cAMP]_i$ and activates the CFTR Cl^- channel.

Salivary duct cell function is also regulated by the mineralocorticoid hormone **aldosterone**, which stimulates the absorption of NaCl and secretion of K^+ by salivary duct cells in several species. Although its role has not been well examined in salivary duct cells, aldosterone in other Na^+-absorbing epithelia (e.g., kidney and colon) stimulates Na^+ transport by increasing both ENaC and Na-K pump activity (see ⊙ 35-6).

COMPOSITION, FUNCTION, AND CONTROL OF SALIVARY SECRETION

Depending on protein composition, salivary secretions can be serous, seromucous, or mucous

Most saliva (~90%) is produced by the major salivary glands: the parotid, the sublingual, and the submandibular glands (Fig. 43.7A). The remaining 10% of saliva comes from numerous minor salivary glands that are scattered throughout the submucosa of the oral cavity. Each salivary gland produces either a serous, a seromucous, or a mucous secretion; the definition of these three types of saliva is based on the glycoprotein content of the gland's final secretory product. In humans, the parotids produce a serous secretion (i.e., low glycoprotein content), the sublingual and submandibular glands produce a seromucous secretion, and the minor salivary glands produce a mucous secretion.

Serous secretions are enriched in α-amylase, and mucous secretions are enriched in mucin. However, the most abundant proteins in parotid and submandibular saliva are members of the group of **proline-rich proteins,** in which one third of all amino acids are proline. These proteins exist in acidic, basic, and glycosylated forms. They have antimicrobial properties and may play an important role in neutralizing dietary tannins, which can damage epithelial cells. In addition to serving these protective functions, proline-rich salivary proteins contribute to the lubrication of ingested foods and may enhance tooth integrity through their interactions with Ca^{2+}

TABLE 43.5 Major Organic Components of Mammalian Saliva

COMPONENTS	CELL TYPE	GLANDS	POSSIBLE FUNCTION
Proline-rich proteins	Acinar	P, SM	Enamel formation Ca^{2+} binding Antimicrobial Lubrication
Mucin glycoproteins	Acinar	SL, SM	Lubrication
Enzymes			
α-amylase	Acinar	P, SM	Starch digestion
Lipase	Acinar	SL	Fat digestion
Ribonuclease	Duct	SM	RNA digestion
Kallikrein	Duct	P, SM, SL	Unknown
Miscellaneous			
Lactoperoxidase	Acinar	SM	Antimicrobial
Lactoferrin	Acinar	Unknown	Antimicrobial
Lysozyme	Duct	SM	Antimicrobial
IgA receptor	Duct	Unknown	Antimicrobial
IgA secretory component	Duct	Unknown	Antimicrobial
Growth factors	Duct	SM	Unknown

P, Parotid; *SL*, sublingual; *SM*, submandibular.

and hydroxyapatite. Saliva also contains smaller amounts of lipase, nucleases, lysozyme, peroxidases, lactoferrin, secretory IgA, growth factors, regulatory peptides, and vasoactive proteases such as kallikrein and renin (Table 43.5).

Saliva functions primarily to prevent dehydration of the oral mucosa and to provide lubrication for the mastication and swallowing of ingested food. The senses of taste and, to a lesser extent, smell depend on an adequate supply of saliva. Saliva plays a very important role in maintaining proper oral hygiene. It accomplishes this task by washing away food particles, killing bacteria (lysozyme and IgA activity), and contributing to overall dental integrity. Although α-amylase is a major constituent of saliva and digests a significant amount of the ingested starch, salivary amylase does not appear to be essential for effective carbohydrate digestion in the presence of a normally functioning pancreas. The same can be said for lingual lipase. However, in cases of pancreatic insufficiency, these salivary enzymes can partially compensate for the maldigestion that results from pancreatic dysfunction.

Parasympathetic stimulation increases salivary secretion

Humans produce ~1.5 L of saliva each day. Under basal conditions, the salivary glands produce saliva at a rate of ~0.5 mL/min, with a much slower flow rate during sleep. After stimulation, flow increases 10-fold over the basal rate. Although the salivary glands respond to both cholinergic and adrenergic agonists in vitro, the parasympathetic nervous system is the most important physiological regulator of salivary secretion in vivo.

Parasympathetic Control Taste and tactile stimuli from the tongue are transmitted to the brainstem, where their signals can excite the salivatory nuclei and stimulate salivary gland secretion. In addition, central impulses triggered by the sight and smell of food also excite the salivatory nuclei and can induce salivation before food is ingested. These central effects were best illustrated by the classic experiments of Ivan Pavlov, who conditioned dogs to salivate at the sound of a bell.

Parasympathetic fibers stimulate the salivary glands through their release of ACh. The prominent role of the parasympathetic nervous system in salivary function can be readily appreciated by examining the consequences of cholinergic blockage. Disruption of the parasympathetic fibers to the salivary glands can lead to glandular atrophy.

Sympathetic Control Although sympathetic (adrenergic) stimulation increases saliva flow, interruption of sympathetic nerves to the salivary glands has no major effect on salivary gland function in vivo.

CHAPTER 44

INTESTINAL FLUID AND ELECTROLYTE MOVEMENT

Henry J. Binder

FUNCTIONAL ANATOMY

The small intestine and large intestine have many similarities in structure and function. In some cases, different regions of the intestinal tract carry out certain functions in much the same manner. In other cases, however, substantial heterogeneity exists between different intestinal segments (e.g., ileum versus jejunum) or between different mucosal areas (e.g., villus versus crypt) in one intestinal segment.

Both the small and large intestine absorb and secrete fluid and electrolytes, whereas only the small intestine absorbs nutrients

Among mammals, **absorption** of dietary nutrients is an exclusive function of the small intestine. The small intestine absorbs nonelectrolytes after extensive digestion of dietary nutrients by both luminal and brush-border enzymes. In contrast, *both* the small intestine and the large intestine absorb fluid and electrolytes by several different cellular transport processes, which may differ between the small intestine and large intestine and are the subject of this chapter.

Another vitally important function of the intestinal epithelium is the **secretion** of intestinal fluid and electrolytes. In general, the cellular mechanisms of intestinal electrolyte secretion in the small intestine and colon are similar, if not identical.

The small intestine has a villus-crypt organization, whereas the colon has surface epithelial cells with interspersed crypts

Both the small intestine and the large intestine have a specialized epithelial structure that correlates well with epithelial transport function.

The small intestine (Fig. 44.1A) consists of finger-like projections—**villi**—surrounded by the openings of glandular structures called **crypts of Lieberkühn,** or simply crypts. Both villi and crypts are covered by columnar epithelial cells. The cells lining the villi are considered to be the primary cells responsible for both nutrient and electrolyte *absorption,* whereas the crypt cells primarily participate in *secretion.*

The colon (Fig. 44.1B) does not have villi. Instead, the cells lining the large intestine are surface epithelial cells, and interspersed over the colonic surface are numerous apertures of **colonic crypts** (or glands) that are similar in function and structure to the small-intestinal crypts. Not surprisingly, the surface epithelial cells of the colon are the primary cells responsible for colonic electrolyte *absorption,* whereas colonic gland cells are generally believed to mediate ion *secretion.*

The intestinal mucosa is a dynamic organ with continuous cell proliferation and migration. The zone of cell proliferation is at the base of the crypt in both the small and large intestine, and the program of events is similar in both organs. The **progenitor cell** is a stem cell that differentiates into several specialized cells (e.g., vacuolated, goblet, and Paneth cells) that line the villi and crypts in the small intestine and the surface and glands in the colon. In the small intestine, these villous cells migrate until they reach the tips of the villi, undergo apoptosis, and then slough into the lumen of the intestine. The overall period from the initiation of cell proliferation to sloughing is ~48 to 96 hours.

The surface area of the small intestine is amplified by folds, villi, and microvilli; amplification is less marked in the colon

An additional hallmark of both the small and large intestine is the presence of structures that amplify function by increasing the luminal surface area. These structures exist at three levels. In the small intestine, the first level consists of the macroscopic **folds of Kerckring.** The second level consists of the microscopic **villi** and **crypts** that we have already discussed. The third level is the submicroscopic **microvilli** on the apical surfaces of the epithelial cells. Thus, if the small intestine is thought of as a hollow cylinder, the net increase in total surface area of the small intestine (versus that of a smooth cylinder) is 600-fold. The total surface area of the human small intestine is ~200 m^2, or the surface area of a doubles tennis court (Table 44.1). The colonic surface area is also amplified, but to a more limited extent. Because the colon lacks villi, amplification is a result of only the presence of colonic folds, crypts, and microvilli.

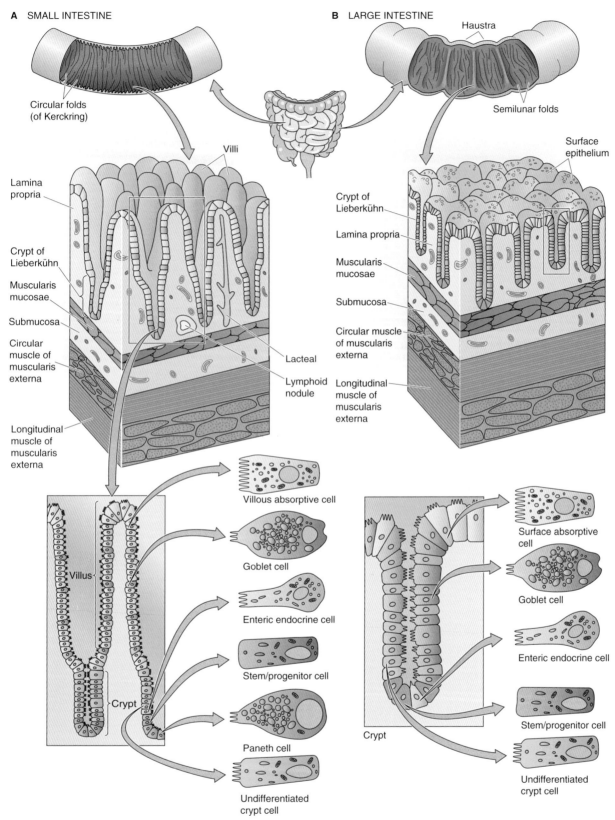

A SMALL INTESTINE

Circular folds
(of Kerckring)

Villi

Lamina
propria

Crypt of
Lieberkühn

Muscularis
mucosae

Submucosa

Circular
muscle of
muscularis
externa

Longitudinal
muscle of
muscularis
externa

Lacteal

Lymphoid
nodule

Villus

Crypt

Villous absorptive cell

Goblet cell

Enteric endocrine cell

Stem/progenitor cell

Paneth cell

Undifferentiated
crypt cell

B LARGE INTESTINE

Haustra

Semilunar folds

Surface
epithelium

Crypt of
Lieberkühn

Lamina propria

Muscularis
mucosae

Submucosa

Circular muscle
of muscularis
externa

Longitudinal
muscle of
muscularis
externa

Crypt

Surface absorptive
cell

Goblet cell

Enteric endocrine cell

Stem/progenitor cell

Undifferentiated
crypt cell

Figure 44.1 Microscopic view of the anatomy of the small and large intestine.

TABLE 44.1 Structural and Functional Differences Between the Small and Large Intestine

	SMALL INTESTINE	LARGE INTESTINE
Length (m)	6	2.4
Area of apical plasma membrane (m²)	~200	~25
Folds	Yes	Yes
Villi	Yes	No
Crypts or glands	Yes	Yes
Microvilli	Yes	Yes
Nutrient absorption	Yes	No
Active Na⁺ absorption	Yes	Yes
Active K⁺ secretion	No	Yes

OVERVIEW OF FLUID AND ELECTROLYTE MOVEMENT IN THE INTESTINES

The small intestine absorbs ~6.5 L/day of an ~8.5-L fluid load that is presented to it, and the colon absorbs ~1.9 L/day

The fluid content of the average diet is typically 1.5 to 2.5 L/day. However, the fluid load to the small intestine is considerably greater—8 to 9 L/day. The difference between these two sets of figures is accounted for by salivary, gastric, pancreatic, and biliary secretions, as well as the secretions of the small intestine itself (Fig. 44.2). Similarly, the total quantity of electrolytes (Na^+, K^+, Cl^-, and HCO_3^-) that enters the lumen of the small intestine also comes from dietary sources in addition to endogenous secretions.

The small intestine absorbs net amounts of water, Na⁺, Cl⁻, and K⁺ and secretes HCO₃⁻, whereas the colon absorbs net amounts of water, Na⁺, and Cl⁻ and secretes both K⁺ and HCO₃⁻

Net ion movement represents the summation of several events. At the level of the entire small or large intestine, substantial movement of ions occurs from the intestinal lumen into the blood and from the blood into the lumen. The *net* ion movement across the entire epithelium is the difference between these two unidirectional fluxes.

Fluid and electrolyte transport in the intestine varies considerably in two different axes, both along the length of the intestines—**segmental heterogeneity**—and from the bottom of a crypt to the top of a villus or to the surface cells—**crypt-villus/surface heterogeneity.**

In health, the small intestine is a net absorber of water, Na^+, Cl^-, and K^+, but is a net secretor of HCO_3^- (Fig. 44.2). Fluid absorption is isosmotic in the small intestine, similar to that observed in the renal proximal tubule (see ⊙ **35-3**). In general, absorptive processes in the small intestine are enhanced in the postprandial state. The human colon carries out net absorption of water, Na^+, and Cl^- with few exceptions, but it carries out net secretion of K^+ and HCO_3^-.

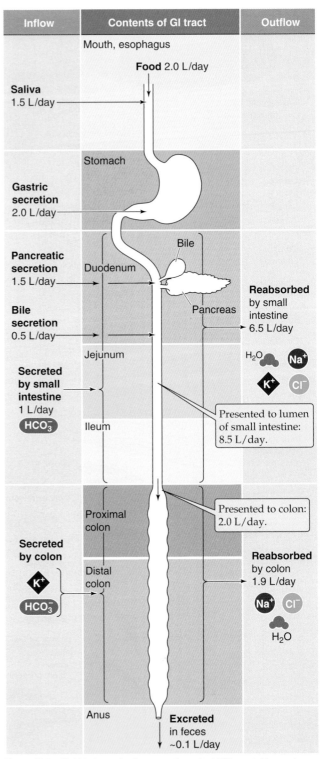

Figure 44.2 Fluid balance in the gastrointestinal (GI) tract. For each segment of the GI tract, the figure shows substances flowing into the lumen on the *left* and substances flowing out of the lumen on the *right*. Of the ~8.5 L/day that are presented to the small intestine, the small intestine removes ~6.5 L/day, delivering ~2/day to the colon. The large intestine removes ~1.9 L/day, leaving ~0.1 L/day in the feces.

Intestinal fluid movement is always coupled to solute movement, and sometimes solute movement is coupled to fluid movement by solvent drag

Fluid movement is always coupled to active solute movement. It is likely that the water movement occurs predominantly by a paracellular route rather than by a transcellular route.

Solute movement is the driving force for fluid movement. However, the converse may also be true: solute movement may be coupled to fluid movement by **solvent drag,** a phenomenon in which the dissolved solute is swept along by bulk movement of the solvent, that is water (see ◉ 20-8). Solvent drag occurs through the paracellular route, and it depends on the permeability properties of the tight junctions and the magnitude of the convective water flow. Thus, solvent drag contributes primarily to the absorption of relatively small, water-soluble molecules, such as urea and Na^+.

The next three major divisions of this chapter discuss the mechanisms of intestinal transport of three major solutes: Na^+, Cl^-, and K^+.

CELLULAR MECHANISMS OF Na⁺ ABSORPTION

Both the small intestine and the large intestine absorb large amounts of Na^+ and Cl^- daily, but different mechanisms are responsible for this extremely important physiological process in different segments of the intestine. The villous epithelial cells in the small intestine and the surface epithelial cells in the colon are responsible for absorbing most of the Na^+. Absorption of Na^+ is the result of a complex interplay of both apical and basolateral membrane transport processes. Fig. 44.3 summarizes the four fundamental mechanisms by which Na^+ may enter the cell across the apical membrane. In each case, the Na-K pump is responsible, at least in part, for the movement of Na^+ from cell to blood. Also in each case, the driving force for apical Na^+ entry is provided by the large, inwardly directed electrochemical gradient for Na^+, which in turn is provided by the Na-K pump.

The following four sections describe these four apical membrane transport processes.

Na/glucose and Na/amino-acid cotransport in the small intestine is a major mechanism for postprandial Na⁺ absorption

"Nutrient-coupled" Na^+ absorption (Fig. 44.3A) occurs throughout the small intestine. Glucose- and amino acid–coupled Na^+ absorption occurs only in villous epithelial cells and not in crypt epithelial cells (Fig. 44.1A). This process is the primary mechanism for Na^+ absorption after a meal.

Glucose- and amino acid–coupled Na^+ absorption is mediated by specific apical membrane transport proteins. The Na/glucose cotransporter is responsible for glucose uptake across the apical membrane, and several distinct Na/amino-acid cotransporters are responsible for the Na^+-coupled uptake of amino acids across the apical membrane (see ◉ 5-12). The glucose and amino acid–coupled uptake of Na^+ entry across the apical membrane increases $[Na^+]_i$, which in turn increases Na^+ extrusion across the basolateral membrane through the Na-K pump.

Electroneutral Na-H exchange in the duodenum and jejunum is responsible for Na⁺ absorption that is stimulated by luminal alkalinity

Luminal HCO_3^- —the result of pancreatic, biliary, and duodenal secretion—increases Na^+ absorption in the proximal portion of the small intestine by stimulating apical membrane Na-H exchange (Fig. 44.3B). The Na-H exchanger couples Na^+ uptake across the apical membrane to proton extrusion into the intestinal lumen, a process that is enhanced by both decreases in intracellular pH (pH_i) and increases in luminal pH. The energy for Na-H exchange comes from the Na^+ gradient.

Parallel Na-H and Cl-HCO₃ exchange in the ileum and proximal part of the colon is the primary mechanism of Na⁺ absorption during the interdigestive period

Electroneutral NaCl absorption occurs in portions of both the small and large intestine (Fig. 44.3C). Electroneutral NaCl absorption is the result of parallel apical membrane Na-H and $Cl-HCO_3$ exchangers that are closely linked by small changes in pH_i. This mechanism of NaCl absorption, which is the primary method of Na^+ absorption between meals (i.e., the interdigestive period), occurs in the ileum and throughout the large intestine, with the exception of the most distal segment.

Epithelial Na⁺ channels are the primary mechanism of "electrogenic" Na⁺ absorption in the distal part of the colon

In the distal part of the colon, Na^+ entry across the apical membrane occurs through epithelial Na^+ channels (ENaCs) that are highly specific for Na^+ (Fig. 44.3D). Because this segment of the colon is capable of absorbing Na^+ against large concentration gradients, it plays an important role in Na^+ conservation. Na^+ movement via electrogenic Na^+ absorption is markedly enhanced by mineralocorticoids (e.g., aldosterone).

Aldosterone increases electrogenic Na^+ absorption by increasing Na^+ entry through the apical Na^+ channel and by stimulating activity of the Na-K pump.

CELLULAR MECHANISMS OF Cl⁻ ABSORPTION AND SECRETION

Cl^- absorption occurs throughout the small and large intestine and is often closely linked to Na^+ absorption. Cl^- and Na^+ absorption may be coupled through either an electrical potential difference or by pH_i. However, sometimes *no* coupling takes place, and the route of Cl^- movement may be either paracellular or transcellular.

Voltage-dependent Cl⁻ absorption represents coupling of Cl⁻ absorption to electrogenic Na⁺ absorption in both the small intestine and the large intestine

Cl^- absorption can be a purely passive process (Fig. 44.4A), driven by the electrochemical gradient for Cl^- either across the tight junctions (paracellular route) or across the individual membranes of the epithelial cell (transcellular route). This process is referred to as *voltage-dependent Cl^- absorption.*

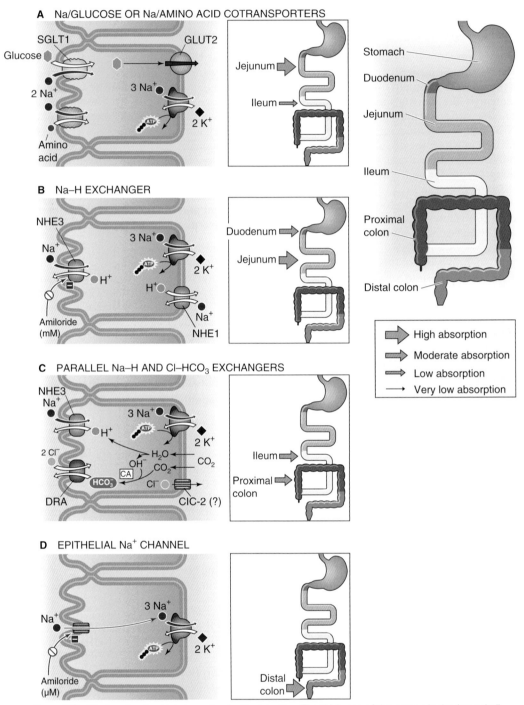

Figure 44.3 Modes of active Na⁺ absorption by the intestine. The thickness of the *arrows* in the *insets* indicates the relative magnitudes of different mechanisms of Na⁺-absorptive fluxes in different segments. *CA,* Carbonic anhydrase.

Electroneutral Cl-HCO₃ exchange results in Cl⁻ absorption and HCO₃⁻ secretion in the ileum and colon

Electroneutral Cl-HCO₃ exchange, in the absence of parallel Na-H exchange, occurs in villous cells in the ileum and in surface epithelial cells in the large intestine (Fig. 44.4B). A Cl-HCO₃ exchanger in the apical membrane is responsible for the 1:1 exchange of apical Cl⁻ for intracellular HCO₃⁻ . The details

of Cl⁻ movement across the *basolateral* membrane are not well understood, but the process may involve a ClC-2 Cl⁻ channel.

Parallel Na-H and Cl-HCO₃ exchange in the ileum and the proximal part of the colon mediates Cl⁻ absorption during the interdigestive period

Electroneutral NaCl absorption mediates Cl⁻ absorption in the ileum and proximal part of the colon (Fig. 44.4C). The apical

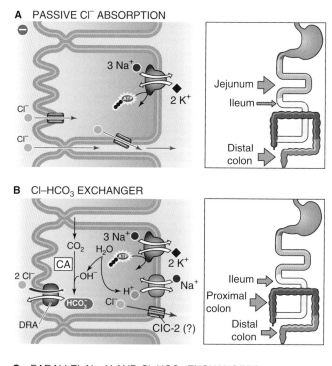

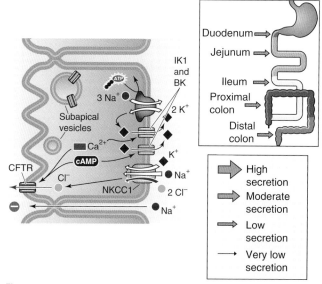

Figure 44.5 Cellular mechanism of electrogenic Cl⁻ secretion by crypt cells. The thickness of the *arrows* in the *inset* indicates the relative magnitudes of Cl⁻ secretory fluxes in different segments.

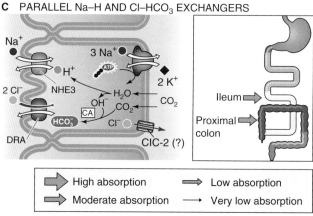

Figure 44.4 Modes of Cl⁻ absorption by the intestine. The thickness of the *arrows* in the *insets* indicates the relative magnitudes of different mechanisms of Cl⁻ absorptive fluxes in different segments. *CA,* Carbonic anhydrase.

step of Cl⁻ absorption by this mechanism is mediated by parallel Na-H exchange (NHE3) and Cl-HCO₃ exchange (DRA; down-regulated in adenoma), which are coupled through pH$_i$.

Electrogenic Cl⁻ secretion occurs in crypts of both the small and the large intestine

The small intestine and the large intestine are also capable of active Cl⁻ secretion.

The cellular model of active Cl⁻ secretion is outlined in Fig. 44.5 and includes three transport pathways on the basolateral membrane: (1) an Na-K pump, (2) an Na/K/Cl cotransporter (NKCC1), and (3) two types of K⁺ channels (IK1 and BK). In addition, a Cl⁻ channel (cystic fibrosis transmembrane conductance regulator [CFTR]) is present on the apical membrane. This complex Cl⁻ secretory system is energized by the Na-K pump, which generates a low [Na⁺]$_i$ and provides the

driving force for Cl⁻ entry across the basolateral membrane through Na/K/Cl cotransport. As a result, [Cl⁻]$_i$ is raised sufficiently that the Cl⁻ electrochemical gradient favors the passive efflux of Cl⁻ across the apical membrane.

Cl⁻ secretion requires stimulation by any of several **secretagogues,** including (1) bacterial exotoxins (i.e., enterotoxins), (2) hormones and neurotransmitters, (3) products of cells of the immune system (e.g., histamine), and (4) laxatives (Table 44.2). These secretagogues act by increasing intracellular levels of cyclic nucleotides or Ca²⁺.

The resulting activation of one or more protein kinases—by any of the aforementioned pathways—increases the Cl⁻ conductance of the apical membrane either by activating pre-existing Cl⁻ channels or by inserting into the apical membrane Cl⁻ channels that—in the unstimulated state—are stored in subapical membrane vesicles. The net result is the initiation of active Cl⁻ secretion across the epithelial cell.

The induction of apical membrane Cl⁻ channels is extremely important in the pathophysiology of many diarrheal disorders, including the secretory diarrhea known as **cholera.** A central role in **cystic fibrosis** has been posited for the CFTR Cl⁻ channel in the apical membrane.

CELLULAR MECHANISMS OF K⁺ ABSORPTION AND SECRETION

Overall net transepithelial K⁺ movement is absorptive in the small intestine and secretory in the colon

Dietary K⁺ furnishes 70 to 120 mmol/day, whereas stool K⁺ output is only ~10 mmol/day. The kidney is responsible for disposal of the remainder of the daily K⁺ intake (see Fig. 37.1). Substantial quantities of K⁺ are secreted in gastric, pancreatic, and biliary fluid. Therefore, the total K⁺ load presented to the small intestine is considerably greater than that represented by the diet. The concentration of K⁺

TABLE 44.2 Mode of Action of Secretagogues

CATEGORY	SECRETAGOGUE	SECOND MESSENGER
Bacterial enterotoxins	Cholera toxin	cAMP
	Escherichia coli toxins: heat labile	cAMP
	E. coli toxins: heat stable	cGMP
	Yersinia toxin	cGMP
	Clostridium difficile toxin	Ca²⁺
Hormones and neurotransmitters	VIP	cAMP
	Guanylin	cGMP
	Acetylcholine	Ca²⁺
	Bradykinin	Ca²⁺
	Serotonin (5-HT)	Ca²⁺
Immune cell products	Histamine	cAMP
	Prostaglandins	cAMP
Laxatives	Bile acids	Ca²⁺

in stool is frequently >100 mM. This high stool $[K^+]$ is the result of several factors, including both colonic K^+ secretion and water absorption, especially in the distal part of the colon.

⊙ 44-1 K⁺ absorption in the small intestine probably occurs via solvent drag

K^+ is *absorbed* in the jejunum and ileum of the small intestine and is *secreted* in the large intestine. K^+ absorption in the small intestine is probably passive, most likely a result of **solvent drag** (i.e., pulled along by bulk water movement), as illustrated in Fig. 44.6A.

Passive K⁺ secretion is the primary mechanism for net colonic secretion

The human colon is a net *secretor* of K^+. This secretion occurs by two mechanisms: a passive transport process and an active process.

Passive K⁺ secretion, which is the pathway that is primarily responsible for overall net colonic K^+ secretion, is driven by the lumen-negative V_{te} of 15 to 25 mV. The route of passive K^+ secretion is predominantly paracellular, not transcellular (Fig. 44.6B).

Active K⁺ secretion is also present throughout the large intestine and is induced both by aldosterone and by cAMP

Active K^+ *secretion* occurs throughout the colon, but active K^+ *absorption* is present only in the distal segments of the large intestine.

The general paradigm of active K^+ transport in the colon is a "pump-leak" model (Fig. 44.6C). Uptake of K^+ across the basolateral membrane is a result of both the Na-K pump and the Na/K/Cl cotransporter (NKCC1), which is energized by the low $[Na^+]_i$ that is created by the Na-K pump. Once K^+ enters the cell across the basolateral membrane, it may exit either across the apical membrane (K^+ secretion) or across the basolateral membrane (K^+ recycling). The cell controls the extent to which secretion occurs, in part by K^+ channels present in both the apical and the basolateral membranes. When apical K^+ channel activity is less than basolateral channel activity, K^+ recycling dominates. Indeed, in the basal state, the rate of active K^+ secretion is low because the apical K^+ channel activity is minimal in comparison with the K^+ channel activity in the basolateral membrane.

It is likely that aldosterone stimulates active K^+ secretion in surface epithelial cells of the large intestine, whereas cAMP enhances active K^+ secretion in crypt cells. In both cases, the rate-limiting step is the apical BK K^+ channel, and both secretagogues act by increasing K^+ channel activity.

Aldosterone The mineralocorticoid aldosterone enhances overall net K^+ secretion by two mechanisms. First, it increases **passive** K^+ secretion by increasing Na-K pump activity. The net effects are to increase the lumen-negative V_{te} and to enhance passive paracellular K^+ secretion (Fig. 44.6B). Second, aldosterone stimulates **active** K^+ secretion by increasing the activity of both apical K^+ channels and basolateral Na-K pumps (Fig. 44.6C).

cAMP and Ca²⁺ VIP and cholera enterotoxin both increase $[cAMP]_i$ and thus stimulate K^+ secretion. Increases in $[Ca^{2+}]_i$—induced, for example, by serotonin (or 5-hydroxytryptamine [5-HT])—also stimulate active K^+ secretion.

⊙ 44-2 Active K⁺ absorption takes place only in the distal portion of the colon and is energized by an apical H-K pump

As noted above, not only does the distal end of the colon actively secrete K^+, it also actively absorbs K^+. The balance between the two processes plays a role in overall K^+ homeostasis. Increases in dietary K^+ enhance both passive and active K^+ *secretion* (Fig. 44.6B and C). However, dietary K^+ depletion enhances active K^+ *absorption* (Fig. 44.6D). The mechanism of active K^+ absorption appears to be an exchange of luminal K^+ for intracellular H^+ across the apical membrane, mediated by an H-K pump (see ⊙ 5-9).

REGULATION OF INTESTINAL ION TRANSPORT

Chemical mediators from the enteric nervous system, endocrine cells, and immune cells in the lamina propria may be either secretagogues or absorptagogues

Numerous chemical mediators from several different sources regulate intestinal electrolyte transport. Some of these agonists are important both in health and in diarrheal disorders, and at times only quantitative differences separate normal regulatory control from the pathophysiology of diarrhea. These mediators may function in one or more modes: neural,

A PASSIVE K⁺ ABSORPTION

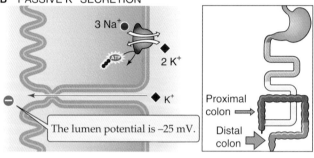

B PASSIVE K⁺ SECRETION

The lumen potential is –25 mV.

C ACTIVE K⁺ SECRETION

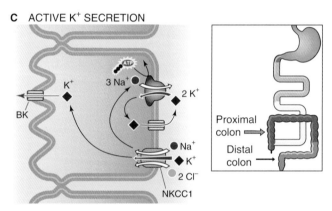

D ACTIVE K⁺ ABSORPTION

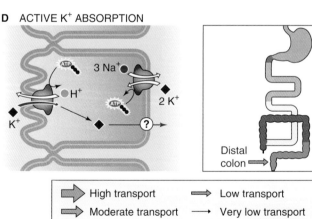

| ⇒ High transport | ⇒ Low transport |
| ⇒ Moderate transport | → Very low transport |

Figure 44.6 Cellular mechanisms of K⁺ secretion and absorption. The thickness of the *arrows* in the *insets* indicates the relative magnitude of different mechanisms of K⁺ flux in different segments.

TABLE 44.3 **Products of Lamina Propria Cells That Affect Intestinal Ion Transport**

CELL	PRODUCT
Macrophages	Prostaglandins O₂ radicals
Mast cells	Histamine
Neutrophils	Eicosanoids Platelet-activating factor
Fibroblasts	Eicosanoids Bradykinin

endocrine, paracrine, and perhaps autocrine. Most of these agonists (i.e., secretagogues) promote secretion, whereas some others (i.e., absorptagogues) enhance absorption.

The **enteric nervous system (ENS)** is important in the normal regulation of intestinal epithelial electrolyte transport. Activation of enteric secretomotor neurons results in the release of acetylcholine from mucosal neurons and in the induction of active Cl⁻ secretion (Fig. 44.5). Additional neurotransmitters, including VIP, 5-HT, and histamine, mediate ENS regulation of epithelial ion transport.

An example of regulation mediated by the **endocrine system** is the renin-angiotensin-aldosterone axis (see ⊙ 40-2). Both angiotensin and aldosterone regulate total-body Na⁺ homeostasis by stimulating Na⁺ absorption, angiotensin in the small intestine, and aldosterone in the colon.

The response of the intestine to angiotensin and aldosterone represents a classic endocrine feedback loop: dehydration results in increased levels of angiotensin and aldosterone, the primary effects of which are to stimulate fluid and Na⁺ absorption by both the renal tubules (see ⊙ 35-5) and the intestines. The result is restoration of total-body fluid and Na⁺ content.

Regulation of intestinal transport also occurs by **paracrine effects.** Endocrine cells constitute a small fraction of the total population of mucosal cells in the intestines. These endocrine cells contain several peptides and bioactive amines that are released in response to various stimuli. Relatively little is known about the biology of these cells, but gut distention can induce the release of one or more of these agonists (e.g., 5-HT). The effect of these agonists on adjacent surface epithelial cells represents a paracrine action.

Another example of paracrine regulation of intestinal fluid and electrolyte transport is the influence of **immune cells** in the *lamina propria* (Fig. 44.1). Table 44.3 lists these immune cells and some of the agonists that they release. The same agonist may be released from more than one cell, and individual cells produce multiple agonists. These agonists may activate epithelial cells directly or may activate other immune cells or enteric neurons.

Secretagogues can be classified by their type and by the intracellular second-messenger system that they stimulate

Several agonists induce the accumulation of fluid and electrolytes in the intestinal lumen (i.e., net secretion). These secretagogues are a diverse, heterogeneous group of compounds, but they can be effectively classified in two different ways: by the type of secretagogue and by the intracellular second messenger that these agonists activate.

Grouped according to type, the secretagogues fall into four categories: (1) bacterial exotoxins (i.e., enterotoxins), (2) hormones and neurotransmitters, (3) products of cells of the immune system, and (4) laxatives. Table 44.2 provides a partial list of these secretagogues. A **bacterial exotoxin** is a peptide that is produced and excreted by bacteria that can produce effects independently of the bacteria. An **enterotoxin** is an exotoxin that induces changes in intestinal fluid and electrolyte movement. For example, *E. coli* produces two distinct enterotoxins—the so-called **heat-labile** and **heat-stable toxins**—that induce fluid and electrolyte secretion via two distinct receptors and second-messenger systems.

We can also classify secretagogues according to the signal-transduction system that they activate after binding to a specific membrane receptor. As summarized in Table 44.2, the second messengers of these signal-transduction systems include cAMP, cGMP, and Ca^{2+}.

Although the secretagogues listed in Table 44.2 stimulate fluid and electrolyte secretion via one of three distinct second messengers (i.e., cAMP, cGMP, and Ca^{2+}), the *end effects* are quite similar. All three second-messenger systems stimulate active Cl^- secretion (Fig. 44.5) and inhibit electroneutral NaCl absorption (Fig. 44.3C). Both stimulation of Cl^- secretion and inhibition of electroneutral NaCl absorption have the same overall effect: *net secretion of fluid and electrolytes.*

CHAPTER 45

NUTRIENT DIGESTION AND ABSORPTION

Henry J. Binder and Charles M. Mansbach II[†]

The **digestive process**—the enzymatic conversion of complex dietary substances to a form that can be absorbed—is initiated by the sight, smell, and taste of food. Although some digestion (that of carbohydrates) begins in the mouth, most digestive processes occur in the small intestine. Digestion within the small intestine occurs in the *lumen,* mediated by pancreatic enzymes; at the small-intestinal *brush-border membrane* (membrane digestion), mediated by brush-border enzymes; and within the cytosol of intestinal epithelial cells (Fig. 45.1).

Multiple diseases can alter these digestive-absorptive processes and can thereby impair nutrient **assimilation.** Because of the substantial segmental distribution of nutrient absorption along the gastrointestinal tract (Fig. 45.2), the clinical manifestations of disease often reflect these segmental differences.

CARBOHYDRATE DIGESTION

Carbohydrates provide ~45% of total energy needs of Western diets and require hydrolysis to monosaccharides before absorption

We can classify dietary carbohydrates into two major groups: (1) the **monosaccharides** (monomers), and (2) the **oligosaccharides** (short polymers) and **polysaccharides** (long polymers). The small intestine can directly absorb the monomers but not the polymers. Some polymers are **digestible,** that is, the body can digest them to form the monomers that the small intestine can absorb. Other polymers are **nondigestible,** or "fiber." Approximately 45% to 60% of dietary carbohydrate is in the form of **starch,** which is a polysaccharide.

Most dietary oligosaccharides are the disaccharides sucrose and lactose, which represent 30% to 40% of dietary carbohydrates. **Sucrose** is table sugar, derived from sugar cane and sugar beets, whereas **lactose** is the sugar found in milk. The remaining carbohydrates are the monosaccharides **fructose** and **glucose,** which make up 5% to 10% of total carbohydrate intake. Because the small intestine can absorb only *monosaccharides,* all dietary carbohydrate must be digested to monosaccharides before absorption. The colon cannot absorb monosaccharides.

As we discuss below, the digestive process for dietary carbohydrates has two steps: (1) **intraluminal hydrolysis** of starch to oligosaccharides by salivary and pancreatic amylases (Fig. 45.3), and (2) so-called **membrane digestion** of oligosaccharides to monosaccharides by brush-border disaccharidases. The resulting carbohydrates are absorbed

by transport processes that are specific for certain monosaccharides. These transport pathways are located in the apical membrane of the small-intestinal villous epithelial cells.

Luminal digestion begins with the action of salivary amylase and finishes with pancreatic amylase

Acinar cells from both the salivary glands and pancreas synthesize and secrete α-amylases. Salivary and pancreatic amylases are secreted in an active form.

Salivary α-**amylase** in the mouth initiates starch digestion. Salivary amylase is inactivated by gastric acid but can be partially protected by complexing with oligosaccharides.

Pancreatic α-**amylase** completes starch digestion in the lumen of the small intestine. α-Amylase is an **endoenzyme** that hydrolyzes starch to **maltose, maltotriose,** and α-**limit dextrins.**

The intestine cannot absorb these products of amylase digestion of starch, and thus further digestion is required to produce substrates (i.e., monosaccharides) that the small intestine can absorb.

"Membrane digestion" involves hydrolysis of oligosaccharides to monosaccharides by brush-border disaccharidases

The human small intestine has three brush-border proteins with oligosaccharidase activity: lactase, glucoamylase (most often called maltase), and sucrase-isomaltase. These are all integral membrane proteins whose catalytic domains face the intestinal lumen. Sucrase-isomaltase is actually two enzymes—sucrase and isomaltase—bound together. Thus, four oligosaccharidase entities are present at the brush border (Fig. 45.3B).

The action of the four oligosaccharidases generates several monosaccharides. Whereas the hydrolysis products of maltose are two glucose residues, those of sucrose are glucose and fructose. The hydrolysis of lactose by lactase yields glucose and galactose.

The oligosaccharidases have a varying spatial distribution throughout the small intestine. In general, the abundance and activity of oligosaccharidases peak in the proximal jejunum and are considerably less in the duodenum and distal ileum. Oligosaccharidases are absent in the large intestine.

CARBOHYDRATE ABSORPTION

The three monosaccharide products of carbohydrate digestion—**glucose, galactose,** and **fructose**—are absorbed by

---

[†]Deceased.

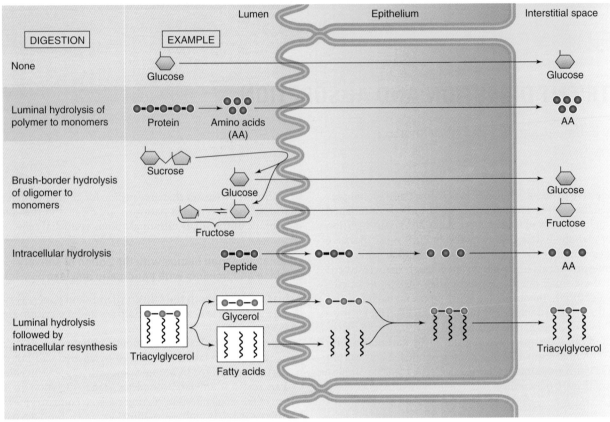

Figure 45.1   General mechanisms of digestion and absorption.

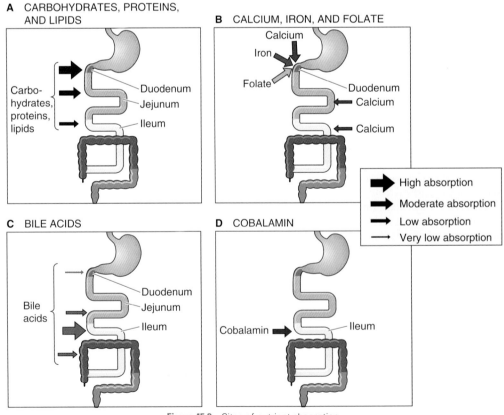

Figure 45.2   Sites of nutrient absorption.

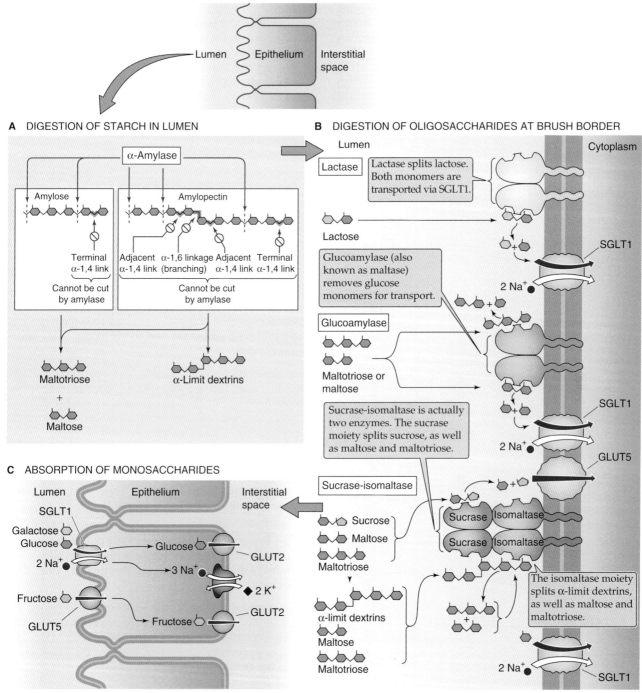

Figure 45.3 Digestion of carbohydrates to monosaccharides.

the small intestine in a two-step process involving their uptake across the apical membrane into the epithelial cell and their coordinated exit across the basolateral membrane (Fig. 45.3C). Na/glucose transporter 1 (SGLT1) is the membrane protein responsible for glucose and galactose uptake at the *apical membrane.* The exit of all three monosaccharides across the *basolateral membrane* uses a facilitated sugar transporter (GLUT2). Because SGLT1 cannot carry fructose, the apical step of fructose absorption occurs by the facilitated diffusion of fructose via GLUT5. Thus, although two different apical membrane transport mechanisms exist for glucose

and fructose uptake, a single transporter (GLUT2) is responsible for the movement of both monosaccharides across the basolateral membrane.

PROTEIN DIGESTION

Proteins require hydrolysis to oligopeptides or amino acids before absorption in the small intestine

With the exception of antigenic amounts of dietary protein that are absorbed intact, proteins must first be digested into their constituent oligopeptides and amino acids before being taken up by the enterocytes. Digestion-absorption occurs through four major pathways. First, several *luminal* enzymes (i.e., proteases) from the stomach and pancreas may hydrolyze proteins to peptides and then to amino acids, which are then absorbed (Fig. 45.4). Second, *luminal* enzymes may digest proteins to peptides, but enzymes present at the *brush border* digest the peptides to amino acids, which are then absorbed. Third, *luminal* enzymes may digest proteins to peptides, which are themselves taken up as oligopeptides by the enterocytes. Further digestion of the oligopeptides by cytosolic enzymes yields intracellular amino acids, which are moved by transporters across the basolateral membrane into the blood. Fourth, luminal enzymes may digest dietary proteins to oligopeptides, which are taken up by enterocytes via an endocytotic process and moved directly into the blood. Overall, protein digestion-absorption is very efficient; <4% of ingested nitrogen is excreted in the stool.

The protein that is digested and absorbed in the small intestine comes from both dietary and endogenous sources. Dietary protein in developed countries amounts to 70 to 100 g/day. This amount is far in excess of minimum daily requirements and represents 10% to 15% of energy intake.

In addition to protein from dietary sources, significant amounts of endogenous protein are secreted into the gastrointestinal tract, then conserved by protein digestion and absorption. Such endogenous sources represent ~50% of the total protein entering the small intestine and include enzymes, hormones, and immunoglobulins present in salivary, gastric, pancreatic, biliary, and jejunal secretions. A second large source of endogenous protein is desquamated intestinal epithelial cells as well as plasma proteins that the small intestine secretes.

Luminal digestion of protein involves both gastric and pancreatic proteases and yields amino acids and oligopeptides

Five pancreatic enzymes (Table 45.1) participate in protein digestion and are secreted as inactive proenzymes. Trypsinogen is initially activated by a jejunal brush-border enzyme, enterokinase (enteropeptidase), by the cleavage of a hexapeptide, thereby yielding trypsin. **Trypsin** not only autoactivates trypsinogen, but also activates the other pancreatic proteolytic proenzymes. The secretion of proteolytic enzymes as proenzymes, with subsequent luminal activation, prevents pancreatic **autodigestion** before enzyme secretion into the intestine.

⦿ 45-1 Brush-border peptidases fully digest some oligopeptides to amino acids, whereas cytosolic peptidases digest oligopeptides that directly enter the enterocyte

Small peptides present in the small-intestinal lumen after digestion by gastric and pancreatic proteases undergo further hydrolysis by peptidases at the brush border (Fig. 45.4). Multiple peptidases are present both on the brush border and in the cytoplasm of villous epithelial cells.

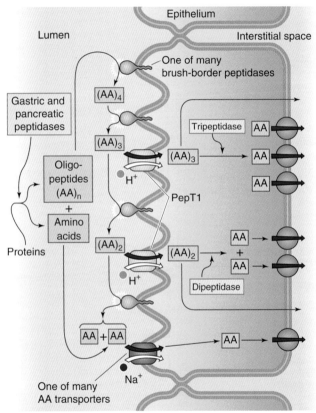

Figure 45.4 Action of luminal, brush-border, and cytosolic peptidases. *AA,* Single amino acids; *(AA)ₙ,* oligopeptides.

TABLE 45.1 Pancreatic Peptidases

PROENZYME	ACTIVATING AGENT	ACTIVE ENZYME	ACTION	PRODUCTS
Trypsinogen	Enteropeptidase (i.e., enterokinase from jejunum) and trypsin	Trypsin	Endopeptidase	Oligopeptides (2–6 amino acids)
Chymotrypsinogen	Trypsin	Chymotrypsin	Endopeptidase	Oligopeptides (2–6 amino acids)
Proelastase	Trypsin	Elastase	Endopeptidase	Oligopeptides (2–6 amino acids)
Procarboxypeptidase A	Trypsin	Carboxypeptidase A	Exopeptidase	Single amino acids
Procarboxypeptidase B	Trypsin	Carboxypeptidase B	Exopeptidase	Single amino acids

A transporter PepT1 on the apical membrane of enterocytes can take up small oligopeptides, primarily dipeptides and tripeptides. Once inside the cell, these oligopeptides may be further digested by *cytoplasmic* peptidases.

⊙ 45-2 PROTEIN, PEPTIDE, AND AMINO-ACID ABSORPTION

Absorption of whole protein by apical endocytosis occurs primarily during the neonatal period

During the postnatal period, intestinal epithelial cells absorb protein by endocytosis (Fig. 45.5), a process that provides a mechanism for transfer of passive immunity from mother to child. The uptake of intact protein by the epithelial cell ceases by the sixth month; the cessation of this protein uptake, called *closure,* is hormonally mediated. For example, administration of corticosteroids during the postnatal period induces closure and reduces the time that the intestine can absorb significant amounts of whole protein.

The adult intestine can absorb finite amounts of intact protein and polypeptides. Uncertainty exists regarding the cellular route of absorption, as well as the relationship of the mechanism of protein uptake in adults to that in neonates. Enterocytes can take up by endocytosis a small amount of intact protein, most of which is degraded in lysosomes (Fig. 45.5). However, a small amount of intact protein appears in the interstitial space. The uptake of intact protein also occurs through a second, more specialized route via **M cells.** M cells have limited ability for lysosomal protein degradation; rather, they package ingested proteins (i.e., antigens) in clathrin-coated vesicles, which they secrete at their basolateral membranes into the lamina propria. There, immunocompetent cells process the target antigens and transfer them to lymphocytes to initiate an immune response. Although protein uptake in adults may not have nutritional value, such uptake is clearly important in mucosal immunity and probably is involved in one or more disease processes.

The apical absorption of dipeptides, tripeptides, and tetrapeptides occurs via an H⁺-driven cotransporter

Virtually all absorbed protein products exit the villous epithelial cell and enter the blood as individual amino acids. Substantial portions of these amino acids are released in the lumen of the small intestine by luminal proteases and brush-border peptidases and move across the apical membranes of enterocytes via several amino-acid transport systems (Fig. 45.4). However, substantial amounts of protein are absorbed from the intestinal lumen as dipeptides, tripeptides, or tetrapeptides and then hydrolyzed to amino acids by intracellular peptidases. The transporter responsible for the uptake of luminal oligopeptides is distinct from the various amino-acid transporters.

Oligopeptide uptake is an active process driven by a proton gradient. Oligopeptide uptake occurs via an apical **H/oligopeptide cotransporter** known as **PepT1.** PepT1 also contributes to the intestinal uptake of certain dipeptide-like antibiotics (e.g., oral amino-substituted cephalosporins).

⊙ 45-3 Enterocytes absorb amino acids via group-specific apical and basolateral transporters

The absorption of amino acids across the small intestine requires sequential movement across both the apical and basolateral membranes of the villous epithelial cell. Although the amino-acid transport systems have overlapping affinities for various amino acids, the consensus is that at least seven distinct transport systems are present at the apical membrane.

At the basolateral membrane, amino acids exit enterocytes via Na⁺-independent transporters.

⊙ 45-4 LIPID DIGESTION

Natural lipids of biological origin are sparingly soluble in water

Lipids in the diet are derived from animals or plants and are composed of carbon, hydrogen, and a smaller amount of oxygen. Some lipids also contain small but functionally important amounts of nitrogen and phosphorus (Fig. 45.6).

⊙ 45-5 Dietary lipids are predominantly triacylglycerols

Of the fat in an adult diet, >90% are **triacylglycerols (TAGs),** which are commonly long-chain fatty acyl esters of glycerol. Typical adult Western diets contain ~140 g of fat per day (providing ~60% of the energy), which is more than the recommended intake of less than ~70 g of fat per day (<30% of total dietary calories).

Approximately 5% (4 to 6 g/day) of dietary lipids come from cell membranes and are **phospholipids.** The typical Western diet contains ~0.5 g of unesterified **cholesterol.** Traces of **lipovitamins** and **provitamins** (e.g., carotene) are present in dietary fat, which may also contain lipid-soluble toxins and carcinogens from the environment.

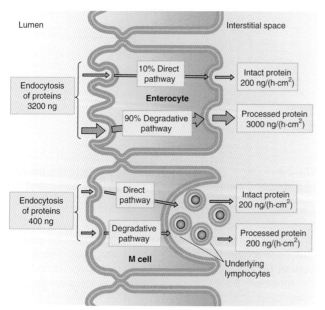

Figure 45.5 Absorption of whole proteins by enterocytes and specialized M cells.

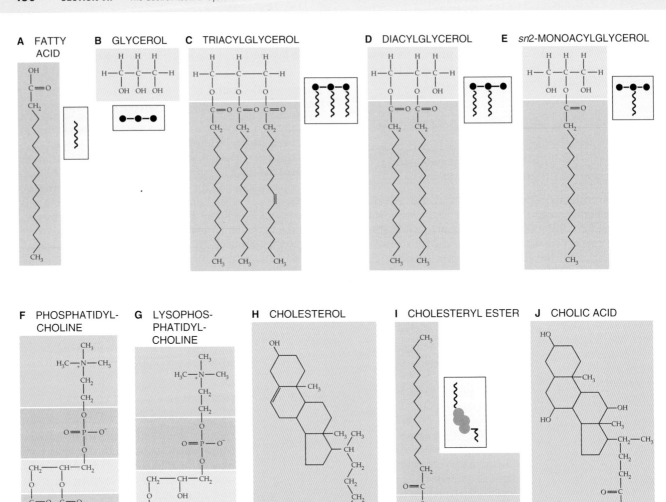

Figure 45.6 Chemical formulas of some common lipids.

Endogenous lipids are phospholipids and cholesterol from bile and membrane lipids from desquamated intestinal epithelial cells

The bile secreted into the intestine plays a key role in the assimilation of dietary lipids. This bile contains phospholipid (10 to 15 g/day)—predominantly phosphatidylcholine—and unesterified cholesterol (1 to 2 g/day). Quantitatively, these biliary lipids exceed those present in the diet by 2- to 4-fold. Membrane lipids from desquamated intestinal cells account for a further 2 to 6 g of lipid for digestion. Dead bacteria contribute ~10 g/day of lipids, mainly in the colon.

The mechanical disruption of dietary lipids in the mouth and stomach produces an emulsion of lipid particles

The central process in the digestion of lipids is their hydrolysis in the aqueous milieu of the intestinal lumen. Lipid hydrolysis is catalyzed by **lipases** secreted by the glands and cells of the upper gastrointestinal tract. The products of lipolysis diffuse through the aqueous content of the intestinal lumen and enter the enterocyte for further processing.

A key step preliminary to lipid digestion is the transformation of ingested solid fat and oil masses into an emulsion of fine oil droplets in water. The **emulsification** of dietary fats begins with food preparation (grinding, marinating, blending, and cooking), followed by chewing and gastric churning caused by antral peristalsis against a closed pylorus. Emulsification of ingested lipids is enhanced when muscular movements of the stomach intermittently squirt the gastric contents into the duodenum and, conversely, when peristalsis of the duodenum propels the duodenal contents in retrograde fashion into the stomach through the narrow orifice of a contracted pylorus. The grinding action of the antrum also mixes food with the various digestive enzymes derived from the mouth and stomach. Intestinal peristalsis mixes luminal contents with pancreatic and biliary secretions. Together, these mechanical processes reduce the size of the lipid droplets.

In the stomach, both **lingual lipase** that is swallowed and a gastric lipase secreted by gastric chief cells digest substantial amounts of lipid. The process of fat digestion that begins in the stomach is completed in the proximal small intestine, predominantly by enzymes synthesized and secreted by pancreatic acinar cells.

Once the fatty acids generated in the stomach reach the duodenum, they trigger the release of **CCK** and gastric inhibitory polypeptide (GIP) from the duodenal mucosa. CCK stimulates the *flow of bile* into the duodenum by causing the gallbladder to contract and the sphincter of Oddi to relax. CCK also stimulates the *secretion of pancreatic enzymes,* including lipases and esterases. As we discuss below, LCFAs also facilitate the lipolytic action of pancreatic lipase.

The major lipolytic enzyme of pancreatic juice is **pancreatic (alkaline) lipase,** sometimes referred to as colipase-dependent pancreatic lipase. Full lipolytic activity of pancreatic lipase requires the presence of the small (10-kDa) protein cofactor called **colipase,** as well as an alkaline pH, Ca^{2+}, bile salts, and fatty acids. The pancreas secretes colipase in the pro form (i.e., procolipase). Trypsin cleaves procolipase into colipase

The pancreas secretes other enzymes that hydrolyze lipid esters. **Carboxyl ester hydrolase** is a pancreatic enzyme that is active against a wide range of esters. Among the many products of reactions catalyzed by this enzyme are free cholesterol and free glycerol.

The pancreas also secretes **phospholipase A_2 (PLA$_2$),** which is active against glycerophospholipids. Pancreatic PLA$_2$, secreted as a trypsin-activatable proenzyme, is effective at alkaline pH and requires bile salts and Ca^{2+} for activity.

⊙ 45-6 LIPID ABSORPTION

Products of lipolysis enter the bulk water phase of the intestinal lumen as vesicles, mixed micelles, and monomers

After their secretion in pancreatic juice and bile, respectively, the various activated pancreatic lipases and biliary bile salts, along with phosphatidylcholine and cholesterol adsorb to the surface of the **emulsion droplets** arriving from the stomach (Fig. 45.7A). A multilamellar liquid crystalline layer of fatty acids, monoacylglycerols (MAGs), lysophosphatidylcholine,

cholesterol (see Fig. 45.6), and possibly bile salts builds up on the surface of the emulsion particle. This liquid crystalline layer buds off as a **multilamellar liquid crystal vesicle** (Fig. 45.7B). Bile-salt micelles transform these multilamellar vesicles into **unilamellar vesicles** (Fig. 45.7C), which are single-lipid bilayers, and then into **mixed micelles** (Fig. 45.7D) composed of bile salts and mixed lipids (i.e., fatty acids, MAGs, lysophospholipids, and cholesterol).

Lipids diffuse as mixed micelles and monomers through unstirred layers before crossing the jejunal enterocyte brush border

To reach the interior of the enterocyte, lipolytic products must cross several barriers. These include (1) the mucous gel layer that lines the intestinal epithelial surface, (2) the unstirred water layer (disequilibrium zone) contiguous with the enterocyte's apical membrane, and (3) the apical membrane itself.

When the fatty-acid/bile-salt mixed micelles reach the enterocyte surface, they encounter an acidic microclimate generated by Na-H exchange at the brush-border membrane. It is postulated that fatty acids now become protonated and leave the mixed micelle to enter the enterocyte. At least three integral membrane proteins promote the uptake of fatty acids (Fig. 45.8): **fatty-acid translocase (FAT),** the plasma-membrane **fatty acid–binding protein (FABPpm),** and **fatty-acid transport proteins (FATPs).** Similarly, unesterified cholesterol and lysophospholipids must leave the micelle carrier to enter the enterocyte as monomers. The bile salts are absorbed via active transport by the apical, Na^+-dependent bile-acid transporter (ASBT) in the distal ileum (see Fig. 46.9).

The enterocyte re-esterifies lipid components and assembles them into chylomicrons

The assimilation of fats, as described thus far, has been a process of disassembly of energy-dense, water-insoluble lipid macromolecular aggregates into monomers for intestinal absorption. The enterocyte elegantly reverses this process in the formation of chylomicrons (Fig. 45.9).

⊙ 45-7 The enterocyte secretes chylomicrons into the lymphatics during feeding and secretes VLDLs during fasting

Chylomicrons are the largest of the five lipoprotein particles in the bloodstream. Vesicles carrying mature chylomicrons discharge their contents from the enterocyte into the lamina propria via exocytosis at the basolateral membrane. Chylomicrons are too large to pass through the fenestrae of blood capillaries, and thus they enter **lymph** through the larger interendothelial channels of the lymphatic capillaries. In both the fed and fasted states, the intestine also secretes into the lymph **VLDLs,** which are smaller (30 to 80 nm) than chylomicrons. VLDLs have a protein and lipid composition similar to that of chylomicrons (see Table 46.1) but are synthesized independently and carry mainly endogenous (as opposed to dietary) lipids.

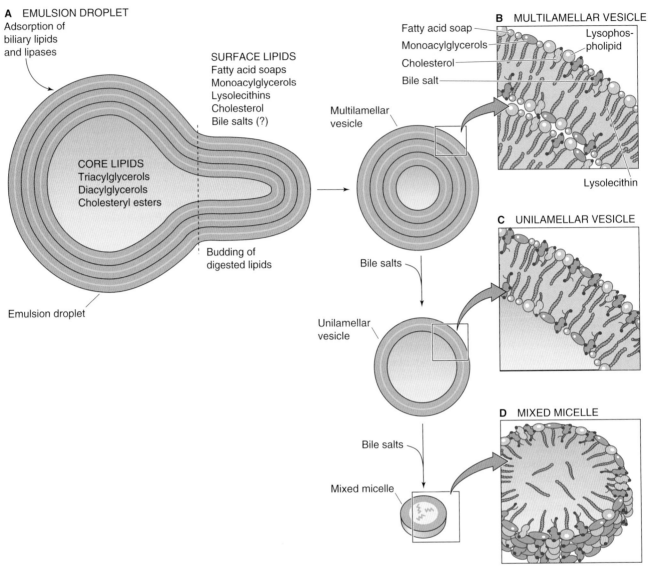

A   EMULSION DROPLET

Adsorption of biliary lipids and lipases

SURFACE LIPIDS
Fatty acid soaps
Monoacylglycerols
Lysolecithins
Cholesterol
Bile salts (?)

CORE LIPIDS
Triacylglycerols
Diacylglycerols
Cholesteryl esters

Budding of digested lipids

Emulsion droplet

B   MULTILAMELLAR VESICLE

Fatty acid soap
Monoacylglycerols
Cholesterol
Bile salt

Lysophos-pholipid

Multilamellar vesicle

Lysolecithin

C   UNILAMELLAR VESICLE

Bile salts

Unilamellar vesicle

D   MIXED MICELLE

Bile salts

Mixed micelle

Figure 45.7   Breakdown of emulsion droplets to mixed micelles.

DIGESTION AND ABSORPTION OF VITAMINS AND MINERALS

⊙ 45-8 Intestinal absorption of fat-soluble vitamins follows the pathways of lipid absorption and transport

Table 45.2 summarizes some characteristics of the 13 recognized vitamins.

The fat-soluble vitamins A, D, E, and K represent a class of vitamins, the absorption of which relies on the lipid-absorption process discussed in the preceding subchapter.

After ingestion, fat-soluble vitamins are released from their association with proteins by the acidity of gastric juice or by proteolysis. In the proximal small intestine, fat-soluble vitamins incorporate with other lipid products into emulsion droplets, vesicles, and mixed micelles, which ferry them to the enterocyte surface for uptake.

Enterocytes take up fat-soluble vitamins by simple diffusion or via transporters. After entry into the enterocyte, fat-soluble vitamins diffuse to the SER attached to carrier proteins. In the SER, the vitamins associate with lipid droplets that form nascent chylomicrons and VLDLs, which then translocate through the Golgi and secretory vesicles for exocytosis into lymph.

Once in the systemic blood circulation, the fat-soluble vitamins A, D, E, and K enter the liver by receptor-mediated endocytosis of chylomicrons or remnant chylomicrons.

Ca^{2+} absorption, regulated primarily by vitamin D, occurs by active transport in the duodenum and by diffusion throughout the small intestine

⊙ 45-9 Table 45.3 summarizes some characteristics of 11 essential minerals.

The physiological importance and complex regulation of Ca^{2+} and vitamin D are discussed in Chapter 52. The Ca^{2+} load presented to the small intestine is derived from dietary sources and digestive secretions. Most of the dietary Ca^{2+} (~1000 mg/day) comes from milk and milk products (see Fig. 52.1). However, not all of this ingested Ca^{2+} is bioavailable. The small intestine absorbs ~500 mg/day of Ca^{2+}, but also secretes ~325 mg/day of Ca^{2+}. Thus, the net uptake is ~175 mg/day.

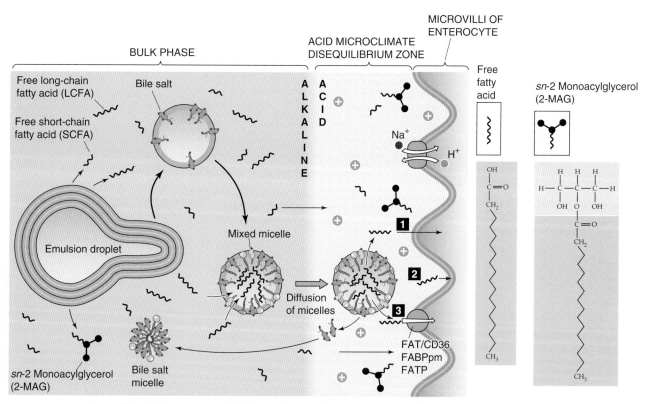

Figure 45.8 Micellar transport of lipid breakdown products to the surface of the enterocyte. Mixed micelles carry lipids through the acidic unstirred layer to the surface of the enterocyte. The lipids enter the enterocyte by (1) nonionic diffusion, (2) incorporation into the enterocyte membrane ("collision"), or (3) carrier-mediated transport.

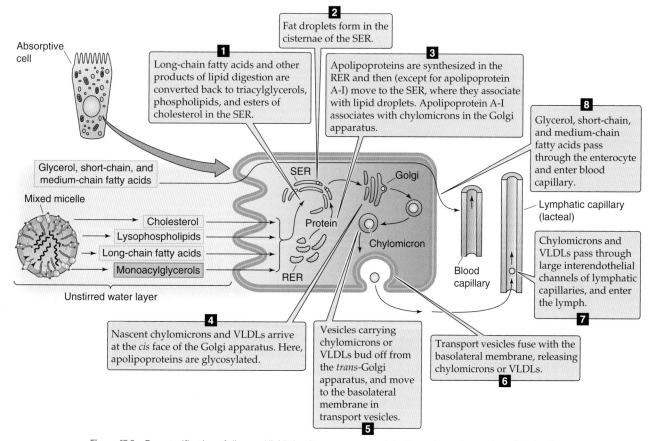

Figure 45.9 Re-esterification of digested lipids by the enterocyte and the formation and secretion of chylomicrons. *RER*, Rough endoplasmic reticulum; *SER*, smooth endoplasmic reticulum.

TABLE 45.2 Vitamins

VITAMIN	ROLE	RDA	EFFECT OF DEFICIENCY
A (retinol)	Retinal pigment	Male: 1000 µg Female: 800 µg	Follicular hyperkeratosis, night blindness
B_1 (thiamine)	Coenzyme in decarboxylation of pyruvate and α-keto acids	Male: 1.5 mg Female: 1.1 mg	Beriberi
B_2 (riboflavin)	Component of coenzymes FAD and FMN, H carriers in mitochondria	Male: 1.7 mg Female: 1.3 mg	Hyperemia of nasopharyngeal mucosa, normocytic anemia
B_3 (niacin, nicotinic acid)	Component of coenzymes NAD and NADP, H carriers in mitochondria	Male: 19 mg Female: 15 mg	Pellagra
B_6 (pyridoxine)	Coenzyme in transamination for synthesis of amino acids	Male: 2 mg Female: 1.6 mg	Stomatitis, glossitis, normocytic anemia
B_{12} (cobalamin)	Coenzyme in reduction of ribonucleotides to deoxyribonucleotides. Promotes formation of erythrocytes, myelin	2 µg	Pernicious anemia (a megaloblastic anemia)
C (ascorbic acid)	Coenzyme in formation of hydroxyproline used in collagen	60 mg	Scurvy
D (1,25-dihydroxy-cholecalciferol; see ◉ 52-8)	Ca^{2+} absorption	5–10 µg	Rickets
E (α-tocopherol)	Antioxidant: thought to prevent oxidation of unsaturated fatty acids	Male: 10 mg Female: 8 mg	Peripheral neuropathy
K (K_1 = phylloquinone, K_2 = various menaquinones)	Clotting: necessary for synthesis by liver of prothrombin and factors VII, IX, and X (see Table 18.3)	Male: 70–80 µg Female: 60–65 µg	Hemorrhagic disease
Folate	Backbone used to synthesize purines and thymine	Male: 200 µg Female: 180 µg Pregnancy: 400 µg	Megaloblastic anemia
Biotin	Coenzyme in reactions	30–100 µg[a]	Neurological changes
Pantothenic acid	Component of CoA; necessary for carbohydrate and fat metabolism involving acetyl CoA; amino-acid synthesis	4–7 mg[a]	Abdominal pain, vomiting, neurological signs

[a]Safe and allowable range.

FAD, Flavin adenine dinucleotide; *FMN,* flavin mononucleotide; *NAD,* nicotinamide adenine dinucleotide; *NADP,* nicotinamide adenine dinucleotide phosphate.

◉ **45-10** Active transcellular uptake of Ca^{2+} occurs only in the epithelial cells of the duodenum, but Ca^{2+} is absorbed by passive paracellular diffusion throughout the small intestine. The *active* transport of Ca^{2+} across the villous epithelial cells of the duodenum is transcellular and is under the control of vitamin D—primarily via genomic effects (see ◉ 3-28). Transcellular Ca^{2+} absorption involves three steps (Fig. 45.10). The uptake of Ca^{2+} across the apical membrane occurs via **TRPV6 Ca^{2+} channels,** driven by the electrochemical gradient between the lumen and the cell. Cytosolic Ca^{2+} then binds to a protein called **calbindin,** which buffers intracellular Ca^{2+}. This step is important because it allows levels of unbound (i.e., free) intracellular Ca^{2+} to remain rather low despite large transcellular

fluxes of Ca^{2+}. A **Ca pump** and an **Na-Ca exchanger** on the basolateral membrane then extrude the Ca^{2+} from the cell into the interstitial fluid. The active form of vitamin D—1,25-dihydroxyvitamin D—stimulates all three steps of the transcellular pathway, but its most important effect is to enhance the second step by increasing the synthesis of calbindin.

The *passive* absorption of Ca^{2+} throughout the small intestine occurs via the paracellular pathway, which is *not* under the control of vitamin D.

Vitamin D itself is a fat-soluble vitamin that is absorbed mainly in the jejunum. In addition, the skin synthesizes vitamin D_3 from cholesterol in a process that requires ultraviolet light (see ◉ 52-8).

TABLE 45.3 Essential Minerals

MINERAL	ROLE	RDA
Ca	Bone mineralization (see ⊙ **52-1**), intracellular signaling (see ⊙ **3-14**)	800–1200 mg
Cr	Possibly a cofactor in metabolism of carbohydrates, protein, lipids	50–200 μg
Cu	Enzyme cofactor (e.g., superoxide dismutase)	1.5–3 mg
Fe	Constituent of hemoglobin (see ⊙ **29-1**) and cytochromes (see ⊙ **46-2**)	Male: 10 mg Female (childbearing age): 15 mg
I	Constituent of thyroid hormones (see ⊙ **49-1**)	150 μg
Mg	Complexes with ATP	Male: ~350 mg Female: ~280 mg
Mn	Antioxidant	2–5 mg
Mo	Cofactor in carbon, nitrogen, and sulfur metabolism	75–250 μg
P	Bone mineralization (see ⊙ **52-1**)	800–1000 mg
Se	Antioxidant	Male: 70 μg Female: 55 μg
Zn	Antioxidant, component of transcription factors, enzyme cofactor	Male: 15 mg Female: 12 mg

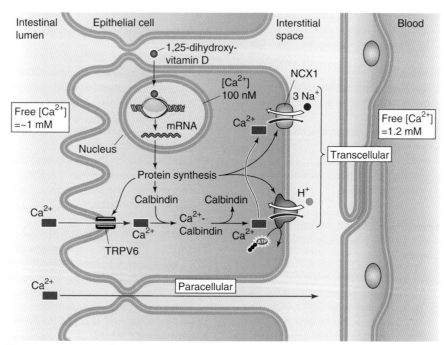

Figure 45.10 Active Ca^{2+} uptake in the duodenum.

CHAPTER 46

HEPATOBILIARY FUNCTION

Frederick J. Suchy

OVERVIEW OF LIVER PHYSIOLOGY

The liver weighs between 1200 and 1500 g, and is strategically situated in the circulatory system to receive the portal blood that drains the stomach, small intestine, large intestine, pancreas, and spleen. In this position, the liver plays a key role in handling foodstuffs assimilated by the small intestine. In addition, the liver serves as a chemical factory, an excretory system, an exocrine gland, and an endocrine gland.

The liver biotransforms and degrades substances taken up from blood and either returns them to the circulation or excretes them into bile

A major function of the liver is to metabolize, detoxify, and inactivate both endogenous compounds (e.g., steroids and other hormones) and exogenous substances (e.g., drugs and toxins). In addition, the phagocytic Kupffer cells provide an important mechanism to remove bacteria, endotoxins, parasites, and aging red blood cells.

The liver has the capacity to convert important hormones and vitamins into a more active form (e.g., hydroxylation of vitamin D).

Bile is a complex secretory product produced by the liver. Biliary secretion has two principal functions: (1) elimination of many endogenous and exogenous waste products, such as bilirubin and cholesterol, and (2) promotion of digestion and absorption of lipids from the intestine.

The liver stores carbohydrates, lipids, vitamins, and minerals; it synthesizes carbohydrates, protein, and intermediary metabolites

The liver avidly extracts carbohydrates, peptides, vitamins, and some lipids from portal blood. Depending on the metabolic requirements of the body, these substrates may be stored by the hepatocytes or released into the bloodstream either unbound (e.g., glucose) or associated with a carrier molecule (e.g., a triacylglycerol molecule complexed to a lipoprotein).

The liver also synthesizes many substances that are essential to the metabolic demands of the body. These substances include albumin, coagulation factors, and other plasma proteins; glucose; cholesterol; fatty acids for triacylglycerol biosynthesis; and phospholipids. The liver also produces ketone bodies, which can be used by the central nervous system during periods of fasting.

FUNCTIONAL ANATOMY OF THE LIVER AND BILIARY TREE

Hepatocytes are secretory epithelial cells separating the lumen of bile canaliculi from the fenestrated endothelium of sinusoids

A classic hepatic lobule is a hexagon in cross section (Fig. 46.1A) with a branch of the hepatic vein at its center and, at each of the six corners, triads composed of branches of the hepatic artery, portal vein, and bile duct. Hepatocytes account for ~80% of the parenchymal volume in human liver. Hepatocytes form an epithelium, one cell thick, that constitutes a functional barrier between two fluid compartments: the **canalicular lumen** containing bile, and the **sinusoid** containing blood (Fig. 46.1B). Hepatocytes significantly alter the composition of these fluids by vectorial transport of solutes across the hepatocyte. This vectorial transport depends on the polarized distribution of specific transport mechanisms and receptors that are localized to the **apical membrane** that faces the canalicular lumen and the **basolateral membrane** that faces the pericellular space between hepatocytes and the blood-filled sinusoid (Fig. 46.1B and C).

The **space of Disse** (Fig. 46.1B), or perisinusoidal space, is the extracellular gap between the endothelial cells lining the sinusoids and the basolateral membranes of the hepatocytes. These basolateral membranes have microvilli that greatly amplify the surface area, and project into the space of Disse to facilitate contact with the solutes in sinusoidal blood.

The bile canaliculi, into which bile is initially secreted, are formed by the apical membranes of adjoining hepatocytes (Fig. 46.1B and C). Two adjacent hepatocytes form a canaliculus, ~1 μm, in diameter by juxtaposing their groove-like apical membranes along their common face. The canaliculi run along the contiguous surfaces of hepatocytes and communicate to form a three-dimensional tubular network. Its extensive microvillous structure greatly amplifies its surface area.

The seal that joins the apical membranes of two juxtaposed hepatocytes and separates the canalicular lumen from the pericellular space comprises several elements, including **tight junctions** (Fig. 46.1D) and desmosomes (see ⊙ 2-20). Specialized structures called *gap junctions* (see ⊙ 2-19) allow functional communication between adjacent hepatocytes.

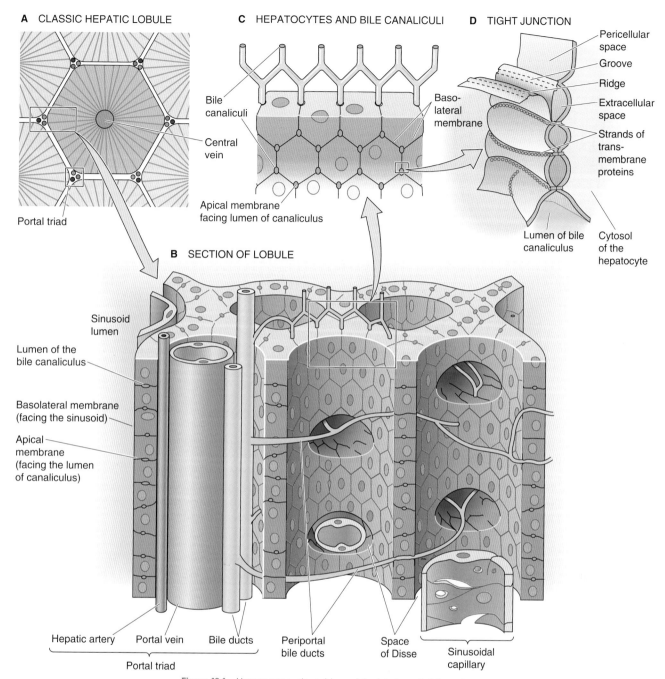

A CLASSIC HEPATIC LOBULE

Portal triad

Central vein

C HEPATOCYTES AND BILE CANALICULI

Bile canaliculi

Baso-lateral membrane

Apical membrane facing lumen of canaliculus

D TIGHT JUNCTION

Pericellular space

Groove

Ridge

Extracellular space

Strands of trans-membrane proteins

Lumen of bile canaliculus

Cytosol of the hepatocyte

B SECTION OF LOBULE

Sinusoid lumen

Lumen of the bile canaliculus

Basolateral membrane (facing the sinusoid)

Apical membrane (facing the lumen of canaliculus)

Hepatic artery   Portal vein   Bile ducts

Portal triad

Periportal bile ducts

Space of Disse

Sinusoidal capillary

Figure 46.1   Hepatocytes, sinusoids, and the intrahepatic bile system.

⊙ 46-1 The liver has a dual blood supply, but a single venous drainage system

The blood supply to the liver has two sources. The **portal vein** contributes ~75% of the total circulation to the liver; the **hepatic artery** contributes the other 25%. Blood from portal venules and hepatic arterioles combines in a complex network of hepatic sinusoids. Blood from these sinusoids converges on terminal hepatic venules (or **central veins;** Fig. 46.1A), which, in turn, join to form the **hepatic veins.** Branches of the portal vein, hepatic artery, and a bile duct—the "portal triad" (Fig. 46.1A and B)—as well as lymphatics and nerves, travel together as a **portal tract.**

Bile drains from canaliculi into small terminal ductules, then into larger ducts, and eventually, via a single common duct, into the duodenum

The adult human liver has >2 km of bile ductules and ducts, with a volume of ~20 cm^3 and a macroscopic surface area of ~400 cm^2. Microvilli at the apical surface magnify this area by ~5.5-fold.

The **canaliculi** into which bile is secreted form a three-dimensional polygonal meshwork of tubes between hepatocytes, with many anastomotic interconnections (Fig. 46.1). From the canaliculi, the bile enters the small terminal bile **ductules** (i.e., **canals of Hering**), which have a basement membrane and in cross section are surrounded by three to six

A DUCTULES AND SMALL DUCTS   **B** LARGE DUCTS AND GALLBLADDER

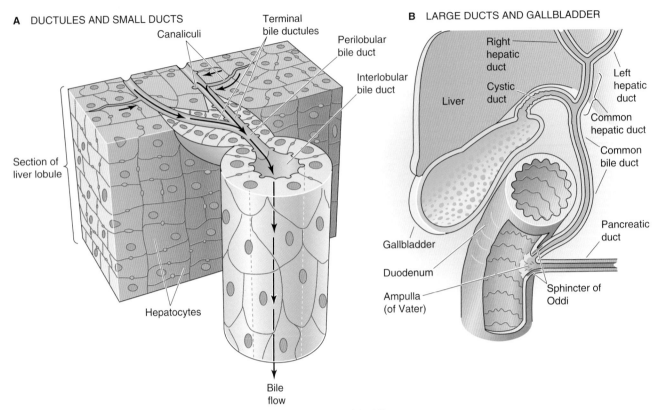

Figure. 46.2 Structure of the biliary tree.

ductal epithelial cells or hepatocytes (Fig. 46.2A). The canals of Hering then empty into a system of **perilobular ducts,** which, in turn, drain into interlobular bile ducts. The **interlobular bile ducts** form a richly anastomosing network that closely surrounds the branches of the portal vein. These bile ducts are lined by a layer of cuboidal or columnar epithelium that has microvillous architecture on its luminal surface.

The interlobular bile ducts unite to form larger and larger ducts, first the septal ducts and then the lobar ducts, two hepatic ducts, and finally a common hepatic duct (Fig. 46.2B). Along the biliary tree, the biliary epithelial cells, or **cholangiocytes,** are similar in their fine structure except for size and height. Tight junctions between cholangiocytes limit the exchange of water and solutes between plasma and bile.

The **common hepatic duct** emerges from the union of the right and left hepatic ducts. It merges with the cystic duct emanating from the gallbladder to form the common bile duct. In adults, the **common bile duct** is quite large, ~7 cm in length and ~0.5 to 1.5 cm in diameter. In most individuals, the common bile duct and the pancreatic duct merge before forming a common antrum known as the **ampulla of Vater.** At the point of transit through the duodenal wall, this common channel is surrounded by longitudinal and circular layers of smooth muscle, the so-called **sphincter of Oddi.** This sphincter constricts the lumen of the bile duct and thus regulates the flow of bile into the duodenum. The hormone cholecystokinin (CCK) relaxes the sphincter of Oddi via a non-adrenergic, non-cholinergic neural pathway (see ⊙ **14-8**) involving vasoactive intestinal peptide (VIP).

The **gallbladder** has a capacity of 30 to 50 mL in adults. The gallbladder is connected at its neck to the **cystic duct,** which empties into the common bile duct (Fig. 46.2B). The cystic duct maintains continuity with the surface columnar epithelium, lamina propria, muscularis, and serosa of the gallbladder. Instead of a sphincter, the gallbladder has, at its neck, a spiral valve—**the valve of Heister**—which regulates flow into and out of the gallbladder.

UPTAKE, PROCESSING, AND SECRETION OF COMPOUNDS BY HEPATOCYTES

The liver metabolizes an enormous variety of compounds that are brought to it by the portal and systemic circulations. The hepatocyte handles these molecules in four major steps (Fig. 46.3A): (1) the hepatocyte imports the compound from the blood across its basolateral (i.e., sinusoidal) membrane, (2) the hepatocyte transports the material within the cell, (3) the hepatocyte may chemically modify or degrade the compound intracellularly, and (4) the hepatocyte excretes the molecule or its product or products into the bile across the apical (i.e., canalicular) membrane.

An Na-K pump at the basolateral membranes of hepatocytes provides the energy for transporting a wide variety of solutes via channels and transporters

The hepatocyte is endowed with a host of transporters that are necessary for basic housekeeping functions. To the extent that these transporters are restricted to either the apical or basolateral membrane, they have the potential of participating in net transepithelial transport.

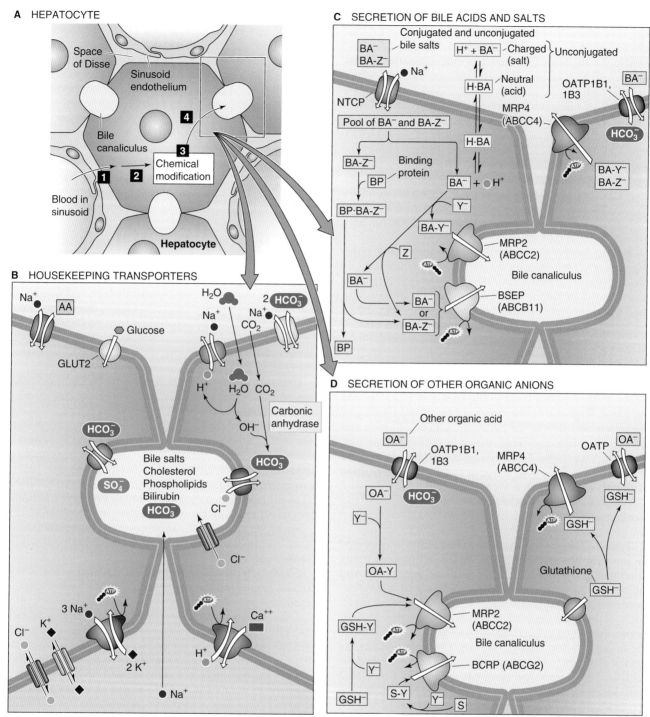

Figure 46.3 Transporters in hepatocyte. (C) Bile acids can enter the hepatocyte in any of several forms: the unconjugated salt (BA⁻); the neutral, protonated bile acid (H · BA); or the bile salt conjugated to taurine or glycine (BA-Z⁻, where Z represents taurine or glycine). Some bile acids are conjugated to sulfate or glucuronate (Y⁻). (D) Organic anions (OA), including bile acids and bilirubin, may enter across the basolateral membrane via an OATP. *AA*, Amino acid.

Hepatocytes take up bile acids, other organic anions, and organic cations across their basolateral (sinusoidal) membranes

Bile Acids and Salts Most bile-acid molecules are neutral **bile acids** (H · BA) and not very water soluble. Some of these molecules are deprotonated and hence are **bile salts** (BA⁻). The liver may conjugate the primary bile acids and salts to

glycine or taurine (Z in Fig. 46.3C), as well as to sulfate or glucuronate (Y⁻ in Fig. 46.3C). Most of the bile acids that the liver secretes into the bile are conjugated, such as taurocholate (the result of conjugating cholic acid to taurine). These conjugated derivatives have a negative charge and hence they, too, are *bile salts* (BA-Z⁻ and BA-Y⁻). Bile salts are far more water soluble than the corresponding bile acids.

Because the small intestine absorbs some bile acids and salts, they appear in the blood plasma, mainly bound to albumin, and are presented to the hepatocytes for re-uptake. This recycling of bile acids, an example of **enterohepatic circulation** (see ⊙ 46-6, below). Dissociation from albumin occurs before uptake.

Uptake of bile acids occurs predominantly by an Na^+-coupled transporter known as **Na/taurocholate cotransporting polypeptide** or **NTCP** (a member of the SLC10A1 family; Fig. 46.3C). NTCP has a particularly high affinity for conjugated bile acids it. Although NTCP also carries unconjugated bile acids, as much as 50% of these *unconjugated* bile acids may enter the hepatocyte by passive nonionic diffusion (Fig. 46.3B).

Conjugation of bile acids enhances their hydrophilicity (taurine more so than glycine).

Organic Anions The **organic anion-transporting polypeptides (OATPs)** mediate the Na^+-independent uptake of a wide spectrum of endogenous and exogenous amphipathic compounds—including bile acids, bilirubin, eicosanoids, steroid and thyroid hormones, prostaglandins, statin drugs, methotrexate, bromosulfophthalein, and many xenobiotics. OATPs appear to exchange organic anions for intracellular HCO_3^- (Fig. 46.3C and D).

Bilirubin Senescent erythrocytes are taken up by macrophages in the reticuloendothelial system, where the degradation of hemoglobin leads to the release of bilirubin into the blood (Fig. 46.4A). As evidenced by yellow staining of the sclerae and skin in the jaundiced patient, bilirubin can leave the circulation and enter tissues by diffusion. However, uptake of *unconjugated* bilirubin by the hepatocyte is faster than can occur by diffusion and is consistent with electroneutral or electrogenic transport (Fig. 46.4B).

OATP1B1 and OATP1B3 can transport *conjugated* (and possibly unconjugated) bilirubin (Fig. 46.4A).

Organic Cations The major organic cations transported by the liver are aromatic and aliphatic amines, including important drugs such as cholinergics, local anesthetics, and antibiotics, as well as endogenous solutes such as choline, thiamine, and nicotinamide (Fig. 46.5). At physiological pH, ~40% of drugs are organic cations, in equilibrium with their respective conjugate weak bases (see ⊙ 28-1). Members of the **organic cation transporter (OCT)** family mediate the uptake of a variety of structurally diverse lipophilic organic cations of endogenous or xenobiotic origin. OCT-mediated transport is electrogenic, independent of an Na^+ ion or proton gradient, and may occur in either direction across the plasma membrane. In addition to the OCTs, members of the OATP family as well as an electroneutral proton-cation exchanger may contribute to organic cation uptake across the basolateral membrane.

Inside the hepatocyte, the basolateral-to-apical movement of many compounds occurs by protein-bound or vesicular routes

Bile Salts Some compounds traverse the cell while bound to **intracellular "binding" proteins** (Fig. 46.3C). For bile salts, three such proteins have been identified. In humans, the main bile acid-binding protein appears to be the hepatic **dihydrodiol dehydrogenase.** The two others are **glutathione-S-transferase B** and **fatty acid-binding protein.** Intracellular sequestration of bile salts by these proteins may serve an important role in bile acid transport or regulation of bile acid synthesis. Transcellular diffusion of bile salts bound to proteins may be the primary mode of cytoplasmic transport under basal conditions. Free, unbound bile acids may also traverse the hepatocyte by rapid diffusion.

Bilirubin After uptake at the basolateral membrane, unconjugated bilirubin is transported to the endoplasmic reticulum (ER), where it is conjugated to glucuronic acid (Fig. 46.4). Direct membrane-to-membrane transfer may be the principal mode of bilirubin transport within the hepatocyte.

In phase I of the biotransformation of organic anions and other compounds, hepatocytes use mainly cytochrome P-450 enzymes

The liver is responsible for the metabolism and detoxification of many endogenous and exogenous compounds. Some compounds taken up by hepatocytes (e.g., proteins and other ligands) are completely digested within lysosomes. Specific carriers exist for the lysosomal uptake of sialic acid, cysteine, and vitamin B_{12}.

Hepatocytes handle other compounds by biotransformation reactions that usually occur in three phases. Phase I reactions represent oxidation or reduction reactions in large part catalyzed by the P-450 cytochromes. The common feature of all of these reactions is that one atom of oxygen is inserted into the substrate. Hence, these monooxygenases make the substrate (RH) a more polar compound (ROH), poised for further modification by a phase II reaction, which is usually represented by conjugation to a highly hydrophilic compound such as glucuronate, sulfate, or glutathione.

Finally, in phase III, the conjugated compound moves out of the liver via transporters on the sinusoidal and canalicular membranes.

⊙ 46-2 The **P-450 cytochromes**—colored proteins that contain heme—are the major enzymes involved in phase I reactions.

P-450 oxidases are present in two sets of organs. In cells that synthesize *steroid hormones*—the adrenal cortex (see ⊙ 50-2) testes, ovary, and placenta—the P-450 oxidases are localized either in the mitochondria or in the ER, where they catalyze various steps in steroidogenesis. In the liver, these enzymes are located in the ER, where they catalyze a vast array of hydroxylation reactions involving the metabolism of drugs and chemical carcinogens, bile acid synthesis, and the activation and inactivation of vitamins.

In phase II of biotransformation, conjugation of phase I products makes them more water soluble for secretion into blood or bile

In phase II, the hepatocyte conjugates the metabolites generated in phase I to produce more hydrophilic compounds, such as glucuronides, sulfates, and mercapturic acids. These phase II products are readily secreted into the blood or bile. Conjugation reactions are generally considered to be the critical step in detoxification.

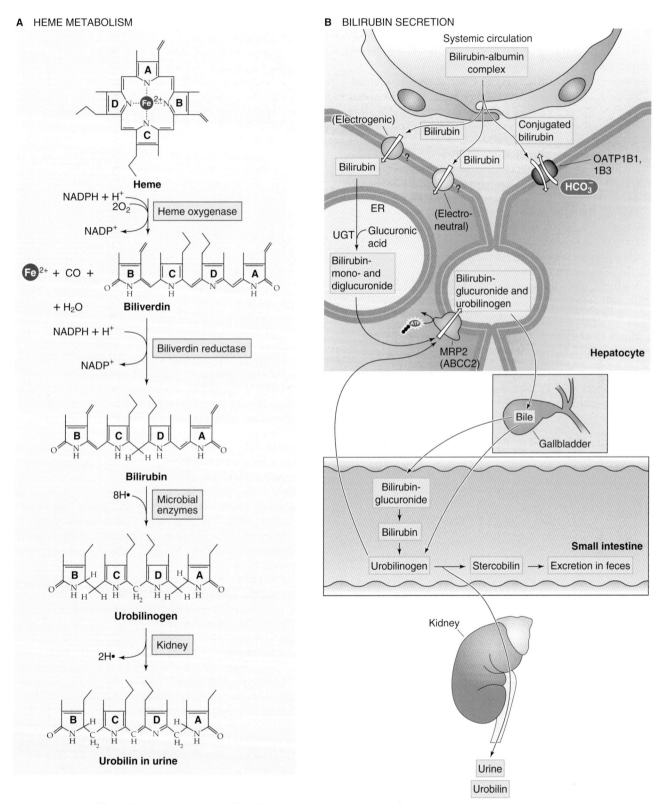

Figure 46.4 Excretion of bilirubin. (A) Macrophages phagocytose senescent red blood cells and break the heme down to bilirubin, which travels in the blood, linked to albumin, to the liver. The conversion to the colorless urobilinogen occurs in the terminal ileum and colon, whereas the oxidation to the yellowish urobilin occurs in the urine.

Hepatocytes use three major conjugation reactions:

1. **Conjugation to glucuronate.** ⊙ **46-3** The uridine diphosphate-glucuronosyltransferases (UGTs), which reside in the smooth endoplasmic reticulum (SER) of the liver, are divided into two families based on their substrate specificity.

2. **Conjugation to sulfate.** ⊙ **46-4** The sulfotransferases—which are located in the cytosol rather than in the SER—catalyze the sulfation of steroids, catechols, and foreign compounds such as alcohol and metabolites of carcinogenic hydrocarbons.

3. **Conjugation to glutathione.** ⊙ **46-5** Hepatocytes also conjugate a range of compounds to **reduced glutathione (GSH)** for excretion and later processing in either the bile ducts or kidney. In some cases, the conjugates are secreted into bile. In other cases, the glutathione conjugates are secreted into plasma and are filtered by the kidney and excreted in the urine.

Other forms of conjugation include methylation (e.g., catechols, amines, and thiols), acetylation (e.g., amines and hydrazines), and conjugation (e.g., bile acids) with amino acids such as taurine, glycine, or glutamine.

In phase III of biotransformation, hepatocytes excrete products of phase I and II into bile or sinusoidal blood

Phase III involves multidrug transporters located on the *canalicular membrane.* These transporters have broad substrate specificity and play an important role in protecting tissues from toxic xenobiotics and endogenous metabolites.

The interactions of xenobiotics with nuclear receptors control phase I, II, and III

The nuclear receptors (NRs, see Table 3.3) for xenobiotics, the steroid and xenobiotic receptor (SXR, also known as the pregnane X receptor, or PXR), the constitutive androstane receptor (CAR), and the aryl hydrocarbon receptor (AhR) coordinately induce genes involved in the three phases of xenobiotic biotransformation.

Hepatocytes secrete bile acids, organic anions, organic cations, and lipids across their apical (canalicular) membranes

At the apical membrane, the transport of compounds is generally unidirectional, from cell to canalicular lumen. An exception is certain precious solutes, such as amino acids and adenosine, which are reabsorbed from bile by Na^+-dependent secondary active transport systems.

Bile Salts Bile-salt transport from hepatocyte to canalicular lumen (Fig. 46.3C) occurs via an ATP-dependent transporter called the **bile-salt export pump** (**BSEP** or ABCB11). BSEP has a very high affinity for bile salts. Secretion of bile salts occurs against a significant cell-to-canaliculus concentration gradient, which may range from 1:100 to 1:1000.

Organic Anions Organic anions that are *not bile salts* move from the cytoplasm of the hepatocyte to the canalicular lumen largely via **MRP2** (ABCC2, Fig. 46.3D). MRP2

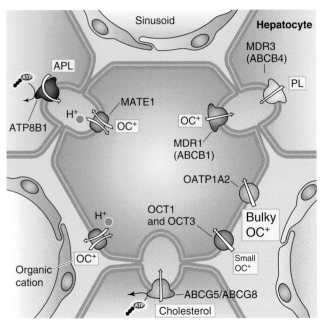

Figure 46.5 Excretion of organic cations and lipids. *APL,* Aminophospholipid; *C,* cholesterol; *PL,* phospholipid.

is electrogenic, ATP dependent, and has a broad substrate specificity. Its substrates include bilirubin diglucuronide (Fig. 46.5B), sulfated bile acids, glucuronidated bile acids (Fig. 46.3C), and several xenobiotics. MRP2 is critical for the transport of GSH conjugates across the canalicular membrane into bile.

Organic Cations Biliary excretion of organic cations is thought to occur via the **MDR1** (ABCB1) transporter present in the canalicular membrane.

Other pathways for organic cations excretion into the canaliculus include the **multidrug and toxin extrusion 1 (MATE1)** transporters (Fig. 46.5). Thus, transcellular cation movement in liver is mediated by the combined action of electrogenic OCT-type uptake systems and MATE-type efflux systems.

Biliary Lipids Phospholipid is a major component of bile. **MDR3** (ABCB4) is a flippase that promotes the active translocation of **phosphatidylcholine (PC)** from the inner to the outer leaflet of the canalicular membrane (Fig. 46.5).

Lipid asymmetry in the canalicular membrane is essential for protection against the detergent properties of bile salts. The **P-type ATPase ATP8B1** in the canalicular membrane translocates aminophospholipids—such as phosphatidylserine (PS) and phosphatidylethanolamine (PE)—from the *outer* to the *inner* leaflet of the bilayer, thereby leaving behind an outer leaflet that is depleted of PC, PS, and PE but enriched in sphingomyelin and cholesterol (Fig. 46.5). The resulting lipid asymmetry renders the membrane virtually detergent insoluble and helps to maintain the functional complement of enzymes and transporters within the lipid bilayer.

Bile is also the main pathway for elimination of **cholesterol.** A heterodimer composed of the "half" ABC transporters **ABCG5** and **ABCG8** is located on the canalicular membrane and is responsible for the secretion of cholesterol into bile (Fig. 46.5).

HEPATOCYTES TAKE UP PROTEINS ACROSS THEIR BASOLATERAL MEMBRANES BY RECEPTOR-MEDIATED ENDOCYTOSIS AND FLUID-PHASE ENDOCYTOSIS

The hepatocyte takes up macromolecules, such as plasma proteins, from the blood plasma through endocytosis, transports these molecules across the cytoplasm, and then secretes them into the bile through exocytosis. Three forms of endocytosis have been identified in the basolateral (sinusoidal) membrane: fluid-phase endocytosis (nonspecific), adsorptive endocytosis (nonspecific), and receptor-mediated endocytosis (specific).

Fluid-phase endocytosis involves the uptake of a small amount of extracellular fluid with its solutes and is a result of the constitutive process of membrane invagination and internalization. The process is nondiscriminatory and inefficient.

Adsorptive endocytosis involves nonspecific binding of the protein to the plasma membrane before endocytosis, and it results in more efficient protein uptake.

Receptor-mediated endocytosis is quantitatively the most important mechanism for the uptake of macromolecules. After endocytosis, the receptor recycles to the plasma membrane, and the ligand may be excreted directly into bile by exocytosis or delivered to lysosomes for degradation.

BILE FORMATION

The secretion of canalicular bile is active and isotonic

The formation of bile occurs in three discrete steps. First, the hepatocytes actively secrete bile into the bile canaliculi. Second, intrahepatic and extrahepatic bile ducts transport this bile and secrete into it a watery, HCO_3^--rich fluid. These first two steps may produce ~900 mL/day of so-called hepatic bile. Third, between meals, approximately half the hepatic bile is diverted to the gallbladder, which stores the bile and isosmotically removes salts and water. The result is that the gallbladder concentrates bile salts, bilirubin, cholesterol, and lecithin by 10- to 20-fold. The 500 mL/day of bile that reaches the duodenum through the ampulla of Vater is thus a mixture of relatively "dilute" hepatic bile and "concentrated" gallbladder bile.

Bile formation by hepatocytes requires the active, energy-dependent secretion of inorganic and organic solutes into the canalicular lumen, followed by the passive movement of water.

Canalicular bile is an isosmotic fluid. Water movement into the bile canaliculus can follow both paracellular and transcellular pathways. As far as the *paracellular* pathway is concerned, the movement of water through the tight junctions between hepatocytes carries with it solutes by solvent drag.

As far as the *transcellular* pathway is concerned, water enters hepatocytes via aquaporin 9 (AQP9), found exclusively on the sinusoidal membrane. AQP9 also allows the passage of a wide variety of neutral solutes such as urea, glycerol, purines, and pyrimidines. The canalicular membrane expresses AQP8. Under basal conditions, AQP8 is predominantly localized to intracellular vesicles so that water permeability in the canalicular membrane is lower than that in the sinusoidal membrane and is rate limiting for transcellular water transport. Upon cAMP stimulation, AQP8 from the intracellular pool inserts into the canalicular membrane substantially increasing the water permeability of this membrane. The transcellular pathway accounts for most of the water entering the bile canaliculus during choleresis.

Major organic molecules in bile include bile acids, cholesterol, and phospholipids

Bile has two important functions: (1) it provides the excretory route for many solutes that are not excreted by the kidney, and (2) it secretes stored bile salts and acids required for normal lipid digestion (see ◉ 45-4) and absorption (see ◉ 45-6).

Bile acids promote dietary lipid absorption through their micelle-forming properties (see ◉ 45-6). As shown in Fig. 46.6, hepatocytes synthesize the **primary bile acids**—cholic acid and chenodeoxycholic acid—from cholesterol. Biliary excretion of cholesterol and conversion of **cholesterol** to bile acids are the principal routes of cholesterol excretion and catabolism. **Secondary bile acids** are the products of bacterial dehydroxylation in the terminal ileum and colon. After being absorbed and returning to the liver through the enterohepatic circulation, these secondary bile acids may also undergo conjugation reactions (Fig. 46.6).

Phospholipids in bile help to solubilize cholesterol as well as diminish the cytotoxic effects of other bile acids on hepatocytes and bile duct cells. **IgA** inhibits bacterial growth in bile.

Excretory or **waste products** found in bile include cholesterol, bile pigments, trace minerals, plant sterols, lipophilic drugs and metabolites, antigen-antibody complexes, and oxidized glutathione, as well as compounds that do not readily enter the renal glomerular filtrate, either because they are associated with proteins such as albumin or because they are associated with formed elements in blood. Some bile acids are only partly bound to serum albumin and may therefore enter the glomerular filtrate. However, they are actively reabsorbed by the renal tubule, and are virtually absent from the urine.

Canalicular bile flow has a constant component driven by the secretion of small organic molecules and a variable component driven by the secretion of bile acids

Total bile flow is the sum of the bile flow from hepatocytes into the canaliculi (canalicular flow) and the additional flow from cholangiocytes into the bile ducts (ductular flow). Canalicular bile flow is the sum of two components: (1) a "constant" component that is independent of bile acid secretion (bile acid-*in*dependent flow), and (2) a rising component that increases linearly with bile acid secretion (bile acid-*dependent* flow). In humans, most of the canalicular bile flow is bile acid dependent. If we now add the **ductular secretion,** which is also "constant," we have the **total bile flow.**

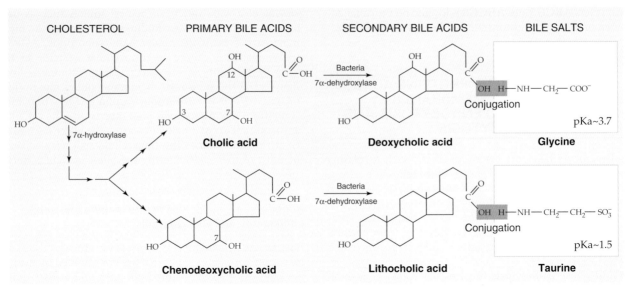

Figure 46.6   Synthesis of bile acids.

Secretin stimulates the cholangiocytes of ductules and ducts to secrete a watery, HCO_3^--rich fluid

Biliary epithelial cells, or **cholangiocytes,** are the second major source of the fluid in hepatic bile. These cholangiocytes (Fig. 46.7) have 6 of the 13 known human aquaporins, an apical Cl-HCO_3 exchanger AE2, and several apical Cl⁻ channels, including the cystic fibrosis transmembrane conductance regulator (CFTR). The Cl-HCO_3 exchanger, in parallel with the Cl⁻ channels for Cl⁻ recycling, can secrete an HCO_3^--rich fluid. AQP1, CFTR, and AE2 colocalize to intracellular vesicles in cholangiocytes; secretory agonists cause all three to co-redistribute to the apical membrane.

A complex network of hormones, mainly acting via cAMP, regulates cholangiocyte secretory function. Secretin receptors (see ⊙ 43-3) are present on the cholangiocyte basolateral membrane, a fact that explains why **secretin** produces a watery choleresis—that is, a bile rich in HCO_3^- (i.e., alkaline) but poor in bile acids. The hormones **glucagon** (see ⊙ 51-11) and **vasoactive intestinal peptide** (**VIP;** see Fig. 13.7) have similar actions. These choleretic hormones raise [cAMP]ᵢ and stimulate apical Cl⁻ channels and the Cl-HCO_3 exchanger. A Ca^{2+}-activated Cl⁻ channel is also present in the apical membrane.

Cholangiocytes are also capable of reabsorbing fluid and electrolytes, as suggested by the adaptation that occurs after removal of the gallbladder (i.e., cholecystectomy).

The hormone **somatostatin** inhibits bile flow by lowering [cAMP]ᵢ, an effect opposite that of secretin. This inhibition may be caused by enhancing fluid reabsorption by bile ducts or by inhibiting ductular secretion of the HCO_3^--rich fluid discussed above.

Solutes reabsorbed from bile by cholangiocytes are recycled and returned to the hepatocytes for repeat secretion, a process that induces significant choleresis.

The gallbladder stores bile and delivers it to the duodenum during a meal

The gallbladder is not an essential structure of bile secretion. Tonic contraction of the sphincter of Oddi facilitates gallbladder filling by maintaining a positive pressure within the common bile duct. As we noted above, up to 50% of hepatic bile is diverted to the gallbladder during fasting. The remaining ~450 mL/day passes directly into the duodenum.

Gallbladder emptying and filling is under feedback control. During feeding, CCK secreted by duodenal I cells (see Table 41.1) causes gallbladder contraction and the release of bile into the duodenum, where the bile promotes fat digestion and suppresses further CCK secretion. On reaching the ileum, bile acids induce synthesis of fibroblast growth factor 19 (FGF19); FGF19, after transit in portal blood, causes relaxation of gallbladder smooth muscle, which allows gallbladder refilling.

During the interdigestive period, the gallbladder concentrates bile acids up to 10- or even 20-fold within the gallbladder lumen (Fig. 46.8). The apical step of NaCl uptake and transport is electroneutral and is mediated by parallel Na-H and Cl-HCO_3 exchangers. At the basolateral membrane, Na⁺ exits through the Na-K pump, whereas Cl⁻ most likely exits by Cl⁻ channels. Both water and HCO_3^- move passively from lumen to blood through the tight junctions. Water can also move through the cell via AQP1 (expressed on apical and basolateral membranes) and AQP8 (found only apically). The net transport is isotonic, which leaves behind gallbladder bile that is also isotonic but has a higher concentration of bile salts, K⁺, and Ca^{2+}. Net fluid and electrolyte transport across the gallbladder epithelium is under hormonal regulation. Both VIP (released from neurons innervating the gallbladder) and serotonin inhibit net fluid and electrolyte absorption. Conversely, α-adrenergic blockade of neuronal VIP release increases fluid absorption.

Although the gallbladder reabsorbs NaCl by parallel Na-H and Cl-HCO_3 exchange at the apical membrane, Na-H exchange outstrips Cl-HCO_3 exchange; the end result is net secretion of **H⁺ ions.** This action neutralizes HCO_3^- the and acidifies the bile. The H⁺ secreted by the gallbladder protonates the intraluminal contents. This action greatly increases the solubility of calcium salts in bile and reduces the likelihood of calcium salt precipitation and **gallstone formation.** Common "pigment gallstones" contain one or more of several calcium salts, including carbonate, bilirubinate, phosphate,

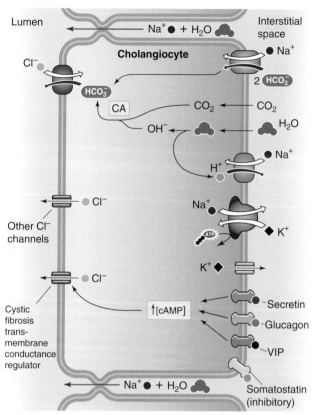

Figure 46.7   Secretion of an HCO_3^--rich fluid by cholangiocytes.

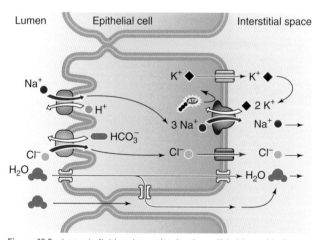

Figure 46.8   Isotonic fluid reabsorption by the gallbladder epithelium.

and fatty acids. The solubility of each of these compounds is significantly increased by the acidification of bile.

Mucus secretion by gallbladder epithelial cells results in the formation of a polymeric gel that protects the apical surface of the gallbladder epithelium from the potentially toxic effects of bile salts.

The relative tones of the gallbladder and sphincter of Oddi determine whether bile flows from the common hepatic duct into the gallbladder or into the duodenum

Bile exiting the liver and flowing down the common hepatic duct reaches a bifurcation that permits flow either into the

cystic duct and then into the gallbladder or into the common bile duct, through the sphincter of Oddi, and into the duodenum (see Fig. 46.2).

The sphincter of Oddi—which also controls the flow of pancreatic secretions into the duodenum—corresponds functionally to a short (4- to 6-mm) zone within the wall of the duodenum.

Both hormonal and cholinergic mechanisms appear to be involved in gallbladder emptying. Dietary lipid stimulates the release of CCK from duodenal I cells (see ⊙ 43-4). This CCK not only stimulates pancreatic secretion but also causes smooth-muscle contraction and evacuation of the gallbladder. The coordinated response to CCK also includes relaxation of the sphincter of Oddi, which enhances bile flow into the duodenum.

⊙ 46-6 ENTEROHEPATIC CIRCULATION OF BILE ACIDS

The enterohepatic circulation of bile acids is a loop consisting of secretion by the liver, reabsorption by the intestine, and return to the liver in portal blood for repeat secretion into bile

Bile acids are important for promoting the absorption of dietary lipids in the intestine. The quantity of bile acid that the liver normally *secretes* in a day varies with the number of meals and the fat content of these meals, but it typically ranges between 12 and 36 g. The liver's basal rate of *synthesis* of bile acids from cholesterol (Fig. 46.6) is only ~600 mg/day in healthy humans, sufficient to replace the equivalent losses of bile acid in the feces. The gastrointestinal tract has an extremely efficient mechanism for recycling the bile acids secreted by the liver (Fig. 46.9). This recycling, known as the **enterohepatic circulation**, occurs as the terminal ileum and colon reabsorb bile acids and return them to the liver in the portal blood.

Efficient intestinal conservation of bile acids depends on active apical absorption in the terminal ileum and passive absorption throughout the intestinal tract

Most of the bile secreted into the duodenum is in the conjugated form. Very little of these bile salts is reabsorbed into the intestinal tract until they reach the terminal ileum, an arrangement that allows the bile salts to remain at high levels throughout most of the small intestine, where they can participate in lipid digestion (see ⊙ 45-4) and absorption (see ⊙ 45-6). The enterohepatic circulation reclaims 95% or more of these secreted bile salts. Some of the absorption of bile acids by the intestines is passive and occurs along the entire small intestine and colon. The major component of bile acid absorption is active and occurs only in the terminal ileum (Fig. 46.9).

Passive absorption of bile acids occurs along the entire small intestine and colon (Fig. 46.9), but it is less intensive than active absorption. The mechanism of bile acid uptake across the apical membrane may consist of either **ionic** or **nonionic diffusion**. Nonionic diffusion—or passive diffusion of the protonated or neutral form of the bile acid—is 10-fold greater than ionic diffusion.

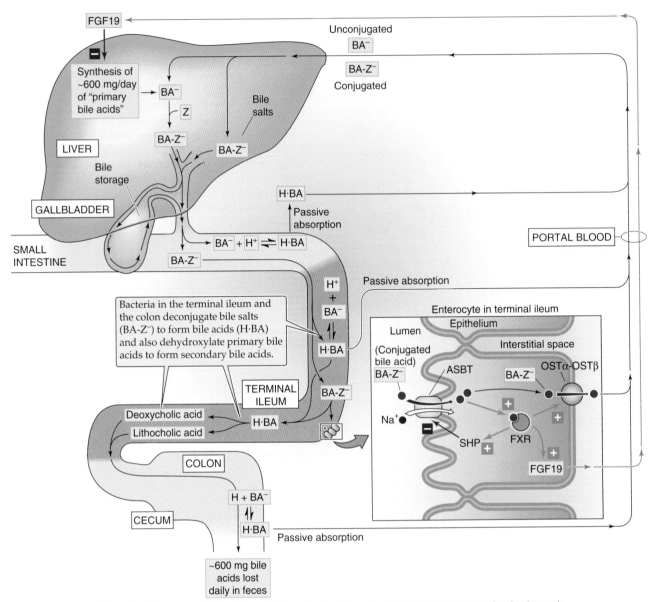

Figure 46.9 Enterohepatic circulation of bile acids. The bile acids that the liver delivers to the duodenum in the bile are primarily conjugated to taurine or glycine (BA-Z⁻), and these conjugates enter the portal blood in the terminal ileum to return to the liver. Some unconjugated bile acids and secondary bile acids also return to the hepatocyte for resecretion.

Active absorption of bile acids in the intestine is restricted to the *terminal ileum* (Fig. 46.9). This active process preferentially absorbs the negatively charged *conjugated* bile salts. Active uptake of bile salts requires Na^+. The Na^+-dependent transporter responsible for the apical step of active absorption is known as the **apical Na/bile-salt transporter (ASBT).** After bile salts enter ileal enterocytes across the apical membrane, they exit across the basolateral membrane via the heteromeric **organic solute transporter OSTα-OSTβ.**

Because the most polar bile salts are poorly absorbed by nonionic diffusion, the ASBT in the apical membrane of the enterocytes of the terminal ileum has the highest affinity and maximal transport rates for these salts.

On their entry into portal blood, the bile acids are predominantly bound to albumin and, to a lesser extent, lipoproteins. The liver removes or clears these bile acids from portal blood by the transport mechanisms outlined above in Fig. 46.3C.

The small fraction of bile acids that escapes active or passive absorption in the small intestine is subject to *bacterial modification* in the *colon*. This bacterial modification takes two forms. First, the bacteria deconjugate the bile. Second, the bacteria perform a 7α-dehydroxylation reaction with the formation of *secondary bile acids*. These secondary bile acids include **deoxycholate** and **lithocholate** (Fig. 46.6). The deconjugated secondary bile acids may then be either absorbed passively in the colon or excreted in the feces. The secondary bile acids formed by colonic bacteria and recycled back to the liver may undergo biotransformation through conjugation to glycine and taurine.

Thus, the enterohepatic circulation of bile acids is driven by two *mechanical* pumps: (1) the motor activity of the gallbladder, and (2) peristalsis of the intestines to propel the bile acids to the terminal ileum and colon. It is also driven by two *chemical* pumps: (1) energy-dependent transporters located in the terminal ileum, and (2) energy-dependent transporters in the hepatocyte.

The **bile acid receptor FXR,** a member of the nuclear receptor family (see Table 3.3), controls multiple components of the enterohepatic circulation of bile acids, coordinating bile acid synthesis and transport by the liver and intestine. Primary bile acids are potent agonists of FXR, which transcriptionally regulates several genes involved in bile acid homeostasis, producing negative feedback.

THE LIVER AS A METABOLIC ORGAN

The liver is a metabolically active and highly aerobic organ. It receives ~28% of the total blood flow and extracts ~20% of the oxygen used by the body. The liver is responsible for the synthesis and degradation of carbohydrates, proteins, and lipids. The small molecules that are products of digestion are efficiently sorted in the liver for metabolism, storage, or distribution to extrahepatic tissues for energy. The liver provides energy to other tissues mainly by exporting two substrates that are critical for oxidization in the peripheral tissues, glucose and ketone bodies (e.g., acetoacetate).

The liver can serve as either a source or a sink for glucose

The liver is one of the key organs that maintain blood glucose concentrations within a narrow range (4 to 5 mM), in a dynamic process involving endogenous glucose production and glucose utilization. The de novo synthesis of glucose from lactate, pyruvate, and amino acids—**gluconeogenesis** (see ◉ 58-4)—is one of the liver's most important functions; it is essential for maintaining a normal plasma concentration of glucose, which is the primary energy source for most tissues.

The second way in which the liver delivers glucose to blood plasma is by **glycogenolysis** (see ◉ 58-10). Stored glycogen may account for as much as 7% to 10% of the total weight of the liver. Glycogenolysis in the *liver* yields glucose as its major product.

After a meal, when serum levels of insulin are relatively high, the liver does just the opposite: it acts as a sink for glucose by taking it up from the portal blood and either breaking it down to pyruvate or using it to synthesize glycogen (see ◉ 58-6). Glucose oxidation has two phases. In the anaerobic phase, glucose is broken down to pyruvic acid **(glycolysis).** In the aerobic phase, pyruvic acid is completely oxidized to H_2O and CO_2 through the citric acid cycle.

The liver also consumes glucose by using it for **glycogen synthesis.** Carbohydrate that is not stored as glycogen or oxidized is metabolized to **fat.**

The liver synthesizes a variety of important plasma proteins (e.g., albumin, coagulation factors, and carriage proteins) and metabolizes dietary amino acids

Protein Synthesis The liver produces a wide array of proteins for export to the blood plasma. These products include major plasma proteins that are important for maintaining the colloid osmotic pressure of plasma (see ◉ 20-15). Other products include factors involved in hemostasis (blood clotting) and fibrinolysis (breakdown of blood clots), carriage proteins that bind and transport hormones and other substances in the blood, prohormones, and lipoproteins. The liver synthesizes plasma proteins at a maximum rate of 15 to 50 g/day.

Amino-Acid Uptake A major role of the liver is to take up and metabolize dietary amino acids that are absorbed by the gastrointestinal tract (see ◉ 45-3) and are transported to the liver in portal blood. These amino acids are taken up by both Na$^+$-*dependent* and Na$^+$-*in*dependent transporters. An unusual feature of the liver is that, the same amino-acid transporter may be located on *both* the basolateral and apical membranes.

Amino-Acid Metabolism Under physiological conditions, total and individual plasma concentrations of amino acids are tightly regulated. The liver controls the availability of amino acids in the systemic blood, activating ureagenesis after a high-protein meal and repressing it during fasting or low protein intake. Unlike glucose, which can be stored, amino acids must either be used immediately (e.g., for the synthesis of proteins) or broken down. The breakdown of α-amino acids occurs by deamination to α-keto acids and NH_4^+ (Fig. 46.10). The α-keto acids are metabolized to pyruvate, various intermediates of the citric acid cycle, acetyl coenzyme A (acetyl CoA), or acetoacetyl CoA. The liver detoxifies ~95% of the NH_4^+ through a series of reactions known as the urea cycle (Fig. 46.10); the liver can also use NH_4^+—together with glutamate—to generate glutamine. The urea generated by the urea cycle exits the hepatocyte via AQP9, which acts as a urea channel. The urea then enters the blood and is ultimately excreted by the kidneys (see ◉ 36-1). The glutamine synthesized by the liver also enters the blood. Some of this glutamine is metabolized by the kidney to yield glutamate and NH_4^+, which is exported in the urine (see ◉ 39-2).

The liver is also the main site for the synthesis and secretion of **glutathione.** GSH is critical for detoxification (in conjugation reactions in the liver) and for protection against oxidative stress in multiple organs.

The liver obtains dietary triacylglycerols and cholesterol by taking up remnant chylomicrons via receptor-mediated endocytosis

Enterocytes in the small intestine process fatty acids consumed as dietary triacylglycerols and secrete them into the lymph primarily in the form of extremely large proteolipid aggregates called chylomicrons (Fig. 46.11). These **chylomicrons**—made up of triacylglycerols, phospholipids, cholesterol, and several apolipoproteins (Table 46.1)—are synthesized in the intestine and pass from the lymph to the blood via the thoracic duct. **Lipoprotein lipase (LPL)** on the walls of the capillary endothelium in adipose tissue and muscle partially digests the triacylglycerols in these chylomicrons, generating glycerol, fatty acids, and smaller or "remnant" chylomicrons, which are triacylglycerol depleted and enriched in cholesterol. The glycerol and fatty acids generated by LPL enter adipocytes and muscle

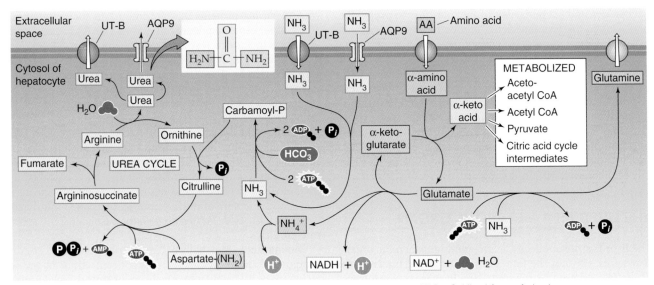

Figure 46.10 Amino-acid metabolism and urea formation in hepatocytes. *NAD+*, Oxidized form of nicotinamide adenine dinucleotide; *NADH*, reduced form of nicotinamide adenine dinucleotide; *P_i*, inorganic phosphate; *UT-B*, urea transporter B.

TABLE 46.1 Major Classes of Lipoproteins

	CHYLOMICRONS	VLDL	IDL	LDL	HDL
Density (g/cm³)	<0.95	<1.006	1.006–1.019	1.019–1.063	1.063–1.210
Diameter (nm)	75–1200	30–80	25–35	18–25	50–120
Mass (kDa)	400,000	10,000–80,000	5000–10,000	2300	175–360
% Protein (surface)	1.5–2.5	5–10	15–20	20–25	40–55
% Phospholipid (surface)	6–12	15–20	22	15–20	20–35
% Free cholesterol (surface)	1–3	5–10	8	7–10	3–4
% Triacylglycerols (core)	85–92	50–65	22	7–10	3–5
% Cholesteryl esters (core)	3–5	10–15	30	35–40	12
Major apolipoproteins	A-I, A-II, B-48, C-I, C-II, C-III, E (1%-2%)	B-100, C-I, C-II, C-III, E	B-100, C-III, E	B-100	A-I, A-II, C-I, C-II, C-III, D, E

Adapted from Voet D, Voet JG: Biochemistry, 2nd ed. New York, John Wiley & Sons, 1995, p 317.

cells. The cholesterol-rich **remnant chylomicrons** remain in the blood and reach the liver, where they enter hepatocytes by basolateral receptor-mediated endocytosis. After entry, the chylomicron remnants undergo degradation in lysosomes. Thus, chylomicrons transport dietary triacylglycerols to adipose tissue and muscle, whereas their remnants transport dietary triglycerides and cholesterol to hepatocytes.

Using various transporter proteins, the hepatocyte can also take up across its basolateral membrane the **long-chain fatty acids (LCFAs)** liberated by LPL but not used by other tissues.

To derive energy from the neutral fats in the remnant chylomicrons, hepatocytes must first split the triacylglycerols into glycerol and fatty acids. The fatty acids derived from remnant chylomicrons, and those that enter the hepatocyte directly, mainly undergo β-oxidation in mitochondria (see ⊙ 58-13).

⊙ **46-7** Fatty acids in the liver can also undergo re-esterification to glycerol to form triacylglycerols that can either be stored or exported as **very-low-density lipoproteins (VLDLs)** and released into the circulation for use by peripheral tissues.

Cholesterol, synthesized primarily in the liver, is an important component of cell membranes and serves as a precursor for bile acids and steroid hormones

The body's major pools of cholesterol include the cholesterol and cholesterol derivatives in bile, cholesterol in membranes,

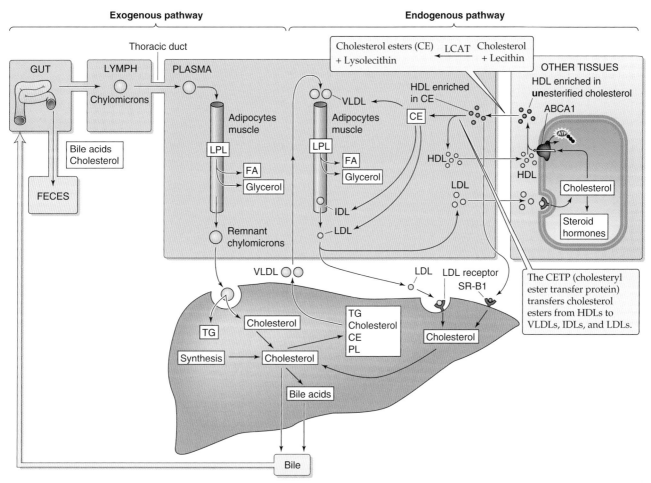

Figure 46.11 Cholesterol metabolism. *FA*, Fatty acid; *PL*, phospholipid; *TG*, triacylglycerol.

cholesterol carried as lipoproteins in blood (Table 46.1), and cholesterol-rich tissues. Cholesterol is present in membranes and bile mainly as free cholesterol. In plasma and in some tissues, cholesterol is esterified with LCFAs. The major *sources* of cholesterol are dietary uptake of cholesterol and de novo synthesis of cholesterol by various cells. The major *fates* of cholesterol are secretion into bile, excretion in the feces when intestinal cells are sloughed, sloughing of skin, and synthesis of steroid hormones. In mammals, the most important route for the elimination of cholesterol is the hepatic conversion of cholesterol into bile acids. In the steady state, the liver must excrete an amount of sterol (as cholesterol and bile acids) that equals the amount of cholesterol that is synthesized in the various organs and absorbed from the diet.

 ◉ **46-8** The liver is the major organ for controlling cholesterol metabolism (Fig. 46.11). The liver obtains cholesterol from three major sources: (1) The intestine packages dietary cholesterol as chylomicrons. The cholesterol-enriched remnant chylomicrons resulting from the removal of fatty acids and glycerol via LPL activity in muscle and adipocytes are delivered as cholesterol to the liver. (2) The liver synthesizes cholesterol de novo. (3) The liver takes up cholesterol in the form of **low-density lipoproteins (LDLs).** The liver exports cholesterol in two major ways: (1) through the bile in the form of synthesized bile acids together with cholesterol and cholesteryl esters, and (2) as circulating VLDLs.

Synthesis of Cholesterol ◉ **46-9** The de novo synthesis of cholesterol occurs in many extrahepatic tissues, as well as in the intestine and liver. The synthesis of cholesterol proceeds from acetyl CoA in a multistep process that takes place in the SER and cytosol. The hepatic synthesis of cholesterol is inhibited by dietary cholesterol and by fasting, and is increased with bile drainage and bile duct obstruction. The rate-limiting step in cholesterol synthesis is the reaction catalyzed by the enzyme HMG-CoA reductase, the level of which is decreased (negative feedback by cholesterol levels in the cell). The most potent cholesterol-lowering agents clinically available today—the "statins"—inhibit HMG-CoA reductase.

The liver is the central organ for cholesterol homeostasis and for the synthesis and degradation of LDL

The liver takes up dietary cholesterol as remnant chylomicrons and exports cholesterol and cholesterol metabolites into bile. The liver also exports cholesterol and other lipids as VLDLs and takes them up from the blood as LDLs. Table 46.1 summarizes the properties of these lipoproteins, as well as of two others: the **intermediate-density lipoproteins (IDLs)** and the **high-density lipoproteins (HDLs).**

Regardless of the source of the cholesterol, the liver can package cholesterol along with other lipids and apolipoproteins as **VLDLs.** VLDLs enter the bloodstream from the liver (Fig. 46.11) and eventually make their way to the blood vessels of adipose tissue and muscle, where the same LPL that degrades chylomicrons degrades the VLDLs on the luminal surface of blood vessel endothelial cells. In the process, fatty acids are released to the tissues. As a result of the LPL activity, the large VLDLs rapidly shrink to become the smaller **IDLs** and the even smaller LDLs. The half-life of VLDLs is less than an hour. In plasma, only minute amounts of IDLs are present.

Both the liver and extrahepatic tissue can take up LDLs via receptor-mediated endocytosis. **LDLs** are the major carriers of cholesterol in plasma. The half-life of LDLs is 2 to 3 days. The liver degrades ~40% to 60% of LDLs, and no other tissue takes up more than ~10%. LDL uptake by other tissues provides a mechanism for the delivery of cholesterol that can be used for the synthesis of cell membranes and steroid hormones or for storage as cholesteryl ester droplets.

The other major player in cholesterol metabolism is **HDL,** which is composed of cholesterol, phospholipids, triacylglycerols, and apolipoproteins. As LPL digests VLDLs on endothelial cells, some excess surface material (i.e., cholesterol and phospholipids) of these rapidly shrinking particles is transferred to the HDLs. An enzyme that is associated with HDL, **lecithin-cholesterol acyltransferase (LCAT)**—synthesized in the liver, then takes an acyl group from lecithin and esterifies it to cholesterol to produce a **cholesterol ester (CE).**

When the CE-enriched HDL (HDL-CE) reaches the liver, it binds to **scavenger receptor class B type 1 (SR-B1),** which mediates selective uptake of HDL-CE. The cholesterol moiety is targeted for biliary excretion.

Cholesteryl ester transfer protein (CETP) in blood plasma can mediate the transfer of CE from HDL-CE to VLDLs, IDLs, and LDLs—all of which contain apolipoprotein B-100. These less-dense lipoproteins can now move to the liver for uptake by the LDL receptor. The HDL-mediated removal of cholesterol from peripheral tissues via both SR-B1 and CETP for transport to the liver and excretion in bile is known as **reverse cholesterol transport.**

The liver is the prime site for metabolism and storage of the fat-soluble vitamins A, D, E, and K

We discuss the intestinal uptake of the fat-soluble vitamins in Chapter 45 (see ◉ 45-8).

Vitamin A Vitamin A (retinol and its derivatives)—like dietary vitamin D, as well as vitamins E and K—is absorbed from the intestine and transported in newly synthesized chylomicrons or VLDLs. As the remnant chylomicrons are taken up by the hepatocyte, retinyl esters may be hydrolyzed to release free retinol, which can then be transported into the sinusoids bound to **retinol-binding protein (RBP)** and prealbumin in the blood. Alternatively, retinyl esters may be stored in the liver.

Vitamin D Skin cells—under the influence of ultraviolet light—synthesize vitamin D_3 (see ◉ 52-8). Dietary vitamin D can come from either animal sources (D_3) or plant sources (D_2). In either case, the first step in activation of vitamin D is the 25-hydroxylation of vitamin D in the liver. This hydroxylation is followed by 1-hydroxylation in the kidney to yield 1,25-dihydroxyvitamin D. Termination of the activity of 1,25-dihydroxyvitamin D also occurs in the liver by hydroxylation at carbon 24.

Vitamin E The fat-soluble vitamin E is absorbed from the intestine primarily in the form of α- and γ-tocopherol. It is incorporated into chylomicrons and VLDLs with other products of dietary lipid digestion. As these particles undergo triacylglycerol hydrolysis, some vitamin E is transferred to other tissues. The α- and γ-tocopherol remaining in the remnant chylomicrons is transported into the liver, which secretes the α-tocopherol as a component of hepatically derived VLDL and perhaps HDL, but metabolizes or excretes the γ-tocopherol.

Vitamin K Vitamin K is a fat-soluble vitamin produced by intestinal bacteria. This vitamin is essential for the γ-carboxylation of certain glutamate residues in coagulation factors II, VII, IX, and X as well as anticoagulants protein C and protein S (see Table 18.3) and other proteins. Intestinal absorption and handling of vitamin K are similar to those of the other fat-soluble vitamins, A, D, and E.

The liver stores copper and iron

Copper The trace element copper is essential for the function of cuproenzymes such as cytochrome C oxidase and superoxide dismutase (see ◉ 62-2). Approximately half the copper in the diet (recommended dietary allowance, 1.5 to 3 mg/day) is absorbed in the jejunum and reaches the liver in the portal blood, mostly bound to albumin. A small fraction is also bound to amino acids, especially histidine.

High-affinity copper import across the hepatocyte basolateral membrane is mediated by the copper transport protein CTR1. Copper then binds to members of a family of intracellular metallochaperones that direct the metal to the appropriate pathway for incorporation into cuproenzymes or for excretion across the canalicular membrane into the bile. More than 80% of the copper absorbed each day is excreted in bile, for a total of 1.2 to 2.4 mg/day. Processes that impair the biliary excretion of copper result in the accumulation of copper, initially in the lysosomal fraction of hepatocytes, with subsequent elevation of plasma copper levels.

Ceruloplasmin, an α_2-globulin synthesized by the liver, binds 95% of copper present in the systemic circulation.

Iron Dietary iron is absorbed by the duodenal mucosa and then transported through the blood bound to transferrin, a protein synthesized in the liver. The liver also takes up, secretes, and stores iron. Entry of iron into hepatocytes is mediated through specific cell-surface transferrin receptors. Within the cell, a small pool of soluble iron is maintained for intracellular enzymatic reactions, primarily for those involved in electron transport. Because iron is toxic to the cell at high concentrations, most intracellular iron is complexed to ferritin.

Hepatocytes also synthesizes **hepcidin,** which down-regulates the iron-efflux pump FPN1 in the intestine and macrophages, thereby blocking the release of iron into the circulation and lowering plasma iron levels.

THE ENDOCRINE SYSTEM

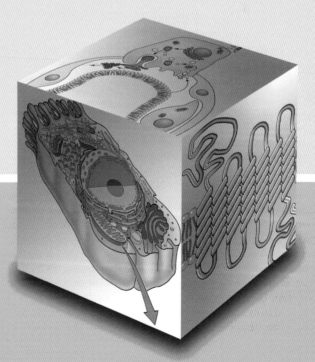

CHAPTER 47

ORGANIZATION OF ENDOCRINE CONTROL

Eugene J. Barrett

Multicellular organisms evolved two major systems to communicate and to coordinate body functions:

1. The **nervous system** integrates tissue functions by a network of cells and cell processes that constitute the nervous system and all subdivisions, as discussed in Chapters 10 through 16.
2. The **endocrine system** integrates organ function via chemicals that are secreted from endocrine tissues or "glands" into the extracellular fluid. These chemicals, called **hormones,** are carried through the blood to distant target tissues, where they are recognized by specific high-affinity receptors. As discussed in Chapter 3, these receptors may be located on the surface of the target tissue, within the cytosol, or in the target cell's nucleus. These receptor molecules allow the target cell to recognize a unique hormonal signal from among the numerous chemicals that are carried through the blood and bathe the body's tissues. The accuracy and sensitivity of this recognition are remarkable in view of the very low concentration (10^{-9} to 10^{-12} M) at which many hormones circulate.

Once a hormone is recognized by its target tissue or tissues, it can exert its biological action by a process known as **signal transduction** (see Chapter 3). Some hormones elicit responses within seconds (e.g., the increased heart rate provoked by epinephrine or the stimulation of hepatic glycogen breakdown caused by glucagon), whereas others may require many hours or days (e.g., the changes in salt retention elicited by aldosterone or the increases in protein synthesis caused by growth hormone [GH]).

PRINCIPLES OF ENDOCRINE FUNCTION

Chemical signaling can occur through endocrine, paracrine, or autocrine pathways

As shown in Fig. 3.1A, in classic endocrine signaling, a hormone carries a signal from a secretory gland across a large distance to a target tissue. Hormones secreted into the extracellular space can also regulate nearby cells without ever passing through the systemic circulation. This regulation is referred to as paracrine action of a hormone (see Fig. 3.1B). Finally, chemicals can also bind to receptors on or in the cell that is actually secreting the hormone and thus affect the function of the hormone-secreting cell itself. This action is referred to as autocrine regulation (see Fig. 3.1C). At the outset, it can be appreciated that summation of the endocrine,

paracrine, and autocrine actions of a hormone can provide the framework for a complex regulatory system.

Endocrine Glands The major hormones of the human body are produced by one of seven classic endocrine glands or gland pairs: the pituitary, the thyroid, the parathyroids, the testes, the ovaries, the adrenals (cortex and medulla), and the endocrine pancreas. In addition, other tissues that are not classically recognized as part of the endocrine system produce hormones. These tissues include the central nervous system (CNS), particularly the hypothalamus, as well as the gastrointestinal tract, adipose tissue, liver, heart, and kidney.

Paracrine Factors Numerous specialized tissues that are not part of the classic endocrine system release "factors" into the extracellular fluid that can signal neighboring cells to effect a biological response. The interleukins, or lymphokines, are an example of such paracrine factors, as are several of the growth factors, such as platelet-derived growth factor (PDGF), fibroblast growth factor, and others. These signaling molecules share many properties of the classic peptide and amine hormones in that they bind to surface receptors and regulate one or more of the specific intracellular signaling mechanisms described in Chapter 3.

Hormones may be peptides, metabolites of single amino acids, or metabolites of cholesterol

Table 47.1 is a list of many of the recognized classic mammalian hormones, divided into three groups based on chemical structure.

Several glands make two or more hormones. Examples are the pituitary, the pancreatic islets, and the adrenal glands. However, for the most part, individual cells within these glands are specialized to secrete a single hormone. One exception is the gonadotropin-producing cells of the pituitary, which secrete both FSH and LH.

Hormones can circulate either free or bound to carrier proteins

Once secreted, many hormones circulate freely in the blood until they reach their target tissue. Others form complexes with a circulating **binding protein;** this use of binding proteins is particularly applicable for thyroid hormones (thyroxine [T_4] and triiodothyronine [T_3]), steroid hormones, insulin-like growth factor types 1 and 2 (IGF-1 and IGF-2), and GH.

TABLE 47.1 Chemical Classification of Selected Hormones

Peptide Hormones

Adrenocorticotropic hormone (ACTH)

Atrial natriuretic peptide (ANP)

Arginine vasopressin (AVP), also known as antidiuretic hormone (ADH)

Calcitonin

Cholecystokinin (CCK)

Corticotropin-releasing hormone (CRH)

Follicle-stimulating hormone (FSH)

Glucagon

Gonadotropin-releasing hormone (GnRH)

Growth hormone (GH)

Growth hormone–releasing hormone (GHRH)

Inhibin

Insulin

Insulin-like growth factors 1 and 2 (IGF-1 and IGF-2)

Luteinizing hormone (LH)

Oxytocin (OT)

Parathyroid hormone (PTH)

Prolactin (PRL)

Secretin

Somatostatin (SST)

Thyrotropin (TSH)

Thyrotropin-releasing hormone (TRH)

Vasoactive intestinal peptide (VIP)

Amino Acid–Derived Hormones

Dopamine (DA)

Epinephrine (Epi), also known as adrenaline

Norepinephrine (NE), also known as noradrenaline

Serotonin, also known as 5-hydroxytryptamine (5-HT)

Thyroxine (T_4)

Triiodothyronine (T_3)

Steroid Hormones

Aldosterone

Cortisol

Estradiol (E2)

Progesterone

Testosterone

Formation of a complex between a hormone and a circulating binding protein serves several functions. First, it provides the blood with a reservoir or pool of the hormone and thus minimizes minute-to-minute fluctuations in hormone concentration. Second, it extends the half-life of the hormone in the circulation. The hormones bound to plasma binding proteins appear to be those whose actions are *long term*—in particular, those involving induction of the synthesis of new protein in target tissues. Hormones that play a major *short-term* role in the regulation of body metabolism (e.g., catecholamines, many peptide hormones) circulate freely without associated binding proteins.

The presence of plasma binding proteins can affect the total circulating concentration of a hormone without necessarily affecting the concentration of unbound or **free hormone** in the blood.

Immunoassays allow measurement of circulating hormones

The body's immune system can react to endogenous compounds; therefore, autoimmunity or reaction to self-antigens does occur. Autoimmune endocrine diseases include type 1 diabetes mellitus, autoimmune hypothyroidism, Graves disease (a common form of autoimmune hyperthyroidism), and Addison disease (one form of adrenal insufficiency).

It is often possible to obtain antibodies that are highly specific for hormones and are of sufficiently high affinity that they can bind even the often-minute amounts of hormone that circulate in blood. **Immunoassays** are now used for the measurement of virtually all hormones, as well as many drugs, viruses, and toxins.

Hormones can have complementary and antagonistic actions

Regulation of many complex physiological functions necessitates the **complementary action** of several hormones. This principle is true both for minute-to-minute homeostasis and for more long-term processes. For example, epinephrine (adrenaline), cortisol, and glucagon each contribute to the body's response to a short-term bout of exercise. On a longer time scale, GH, insulin, IGF-1, thyroid hormone, and sex steroids are all needed for normal growth. Deficiency of GH, IGF-1, or thyroid hormone results in dwarfism. Deficiency of sex steroids, cortisol, or insulin produces less severe disturbances of growth.

Integration of hormone action can also involve hormones that exert **antagonistic actions.** In this case, the overall effect on an end organ depends on the balance between opposing influences. One example is the counterpoised effects of insulin and glucagon on blood glucose levels. Insulin lowers glucose levels by *inhibiting* glycogenolysis and gluconeogenesis in the liver and by stimulating glucose uptake into muscle and adipose tissue. Glucagon, in contrast, *stimulates* hepatic glycogenolysis and gluconeogenesis.

Endocrine regulation occurs through feedback control

The key to any regulatory system is its ability to sense when it should increase or decrease its activity. For the endocrine system, this function is accomplished by **feedback control** of hormone secretion (Fig. 47.1A). The hormone-secreting cell functions as a "sensor" that continually monitors the circulating concentration of some regulated variable. This variable may be a metabolic factor (e.g., glucose concentration)

A SIMPLE FEEDBACK LOOP   **B** HIERARCHICAL CONTROL

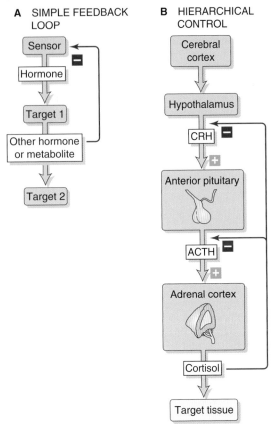

Figure 47.1 Feedback control of hormone secretion.

or the activity of another hormone. When the endocrine gland senses that too much (or too little) of the regulated variable is circulating in blood, it responds by decreasing (or increasing) the rate of hormone secretion. This response in turn affects the metabolic or secretory behavior of the target tissue, which may either directly feed back to the sensing cell or stimulate some other cell that eventually signals the sensor regarding whether the altered function of the endocrine gland has been effective.

Endocrine regulation can involve hierarchic levels of control

Faced with a stress (e.g., a severe infection or extensive blood loss), the cerebral cortex stimulates the hypothalamus to release a neuropeptide called corticotropin-releasing hormone (CRH; Fig. 47.1B). Carried by the pituitary portal system (blood vessels that connect the hypothalamus to the anterior pituitary), CRH stimulates the anterior pituitary to release another hormone, ACTH, which in turn stimulates the adrenal cortical cells to synthesize cortisol. Cortisol regulates vascular tone as well as metabolic and growth functions in a variety of tissues.

This *stress response* therefore involves the cerebral cortex, specialized *neuroendocrine tissue* in the **hypothalamus,** as well as two glands, the pituitary and the adrenal cortex. This hierarchic control is regulated by feedback, just as in the simple feedback between plasma [glucose] and insulin. Within this CRH-ACTH-cortisol axis, feedback can occur at several

levels. Cortisol inhibits the production of CRH by the hypothalamus as well as the sensitivity of the pituitary to a standard dose of CRH, which directly reduces ACTH release.

◉ **47-1** Among the classic endocrine tissues, the **pituitary** (also known as the hypophysis) plays a special role (Fig. 47.2). Located at the base of the brain, just below the hypothalamus, the human pituitary is composed of both an anterior lobe and a posterior lobe. Through vascular and neural connections, the pituitary bridges and integrates neural and endocrine mechanisms of homeostasis. The pituitary is a highly vascular tissue. The posterior pituitary receives arterial blood, whereas the anterior pituitary receives only portal venous inflow from the median eminence. The pituitary portal system is particularly important in carrying neuropeptides from the hypothalamus and pituitary stalk to the anterior pituitary.

The anterior pituitary regulates reproduction, growth, energy metabolism, and stress responses

◉ **47-2** Glandular tissue in the anterior lobe of the pituitary synthesizes and secretes six peptide hormones: GH, TSH, ACTH, LH, FSH, and PRL. In each case, secretion of these hormones is under the control of hypothalamic releasing hormones (Table 47.2). The sources of these releasing hormones are small-diameter neurons located mainly in the "periventricular" portion of the hypothalamus that surrounds the third ventricle (see ◉ 11-1). These small-diameter neurons synthesize the releasing hormones and discharge them into the median eminence and neural stalk (Fig. 47.2), where they enter leaky capillaries—which are not part of the blood-brain barrier (see ◉ 11-3). The releasing hormones then travel via the pituitary portal veins to the anterior pituitary. Once in the anterior pituitary, a releasing factor (e.g., GHRH) stimulates specialized cells to release a particular peptide hormone (e.g., GH) into the systemic bloodstream. The integrative function of the anterior pituitary can be appreciated by realizing that the main target for four of the anterior pituitary hormones (i.e., TSH, ACTH, and LH/FSH) is other endocrine tissue. Thus, these four anterior pituitary hormones are themselves "releasing hormones" that trigger the secretion of specific hormones.

◉ 47-3 The posterior pituitary regulates water balance and uterine contraction

Unlike the anterior pituitary, the posterior lobe of the pituitary is actually part of the brain. The posterior pituitary (or neurohypophysis) contains the nerve endings of *large*-diameter neurons whose cell bodies are in the supraoptic and paraventricular nuclei of the hypothalamus (Fig. 47.2). The large-diameter hypothalamic neurons synthesize arginine vasopressin (AVP) and oxytocin and then transport these hormones along their axons to the site of release in the posterior pituitary. As in the anterior pituitary, release of these hormones is under ultimate control of the hypothalamus. However, the hypothalamic axons traveling to the posterior pituitary replace both the transport of releasing factors by the portal system of the anterior pituitary and the synthesis of hormones by the anterior pituitary "troph" cells.

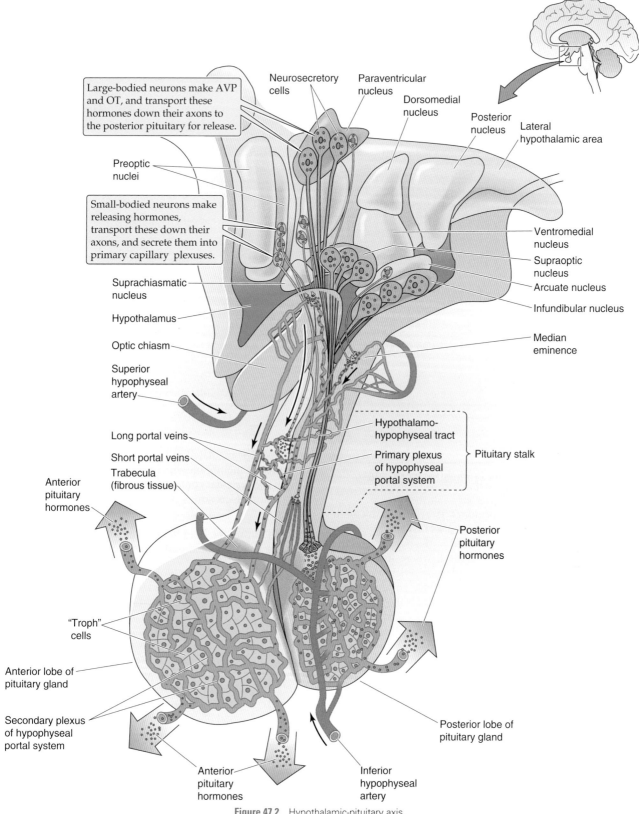

Large-bodied neurons make AVP and OT, and transport these hormones down their axons to the posterior pituitary for release.

Neurosecretory cells

Paraventricular nucleus

Dorsomedial nucleus

Posterior nucleus

Lateral hypothalamic area

Preoptic nuclei

Small-bodied neurons make releasing hormones, transport these down their axons, and secrete them into primary capillary plexuses.

Ventromedial nucleus

Supraoptic nucleus

Arcuate nucleus

Suprachiasmatic nucleus

Infundibular nucleus

Hypothalamus

Optic chiasm

Median eminence

Superior hypophyseal artery

Long portal veins

Short portal veins

Trabecula (fibrous tissue)

Hypothalamo-hypophyseal tract

Primary plexus of hypophyseal portal system

Pituitary stalk

Anterior pituitary hormones

Posterior pituitary hormones

"Troph" cells

Anterior lobe of pituitary gland

Secondary plexus of hypophyseal portal system

Posterior lobe of pituitary gland

Anterior pituitary hormones

Inferior hypophyseal artery

Figure 47.2 Hypothalamic-pituitary axis.

AVP (or antidiuretic hormone, ADH) is a neuropeptide hormone that acts on the collecting duct of the kidney to increase water reabsorption (see ◉ **38-2**). **Oxytocin (OT)** is the other neuropeptide secreted by the posterior pituitary. However, its principal biological action relates to stimulation of smooth-muscle contraction by the uterus during parturition (see ◉ **56-3**) and by the mammary gland during suckling (see ◉ **56-4**).

TABLE 47.2 Hypothalamic and Pituitary Hormones

ANTERIOR PITUITARY			
RELEASING (INHIBITORY) FACTOR MADE BY HYPOTHALAMUS	**TARGET CELL IN ANTERIOR PITUITARY**	**HORMONE RELEASED BY ANTERIOR PITUITARY**	**TARGET OF ANTERIOR PITUITARY HORMONE**
GHRH (inhibited by somatostatin)	Somatotroph	GH	Stimulates IGF-1 production by multiple somatic tissues, especially liver
TRH	Thyrotroph	TSH	Thyroid follicular cells, stimulated to make thyroid hormone
CRH	Corticotroph	ACTH	Fasciculata and reticularis cells of the adrenal cortex, to make corticosteroids
GnRH	Gonadotroph	FSH	Ovarian follicular cells, to make estrogens and progestins Sertoli cells, to initiate spermatogenesis
GnRH	Gonadotroph	LH	Leydig cells, to make testosterone
(inhibited by dopamine)	Lactotroph	PRL	Mammary glands, initiates and maintains milk production

POSTERIOR PITUITARY		
HORMONE SYNTHESIZED IN HYPOTHALAMUS	**HORMONE RELEASED INTO POSTERIOR PITUITARY**	**TARGET OF POSTERIOR PITUITARY HORMONE**
AVP	AVP	Collecting duct, to increase water permeability
OT	OT	Uterus, to contract Mammary gland, to eject milk

GnRH, Gonadotropin-releasing hormone; *OT*, oxytocin.

PEPTIDE HORMONES

Specialized endocrine cells synthesize, store, and secrete peptide hormones

Transcription of peptide hormones is regulated by both *cis*- and *trans*-acting elements (see ◉ 4-1). When transcription is active, the mRNA is processed in the nucleus and the capped message moves to the cytosol, where it associates with ribosomes on the rough endoplasmic reticulum. These peptides are destined for secretion because an amino-acid **signal sequence** on the nascent protein targets the ribosome-mRNA complex to the rough ER.

The **secretory pathway** is responsible for the synthesis, processing, storage, and secretion of peptides by a wide variety of endocrine tissues. Once the protein is in the lumen of the endoplasmic reticulum, processing (e.g., glycosylation or further proteolytic cleavage) yields the mature, biologically active hormone. This processing occurs in a very dynamic setting. The protein is first transferred to the *cis*-Golgi domain, then through to the *trans*-Golgi domain, and finally to the membrane-bound secretory vesicle or granule in which the mature hormone is stored before secretion. This pathway is referred to as the **regulated pathway** of hormone synthesis because external stimuli can trigger the cell to release hormone that is stored in the secretory granule as well as to increase synthesis of additional hormone.

A second pathway of hormone synthesis is the **constitutive pathway.** Here, secretion occurs more directly from the endoplasmic reticulum or vesicles formed in the *cis* Golgi. Secretion of hormone, both mature and partially processed, by the constitutive pathway is less responsive to secretory stimuli than is secretion by the regulated pathway.

In both the regulated and constitutive pathways, fusion of the vesicular membrane with the plasma membrane—exocytosis of the vesicular contents—is the final common pathway for hormone secretion.

Peptide hormones bind to cell-surface receptors and activate a variety of signal-transduction systems

Once secreted, most peptide hormones exist free in the circulation. As noted above, this lack of binding proteins contrasts with the situation for steroid and thyroid hormones, which circulate bound to plasma proteins.

While traversing the circulation, peptide hormones encounter receptors on the surface of target cells. These receptors are intrinsic membrane proteins that bind the hormone with very high affinity (typically, K_D ranges from 10^{-8} to 10^{-12} M). Occupancy of the receptor can activate many different intracellular signal-transduction systems (Table 47.3) that transfer the signal of cell activation from the internal surface of the membrane to intracellular targets. The receptor provides the link between a specific extracellular hormone and the activation of a specific signal-transduction system.

G Proteins Coupled to Adenylyl Cyclase Binding of the appropriate hormone (e.g., PTH) to its receptor initiates a cascade of events (see ◉ 3-8): (1) activation of a heterotrimeric G protein (α_s or α_i); (2) activation (by α_s) or inhibition (by α_i) of a membrane-bound adenylyl cyclase; (3) formation of intracellular cAMP from ATP, catalyzed by adenylyl cyclase; (4) binding of cAMP to the enzyme protein kinase A (PKA); (5) separation of the two catalytic subunits of PKA from the two regulatory subunits; (6) phosphorylation of *serine* and *threonine* residues on a variety of cellular

TABLE 47.3 **Peptide Hormones and Their Signal-Transduction Pathways**

AGONISTS	RECEPTOR	LINKED ENZYME	SECOND MESSENGER
PTH	Coupled to $G\alpha_s$	Adenylyl cyclase	cAMP
ANG II	Coupled to $G\alpha_i$	Adenylyl cyclase (inhibited)	cAMP
AVP, ANG II, TRH	Coupled to $G\alpha_q$	PLC	IP_3 and DAG
ANG II	Coupled to G_i/G_o	PLA_2	Arachidonic acid metabolites
ANP	Guanylyl cyclase	Guanylyl cyclase	cGMP
Insulin, IGF-1, IGF-2, EGF, PDGF	Tyrosine kinase	Tyrosine kinase	Phosphoproteins
GH, erythropoietin, LIF	Associated with tyrosine kinase	JAK/STAT family of tyrosine kinases	Phosphoproteins

ANG II, Angiotensin II; *ANP,* atrial natriuretic peptide; *EGF,* epidermal growth factor; *LIF,* leukemia inhibitory factor; *STAT,* signal transducer and activator of transcription.

enzymes and other proteins by the free catalytic subunits of PKA that are no longer restrained; and (7) modification of cellular function by these phosphorylations. The activation is terminated in two ways. First, phosphodiesterases in the cell degrade cAMP. Second, *serine/threonine*-specific phosphoprotein phosphatases can dephosphorylate enzymes and proteins that had previously been phosphorylated by PKA.

G Proteins Coupled to Phospholipase C Binding of the appropriate peptide hormone (e.g., AVP) to its receptor initiates the following cascade of events (see ⊙ 3-12): (1) activation of $G\alpha_q$; (2) activation of a membrane-bound phospholipase C (PLC); and (3) cleavage of phosphatidylinositol 4,5-bisphosphate (PIP_2) by this PLC, with the generation of *two* signaling molecules, inositol 1,4,5-trisphosphate (IP_3) and diacylglycerol (DAG).

The IP_3 fork of the pathway includes (4a) binding of IP_3 to a receptor on the cytosolic surface of the endoplasmic reticulum; (5a) release of Ca^{2+} from internal stores, which causes $[Ca^{2+}]_i$ to rise by several-fold; and (6a) activation of Ca^{2+}-dependent kinases (e.g., Ca^{2+}-calmodulin–dependent protein kinases, protein kinase C [PKC]) by the increases in $[Ca^{2+}]_i$.

The DAG fork of the pathway includes (4b) allosteric activation of PKC by DAG (the activity of this enzyme is also stimulated by the increased $[Ca^{2+}]_i$), and (5b) phosphorylation of a variety of proteins by PKC, which is activated in the plane of the cell membrane. An example of a hormone whose actions are in part mediated by DAG is TSH.

G Proteins Coupled to Phospholipase A_2 Some peptide hormones (e.g., TRH) activate phospholipase A_2 (PLA_2) through the following cascade (see ⊙ 3-18): (1) activation of $G\alpha_q$ or $G\alpha_{11}$, (2) stimulation of membrane-bound PLA_2 by the activated $G\alpha$, (3) cleavage of membrane phospholipids by PLA_2 to produce lysophospholipid and arachidonic acid, and (4) conversion—by several enzymes—of arachidonic acid into a variety of biologically active eicosanoids (e.g., prostaglandins, prostacyclins, thromboxanes, and leukotrienes).

Guanylyl Cyclase Other peptide hormones (e.g., atrial natriuretic peptide) bind to a receptor that is itself a guanylyl cyclase that converts cytoplasmic GTP to cGMP (see ⊙ 3-21). In turn, cGMP can activate cGMP-dependent kinases, phosphatases, or ion channels.

Receptor Tyrosine Kinases For some peptide hormones, notably insulin and IGF-1 and IGF-2, the hormone receptor itself possesses tyrosine kinase activity (see ⊙ 3-24).

Occupancy of the receptor by the appropriate hormone increases kinase activity. For the insulin and IGF-1 receptors, the kinases autophosphorylate tyrosines within the hormone receptor, as well as substrates within the cytosol, thus initiating a cascade of phosphorylation reactions.

Tyrosine Kinase–Associated Receptors Some peptide hormones (e.g., GH) bind to a receptor that, when occupied, activates a cytoplasmic tyrosine kinase (see ⊙ 3-27). As for the receptor tyrosine kinases, activation of these receptor-associated kinases initiates a cascade of phosphorylation reactions.

AMINE HORMONES

Amine hormones are made from tyrosine and tryptophan

Four major amine hormones are recognized. The adrenal medulla makes the catecholamine hormones **epinephrine** and **norepinephrine** from the amino acid tyrosine (see Fig. 13.6C). These hormones are the principal active amine hormones made by the endocrine system. In addition to acting as a hormone, norepinephrine also serves as a neurotransmitter in the CNS (see ⊙ 13-2) and in postganglionic sympathetic neurons (see ⊙ 14-6). **Dopamine,** which is also synthesized from tyrosine, acts as a neurotransmitter in the CNS (see ⊙ 13-4). Finally, the hormone **serotonin** is made from tryptophan (see Fig. 13.6B) by endocrine cells that are located within the gut mucosa. Serotonin appears to act locally to regulate both motor and secretory function in the gut, and also acts as a neurotransmitter in the CNS (see ⊙ 13-3).

The human **adrenal medulla** secretes principally epinephrine (see ⊙ 50-9). The final products are stored in vesicles called **chromaffin granules.** Secretion of catecholamines by the adrenal medulla appears to be mediated entirely by stimulation of the sympathetic division of the autonomic nervous system (see ⊙ 14-7). Unlike other peptide hormones, in which the circulating concentration of the hormone (e.g., TSH) negatively feeds back on secretion of the releasing hormone (e.g., TRH), the feedback of amine hormones is indirect. The higher control center does not sense circulating levels of the amine hormones (e.g., epinephrine) but rather a physiological end effect of that amine hormone (e.g., blood pressure; see ⊙ 23-1). The sensor of the end effect may be a peripheral receptor (e.g., stretch receptor) that communicates to the higher center (e.g., the CNS), and the efferent limb is the sympathetic outflow that determines release of the amine.

Amine hormones act via surface receptors

Once secreted, circulating epinephrine is free to associate with specific adrenergic receptors, or **adrenoceptors,** located on the surface membranes of target cells. Numerous types of adrenoceptors exist and are generically grouped as α or β, each of which has several subtypes (see Table 14.2). Epinephrine has a greater affinity for β-adrenergic receptors than for α-adrenergic receptors, whereas norepinephrine acts predominantly through α-adrenergic receptors. β-adrenergic stimulation occurs through the adenylyl cyclase system. The α_2 receptor also usually acts through adenylyl cyclase. However, α_1-adrenergic stimulation is linked to $G\alpha_q$, which activates a membrane-associated PLC that liberates IP_3 and DAG. IP_3 can release Ca^{2+} from intracellular stores, and DAG directly enhances the activity of PKC. Combined, these actions enhance the cellular activity of Ca^{2+}-dependent kinases, which produce a metabolic response that is characteristic of the specific cell.

STEROID AND THYROID HORMONES

Cholesterol is the precursor for the steroid hormones: cortisol, aldosterone, estradiol, progesterone, and testosterone

Members of the family of hormones called **steroids** share a common biochemical parentage: all are synthesized from cholesterol. Only two tissues in the body possess the enzymatic apparatus to convert cholesterol to active hormones. The **adrenal cortex** makes cortisol (the main glucocorticoid hormone), aldosterone (the principal mineralocorticoid in humans), and androgens. The **gonads** make either estrogen and progesterone (ovary) or testosterone (testis). In each case, production of steroid hormones is regulated by trophic hormones released from the pituitary. For aldosterone, the renin-angiotensin system also plays an important regulatory role.

⊙ **47-4** The pathways involved in steroid synthesis are summarized in Fig. 47.3. Cells that produce steroid hormones can use, as a starting material for hormone synthesis, the cholesterol that is circulating in the blood in association with low-density lipoprotein (LDL; see ⊙ **46-8**). Alternatively, these cells can synthesize cholesterol de novo from acetate. The cell takes up this LDL particle via the LDL receptor and receptor-mediated endocytosis into clathrin-coated vesicles. Lysosomal hydrolases then act on the cholesteryl esters to release free cholesterol. The cholesterol nucleus, whether taken up or synthesized de novo, subsequently undergoes a series of reactions that culminate in the formation of **pregnenolone,** the common precursor of all steroid hormones. Via divergent pathways, pregnenolone is then further metabolized to the major steroid hormones: the mineralocorticoid aldosterone (see Fig. 50.2), the glucocorticoid cortisol (see Fig. 50.2), the androgen testosterone (see Fig. 54.4), and the estrogen estradiol (see Fig. 55.6).

Steroid hormones are not stored in secretory vesicles before their secretion (Table 47.4). For these hormones, synthesis and secretion are very closely linked temporally. Steroid-secreting cells are capable of increasing the secretion of steroid hormones many-fold within several hours. Furthermore, steroid hormones mediate nearly all their actions on target tissues by regulating gene transcription. As a result, the response of target tissues to steroids typically occurs over hours to days.

On their release into the circulation, some steroid hormones associate with specific binding proteins (e.g., cortisol-binding globulin) that transport the steroid hormones through the circulatory system to their target tissues.

Steroid hormones bind to intracellular receptors that regulate gene transcription

⊙ **47-5** Steroid hormones appear to enter their target cell by simple diffusion across the plasma membrane (Fig. 47.4). Once within the cell, steroid hormones are bound with high affinity (K_D in the range of 1 nM) to receptor proteins located in the cytosol or the nucleus. As detailed in Chapter 4, binding of steroid hormone to its receptor results in a change in the receptor conformation so that the "active" receptor-hormone complex now binds with high affinity to specific DNA sequences called **hormone response elements** (see ⊙ **4-4**) or **steroid response elements (SREs),** also called sterol regulatory elements.

Steroid receptors are monomeric phosphoproteins with a molecular weight that is between 80 and 100 kDa. A remarkable similarity is seen among receptors for the glucocorticoids, sex steroids, retinoic acid, the steroid-like vitamin 1,25-dihydroxyvitamin D, and thyroid hormone. The genes encoding the receptors for these diverse hormones are considered part of a gene superfamily (see ⊙ **3-28**).

Steroid hormone receptors dimerize on binding to their target sites on DNA. Because the specificity with which genes are regulated by a specific steroid receptor arises from the specificity of the DNA-binding domain, mutations in this region can greatly alter hormone function.

The activated steroid receptor, binding as a dimer to SREs in the 5′ region of a gene, regulates the rate of transcription of that gene. Each response element is identifiable as a consensus sequence of nucleotides, or a region of regulatory DNA in which the nucleotide sequences are preserved through different cell types.

The activated steroid hormone receptors recognize these SREs from their specific consensus sequences. The specificity of the response thus depends on the cell's expression of particular steroid receptors, not simply the consensus sequence.

From the foregoing it should be apparent that the specificity of response of a tissue to steroid hormones depends on the abundance of specific steroid receptors expressed within a cell.

Within a given tissue, several factors control the concentration of steroid hormone receptors. In the cytosol of all steroid-responsive tissues, steroid receptor levels usually drop dramatically immediately after exposure of the tissue to the agonist hormone. This decrease in receptor level is the result of net movement of the agonist-receptor complex to the nucleus. Eventually, the cytosolic receptors

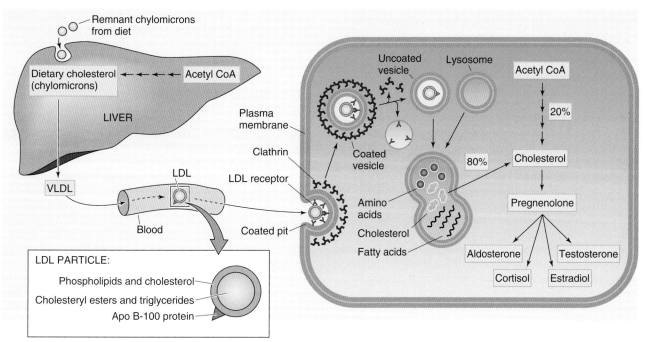

Figure 47.3 Uptake of cholesterol and synthesis of steroid hormones from cholesterol.

TABLE 47.4 Differences Between Steroid and Peptide/Amine Hormones

PROPERTY	STEROID HORMONES	PEPTIDE/AMINE HORMONES
Storage pools	None	Secretory vesicles
Interaction with cell membrane	Diffusion through cell membrane	Binding to receptor on cell membrane
Receptor	In cytoplasm or nucleus	On cell membrane
Action	Regulation of gene transcription (primarily)	Signal-transduction cascade(s) that affect a variety of cell processes
Response time	Hours to days (primarily)	Seconds to minutes

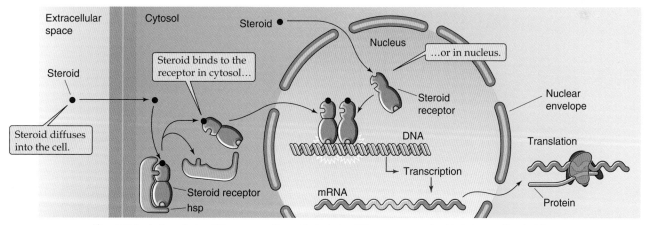

Figure 47.4 Action of steroid hormones. The activated steroid hormone receptor binds to specific stretches of DNA called steroid response elements (SREs), which stimulates the transcription of appropriate genes. *hsp,* Heat shock protein.

are repopulated. Depending on the tissue, this repopulation may involve new synthesis of steroid hormone receptors or simply recycling of receptors from the nucleus after dissociation of the agonist from the receptor. The genes for steroid receptor proteins do *not* appear to have SREs in their 5′ flanking region. Thus, this regulation of receptor number probably involves *trans*-acting transcriptional factors other than the steroid hormones themselves.

Thyroid hormones bind to intracellular receptors that regulate metabolic rate

The thyroid gland and thyroid hormone are unique among the classic endocrine axes. Neither of the two thyroid hormones secreted into the circulation—T_4 nor T_3—is free in the follicular fluid at the center of the thyroid follicle. These hormones are formed by the iodination of tyrosine residues within the primary structure of the thyroglobulin molecule that represents the principal component of the follicular fluid.

T_4 and T_3 remain part of the thyroglobulin molecule in the follicle lumen until thyroid secretion is stimulated. The entire thyroglobulin molecule then undergoes endocytosis by the follicular cell and is degraded within the lysosomes of these cells. Finally, the follicular cell releases the free T_4 and T_3 into the circulation. Once secreted, T_4 is tightly bound to one of several binding proteins. It is carried to its sites of action, which include nearly all the cells in the body. In the process of this transport, the liver and other tissues take up some of the T_4 and partially deiodinate it to T_3; this T_3 can then re-enter the circulation.

Both T_3 and T_4 enter target cells and bind to cytosolic and nuclear receptors (see ⊙ 3-28). T_3 has higher affinity than T_4 for the thyroid hormone receptor. T_3 is probably the main effector of thyroid hormone signaling. The activated thyroid hormone receptor binds to thyroid hormone response elements in the 5′ region of responsive genes and regulates the transcription of multiple target genes.

Thyroid hormone receptors are present in many tissues, including the heart, vascular smooth muscle, skeletal muscle, liver, kidney, skin, and CNS. A major role for thyroid hormone is overall regulation of metabolic rate.

⊙ 47-6 Steroid and thyroid hormones can also have nongenomic actions

A central dogma has been that all the diverse actions of steroid and thyroid hormones are due to genomic regulation. However, the very rapid onset of some effects (occurring within 2 to 15 minutes) appear incompatible with a mechanism requiring new protein synthesis. Such accumulating evidence suggests that steroid and thyroid hormones can bind to receptors that modulate the activity of cytosolic proteins and thereby regulate their activity or behavior via a *nongenomic* action. An example is the binding of extracellular estrogen or aldosterone to the GPCR called **GPR30,** also known as the G-protein-coupled estrogen receptor (GPER). Receptor occupancy rapidly activates $G\alpha_s$ and then adenylyl cyclase (see ⊙ 3-8), thereby raising $[cAMP]_i$ and stimulating PKA (see ⊙ 3-9). In addition, GPR30 indirectly activates the epidermal growth factor receptor (EGFR), a receptor tyrosine kinase (see ⊙ 3-24), and some of its downstream effectors, such as **phosphatidylinositol 3-kinase (PI3K;** see ⊙ 3-26) and the **mitogen-activated protein kinases (MAPKs;** see ⊙ 3-25). Besides estrogen and aldosterone, other ligands of nuclear receptors have nongenomic actions: thyroid hormones, testosterone, and glucocorticoids.

CHAPTER 48

ENDOCRINE REGULATION OF GROWTH AND BODY MASS

Eugene J. Barrett

In this chapter, we will focus on nutritional and hormonal processes in which physiological regulation appears to play an important role across individuals. The impact of environmental and nutritional factors, such as emotional or nutritional deprivation, on growth is most profound when it occurs during periods of tissue hyperplasia, most critically during the first 2 years of life.

◉ **48-1** The first two subchapters deal with factors that affect **linear growth,** whereas the third deals with factors that regulate **body mass.** The control of linear growth in humans depends on multiple hormones, including growth hormone (GH), insulin-like growth factors 1 and 2 (IGF-1 and IGF-2), insulin, thyroid hormones, glucocorticoids, androgens, and estrogens. Among these, GH and IGF-1 have been implicated as the major determinants of growth in normal postuterine life. Deficiencies (or excesses) of each of the other hormones can seriously affect the normal growth of the musculoskeletal system as well as the growth and maturation of other tissues.

◉ 48-2 GROWTH HORMONE

GH, secreted by somatotrophs in the anterior pituitary, is the principal endocrine regulator of growth

Individuals with excessive GH secretion during childhood develop **gigantism,** and those with a deficiency of GH develop **pituitary dwarfism.** It is thus quite clear that GH profoundly affects somatic size. Children with GH deficiency are of normal size at birth and only subsequently fall behind their peers in stature.

A deficiency of GH beginning in adult life does not result in any major clinical illness. However, it is now appreciated that *replacement* of GH in adults with **GH deficiency** leads to increased lean body mass, decreased body fat, and perhaps an increased sense of vigor or well-being. An *excess* of GH after puberty results in the clinical syndrome of **acromegaly.** This condition is characterized by the growth of bone and many other somatic tissues, including skin, muscle, heart, liver, and the gastrointestinal (GI) tract. The lengthening of long bones is not part of the syndrome because the epiphyseal growth plates close at the end of puberty. Thus, acromegaly causes a progressive thickening of bones and soft tissues of the head, hands, feet, and other parts of the body.

GH is made by **somatotrophs** throughout the anterior pituitary (see ◉ 47-2). GH is synthesized as a larger "prehormone." During processing through the endoplasmic reticulum and Golgi system, several small peptides are removed. GH exists in at least three molecular forms, of which the predominant form is a 22-kDa polypeptide with two intramolecular sulfhydryl bonds. Once synthesized, GH is stored in secretory granules in the cytosol of the somatotrophs until secreted.

Growth hormone is in a family of hormones with overlapping activity

GH appears to be a single-copy gene, but four other hormones have significant homology to GH: placental-variant GH (pvGH), human chorionic somatomammotropins 1 and 2 (hCS1 and hCS2), and human prolactin (PRL).

Somatotrophs secrete growth hormone in pulses

Whereas growth occurs slowly over months and years, the secretion of GH is highly episodic, varying on a minute-to-minute basis. Physiologically, normal children experience episodes or bursts of GH secretion throughout the day, prominently within the first several hours of sleep. Underlying each peak in plasma levels of GH, in Fig. 48.1, are bursts of many hundreds of pulses of GH secretion by the somatotrophs in the anterior pituitary. With the induction of slow-wave sleep, several volleys of GH pulses may occur. This pulsatile secretion underlines the prominent role of the CNS in the regulation of GH secretion and growth. The pattern of bursts depends on sleep-wake patterns. Exercise, stress, high-protein meals, and fasting also cause a rise in the mean GH level in humans. In circumstances in which GH secretion is stimulated (e.g., fasting or consumption of a high-protein diet), the increased GH output results from an increase in the frequency of pulses of GH secretion by the somatotrophs.

◉ 48-3 GH secretion is under hierarchical control by GH–releasing hormone and somatostatin

The coordination of GH secretion by the somatotrophs during a secretory pulse presumably occurs in response to both positive and negative hypothalamic control signals.

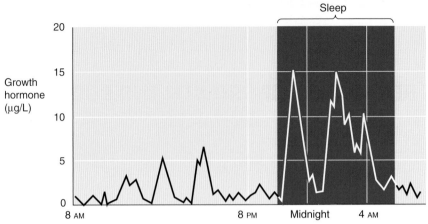

Figure 48.1 Bursts in plasma levels of GH, sampled in the blood plasma of a 23-year-old woman. Data from Hartman ML, Veldhuis JD, Vance ML, et al: Somatotropin pulse frequency and basal concentrations are increased in acromegaly and are reduced by successful therapy. J Clin Endocrinol Metab 70:1375, 1990.

Growth Hormone–Releasing Hormone Small-diameter neurons in the arcuate nucleus of the hypothalamus secrete **growth hormone–releasing hormone (GHRH)**, a 43–amino-acid peptide that reaches the somatotrophs in the anterior pituitary via the hypophyseal portal blood (Fig. 48.2).

Growth Hormone–Releasing Hormone Receptor GHRH binds to a G protein–coupled receptor (GPCR) on the somatotrophs and activates $G\alpha_s$, which in turn stimulates adenylyl cyclase (see ⊙ 3-8). The subsequent rise in $[cAMP]_i$ causes increased gene transcription and synthesis of GH. In addition, the rise in $[cAMP]_i$ opens Ca^{2+} channels in the plasma membrane and causes $[Ca^{2+}]_i$ to rise. This increase in $[Ca^{2+}]_i$ stimulates the release of preformed GH.

Ghrelin ⊙ **48-4** Distinct endocrine cells within the mucosal layer of the stomach release ghrelin in response to fasting. Endocrine cells throughout the GI tract also make ghrelin, although the highest ghrelin concentrations are in the fundus of the stomach. The arcuate nucleus of the hypothalamus also makes small amounts of ghrelin. Ghrelin appears to be involved in the postmeal stimulation of growth hormone secretion. Ghrelin also is orexigenic (i.e., it stimulates appetite; see ⊙ **48-12**), thereby contributing to body mass regulation as well as linear growth.

Ghrelin Receptor ⊙ **48-5** The hormone ghrelin binds to a GPCR designated GH secretagogue receptor 1a (GHSR1a). This receptor is like the GHRH receptor (GHRHR); however, GHSR1a does not bind GHRH.

Somatostatin ⊙ **48-6** The hypothalamus also synthesizes **SST**, a 14–amino-acid neuropeptide. SST is made in the periventricular region of the hypothalamus and is secreted into the hypophyseal portal blood supply. It is a potent inhibitor of GH secretion.

It appears that the primary regulation of GH secretion is stimulatory, because sectioning the pituitary stalk, and thereby interrupting the portal blood flow from the hypothalamus to the pituitary, leads to a decline in GH secretion. It also appears that the pulses of GH secretion are entrained by the pulsatile secretion of GHRH (as opposed to the periodic loss of SST inhibition).

SST Receptor SS binds to a GPCR called SSTR found on somatotrophs and activates $G\alpha_i$, which inhibits adenylyl cyclase. As a result, $[Ca^{2+}]_i$ decreases, which diminishes the responsiveness of the somatotroph to GHRH. When somatotrophs are exposed to both GHRH and SST, the inhibitory action of SST prevails.

⊙ 48-7 Both GH and IGF-1 negatively feed back on GH secretion by somatotrophs

Somatotroph secretion of GH is under negative-feedback control via IGF-1. GH triggers the secretion of IGF-1 from GH target tissues throughout the body (Fig. 48.3, No. 1). Indeed, IGF-1 mediates many of the growth-promoting actions of GH. IGF-1 synthesized in tissues such as muscle, cartilage, and bone may act in a **paracrine** or **autocrine** fashion to promote local tissue growth. In contrast, circulating IGF-1, largely derived from hepatic secretion, exerts **endocrine** effects. Circulating IGF-1 suppresses GH secretion through both direct and indirect mechanisms.

First, circulating IGF-1 exerts a *direct* action on the pituitary to suppress GH secretion by the somatotrophs (Fig. 48.3, No. 2). In its peripheral target cells, IGF-1 acts through a receptor tyrosine kinase (see ⊙ 3-24) and not by either the Ca^{2+} or cAMP messenger systems. IGF-1 presumably acts by this same mechanism to inhibit GH secretion in somatotrophs.

Second, circulating IGF-1 inhibits GH secretion via two *indirect* feedback pathways, both targeting the hypothalamus. IGF-1 suppresses GHRH release (Fig. 48.3, No. 3) and also increases SST secretion (Fig. 48.3, No. 4).

GH itself appears to inhibit GH secretion in a short-loop feedback system (Fig. 48.3, No. 5).

GH has short-term anti-insulin metabolic effects as well as long-term growth-promoting effects mediated by IGF-1

Once secreted, most GH circulates free in the plasma. However, a significant fraction (~40% for the 22-kDa GH) is

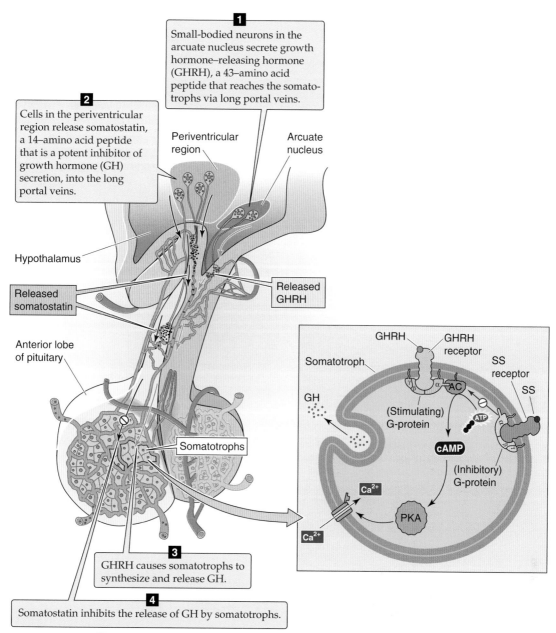

1 Small-bodied neurons in the arcuate nucleus secrete growth hormone–releasing hormone (GHRH), a 43–amino acid peptide that reaches the somatotrophs via long portal veins.

2 Cells in the periventricular region release somatostatin, a 14–amino acid peptide that is a potent inhibitor of growth hormone (GH) secretion, into the long portal veins.

Periventricular region

Arcuate nucleus

Hypothalamus

Released somatostatin

Released GHRH

Anterior lobe of pituitary

Somatotrophs

3 GHRH causes somatotrophs to synthesize and release GH.

4 Somatostatin inhibits the release of GH by somatotrophs.

GHRH   GHRH receptor

Somatotroph   SS receptor

SS

GH   α   AC

(Stimulating) G-protein   ATP

cAMP   (Inhibitory) G-protein

Ca²⁺   PKA

Ca²⁺

Figure 48.2 Synthesis and release of GHRH and SS, and the control of GH release.

complexed to a **GH-binding protein** formed by proteolytic cleavage of the extracellular domain of GH receptors in GH target tissues. This protein fragment binds to GH with high affinity, thereby increasing the half-life of GH and competing with GH target tissues for GH. In the circulation, GH has a half-life of ~25 minutes.

Growth Hormone Receptor GH binds to a receptor (GHR) on the surface of multiple target tissues. GHR is a **tyrosine kinase–*associated* receptor** (see ◉ 3-27). When one GH molecule simultaneously binds to sites on two GHR monomers and acts as a bridge, the monomers dimerize (see Fig. 3.10D). Receptor occupancy increases the activity of a tyrosine kinase (JAK2 family) that is associated with the GH receptor. This tyrosine kinase triggers a series of protein phosphorylations that modulate target cell activity.

Short-Term Effects of Growth Hormone GH has certain short-term (minutes to hours) actions on muscle, adipose

tissue, and liver that may not necessarily be related to the more long-term growth-promoting actions of GH. These acute metabolic effects (Table 48.1) include stimulation of lipolysis in adipose tissue, inhibition of glucose uptake by muscle, and stimulation of gluconeogenesis by hepatocytes. These actions oppose the normal effects of insulin (see ◉ 51-2) on these same tissues and have been termed the **anti-insulin** or **diabetogenic** actions of GH.

Long-Term Effects of Growth Hormone via IGF-1 Distinct from these acute actions of GH is its action to promote tissue growth by stimulating target tissues to produce another circulating factor that mediates further actions of GH. This intermediate, termed **somatomedin** because it mediates the somatic effects of GH, is in fact two peptides resembling proinsulin and thus termed **insulin-like growth factors 1** and **2**. Indeed, the IGFs exert insulin-like actions in isolated adipocytes and can produce hypoglycemia in animals and humans. IGF-1 and IGF-2 are

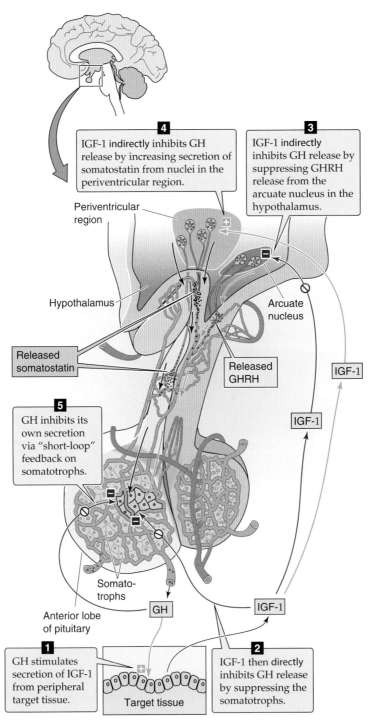

4 IGF-1 indirectly inhibits GH release by increasing secretion of somatostatin from nuclei in the periventricular region.

3 IGF-1 indirectly inhibits GH release by suppressing GHRH release from the arcuate nucleus in the hypothalamus.

Periventricular region

Hypothalamus

Arcuate nucleus

Released somatostatin

Released GHRH

IGF-1

IGF-1

5 GH inhibits its own secretion via "short-loop" feedback on somatotrophs.

Somato-trophs

Anterior lobe of pituitary

GH

IGF-1

1 GH stimulates secretion of IGF-1 from peripheral target tissue.

Target tissue

2 IGF-1 then directly inhibits GH release by suppressing the somatotrophs.

Figure 48.3 GH and IGF-1 (also called somatomedin C) negative-feedback loops. Both GH and IGF-1 feed back—either directly or indirectly—on the somatotrophs in the anterior pituitary to decrease GH secretion.

TABLE 48.1 Diabetogenic Effects of GH

TARGET	EFFECT
Muscle	↓ Glucose uptake
Fat	↑ Lipolysis
Liver	↑ Gluconeogenesis
Muscle, fat, and liver	Insulin resistance

made in various tissues, including the liver, kidney, muscle, cartilage, and bone. The liver produces most of the circulating IGF-1, which more closely relates to GH secretion than does IGF-2.

GROWTH-PROMOTING HORMONES

IGF-1 is the principal mediator of the growth-promoting action of GH

The synthesis of IGF-1 and, to a lesser extent, IGF-2 depends on circulating GH. The periodic nature of GH secretion results in a wide range of plasma GH concentrations. In contrast, plasma [IGF-1] does not vary by more than ~2-fold over a 24-hour period. The plasma [IGF-1] in effect integrates the pulsatile, highly fluctuating GH concentration. The reason is that IGF-1 circulates bound to several **IGF-1–binding proteins.** These binding proteins are made principally in the liver, but they are also manufactured by other tissues. At least six distinct IGF-binding proteins have been identified. The local free fraction of IGF-1 is probably the more biologically active component that binds to the receptor and stimulates tissue growth.

IGF-1 and IGF-2 are secreted into the extracellular space, where they may act locally in a paracrine fashion. In the extracellular space, the IGFs encounter binding proteins that may promote local retention of the secreted hormone by increasing the overall molecular size of the complex.

◉ **48-8** Whether made locally or reaching tissues through the circulation, IGF-1 acts via a specific **receptor tyrosine kinase** (see ◉ 3-24), a heterotetramer that is structurally related to the insulin receptor (Fig. 48.4). Like the insulin receptor (see ◉ 51-6) the **IGF-1 receptor (IGF1R)** has two extracellular α chains and two transmembrane β chains. The β chains have intrinsic tyrosine kinase activity. Binding of IGF-1 to its receptor enhances receptor autophosphorylation as well as phosphorylation of downstream

effectors. The structural homology between the insulin and IGF-1 receptors is sufficiently high that insulin can bind to the IGF-1 receptor, although with an affinity that is about two orders of magnitude less than that for IGF-1. The same is true for the binding of IGF-1 to insulin receptors. The homology between the insulin and IGF-1 receptors is so strong that hybrid receptors containing one α-β chain of the insulin receptor and one α-β chain of the IGF-1 receptor are present in many tissues. These hybrid receptors bind both insulin and IGF-1, but their affinity for IGF-1 is greater.

IGF-1 is less effective in mimicking insulin's action on adipose and liver tissue; in humans, these tissues have few IGF-1 receptors. In muscle, IGF-1 promotes the uptake of amino acids and stimulates protein synthesis at concentrations that do not stimulate glucose uptake. Thus, IGF-1 promotes growth at lower circulating concentrations than those required to produce hypoglycemia.

IGF-2 acts similarly to IGF-1 but is less dependent on GH

The physiology of IGF-2 differs from that of IGF-1 both in terms of control of secretion and receptor biology. Regarding control of secretion, IGF-2 levels depend less on circulating GH than do IGF-1 levels.

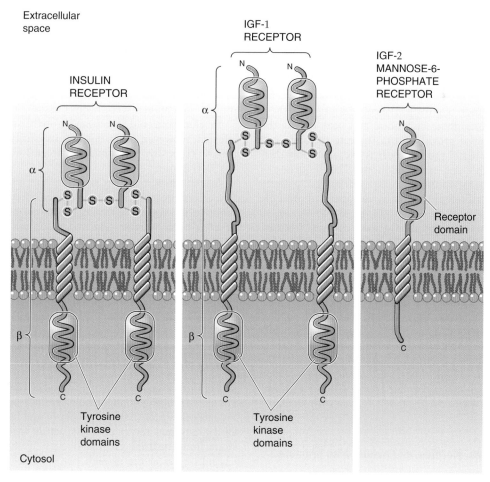

Figure 48.4 Comparison of insulin, IGF-1, and IGF-2 receptors.

Regarding receptor biology, although IGF-2 binds to the IGF-1 receptor, it preferentially binds to the so-called **IGF-2 receptor (IGF2R).** This IGF-2 receptor is a single-chain polypeptide that is structurally very distinct from the IGF-1 receptor and is not a receptor tyrosine kinase (Fig. 48.4).

IGF-2 shares with IGF-1 (and also with insulin) the ability to promote tissue growth and to cause acute hypoglycemia.

Growth rate parallels plasma levels of IGF-1 except early and late in life

During puberty, the greatest growth rates are observed at times when plasma [IGF-1] is highest. A similar comparison can be made using GH, provided care is taken to obtain multiple measurements at each age and thereby account for the pulsatile secretion and marked diurnal changes that occur in plasma [GH].

During puberty, growth rate parallels plasma [IGF-1]. The two parameters diverge at both younger and older ages. A first period of life for this divergence is very early childhood, which is characterized by a very rapid longitudinal growth rate, but quite low IGF-1 levels. Children with complete GH deficiency have very low plasma [IGF-1] levels but are of normal length and weight at birth. This observation suggests that during intrauterine life, factors other than GH and IGF-1 are important regulators of growth. One of these additional factors may be insulin. Another may be that IGF-2 is an important mediator of intrauterine growth. Plasma [IGF-2] is greater during fetal life than later and peaks just before birth. Plasma [IGF-2] plummets soon after birth, but then it gradually doubles between birth and age 1 year, and remains at this level until at least the age of 80 years.

By age 3 or 4 years, GH and IGF-1 begin to play major roles in the regulation of growth. The concentrations of these hormones rise throughout childhood and peak during the time of the pubertal growth spurt. The rate of long-bone growth in the pubertal growth spurt is exceeded only during intrauterine life and early childhood. The frequency of pituitary GH secretory pulses increases markedly at puberty because both estradiol and testosterone appear to promote GH secretion.

During adulthood, longitudinal growth essentially ceases, yet secretion of GH and of IGF-1 continues to be highly regulated, although the circulating concentrations of both hormones decline during aging. GH and IGF-1 remain important regulators of body composition and appear to promote anabolic actions in muscle. Some investigators have suggested that supplementing normal adults with GH or IGF-1 may reverse some of the effects of aging, including loss of muscle mass, negative nitrogen balance, and osteoporosis.

Nutritional factors also modulate both GH secretion and IGF-1 production. In both children and adults, GH secretion is triggered by high dietary protein intake. Conversely, **fasting,** is associated with a decline in IGF-1 even with increased GH.

Thyroid hormones, steroids, and insulin also promote growth

GH and the GH-induced growth factors are modulators of somatic growth. Hence, we could regard them as necessary but not sufficient agents for normal growth as other hormones are certainly required. Much of our understanding of endocrine regulation of normal growth derives from observations of abnormal growth as it occurs in clinical syndromes of endocrine excess or deficiency.

Thyroid Hormones Next to GH, perhaps the most prominent among the growth-promoting hormones are the thyroid hormones thyroxine and triiodothyronine. In humans, severe deficiency of thyroid hormones early in life causes dwarfism and mental retardation (cretinism; see ⊙ 49-5). In children with normal thyroid function at birth, development of hypothyroidism at any time before epiphyseal fusion leads to growth retardation or arrest. Much of the loss in height that occurs can be recovered through thyroid hormone treatment, a phenomenon called *catch-up growth.*

Sex Steroids Androgen or estrogen excess occurring before the pubertal growth spurt accelerates bone growth. However, the sex steroids also accelerate the rate at which the skeleton matures and thus shorten the time available for growth before epiphyseal closure occurs.

Glucocorticoids An *excess* of adrenal glucocorticoids inhibits growth. Growth ceases in children who produce too much cortisol, as a result of either adrenal or pituitary tumors. The use of synthetic glucocorticoids in treating various serious illnesses (e.g., asthma, organ transplantation, various chronic autoimmune processes) also can arrest growth. Restoration of normal growth does not occur until the glucocorticoid levels return toward normal. Because linear growth is related to cartilage and bone synthesis at the growth plates, glucocorticoids presumably are acting at least in part at these sites to impair growth. In adults, as in children, glucocorticoid excess impairs tissue anabolism and thus may manifest as wasting in some tissues (e.g., bone, muscle, subcutaneous connective tissue).

In glucocorticoid *deficiency,* growth is not substantially affected. However, other deleterious effects of cortisol deficiency (e.g., hypoglycemia, hypotension, weakness; see ⊙ 50-4) dominate.

Insulin Insulin is also an important growth factor, particularly in utero. Women with diabetes frequently have high blood levels of glucose during pregnancy and deliver babies of high birth weight (fetal macrosomia). The developing fetus exposed to glucose concentrations that are higher than normal secretes additional insulin. Hyperinsulinemia results in increased fetal growth.

Conversely, infants born with pancreatic agenesis or with one of several forms of severe insulin resistance are very small at birth.

The musculoskeletal system responds to growth stimuli of the GHRH–GH–IGF-1 axis

Longitudinal growth involves lengthening of the somatic tissues (including bone, muscle, tendons, and skin) through a combination of tissue hyperplasia and hypertrophy. Each of these tissues remodels its structure throughout life. For bone, **longitudinal growth** occurs by the hyperplasia of chondrocytes at the growth plates of the long bones, followed by endochondral ossification. The calcified cartilage is remodeled as it moves toward the metaphyses of the bone, where it is eventually replaced by cortical bone and trabecular bone (see ◉ 52-2). This process continues until epiphyseal closure occurs toward the completion of puberty.

In most children, growth ceases within several years after completion of puberty, when the chondrocytes at the growth plates of the long bones cease dividing and calcify the previously cartilaginous surrounding matrix. After puberty, **radial growth** occurs as bones increase their *diameter* through a process of endosteal bone resorption and periosteal bone deposition. This process occurs at both the periosteal and endosteal surfaces.

GH and IGF-1 clearly play important roles in mediating longitudinal bone growth and also modulate growth of other tissues. Thus, proportional growth of muscle occurs as bones elongate, and the visceral organs enlarge as the torso increases in size.

REGULATION OF BODY MASS

The multiple hormonal factors that influence longitudinal growth are responsive to the nutritional intake of a growing individual. For example, amino acids and carbohydrates promote insulin secretion, and amino acids stimulate GH secretion. The availability of an adequate balanced nutrient supply likely exerts both direct and indirect influences to promote tissue growth. Independent of any hormonal factors, glucose, fatty acids, and amino acids can each influence the transcription of specific genes. Amino acids can directly activate the signaling pathways involved in regulating messenger RNA (mRNA) translation.

◉ 48-9 Beyond the effects of macronutrients, the effects of micronutrients can be similarly important in regulating cell growth and, by extension, growth of the organism. An example is iodine, a deficiency of which can produce dwarfism. Nutritional deprivation early in life (see ◉ 48-1) can markedly limit longitudinal growth. Also, it appears to predispose affected individuals to *obesity* when they reach middle age.

The balance between energy intake and expenditure determines body mass

At any age or stage of life the factors that govern body mass accretion relate specifically to the energy balance between intake and expenditure. If energy intake exceeds expenditure over time— **positive energy balance** (see ◉ 58-3)—body mass will increase. Small positive deviations from a perfect energy balance, over time, contribute to the major increase in body weight—the "obesity epidemic"—that affects many middle-aged adults, and increasingly adolescents, in developed societies.

Many adults maintain a consistent body weight for decades in the absence of conscious effort. Thus, a finely tuned regulatory system must "monitor" one or more aspects of body mass, direct the complex process of feeding (appetite and satiety) to replete perceived deficiencies, and yet avoid excesses.

Energy expenditure comprises resting metabolic rate, activity-related energy expenditure, and diet-induced thermogenesis

We can group energy expenditure into three components:

1. **Resting metabolic rate (RMR).** The metabolism of an individual who is doing essentially nothing (e.g., sleeping) is known as the RMR (see ◉ 58-1), which amounts to ~2100 kcal/day for a young 70-kg adult.
2. **Activity-related energy expenditure.** As we wake up in the morning and begin to move about, we expend more energy than resting metabolism. Exercise or physical work can have a major impact on total daily energy expenditure and varies widely across individuals, and within an individual on a day-to-day basis. Additional energy expenditure occurs through **non–exercise-associated thermogenesis (NEAT)**. Such energy expenditures can vary 3- to 10-fold across individuals and can account for 500 kcal or more of daily energy expenditure.
3. **Diet-induced thermogenesis.** Eating requires an additional component of energy expenditure for digesting, absorbing, and storing food. Typically, diet-induced thermogenesis accounts for 10% of daily energy expenditure. Proteins have a higher *thermic effect* than either carbohydrates or fats (i.e., the metabolism and storage of proteins require more energy).

Hypothalamic centers control the sensations of satiety and hunger

◉ 48-10 Specific brain regions in the hypothalamus are important for controlling eating. A **satiety center** is located in the ventromedial nucleus (VMN; see Fig. 47.2). Stimulation of the satiety center elicits sensations of satiety. Conversely, a lesion of the satiety center causes continuous food intake *(hyperphagia)* even in the absence of need. A **hunger** (or feeding) **center** is located in the lateral hypothalamic area (see Fig. 47.2). Stimulation of this center elicits a voracious appetite, even after an animal has ingested adequate amounts of food. A lesion of the hunger center causes complete and lasting cessation of food intake *(aphagia)*.

◉ 48-11 Leptin tells the brain how much fat is stored

Ob/Ob strain of hyperphagic mice develop morbid obesity; affected mice typically weigh >100% more than unaffected animals of the same strain. In parabiosis experiments in which an Ob/Ob mouse was surgically connected to a wild-type mouse, the Ob/Ob mouse lost weight, which suggests that such mice lack a blood-borne factor. Another model of monogenic obesity is the (Db/Db) mouse, named Db because it secondarily develops type 2 diabetes. Like Ob/Ob mice, Db/Db mice are hyperphagic, with adult body weights ~100% greater than those of lean littermates. However, in parabiosis experiments connecting a Db/Db and a wild-type mouse, the wild-type mouse starved. Finally, in parabiosis experiment connecting an Ob/Ob to a Db/Db mouse, the Ob mouse lost weight but the Db mouse remained obese. These results indicate the following:

1. The Db mouse makes an excess of the blood-borne factor that cures the Ob mouse.
2. The Db mouse lacks the receptor for this factor.
3. Absence of the receptor in the Db mouse removes the negative feedback, which leads to high levels of the blood-borne factor.

Leptin is the blood-borne factor lacked by Ob mice. Leptin is a 17-kDa protein made almost exclusively in adipocytes. The replacement of leptin in Ob/Ob mice leads to rapid weight loss. The deficiency in **leptin receptor (LEP-R)** in Db mice makes them leptin resistant. LEP-R is a tyrosine kinase–associated receptor (see Fig. 3.10D) that signals through JAK2 and STAT (see Fig. 4.7).

Leptin acts on numerous tissues and, after crossing the blood-brain barrier (see ⊙ 11-3), modulates neurons in the arcuate nucleus of the hypothalamus that secrete pro-opiomelanocortin and suppresses appetite. These same neurons also have insulin receptors. Plasma leptin levels in humans appear to rise in proportion to the mass of adipose tissue. Conversely, the absence of leptin produces extreme hyperphagia, as in Ob/Ob mice. It appears that leptin acts as an *intermediate-* to *long-term regulator* of CNS feeding behavior, whereas insulin (in addition to intestinal hormones like glucagon-like peptide 1 [GLP-1] and cholecystokinin [CCK]) is a *short-term regulator* of the activity of hypothalamic feeding centers.

Leptin and insulin are anorexigenic (i.e., satiety) signals for the hypothalamus

At least two classes of neurons within the arcuate nucleus contain receptors for leptin and insulin. These neurons, in turn, express neuropeptides. One class of neurons produces pro-opiomelanocortin (POMC), whereas the other produces neuropeptide Y (NPY) and agouti-related protein (AgRP).

Pro-opiomelanocortin Neurons Insulin and leptin each stimulate largely distinct subgroups of **POMC-secreting neurons** (Fig. 48.5), which produce POMC. At their synapses, POMC neurons release the melanocortin α-melanocyte–stimulating hormone (α-MSH), which in turn binds to MC3R and MC4R **melanocortin receptors** on second-order neurons. Stimulation of these receptors not only promotes satiety and decreases food intake—thus, α-MSH is **anorexigenic**—but also increases energy expenditure via activation of descending sympathetic pathways. Approximately 4% of individuals with severe, early-onset obesity have mutations in MC3R or MC4R.

NPY/AgRP Neurons In addition to stimulating POMC neurons, both insulin and leptin can also suppress neurons in the arcuate nucleus that release **NPY** and **AgRP** at their synapses (Fig. 48.5). NPY activates NPY receptors on secondary neurons, thereby stimulating eating behavior. AgRP binds to and *inhibits* MC4R melanocortin receptors on the secondary neurons in the POMC pathway, thereby inhibiting the anorexigenic effect of α-MSH. Thus, both NPY and AgRP are **orexigenic**. The **agouti mouse** overexpresses the agouti protein, which inhibits melanocortin receptors and thus makes the mouse yellow. Moreover, overinhibition of MC3R and MC4R on anorexigenic neurons blocks the action of α-MSH and causes obesity.

Secondary Neurons The POMC/CART and NPY/AgRP neurons project to secondary neurons in five major locations (Fig. 48.5; see also Fig. 47.2):

1. **Lateral hypothalamic area (LHA).** In this hunger center (see ⊙ 48-10) NPY/AgRP neurons stimulate—but POMC neurons *inhibit*—secondary neurons. These project throughout the brain and release the orexigenic peptides **melanin-concentrating hormone (MCH)** or **orexins A** and **B.**
2. **Ventromedial hypothalamic nucleus (VMN).** This nucleus is a satiety center (see ⊙ 48-10).
3. **Dorsomedial hypothalamic nucleus (DMN).**
4. **Paraventricular nucleus (PVN).** This nucleus contains neurons that in turn project to both cerebral cortex and areas of the brainstem (see Fig. 47.2).
5. **Nucleus tractus solitarii (NTS).** This nucleus (see ⊙ 14-11) integrates sensory information from the viscera and also receives input from paraventricular neurons.

⊙ 48-12 Ghrelin is an orexigenic signal for the hypothalamus

Signals originating from the periphery can be *anorexigenic* (i.e., promoting satiety)—as in the case of leptin (from adipose tissue) and insulin (from the pancreas)—or *orexigenic* (i.e., promoting appetite). One signal is **ghrelin** (see ⊙ 48-4) made in response to fasting by specialized endocrine cells in the gastric mucosa. Systemically administered ghrelin acutely increases food intake when it is given at physiological doses in humans. Gastric bypass procedures in morbidly obese patients also cause a dramatic decline in ghrelin levels, along with a decline in body weight and food consumption.

Ghrelin binds to GHSR1a (see ⊙ 48-5), which is present in neurons of the arcuate nucleus as well as vagal afferents. It is not clear to what extent circulating ghrelin promotes appetite via vagal afferents versus hypothalamic receptors.

Plasma nutrient levels and enteric hormones are short-term factors that regulate feeding

Various theories may explain the *short-term* regulation of food intake. For example, hypoglycemia produces hunger and also increases the firing rate of glucose-sensitive neurons in the hunger center in the LHA, but decreases the firing rate of glucose-sensitive neurons in the satiety center in the VMN. Hypoglycemia also activates orexin-containing neurons in the LHA.

Feedback from the GI tract also controls the short-term desire for food (Fig. 48.5). For example, GI distention triggers vagal afferents that, via the NTS (see ⊙ 14-11), suppress the hunger center. Moreover, several GI peptide hormones (see Table 41.1) normally released in response to a meal—gastrin-releasing peptide (GRP), CCK, peptide YY (PYY), SST, as well as glucagon (see ⊙ 51-11) and GLP-1 (see ⊙ 51-5)—reduce meal size (i.e., these substances are anorexigenic). Additionally, an oropharyngeal reflex responds to chewing and swallowing; it may meter food intake, thus inhibiting further eating after a threshold.

Two other factors that influence body mass are cortical control (e.g., "willpower") and environment (e.g., the availability of high-calorie foods).

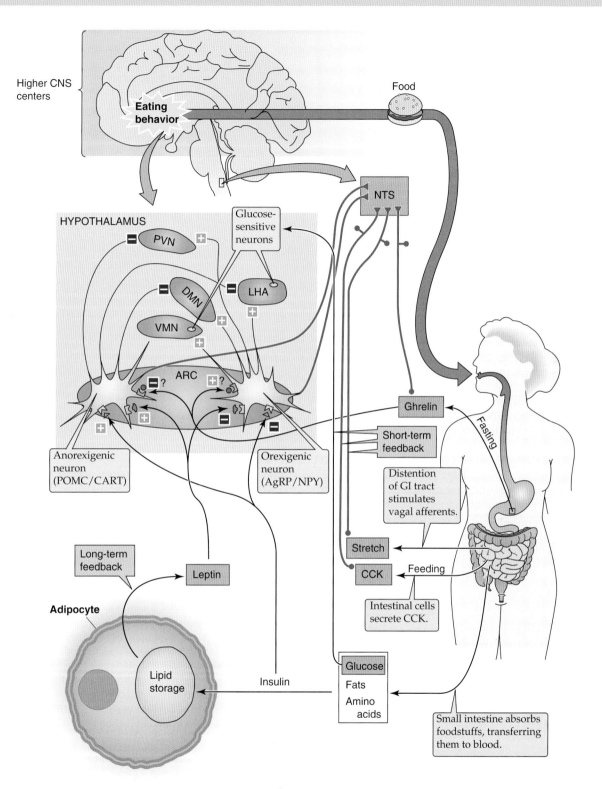

Figure 48.5 Control of appetite. *ARC,* Arcuate nucleus; *CART,* cocaine- and amphetamine-regulated transcript; *DMN,* dorsomedial hypothalamic nucleus; *LHA,* lateral hypothalamic area; *NTS,* nucleus tractus solitarii; *PVN,* paraventricular nucleus; *VMN,* ventromedial hypothalamic nucleus.

CHAPTER 49

THE THYROID GLAND

Eugene J. Barrett

The thyroid gland is located in the anterior neck, across the front of the trachea. It is composed of left and right lobes and a small connecting branch, or isthmus, and can be palpated in the course of a routine clinical examination. At the biochemical level, the thyroid hormones are the only ones that require an essential trace element, iodine, for the production of active hormone. Another unusual feature of thyroid hormone physiology is that the hormone is stored in an extracellular site within a highly proteinaceous material called *thyroid colloid*. The major protein within this material is thyroglobulin, which contains—as part of its primary structure—the thyroid hormones **tetraiodothyronine (T_4 or thyroxine)** and **triiodothyronine (T_3).** Thyroglobulin, the sequestered prohormone, is entirely surrounded by thyroid follicular cells, which are responsible for the synthesis of thyroid hormones (Fig. 49.1).

Although derived from a large protein (i.e., thyroglobulin), T_4 and T_3 are single amino acids, with no cell membrane receptors. Thyroid hormones act principally by binding to *nuclear* receptors (see ◉ 3-28) and regulate the transcription of cell proteins. T_4 and T_3 act on multiple tissues and are essential for normal development, growth, and metabolism.

The **C cells** (parafollicular cells) of the thyroid, which are not part of the follicular unit, synthesize another hormone, calcitonin (Fig. 49.1).

SYNTHESIS OF THYROID HORMONES

T_4 and T_3, made by iodination of tyrosine residues on thyroglobulin, are stored as part of thyroglobulin molecules in thyroid follicles

The structures of T_4 and T_3, the two active thyroid hormones, are shown in Fig. 49.2. T_3 is far more active than T_4. Also shown is **reverse T_3 (rT_3),** which has no known biological activity. It has two iodines on its *outer* benzyl ring, rather than two on its *inner* ring, as is the case for T_3.

◉ **49-1** The synthesis of thyroid hormones begins with the trapping of iodine by the thyroid gland. The iodide anion (I^-) is rapidly absorbed by the gastrointestinal (GI) tract and is actively taken up via a specialized **Na/I cotransporter** or **symporter** (**NIS**, located at the basolateral membrane [i.e., facing the blood] of the thyroid **follicular cell** [Fig. 49.3]). NIS moves two Na^+ and one I^- into the follicular cell against the I^- electrochemical gradient, fueled by the energy of the Na^+ electrochemical gradient (see ◉ 5-12). Several other anions (e.g., perchlorate, pertechnetate, and thiocyanate) can compete with I^- for uptake by the thyroid. Iodide leaves the follicular cell and enters the lumen of the follicle across the apical membrane. The Cl-I exchanger **pendrin** is present on the apical membrane, where it contributes to I^- secretion. Mutations in this protein can lead to a congenital syndrome typically characterized by a large thyroid gland (goiter) and hearing loss. The thyroid enlarges because of deficient I^- delivery to the follicular colloid, just as it would with an I^--deficient diet.

In parallel with the secretion of I^- into the follicle lumen, the follicular cell secretes **thyroglobulin (Tg)** into the lumen; Tg contains the tyrosyl groups to which the I^- will ultimately attach. The Tg molecule is a glycoprotein synthesized within the follicular cell and exported to the follicular lumen via the secretory pathway. It has relatively few tyrosyl residues (~100 per molecule of Tg), and only a few of these (<20) are subject to iodination. The secretory vesicles that contain Tg also carry the enzyme **thyroid peroxidase (TPO)**—an integral membrane protein, with the catalytic domain facing the vesicle lumen. As the secretory vesicles fuse with the apical membrane, the catalytic domain faces the follicular lumen and catalyzes the oxidation of I^- to I^0. This reaction requires H_2O_2, provided by another apical membrane protein, **dual-oxidase 2 (DUOX2).** As the Tg is entering the lumen of the thyroid follicle by the process of exocytosis, its tyrosyl groups react with I^0.

One or two oxidized iodine atoms incorporate selectively into specific tyrosyl residues of Tg. TPO in the presence of H_2O_2 catalyzes the coupling of two iodinated tyrosyl residues within the Tg molecule to form a single iodothyronine as well as a remnant dehydroalanine. Because only a few tyrosyl groups become iodinated, something specific about the structure of the protein near these residues probably facilitates both iodination and conjugation. The thyroid hormones, although still part of the Tg molecule, are stored as colloid in the thyroid follicle.

Follicular cells take up iodinated thyroglobulin, hydrolyze it, and release T_4 and T_3 into the blood for binding to plasma proteins

Thyroid hormones, attached to Tg in the follicular lumen (Fig. 49.1), remain inactive until the iodinated Tg is hydrolyzed (Fig. 49.3). Before this proteolysis can begin, the follicular cells must resorb Tg from the follicular lumen by fluid-phase endocytosis. As the endocytic vesicle containing the colloid droplet moves from the apical toward the basolateral membrane, it fuses with lysosomes to form a lysoendosome. Inside this vesicle, lysosomal enzymes hydrolyze the

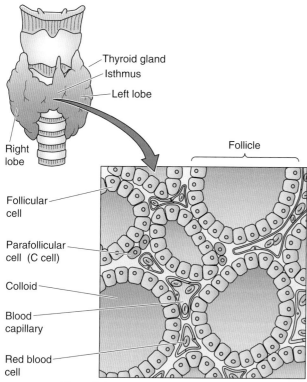

Figure 49.1 Structure of the thyroid gland.

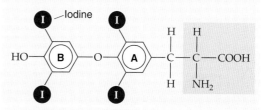

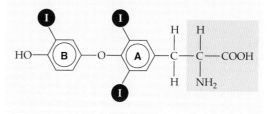

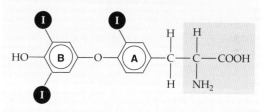

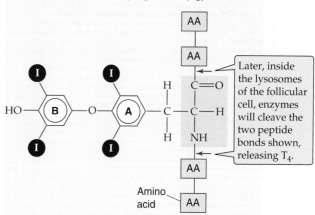

Figure 49.2 Structure of T_4, T_3, and rT_3. *AA*, Amino acid.

Tg and form T_4 and T_3, as well as diiodothyronine (DIT) and monoiodothyronine (MIT). The vesicle releases both T_4 and T_3 near the basolateral membrane, and these substances exit the cell into the blood by an unknown mechanism. Approximately 90% of the thyroid hormone secreted by the thyroid is released as T_4, and 10% is released as T_3. The thyroid releases very little rT_3 into the blood. Nonthyroidal tissues metabolize the T_4 released by the thyroid into T_3 and rT_3.

In the circulation, both T_4 and T_3 are highly bound to plasma proteins. **Thyroid-binding globulin (TBG),** albumin, and **transthyretin (TTR)** account for most of this binding. The affinity of these binding proteins is sufficiently high that ~99.98% of T_4 and ~99.5% of T_3 circulates tightly bound to protein.

◉ **49-2** The liver makes each of the thyroid-binding proteins. The extensive binding of thyroid hormones to plasma proteins serves several functions. It provides a large buffer pool of thyroid hormones in the circulation, so that the active concentrations of hormone in the circulation change very little on a minute-to-minute basis. The binding to plasma proteins markedly prolongs the half-lives of both T_4 and T_3. Because much of the T_3 in the circulation is formed by the conversion of T_4 to T_3 in extrathyroidal tissues, the presence of a large pool of T_4 in the plasma provides a reserve of prohormone available for synthesis of T_3.

Peripheral tissues deiodinate T_4 to produce T_3

The thyroid synthesizes and stores much more T_4 than T_3, and this is reflected in the ~10:1 ratio of T_4 to T_3 secreted by the thyroid. However, certain tissues in the body have the capacity to selectively deiodinate T_4, thereby producing either T_3 or rT_3. Both iodine atoms on the inner ring, and at least one iodine

atom on the outer ring, appear essential for biological activity. Similarly, the loss of the amino group renders T_4 or T_3 inactive.

The regulated conversion of T_4 to T_3 in peripheral tissues is under the control of three **deiodinases.** Two deiodinases are 5'/3'-deiodinases that remove an I from the *outer* ring and thereby convert T_4 to T_3. The first of these 5'/3'-deiodinases—**type 1 deiodinase**—is present at high concentrations in the liver, kidneys, skeletal muscle, and thyroid. It appears to be responsible for generating most of the T_3 that

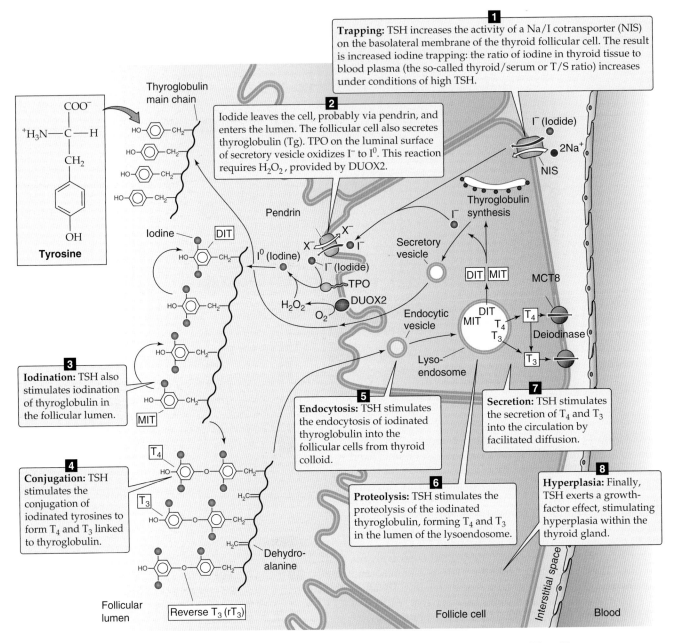

Tyrosine

1

Trapping: TSH increases the activity of a Na/I cotransporter (NIS) on the basolateral membrane of the thyroid follicular cell. The result is increased iodine trapping: the ratio of iodine in thyroid tissue to blood plasma (the so-called thyroid/serum or T/S ratio) increases under conditions of high TSH.

2

Iodide leaves the cell, probably via pendrin, and enters the lumen. The follicular cell also secretes thyroglobulin (Tg). TPO on the luminal surface of secretory vesicle oxidizes I^- to I^0. This reaction requires H_2O_2, provided by DUOX2.

3

Iodination: TSH also stimulates iodination of thyroglobulin in the follicular lumen.

4

Conjugation: TSH stimulates the conjugation of iodinated tyrosines to form T_4 and T_3 linked to thyroglobulin.

5

Endocytosis: TSH stimulates the endocytosis of iodinated thyroglobulin into the follicular cells from thyroid colloid.

6

Proteolysis: TSH stimulates the proteolysis of the iodinated thyroglobulin, forming T_4 and T_3 in the lumen of the lysoendosome.

7

Secretion: TSH stimulates the secretion of T_4 and T_3 into the circulation by facilitated diffusion.

8

Hyperplasia: Finally, TSH exerts a growth-factor effect, stimulating hyperplasia within the thyroid gland.

Figure 49.3 The follicular cell and its role in the synthesis of T_4 and T_3. The synthesis and release of T_4 and T_3 occurs in seven steps. *MCT8*, Monocarboxylate transporter 8.

reaches the circulation. The second 5′/3′-deiodinase—**type 2 deiodinase**—is found predominantly in the pituitary, central nervous system (CNS), and placenta, and is involved in supplying those tissues with T_3 by local generation from plasma-derived T_4. The type 2 enzyme in the pituitary is of particular importance because the T_3 that is generated there is responsible for the feedback inhibition of the release of **thyrotropin** (or **thyroid-stimulating hormone, TSH**). Because the 3′ and 5′ positions in T_4 are equivalent stereochemically, removing either of these by type 1 or type 2 deiodinase yields T_3.

A third 5/3-deiodinase—**type 3 deiodinase**—removes an I from the *inner* ring, thereby converting T_4 to the inactive rT_3.

ACTION OF THYROID HORMONES

Thyroid hormones act through nuclear receptors in target tissues

Thyroid hormones act on many body tissues to exert both metabolic and developmental effects. Once T_4 and T_3 leave the plasma, they enter the cell either by diffusing through the lipid of the cell membrane or by carrier-mediated transport (Fig. 49.4). Thyroid hormones bind to and activate **nuclear receptors** (see ⊙ 3-28). There are two **thyroid hormone receptors (TRs)** genes, α and β, and at least two variants of TRβ. The expression of these receptor

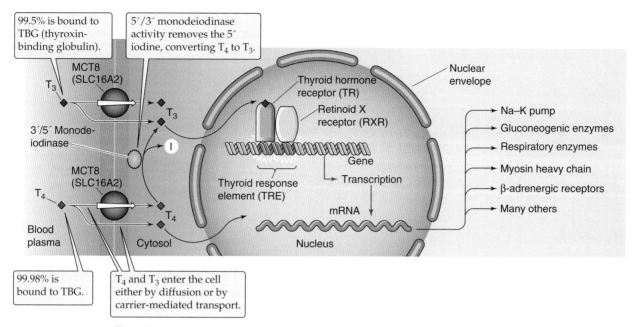

Figure 49.4 Action of thyroid hormones on target cells. *MCT8,* Monocarboxylate transporter 8.

genes is tissue specific and varies with time of development. The liver expresses TRβ, whereas TRα predominates in the brain. Both receptors bind to DNA response elements, predominantly as heterodimers in association with the **retinoid X receptor** (**RXR;** see Table 3.3). When T_3 or T_4 binds to the TR in the nucleus, the hormone-bound receptor either activates or represses the transcription of specific genes.

Biologically, T_3 is much more important than T_4 for three reasons. First, T_4 is bound (only 0.01 to 0.02% is *free*) more tightly to plasma proteins than is T_3 (0.50% is *free*). Second, because the target cell converts some T_4—once it has entered the cell—to T_3, it turns out that T_4 and T_3 are present at similar concentrations in the cytoplasm of target cells. Third, the TR in the nucleus has ~10-fold greater affinity for T_3 than for T_4, so that T_3 is more potent on a molar basis. As a result, T_3 is responsible for ~90% of the occupancy of TRs in the euthyroid state.

Thyroid hormones can also act by nongenomic pathways

In addition to binding to receptors in the nucleus, T_4 and T_3 bind to sites in the cytosol, microsomes, and mitochondria. This observation has raised the issue of whether thyroid hormones exert actions through mechanisms *not* involving transcriptional regulation. For example, thyroid hormones can act via nongenomic pathways to enhance mitochondrial oxidative phosphorylation.

⊙ 49-3 Thyroid hormones increase basal metabolic rate by stimulating futile cycles of catabolism and anabolism

Excess thyroid hormone raises the **basal metabolic rate** (**BMR**) as measured by either heat production (direct calorimetry) or O_2 consumption (indirect calorimetry) (see ⊙

58-1). Conversely, thyroid hormone deficiency is accompanied by a decrease in BMR. Table 49.1 summarizes the effect of the thyroid hormones on several parameters.

Carbohydrate Metabolism Thyroid hormones raise the rate of hepatic glucose production, principally by increasing hepatic gluconeogenic activity (see ⊙ 58-4). Thyroid hormones also enhance the availability of the starting materials required for increased gluconeogenic activity (i.e., amino acids and glycerol), and they specifically induce the expression of several key gluconeogenic enzymes, including phosphoenolpyruvate carboxykinase, pyruvate carboxylase, and glucose 6-phosphatase.

Protein Metabolism The amino acids required for increased hepatic gluconeogenesis stimulated by thyroid hormones come from increased proteolysis, predominantly in muscle. Thyroid hormones also increase protein synthesis. Because the increases in protein degradation usually outweigh the increases in synthesis, a net loss of muscle protein occurs.

Lipid Metabolism Thyroid hormones increase the degradation of stored triacylglycerols in adipose tissue, releasing fatty acids (FAs) and glycerol. The FAs provide fuel for the liver to support the energy demand of gluconeogenesis, and the glycerol provides some of the starting material for gluconeogenesis. Thyroid hormones not only increase lipolysis but also enhance lipogenesis. Indeed, modest amounts of thyroid hormones are needed for the normal synthesis of FAs by liver.

By accelerating the rates of glucose production, protein synthesis and degradation, as well as lipogenesis and lipolysis, the thyroid hormones stimulate energy consumption. Therefore, to the extent that thyroid hormones stimulate both synthesis and degradation, they promote **futile cycles** that contribute significantly to the increased O_2 consumption seen in thyrotoxicosis (hyperthyroidism).

TABLE 49.1 Physiological Effects of the Thyroid Hormones (T$_3$ and T$_4$)

PARAMETER	LOW LEVEL OF THYROID HORMONES (HYPOTHYROID)	HIGH LEVEL OF THYROID HORMONES (HYPERTHYROID)
Basal metabolic rate	↓	↑
Carbohydrate metabolism	↓ Gluconeogenesis ↓ Glycogenolysis Normal serum [glucose]	↑ Gluconeogenesis ↑ Glycogenolysis Normal serum [glucose]
Protein metabolism	↓ Synthesis ↓ Proteolysis	↑ Synthesis ↑ Proteolysis Muscle wasting
Lipid metabolism	↓ Lipogenesis ↓ Lipolysis ↑ Serum [cholesterol]	↑ Lipogenesis ↑ Lipolysis ↓ Serum [cholesterol]
Thermogenesis	↓	↑
Autonomic nervous system	Normal levels of serum catecholamines	↑ Expression of β adrenoceptors (increased sensitivity to catecholamines, which remain at normal levels)

Na-K Pump Activity In muscle, liver, and kidney, thyroid hormone–induced increases in oxygen consumption are paralleled by increases in the activity of the **Na-K pump** in the plasma membrane (see ◉ 5-6). This increase in transport is the result, at least in part, of an increase in the synthesis of new transporter units that are inserted into the plasma membrane. T$_3$ stimulates the transcription of the genes for both the α and β subunits of the Na-K pump. Increases in pump activity consume additional ATP, which results in increased O$_2$ consumption and heat generation. Overall, the increased activity of the Na-K pump (with an accompanying cation leak) would result in a futile cycle in which energy was consumed without useful work.

Thermogenesis ◉ **49-4** Brown fat expresses a mitochondrial **uncoupling protein (UCP)**, or **thermogenin**, that dissociates **oxidative phosphorylation** from ATP generation. Thus, mitochondria consume O$_2$ and produce heat without generating ATP. Both T$_3$ and β-adrenergic stimulation (acting through the β$_3$ receptor) enhance respiration in brown adipose tissue by stimulating this uncoupling mechanism.

Thyroid hormones also increase the BMR by increasing the thermogenic effects of other processes. In humans, plasma *concentrations* of catecholamines are normal in states of both excess and deficient T$_3$ and T$_4$. However, excess thyroid hormone raises the *sensitivity* of tissues to the action of adrenergic hormones.

◉ 49-5 Thyroid hormones are essential for normal growth and development

Thyroid hormones are essential for normal human development as well, as starkly illustrated by the unfortunate condition of cretinism in regions of endemic iodine deficiency. **Cretinism** is characterized by profound mental retardation, short stature, delay in motor development, coarse hair, and a protuberant abdomen. If hypothyroidism is recognized and corrected within 7 to 14 days after birth,

development—including mental development—can proceed almost normally. Once the clinical signs of congenital hypothyroidism become apparent, the developmental abnormalities in the CNS are irreversible.

Typically overshadowed by the impaired cognitive development that occurs in cretinism is the **dwarfism** that results from the effects of thyroid hormone deficiency on human growth. Much of the loss in height that occurs can be recovered after thyroid hormone treatment begins, a phenomenon called *catch-up growth*. If the diagnosis and treatment of hypothyroidism are delayed, loss of potential growth may occur.

Mental development does not catch up unless the treatment begins within 7 to 14 days of birth. In general, the longer the duration of congenital hypothyroidism, the more profound is the mental retardation.

Hypothalamic-Pituitary-Thyroid Axis

The pituitary regulates the synthesis and secretion of thyroid hormones through the release of **thyrotropin**—also known as **thyroid-stimulating hormone (TSH)**—from the anterior pituitary. The hypothalamus, in turn, stimulates the release of TSH through **thyrotropin-releasing hormone (TRH)**. Finally, circulating thyroid hormones exert feedback control on both TRH and TSH secretion.

TRH from the hypothalamus stimulates thyrotrophs of the anterior pituitary to secrete TSH, which stimulates T$_4$/T$_3$ synthesis

Thyrotropin-Releasing Hormone TRH is a tripeptide pyro-Glu-His-Pro containing the modified amino acid pyro-Glu. The arcuate nucleus and the median eminence of the **hypothalamus** appear to be the major sources of the TRH that stimulates TSH synthesis and secretion (Fig. 49.5). TRH released by neurons in the hypothalamus travels to the anterior pituitary through the hypophyseal portal system (see ◉ 47-1).

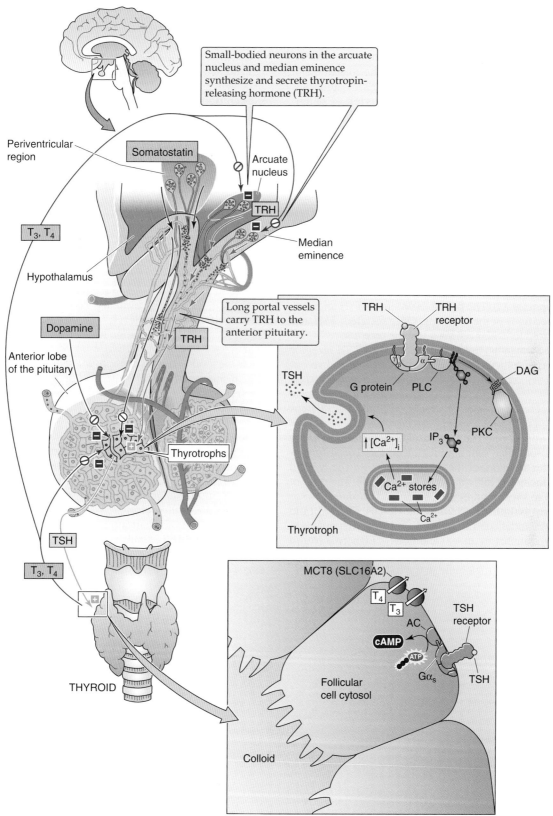

Figure 49.5 Hypothalamic-pituitary-thyroid axis. *AC,* Adenylyl cyclase; *MCT8,* monocarboxylate transporter 8; *PKC,* protein kinase C; *PLC,* phospholipase C.

Thyrotropin-Releasing Hormone Receptor Once it reaches the thyrotrophs in the anterior pituitary, TRH binds to the TRH receptor, a G protein–coupled receptor on the cell membranes of the thyrotrophs. TRH binding triggers the phospholipase C pathway (see ◉ 3-13). The formation of diacylglycerols (DAGs) stimulates protein kinase C and leads to protein phosphorylation. The simultaneous release of inositol trisphosphate (IP_3) triggers Ca^{2+} release from internal stores, raising $[Ca^{2+}]_i$. The result is an increase in both the synthesis and release of TSH, which is stored in secretory granules. TRH produces some of its effects by activating phospholipase A_2, a process leading to the release of arachidonic acid and the formation of a variety of biologically active eicosanoids (see ◉ 3-18).

Thyrotropin The thyrotrophs represent a relatively small number of cells in the **anterior pituitary**. The TSH that they release is a 28-kDa glycoprotein with α and β chains. The α chain of TSH is identical to that of the other glycoprotein hormones: the gonadotropins luteinizing hormone (LH), follicle-stimulating hormone (FSH), and human chorionic gonadotropin (hCG). The β chain is unique to TSH and confers the specificity of the hormone. Once secreted, TSH acts on the thyroid follicular cell via a specific receptor.

Thyroid-Stimulating Hormone Receptor The TSH receptor on the thyroid follicular cells is a G protein–coupled receptor. The TSH receptor, via $G\alpha_s$, activates adenylyl cyclase (see ◉ 3-4). The rise in $[cAMP]_i$ stimulates a diverse range of physiological processes or events—including all 8 steps summarized in Fig. 49.3, except #2:

1. **Iodide uptake** by NIS on the basolateral membrane of the thyroid follicular cell. Stimulation of this cotransporter allows for trapping of dietary iodine within the thyroid gland (including follicular cells and colloid). The ratio of thyroid to serum iodine (the so-called thyroid/serum or T/S ratio) is 30:1 in euthyroid individuals. The T/S ratio decreases under conditions of low TSH (e.g., hypophysectomy) and increases under conditions of high TSH (e.g., a TSH-secreting pituitary adenoma).
2. **Iodination** of thyroglobulin in the follicular lumen.
3. **Conjugation** of iodinated tyrosines to form T_4 and T_3 within the thyroglobulin molecule.
4. **Endocytosis** of iodinated thyroglobulin into the follicular cells from thyroid colloid.
5. **Proteolysis** of the iodinated thyroglobulin in the follicular cell.
6. **Secretion** of T_4 and T_3 into the circulation.
7. **Hyperplasia** of the thyroid gland because of the growth-promoting effects of TSH.

When TSH concentrations are elevated for a prolonged period and stimulate an otherwise normal thyroid gland, the result may be a **goiter.** Hyperplasia of the thyroid gland also occurs in Graves disease because of stimulation of the TSH receptor by a thyroid-stimulating immunoglobulin.

T_3 exerts negative feedback on thyroid-stimulating hormone secretion

Circulating *free* T_4 and T_3 inhibit both the synthesis of TRH by hypothalamic neurons and the release of TSH by the thyrotrophs in the anterior pituitary. Plasma [TSH] is very sensitive to alteration in the levels of free T_4 and T_3. Conversely, an excess of thyroid hormone leads to a decrease in plasma [TSH].

At the level of the thyrotroph, the sensor in this feedback system monitors the concentration of T_3 *inside* the thyrotroph (Fig. 49.5). Either T_3 can enter directly from the blood plasma, or T_3 can form inside the thyrotroph by deiodination of T_4. The negative feedback of T_4 and T_3 on TSH release occurs at the level of the pituitary thyrotroph by both indirect and direct mechanisms. In the **indirect feedback pathway,** intracellular T_3 decreases the number of TRH receptors on the surface of the thyrotroph. In the **direct feedback pathway,** intracellular T_3 inhibits the synthesis of both the α and the β chains of TSH.

Free T_4 and T_3 concentrations in the plasma, which determine intracellular T_3 levels in the thyrotroph, are relatively constant over the course of 24 hours, a finding reflecting the long half-lives of both T_4 and T_3 (see ◉ 49-2).

CHAPTER 50

THE ADRENAL GLAND

Eugene J. Barrett

The human adrenal glands are located above the upper pole of each kidney in the retroperitoneal space. Each adrenal gland is composed of an inner medulla and an outer cortex (Fig. 50.1). The cortex produces two principal steroid hormones, cortisol and aldosterone, as well as several androgenic steroids. The medulla produces epinephrine and norepinephrine.

The **adrenal cortex** can be further divided into three cellular layers: the *glomerulosa* layer near the surface, the *fasciculata* layer in the midcortex, and the *reticularis* layer near the cortical-medullary junction. **Aldosterone** is made in the glomerulosa cell layer. **Cortisol** is made in the fasciculata and, to a small extent, in the reticularis layer. The **adrenal androgens**—dehydroepiandrosterone (DHEA) and its sulfated form, DHEAS—are made in the reticularis layer. Cortisol is considered a **glucocorticoid** because it was recognized early on to increase plasma glucose levels; deficiency of cortisol can result in hypoglycemia. Aldosterone is considered a **mineralocorticoid** because it promotes salt and water retention by the kidney. DHEA and DHEAS are weak androgens (compared to testosterone or dihydrotestosterone) and little is known about the regulation of their secretion.

In the **adrenal medulla,** chromaffin cells produce **epinephrine** (or adrenaline), a catecholamine that is synthesized from the amino acid tyrosine and variable amounts of the epinephrine precursor **norepinephrine.**

THE ADRENAL CORTEX: CORTISOL

Cortisol is the primary glucocorticoid hormone in humans

◉ 50-1 Steroid hormones are divided into three major classes based on their actions: glucocorticoids, mineralocorticoids, and sex steroids. **Cortisol** is the primary glucocorticoid.

The structures of cortisol and aldosterone (Fig. 50.2) differ only slightly: aldosterone lacks the -OH group at position 17 and has an aldehyde (aldo) group at position 18.

Target Tissues In addition to the principal glucose-regulatory tissues, namely, the liver, fat, and muscle, cortisol affects bone, skin, other viscera, hematopoietic and lymphoid tissue, and the central nervous system (CNS).

Actions Glucocorticoids have numerous actions other than their ability to raise plasma glucose levels, including potent immunosuppressive and anti-inflammatory activity, effects on protein and fat metabolism, behavioral effects due to actions on the CNS, and important effects on calcium and bone metabolism. The multiple actions of glucocorticoids, in particular, their "anti-inflammatory" action on leukocytes, has led to the development of numerous synthetic analogs.

Most of the well-characterized actions of glucocorticoids result from their genomic actions to influence (either positively or negatively) the transcription of a variety of genes through glucocorticoid response elements (see ◉ 47-5).

The adrenal zona fasciculata converts cholesterol to cortisol

Synthesis of cortisol starts with cholesterol (Fig. 50.2). The adrenal gland has two sources of cholesterol (see ◉ 47-4): (1) it can import cholesterol from circulating cholesterol-containing low-density lipoprotein (LDL) cholesterol by means of LDL receptor-mediated endocytosis, or (2) it can synthesize cholesterol de novo from acetate.

◉ 50-2 In the adrenal gland, cholesterol is metabolized through a series of five reactions—via alternative pathways (Fig. 50.2)—to make cortisol. All relevant enzymes are located in either the mitochondria or smooth endoplasmic reticulum (SER), and except for 3β-hydroxysteroid dehydrogenase (3β-HSD), belong to the family of **cytochrome P-450 oxidases.**

◉ 50-3 The cells of the reticularis layers are principally responsible for androgen synthesis (Fig. 50.2). These cells convert 17α-hydroxypregnenolone and 17α-hydroxyprogesterone into the *adrenal androgens* **dehydroepiandrosterone** and **androstenedione.** The enzyme that catalyzes this reaction is called 17,20-desmolase. The androgens formed by the adrenal are far less potent than either testosterone or dihydrotestosterone.

The cortisol synthesized by the adrenal cortex diffuses out of the cells and into the blood plasma. There, ~90% of the cortisol is transported bound to **corticosteroid-binding globulin (CBG),** also known as transcortin, which is made in the liver. An additional ~7% of the circulating cortisol is bound to albumin. Thus, only 3% to 4% of the circulating cortisol is free.

The clearance of cortisol from the body depends principally on the liver and kidney. An early step is the formation of an inactive metabolite, cortisone, by the action of either of two **11β-hydroxysteroid dehydrogenases (11β-HSDs).** 11β-HSD1 is highly expressed in certain glucocorticoid *target tissues,* including liver and both subcutaneous and

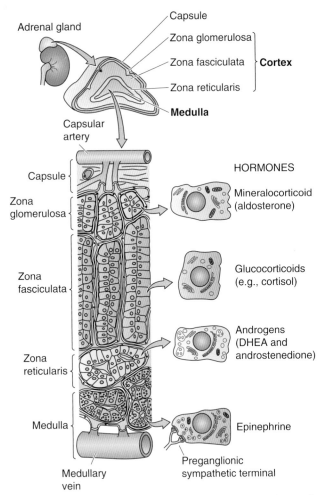

Figure 50.1 Anatomy of the adrenal gland. An adrenal gland—actually two glands, cortex and medulla—sits upon each kidney.

visceral adipose tissue. The body must convert cortisone to cortisol, which is the biologically active agent.

The second **11β-HSD isozyme (11β-HSD2)** is expressed in the adrenal cortex. 11β-HSD2 is highly expressed in the renal distal tubule and collecting duct (see ⊙ **35-8**), where it catalyzes an essentially *irreversible* conversion of cortisol to cortisone. This breakdown of cortisol allows aldosterone to regulate the relatively nonspecific mineralocorticoid receptor (MR) without interference from cortisol.

Cortisol binds to a cytoplasmic receptor that translocates to the nucleus and modulates transcription in multiple tissues

Cortisol, like all steroid hormones, binds to intracellular receptors within target cells (see ⊙ **3-28**). Virtually all nucleated tissues in the body contain receptors for glucocorticoids. The glucocorticoid receptor (GR) is primarily located in the cytoplasm, where in its unbound form it is complexed to a chaperone protein (i.e., the heat shock protein hsp90; see Fig. 4.15A). Binding of cortisol causes the chaperone to dissociate from the GR, and this allows the cortisol-GR complex to translocate to the nucleus. There, the cortisol-receptor complex associates with **glucocorticoid response elements (GREs)** on the 5′ untranslated region of multiple genes to either enhance or diminish gene expression (see ⊙ **4-4**).

Activity of the glucocorticoid-receptor complex requires dimerization of two identical receptor complexes (i.e., the GR functions as a *homodimer*). Glucocorticoids mainly act by modulating gene transcription. One exception is the acute feedback effect of cortisol to block the release of preformed **adrenocorticotropic hormone (ACTH)** in the secretory granules of pituitary corticotrophs.

⊙ **50-4** In **liver,** cortisol induces the synthesis of enzymes involved in gluconeogenesis and amino-acid metabolism in support of gluconeogenesis, thus enhancing hepatic glucose production. In **muscle,** cortisol stimulates the breakdown of muscle protein, which releases amino acids for uptake by the liver. Similarly, cortisol promotes lipolysis in **adipose tissue.**

Glucocorticoids also act on the cellular elements of trabecular bone (see ⊙ **52-11**), decreasing the ability of osteoblasts to synthesize new bone. They also interfere with absorption of Ca^{2+} from the gastrointestinal tract. As a result, long-term glucocorticoid use causes osteoporosis. In addition, glucocorticoids act on the CNS and can cause a variety of effects, including alterations in mood and cognition.

Corticotropin-releasing hormone from the hypothalamus stimulates anterior pituitary corticotrophs to secrete ACTH, which stimulates the adrenal cortex to synthesize and secrete cortisol

As summarized in Fig. 50.3, regulation of the synthesis and secretion of cortisol begins with the release of **corticotropin-releasing hormone (CRH)** from hypothalamic neurons as part of either a normal daily circadian rhythm or a centrally driven stress response. CRH stimulates the release of ACTH, also called corticotropin, from the anterior pituitary. ACTH directly stimulates the adrenal fasciculata layers to synthesize and secrete cortisol. Circulating cortisol exerts negative-feedback control on the release of both ACTH and CRH.

Corticotropin-Releasing Hormone ⊙ **50-5** Small-bodied neurons in the paraventricular nucleus of the **hypothalamus** (see Fig. 47.2) secrete CRH (Fig. 50.3). The hypothalamic neurons synthesize and release CRH via the classic secretory pathway. Neurons store CRH in secretory vesicles located in synaptic terminals in the median eminence of the hypothalamus and can release CRH acutely in the absence of new synthesis. After release into the interstitial fluid of the median eminence, CRH enters the hypophyseal portal venous plexus (see ⊙ **47-1**) and travels to the anterior pituitary.

Corticotropin-Releasing Hormone Receptor CRH arriving in the anterior pituitary binds to CRH-R1, a G protein–coupled receptor (GPCR) on the cell membrane of corticotroph cells. Hormone binding activates $G\alpha_s$, which in turn stimulates adenylyl cyclase and raises $[cAMP]_i$ (see ⊙ **3-4**). Subsequent stimulation of protein kinase A (PKA) activates L-type Ca^{2+} channels, leading to an increase in $[Ca^{2+}]_i$, which stimulates the exocytosis of preformed ACTH. Over a much longer time, CRH receptor activation also leads to increased gene transcription and synthesis of the ACTH precursor.

Arginine Vasopressin Although CRH is the major regulator of ACTH secretion, the paraventricular nuclei also make another hormone, arginine vasopressin (AVP; see Fig. 40.4). AVP is also a potent ACTH secretagogue and probably plays a physiological role in the regulation of ACTH secretion during stresses like dehydration or trauma.

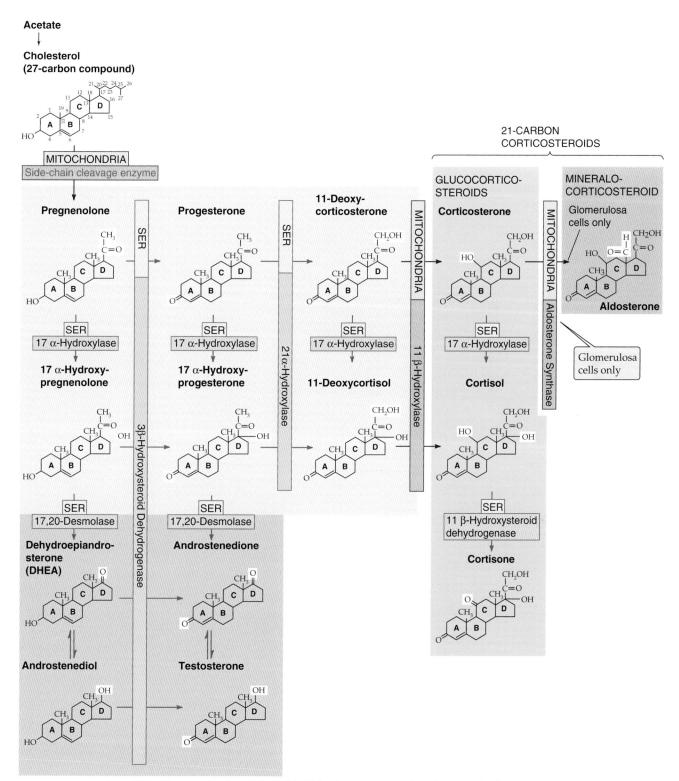

Figure 50.2 Biosynthesis of adrenal steroids. This schematic summarizes the synthesis of the adrenal steroids—the mineralocorticoid *aldosterone* and the glucocorticoid *cortisol*—from cholesterol. The individual enzymes are shown in the horizontal and vertical boxes; they are located in either the SER or the mitochondria.

Adrenocorticotropic Hormone Pituitary corticotrophs synthesize ACTH by complex post-translational processing of a large precursor protein (i.e., a preprohormone) called **pro-opiomelanocortin (POMC).** POMC is the precursor not only for ACTH, but also for a variety of peptide hormones.

Adrenocorticotropic Hormone Receptor ⊚ 50-6 In the adrenal cortex, ACTH binds to the **melanocortin 2 receptor MC2R** on the plasma membranes of all three steroid-secreting cell types (Fig. 50.3). However, because only the cells in the fasciculata and reticularis layers have the 17α-hydroxylase needed for synthesizing cortisol (Fig. 50.2),

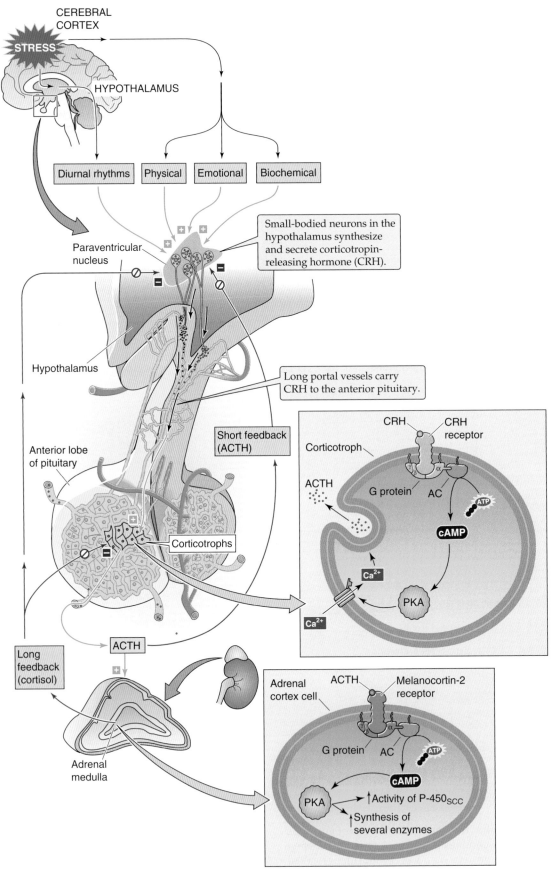

CEREBRAL CORTEX

STRESS

HYPOTHALAMUS

Diurnal rhythms   Physical   Emotional   Biochemical

Paraventricular nucleus

Small-bodied neurons in the hypothalamus synthesize and secrete corticotropin-releasing hormone (CRH).

Hypothalamus

Long portal vessels carry CRH to the anterior pituitary.

Short feedback (ACTH)

Anterior lobe of pituitary

Corticotrophs

CRH   CRH receptor

Corticotroph

ACTH

G protein   AC

ATP

cAMP

Ca^{2+}

Ca^{2+}

PKA

ACTH

Long feedback (cortisol)

Adrenal medulla

Adrenal cortex cell   ACTH   Melanocortin-2 receptor

G protein   AC

ATP

cAMP

PKA   →↑Activity of P-450$_{SCC}$

↑Synthesis of several enzymes

Figure 50.3   Hypothalamic-pituitary-adrenocortical axis.

these cells are the only ones that secrete cortisol in response to ACTH. MC2R is coupled to a heterotrimeric G protein and stimulates adenylyl cyclase (see ⊙ 3-8). The resulting increase in [cAMP]$_i$ activates PKA, which phosphorylates a variety of proteins. A rapid effect of ACTH is to stimulate the conversion of cholesterol to pregnenolone via the **side-chain-cleavage** (SCC) enzyme. In addition, ACTH increases the synthesis of several proteins needed for cortisol synthesis.

In the absence of pituitary ACTH, the fasciculata and reticularis layers of the adrenal cortex atrophy. The glomerulosa layer does not atrophy under these conditions because in addition to ACTH, angiotensin II (ANG II) and high levels of K$^+$ are trophic factors that act on the glomerulosa layer. The atrophy of the fasciculata and reticularis layers occurs routinely in people treated with glucocorticoid drugs and leaves the person with an iatrogenic form of adrenal insufficiency when use of the drug is abruptly discontinued. Conversely, chronic stimulation of the adrenals by ACTH, such as can occur with pituitary tumors (Cushing disease) or with the simple physiological ACTH excess that can occur with chronic stress, can increase the weight of the adrenals several-fold.

Cortisol exerts negative feedback on CRH and ACTH secretion, whereas stress acts through higher CNS centers to stimulate the axis

Cortisol exerts negative-feedback control on the very axis that stimulates its secretion (Fig. 50.3), and it does so at the level of both the anterior pituitary and hypothalamus.

Feedback to the Anterior Pituitary In the corticotrophs of the anterior pituitary, cortisol acts by binding to a cytosolic receptor, which then moves to the nucleus, where it binds to GREs and modulates gene expression and thus inhibits the synthesis of both the CRH receptor and ACTH. In addition, elevated levels of cortisol in plasma inhibit the release of pre-synthesized ACTH stored in vesicles.

Feedback to the Hypothalamus The negative feedback of cortisol on the CRH-secreting neurons of the hypothalamus is less important than that on the corticotrophs discussed above. Plasma cortisol decreases the mRNA and peptide levels of CRH in paraventricular hypothalamic neurons. Cortisol also inhibits the release of presynthesized CRH. Synthetic glucocorticoids have a similar action.

Control by a Higher CNS Center CRH-secreting neurons in the hypothalamus are under higher CNS control. The pituitary secretes ACTH with a **circadian rhythm.** The suprachiasmatic nucleus of the hypothalamus controls the circadian rhythms of the body. Input from hypothalamic nuclei to the corticotrophs—via both CRH and AVP—appears to modulate the circadian secretion of ACTH and thus the circadian secretion of cortisol as well. CRH is released in pulses. As a result, superimposed on the circadian rhythm of ACTH is the **pulsatile secretion** of ACTH. ACTH secretory activity is greatest in the early morning and diminishes late in the afternoon and early evening.

The increase in ACTH secretion that occurs nocturnally and with stress appears to result from an increased amplitude of the secretory CRH burst rather than an increased frequency of secretion episodes. Because the half-life of cortisol is much longer than that of ACTH, the period of the pulsatile

changes in cortisol is longer and the magnitude of the excursions is damped in comparison with those of ACTH.

THE ADRENAL CORTEX: ALDOSTERONE

The mineralocorticoid aldosterone is the primary regulator of salt balance and extracellular volume

Aldosterone determines extracellular volume by controlling the extent to which the kidney excretes or reabsorbs the Na$^+$ filtered at the renal glomerulus. Na$^+$ in the extracellular space retains water determines the volume of extracellular fluid (see ⊙ 5-16). The extracellular volume is itself a prime determinant of arterial blood pressure (see ⊙ 23-26), and therefore aldosterone plays an important role in the maintenance of blood pressure.

The glomerulosa cells of the adrenal cortex synthesize aldosterone from cholesterol via progesterone

The adrenal cortex synthesizes aldosterone from cholesterol by using P-450 enzymes in five steps (Fig. 50.2). The initial steps in the synthesis of aldosterone from cholesterol follow the same synthetic pathway that cortisol-secreting cells use to generate **progesterone.** Because glomerulosa cells are the only ones that contain aldosterone synthase, these cells are the exclusive site of aldosterone synthesis.

As with cortisol, no storage pool of presynthesized aldosterone is available in the glomerulosa cell for rapid secretion. Thus, secretion of aldosterone by the adrenal is limited by the rate at which the glomerulosa cells can synthesize the hormone. Although ACTH also stimulates the production of aldosterone in the glomerulosa cell, increases in extracellular [K$^+$] and the peptide hormone ANG II are physiologically more important secretagogues.

Once secreted, ~37% of circulating aldosterone remains free in plasma. The rest weakly binds to CBG (~21%) or albumin (~42%).

Aldosterone stimulates Na$^+$ reabsorption and K$^+$ secretion by the renal tubule

The major action of aldosterone is to stimulate the kidney to reabsorb Na$^+$ and water and enhance K$^+$ secretion. Aldosterone has similar actions on salt and water transport in the colon, salivary glands, and sweat glands.

Aldosterone, like all the other steroid hormones, acts principally by modulating gene transcription (see ⊙ 4-4). In the kidney, aldosterone binds to both low- and high-affinity receptors. The low-affinity receptor appears to be identical to the **GR.** The high-affinity receptor is a distinct **MR.** Surprisingly, MR in the kidney has a similar affinity for aldosterone and cortisol.

However, the cells that are targets for aldosterone—particularly in the initial collecting tubule and cortical collecting tubule of the kidney (see ⊙ 35-8)—contain 11β-HSD2, which converts cortisol to cortisone, a steroid with a very low affinity for MR. As a result, within the target cell, the cortisol-to-aldosterone ratio is much smaller than the cortisol dominance seen in plasma. Thus, the presence of 11β-HSD2 effectively confers aldosterone specificity on the MR.

In the target cells of the renal tubule, aldosterone increases the activity of several key proteins involved in Na$^+$ transport (see ◉ 35-6). It increases transcription of the Na-K pump, thus augmenting distal Na$^+$ reabsorption. Aldosterone also raises the expression of apical Na$^+$ channels and of an Na/K/Cl cotransporter. The net effect of these actions is to increase Na$^+$ reabsorption and K$^+$ secretion.

Loss of aldosterone-mediated Na$^+$ reabsorption can result in significant electrolyte abnormalities, including life-threatening hyperkalemia and, in the absence of other compensatory mechanisms, hypotension. Conversely, excess aldosterone secretion produces hypokalemia and hypertension (see ◉ 50-7).

Angiotensin II, K$^+$, and ACTH all stimulate aldosterone secretion

Three secretagogues control aldosterone synthesis by the glomerulosa cells of the adrenal cortex. The most important is ANG II, which is a product of the renin-angiotensin cascade. An increase in plasma [K$^+$] is also a powerful stimulus for aldosterone secretion and augments the response to ANG II. Third, just as ACTH promotes cortisol secretion, it also promotes the secretion of aldosterone, although this effect is weak.

Angiotensin II We introduced the renin-angiotensin-aldosterone axis in Chapter 40 (see ◉ 40-2). The liver synthesizes and secretes a very large protein called **angiotensinogen** (Fig. 50.4). **Renin,** which is synthesized by the granular (or juxtaglomerular) cells of the juxtaglomerular apparatus (JGA) in the kidney (see ◉ 33-1), is the enzyme that cleaves this angiotensinogen to form **ANG I,** a decapeptide. Finally, angiotensin-converting enzyme (ACE) cleaves ANG I to form the octapeptide **ANG II.** ACE is present in both the vascular endothelium of the lung (~40%) and elsewhere (~60%). In addition to acting as a potent secretagogue for aldosterone, ANG II exerts powerful vasoconstrictor actions on vascular smooth muscle.

On the plasma membrane of the glomerulosa cell, ANG II binds to the **AT$_1$ receptor** (type 1 ANG II receptor), which couples through the Gα_q-mediated pathway to phospholipase C (PLC). Stimulation of PLC leads to the formation of diacylglycerol (DAG) and inositol 1,4,5-trisphosphate (IP$_3$; see ◉ 3-13). DAG activates protein kinase C (PKC). IP$_3$ triggers the release of Ca^{2+} from intracellular stores, thus causing a rise in [Ca^{2+}]$_i$, which activates Ca^{2+}-dependent enzymes such as PKC and Ca^{2+}-calmodulin-dependent protein kinases. These changes lead to depolarization of the glomerulosa cell's plasma membrane, opening of voltage-activated Ca^{2+} channels, and a *sustained* increase in Ca^{2+} influx from the extracellular space. This rise in [Ca^{2+}]$_i$ is primarily responsible for triggering the synthesis (i.e., secretion) of aldosterone. Aldosterone secretion increases because the rise in [Ca^{2+}]$_i$ facilitates the production of pregnenolone either by directly increasing the activity of SCC or by enhancing the delivery of cholesterol to the SCC enzyme in the mitochondria (Fig. 50.2). In addition, increased [Ca^{2+}]$_i$ also stimulates aldosterone synthase, enhancing the conversion of corticosterone to aldosterone.

Potassium An increase in extracellular K$^+$ ([K$^+$]$_o$) has a direct action on the glomerulosa cell (Fig. 50.4). Several K$^+$

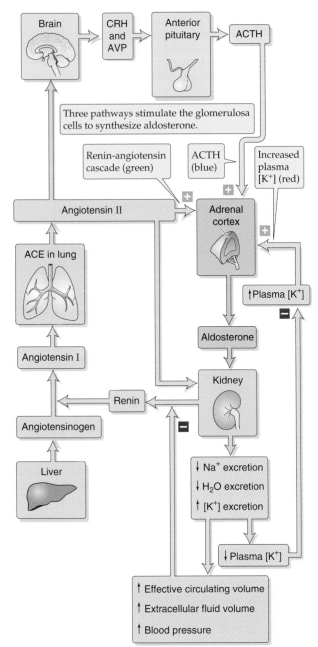

Figure 50.4 Control of aldosterone secretion. Three pathways (shown in three different colors) stimulate the glomerulosa cells of the adrenal cortex to secrete aldosterone.

channels maintain the normal resting potential of these cells. Thus, high [K$^+$]$_o$ depolarizes the plasma membrane and opens voltage-gated Ca^{2+} channels. The result is an influx of Ca^{2+} and a rise in [Ca^{2+}]$_i$ that stimulates the same two steps as ANG II—production of pregnenolone from cholesterol and conversion of corticosterone to aldosterone. Because increased [K$^+$]$_o$ and ANG II both act by raising [Ca^{2+}]$_i$, they can act synergistically on glomerulosa cells.

Adrenocorticotropic Hormone ACTH stimulates aldosterone secretion via the MC2R receptor in glomerulosa cells, which is coupled via a heterotrimeric G protein to adenylyl cyclase. Increases in ACTH raise [cAMP]$_i$ and activate PKA, which phosphorylates large numbers of cytosolic proteins. It is unclear how these changes stimulate Ca^{2+} influx across

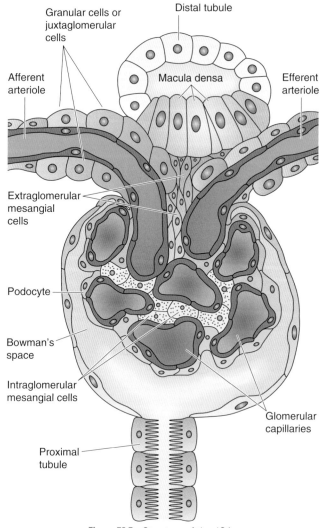

Granular cells or juxtaglomerular cells

Distal tubule

Afferent arteriole

Macula densa

Efferent arteriole

Extraglomerular mesangial cells

Podocyte

Bowman's space

Intraglomerular mesangial cells

Glomerular capillaries

Proximal tubule

Figure 50.5 Structure of the JGA.

the plasma membrane and enhance the synthesis and secretion of aldosterone. ACTH also enhances mineralocorticoid activity by a second mechanism: stimulation of the fasciculata cells to secrete cortisol, corticosterone, and DOC, all of which have weak mineralocorticoid activity.

Aldosterone exerts indirect negative feedback on the renin-angiotensin axis by increasing effective circulating volume and by lowering plasma [K⁺]

The feedback regulation exerted by aldosterone is indirect and occurs through its effects of both increasing salt retention (i.e., extracellular volume) and decreasing $[K^+]_o$.

Renin-Angiotensin Axis A decrease in effective circulating volume stimulates the granular cells of the JGA of the kidney to increase their synthesis and release of renin, which increases the generation of ANG II and, therefore, aldosterone (Fig. 50.4). The **JGA** is located at the glomerular pole of the nephron, between the afferent and efferent arterioles, where the early distal tubule comes in close proximity to its own glomerulus (Fig. 50.5). The JGA comprises specialized epithelial cells of the distal tubule called **macula densa cells,** as well as specialized smooth-muscle cells of the *afferent*

arteriole, which are called granular cells or juxtaglomerular cells. Macula densa cells and granular cells communicate through the extracellular matrix.

Decreases in effective circulating volume—or the associated decreases in systemic arterial pressure—stimulate renin release from the **granular cells** of the JGA in three ways discussed in Chapter 40 (see ⊙ **40-4**). Enhanced renin release leads to increased levels of ANG II and aldosterone. ANG II negatively feeds back on renin release *directly* by inhibiting renin release by granular cells (short-loop feedback). ANG II also negatively feeds back on renin release *indirectly* by acutely increasing systemic arterial pressure (see ⊙ **23-23**), thereby reducing the stimuli to release renin (see ⊙ **40-4**). Finally, aldosterone negatively feeds back on renin release more slowly by enhancing renal Na⁺ reabsorption (see ⊙ **35-6**) and thus increasing effective circulating blood volume and blood pressure. Therefore, ANG II and aldosterone complete the regulatory feedback circuit that governs the secretion of aldosterone.

Potassium High plasma [K⁺] stimulates the glomerulosa cell in the adrenal cortex to synthesize and release aldosterone, which in turn stimulates the principal cells of the renal collecting duct to reabsorb more Na⁺ and excrete more K⁺ (Fig. 50.4). This excretion of K⁺ causes plasma [K⁺] to fall toward normal. As a result, stimulation of glomerulosa cells declines, aldosterone secretion falls, and the negative-feedback loop is completed.

Role of Aldosterone in Normal Physiology The salt- and water-retaining properties of aldosterone are of greatest value in meeting the environmental stresses associated with limited availability of salt, water, or both. In healthy, normotensive humans, blockade of aldosterone generation with ACE-inhibiting drugs reduces ANG II production and markedly decreases plasma aldosterone, but it causes only slight decreases in total-body Na⁺ and blood pressure. In contrast to the minor effects of low aldosterone on blood pressure and *Na⁺* balance in physiologically normal people, the effects of blocking aldosterone production can result in life-threatening hyperkalemia. Potassium levels are carefully followed in patients receiving aldosterone antagonists, ACE inhibitors, angiotensin receptor blockers (ARBs), and renin inhibitors.

Role of Aldosterone in Disease Aldosterone does play important roles in several pathological conditions. For example, in many patients with *hyper*tension, ACE inhibitors or ARBs are effective in reducing blood pressure, a finding implying that their renin-angiotensin-aldosterone axis was overactive. In *hypo*tension, as occurs with hemorrhage or dehydration, aldosterone secretion increases, thus raising effective circulating volume and blood pressure.

⊙ **50-7** Hyperaldosteronism was long thought to be an uncommon cause of hypertension. Now we recognize that hyperaldosteronism is responsible for ~10% of hypertension and for an even greater fraction of treatment-resistant hypertension. **Primary hyperaldosteronism** can result from either an isolated adrenal adenoma or bilateral adrenal hyperplasia; more rarely, adrenal carcinoma can produce excess aldosterone. In patients with adenomas of the glomerulosa cell, the disorder is called **Conn syndrome.** Hypertension and hypokalemia frequently develop in these patients. As would be expected from feedback regulation of the renin-angiotensin-aldosterone system, the plasma renin concentration is characteristically suppressed in this form of hypertension.

THE ADRENAL MEDULLA

⊙ 50-8 The adrenal medulla bridges the endocrine and sympathetic nervous systems

The cells of the medulla, termed **chromaffin cells,** derive from neural crest cells and migrate into the center of the adrenal cortex, which is derived from the mesoderm. The adrenomedullary cells synthesize and secrete epinephrine and—to a lesser extent—norepinephrine. Norepinephrine is the neurotransmitter of the sympathetic division of the autonomic nervous system (see ⊙ 14-6). Both the norepinephrine and epinephrine made in the adrenal medulla enter the circulation and act on distal tissues just like other hormones.

Chromaffin cells are the structural and functional equivalents of the **postganglionic** neurons in the sympathetic nervous system (see ⊙ 14-7). The preganglionic sympathetic fibers of the splanchnic nerves, which release acetylcholine (ACh), are the principal regulators of adrenomedullary hormone secretion.

The vascular supply to the adrenal medulla is also unusual. The medulla receives vascular input from vessels that begin in a subcapsular plexus of the adrenal cortex. The vessels then branch into a capillary network in the cortex only to merge into small venous vessels that branch into a second capillary network within the medulla. This **portal blood supply** (originating at the entrance to the adrenal) exposes the adrenal medulla to the highest concentrations of glucocorticoids and mineralocorticoids of all somatic tissues.

⊙ 50-9 Only chromaffin cells of the adrenal medulla have the enzyme for epinephrine synthesis

Catecholamines (Fig. 50.6A)—L-dopa, dopamine, norepinephrine, and epinephrine—are all made in the adrenal medulla. Although **norepinephrine** is found in many other somatic tissues, it is not made there but is derived from the sympathetic nerve endings in them. Virtually all the circulating **epinephrine,** the principal product of the adrenal medulla, comes from the adrenal medulla.

Dopamine, norepinephrine, and epinephrine are all synthesized from the amino acid tyrosine. Fig. 50.6A summarizes the four enzymatic reactions involved in the synthesis of epinephrine. Fig. 50.7 illustrates the cellular localization of these four reactions, as well as the three critical transport steps that shuttle the reactants and products to their proper location.

Epinephrine synthesis is under the control of the CRH-ACTH-cortisol axis at two levels. First, ACTH stimulates the synthesis of L-dopa and norepinephrine. Second, cortisol transported from the adrenal cortex by the portal circulation to the medulla upregulates **phenylethanolamine-N-methyltransferase (PNMT)** in chromaffin cells. The result is synergy between the CRH-ACTH-cortisol axis and the sympathetic-epinephrine axis.

The secretory granules of the adrenal medulla contain very high concentrations of catecholamines (as high as 0.5 M). These catecholamines bind to granular proteins

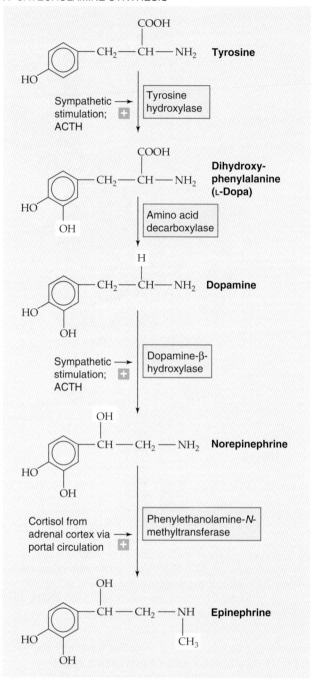

A CATECHOLAMINE SYNTHESIS

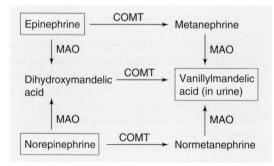

B DEGRADATIVE METABOLISM OF CATECHOLAMINES

Figure 50.6 Synthesis and degradation of catecholamines. In (A) the *horizontal arrows* indicate enhancement of the reaction. *MAO,* Monoamine oxidase.

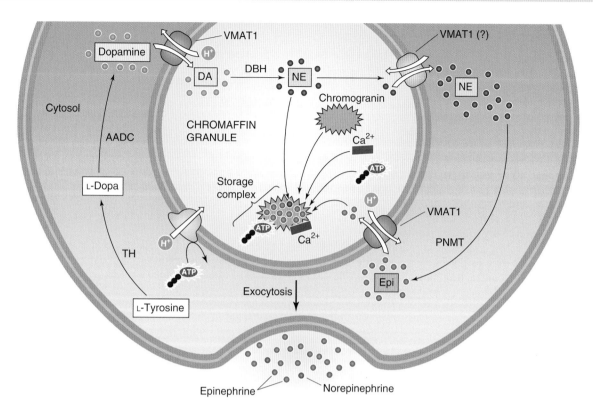

Figure 50.7 Cellular view of catecholamine synthesis. The chromaffin cell synthesizes and stores epinephrine in a sequence of four enzymatic reactions and three transport steps. *AADC*, Amino-acid decarboxylase; *DA*, dopamine; *DBH*, dopamine β-hydroxylase; *Epi*, epinephrine; *NE*, norepinephrine; *PNMT*, phenylethanolamine-*N*-methyltransferase; *TH*, tyrosine hydroxylase.

called **chromogranins** and thus are not osmotically active in these storage vesicles. The release of catecholamines is initiated by CNS control. ACh released from preganglionic neurons in the splanchnic nerves acts on nicotinic ACh receptors to depolarize the postganglionic chromaffin cells. This depolarization triggers the opening of voltage-gated Ca^{2+} channels, raises $[Ca^{2+}]_i$, and triggers the exocytotic release of epinephrine.

In the fight-or-flight response to stress (see ⊚ **14-10**), an organism responds with centrally driven release of adrenal hormones, as well as activation of other aspects of the sympathetic nervous system. This response includes increases in heart rate and contractility, mobilization of fuel stores from muscle and fat, piloerection, pupillary dilatation, and increased sphincter tone of the bowel and bladder.

The biological actions of catecholamines are very brief, lasting only ~10 seconds in the case of epinephrine. Circulating catecholamines are degraded first by the enzyme **catechol-O-methyltransferase (COMT),** which is present in high concentrations in endothelial cells and the heart, liver, and kidneys (Fig. 50.6B). COMT converts epinephrine to metanephrine, as well as norepinephrine to normetanephrine. A second enzyme, **monoamine oxidase,** converts these metabolites to vanillylmandelic acid (VMA). The liver and also the gut then conjugate these compounds to sulfate (see ⊚ **46-4**) or glucuronide (see ⊚ **46-3**) to form derivatives that the kidney excretes in the urine. Determination of the concentration of catecholamines, metanephrines, and VMA in the urine provides a measure of the total adrenal catecholamine production by both the adrenal medulla and the sympathetic system.

Catecholamines bind to α and β adrenoceptors on the cell surface and act through heterotrimeric G proteins

Epinephrine and norepinephrine can each bind to more than one type of adrenergic receptor, or **adrenoceptor,** all of which are GPCRs.

Epinephrine and epinephrine analogs produce both excitatory and inhibitory effects, depending on the tissue. This property led to the designation of α-adrenergic receptors (mostly associated with stimulation) and β-adrenergic receptors (mostly associated with inhibition). Moreover, certain drugs could selectively block the α and β effects.

It is now clear that at least three types of β and two types of α receptors exist (see Table 14.2), as well as subtypes within these major classes. These receptors differ in primary structure and in the types of G proteins that associate with the receptor. The several β receptors are coupled to stimulatory heterotrimeric G proteins ($G\alpha_s$) that *stimulate* adenylyl cyclase and thus increase levels of cAMP (see ⊚ **3-4**), the principal intracellular mediator of β activation. The α_2 adrenoceptors are coupled to other G proteins ($G\alpha_i$) that *inhibit* adenylyl cyclase and thus lower $[cAMP]_i$ in target tissues. The α_1 receptors are coupled to yet another heterotrimeric G protein ($G\alpha_q$) that activates PLC (see ⊚ **3-13**) and thereby increases $[IP_3]_i$ and $[Ca^{2+}]_i$ in target tissues.

The CNS-epinephrine axis provides integrated control of multiple functions

The actions of the sympathetic nervous system in the control of blood pressure (see ⊚ **23-9**), heart rate (see ⊚ **23-8**), sweating (see ⊙ **60-4**), micturition (see ⊙ **33-3**), and airway resistance (see ⊙ **27-8**) are discussed in more detail in other chapters, as indicated. Here, we mention only some of the unique actions attributed to adrenal catecholamine release that integrate several bodily functions as part of the stress response. These adrenal-mediated activities do not occur in isolation but are usually accompanied by generalized noradrenergic sympathetic discharge.

In response to the stress of simple **exercise** (see ⊙ **25-4**), blood flow to muscle is increased; circulating epinephrine appears to be important in this response. Circulating epinephrine also relaxes bronchial smooth muscle to meet the demand for increased ventilation and, when combined with the increased blood flow, increases oxygen delivery to the exercising muscle. Similarly, early in exercise, epinephrine acting via the β adrenoceptor activates the degradation of muscle glycogen to provide a ready fuel source for the contracting muscle (see ⊙ **58-10**).

Epinephrine also activates lipolysis in adipose tissue (see ⊙ **58-12**) to furnish fatty acids for more sustained muscular activity if needed. In liver, as in muscle, epinephrine activates glycogenolysis, so that the supply of glucose is maintained in the blood.

In addition to enhancing blood flow and ventilation, the integrated response to exercise increases fuel availability by decreasing insulin levels. Circulating epinephrine, acting through a β adrenoceptor, *stimulates* the secretion of insulin (see ⊙ **51-4**). However, during exercise, local autonomic innervation, acting by means of an α adrenoceptor of the pancreas, *inhibits* this effect so that insulin levels fall. The net effects are to promote glycogenolysis and to allow muscle to increase its work while maintaining glycemia so that brain function is not impaired.

Unlike in other glandular tissue, no endocrine feedback loop governs the secretion of adrenal medullary hormones. Control of catecholamine secretion resides within the CNS.

CHAPTER 51

THE ENDOCRINE PANCREAS

Eugene J. Barrett

The islets of Langerhans are endocrine and paracrine tissue

The pancreas contains two types of glands: (1) exocrine glands, which secrete digestive enzymes (see ⊙ 43-1) and HCO_3^- (see ⊙ 43-2) into the intestinal lumen, and (2) endocrine glands, called the *islets of Langerhans.* The islets are spread throughout the pancreas and in aggregate compose only 1% to 2% of its tissue mass.

⊙ **51-1** The normal human pancreas contains between 500,000 and several million islets. Islets contain at least four types of secretory cells—α cells, β cells, δ cells, and F cells—in addition to various vascular and neural elements. β **cells** secrete insulin, proinsulin, C peptide, and a newly described protein, amylin (or IAPP for islet amyloid polypeptide). β cells are the most numerous type of secretory cell within the islets; they are located throughout the islet, but are particularly numerous in the center. α **cells** principally secrete glucagon, δ **cells** secrete somatostatin, and **F cells** (also called pancreatic polypeptide cells) secrete pancreatic polypeptide.

The islets are richly perfused (blood flow per gram of tissue is >5 times that of the myocardium) and receive both sympathetic and parasympathetic innervation. These cells also can communicate with each other and influence each other's secretion. We can group these communication links into three categories:

1. **Humoral communication.** Cells within a given islet can influence the secretion of other cells as the blood supply courses from the center, outward through the islet, carrying with it the secreted hormonal product of each cell type.
2. **Cell-cell communication.** Both gap and tight junctional structures connect islet cells with one another.
3. **Neural communication.** Both the sympathetic and parasympathetic divisions of the autonomic nervous system (ANS) regulate islet secretion.

⊙ 51-2 INSULIN

Following the identification of insulin, the physiology of the synthesis, secretion, and action of the hormone has been studied more extensively than that of any other hormone.

Insulin replenishes fuel reserves in muscle, liver, and adipose tissue

Insulin efficiently integrates body fuel metabolism both during periods of fasting and during feeding (Table 51.1). When an individual is *fasting,* the β cell secretes less insulin. When insulin levels decrease, lipids are mobilized from adipose tissue and amino acids are mobilized from body protein stores within muscle and other tissues. These lipids and amino acids provide fuel for oxidation and serve as precursors for hepatic ketogenesis and gluconeogenesis, respectively. During *feeding,* insulin secretion increases promptly, which diminishes the mobilization of endogenous fuel stores and stimulates the uptake of carbohydrates, lipids, and amino acids by insulin-sensitive target tissues.

As a result of its ability to regulate the mobilization and storage of fuels, insulin maintains plasma [glucose] within narrow limits. Such regulation provides the central nervous system (CNS) with a constant supply of glucose needed to fuel cortical function. In higher organisms, if plasma [glucose] (normally ≅ 5 mM) declines to <2 to 3 mM (hypoglycemia) for even a brief period, confusion, seizures, and coma may result. Conversely, persistent elevations of plasma [glucose] are characteristic of the diabetic state. Severe *hyper*glycemia (plasma glucose levels > 15 mM) produces an osmotic diuresis that, when severe, can lead to dehydration, hypotension, and vascular collapse.

β cells synthesize and secrete insulin

The Insulin Gene Circulating insulin comes only from the β cells of the pancreatic islet. It is encoded by a single gene on the short arm of chromosome 11. Exposing islets to glucose stimulates insulin synthesis and secretion.

Insulin Synthesis Transcription of the insulin gene product and subsequent processing produces full-length messenger RNA (mRNA) that encodes **preproinsulin.** Insulin is a *secretory protein.* As the preprohormone is synthesized, the leader sequence of ~24 amino acids is cleaved from the nascent peptide as it enters the rough endoplasmic reticulum. The result is **proinsulin,** which consists of domains B, C, and A. As the *trans* Golgi packages the proinsulin and creates secretory granules, proteases excise the C peptide, resulting in the mature insulin

TABLE 51.1 Effects of Nutritional States

PARAMETER	AFTER A 24-HOUR FAST	2 HOURS AFTER A MIXED MEAL
Plasma [glucose], mg/dL	60–80	100–140
mM	3.3–4.4	5.6–7.8
Plasma [insulin], µU/mL	3–8	50–150
Plasma [glucagon], pg/mL	40–80	80–200
Liver	↑ Glycogenolysis ↑ Gluconeogenesis	↓ Glycogenolysis ↓ Gluconeogenesis ↑ Glycogen synthesis
Adipose tissue	Lipids mobilized for fuel	Lipids synthesized
Muscle	Lipids metabolized Protein degraded and amino acids exported	Glucose oxidized or stored as glycogen Protein preserved

molecule, composed of two peptide chains (the **A and B chains**), joined by two disulfide linkages. The secretory vesicle contains this insulin, as well as proinsulin and C peptide. All three are released into the portal blood when glucose stimulates the β cell.

Secretion of Insulin, Proinsulin, and C Peptide C peptide has no established biological action. Yet because it is secreted in a 1:1 molar ratio with insulin, it is a useful marker for insulin secretion. Proinsulin does have modest insulin-like activities.

Most of the insulin (~60%) that is secreted into the portal blood is removed in a first pass through the liver. In contrast, C peptide is not extracted by the liver at all, but is eventually excreted in the urine. The quantity of C peptide excreted in a 24-hour period is a rough measure of the amount of insulin released.

Glucose is the major regulator of insulin secretion

In healthy individuals, the **plasma [glucose] concentration** remains within a remarkably narrow range. After an overnight fast, it typically averages between 4 and 5 mM; the plasma [glucose] rises after a meal, but even with a very large meal it does not exceed 10 mM. Modest increases in plasma [glucose] provoke marked increases in the secretion of insulin and C peptide and hence raise plasma [insulin], as illustrated by the results of an **oral glucose tolerance test (OGTT)** in Fig. 51.1A. Conversely, a decline in plasma [glucose] of only 20% markedly lowers plasma [insulin]. The change in the concentration of plasma glucose that occurs in response to feeding or fasting is the main determinant of insulin secretion. In a patient with type 1 diabetes mellitus caused by destruction of pancreatic islets, an oral glucose challenge evokes either no response or a much smaller insulin response, but a much larger increment in plasma [glucose] that lasts for a much longer time (Fig. 51.1B).

A glucose challenge of 0.5 g/kg body weight given *as an intravenous bolus* raises the plasma glucose concentration more rapidly than glucose given *orally*. Such a rapid rise in plasma glucose concentration leads to two distinct phases of insulin secretion (Fig. 51.1C). The acute-phase

or first-phase insulin response lasts only 2 to 5 minutes, whereas the second-phase insulin response persists as long as the blood glucose level remains elevated. The insulin released during the acute-phase insulin response to intravenous glucose arises from preformed insulin that had been packaged in secretory vesicles docked at, or residing near, the β-cell plasma membrane. The second-phase insulin response also comes from preformed insulin within the vesicles with some contribution from newly synthesized insulin. One of the earliest detectable metabolic defects that occurs in both type 1 and type 2 diabetes is loss of the first phase of insulin secretion, as determined by an **intravenous glucose tolerance test.** If a subject consumes glucose or a mixed meal, plasma [glucose] rises much more slowly—as in Fig. 51.1A—because the appearance of glucose in plasma depends on gastric emptying and intestinal absorption. Given that plasma [glucose] rises so slowly, the acute-phase insulin response can no longer be distinguished from the chronic response, and only a single phase of insulin secretion is apparent. However, the total insulin response to an oral glucose challenge exceeds the response observed when comparable changes in plasma [glucose] are produced by intravenously administered glucose (Fig. 51.1A). This difference is referred to as the *incretin effect*, discussed below.

◉ 51-3 Metabolism of glucose by the β cell triggers insulin secretion

The pancreatic β cells take up and metabolize glucose, galactose, and mannose, and each can provoke insulin secretion by the islet. Although glucose itself is the best secretagogue, some amino acids (especially arginine and leucine) and small keto acids (e.g., α-ketoisocaproate, α-ketoglutarate), as well as ketohexoses (fructose), can also weakly stimulate insulin secretion. It appears that the ATP generated from the metabolism of these varied substances plays a role in insulin secretion.

Key to this picture is the presence in the islet of an ATP-sensitive K⁺ channel and a **voltage-gated Ca²⁺ channel** in the plasma membrane (Fig. 51.2). The **K⁺ channel (K$_{ATP}$;** see ◉ 7-10) is an octamer of four Kir6.2 channels (see ◉ 7-8)

A NORMAL SUBJECT UNDERGOING SAME CHANGES IN PLASMA [GLUCOSE] FOLLOWING ORAL VS. IV GLUCOSE CHALLENGES

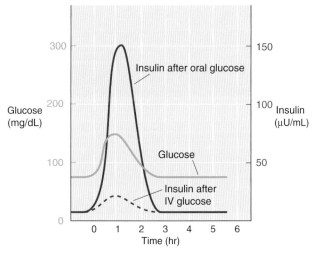

B DIABETES SUBJECT RECEIVING ORAL GLUCOSE

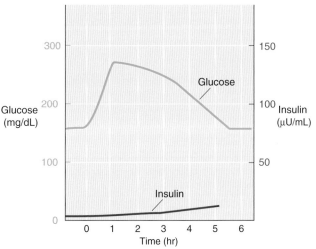

C NORMAL SUBJECT RECEIVING A HIGHER DOSE OF IV GLUCOSE THAN IN PANEL A

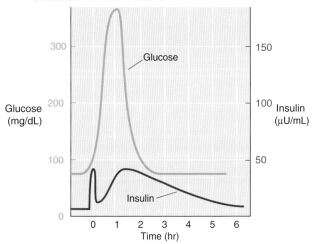

Figure 51.1 Glucose tolerance test results.

and four **sulfonylurea receptors** (**SURs**; see ⊙ 7-10). Glucose triggers insulin release in a seven-step process, summarized in Fig. 51.2.

Neural and humoral factors modulate insulin secretion

⊙ **51-4** The islet is richly innervated by both the sympathetic and the parasympathetic divisions of the ANS. Neural signals appear to play an important role in the β-cell response in several settings. β-**adrenergic** stimulation augments islet insulin secretion, whereas α-**adrenergic** stimulation inhibits it (Fig. 51.2). In contrast to α-adrenergic stimulation, **parasympathetic** stimulation via the vagus nerve, which releases acetylcholine, causes an increase in insulin release.

Exercise The effect of sympathetic regulation on insulin secretion may be particularly important during exercise, when adrenergic stimulation of the islet increases. α-adrenergic *inhibition* of insulin secretion during exercise prevents hypoglycemia.

Feeding Another important setting in which neural and humoral factors regulate insulin secretion is during feeding. Food ingestion triggers a complex series of neural, endocrine, and nutritional signals to many body tissues. The *cephalic phase* (see ⊙ 42-4 and ⊙ 43-5) of eating, which occurs before food is ingested, results in stimulation of gastric acid secretion and a small rise in plasma insulin level.

⊙ **51-5** After a subject drinks a glucose solution, the total amount of insulin secreted is greater than when the same amount of glucose is administered intravenously (Fig. 51.1A). This observation has led to identification of enteric factors or **incretins** that augment the islet β-cell response to an oral glucose stimulus. Currently, we know of three peptides released by intestinal cells in response to feeding that enhance insulin secretion: **cholecystokinin** from I cells, **glucagon-like peptide 1** (**GLP-1**) from L cells, and **gastric inhibitory polypeptide** (**GIP**, also called glucose-dependent insulinotropic peptide) from K cells.

The presence of these incretins in the gut mucosa gives the islets advance notice that nutrients are being absorbed and "primes" the β cells to amplify their response to glucose. In addition, vagal stimulation of the β cells primes the islets for an amplified response.

⊙ 51-6 The insulin receptor is a receptor tyrosine kinase

Once insulin is secreted into the portal blood, it first travels to the liver, where more than half is bound and removed from the circulation. The insulin that escapes the liver is available to stimulate insulin-sensitive processes in other tissues. At each target tissue, the first action of insulin is to bind to a specific receptor tyrosine kinase on the plasma membrane (Fig. 51.3).

The insulin receptor is a heterotetramer, with two identical α chains and two identical β chains. The chains are joined by disulfide linkages in the sequence β-α-α-β. The insulin receptor shares considerable structural similarity with the IGF-1 receptor (see ⊙ 48-8). Because of this similarity, very high concentrations of insulin can stimulate the IGF-1 receptor and vice versa.

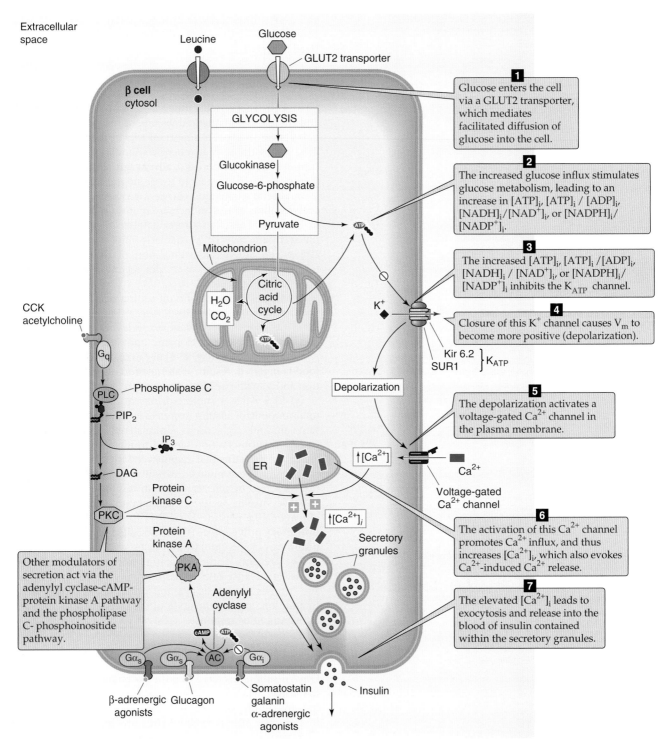

Figure 51.2 Mechanism of insulin secretion by the pancreatic β cell. Increased levels of extracellular glucose trigger the β cell to secrete insulin in the seven steps outlined in this figure. Metabolizable sugars (e.g., galactose and mannose) and certain amino acids (e.g., arginine and leucine) can also stimulate the fusion of vesicles that contain previously synthesized insulin. In addition to these fuel sources, certain hormones (e.g., glucagon, somatostatin, cholecystokinin [CCK]) can also modulate insulin secretion. *DAG,* Diacylglycerol; *ER,* endoplasmic reticulum; *IP₃,* inositol 1,4,5-trisphosphate; *PKC,* protein kinase C; *PLC,* phospholipase C.

The intracellular domain of the β chain possesses tyrosine kinase activity, which increases markedly when insulin binds to sites on the α chains of the receptor. The insulin receptor can phosphorylate both itself and other intracellular substrates at tyrosine residues (see ◉ 3-24). The targets of tyrosine phosphorylation (beyond the receptor itself) include a family of cytosolic proteins known as **insulin-receptor substrates** (**IRS-1, IRS-2, IRS-3,** and **IRS-4**) as well as **S**rc **h**omology **C** **terminus** (**SHC**), as illustrated in Fig. 51.3. This phosphorylation mechanism appears to be the

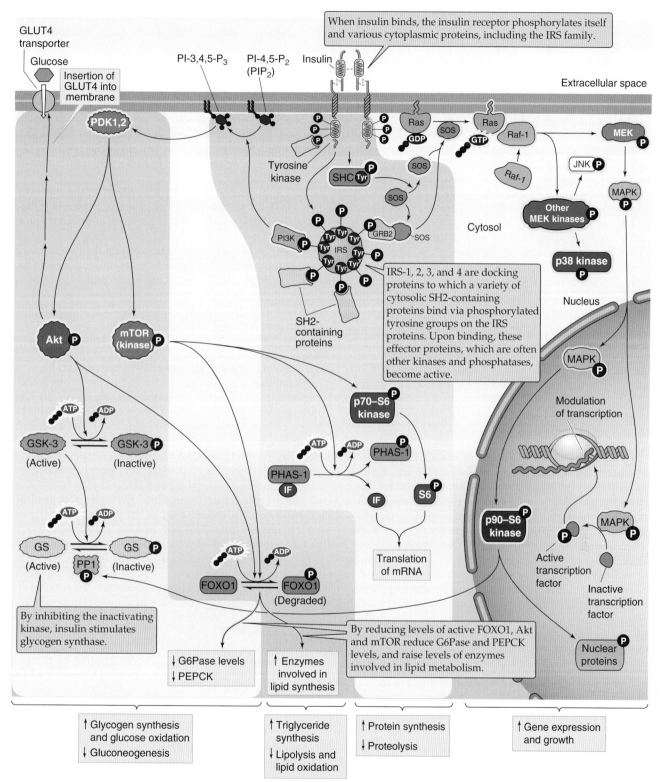

Figure 51.3 Insulin signal-transduction system. *mTOR*, Target of rapamycin.

major one by which insulin transmits its signal across the plasma membrane of insulin target tissues.

The IRS proteins are *docking proteins* to which various downstream effector proteins bind and thus become activated. IRS-1 has at least eight tyrosines within specific motifs that generally bind proteins containing SH2 (Src homology

domain 2) domains (see ⊙ **3-11**), so that a single IRS molecule simultaneously activates multiple pathways. The IGF-1 receptor, which is closely related to the insulin receptor, also acts through IRS proteins.

⊙**51-7** Fig. 51.3 illustrates three major signaling pathways triggered by the aforementioned tyrosine phosphorylations.

The first begins when **phosphatidylinositol 3-kinase (PI3K)** binds to phosphorylated IRS and becomes activated. PI3K phosphorylates a membrane lipid phosphatidylinositol 4,5-bisphosphate (PIP$_2$) to form phosphatidylinositol 3,4,5-trisphosphate (PIP$_3$), and it leads to major changes in glucose and protein metabolism.

The second signaling pathway begins in one of two ways: (1) the insulin receptor phosphorylates SHC, or (2) growth factor receptor–bound protein 2 (GRB2; see Fig. 3.11) binds to an IRS and becomes activated. As illustrated in Fig. 51.3, both phosphorylated SHC and activated GRB2 trigger the Ras signaling pathway, leading through mitogen-activated protein kinase kinase (MEK) and mitogen-activated protein kinase (MAPK; see ⊙ 3-25) to increased gene expression and growth.

The third signaling pathway begins with the binding of SH2-containing proteins—other than PI3K and GRB2, already discussed—to specific phosphotyrosine groups on either the insulin receptor or IRS proteins. This binding activates the SH2-containing protein.

High levels of insulin lead to downregulation of insulin receptors

The number of insulin receptors expressed on the cell surface is far greater than that needed for the maximal biological response to insulin. For example, in the adipocyte, the glucose response to insulin is maximal when only ~5% of the receptors are occupied; that is, the target cells have many "spare" receptors for insulin.

The number of insulin receptors present on the membrane of a target cell is determined by the balance among three factors: (1) receptor synthesis, (2) endocytosis of receptors followed by recycling of receptors back to the cell surface, and (3) endocytosis followed by degradation of receptors. Cells chronically exposed to high concentrations of insulin have fewer surface receptors than do those exposed to lower concentrations. This dynamic ability of cells to decrease the number of specific receptors on their surface is called *downregulation*. Insulin downregulates insulin receptors by decreasing receptor synthesis and increasing degradation. Downregulation of insulin receptors results in a decrease in the sensitivity of the target tissue to insulin without diminishing insulin's maximal effect.

In liver, insulin promotes conversion of glucose to glycogen stores or to triacylglycerols

Insulin's actions on cellular targets frequently involve numerous tissue-specific enzymatic and structural processes. The three principal targets for insulin action are liver, muscle, and adipose tissue.

Because the pancreatic veins drain into the portal venous system, all hormones secreted by the pancreas must traverse the liver before entering the systemic circulation. For insulin, the liver is both a target tissue for hormone action and a major site of degradation.

After feeding, the plasma [insulin] rises, triggered by glucose and by neural and incretin stimulation of β cells. In the liver, this insulin rise acts on four main processes involved in fuel metabolism (Fig. 51.4).

Glycogen Synthesis and Glycogenolysis Physiological increases in plasma [insulin] decrease the breakdown and utilization of glycogen and promote the formation of glycogen from plasma glucose.

Glucose enters the hepatocyte from the blood via GLUT2, which mediates the facilitated diffusion of glucose. GLUT2 is present in abundance in the liver plasma membrane, and its activity is not influenced by insulin. Insulin stimulates glycogen synthesis from glucose by activating **glucokinase** (numbered *box 1* in Fig. 51.4) and **glycogen synthase** (*box 2*). The latter enzyme contains multiple serine phosphorylation sites. Insulin causes a net dephosphorylation of the protein, thus increasing the enzyme's activity. At the same time that glycogen synthase is being activated, increases in both insulin and glucose diminish the activity of **glycogen phosphorylase** (*box 3*). This enzyme is rate limiting for the breakdown of glycogen. The same enzyme that dephosphorylates (and thus *activates*) glycogen synthase also dephosphorylates (and thus *inhibits*) phosphorylase. Thus, insulin has opposite effects on the opposing enzymes, with the net effect that it promotes glycogen formation. Insulin also inhibits **glucose-6-phosphatase (G6Pase;** *box 4*), which otherwise converts glucose-6-phosphate (derived either from glycogenolysis or gluconeogenesis) to glucose. Glycogen is an important storage form of carbohydrate in both liver and muscle.

Glycolysis and Gluconeogenesis Insulin promotes the conversion of some of the glucose taken up by the liver into pyruvate and diminishes the use of pyruvate and other three-carbon compounds for gluconeogenesis. Insulin induces transcription of the **glucokinase** gene (numbered *box 1* in Fig. 51.4) and thus results in increased synthesis of this enzyme, which is responsible for phosphorylating glucose to glucose-6-phosphate and initiating the metabolism of glucose. In acting to promote glycolysis and diminish gluconeogenesis, insulin induces the synthesis of a glucose metabolite, fructose-2,6-bisphosphate. This compound is a potent allosteric activator of **phosphofructokinase** (*box 5*), a key regulatory enzyme in glycolysis. Insulin also stimulates **pyruvate kinase** (*box 6*), which forms pyruvate, and stimulates **pyruvate dehydrogenase** (*box 8*), which catalyzes the first step in pyruvate oxidation. Finally, insulin promotes glucose metabolism by the **hexose monophosphate shunt** (*box 7*).

In addition, insulin also inhibits gluconeogenesis at several steps. Insulin diminishes transcription of the gene encoding **phosphoenolpyruvate carboxykinase (PEPCK;** numbered *box 9* in Fig. 51.4), thus reducing the synthesis of a key regulatory enzyme required to form phosphoenolpyruvate from oxaloacetate early in the gluconeogenic pathway. The increased levels of fructose-2,6-bisphosphate also inhibit the activity of **fructose-1,6-bisphosphatase** (*box 10*), which is also part of the gluconeogenic pathway.

Lipogenesis Insulin promotes the storage of fats and inhibits the oxidation of fatty acids (see Fig. 58.4) through allosteric and covalent modification of key regulatory enzymes, as well as by transcription of new enzymes (*numbered boxes* in Fig. 51.4). The pyruvate that is now available from glycolysis can be used to synthesize fatty acids. Insulin promotes dephosphorylation of **acetyl coenzyme A (CoA) carboxylase 2 (ACC2;** *box 11*), the first committed step in fatty-acid synthesis in the liver. This dephosphorylation

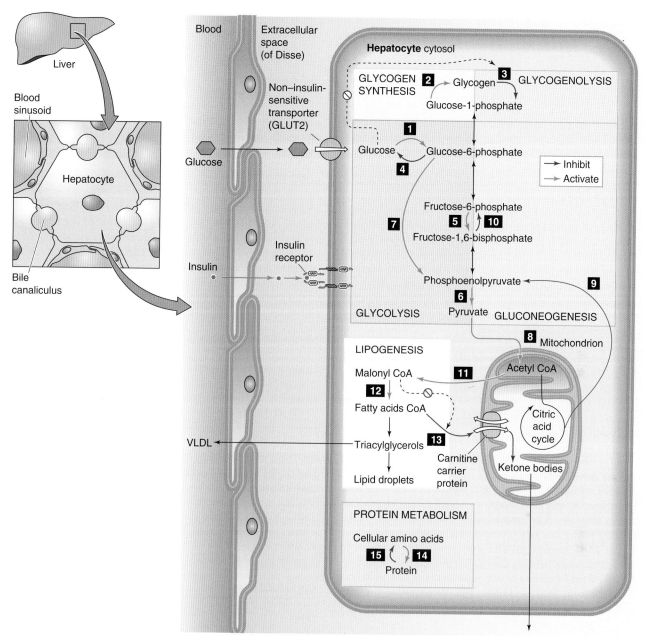

Figure 51.4 Effect of insulin on hepatocytes.

leads to increased synthesis of malonyl CoA, which allosterically inhibits **carnitine acyltransferase I** (**CAT I;** *box 13*). This enzyme converts acyl CoA and carnitine to acylcarnitine, a reaction necessary for long-chain fatty acids to cross the inner mitochondrial membrane, where they can be oxidized. Thus, malonyl CoA inhibits fatty-acid transport and fat oxidation. At the same time, insulin stimulates **fatty-acid synthase** (*box 12*), which generates fatty acids. Because insulin promotes the formation of malonyl CoA and fatty acids but inhibits fatty-acid oxidation, this hormone favors esterification of the fatty acids with glycerol within the liver to form **triacylglycerols (TAGs).** The liver can either store these TAGs in lipid droplets or export them as very-low-density lipoprotein (VLDL) particles (see ⊙ 46-7). Insulin also induces the synthesis of several of the **apoproteins** that are packaged with the VLDL particle. The hepatocyte then

releases these VLDLs, which leave the liver via the hepatic vein. Muscle and adipose tissue subsequently take up the lipids in these VLDL particles and either store them or oxidize them for fuel. Thus, by regulation of transcription, by allosteric activation, and by regulation of protein phosphorylation, insulin acts to promote the synthesis and storage of fat and diminish its oxidation in liver.

Protein Metabolism Insulin stimulates the synthesis of protein and simultaneously reduces the degradation of protein within the liver (*numbered boxes* in Fig. 51.4). The general mechanisms by which insulin stimulates protein synthesis (*box 14*) and restrains proteolysis (*box 15*) by the liver are less well understood.

In summary, in the above four pathways, insulin modulates the activity of multiple regulatory enzymes that are responsible for the hepatic metabolism of carbohydrates, fat, and protein. The ultimate result is that insulin causes the liver, as well as other body tissues, to burn carbohydrates preferentially.

In muscle, insulin promotes the uptake of glucose and its storage as glycogen

Muscle is a major insulin-sensitive tissue and the principal site of insulin-mediated glucose disposal. Insulin has four major effects on muscle.

⦿ **51-8** First, in muscle, unlike in the liver, glucose crosses the plasma membrane principally via **GLUT4**, an *insulin-sensitive* glucose transporter. GLUT4, which is found virtually exclusively in striated muscle and adipose tissue, belongs to a family of proteins that mediate the facilitated diffusion of glucose (see ⦿ **5-5**). Insulin markedly stimulates GLUT4 in both muscle (Fig. 51.5) and fat (see below) by a process involving recruitment of preformed transporters from a membranous compartment in the cell cytosol out to the plasma membrane. Recruitment places additional glucose transporters in the plasma membrane, thereby increasing glucose transport into muscle and increasing the flow of glucose from the interstitial fluid to the cytosol.

The *enzymatic* steps regulated by insulin are indicated by numbered boxes in Fig. 51.5.

The second effect of insulin on muscle is to enhance the conversion of glucose to glycogen by activating **hexokinase** (*box 1* in Fig. 51.5)—different from the glucokinase in liver—and **glycogen synthase** (*box 2*).

Third, insulin increases glycolysis and oxidation by increasing the activity of **phosphofructokinase** (*box 3*) and **pyruvate dehydrogenase** (*box 4*).

Fourth, insulin stimulates the synthesis of protein in skeletal muscle (*box 5*) and slows the degradation of existing proteins (*box 6*). The result is preservation of muscle protein mass, which has obvious beneficial effects in preserving strength and locomotion. The insulin-induced increase in glucose utilization permits the muscle to diminish fat utilization and allows it to store as TAGs some of the fatty acid that it removes from the circulation. The stored TAGs and glycogen are major sources of energy that muscle can use later when called on to exercise or generate heat.

In muscle, as in the liver, insulin directs the overall pattern of cellular fuel metabolism by acting at multiple sites. In both tissues, insulin increases the oxidation of carbohydrate, thus preserving body protein and fat stores.

In adipocytes, insulin promotes glucose uptake and conversion to TAGs for storage

Adipose tissue is the third major insulin-sensitive tissue involved in the regulation of body fuel. Again, insulin has several sites of action in adipocytes. All begin with the same receptor-mediated action of insulin to stimulate several cellular effector pathways. Insulin has four major actions on adipocytes.

First, like muscle, adipose tissue contains the insulin-sensitive GLUT4 glucose transporter. In insulin-stimulated cells, preformed transporters are recruited from an intracellular compartment to the cell membrane, which markedly accelerates the entry of glucose into the cell.

Second, insulin promotes the breakdown of glucose to metabolites that will eventually be used to synthesize TAGs. Unlike in muscle or liver, little of the glucose taken up is stored as glycogen. Instead, the adipocyte glycolytically metabolizes much of the glucose to α-glycerol phosphate, which it uses to esterify long-chain fatty acids into TAGs. The glucose not used for esterification goes on to form acetyl CoA and then malonyl CoA and fatty acids. Insulin enhances this flow of glucose to fatty acids by stimulating **pyruvate dehydrogenase** (*box 1* in Fig. 51.6) and **acetyl CoA carboxylase** (*box 2*).

⦿ **51-9** Third, insulin promotes the formation of TAGs by simple mass action; the increased levels of α-glycerol phosphate increase its esterification with fatty acids (principally C-16 and C-18) to yield TAGs. Some of the fatty acids are a result of the glucose metabolism noted above. Most of the fatty acids, however, enter the adipocyte from chylomicrons and VLDLs (see Table 46.1) in the blood. The cell sequesters these TAGs in lipid droplets, which form most of the mass of the adipose cell. Conversely, insulin restrains the activity of **adipose triacylglycerol lipase** (**ATGL;** see ⦿ **58-9**) which converts TAGs to diacylglycerols (DAGs), and **hormone-sensitive lipase** (**HSL**), which converts DAGs to monoacylglycerols (MAGs). In adipocytes, these enzymes (numbered *box 3* in Fig. 51.6) mediate the conversion of stored TAGs to fatty acids and glycerol for export to other tissues.

⦿ **51-10** Fourth, insulin induces the synthesis of a different enzyme—**lipoprotein lipase** (**LPL**). The adipocyte exports the LPL to the endothelial cell, where it resides on the extracellular surface of the endothelial cell, facing the blood and anchored to the plasma membrane. In this location, the LPL acts on TAGs in chylomicrons and VLDLs and cleaves them into glycerol and fatty acids. These fatty acids are then available for uptake by nearby adipocytes, which esterify them with glycerol phosphate to form TAGs.

GLUCAGON

⦿ **51-11** Glucagon is the other major pancreatic islet hormone that is involved in the regulation of body fuel metabolism. Ingestion of protein appears to be the major physiological stimulus for secretion of glucagon. Glucagon's principal target tissue is the liver. Like insulin, glucagon is secreted first into the portal blood and is therefore anatomically well positioned to regulate hepatic metabolism.

Although the *amino acids* released by digestion of a protein meal appear to be the major glucagon secretagogue, glucagon's main actions on the liver appear to involve the regulation of *carbohydrate* and *lipid* metabolism. Glucagon is particularly important in stimulating glycogenolysis, gluconeogenesis, and ketogenesis. Glucagon has glycogenolytic action on cardiac and skeletal muscle, lipolytic action on adipose tissue, and proteolytic actions on several tissues at pharmacological concentrations whereas, at more physiological concentrations, the liver is the major target tissue.

In many circumstances, glucagon's actions on liver antagonize those of insulin, and the mechanism of glucagon action is understood in considerable detail.

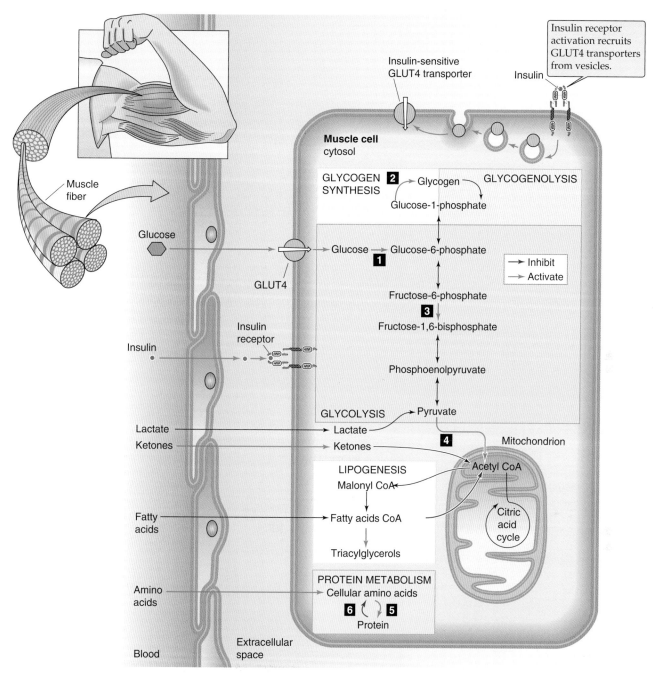

Figure 51.5 Effect of insulin on muscle.

Pancreatic α cells secrete glucagon in response to ingested protein

Glucagon is a 31–amino-acid peptide synthesized by α cells in the islets of Langerhans. The initial gene product is the mRNA encoding preproglucagon. As is the case for insulin, a peptidase removes the signal sequence of preproglucagon during translation of the mRNA in the rough endoplasmic reticulum to yield proglucagon. Proteases in the α cells subsequently cleave the proglucagon into the mature glucagon molecule and several biologically active peptides.

Pancreatic α Cells The mature glucagon molecule is the major secretory product of the α cell. As with insulin, the fully processed glucagon molecule is stored in secretory vesicles within the cell's cytosol. Although amino acids are the major secretagogues, the concentrations of amino acids required to provoke secretion of glucagon in vitro are higher than those generated in vivo. This observation suggests that other neural or humoral factors amplify the response in vivo, in a manner analogous to the effects of incretin on insulin secretion. However, the best studied incretin (GLP-1) *inhibits* glucagon secretion. Whereas both glucose and several amino acids stimulate insulin secretion by β cells, only amino acids stimulate glucagon secretion by α cells; glucose inhibits glucagon secretion.

Glucagon, like the incretins, is a potent insulin secretagogue. However, because most of the α cells are located downstream from the β cells (recall that the circulation of

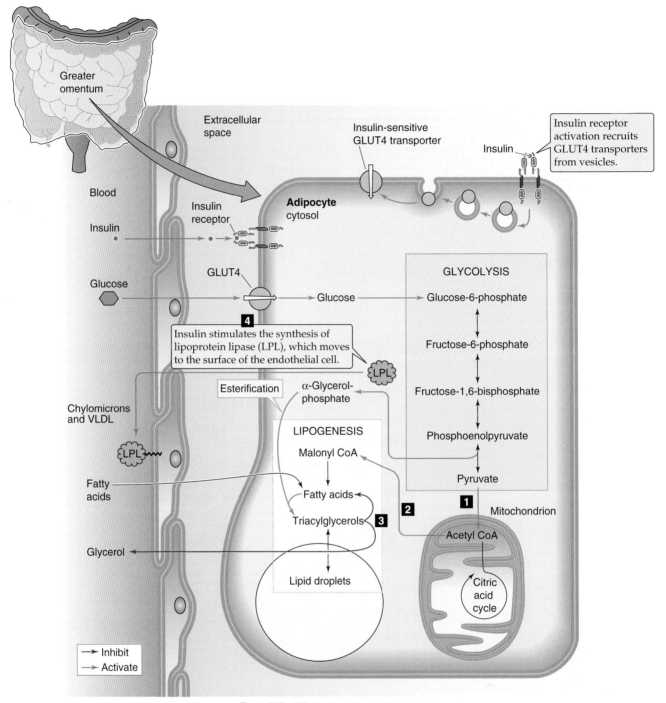

Figure 51.6 Effect of insulin on adipocytes.

blood proceeds from the β cells and then out past the α cells), it is unlikely that glucagon exerts an important paracrine effect on insulin secretion.

Intestinal L Cells Proteases in neuroendocrine cells in the intestine process proglucagon differently than do α cells. L cells produce four peptide fragments: glicentin, GLP-1, intervening peptide 2 (IP-2), and GLP-2. **Glicentin** contains the amino-acid sequence of glucagon but does not bind to glucagon receptors. Both GLP-1 and GLP-2 are glucagon-like in that they cross-react with some antisera directed to glucagon, but GLP-1 and GLP-2 have very weak biological

activity as glucagon analogs. However, GLP-1—released by the gut into the circulation in response to carbohydrate or protein ingestion—is one of the most potent incretins, stimulating insulin secretion.

Glucagon, acting through cAMP, promotes the synthesis of glucose by the liver

Glucagon is an important regulator of hepatic glucose production and ketogenesis in the liver. As shown in Fig. 51.7, glucagon binds to a receptor that activates the heterotrimeric

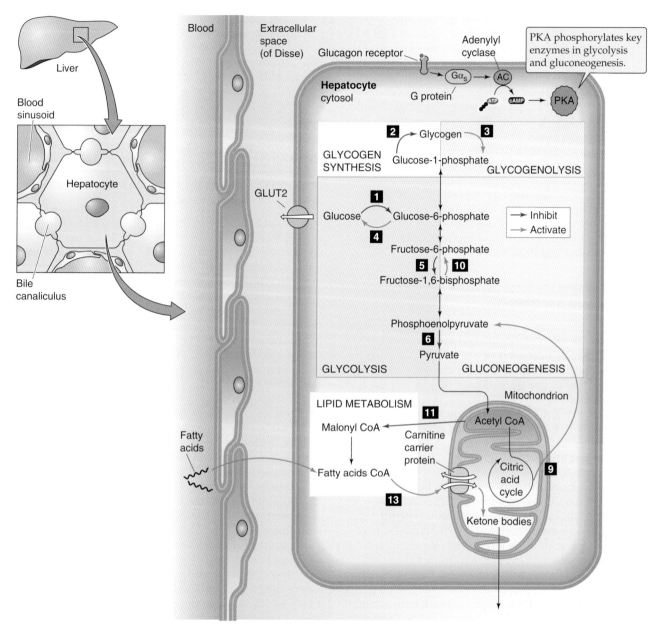

Figure 51.7 Glucagon signal transduction.

G protein $G\alpha_s$, which stimulates membrane-bound adenylyl cyclase (see ⊚ 3-4). The cAMP formed by the cyclase in turn activates PKA, which phosphorylates numerous regulatory enzymes and other protein substrates, thus altering glucose and fat metabolism in the liver. Whereas insulin leads to the dephosphorylation of certain key enzymes (i.e., glycogen synthase, acetyl CoA carboxylase, phosphorylase), glucagon leads to their phosphorylation.

A particularly clear example of the opposing actions of insulin and glucagon involves the activation of **glycogenolysis** (see ⊚ 58-11). PKA phosphorylates the enzyme **phosphorylase kinase** (see Fig. 58.3), thus increasing the activity of phosphorylase kinase and allowing it to increase the phosphorylation of its substrate, **glycogen phosphorylase *b***. The addition of a single phosphate residue to phosphorylase *b* converts it to phosphorylase *a*. In addition to converting phosphorylase *b* to the active phosphorylase

a form, PKA also phosphorylates a peptide called **inhibitor I** (see Fig. 3.5). In its phosphorylated form, inhibitor I decreases the activity of phosphoprotein phosphatase 1 (PP1), which otherwise would dephosphorylate both phosphorylase kinase and phosphorylase *a* (converting them to their *inactive* forms). PP1 also activates glycogen synthase. Thus, via inhibitor I, glucagon modulates several of the enzymes involved in hepatic glycogen metabolism to provoke *net glycogen breakdown*. As a result of similar actions on the pathways of gluconeogenesis and lipid oxidation, glucagon also stimulates these processes. Conversely, glucagon restrains glycogen synthesis, glycolysis, and lipid storage.

Glucagon also enhances gluconeogenesis by genomic effects, acting synergistically with glucocorticoids (see ⊚ 50-4). The genomic effects of glucagon occur as PKA phosphorylates the transcription factor cAMP response element–binding protein (CREB; see ⊙ **4-3**), which interacts with the cAMP response elements (CREs; see ⊙ **4-3**), increasing the expression of key gluconeogenic enzymes (e.g., G6Pase and PEPCK). Phosphorylated CREB also increases the expression of peroxisome proliferator–activated receptor-γ coactivator-1α (PGC-1α), which also enhances the expression of key gluconeogenic enzymes. Insulin restrains the transcription of these two enzymes in two ways, both via the PI3K/Akt pathway (Fig. 51.3). First, insulin increases the release of the transcription-factor domain of sterol regulatory element–binding protein 1 (SREBP-1), which antagonizes the transcription of mRNA encoding the two enzymes. Second, insulin increases the phosphorylation of the transcription factor FOXO1, thereby promoting its movement out of the nucleus and subsequent degradation; this action prevents FOXO1 from binding to the promoter regions of G6Pase and PEPCK.

⊙ 51-12 Glucagon promotes oxidation of fat in the liver, which can lead to ketogenesis

Glucagon plays a major regulatory role in hepatic lipid metabolism. The liver can esterify fatty acids with glycerol to form TAGs, which it can store or export as VLDL particles. Alternatively, the liver can partially oxidize fatty acids—and form **ketone bodies** (see ⊙ **58-16**)—or fully oxidize them to CO_2.

Glucagon stimulates fat oxidation indirectly by increasing the activity of **CAT I** (see ⊙ **58-13**), which mediates the transfer of fatty acids across the outer mitochondrial membrane. Glucagon produces this stimulation by inhibiting acetyl CoA carboxylase, which generates malonyl CoA, the first committed intermediate in the synthesis of fatty acids by the liver. Malonyl CoA is also an inhibitor of the CAT system. By inhibiting acetyl CoA carboxylase, glucagon lowers the concentration of malonyl CoA, releases the inhibition of CAT I, and allows fatty acids to be transferred into the mitochondria. These fatty acids are oxidized to furnish ATP to the liver cell. If the rate of fatty-acid transport into the mitochondria exceeds the need of the liver to phosphorylate ADP, the fatty acids will be only *partially oxidized;* the result is the accumulation of the keto acids β-**hydroxybutyric acid** and **acetoacetic acid,** which are two of the three ketone bodies. These keto acids can exit the mitochondria and the liver to be used by other tissues as oxidative fuel.

During fasting, the decline in insulin and the increase in glucagon promote ketogenesis (see ⊙ **58-16**); this process is of vital importance to the CNS, which can use keto acids but not fatty acids as fuel.

In addition to its effects on hepatic glucose and lipid metabolism, glucagon also has the extrahepatic actions of accelerating **lipolysis** in adipose tissue and **proteolysis** in muscle.

SOMATOSTATIN

Somatostatin inhibits the secretion of growth hormone, insulin, and other hormones

Somatostatin is made in the δ cells of the pancreatic islets, as well as in the D cells of the gastrointestinal tract (see ⊙ **42-2**), in the hypothalamus, and in several other sites in the CNS (see ⊙ **48-6**). Somatostatin *suppresses* the release of growth hormone; growth hormone had also been called somatotropin, which accounts for the name somatostatin. In both pancreatic δ cells and the hypothalamus, somatostatin exists as both 14– and 28–amino-acid peptides. In the hypothalamus, the 14–amino-acid form is predominant, whereas in the gastrointestinal tract (including the δ cells), the 28–amino-acid form predominates. The 14–amino-acid form is the C-terminal portion of the 28–amino-acid form. The biological activity of somatostatin resides in these 14 amino acids.

Somatostatin inhibits the secretion of multiple hormones, including growth hormone, insulin, glucagon, gastrin, vasoactive intestinal peptide (VIP), and thyroid-stimulating hormone. This property has led to therapeutic use of a long-acting somatostatin analog (octreotide) in some difficult-to-treat endocrine tumors, including those that produce growth hormone (acromegaly), insulin (insulinoma), or serotonin (carcinoid), among others. The concentration of somatostatin found in pancreatic venous drainage is sufficiently high to inhibit basal insulin secretion. Blood flows from the center of each islet—which is where the bulk of the β cells are—to the periphery of the islet—which is where the δ cells tend to be located. This spatial arrangement minimizes the effect of somatostatin on the islet from which it is secreted. Whether somatostatin has important paracrine actions on some β cells or on α cells remains controversial.

CHAPTER 52

THE PARATHYROID GLANDS AND VITAMIN D

Eugene J. Barrett and Paula Q. Barrett

CALCIUM AND PHOSPHATE BALANCE

Calcium and phosphate homeostasis are intimately tied to each other for two reasons. First, calcium and phosphate are the principal components of hydroxyapatite crystals $[Ca_{10}(PO_4)_6(OH)_2]$, which by far constitute the major portion of the mineral phase of bone. Second, they are regulated by the same hormones, primarily parathyroid hormone (PTH) and 1,25-dihydroxyvitamin D (calcitriol) and, to a lesser extent, the hormone calcitonin. These hormones act on three organ systems—bone, kidneys, and gastrointestinal (GI) tract—to control the levels of calcium and phosphate in plasma. Figs. 52.1 and 52.2 depict the overall daily balance of calcium and phosphate for an individual in a steady state.

The gut, kidneys, and bone regulate calcium balance

In plasma, calcium exists: (1) as a free ionized species (Ca^{2+}), (2) bound to (more accurately, associated with) anionic sites on serum proteins (especially albumin), and (3) complexed with low-molecular-weight organic anions (e.g., phosphate, citrate, and oxalate). The **total concentration** of all three forms in the plasma is normally 2.2 to 2.6 mM (8.8 to 10.6 mg/dL). In healthy individuals, ~45% of calcium is free, 45% is bound to protein, and 10% is bound to small anions. The body tightly regulates the ionized form of Ca^{2+} between 1.0 and 1.3 mM (4.0 and 5.2 mg/dL).

Most total-body calcium is located within bone, ~1 kg (Fig. 52.1). The total amount of calcium in the extracellular pool is only a tiny fraction of this amount, ~1 g or 1000 mg. The typical daily dietary intake of calcium is ~800 to 1200 mg. Although the intestines absorb approximately one half the dietary calcium (~500 mg/day), they also secrete calcium for removal from the body (~325 mg/day), and, therefore, the *net* intestinal uptake of calcium is only ~175 mg/day. The second major organ governing calcium homeostasis is bone, which in the steady state deposits ~280 mg/day of calcium and resorbs an equal amount. The third organ system involved, the kidney, filters ~10 times the total extracellular pool of calcium per day, ~10,000 mg/day. The kidneys reabsorb ~99% of this Ca^{2+}, so that the net renal excretion of Ca^{2+} is ~1% of the filtered load (see Fig. 36.10). In a person in Ca^{2+} balance, urinary excretion (~175 mg/day) matches net absorption by the GI tract.

The gut, kidneys, and bone also regulate phosphate balance

The concentration of total phosphate in adult plasma—predominantly inorganic phosphate in the form of $H_2PO_4^-$ and HPO_4^{2-}—ranges from 0.8 to 1.5 mM, a variation of 80%. Between 85% and 90% of the circulating inorganic phosphate is filterable by the kidneys, either ionized (50%) or complexed to Na^+, Ca^{2+}, or Mg^{2+} (40%); only a small proportion (10% to 15%) is protein bound.

Like calcium, most total-body phosphate is present in bone, which contains ~0.6 kg of elemental phosphorus (Fig. 52.2). A smaller amount of phosphorus (0.1 kg) resides in the soft tissues, mainly as organic phosphates, such as phospholipids, phosphoproteins, nucleic acids, and nucleotides. An even smaller amount (~500 mg) is present in the extracellular fluid (ECF) as inorganic phosphate. The net absorption of phosphate by the intestines is ~900 mg/day. In the steady state, bone has relatively small phosphate turnover, ~210 mg/day. The kidneys filter ~14 times the total extracellular pool of phosphate per day (~7000 mg/day) and reabsorb ~6100 mg/day. Hence, the net renal excretion of phosphorus is ~900 mg/day, the same as the net absorption by the GI tract.

⊙ 52-1 PHYSIOLOGY OF BONE

Dense cortical bone and the more reticulated trabecular bone are the two major bone types

Bone consists largely of an extracellular matrix composed of proteins and hydroxyapatite crystals, in addition to a small population of cells. The matrix provides strength and stability. The cellular elements continually remodel bone to accommodate growth and allow bone to reshape itself in response to varying loading stresses. **Osteoblasts** promote bone formation. Osteoblasts and preosteoblasts are the principal target cells for PTH's action to stimulate bone growth. **Osteoclasts** promote bone resorption and are found on the growth surfaces of bone. Their activity is increased by cytokines, with RANK ligand being particularly important. **Osteocytes** are found within the bony matrix and are derived from osteoblasts that have encased themselves within bone. Osteocytes play a role in the transfer of mineral from the interior of bone to the growth surfaces. Bone remodeling consists of a carefully coordinated interplay of osteoblastic, osteocytic, and osteoclastic activities.

Cortical (also called **compact** or **lamellar**) **bone** represents ~80% of the total bone mass. Cortical bone is the outer layer (the cortex) of all bones and forms the bulk of the long bones of the body. Osteocytes are interconnected with one another and with the osteoblasts on the surface of the bone by canaliculi. These connections permit the transfer of Ca^{2+} from the interior of the bone to the surface, a process called *osteocytic osteolysis*.

⊙ **52-2 Trabecular** (or **cancellous** or **medullary**) bone constitutes ~20% of the total bone mass. It is found in the

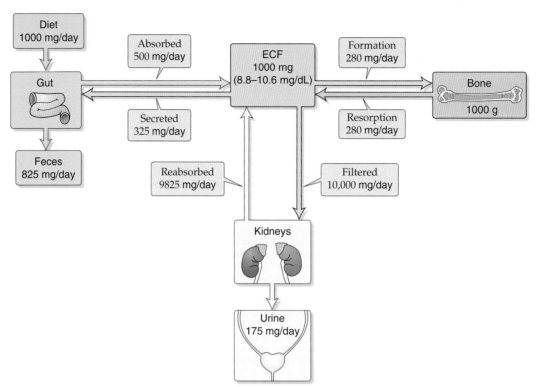

Figure 52.1 Calcium distribution and balance. Note that all values are examples for a 70-kg human, expressed in terms of elemental calcium. These values can vary depending on factors such as diet.

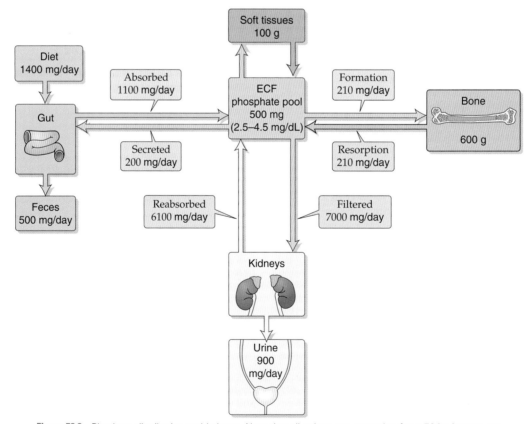

Figure 52.2 Phoshate distribution and balance. Note that all values are examples for a 70-kg human, expressed in elemental phosphorus. These values can vary depending on factors such as diet.

interior of bones and is especially prominent within the vertebral bodies. It is composed of thin spicules of bone that extend from the cortex into the medullary cavity.

The extracellular matrix forms the nidus for the nucleation of hydroxyapatite crystals

Collagen and the other extracellular matrix proteins that form the protein matrix of bone are called osteoid. **Osteoid** provides sites for the nucleation of hydroxyapatite crystals, the mineral component of bone. Osteoid is not a single compound, but a highly organized matrix of proteins synthesized principally by osteoblasts. Type I collagen accounts for ~90% of the protein mass of osteoid. Collagen fibers are arranged in the osteoid in a highly ordered manner and act as a nidus for nucleation of bone mineralization. Within the collagen fibers, the crystals of hydroxyapatite are arranged with their long axis aligned with the long axis of the collagen fibers.

Several other osteoblast-derived proteins are important to the mineralization process. **Osteocalcin** is a 6-kDa protein synthesized by osteoblasts at sites of new bone formation. 1,25-Dihydroxyvitamin D induces the synthesis of osteocalcin. Osteocalcin binds Ca^{2+} avidly. **Osteonectin**, a 35-kDa protein, is another osteoblast product that binds to hydroxyapatite. It also binds to collagen fibers and facilitates the mineralization of collagen fibers in vitro.

⊙ 52-3 Bone remodeling depends on the closely coupled activities of osteoblasts and osteoclasts

In addition to providing the proteins for the osteoid, osteoblasts promote mineralization by exporting Ca^{2+} and PO_4^{-3} from intracellular vesicles that have accumulated these minerals. Exocytosis of Ca^{2+} and PO_4^{-3} raises the local extracellular concentration of these ions around the osteoblast to levels that are higher than in the bulk ECF, which promotes crystal **nucleation** and growth (Fig. 52.3).

Vitamin D and PTH stimulate osteoblastic cells to secrete factors—such as macrophage colony-stimulating factor (M-CSF; see ⊙ 18-4)—that cause osteoclast precursors to proliferate (Fig. 52.3) and differentiate into mononuclear. Stimulation by RANK ligand promotes formation of multinucleated osteoclasts. **Osteoclasts** resorb bone in discrete areas (Fig. 52.4). The osteoclast closely attaches to the bone matrix and secretes acid and proteases across its ruffled border membrane into a confined resorption space (the lacuna). The acid secretion is mediated by a V-type H pump and Cl^- channels. The acidic environment beneath the osteoclast dissolves bone mineral and allows acid proteases to hydrolyze the exposed matrix proteins. Having reabsorbed some of the bone in a very localized area, the osteoclast moves away from the pit that it has created. Osteoblastic cells replace the osteoclast and now build new bone matrix and promote its mineralization.

⊙ **52-4 RANK ligand (RANKL)** is a major stimulator of the differentiation of preosteoclasts to osteoclasts (Fig. 52.3) and the

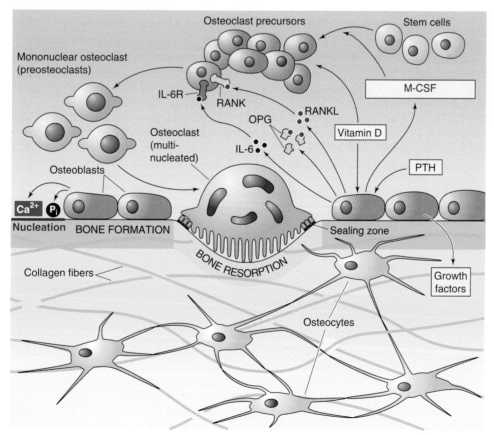

Figure 52.3 Bone formation and resorption.

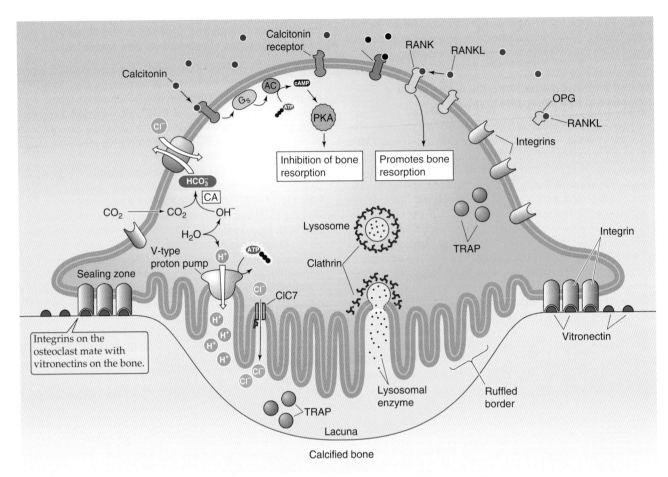

Figure 52.4 Bone resorption by the osteoclast. *AK,* Adenylyl cyclase; *IL-6R,* interleukin-6 receptor; *PKA,* protein kinase A; *TRAP,* tartrate-resistant acid phosphatase.

activity of mature osteoclasts (Fig. 52.4). RANKL binds to and stimulates a membrane-bound receptor of the osteoclast called **RANK** (receptor for activation of nuclear factor κB). The interaction is essential for the formation of mature osteoclasts.

52-5 The activity of RANKL is under the control of a soluble member of the TNF receptor family called **osteoprotegerin (OPG).** Like RANKL, OPG is produced by osteoblastic and stromal cells (Fig. 52.3). By scavenging RANKL, OPG limits osteoclastogenesis, thereby protecting bone from osteoclastic activity. The balance between OPG and RANKL production by the osteoblast/stromal cell appears to be a very important factor in the development of osteoporosis from either estrogen deficiency or glucocorticoid excess. In both cases, RANKL production rises and OPG production falls.

PARATHYROID HORMONE

Plasma Ca²⁺ regulates the synthesis and secretion of parathyroid hormone

Humans have four parathyroid glands, two located on the posterior surface of the left lobe of the thyroid and two more on the right. The glands are composed largely of **chief cells,** which are responsible for the synthesis and secretion of PTH. The major regulator of PTH secretion is ionized plasma Ca²⁺,

although vitamin D also plays a role. Both inhibit the synthesis or release of PTH. In contrast, an increase in plasma phosphorus concentration stimulates PTH release.

Parathyroid Hormone Synthesis and Vitamin D The PTH gene possesses upstream regulatory elements in the 5′ region, including response elements for both vitamins D and A (see **4-4**). The vitamin D response element binds a **vitamin D receptor (VDR)** occupied by a vitamin D metabolite, usually 1,25-dihydroxyvitamin D. The VDR forms a heterodimer with the retinoid X receptor (RXR) to act as a transcription factor (see Table 3.3). Binding of the vitamin D–VDR complex to the VDR response element *decreases* the rate of PTH transcription.

Processing of Parathyroid Hormone After transport of the mature PTH messenger RNA (mRNA) to the cytosol, PTH is synthesized on ribosomes of the rough endoplasmic reticulum (RER). PTH is transcribed as a prepro-PTH of 115 amino acids. The 25–amino-acid "pre" fragment targets PTH for transport into the lumen of the RER. This signal sequence is cleaved as PTH enters the RER. During transit through the secretory pathway, the 90–amino-acid pro-PTH is further processed to the mature, active, 84–amino-acid PTH.

Metabolism of Parathyroid Hormone Once secreted, PTH circulates free in plasma and is rapidly metabolized; the half-life of 1-84 PTH—the **intact PTH hormone**—is ~4 minutes. Beginning in the secretory granules inside the parathyroid chief cells and continuing in the circulation, PTH is cleaved into a 33– or 36–amino-acid N-terminal peptide and a larger C-terminal peptide. Virtually all the known biological activity of PTH resides in the N-terminal fragment, which is rapidly hydrolyzed, especially in the kidney.

High plasma [Ca²⁺] inhibits the synthesis and release of parathyroid hormone

Regulation of PTH secretion by plasma Ca²⁺ appears to be a simple negative-feedback loop. The major stimulus for PTH secretion is a *decline* in the concentration of Ca²⁺ in the blood (hypocalcemia) and ECF. Hypocalcemia also stimulates synthesis of new PTH, which is necessary because the parathyroid gland contains only enough PTH to maintain a stimulated secretory response for several hours.

The **Ca²⁺-sensing receptor (CaSR)** that resides in the plasma membrane of the parathyroid cell (Fig. 52.5A) binds Ca²⁺ in a saturable manner. Coupling of the Ca²⁺ receptor—a **G protein–coupled receptor (GPCR; see ◉ 3-3)**—to $G\alpha_q$ activates phospholipase C, which generates inositol 1,4,5-trisphosphate (IP_3) and diacylglycerol (DAG) and results in the release of Ca²⁺ from internal stores and the activation of protein kinase C (PKC; see ◉ 3-17). In the parathyroid, the rise in [Ca²⁺]ᵢ and activation of PKC *inhibit* hormone secretion (Fig. 52.5B).

The PTH receptor couples via G proteins to either adenylyl cyclase or phospholipase C

◉ **52-6** The action of PTH to regulate plasma [Ca²⁺] is secondary to its binding to the **PTH 1R receptor (PTH1R)**. A second PTH receptor, PTH2R, has been identified. Kidney and bone have the greatest abundance of PTH1R. Within the kidney, PTH1R is most abundant in the proximal and distal convoluted tubules. In bone, the preosteoblast and osteoblast appear to be the major target cells. PTH1R is a GPCR (see ◉ 3-3) that binds the biologically active 1-34 peptide, as well as the 1-84 intact PTH molecule. PTH1R also binds PTH-related protein (PTHrP). In contrast, PTH2R is selectively activated by PTH.

Binding of PTH to the receptor stimulates $G\alpha_s$, which in turn activates **adenylyl cyclase** and thus releases cAMP and stimulates protein kinase A. The activated PTH receptor also stimulates $G\alpha_q$, which in turn stimulates **phospholipase C** to generate IP_3 and DAG. The IP_3 releases Ca²⁺ from internal stores, thus increasing [Ca²⁺]ᵢ and activating Ca²⁺-dependent kinases.

In the kidney, PTH promotes Ca²⁺ reabsorption, phosphate loss, and 1-hydroxylation of 25-hydroxyvitamin D

PTH exerts a spectrum of actions on target cells in the kidney and bone, as illustrated for Ca²⁺ in Fig. 52.6A and for phosphate in Fig. 52.6B. In renal tubules, PTH receptors are located on the basolateral membrane. Binding of PTH to its receptors activates dual intracellular signaling systems and in this manner modifies transepithelial transport.

Stimulation of Ca²⁺ Reabsorption A key action of PTH is to promote the reabsorption of Ca²⁺ in the thick ascending limb (TAL) and distal convoluted tubule (DCT) of the kidney (see ◉ 36-6). The distal nephron is responsible for reabsorbing an additional 5% to 10% of the filtered load of Ca²⁺, with ~0.5% of the filtered load left in the urine.

A PARATHYROID Ca²⁺ RECEPTOR

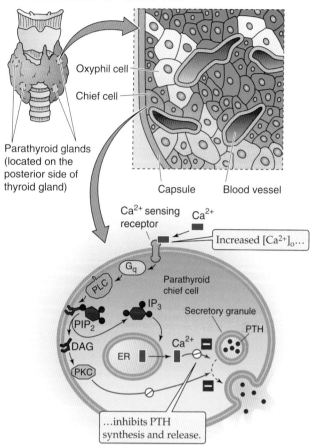

B RESPONSE OF PARATHYROID GLAND TO CHANGES IN PLASMA [Ca²⁺]

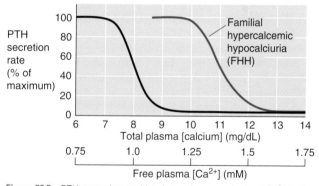

Figure 52.5 PTH secretion and its dependence on ionized Ca²⁺ in the plasma. (B) Small decreases in free plasma [Ca²⁺] greatly increase the rate of PTH release. About half of the total plasma Ca²⁺ is free. In patients with familial hypocalciuric hypercalcemia (FHH), the curve is shifted to the right; that is, plasma [Ca²⁺] must rise to higher levels before inhibiting PTH secretion. As a result, these patients have normal PTH levels, but elevated plasma [Ca²⁺]. *ER*, Endoplasmic reticulum.

Inhibition of Phosphate Reabsorption PTH reduces phosphate reabsorption in the proximal tubule, producing a characteristic phosphaturia and decreasing plasma phosphate levels (Fig. 52.6B). This phosphaturia results from a PTH-induced

A CONTROL OF PLASMA CALCIUM   **B** CONTROL OF PLASMA PHOSPHATE

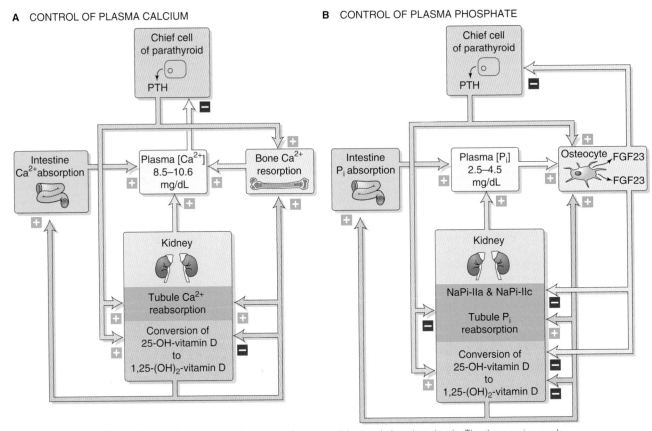

Figure 52.6 Feedback loops in the control of plasma calcium and phosphate levels. The three major regulators are PTH released by parathyroid chief cells; 1,25-dihydroxyvitamin D released by renal proximal-tubule cells; and, in the case of phosphate, FGF23 released by osteocytes. Plasma [Ca²⁺] concentration feeds back on the parathyroid glands, whereas plasma inorganic phosphate (P$_i$) concentration feeds back on osteocytes.

redistribution of **Na/phosphate cotransporters** (**NaPi-IIa** and **NaPi-IIc**; see ⊚ 36-3) away from the apical membrane of the renal proximal tubule and into a pool of subapical vesicles (see ⊚ 36-4). Conversely, a PTH-induced decrease in plasma [P$_i$] inhibits the release of FGF23, which in turn promotes P$_i$ reabsorption, countering the action of PTH.

Stimulation of the Last Step of Synthesis of 1,25-Dihydroxyvitamin D A third important renal action of PTH is to stimulate the 1-hydroxylation of 25-hydroxyvitamin D in the mitochondria of the proximal tubule. The resulting 1,25-dihydroxyvitamin D is the most biologically active metabolite of dietary or endogenously produced vitamin D. Its synthesis by the kidney is highly regulated, and PTH is the primary stimulus to increase 1-hydroxylation. The 1,25-dihydroxyvitamin D formed in the proximal tubule has three major actions: (1) enhancement of renal Ca²⁺ reabsorption, (2) enhancement of Ca²⁺ absorption by the small intestine, and (3) modulation of the movement of Ca²⁺ and phosphate in and out of bone.

In bone, PTH can promote net resorption or net deposition

The second major target tissue for PTH is bone, in which PTH promotes both bone resorption and bone synthesis.

Bone Resorption by Indirect Stimulation of Osteoclasts The net effect of *persistent* increases of PTH on bone is to stimulate

bone *resorption*, thus increasing plasma [Ca²⁺]. Osteoblasts express abundant surface receptors for PTH; osteoclasts do not. Because osteoclasts lack PTH receptors, PTH by itself cannot regulate the coupling between osteoblasts and osteoclasts. Rather, PTH acts on osteoblasts and osteoclast precursors to induce the production of several cytokines that increase both the number and the activity of bone-resorbing osteoclasts. PTH causes osteoblasts to release agents such as M-CSF and stimulates the expression of RANKL, actions that promote the development of osteoclasts (Fig. 52.3). In addition, PTH and vitamin D stimulate osteoblasts to release interleukin-6 (IL-6), which stimulates existing osteoclasts to resorb bone (Fig. 52.4).

Certain lymphocyte-derived proteins strongly activate osteoclastic bone resorption, including RANKL, lymphotoxin, IL-1, and TNF-α.

Bone Resorption by Reduction in Bone Matrix PTH inhibits collagen synthesis by osteoblasts and also promotes the production of proteases that digest bone matrix.

Bone Deposition Whereas persistent increases in PTH favor net resorption, *intermittent* increases in plasma [PTH] have predominately bone-synthetic effects, inducing higher rates of bone formation and mineral apposition. PTH promotes bone synthesis by three mechanisms. First, PTH promotes bone synthesis *directly* by activating Ca²⁺ channels in osteocytes, a process that leads to a net transfer of Ca²⁺ from bone fluid to the osteocyte. The osteocyte then transfers this Ca²⁺ via gap junctions to the osteoblasts at the bone surface. This process is called *osteocytic osteolysis.* The osteoblasts then pump this Ca^{2+} into the extracellular matrix, which contributes to mineralization. Second, PTH decreases the production of **sclerostin** by osteocytes, thereby promoting osteoblastic differentiation and inhibiting osteoblastic apoptosis. Third, PTH stimulates bone synthesis *indirectly* in that osteoclastic bone resorption leads to the release of growth factors trapped within the matrix. Finally, PTH stimulates osteoblasts to produce OPG and thereby interfere with RANKL activation of osteoclasts.

⊙ 52-7 VITAMIN D

The active form of vitamin D is its 1,25-dihydroxy metabolite

Dietary deficiency of a fat-soluble vitamin is responsible for the childhood disease **rickets.** This disorder is characterized clinically by hypocalcemia and multiple skeletal abnormalities. Dietary replacement of vitamin D corrects this disorder.
⊙ **52-8** Vitamin D exists in the body in two forms, vitamin D_3 and vitamin D_2 (Fig. 52.7). **Vitamin D_3** can be synthesized from the 7-dehydrocholesterol that is present in the skin, provided sufficient ultraviolet light is absorbed. Vitamin D_3 is also available from several natural sources, including eggs and fortified milk. **Vitamin D_2** is obtained only from the diet, largely from vegetables.

Vitamin D (i.e., either D_2 or D_3) is fat soluble. Its absorption from the intestine depends on its solubilization by bile salts (see ⊙ **45-8**). In the circulation, vitamin D is found either solubilized with chylomicrons (see ⊙ **45-7**) or associated with a **vitamin D–binding protein.** Most of the body stores of vitamin D are located in body fat. The body's pools of vitamin D are large, and only 1% to 2% of the body's vitamin D is turned over each day.

The principal active form of vitamin D is not vitamin D_2 or D_3, but rather a dihydroxylated metabolite of either. Hydroxylation of vitamin D proceeds in two steps (Fig. 52.7). When circulating levels of 25-hydroxyvitamin D are low, adipocytes release vitamin D into the blood plasma. A cytochrome P-450 mixed-function oxidase in the liver, creates the first hydroxyl group at carbon 25. The second hydroxylation reaction occurs in the renal proximal tubule under the tight control of PTH, vitamin D itself, and FGF23 (see ⊙ **36-5**). PTH stimulates this 1-hydroxylation, whereas FGF23 and 1,25-dihydroxyvitamin D (the reaction product) both inhibit the process (Fig. 52.6).

Vitamin D and its metabolites circulate bound to a vitamin D–binding protein. This binding protein is particularly important for carriage of vitamins D_2 and D_3 in plasma because they are less soluble than their hydroxylated metabolites. Vitamin D and its metabolites arrive at target tissues and, once in the cytosol, associate with the VDR, a nuclear receptor (see ⊙ **3-28** and Table 3.3) that forms a heterodimer with RXR.

The biological actions of 1,25-dihydroxyvitamin D appear to be expressed principally via regulation of the transcription of a variety of proteins. The VDR/RXR complex associates with a regulatory site in the promoter region of the genes coding for certain vitamin D–regulated proteins.

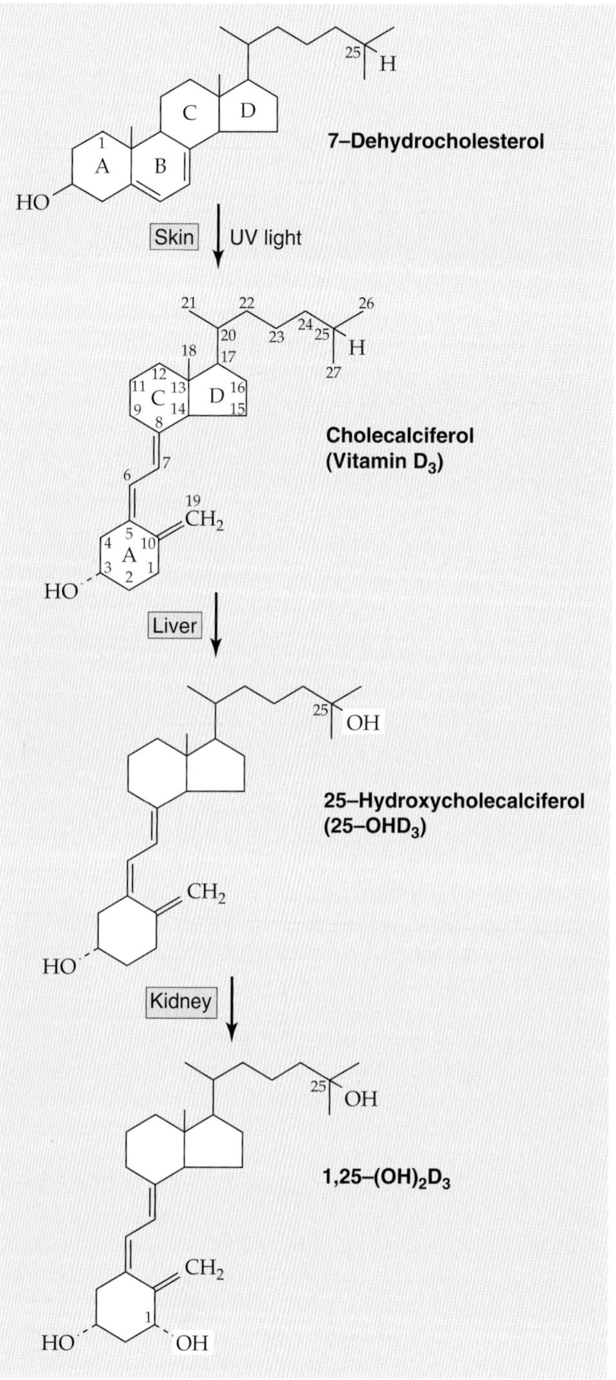

Figure 52.7 Metabolism of vitamin D_3. *UV,* Ultraviolet.

⊙ 52-9 Vitamin D, by acting on the small intestine and kidney, raises plasma $[Ca^{2+}]$ and thus promotes bone mineralization

The actions of vitamin D can be grouped into two categories: actions on target tissues involved in regulating body mineral and skeletal homeostasis, and a more general action that regulates cell growth.

Small Intestine In the duodenum, 1,25-dihydroxyvitamin D increases the production of several proteins that enhance Ca^{2+} absorption. Fig. 45.10 summarizes the intestinal absorption of Ca^{2+}, which moves from the intestinal lumen to the blood by both paracellular and transcellular routes (see ⊙ **45-9**). In the paracellular route, which occurs throughout the small intestine, Ca^{2+} moves *passively* from the lumen to the blood; 1,25-dihydroxyvitamin D does *not* regulate this pathway. The transcellular route, which occurs only in the duodenum, involves three steps. First, Ca^{2+} enters the cell across the apical membrane via TRPV6 Ca^{2+} channels (see ⊙ **45-10**). Second, the entering Ca^{2+} binds to several high-affinity binding proteins, particularly **calbindin.** These proteins, together with the exchangeable Ca^{2+} pools in the RER and mitochondria, effectively buffer the cytosolic Ca^{2+} and maintain a favorable gradient for Ca^{2+} entry across the apical membrane of the enterocyte. Third, the enterocyte extrudes Ca^{2+} across the basolateral membrane by means of both a Ca pump and an Na-Ca exchanger.

Vitamin D promotes intestinal Ca^{2+} absorption primarily by genomic effects that involve induction of the synthesis of epithelial Ca^{2+} channels and pumps and Ca^{2+}-binding proteins, as well as other proteins (e.g., alkaline phosphatase).

The effect of PTH to stimulate intestinal Ca^{2+} absorption is thought to be entirely indirect and mediated by PTH's action to increase the renal formation of 1,25-dihydroxyvitamin D (Fig. 52.6), which then enhances intestinal Ca^{2+} absorption.

Vitamin D also stimulates phosphate absorption by the small intestine. The initial step is mediated by the NaPi cotransporter and appears to be rate limiting for transepithelial transport and subsequent delivery of phosphate to the circulation. 1,25-Dihydroxyvitamin D stimulates the synthesis of this transport protein and thus promotes phosphate entry into the mucosal cell.

Kidney In the kidney, vitamin D appears to act synergistically with PTH to enhance *Ca^{2+} reabsorption* in the DCT (see ⊙ **36-7**). High-affinity Ca^{2+}-binding proteins, similar to those found in the intestinal mucosa, have been specifically localized to this region of the kidney. In addition, vitamin D promotes phosphate *reabsorption* in the kidney. Finally, 1,25-dihydroxyvitamin D directly inhibits the *1-hydroxylation* of vitamin D, establishing a negative-feedback loop.

Bone The actions of vitamin D on bone are complex and are the result of both indirect and direct actions. The overall effect of vitamin D replacement in animals with diet-induced vitamin D deficiency is to increase the flux of Ca^{2+} into bone. The major effects of vitamin D on bone are *indirect:* the action of vitamin D on both the small intestine and the kidneys makes more Ca^{2+} available to mineralize previously unmineralized osteoid. The *direct* effect of vitamin D on bone is via both osteoblasts and osteoclast precursor cells, both of which have VDRs. Vitamin D increases both osteoblastic and osteoclastic differentiation; when these activities are balanced, vitamin D simply increases bone turnover. However, when vitamin D is present in excess, it favors bone resorption because osteoblasts produce certain proteins with matrix-destroying properties (e.g., alkaline phosphatase, collagenase, plasminogen activator) as well as proteins that favor osteoclastogenesis (e.g., RANKL; Fig. 52.3). Thus, vitamin D can directly increase the number of mature osteoclasts, mobilizing Ca^{2+} from bone into the medium.

Calcium ingestion lowers—whereas phosphate ingestion raises—levels of both PTH and 1,25-dihydroxyvitamin D

Calcium Ingestion When an individual ingests a meal containing calcium, the ensuing rise in plasma $[Ca^{2+}]$ inhibits PTH secretion. The decline in PTH causes a decrease in the resorption of Ca^{2+} and phosphorus from bone, thus limiting the postprandial increase in plasma Ca^{2+} and phosphate levels. In addition, the decrease in PTH diminishes Ca^{2+} reabsorption in the kidney and thus facilitates a calciuric response. If dietary Ca^{2+} intake remains high, the lower PTH will result in decreased 1-hydroxylation of 25-hydroxyvitamin D, which will eventually diminish the fractional absorption of Ca^{2+} from the GI tract.

Phosphate Ingestion If one ingests phosphorus much in excess of Ca^{2+}, the rise in plasma [phosphate] will increase the plasma $Ca \times PO_4$ ion product, thereby promoting deposition of mineral in bone and lowering plasma $[Ca^{2+}]$. The low plasma $[Ca^{2+}]$, in turn, increases PTH secretion, provoking a phosphaturia and thus a fall of plasma [phosphate] toward normal. In addition, the PTH mobilizes Ca^{2+} and phosphate from bone by its action. Over longer periods, the action of PTH to increase the 1-hydroxylation of 25-hydroxyvitamin D plays an increasingly important role in defending the plasma $[Ca^{2+}]$ by increasing intestinal Ca^{2+} absorption.

The plasma [phosphate] is thus largely maintained *indirectly* through the actions of PTH in response to $[Ca^{2+}]$.

CALCITONIN AND OTHER HORMONES

Calcitonin inhibits osteoclasts, but its effects are transitory

Calcitonin is a 32–amino-acid peptide hormone made by the clear or C cells of the thyroid gland. C cells (also called parafollicular cells) are derived from neural crest cells of the fifth branchial pouch, which in humans migrate into the evolving thyroid gland.

Calcitonin release is triggered by a rise in the extracellular $[Ca^{2+}]$ above normal. Conversely, a lowering of the extracellular $[Ca^{2+}]$ diminishes calcitonin secretion.

The **calcitonin receptor** is a GPCR that, depending on the target cell, may activate either adenylyl cyclase (see ⊙ **3-4**) or phospholipase C (see ⊙ **3-6**). Within bone, the osteoclast are the principal target of calcitonin. In the osteoclast, calcitonin raises $[cAMP]_i$, which activates effectors such as protein kinases. Calcitonin inhibits the resorptive activity of the osteoclast, thus slowing the rate of bone turnover. It also diminishes osteocytic osteolysis. The hypocalcemic action of calcitonin is particularly effective in circumstances in which bone turnover is accelerated. However, within hours of exposure to high concentrations of calcitonin, osteoclasts desensitize. Thus, the precise role of calcitonin in body Ca^{2+} homeostasis has been difficult to define.

⊙ 52-10 Sex steroid hormones promote bone deposition, whereas glucocorticoids promote resorption

Although PTH and 1,25-dihydroxyvitamin D are the principal hormones involved in modulating bone turnover, other hormones participate in this process. For example, the sex steroids **testosterone** and **estradiol** are needed for maintaining normal bone mass in males and females, respectively. The decline in estradiol that occurs postmenopausally exposes women to the risk of **osteoporosis.**

⊙ 52-11 **Glucocorticoids** also modulate bone mass. This action is most evident in circumstances of glucocorticoid excess, which leads to osteoporosis, as suggested by the effects of glucocorticoids on the production of OPG (see ⊙ 52-5) and RANKL (see ⊙ 52-4).

PTHrP, encoded by a gene that is entirely distinct from that for PTH, can cause hypercalcemia in certain malignancies

Unlike PTH, which is synthesized exclusively by the parathyroid gland, a peptide called **PTH-related protein (PTHrP)** is made in many different normal and malignant tissues. The PTH1R receptor (see ⊙ 52-6) in kidney and bone recognizes PTHrP with an affinity similar to that for intact PTH. PTHrP mimics each of the actions of PTH on kidney and bone. Thus, when present in sufficient concentrations, PTHrP causes hypercalcemia.

The normal physiological roles of PTHrP are largely in regulating endochondral bone and mammary-gland development. The lactating breast also secretes PTHrP, and this hormone is present in very high concentrations in milk. PTHrP may promote the mobilization of Ca^{2+} from maternal bone during milk production. In nonlactating humans, the plasma PTHrP concentration is very low, and PTHrP does not appear to be involved in the day-to-day regulation of plasma $[Ca^{2+}]$.

THE REPRODUCTIVE SYSTEM

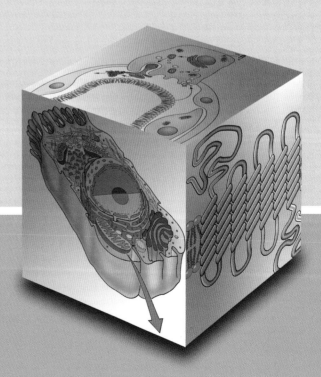

CHAPTER 53

SEXUAL DIFFERENTIATION

Sam Mesiano

Sexual reproduction involves the evolution of two sexually dissimilar individuals belonging to the same species, one male and one female. Each sex produces its own type of sex cell or **gamete,** and the union of male and female gametes generates species-specific progeny. Within each species, the relevant sexual characteristics of each partner have adapted to achieve the most efficient union of the gametes.

The key to successful sexual reproduction is that individuals develop as either male or female. This process is referred to as **sexual differentiation.** It has become abundantly clear that genes determine sexual differentiation and sexual expression and, as a result, mechanisms and patterns of reproduction. Organisms that reproduce sexually normally have a single pair of **sex chromosomes** that are morphologically distinguishable from other chromosomes, the **autosomes.** Each of the sex chromosomes carries genetic information that determines whether the individual functions and appears as male or female.

GENETIC ASPECTS OF SEXUAL DIFFERENTIATION

Meiosis occurs only in germ cells and gives rise to male and female gametes

Gametes (ova or sperm) are derive from a specialized lineage of embryonic cells known as **germ cells** by a process referred to as **gametogenesis.** Germ cells are the only cells that can divide by mitosis and **meiosis** and differentiate into gametes: either sperm or ova.

Except for the gametes, all other nucleated cells in the human body—**somatic cells**—have a **diploid** number (2N) of chromosomes. Human diploid cells have 22 autosome pairs consisting of two homologous chromosomes, one contributed by the father and one by the mother. Diploid cells also contain a single pair of sex chromosomes comprising either XX or XY. Each somatic cell in human females has 44 autosomes (i.e., 22 pairs) plus two X chromosomes, and each somatic cell in males has 44 autosomes plus one X and one Y chromosome. The **karyotype** is the total number of chromosomes and the sex chromosome combination, and thus in normal females is designated 46,XX, and in normal males, 46,XY (Fig. 53.1). Somatic cells divide only by **mitosis** (Fig. 53.2A), which results in the formation of two identical daughter cells, each having the same number of chromosomes (i.e., 46 in humans) and the same DNA content as the original cell. Prior to gametogenesis germ cells also divide by mitosis. Gametes have a **haploid** number (N) of chromosomes and contain either an X or Y sex chromosome. Haploid gamete cells are produced by the process of **meiosis** (Fig. 53.2A and B), which during **gametogenesis,** reduces the number of chromosomes by half, so that each gamete contains one chromosome from each of the original 23 pairs.

Meiosis occurs only in germ cells—**spermatogonia** in males and **oogonia** in females—still with a complement of 2N DNA (N = 23). Germ cells initially multiply by mitosis and then enter meiosis when they begin to differentiate into sperm (Fig. 53.2B) or ova (Fig. 53.2C). This reduction in genetic material from the diploid (2N) to the haploid (N) number involves two divisions referred to as **meiosis I** and **meiosis II.**

Prior to the start of meiosis I, the chromosomes duplicate so that the cells have 23 pairs of duplicated chromosomes (i.e., each chromosome has two chromatids)—or 4N DNA. During prophase of the first meiotic division, homologous pairs of chromosomes—22 pairs of autosomal chromosomes (autosomes) plus a pair of sex chromosomes—exchange genetic material through a process known as **recombination** or **crossing over** at attachment points known as **chiasmata.** This results in a random, but balanced, exchange of DNA between the homologous maternal and paternal chromatids to produce recombinant chromosomes comprising a mix of maternal and paternal DNA. The cells then divide to produce two genetically unique diploid (2N) daughter cells. During meiosis II, no additional duplication of DNA takes place. The chromatids simply separate so that each daughter receives a haploid number of unduplicated chromosomes—1N DNA. Gametes produced by this process are genetically different from each other and from either parent due to the recombination events in meiosis I. The genetic diversity that arises from recombination during meiosis and the combining of gametes from different parental lineages causes significant phenotypic variation within the population, providing an efficient mechanism for adaptation and natural selection.

A major difference between male and female gametogenesis is that one spermatogonium yields four spermatids (Fig. 53.2B), whereas one oogonium yields one mature oocyte and two or three polar bodies (Fig. 53.2C).

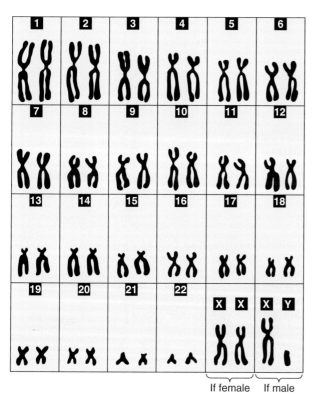

If female   If male

Figure 53.1 Normal human karyotype. The normal human has 22 pairs of autosomal chromosomes (autosomes), as well as a pair of sex chromosomes. Females have two X chromosomes, whereas males have one X and one Y chromosome.

⊙ 53-1 Fertilization of an oocyte by an X- or Y-bearing sperm establishes the zygote's genotypic sex

Fusion of two haploid gametes, a mature spermatozoan from the father and a mature oocyte from the mother—referred to as **fertilization**—produces a new diploid cell with 2N DNA, a **zygote** that will become a new individual. The sex chromosomes that the parents contribute to the offspring determine the **genotypic sex** of that individual.

The genotypic sex determines the **gonadal sex,** which in turn determines the **phenotypic sex** that becomes fully established at puberty.

The potential offspring has a unique complement of chromosomes differing from those of both the mother and the father. The ovum provided by the mother (XX) always provides an X chromosome. Because the male is the heterogenetic (XY) sex, half the spermatozoa are X bearing whereas the other half are Y bearing. Thus, the type of sperm that fertilizes the ovum determines the sex of the zygote. X-bearing sperm produce XX zygotes that develop into females with a 46,XX karyotype, whereas Y-bearing sperm produce XY zygotes that develop into males with a 46,XY karyotype. The genotypic sex of an individual is determined at the time of fertilization. The Y chromosome appears to be the fundamental determinant of sexual development. When a Y chromosome is present, the individual develops as a male; when the Y chromosome is absent, the individual develops as a female.

Compared with males, females have a double dose of X-chromosome genes. To avoid an overdosage of X-derived gene products, each somatic 46,XX cell randomly inactivates either the maternal or paternal X chromosome in a process called **lyonization.** Once inactivated, that X chromosome remains inactivated for the life of the cell and all of its descendants. The inactivated X chromosome is visible as a small dark dot of condensed chromatin in the nucleus known as the **Barr body.** Presence of a Barr body can be used to determine the genotypic sex of a cell as it exists only in female cells.

The testis-determining gene is located on the Y chromosome

A Y chromosome is necessary for normal testicular development. Thus, it stands to reason that the gene that determines organogenesis of the testis is normally located on the Y chromosome. This so-called **testis-determining factor (TDF)** gene has been mapped to the short arm of the Y chromosome and is a single gene called *sex-determining region Y (SRY).*

DIFFERENTIATION OF THE GONADS

Genotypic sex determines differentiation of the indifferent gonad into either an ovary or a testis

⊙ **53-2 Germ cells**—cells that give rise to gametes—play a key role in sexual differentiation by affecting gonad development. The **primordial germ cells (PGCs)** do not originate in the gonad; instead, they migrate to the gonad from the yolk sac along the mesentery of the hindgut at about the fifth week of embryo development. During their journey they divide by mitosis. They eventually take up their position embedded in the gonadal ridges—bilateral swellings adjacent to the developing kidneys, which early in development are identical in males and females and therefore referred to as the **indifferent gonads.** Gonadal development fails to progress normally in the absence of germ cells. The indifferent gonad develops into a testis or ovary depending on genotypic sex.

In embryos with an XY sex chromosome complement (i.e., 46,XY) a testis develops from the indifferent gonad, and in embryos with an XX sex chromosome complement (i.e., 46,XX) an ovary develops from the indifferent gonad. The Y chromosome exerts a powerful testis-determining effect on the indifferent gonad. In the absence of a Y chromosome, the indifferent gonad develops into an ovary.

The primitive testis develops from the medulla of the primordial gonad

In male embryos, germ cells differentiate into sperm and the presence of the SRY gene induces the indifferent gonad to develop into a testis comprising the **seminiferous tubules,** including the Sertoli cells, the **rete testis,** and the **efferent ductules.** These tubular structures establish a pathway from the male gonad to the wolffian duct, which evolves into the outlet for sperm. At the same time, mesenchymal cells take up residence among the seminiferous tubules and eventually become the **Leydig cells** of the testis. At around the 10th week of development, the Leydig cells produce testosterone, which promotes differentiation of the male external genitalia.

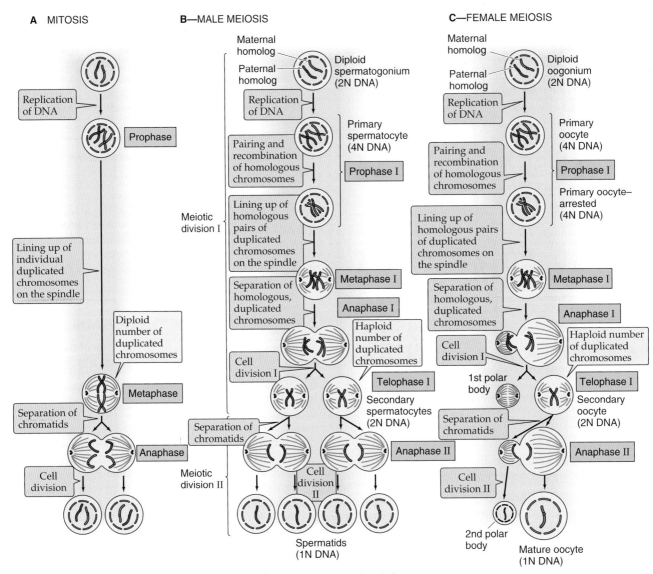

A MITOSIS   **B—MALE MEIOSIS**   **C—FEMALE MEIOSIS**

Figure 53.2 Mitosis and meiosis.

The main cell types within the seminiferous tubules are **Sertoli** cells and male germ cells (**spermatogonia**), which continue to divide by mitosis (albeit slowly) until puberty. At puberty the rate of spermatogonia division increases and a subgroup of spermatogonia begin meiosis and enter the process of spermatogenesis to produce mature sperm. A stem-cell population of spermatogonia is maintained by mitosis throughout the life of the male.

⊙ 53-3 The primitive ovary develops from the cortex of the primordial gonad

In female embryos the germ cells (**oogonia**) form ova (**oocytes**), which—in the absence of the SRY gene—causes the indifferent gonad to develop into an ovary. Unlike gonadogenesis in the male, the entire investment of oogonia reaches the indifferent gonad by mid-gestation and initiates meiosis and the process of oogenesis. At this stage the oocytes become arrested in the early stages of meiosis I and are surrounded by a single layer of granulosa cells to form structures referred to as **primordial follicles**. At birth,

each ovary holds around 1 million primordial follicles, each containing one primary oocyte arrested in meiosis I. Because all the oogonia are depleted at mid-gestation (they either die or become oocytes), the number of primordial follicles formed at that time is all that will be available for reproduction for the rest of the female's life. This process is distinct from spermatogenesis, which occurs continually after puberty due to the replenishment of spermatogonia by mitosis.

PHENOTYPIC SEX

The embryonic gonad determines the development of the internal genitalia and the external sexual phenotype

The hormones produced by the gonad determine the development of the internal genitalia and the external sexual phenotype by affecting the development of internal and external accessory sex organs. In males, the external sex organs are the penis and scrotum; the internal sex organs are the testicles, the epididymis, vas deferens, seminal vesicles, ejaculatory ducts, prostate, and bulbourethral glands. In females, the external organs include the vulva, labia, and clitoris and the internal organs are the vagina, uterus, and fallopian tubes. Other secondary **sex characteristics** are external specializations that are not essential for the production and movement of gametes; instead, they are primarily concerned with sex behavior and with the birth and nutrition of offspring. Examples include pubic hair and breasts. Not only do the sex steroids produced by the gonads affect the accessory sex organs, they also modulate the physiological state of the secondary sex characteristics toward "maleness" in the case of the testes and "femaleness" in the case of the ovaries.

Embryos of both sexes have a double set of embryonic genital ducts

Development of male or female sex structures is under the control of hormones produced by the gonad and, as such, gonadal sex determines phenotypic sex. The internal accessory sex organs develop from embryonic duct systems—the **wolffian ducts** and the **müllerian ducts**—and the external sex organs develop from the urogenital sinus. The genital ducts are an essential part of the genital organs and form the pathway by which the sex cells—ova and spermatozoa—move to the location of fertilization.

In males, the wolffian ducts become the epididymis, vas deferens, seminal vesicles, and ejaculatory duct

In male embryos, the müllerian ducts regress and the **wolffian ducts** develop into the **epididymis,** the **vas deferens,** and the **seminal vesicle.** Moreover, the urogenital sinus masculinizes to give rise to the **ejaculatory duct, prostate gland, bulbourethral gland, penis,** and **scrotum.**

In females, the müllerian ducts become the fallopian tubes, the uterus, and the upper third of the vagina

In female embryos, the wolffian ducts degenerate and the müllerian ducts persist and develop into the fallopian tubes, the **uterus,** including the **cervix,** and the upper third of the **vagina.** The lower two thirds of the vagina and external female genitalia develop from the urogenital sinus, which develops into the female genitalia in the absence of testicular hormones.

⊙ 53-4 In males, antimüllerian hormone causes regression of the müllerian ducts

During embryogenesis in males, the Sertoli cells of the testis produce **antimüllerian hormone (AMH)** that causes degeneration of the müllerian ducts. Testosterone—secreted by the Leydig cells of the testis—stimulates differentiation of the wolffian ducts. In females, who lack Sertoli cells, and therefore AMH, the müllerian ducts differentiate spontaneously in the absence of AMH, and the wolffian ducts involute spontaneously in the absence of testosterone (Fig. 53.3).

DIFFERENTIATION OF THE EXTERNAL GENITALIA

The urogenital sinus develops into the urinary bladder, the urethra, and, in females, the vestibule of the vagina

Both the wolffian and the müllerian ducts empty into this urogenital sinus, from which the external genitalia of both sexes develops.

The external genitalia of both sexes develop from common anlagen

Until about the end of the first trimester of pregnancy, the external genitalia of males and females are anatomically indistinguishable. The phallus undergoes rapid growth in females initially, but its growth slows, and in the absence of androgens, the phallus becomes the relatively small clitoris in females. The paired **urogenital folds** give rise to the ventral aspect of the penis in males. However, in females, the urogenital folds normally remain separate as the labia minora. In males, the **genital** or **labioscrotal swellings** fuse to give rise to the scrotum. In females, however, the labioscrotal swellings fuse anteriorly to give rise to the mons pubis and posteriorly to form the posterior labial commissure. The unfused labioscrotal swellings give rise to the labia majora.

PUBERTY

Although at birth humans have the primary and secondary sex organs necessary for procreation, final sexual maturity occurs only at **puberty,** the transition between the juvenile and adult states when an individual becomes capable of reproducing.

Puberty involves steroid hormones produced by the gonads and the adrenals

Puberty involves two physiological processes: (1) adrenarche, the increased production of the androgenic steroids dehydroepiandrosterone (DHEA), dehydroepiandrosterone sulfate (DHEAS), and androstenedione (A4) by the adrenal cortex (see Fig. 50.2); and (2) gonadarche, the physical and functional maturation of the gonads, such that they produce gametes and sex steroids. **Adrenarche** occurs in both sexes during the prepubertal period (ages 6 to 8 years). The increased levels of adrenal androgens induce **pubarche,** the growth of pubic hair. **Gonadarche** is induced by increased production of the gonadotropic hormones follicle-stimulating hormone (FSH) and luteinizing hormone (LH) by the anterior pituitary (see Figs. 54.2 and 55.3). The gonadal steroids (estrogens in the female and testosterone in the male) produced in response to FSH and LH induce growth and maturation of the genitals and secondary sex organs, and the development of secondary sex characteristics. The gonadal steroids also participate (with growth hormone and insulin-like growth factors) in the adolescent growth spurt. In males gonadarche leads to **spermarche,** the initiation of sperm production by

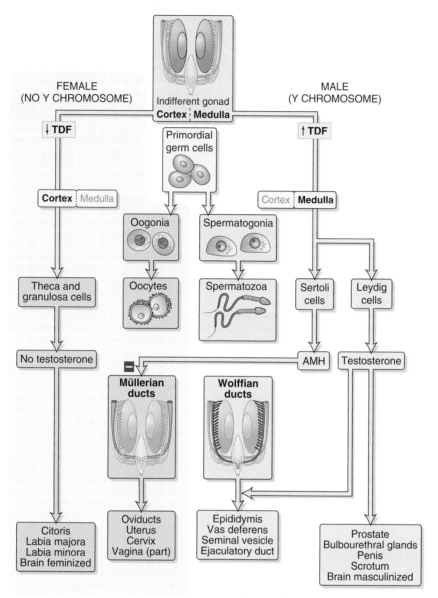

Figure 53.3   Pathways for the hormonal control of sex determination.

the testes, and in females it leads to **folliculogenesis** and **menarche,** the initiation of menstrual cycles, and **thelarche,** development of breasts.

Hypothalamic gonadotropin-releasing hormone secretion controls puberty and reproduction

Gonadotropin production by the anterior pituitary is under the control of gonadotropin-releasing hormone (GnRH), produced in the hypothalamus (see ⊙ 54-1 and ⊙ 55-2). One of the earliest events of puberty in males and females is the onset of pulsatile release of GnRH from the hypothalamus and, in turn, FSH and LH from the anterior pituitary. The appearance of GnRH pulsatility early in puberty is associated with decreased sensitivity of the hypothalamic-pituitary system to the negative feedback of circulating sex steroids. Once a pulsatile pattern of gonadotropin secretion is established, it continues throughout reproductive life.

⊙ 53-5 Multiple factors control the timing of puberty

In girls, adrenarche leads to pubarche, which occurs between 8 and 13 years of age. Gonadarche leads to thelarche, typically followed by menarche, which generally occurs between 12 and 13 years of age. The earliest physical manifestation of puberty in boys is an increase in testicular volume, which usually occurs between 9 and 14 years of age (Table 53.1).

The precise cause of the onset of puberty is not completely understood. Multiple intrinsic (genetic) and extrinsic (environmental) factors play a role. Genetic factors appear to be major determinants of pubertal onset. Other factors, such as nutrition, geographic location, and exposure to light, also play a role. Over the last century, the age of girls at menarche in the United States and Europe has gradually decreased. The reason that menarche now occurs at a younger age is incompletely understood. It could be due to improved nutrition.

TABLE 53.1 Tanner Stages in Male and Female Puberty

STAGE	PUBIC HAIR (BOTH SEXES)	MALE GENITAL DEVELOPMENT	FEMALE BREAST AND GENITAL[a] DEVELOPMENT
1	Preadolescent. No pubic hair is present, only vellus hair, as on the abdomen.	Preadolescent. The penis, scrotum, and testes are the same size—relative to body size—as in a young child.	Preadolescent. Breasts: only papillae are elevated.
2	Pubic hair is sparse, mainly at the base of the penis (boys) or along labia majora (girls).	Scrotum and testes are enlarged.	Breast buds begin to develop. Breasts and papillae are both elevated, and the diameter of the areolae increases.
3	Pubic hair is darker, coarser, and curlier and spreads above the pubis.	Penis is enlarged, predominantly in length. Scrotum and testes are further enlarged.	Breasts and areolae further enlarge. Vagina enlarges and begins producing a discharge. Menstrual periods may begin.
4	Pubic hair is of the adult type, but covers an area smaller than in most adults.	Penis is further enlarged in length and also in diameter. Scrotum and testes are further enlarged.	Areolae and papillae project out beyond the level of the expanding breast tissue. Menstruation and ovulation begin. Periods will most likely be irregular.
5	Adult pattern.	Adult pattern.	With further enlargement of the breast, the areolae are now on the same level as the rest of the breast. Only the papillae project. Adult pattern.

[a]The official Tanner stages for females include pubic hair and breast development.

However, better nutritional status alone cannot completely explain the decreased age of pubertal onset. Proximity to the equator and lower altitudes are also associated with early onset of puberty. A loose correlation is also seen between the onset of menarche in the mother and the onset of menarche in the daughter. The onset of puberty is also related to body composition and to fat deposition. Severe obesity and heavy exercise delay puberty.

Androgens and estrogens influence secondary sex characteristics at puberty

Profound alterations in steroid hormone secretion during the peripubertal period cause changes in the primary sex organs and secondary sex characteristics. In both sexes, the process of puberty can be divided into five developmental stages—referred to as the **Tanner stages**—based on the extent of pubic hair growth and genital and breast development. In males and females, Tanner stage 1 is the prepubertal state and Tanner stage 5 is the adult state (Fig. 53.4 and Table 53.1).

Males The range of onset of normal male puberty extends from 9 to 14 years. Boys complete pubertal development within 2 to 4½ years. In a normal male, the first sign of puberty (Tanner stage 2) is enlargement of the testes to >2.5 cm (Fig. 53.4B). Testicular enlargement is mainly due to growth of the seminiferous tubules with some contribution by Leydig cell growth. In normal boys, pubic hair generally develops 1 to 1½ years after genital development. Pubic hair growth can be due to adrenarche or gonadarche and therefore can occur independently of genital growth.

The changes that occur in male puberty are induced mainly by testosterone secreted by the testes. Testosterone has **androgenic effects;** it stimulates adult maturation of the external genitalia and accessory sex organs, including the

penis, the scrotum, the prostate, and the seminal vesicles. It also induces the male secondary sexual characteristics, which include deepening of the voice, as well as evolving male patterns of hair growth. Testosterone also has **anabolic** effects, including stimulation of linear body growth and muscular development in the adolescent and mature male.

The pubertal growth spurt, a marked increase in growth rate (total body size), occurs late in puberty in boys. The acceleration of growth appears due to the combined effects of increased secretion of growth hormone and testosterone. In boys, height increases by an average of 28 cm during the pubertal spurt. The 10-cm mean difference in adult stature between men and women is due to a greater pubertal growth spurt in boys and to greater height at the onset of peak pubertal height velocity in boys compared with girls. Before puberty, boys and girls have the same mean body mass, skeletal mass, and body fat. However, men have 150% of the average woman's lean and skeletal body mass, and women have 200% of the body fat of men.

Females The first physical sign of puberty in girls is usually the onset of thelarche that begins between 10 and 11 years of age (Fig. 53.4A). During the next 3 to 5 years, the breasts continue to develop under the influence of several hormones. Progesterone is primarily responsible for development of the alveoli of the mammary gland (see Fig. 56.9C). Estrogen is the primary stimulus for development of the duct system of the mammary gland that connects the alveoli to the exterior. Insulin, growth hormone, glucocorticoids, and thyroxin contribute to breast development, but they are incapable of causing breast growth by themselves.

During puberty, the uterus and cervix enlarge, and their secretory functions increase under the influence of estrogens (mainly estradiol). The uterine glands increase in number and length, and the endometrium and stroma proliferate in

A FEMALE PUBERTY (BREAST DEVELOPMENT AND PUBIC HAIR)

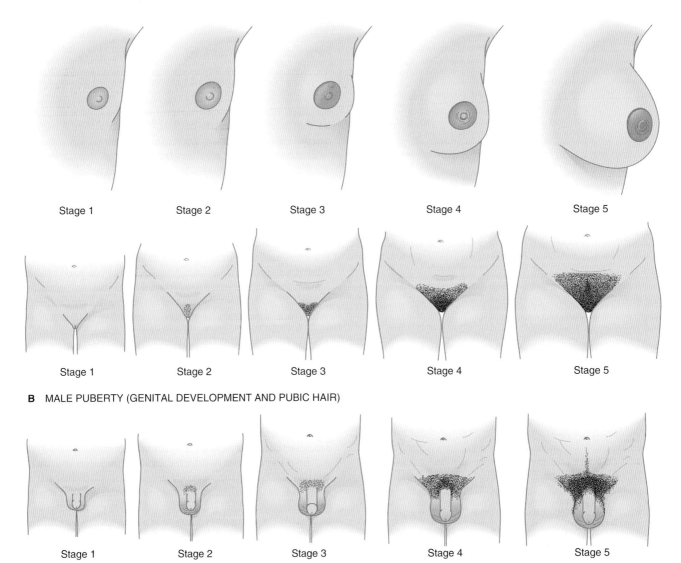

B MALE PUBERTY (GENITAL DEVELOPMENT AND PUBIC HAIR)

Figure 53.4 Tanner stages of puberty based on pubic hair, genital, and breast development in boys and girls. Pubic hair and genital/breast development may not be synchronous and are usually scored separately. For example, a girl may be at breast stage 3 but pubic hair stage 2. (Data from Carel JC, Léger J: Clinical practice. Precocious puberty. N Engl J Med 358:2366, 2008.)

response to estrogens. The mucous membranes of the female urogenital tract respond to hormones, particularly estrogens.

Menarche usually occurs around 2 years after the initiation of thelarche. In the United States, most girls experience menarche between the ages of 11 and 13 years, the average age is 12½ years, and the normal range is between 8 and 16 years. During puberty, a girl's body shape changes in response to rising levels of estradiol. The hips and pelvis widen and the proportion of body fat increases (compared with males) and distributes mainly to the breasts, hips, buttocks, thighs, upper arms, and pubis to produce the typical adult female body shape.

CHAPTER 54

THE MALE REPRODUCTIVE SYSTEM

Sam Mesiano

The male reproductive system consists of: the *gonads* (in this case, the testes) and various glands and ducts that constitute the sex accessory organs (Fig. 54.1A and B).

The **testes** are responsible for the production of gametes, the haploid cells—**spermatozoa,** plural of spermatozoon— necessary for sexual reproduction and for the synthesis and secretion of hormones, including the principal male sex hormone, testosterone, that controls the development and function of the male **secondary sexual characteristics.**

The testes (Fig. 54.1C) are composed mainly of seminiferous tubules (Fig. 54.1D and E) and Leydig cells located in the spaces between the tubules. A seminiferous tubule is an epithelium made up of Sertoli cells (Fig. 54.1E) and is also the site of **spermatogenesis**—the production of the haploid spermatozoa from the diploid germ cells.

The male **sex accessory organs** include the paired epididymides, the vasa deferentia, the seminal vesicles, the ejaculatory ducts, the prostate, the bulbourethral glands, the urethra, and the penis. The primary role of the male sex accessory glands and ducts is to store and transport spermatozoa to the exterior, and thus enable spermatozoa to reach and fertilize female gametes.

HYPOTHALAMIC-PITUITARY-GONADAL AXIS

The hypothalamus secretes GnRH, which acts on gonadotrophs in the anterior pituitary

The hypothalamic-pituitary-gonadal axis (Fig. 54.2) controls two primary functions of reproduction: (1) production of gametes (spermatogenesis in males and oogenesis in females), and (2) gonadal sex steroid biosynthesis (testosterone in males and estradiol and progesterone in females). In both sexes, the hypothalamus produces gonadotropin-releasing hormone (GnRH), which stimulates the gonadotroph cells in the anterior pituitary to secrete the two gonadotropins (hormones that stimulate the growth and function of the gonads), luteinizing hormone (LH), and follicle-stimulating hormone (FSH). Although the names of these hormones reflect their function in the female reproductive system, they play similar roles in controlling gonadal function in both sexes. In the male, LH and FSH control, respectively, the Leydig and Sertoli cells of the testes.

54-1 The hypothalamus secretes GnRH, which acts on gonadotrophs in the anterior pituitary

Gonadotropin-releasing hormone (GnRH), a decapeptide that is synthesized by small-bodied peptidergic neurons in the hypothalamus, stimulates the synthesis, storage, and secretion of gonadotropins by gonadotroph cells in the anterior pituitary. The neurons that synthesize, store, and release GnRH are dispersed throughout the hypothalamus but are principally located in the arcuate nucleus and preoptic area. The hypothalamic-pituitary-portal system (see Fig. 47.2) describes the route by which GnRH and other releasing hormones emanating from the hypothalamus reach the anterior pituitary gland.

GnRH secreted at the axon terminals in response to neuron activation enters the portal vasculature and is transported directly to the anterior pituitary, where it stimulates the release of both FSH and LH from the gonadotroph cells. Because secretion of GnRH is pulsatile, secretion of LH and FSH by the gonadotrophs is also episodic. The frequency of pulsatile LH discharge in men is ~8 to 14 pulses over a 24-hour period. FSH pulses are not as prominent as LH pulses, both because of their lower amplitude and because of the longer half-life of FSH in the circulation.

Under the control of GnRH, gonadotrophs in the anterior pituitary secrete LH and FSH

LH and **FSH** are glycoprotein hormones composed of two polypeptide chains designated α and β, both of which are required for full biological activity. The α subunits of LH and FSH are identical. The β subunits differ and thus confer specific functional characteristics to the intact molecules.

Differential secretion of FSH and LH are under the control of several hormones, including sex steroids and inhibins.

LH stimulates the Leydig cells of the testis to produce testosterone

LH stimulates the synthesis of testosterone by the testes. The interstitial **Leydig cells** are the principal targets for LH and the primary source of testosterone production in the male. The plasma membranes of Leydig cells have a high-affinity LH receptor (LHCGR), a GPCR coupled to $G\alpha_s$ (Fig. 54.3).

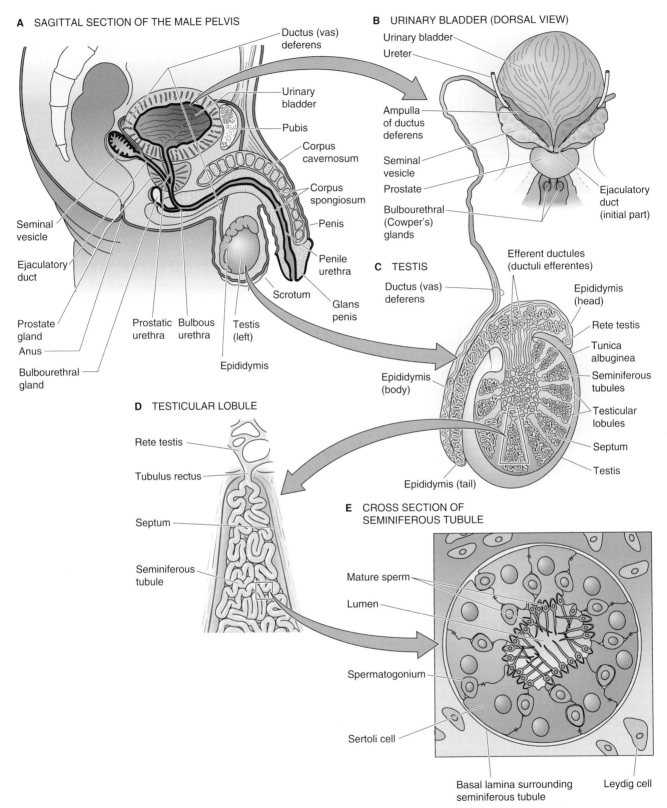

Figure 54.1 Anatomy of the male internal genitalia and accessory sex organs. (A) The two major elements of the male sexual anatomy are the gonads (i.e., testes) and the sex accessories (i.e., epididymis, vas deferens, seminal vesicles, ejaculatory duct, prostate, bulbourethral or Cowper's glands, urethra, and penis). Note that the urethra can be subdivided into the prostatic urethra, the bulbous urethra, and the penile urethra. (B) The vas deferens expands into an ampulla before coursing across the rear of the urinary bladder and merging with the outflow from the seminal vesicle. The merger forms the ejaculatory duct. The left and right ejaculatory ducts penetrate the prostate gland and open into the prostatic urethra. (C) The spermatozoa form in the seminiferous tubules and then flow into the rete testis and from there into the efferent ductules, the epididymis, and the vas deferens. (E) The seminiferous tubule is an epithelium formed by Sertoli cells, with interspersed germ cells. The most immature germ cells (the spermatogonia) are near the periphery of the tubule, whereas the mature germ cells (the spermatozoa) are near the lumen of the tubule. The Leydig cells are interstitial cells that lie between the tubules.

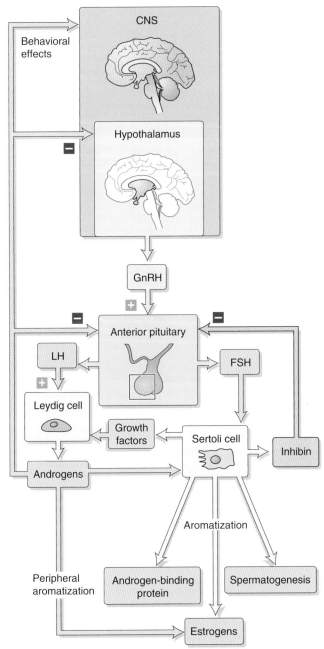

Figure 54.2 Hypothalamic-pituitary-gonadal axis. Small-bodied neurons in the arcuate nucleus and preoptic area of the hypothalamus secrete GnRH, a decapeptide that reaches the gonadotrophs in the anterior pituitary via the long portal veins. Stimulation by GnRH causes the gonadotrophs to synthesize and release LH, which stimulates Leydig cells, and FSH, which stimulates Sertoli cells.

FSH stimulates Sertoli cells to synthesize hormones that influence Leydig cells and spermatogenesis

The Sertoli cells are the primary testicular site of FSH action (Fig. 54.3). FSH also regulates Leydig cell physiology via effects on Sertoli cells. The signaling events after FSH binding are similar to those described above for LH on the Leydig cell. Thus, binding of FSH to its receptor (FSHR, a GPCR) on Sertoli cells activates $G\alpha_s$, thereby increasing the transcription of specific genes, and the synthesis of several proteins important for synthesis and action of steroid hormones,

including androgen-binding protein (ABP), **P-450 aromatase (P-450$_{arom}$)**, several growth factors, and inhibins.

Leydig cells and Sertoli cells engage in **crosstalk** (Fig. 54.3). For example, the Leydig cells make testosterone, which acts on Sertoli cells. Conversely, Sertoli cells affect Leydig cells. For example, Sertoli cells convert testosterone—manufactured by Leydig cells—to estradiol, which decreases the capacity of Leydig cells to produce testosterone in response to LH. In addition, FSH acting on Sertoli cells produces growth factors that may increase the number of LH receptors on Leydig cells.

In summary, optimal spermatogenesis requires two testicular cell types (Leydig cells and Sertoli cells), as well as two gonadotropins (LH and FSH) and one androgen (testosterone).

The hypothalamic-pituitary-testicular axis is under feedback inhibition by testicular steroids and inhibins

Normal circulating levels of **testosterone** inhibit the pulsatile release of GnRH by the hypothalamus and thereby reduce the frequency and amplitude of the LH- and FSH-secretory pulses. Testosterone also has negative-feedback action on LH secretion at the level of the pituitary gonadotrophs.

The **inhibins** also feed back on FSH secretion. FSH specifically stimulates the Sertoli cells to produce inhibin, and inhibin "inhibits" FSH secretion at the level of the anterior pituitary.

The secretion of LH and FSH is under the additional control of neuropeptides, amino acids such as aspartate, corticotropin-releasing hormone (CRH; see ⊙ 50-5), and endogenous opioids. Thus, multiple hormonal signals from various physiologic systems could affect male fertility by altering gonadotropin secretion.

SYNTHESIS OF SEX STEROIDS

Leydig cells convert cholesterol to testosterone

The synthesis of steroid hormones occurs by the metabolism of cholesterol through various intermediates to biologically active steroids. In the testis and ovary LH and FSH induce the expression of genes encoding enzymes that convert cholesterol to androgens and estrogens.

As shown in Fig. 54.4, **Leydig cells** use a series of five enzymes to convert cholesterol to testosterone, along any of four pathways. The preferred pathway for testosterone synthesis in Leydig cells consists of the following five steps:

1. Cholesterol to pregnenolone by the side-chain-cleavage, which is stimulated by LH and is the rate-limiting step in the pathway
2. Pregnenolone to 17-hydroxy-pregnenolone by 17α-hydroxylase
3. 17-hydroxy-pregnenolone to dehydroepiandrosterone (DHEA) by 17,20-desmolase
4. DHEA to androstenedione by 3β-hydroxysteroid dehydrogenase
5. Androstenedione to testosterone by 17β-hydroxysteroid dehydrogenase

Some testosterone target cells convert testosterone, via 5α-reductase, to dihydrotestosterone (DHT), which has much greater androgenic activity than testosterone. DHT

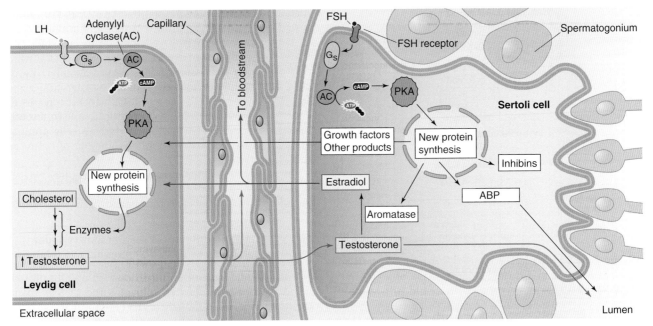

Figure 54.3   Leydig and Sertoli cell physiology. *PKA,* Protein kinase A.

has a higher affinity than testosterone for the **androgen receptor (AR)** and consequently as 30- to 50-fold greater biological activity. The testis can also convert testosterone to DHT. However, extratesticular tissue is responsible for most of the DHT production.

Although testosterone is the major secretory product, the testes also secretes pregnenolone, progesterone, 17-hydroxyprogesterone, androstenedione, androsterone, and DHT. Androstenedione is of major importance because it serves as a precursor for testicular estrogen formation.

Adipose tissue, skin, and the adrenal cortex also produce testosterone and other androgens

Several tissues besides the testes—including adipose tissue, skin, adrenal cortex, brain, and muscle—produce testosterone and several other androgens. These substances may be synthesized de novo from cholesterol or produced by peripheral conversion of precursors.

The adrenal cortex (see ◉ 50-3) is another source of androgen production in both males and females. Normal human adrenal glands synthesize and secrete the weak androgens DHEA, conjugated DHEA sulfate, and androstenedione. Although the adrenal gland contributes significantly to the total androgen milieu in males, it does not appear to have significant effects on stimulation and growth of the male accessory organs. This occurs primarily as a result of DHT production from circulating testosterone.

Testosterone acts on target organs by binding to a nuclear receptor

◉ **54-2** Most testosterone in the circulation is bound to specific binding proteins. About 45% of plasma testosterone binds to **sex hormone–binding globulin (SHBG)** and ~55% binds to serum albumin and corticosteroid-binding globulin (CBG) (see ◉ 50-3). A small fraction (~2%) of the total circulating testosterone circulates free, or unbound, in plasma. The free form of testosterone enters the cell by passive diffusion and subsequently exerts biological actions.

Once it diffuses into the cell, testosterone either binds to a high-affinity AR in the nucleus or undergoes conversion to DHT, which also binds to the AR (see ◉ 3-28). As with other steroid hormone receptors, the AR functions as a ligand-activated transcription factor that binds to hormone response elements on DNA located in the promoter regions of the target genes, leading to changes in gene expression and altered production of specific proteins, which alters cell function.

Whether the active compound in any tissue is DHT or testosterone depends on the presence or absence in that tissue of the microsomal enzyme **5α-reductase,** which converts testosterone to DHT (see Fig. 54.4).

BIOLOGY OF SPERMATOGENESIS AND SEMEN PRODUCTION

Spermatogenesis includes mitotic divisions of spermatogonia, meiotic divisions of spermatocytes to spermatids, and maturation to spermatozoa

Primordial germ cells (see ◉ 53-2) migrate into the gonad during embryogenesis. In males, these cells become the immature stem-cell population of **spermatogonia,** and reside on the inner surface of the seminiferous tubules (Fig. 54.1E). The spermatogonia have the normal diploid complement of 46 chromosomes (2N): 22 pairs of autosomal chromosomes plus one X and one Y chromosome, and after puberty divide by mitosis (Fig. 54.5).

Spermatogonia can be classified into two types: A and B. Type A spermatogonia form the stem-cell population of male germ cells and divide by mitosis. One of the daughter cells renews the stock of type A spermatogonia and the other becomes a type B spermatogonium that undergoes several

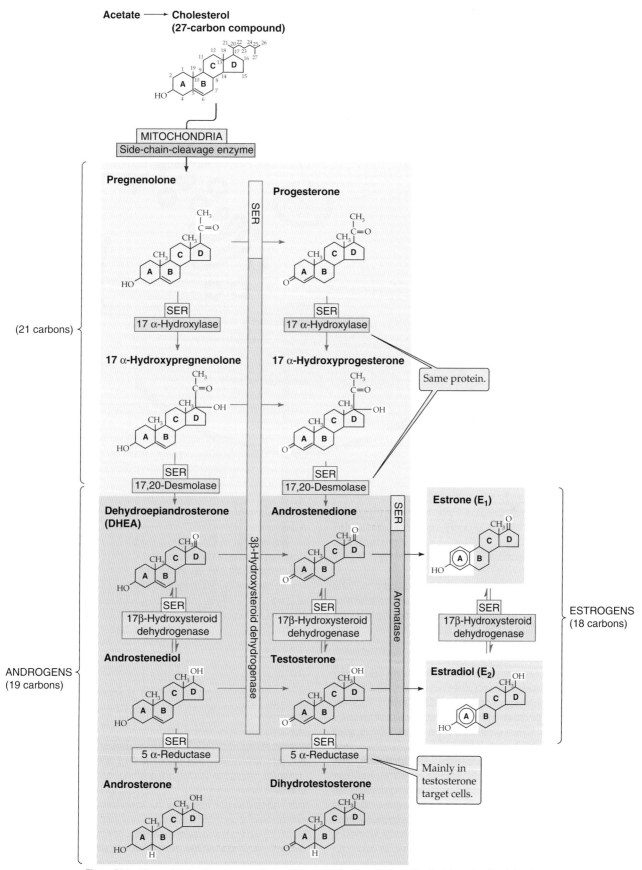

Figure 54.4 Biosynthesis of androgens. Some of these pathways are shared in the biosynthesis of the gluco-corticoids and mineralocorticoids (see Fig. 50.2). *SER*, Smooth endoplasmic reticulum.

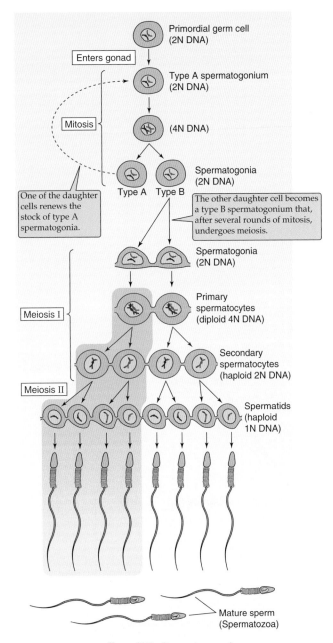

One of the daughter cells renews the stock of type A spermatogonia.

The other daughter cell becomes a type B spermatogonium that, after several rounds of mitosis, undergoes meiosis.

Figure 54.5 Spermatogenesis.

smaller cells called spermatids, which have a *haploid* number of *unduplicated* chromosomes (1N). **Spermatids** form the inner layer of the epithelium and are found in rather discrete aggregates inasmuch as the cells derived from a single spermatogonium tend to remain together—with cytoplasm linked in a syncytium—and differentiate synchronously.

Spermatids transform into **spermatozoa** in a process called **spermiogenesis,** which involves cytoplasmic reduction and differentiation of the body and the tailpieces. Thus, as maturation progresses, developing male gametes decrease in volume. Conversely, maturation leads to an increase in cell number, with each primary spermatocyte producing four spermatozoa, two with an X chromosome and two with a Y chromosome.

When viewed in cross sections of seminiferous tubules (Fig. 54.1E), spermatogonia are located adjacent to the basement membrane, whereas the more differentiated spermatids are located nearest the lumen. Groups of spermatogonia at comparable stages of development undergo mitosis simultaneously. However, spermatogenesis is asynchronous along the seminiferous tubule; different areas along the tubule are at different stages of spermatogenesis. In a continuous process, a young man produces sperm at a rate of ~1000 per second.

The time needed to produce a mature spermatozoon from a diploid germ cell is ~64 days. Healthy 20-year-old men produce sperm at a rate of ~6.5 million sperm per gram of testicular tissue per day. The rate falls progressively with age and averages ~3.8 million sperm per gram per day in men 50 to 90 years old. Among fertile men, those aged 51 to 90 years exhibit a significant decrease in the percentage of morphologically normal and motile spermatozoa.

In summary, three processes occur concurrently in the seminiferous epithelium: (1) the production of cells by mitosis, (2) differentiation of spermatogonia to spermatids with a reduction in the number of chromosomes by meiosis, and (3) the conversion of spermatids to mature sperm by spermiogenesis. Thus, spermatogenesis is a regular, ordered, sequential process resulting in the production of mature male gametes.

The Sertoli cells support spermatogenesis

Sertoli cells are the support or "nurse" cells for the spermatids (Fig. 54.6). Sertoli cells (1) maintain an environment conducive for spermatogenesis; (2) in response to FSH, secrete substances that promote proliferation of spermatogonia and initiate meiosis; (3) secrete androgen-binding protein (SHBG), which concentrates testosterone in the proximity of developing gametes; (4) secrete inhibin, which controls pituitary gland production of FSH; (5) phagocytose excess cytoplasm produced by gametes during spermiogenesis; and (6) produce antimüllerian hormone (see ⊙ 53-4).

Tight junctions connect the adjacent Sertoli cells, forming a **blood-testis barrier**—analogous to the blood-brain barrier—that presumably provides a protective environment for developing germ cells. Release of the spermatozoa from the Sertoli cell is called **spermiation.** Spermatids progressively move toward the lumen of the tubule and eventually lose all contact with the Sertoli cell after spermiation.

additional rounds of mitosis before its progeny initiate meiosis and progress through spermatogenesis (Fig. 54.5). Type B spermatogonia that enter into the first meiotic division become **primary spermatocytes.** At prophase of meiosis I, the chromosomes undergo crossing over. At this stage, each cell has a duplicated set of 46 chromosomes (4N): 22 pairs of duplicated autosomal chromosomes, a duplicated X chromosome, and a duplicated Y chromosome. After this first meiotic division is completed, the daughter cells become **secondary spermatocytes,** which have a haploid number of duplicated chromosomes (2N): 22 duplicated autosomal chromosomes and either a duplicated X or a duplicated Y chromosome. Secondary spermatocytes enter the second meiotic division almost immediately. This division results in

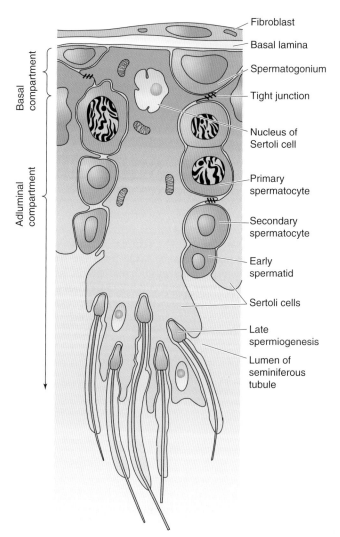

Figure 54.6 Interaction of Sertoli cells and sperm. This figure is an idealized high-magnification view of a portion of the wall of a seminiferous tubule (Fig. 54.1C).

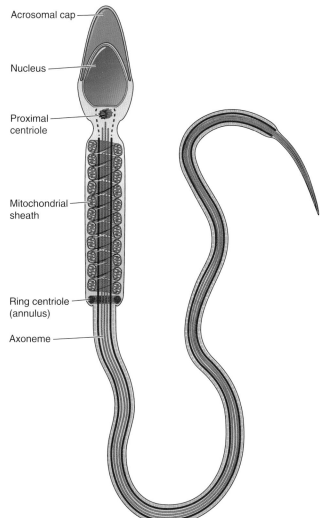

Figure 54.7 Anatomy of a spermatozoon.

Sperm maturation occurs in the epididymis

The seminiferous tubules open into a network of tubules, the **rete testis,** that serves as a reservoir for sperm. The rete testis is connected to the **epididymis,** a highly convoluted single long duct, 4 to 5 m in total length, on the posterior aspect of the testis.

Spermatozoa are essentially immotile on completion of spermiogenesis. Thus, transfer of spermatozoa from the seminiferous tubule to the rete testes and epididymis with assistance by ciliary action of the luminal epithelium. After leaving the testes, sperm take 12 to 26 days to travel through the epididymis and appear in the ejaculate.

Sperm are stored in the epididymis, where they undergo a process of maturation before they are capable of progressive motility and fertilization. Spermatozoa released at ejaculation are fully motile and capable of fertilization, whereas spermatozoa obtained directly from the testis are functionally immature insofar as they cannot penetrate an ovum.

The epididymis empties into the **vas deferens,** which contains well-developed muscle layers that facilitate sperm movement. The vas deferens passes through the inguinal canal, traverses the ureter, and continues medially to the posterior and inferior aspect of the urinary bladder, where it is joined by the duct arising from the **seminal vesicle;** together, they form the ejaculatory duct. The **ejaculatory duct** enters the prostatic portion of the urethra after passing through the prostate. Sperm are stored in the epididymis as well as in the proximal end of the vas deferens. All these accessory structures depend on androgens secreted by the testis for full functional development.

Spermatozoa are the only independently motile cells in the human body

Spermatozoa are highly specialized cells consisting of a head, midpiece, and tail (Fig. 54.7). The **head** contains the nucleus and is essentially devoid of cytoplasm, which is lost during spermatogenesis. Within the nucleus, the haploid number of chromosomes are packaged as tightly coiled chromatin fibers. The anterior segment of the head contains the **acrosome,** which is essentially a large secretory vesicle, containing enzymes that will facilitate penetration of the ovum. The **midpiece** is the engine of sperm. It consists of multiple mitochondria arranged as spirals around a filamentous core. The energy for sperm motility comes from the metabolism of fructose present in the seminal fluid. The filamentous core in the midpiece forms a drive-shaft connection to the tail. The **tail** is a specialized flagellum, powered by the midpiece, that executes rapid lashing movements, propelling the cell forward.

The accessory male sex glands—the seminal vesicles, prostate, and bulbourethral glands—produce the seminal plasma

Only 10% of the volume of **semen** (i.e., seminal fluid) is sperm cells. The normal concentration of sperm cells is >20 million per milliliter and the typical ejaculate volume is >2 mL. The typical ejaculate content varies between 150 and 600 million spermatozoa.

Aside from the sperm cells, the remainder of the semen (i.e., 90%) is **seminal plasma,** the extracellular fluid of semen

TABLE 54.1 Normal Parameter Values for Semen

PARAMETER	VALUE
Volume of ejaculate	2–6 mL
Viscosity	Liquefaction in 1 hr
pH	7–8
Count	≥20 million/mL
Motility	≥50%
Morphology	60% normal

(Table 54.1). The seminal plasma originates primarily from the accessory glands (the seminal vesicles, prostate gland, and bulbourethral glands). The seminal vesicles contribute ~70% of the volume of semen. Aside from the sperm, the remaining ~20% represents epididymal fluids, as well as secretions of the prostate gland and bulbourethral glands.

Human semen coagulates immediately after ejaculation. Coagulation is followed by liquefaction, which is apparently caused by proteolytic enzymes contained in prostatic secretions.

CHAPTER 55

THE FEMALE REPRODUCTIVE SYSTEM

Sam Mesiano

The female reproductive system functions to (1) produce haploid gametes—**ova**, (2) facilitate **syngamy**—or fertilization—between an ovum and a spermatozoon, (3) supply a site for **implantation** of the embryo (if syngamy occurs) and the establishment of pregnancy, (4) provide for the physical environment and nutritional needs of the developing fetus and its timely birth, and (5) nurture the neonate.

The system consists of the gonads (the ovaries), the fallopian tubes, the uterus and cervix, the vagina (Fig. 55.1A), the external genitalia, and the mammary glands, and is controlled by hormones produced in the hypothalamus, pituitary, and ovaries. The principal female sex hormones are estrogens (mainly estradiol) and progesterone, which are produced by the ovaries in a cyclic manner and regulate the growth and function of the female sex accessory structures and the development of secondary sexual characteristics. Function of the female reproductive system is ultimately regulated by hormones produced by the hypothalamic-pituitary-gonadal axis under the control of higher brain centers. The system involves finely tuned neuroendocrine feedback interactions between hormones produced by the hypothalamus and anterior pituitary and hormones produced by the ovaries. The result is the cyclic production of gametes and the preparation of the sex accessory organs for the establishment of pregnancy.

Female reproductive organs include the ovaries and accessory sex organs

The **ovaries** lie on the sides of the pelvic cavity (Fig. 55.1A). Each ovary consists of developing follicles (ovum surrounded by granulosa and theca cells) and corpora lutea (remnant of ruptured follicles after ovulation) in various stages of development (Fig. 55.1B).

The female **sex accessory organs** include the fallopian tubes, the uterus, the vagina, and the external genitalia. The **fallopian tubes** provide a pathway for the transport of ova from the ovary to the uterus. The fimbriae of the fallopian tubes are lined with epithelial cells, most of which have cilia that beat toward the uterus. The cilia facilitate transport of the ovum toward the uterus.

The **uterus** is a pear-shaped, muscular organ composed of a fundus, a corpus, and a narrow caudal portion called the **cervix.** The interior lining, or **endometrium,** of the uterus consists of complex glandular tissue and stroma. The bulk of the uterine wall consists of specialized smooth muscle, **myometrium.** The uterus is continuous with the vagina via the cervical canal. The cervix is composed of dense fibrous connective tissue and smooth-muscle cells.

The human **vagina** is ~10 cm in length and is a single, expandable tube. The **external genitalia** include the clitoris, the labia majora, and the labia minora, as well as the accessory secretory glands (including the glands of Bartholin), which open into the vestibule. The **clitoris** is an erectile organ that is homologous to the penis and mirrors the cavernous ends of the glans penis.

The **breasts** can also be considered as part of the female reproductive system. Breast development (thelarche) begins at puberty in response to ovarian steroid hormones (see ◉ 53-5). The ductal epithelium of the breast is sensitive to ovarian steroids and especially during pregnancy becomes activated to produce milk (**lactation**) that will sustain the newborn infant.

Reproductive function in the human female is cyclic

In humans, **ovulation** occurs in monthly cycles—known as **menstrual cycles**—that are associated with regular episodes of uterine bleeding termed menstruation. Such cyclic reproductive function in females enhances reproductive efficiency by coordinating gamete production with physiological changes that prepare the reproductive tract for sperm and ovum transport, fertilization, implantation, and pregnancy.

THE MENSTRUAL CYCLE

◉ 55-1 The human menstrual cycle coordinates changes in both the ovary and endometrium

The human menstrual cycle involves rhythmic changes in two organs: the ovary and the uterus (Fig. 55.2). Starting with the first day of the menses on day 0, the average menstrual cycle lasts 28 days.

The **ovarian cycle** (Fig. 55.2) includes four key events: (1) folliculogenesis, the growth and development/maturation of follicles; (2) ovulation, rupture of a follicle to release the ovum; (3) formation of the corpus luteum from the remains of the ruptured follicle; and (4) death (atresia) of the corpus luteum. Temporally, the ovarian cycle includes two major phases: the follicular and luteal phases. The **follicular phase** begins soon after the corpus luteum degenerates, lasts 12 to 14 days, and ends at ovulation. The **luteal phase** begins at ovulation, lasts 12 to 14 days, and ends when the corpus luteum degenerates.

A OBLIQUE VIEW OF THE INTERNAL FEMALE SEX ORGANS

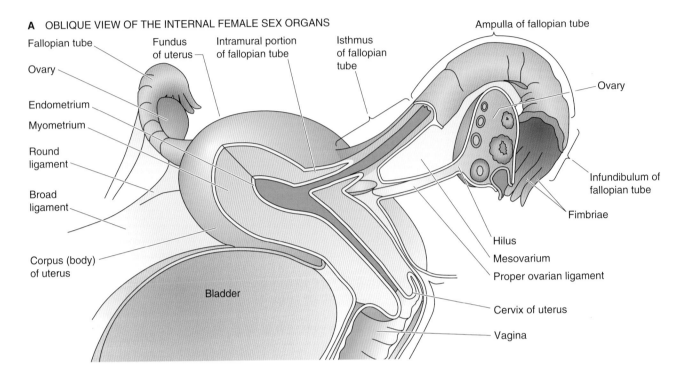

Fallopian tube

Ovary

Endometrium

Myometrium

Round
ligament

Broad
ligament

Corpus (body)
of uterus

Fundus
of uterus

Intramural portion
of fallopian tube

Isthmus
of fallopian
tube

Ampulla of fallopian tube

Ovary

Infundibulum of
fallopian tube

Fimbriae

Hilus

Mesovarium

Proper ovarian ligament

Cervix of uterus

Vagina

Bladder

B CROSS SECTION THROUGH AN OVARY

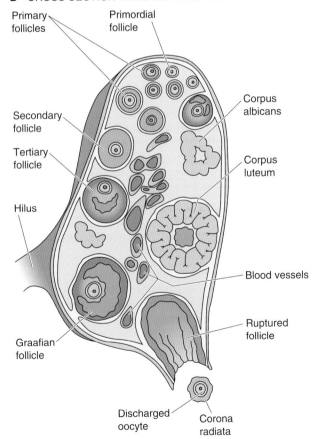

Primary
follicles

Primordial
follicle

Secondary
follicle

Tertiary
follicle

Hilus

Graafian
follicle

Corpus
albicans

Corpus
luteum

Blood vessels

Ruptured
follicle

Discharged
oocyte

Corona
radiata

Figure. 55.1 Anatomy of the female internal genitalia and accessory sex organs.

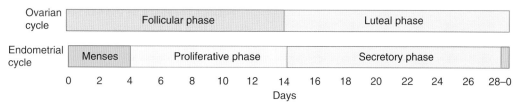

Figure 55.2 Ovarian and endometrial cycles. The menstrual cycle comprises parallel ovarian and endometrial cycles. The follicular phase of the ovarian cycle and the menses start on day 0. In this idealized example, ovulation occurs on day 14, and the entire cycle lasts 28 days.

The **endometrial cycle** (Fig. 55.2) is under the control of steroid hormones, estradiol and progesterone, produced by the ovaries during the follicular and luteal phases and consists of three key events: (1) menstruation (menses), the shedding of the outer layer of the endometrium; (2) endometrial growth and proliferation; and (3) differentiation of the endometrial epithelium into a glandular secretory phenotype. The endometrial cycle is divided into menses, the **proliferative phase** and the **secretory phase.**

Ovarian and endometrial events in the menstrual cycle are integrated into a single sequence as follows.

Follicular/Proliferative Phase The follicular/proliferative phase begins with the initiation of menstruation and averages ~14 days. During this time, **follicle-stimulating hormone (FSH)** and **luteinizing hormone (LH)** stimulate the growth of a cohort of follicles, all of which produce **estradiol.** Consequently, circulating estradiol levels gradually increase during the follicular phase. Because estradiol stimulates rapid growth of the endometrium, this period is the proliferative phase of the *endometrial cycle.* Eventually, a single large, dominant preovulatory follicle develops in one of the ovaries. This follicle becomes the principal source of estradiol as the follicular phase progresses.

Ovulation For most of the follicular phase, estradiol exerts negative feedback on FSH and LH secretion at the level of the hypothalamus and pituitary. However, toward the end of the follicular phase (day 12 to 13), when estradiol levels are maximal, the effect of estradiol on the hypothalamus and pituitary switches from negative to positive feedback. The result is a large transient surge in LH and a small increase in FSH secretion by the gonadotrophs. The LH surge causes the dominant follicle to rupture and releases its oocyte—ovulation. After ovulation the production of estradiol by remaining granulosa cells decreases to a level at which it resumes exerting negative feedback on FSH and LH secretion.

Luteal/Secretory Phase After release of the ovum, the remnants of the dominant follicle transform into a **corpus luteum,** which is why the second half of the *ovarian cycle* is called the luteal phase. Luteal cells produce **progesterone** and small amounts of estradiol in response to LH. Together these steroid hormones stimulate the endometrium to develop secretory glands—hence the term secretory phase of the *endometrial cycle.* The combined effects of progesterone and estradiol produce an endometrial lining that is conducive to embryo implantation and the establishment of pregnancy. If embryo implantation does not occur by day 20 to 22 of the cycle (i.e., midway through the luteal phase), the corpus luteum begins to degenerate and its production of progesterone and estradiol rapidly declines. If pregnancy is established, **human chorionic gonadotropin (hCG)** produced by the placenta maintains the corpus luteum. As a result, the corpus luteum maintains support for the endometrium, and menstruation does not occur.

Menses In the absence of pregnancy, withdrawal of progesterone (and estrogen) due to the demise of the corpus luteum leads to degeneration and shedding of the superficial part of the endometrium known as the **functional layer.** Degeneration of the functional layer is due to necrosis caused by the constriction of blood vessels that supply the endometrium. The necrotic tissue then sloughs away from the uterus and, in conjunction with blood from the underlying vessels and other uterine fluids, is shed as menstrual discharge (i.e., the period). Menstruation usually lasts 4 to 6 days. The decrease in progesterone and estradiol also removes negative feedback of these hormones on the hypothalamus and pituitary, leading to a corresponding increase in FSH (and to a lesser extent LH) secretion. The increase in FSH stimulates recruitment and growth of another cohort of follicles for the next cycle. The first day of the menses (i.e., the first day of the endometrial cycle) is also the first day of the ovarian cycle. Rebuilding of the functional layer resumes when estrogen levels rise as a result of follicle growth during the new follicular phase.

The hypothalamic-pituitary-ovarian axis drives the menstrual cycle

⊙ **55-2** Neurons in the hypothalamus synthesize, store, and release **gonadotropin-releasing hormone (GnRH).** Long portal vessels carry the GnRH to the anterior pituitary, where the hormone binds to receptors on the surface of gonadotrophs. The results are the synthesis and release of both FSH and LH from the gonadotrophs (Fig. 55.3). These trophic hormones, LH and FSH, stimulate the ovary to synthesize and secrete the sex steroids **estrogens** and **progestins** as well as to produce mature gametes. The ovaries also produce peptides called **inhibins** and **activins.** Together, these ovarian steroids and peptides exert both negative and positive feedback on both the hypothalamus and the anterior pituitary. This complex interaction generates a monthly pattern of hormone fluctuations that control endometrial maturation and shedding.

⊙ 55-3 GnRH stimulates gonadotrophs in the anterior pituitary to secrete FSH and LH

GnRH enters the anterior pituitary through the portal system and binds to the **GnRH receptor (GnRHR)** on the surface of the gonadotroph, thus initiating a series of cellular events that result in the synthesis and secretion of gonadotropins (Fig. 55.4). The net effect is an increase in synthesis of the gonadotropins FSH and LH.

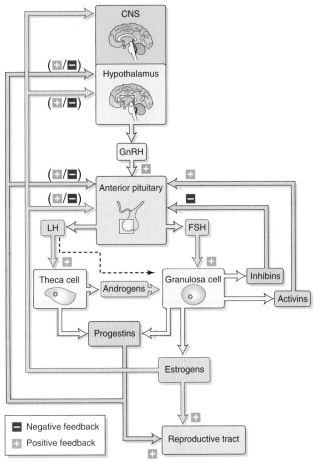

Figure 55.3 Hypothalamic-pituitary-ovarian axis. The androgens enter granulosa cells, which convert androgens to estrogens. The *dashed arrow* indicates that the granulosa cells also have LH receptors. FSH binds to receptors on granulosa cells to increase the production of estrogen as well as activins and inhibins. *CNS,* Central nervous system.

Before ovulation, the LH and FSH act on cells of the developing follicles. The **theca cells** of the follicle have LH receptors (LHCGR), whereas the **granulosa cells** (see ◉ 55-4) have both LH and FSH (FSHR) receptors. After ovulation, LH acts on the cells of the corpus luteum. Both the LH and the FSH receptors are coupled through $G\alpha_s$ to adenylyl cyclase (see ◉ 3-4), which catalyzes the conversion of ATP to cAMP. cAMP stimulates protein kinase A, which increases the expression of genes whose products enhance cell division or the production of peptide and steroid hormones.

The ovarian steroids (estrogens and progestins) feed back on the hypothalamic-pituitary axis

As summarized in Fig. 55.3, the ovarian steroids—primarily estradiol and progesterone—exert both negative and positive feedback on the hypothalamic-pituitary axis.

Negative Feedback by Ovarian Steroids Throughout most of the menstrual cycle, the estradiol and progesterone that are produced by the ovary feed back negatively on both the hypothalamus and the gonadotrophs of the anterior pituitary. The net effect is reduced release of both LH and FSH. Estradiol exerts negative feedback at both low and high concentrations, whereas progesterone is effective only at high concentrations.

Positive Feedback by Ovarian Steroids Although ovarian steroids feed back *negatively* on the hypothalamic-pituitary axis during most of the menstrual cycle, they have the opposite effect at the end of the follicular phase. Levels of estradiol rise gradually during the first half of the follicular phase of the ovarian cycle and then increase steeply during the second half (Fig. 55.5). After the estradiol levels reach a certain threshold for a minimum of 2 days, estradiol now exerts *positive* feedback on the axis. Once high levels of estradiol have properly conditioned the gonadotrophs, rising levels of **progesterone** during the late follicular phase also produce a positive-feedback response and thus facilitate the LH surge.

Ovaries produce peptide hormones—inhibins, activins, and follistatins—that modulate FSH secretion

Inhibins, activins, and follistatins are gonadal peptide hormones that selectively affect the production and secretion of FSH but do not affect LH (Fig. 55.3). **Inhibins** *inhibit* FSH production by gonadotrophs, **activins** *activate* FSH production, and follistatins inhibit FSH production by binding to and thereby inhibiting activins.

Modulation of gonadotropin secretion by positive and negative ovarian feedback produces the normal menstrual rhythm

Fig. 55.5 illustrates the cyclic hormonal changes during the menstrual cycle. The time-averaged records of LH and FSH levels mask their hour-by-hour pulsatility. The **follicular phase** is characterized by a relatively high frequency of GnRH—and thus LH—pulses. Early in the follicular phase, when levels of estradiol are low but rising, the frequency of LH pulses remains unchanged, but their amplitude gradually *increases* with time. Later in the follicular phase, the higher estradiol levels are beginning to feed back positively on the hypothalamic-pituitary axis. The net effect is an increase in the time-averaged circulating levels of LH and FSH.

The **LH surge** is an abrupt and dramatic rise in the LH level that occurs around the 13th to 14th day of the follicular phase in the average woman. The LH surge peaks ~12 hours after its initiation and lasts for ~48 hours. The LH surge is superimposed on the smaller FSH surge. The primary trigger of the gonadotropin surge is a rise in **estradiol** to very high threshold levels just before the LH surge. In addition, gradually increasing levels of LH trigger the preovulatory follicle to increase its secretion of progesterone. These increasing—but still "low"—levels of **progesterone** also have a positive-feedback effect on the hypothalamic-pituitary axis that is synergistic with the positive-feedback effect of the estrogens.

The gonadotropin surge causes ovulation and luteinization. The ovarian follicle ruptures, and expels the oocyte and with it the surrounding cumulus and corona cells. This process is known as **ovulation.** A physiological change—**luteinization**—in the granulosa cells of the follicle causes these cells to secrete progesterone rather than estradiol. The granulosa and theca cells undergo structural changes that transform them into luteal cells—*luteinization*.

As the **luteal phase** of the menstrual cycle begins, circulating levels of LH and FSH rapidly decrease. This fall-off in

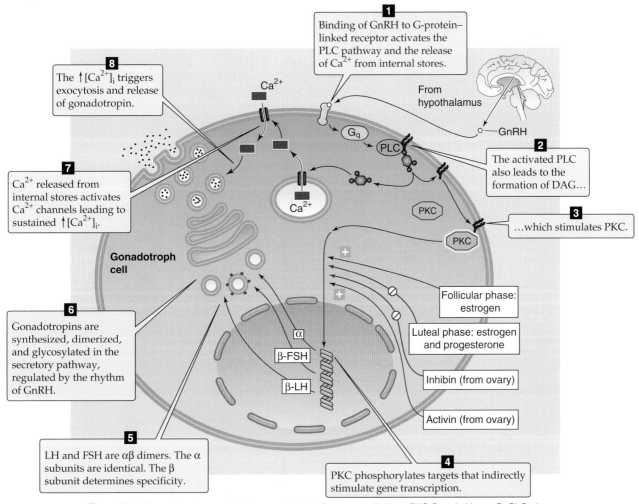

Figure 55.4 Gonadotropin secretion by gonadotrophs in anterior pituitary. *PKC,* Protein kinase C; *PLC,* phospholipase C.

gonadotropin levels reflects *negative* feedback by three ovarian hormones—estradiol, progesterone, and inhibin.

By ~48 hours before onset of the menses, circulating levels of LH slowly fall during the luteal phase. The gradual demise of the corpus luteum leads to decreases in the levels of progesterone, estradiol, and inhibin.

OVARIAN STEROIDS

Starting from cholesterol, the ovary synthesizes estradiol, the major estrogen, and progesterone, the major progestin

The precursor for the biosynthesis of the ovarian steroids is cholesterol. As shown in Fig. 55.6, the side-chain-cleavage enzyme catalyzes the conversion of cholesterol to **pregnenolone.** This reaction is the rate-limiting step in estrogen production. The initial steps of estrogen biosynthesis from pregnenolone follow the same steps as synthesis of the two so-called adrenal androgens **dehydroepiandrosterone (DHEA)** and **androstenedione.** Cells in the ovaries have an **aromatase** that can convert androstenedione to estrone, and testosterone to estradiol. The **estrone** can go on to form the more powerful estrogen **estradiol,** and vice versa. Finally, the liver

can convert both estradiol and estrone into the weak estrogen **estriol.**

The two major **progestins, progesterone** and **17α-hydroxyprogesterone,** form early in the biosynthetic pathway (Fig. 55.6).

Estrogen biosynthesis requires two ovarian cells and two gonadotropins, whereas progestin synthesis requires only a single cell

Because of their unique physiological properties, neither the theca/theca-lutein cells nor the granulosa/granulosa-lutein cells can make estrogens by themselves. Rather, they make estrogens in a cooperative fashion, according to the **two-cell, two-gonadotropin hypothesis** (Fig. 55.7).

⊙ 55-4 The superficial **theca cells** and theca-lutein cells can take up cholesterol and produce DHEA and androstenedione, but they do not have the aromatase necessary for estrogen production. The deeper **granulosa cells** and granulosa-lutein cells have the aromatase, but they lack the enzymes necessary for making DHEA and androstenedione. Another difference between the two cell types is that theca cells have LH receptors, whereas granulosa cells have both LH and FSH receptors.

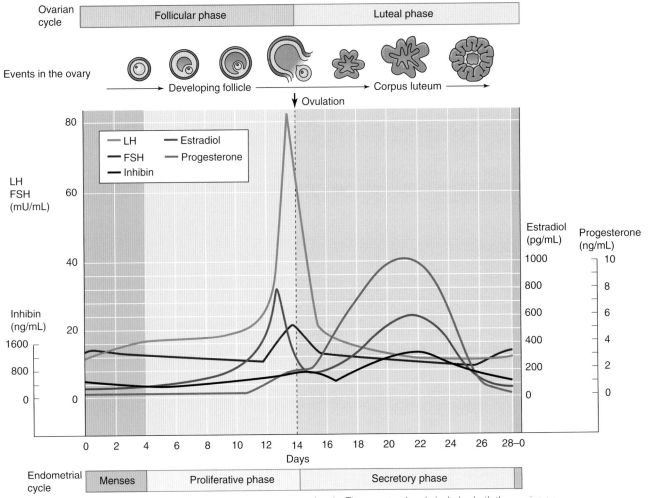

Figure 55.5   Hormonal changes during the menstrual cycle. The menstrual cycle includes both the ovarian cycle—which includes the follicular phase, ovulation, and the luteal phase—and the endometrial cycle—which includes the menstrual, the proliferative, and the secretory phases.

Estrogens stimulate cellular proliferation and growth of sex organs and other tissues related to reproduction

Most estrogens in blood plasma are bound to carrier proteins, including **albumin** and **sex hormone–binding globulin** (**SHBG;** see ⊙ 54-2). The nuclear **estrogen receptors ERα** and **ERβ** function as dimers (see Table 3.3). When bound to estrogen, the ER dimer interacts with steroid response elements on chromatin and induces the transcription of specific genes. Estrogens almost exclusively affect particular target sex organs—including uterus and breasts—that have ERs.

Progesterone, which binds to the dimeric **progesterone receptor (PR),** induces secretory changes in the endometrium, and induces final maturation of the uterine endometrium for reception and implantation of the fertilized ovum.

THE OVARIAN CYCLE: FOLLICULOGENESIS, OVULATION, AND FORMATION OF THE CORPUS LUTEUM

Female reproductive life span is determined by the number of primordial follicles established during fetal life

Unlike the male—which produces large numbers of mature gametes (sperm) continuously beginning at puberty and

for the remainder of the man's life—the female has a limited total number of gametes, determined by the number of oocytes formed during fetal life (see ⊙ 53-3). Oocyte maturation—the production of a haploid female gamete capable of fertilization by a sperm—begins in the fetal ovary. Beginning at around the fourth week of gestation, **primordial germ cells** migrate from the endoderm of the yolk sac to the gonadal ridge, where they develop into **oogonia**—immature germ cells that proliferate by mitosis.

Primary Oocytes ⊙ 55-5 By ~8 weeks' gestation, ~300,000 oogonia are present in each ovary. At around this time, some oogonia enter prophase of meiosis I and become primary oocytes (Fig. 55.8A). By 20 weeks, all the mitotic divisions of the female germ cells have been completed, and the total number of germ cells peaks at 6 to 7 million. All oogonia that have not entered prophase of meiosis I by the 28th to 30th week of gestation die by apoptosis. The oocytes then arrest in the diplotene stage of prophase I. This prolonged state of meiotic arrest lasts until just before ovulation many years later, when the meiosis resumes and the first polar body is extruded.

Primordial Follicles ⊙ 55-6 In the fetal ovary, dictyotene oocytes are surrounded by a single layer of flat, spindle-shaped pregranulosa cells to form a primordial

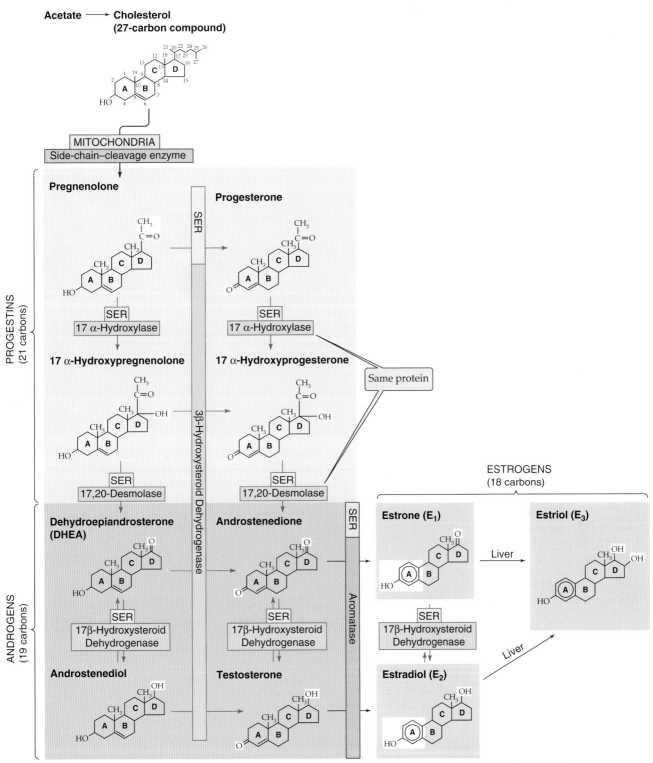

Figure 55.6 Biosynthesis of the ovarian steroids. Certain of these pathways are shared in the biosynthesis of the glucocorticoids and mineralocorticoids (see Fig. 50.2), as well as androgens (see Fig. 54.4).

follicle (Fig. 55.8B). By the 30th week of gestation, the ovaries contain around 5 to 6 million primordial follicles. For the remainder of the female's life, the number of primordial follicles gradually decreases. One reason for the decline is that primordial follicles undergo a relentless process of apoptosis that begins at midgestation and ends at menopause when the endowment of primordial follicles is virtually exhausted. In addition, after puberty, each month a cohort of 10 to 30 primordial follicles is recruited to enter the irreversible process of folliculogenesis, which culminates in either ovulation (rupture of the follicle and expulsion of the ova) or atresia (a

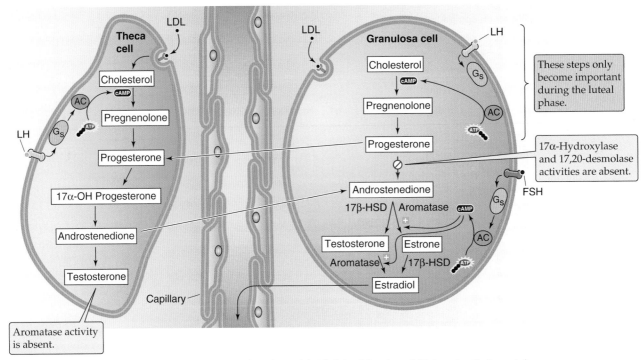

Figure 55.7   Two-cell, two-gonadotropin model. *AC,* Adenylyl cyclase; *LDL,* low-density lipoprotein.

coordinated process in which the oocyte and other follicle cells undergo apoptosis, degeneration, and resorption). Thus, even though the ovaries are invested with ~7 million oogonia at midgestation, the pool of primordial follicles is continually depleted, so that ~1 million exist at birth, ~300,000 remain at puberty, and there are virtually none at menopause. Of the ~300,000 primordial follicles present at puberty, only 400 to 500 are destined for ovulation between puberty and menopause (e.g., 12 per year for 40 years).

The female gametes are stored in the **ovarian follicles**—the primary functional units of the ovary. At any given time, a small proportion of primordial follicles begin a series of changes in size, morphology, and function referred to as **folliculogenesis**—the central event in the human female reproductive system. Folliculogenesis—controlled mainly by the gonadotropins (FSH and LH)—occurs by three processes: (1) enlargement and maturation of the oocyte, (2) differentiation and proliferation of granulosa and theca cells, and (3) formation and accumulation of a fluid.

Primary Follicles   The first step in folliculogenesis is the emergence of a primordial follicle from its quiescent state to become a primary follicle (Fig. 55.8C). In this process the oocyte increases in size and forms the **zona pellucida**—a glycoprotein shell surrounding the plasma membrane of the oocyte—and granulosa cells proliferate.

Secondary Follicles   The further proliferation of granulosa cells and the appearance of the surrounding theca cell layer converts the primary follicle into a secondary follicle (Fig. 55.8D). Secondary follicles contain a primary oocyte surrounded by *several* layers of cuboidal **granulosa cells.** In addition, cells in the ovarian stroma surrounding the follicle

are induced to differentiate into **theca cells.** Progression to secondary follicles also involves the formation of a blood supply from arterioles that terminate in a wreath-like network of capillaries adjacent to the basement membrane surrounding the granulosa cell layer, which remains avascular. The theca cells proliferate and acquire LH receptors, as well as the ability, in response to LH, to synthesize androgens, granulosa cells use to produce estrogen. Gap junctions also form between the oocyte and the adjacent layer of granulosa cells and between granulosa cells. The granulosa cells in this context are analogous to the Sertoli cells in that they nurse the gamete and act as the barrier between the oocyte and the blood supply.

Tertiary Follicles   The next stage of follicular growth is the maturation of secondary follicles into **tertiary follicles** (Fig. 55.8E) as the increasingly abundant granulosa cells secrete fluid into the center of the follicle to form a fluid-filled space called the **antrum.** Follicle development up to this stage is independent of LH and FSH. FSH induces the transition of *preantral* secondary follicles to *antral* tertiary follicles.

Graafian Follicles   As the antrum enlarges, it nearly encircles the oocyte, except for a small mound of granulosa cells that attaches the oocyte to the rest of the follicle. At this stage, the diameter of the follicle increases to 20 to 33 mm and it is called a **preovulatory** or **graafian follicle** (Fig. 55.8F).

The oocyte grows and matures during folliculogenesis

The principal role of folliculogenesis is to produce a mature oocyte that is capable of fertilization and formation of an embryo. The oocyte contributes the majority of the cytoplasmic and nuclear factors needed for embryo development. These factors are not completely established until after the

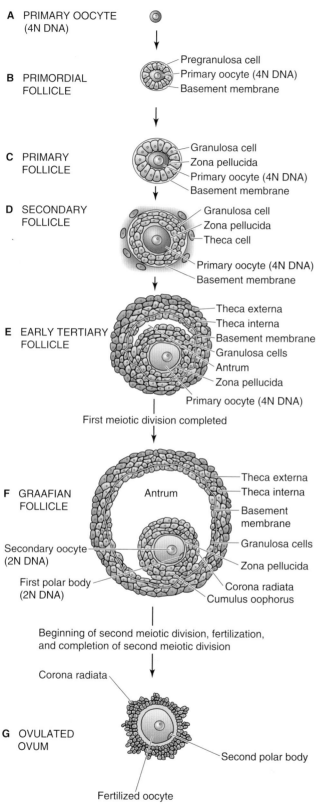

A PRIMARY OOCYTE
(4N DNA)

B PRIMORDIAL
FOLLICLE
- Pregranulosa cell
- Primary oocyte (4N DNA)
- Basement membrane

C PRIMARY
FOLLICLE
- Granulosa cell
- Zona pellucida
- Primary oocyte (4N DNA)
- Basement membrane

D SECONDARY
FOLLICLE
- Granulosa cell
- Zona pellucida
- Theca cell
- Primary oocyte (4N DNA)
- Basement membrane

E EARLY TERTIARY
FOLLICLE
- Theca externa
- Theca interna
- Basement membrane
- Granulosa cells
- Antrum
- Zona pellucida
- Primary oocyte (4N DNA)

First meiotic division completed

F GRAAFIAN
FOLLICLE
Antrum
- Theca externa
- Theca interna
- Basement membrane
- Granulosa cells
- Zona pellucida
- Corona radiata
- Cumulus oophorus

Secondary oocyte (2N DNA)
First polar body (2N DNA)

Beginning of second meiotic division, fertilization, and completion of second meiotic division

Corona radiata

G OVULATED
OVUM
- Second polar body

Fertilized oocyte

Figure 55.8 Maturation of the ovarian follicle.

secondary follicle stage (Fig. 55.8D). Oocyte growth and maturation includes formation of the zona pellucida, formation of increased numbers of mitochondria, acquisition of competence to complete meiosis I.

FSH and LH stimulate the growth of a cohort of follicles

The development of primordial follicles to secondary follicles occurs continually from fetal life until menopause. However, almost all of these follicles undergo **atresia** (death of the ovum, followed by collapse of the follicle and scarring) at some stage in their development.

At the time of puberty, increased levels of FSH and LH stimulate cohorts of secondary follicles to progress to the tertiary and preovulatory stages. Along the course of this development, most follicles undergo atresia until one **dominant graafian follicle** remains at the time of ovulation. The entire developmental process occurs over three to four monthly cycles, so that the graafian follicle of the present ovulatory cycle was part of a cohort of secondary follicles recruited three to four cycles earlier. The other follicles undergo atresia.

Estradiol secretion by the dominant follicle triggers the LH surge and thus ovulation

Estradiol secretion by the dominant follicle increases rapidly near the end of the late follicular phase (Fig. 55.5). This dramatic rise in circulating estradiol switches the *negative*-feedback response of estradiol on the hypothalamus and anterior pituitary to a *positive*-feedback response and also sensitizes the anterior pituitary to GnRH. The result is the LH surge, which generally begins 24 to 36 hours after peak estradiol secretion. Ovulation usually occurs ~36 hours after onset of the LH surge, and ~12 hours after its peak. The LH surge terminates in part as a result of negative feedback caused by rising levels of progesterone produced by the luteal cell that form from the remnants of the ruptured dominant follicle, and in part as a result of loss of the positive feedback derived from estradiol.

At the time of the LH surge, the primary oocyte (4N DNA), which had been arrested in the prophase of its first meiotic division since fetal life (see Fig. 53.2C), now resumes meiosis and completes its first meiotic division several hours before ovulation. The result of this first meiotic division is a small **first polar body,** which degenerates or divides to form nonfunctional cells, and a much larger **secondary oocyte.** Both the first polar body and the secondary oocyte, like secondary spermatocytes (see Fig. 54.5), have a haploid number of duplicated chromosomes (2N DNA): 22 duplicated somatic chromosomes and 1 duplicated X chromosome. This secondary oocyte begins its second meiotic division, but it becomes arrested in metaphase until the time of fertilization. The secondary oocyte is surrounded by the zona pellucida and one or more layers of follicular granulosa cells, the **corona radiata.**

Release of the oocyte from the follicle—**ovulation**—follows thinning and weakening of the follicular wall, probably under the influence of LH, progesterone, and prostaglandins.

The expelled oocyte, with its investment of follicular cells, is guided toward the fallopian tube by the fimbriae that cover the surface of the nearby ovary (Fig. 55.1). The oocyte is then transported through the infundibulum into the ampulla by ciliary movement of the tubal epithelium, as well as by muscular contractions of the tube. Fertilization, if it occurs, takes place in the ampullary portion of the fallopian tube. The resulting zygote resides in

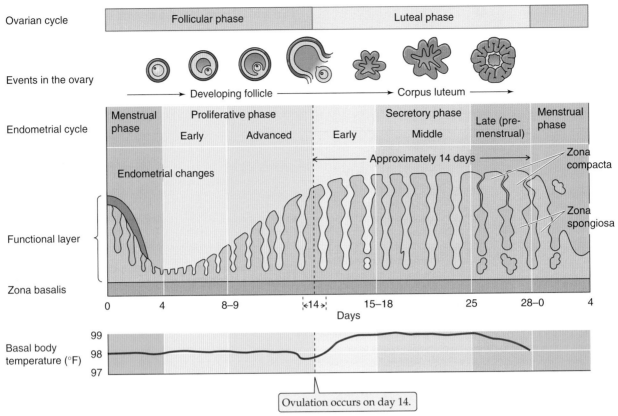

Figure 55.9 Endometrial cycle, which occurs in parallel with the ovarian cycle.

the ampulla for ~72 hours, followed by rapid transport through the isthmus to the uterine cavity, where it floats free for an additional 2 to 3 days before attaching to the endometrium.

After ovulation, theca and granulosa cells of the follicle differentiate into theca-lutein and granulosa-lutein cells of the corpus luteum

After expulsion of the oocyte, the remaining follicular granulosa and theca cells coalesce into folds that occupy the follicular cavity and, under the influence of LH, undergo a phenotypic transformation to form the **corpus luteum**—a temporary endocrine organ whose major product is progesterone. The corpus luteum is highly vascularized, consistent with its primary function as an endocrine organ. During the early luteal phase, progesterone and estradiol produced by the corpus luteum exert negative feedback on the hypothalamic-pituitary axis to suppress gonadotropin secretion and thus inhibit folliculogenesis. If pregnancy is not established, the corpus luteum regresses ~11 days after ovulation.

Growth and involution of the corpus luteum produce the rise and fall in estradiol and progesterone during the luteal phase

Although the corpus luteum produces both estradiol and progesterone, the luteal phase is dominated by progesterone secretion.

Unless rescued by hCG—produced by the syncytial trophoblasts of the embryo (see Fig. 56.4D)—luteal production of progesterone ceases toward the end of the menstrual cycle. If not rescued by pregnancy, the hormone-producing cells of the corpus luteum degenerate, leading to a rapid fall in progesterone levels, which removes negative feedback of gonadotropin secretion, leading to an increase in FSH and resumption of follicle recruitment to initiate the next ovarian cycle.

THE ENDOMETRIAL CYCLE

The ovarian hormones drive the morphological and functional changes of the endometrium during the monthly cycle

The ovarian steroids—primarily estradiol and progesterone—control the cyclic monthly growth and breakdown of the endometrium. The endometrial cycle has three major phases: the menstrual, proliferative, and secretory phases.

The Menstrual Phase If the oocyte was not fertilized and pregnancy did not occur in the previous cycle, a sudden diminution in estradiol and progesterone secretion occurs due to the demise of the corpus luteum. As hormonal support of the endometrium is withdrawn, the vascular and glandular integrity of the endometrium degenerates, the tissue breaks down, and menstrual bleeding ensues; this moment is defined as the start of day 1 of the menstrual cycle (Fig. 55.9). After menstruation, all that remains on the inner surface of most of the uterus is a thin layer of *nonepithelial* stromal cells and some remnant glands.

The Proliferative Phase After menstruation, the endometrium is restored by about the fifth day of the cycle (Fig. 55.9) as a result of proliferation of the basal stromal cells on the denuded surface of the uterus and proliferation of epithelial cells from other parts of the uterus. Cellular hyperplasia and increased extracellular matrix result in thickening of the endometrium during the late proliferative phase. Proliferation and differentiation of the endometrium are stimulated by estrogen that is secreted by the developing follicles.

The Secretory Phase ◉ **55-7** During the early luteal phase of the ovarian cycle, progesterone inhibits the proliferative phase of the endometrial cycle. Instead, progesterone stimulates the glandular components of the endometrium and thus induces secretory changes in the endometrium. The epithelial cells exhibit a marked increase in secretory activity in anticipation of the arrival and implantation of the embryo (blastocyst).

Under the influence of progesterone, spindle-shaped stromal cells of the endometrium become rounded **decidual cells.** Multiple foci of decidual cells spread throughout the upper layer of the endometrium and form a dense layer called the **zona compacta** (Fig. 55.9). Edema of the midzone of the endometrium distinguishes the compact area from the underlying **zona spongiosa,** where the endometrial glands become more prominent.

During the late luteal phase of the menstrual cycle, just before the next menstruation, levels of both estrogens and progestins diminish, and these decreased ovarian steroid levels lead to eventual demise of the upper two thirds of the endometrium leading to menstruation.

The period of endometrial receptivity for implantation of the embryo is estimated to extend from as early as day 16 to as late as day 19 of the menstrual cycle.

◉ 55-8 MENOPAUSE

Menopause signals the termination of reproductive function in women. Cyclic reproductive function ceases, menstruation comes to an end, and childbearing is generally no longer possible. Also occurring are significant physiological changes (Table 55.1) that have a major impact on health.

Only a few functioning follicles remain in the ovaries of a menopausal woman

Progressive loss of ovarian follicular units occurs throughout life (see ◉ **55-6**). In the United States, menarche

TABLE 55.1 **Menopausal Syndrome and Physical Changes in Menopause**

MENOPAUSAL SYNDROME	PHYSICAL CHANGES IN MENOPAUSE
Vasomotor instability	Atrophy of the vaginal
Hot flashes	epithelium
Night sweats	Changes in vaginal pH
Mood changes	Decrease in vaginal secretions
Short-term memory loss	Decrease in circulation to
Sleep disturbances	vagina and uterus
Headaches	Pelvic relaxation
Loss of libido	Loss of vaginal tone
	Cardiovascular disease
	Osteoporosis
	Alzheimer disease

generally occurs at an age of ~12.5 years (see ◉ **53-5**) and menopause at 51.5 years. At menopause and during the ensuing 5 years, the ovary contains only an occasional secondary follicle and a few primary follicles. The massive loss of oocytes over the reproductive life of a woman—from 300,000 at puberty (see ◉ **55-6**) to virtually none at menopause—is the result of the process of atresia during reproductive life.

During menopause, levels of the ovarian steroids fall, whereas gonadotropin levels rise

Because of a gradual decline in the number of follicles, the decreased ovarian production of estradiol reduces the negative feedback to the anterior pituitary and leads to increased levels of FSH. Increased levels of FSH are seen as early as 35 years of age, even though cyclic reproductive function continues.

Because the output of estrogens, progestins, and inhibins from the ovaries falls to very low levels during menopause, negative feedback on the hypothalamic-pituitary-ovarian axis (Fig. 55.3) becomes minimal. As a result, levels of FSH and LH may be higher than the corresponding levels during the midcycle surge in premenopausal women.

During menopause, estradiol and progesterone levels are low and some of the menopausal symptoms may be due to deficiency of ovarian steroid hormones. Hormone replacement therapy is a common approach to alleviate adverse effects of menopause.

CHAPTER 56

FERTILIZATION, PREGNANCY, AND LACTATION

Sam Mesiano

TRANSPORT OF GAMETES AND FERTILIZATION

Cilia and smooth muscle transport the egg and sperm within the female genital tract

Following ovulation, the fimbriae of the fallopian tube sweep over the ovarian surface and pick up the oocyte—surrounded by its complement of cumulus granulosa cells—and deposit it in the fallopian tube. Shortly after ovulation, movements of the cilia and the smooth muscle of fallopian tube propel the oocyte-cumulus complex toward the uterus.

Normally 150 to 600 million sperm cells are deposited into the vagina at the time of ejaculation. Within ~5 minutes, 50 to 100 sperm reach the ampullary portion of the fallopian tube, where fertilization normally occurs.

"Capacitation" of the spermatozoa occurs in the female genital tract

Neither freshly ejaculated sperm nor sperm removed from the epididymis are capable of fertilizing the egg until they have undergone further maturation—capacitation—in the female reproductive tract or in the laboratory. **Capacitation** is a process by which spermatozoa acquire the ability to penetrate the zona pellucida of the ovum. The removal or modification of a protective protein coat from the sperm cell membrane appears to be an important molecular event in the process of capacitation.

Fertilization begins as the sperm cell attaches to the zona pellucida and undergoes the acrosomal reaction, and it ends with the fusion of the male and female pronuclei

After ovulation, the egg in the fallopian tube is in a semidormant state. If it remains unfertilized, the ripe egg will remain quiescent for some time and eventually degenerate. Fertilization causes the egg to awaken (**activation**) and initiates a series of morphological and biochemical events that lead to cell division and differentiation. **Fertilization** occurs in eight steps, numbered in Fig. 56.1.

The fusion of the male and female pronuclei (*step 8* in Fig. 56.1) forms a new cell, the **zygote.** The mingling of chromosomes (syngamy) can be considered as the end of fertilization and the beginning of embryonic development. Thus, fertilization results in a conceptus that bears 46 chromosomes, 23 from the maternal gamete and 23 from the paternal gamete. Fertilization of the ovum by a sperm bearing an X chromosome produces a zygote with XX sex chromosomes; this develops into a female (see ⊙ 53-1). Fertilization with a Y-bearing sperm produces an XY zygote, which develops into a male. Therefore, chromosomal sex is established at fertilization.

IMPLANTATION OF THE DEVELOPING EMBRYO

After fertilization the embryo remains in the fallopian tube for ~72 hours, during which time it develops to the **morula** stage (i.e., a mulberry-shaped solid mass of 12 or more cells).

After the morula moves through the isthmus to the uterine cavity, it floats freely in the lumen of the uterus and transforms into a **blastocyst**—a ball-like structure with a fluid-filled inner cavity (Fig. 56.2). Surrounding the blastocyst is a thin layer of cells—the **trophoectoderm**—that develops into a variety of supporting structures, including the amnion, the yolk sac, and the fetal portion of the placenta. On one side of the blastocyst is an **inner cell mass,** which develops into the embryo proper. The conceptus floats freely in the uterine cavity for ~72 hours before it attaches to the endometrium. Numerous maturational events occur in the conceptus as it travels to the uterus. The embryo must be prepared to draw nutrients from the endometrium on arrival in the uterine cavity, and the endometrium must be prepared to sustain the implantation of the blastocyst. Because of the specific window in time during which implantation can occur, temporal relationships between embryonic and endometrial maturation assume extreme importance.

The presence of an embryo leads to decidualization of the endometrium

During the middle to late secretory phase of the normal endometrial cycle, the endometrium becomes more vascularized and thicker, and the endometrial glands become tortuous and engorged with secretions (see ⊙ 55-7). Beginning 9 to 10 days after ovulation, a process known as **predecidualization** begins near the spiral arteries. If conception fails to occur, the secretory activity of the endometrial glands decreases, followed by regression of the glands 8 to 9 days after ovulation, which is ultimately followed by menstruation.

When pregnancy occurs, the predecidual changes in the endometrium are sustained and extended, which

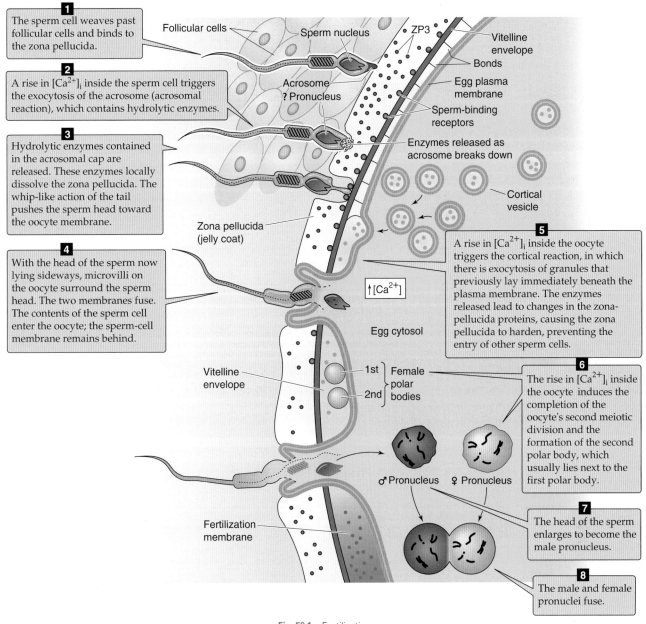

1 The sperm cell weaves past follicular cells and binds to the zona pellucida.

2 A rise in $[Ca^{2+}]_i$ inside the sperm cell triggers the exocytosis of the acrosome (acrosomal reaction), which contains hydrolytic enzymes.

3 Hydrolytic enzymes contained in the acrosomal cap are released. These enzymes locally dissolve the zona pellucida. The whip-like action of the tail pushes the sperm head toward the oocyte membrane.

4 With the head of the sperm now lying sideways, microvilli on the oocyte surround the sperm head. The two membranes fuse. The contents of the sperm cell enter the oocyte; the sperm-cell membrane remains behind.

5 A rise in $[Ca^{2+}]_i$ inside the oocyte triggers the cortical reaction, in which there is exocytosis of granules that previously lay immediately beneath the plasma membrane. The enzymes released lead to changes in the zona-pellucida proteins, causing the zona pellucida to harden, preventing the entry of other sperm cells.

6 The rise in $[Ca^{2+}]_i$ inside the oocyte induces the completion of the oocyte's second meiotic division and the formation of the second polar body, which usually lies next to the first polar body.

7 The head of the sperm enlarges to become the male pronucleus.

8 The male and female pronuclei fuse.

Follicular cells

Sperm nucleus

ZP3

Vitelline envelope

Bonds

Egg plasma membrane

Acrosome

? Pronucleus

Sperm-binding receptors

Enzymes released as acrosome breaks down

Cortical vesicle

Zona pellucida (jelly coat)

$\uparrow [Ca^{2+}]$

Egg cytosol

Vitelline envelope

1st / 2nd Female polar bodies

♂ Pronucleus   ♀ Pronucleus

Fertilization membrane

Fig. 56.1 Fertilization.

completes the process of **decidualization** (Fig. 56.3). The endometrium of pregnancy is known as the **decidua,** a term that refers to the shedding of these tissues at the end of pregnancy, like the shedding of leaves of a deciduous tree.

Uterine secretions nourish the preimplantation embryo, promote growth, and prepare it for implantation

Before the embryo implants, it receives nourishment from uterine secretions. Following conception, the endometrium is under the control of progesterone, which induces the secretion of multiple proteins and nutrients that are important for the nourishment, growth, and implantation of the embryo.

The blastocyst secretes substances that facilitate implantation

If the blastocyst is to survive, it must avoid rejection by the maternal cellular immune system. It does so by releasing immunosuppressive agents. The embryo also synthesizes and secretes macromolecules—including immunoregulatory agents, proteases, and growth factors—that promote implantation, the development of the placenta, and the maintenance of pregnancy.

A key hormone that the early blastocyst secretes is **human chorionic gonadotropin (hCG),** which is closely related to LH. Produced by trophoblast cells, hCG rescues the corpus luteum, thereby sustaining the production of progesterone and preventing menstruation.

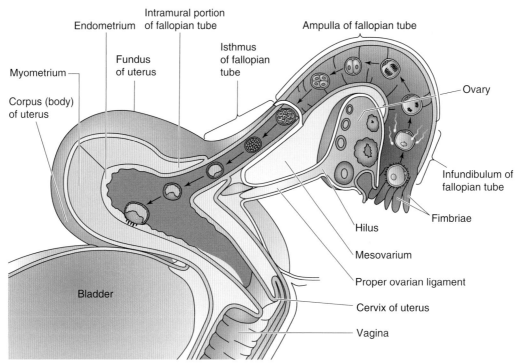

Fig. 56.2   Transport of the conceptus to the uterus.

During implantation, the blastocyst apposes itself to the endometrium, adheres to epithelial cells, and finally invades the stroma

Before the initiation of implantation, the zona pellucida that surrounds the blastocyst must degenerate. This process, known as **hatching** of the embryo (Fig. 56.4A), occurs 6 to 7 days after ovulation. Implantation proceeds in three stages: (1) **apposition** of the blastocyst to the endometrial epithelial cells (Fig. 56.4B), (2) **adhesion** of the blastocyst via the outer trophoblast cells to the endometrial epithelial cells (Fig. 56.4C), and (3) **invasion** of trophoblast cells and the blastocyst proper deep into the endometrial stroma and outer layers of the myometrium (Fig. 56.4D).

As the blastocyst attaches to the endometrial epithelium, the trophoblastic cells rapidly proliferate, and the trophoblast differentiates into two layers: an inner **cytotrophoblast** and an outer syncytiotrophoblast (Fig. 56.4D).

The blastocyst is genetically distinct from maternal tissue. Thus, implantation represents a breach of maternal immune defenses that could lead to immune attack and destruction of the embryo. To avoid attack, trophoblasts that lie at the maternal-fetal interface produce a unique immunogenic molecule, histocompatibility antigen G (HLA-G), on their cell surface, which prevents immunological recognition of the embryo as non-self by the maternal immune cells.

PHYSIOLOGY OF THE PLACENTA

Eventually, almost all the materials that are necessary for fetal growth and development move from the maternal circulation to the fetal circulation across the placenta, either by

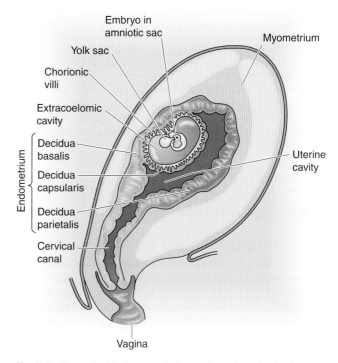

Fig. 56.3   Three decidual zones during early embryonic development (about 13 to 14 days postfertilization). The figure shows a sagittal section through a pregnant uterus, with the anterior side to the right.

passive diffusion or by active transport. The placenta is the major lifeline between the mother and the fetus. It provides nutrients and O_2 to the fetus, and it removes CO_2 and certain waste products from the fetus.

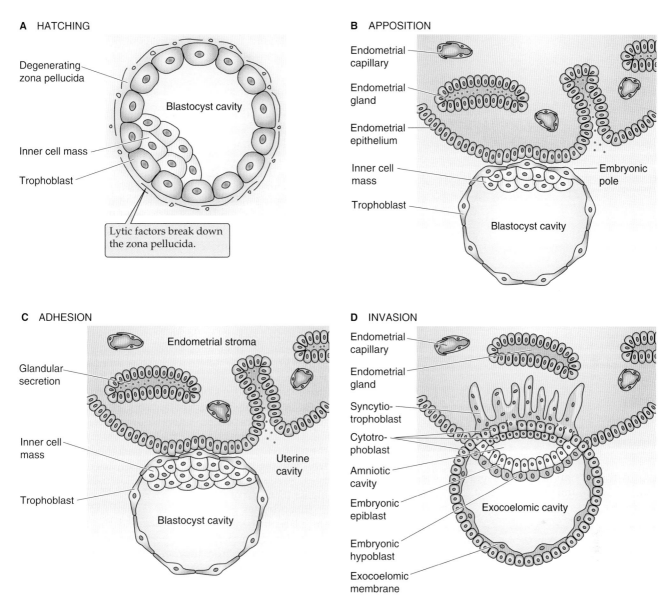

A HATCHING

Degenerating zona pellucida

Blastocyst cavity

Inner cell mass

Trophoblast

Lytic factors break down the zona pellucida.

B APPOSITION

Endometrial capillary

Endometrial gland

Endometrial epithelium

Inner cell mass

Embryonic pole

Trophoblast

Blastocyst cavity

C ADHESION

Endometrial stroma

Glandular secretion

Inner cell mass

Uterine cavity

Trophoblast

Blastocyst cavity

D INVASION

Endometrial capillary

Endometrial gland

Syncytiotrophoblast

Cytotrophoblast

Amniotic cavity

Embryonic epiblast

Embryonic hypoblast

Exocoelomic membrane

Exocoelomic cavity

Fig. 56.4 Embryo hatching, apposition, adhesion, and invasion.

At the placenta, the space between the fetus's chorionic villi and the mother's endometrial wall contains a continuously renewed pool of extravasated maternal blood

Within the syncytium of the invading syncytiotrophoblast cells (Fig. 56.4D), fluid-filled holes called **lacunae** develop 8 to 9 days after fertilization (Fig. 56.5A). Twelve to 15 days after fertilization, the finger-like projections of the syncytiotrophoblast (multinucleated cell formed from the fusion of trophoblast cells) finally penetrate the endothelial layer of small blood vessels in the endometrium. Later, these projections also penetrate the small spiral arteries deeper into the uterine wall. The result is a free communication between the lacunae of the syncytiotrophoblast and the lumina of maternal blood vessels (Fig. 56.5B). Within 12 to 15 days after fertilization, some cytotrophoblasts proliferate and invade the syncytiotrophoblast to form finger-like projections that are the **primary chorionic villi**, which will eventually contain fetal blood vessels.

With further development, mesenchymal cells from the extraembryonic mesoderm invade the primary chorionic villi, now known as **secondary chorionic villi.** Eventually, these mesenchymal cells form fetal blood vessels de novo, at which point the villi are known as **tertiary chorionic villi** (Fig. 56.5C). Continued differentiation and amplification of the surface area of the fetal tissue that is protruding into the maternal blood creates the mature chorionic villi of the placenta. The outer surface of each villus is lined with a very thin layer of syncytiotrophoblast that is in direct contact with maternal blood. Beneath the syncytiotrophoblast lie cytotrophoblasts, mesenchyme, and fetal blood vessels. The lacunae, filled with maternal blood, eventually merge with one another to create one massive, intercommunicating **intervillous space** (Fig. 56.6). Thus, in the mature placenta, fetal blood is separated from maternal blood only by the fetal capillary endothelium, some mesenchyme and cytotrophoblasts, and syncytiotrophoblast.

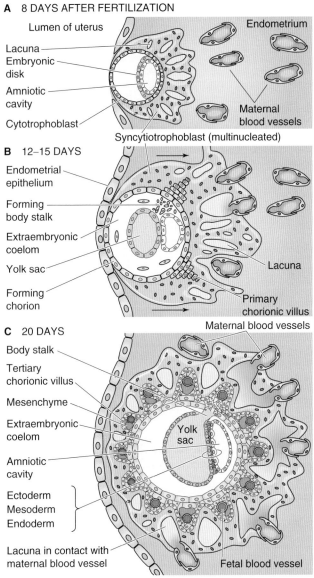

A 8 DAYS AFTER FERTILIZATION

Lumen of uterus
Lacuna
Embryonic disk
Amniotic cavity
Cytotrophoblast
Endometrium
Maternal blood vessels
Syncytiotrophoblast (multinucleated)

B 12–15 DAYS

Endometrial epithelium
Forming body stalk
Extraembryonic coelom
Yolk sac
Forming chorion
Lacuna
Primary chorionic villus

C 20 DAYS

Maternal blood vessels
Body stalk
Tertiary chorionic villus
Mesenchyme
Extraembryonic coelom
Amniotic cavity
Ectoderm
Mesoderm
Endoderm
Yolk sac
Lacuna in contact with maternal blood vessel
Fetal blood vessel

Fig. 56.5 Development of the placenta.

Maternal Blood Flow The maternal arterial blood is discharged into the intervillous space from spiral arteries of the uterine wall. The maternal blood spreads laterally to bathe the chorionic villi, and then drains through venous orifices in the basal plate and ultimately flows into the uterine and other pelvic veins. No capillaries are present between the maternal arterioles and venules; the intervillous space is the functional capillary.

Fetal Blood Flow The fetal blood originates from two **umbilical arteries.** Unlike *systemic* arteries after birth, umbilical arteries carry *deoxygenated* blood. As these umbilical arteries approach the placenta, they branch repeatedly beneath the amnion, penetrate the chorionic plate, and then branch again within the chorionic villi, forming a capillary network. Blood that has obtained a significantly higher O_2 and nutrient content returns to the fetus from the placenta through the single **umbilical vein.**

The **amniotic fluid** that fills the amniotic cavity serves two important functions. First, it serves as a mechanical buffer and thus protects the fetus from external physical insults. Second, it serves as a mechanism by which the fetus excretes many waste products.

Gases and other solutes move across the placenta

The placenta is the major lifeline between the mother and the fetus. It provides nutrients and O_2 to the fetus, and it removes CO_2 and certain waste products from the fetus.

O_2 and CO_2 Transport ⊙ **56-1** The maternal blood coming into the intervillous space has a gas composition similar to that of systemic arterial blood: a partial pressure of oxygen (P_{O_2}) of ~100 mm Hg, a P_{CO_2} of ~40 mm Hg, and a pH of 7.40. However, the diffusion of O_2 from the maternal blood into the chorionic villi of the fetus causes the P_{O_2} of blood in the intervillous space to fall, so the average P_{O_2} is 30 to 35 mm Hg. Given the O_2 dissociation curve of maternal (i.e., adult) hemoglobin (Hb), this P_{O_2} translates to an O_2 saturation of ~65% (see Fig. 29.2). The P_{O_2} of blood in the umbilical vein is even lower. Despite the relatively low P_{O_2} of the maternal blood in the intervillous space, the fetus does not suffer from a lack of O_2. Because fetal Hb has a much higher affinity for O_2 than does maternal Hb, the fetal Hb can extract O_2 from the maternal Hb. Thus, a P_{O_2} of 30 to 35 mm Hg, which yields an Hb saturation of ~65% in the intervillous space in the mother's blood, produces an Hb saturation of ~85% in the umbilical vein of the fetus, assuming that the O_2 fully equilibrates between intervillous and fetal blood. Other mechanisms of ensuring adequate fetal oxygenation include the relatively high cardiac output per unit body weight of the fetus and the increasing O_2-carrying capacity of fetal blood late in pregnancy as the Hb concentration rises to a level 50% higher than that of the adult.

Other Solutes Solutes besides O_2 and CO_2 move across the placenta between the mother and the fetus, availing themselves of numerous transport mechanisms. For example, glucose moves from the mother to the fetus by facilitated diffusion, and amino acids move by secondary active transport (see ⊙ **5-12**). The placenta also transports several other essential substances, such as vitamins and minerals, that are needed for fetal growth and development.

The placenta makes a variety of peptide hormones, including hCG and human chorionic somatomammotropin

The placenta plays a key role in synthesizing a variety of peptide and steroid hormones. Placental hormones may act in a paracrine fashion, controlling the release of local placental hormones, or they may enter the maternal or fetal circulations.

⊙ **56-2** The most important placental peptide hormone is **hCG.** The placenta also produces two **human chorionic somatomammotropins,** hCS1 and hCS2, also called *human placental lactogens* (hPL1, hPL2). hCS1 and hCS2 are polypeptide hormones structurally related to growth hormone (GH) and placental-variant growth hormone (pvGH), as well as to prolactin (PRL). They coordinate the fuel economy of the fetoplacental unit and also promote the development of maternal mammary glands during pregnancy.

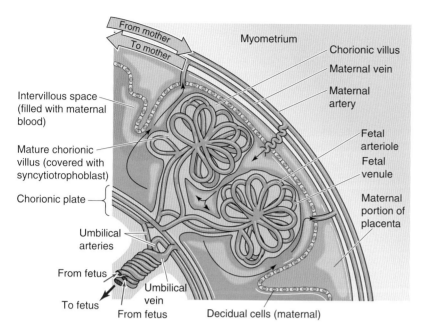

Fig. 56.6 Mature placenta. With further development beyond that shown in Fig. 56.5C, the outer surface of the mature chorionic villus is covered with a thin layer of syncytiotrophoblast. Under this are cytotrophoblasts, mesenchyme, and fetal blood vessels. The lacunae into which the villi project gradually merge into one massive intervillous space. Maternal blood is trapped in this intervillous space, between the endometrium on the maternal side and the villi on the fetal side. In the mature placenta (shown here), spiral arteries from the mother empty directly into the intervillous space, which is drained by maternal veins. The villi look like a thick forest of trees arising from the chorionic plate, which is the analog of the soil from which the trees sprout.

THE MATERNAL-PLACENTAL-FETAL UNIT

During pregnancy, progesterone and estrogens rise to levels that are substantially higher than their peaks in a normal cycle

During pregnancy, maternal levels of progesterone and estrogens (estradiol, estrone, estriol) all increase, reaching levels substantially higher than those achieved during a normal menstrual cycle. These elevated levels are necessary for maintaining pregnancy. For example, progesterone—the progestational hormone—reduces uterine motility and inhibits propagation of contractions. How are these elevated levels of female steroids achieved? Early in the first trimester, hCG that is manufactured by the syncytiotrophoblast rescues the corpus luteum, which is the major source of progesterone and estrogens. However, by itself, the corpus luteum is not adequate to generate the very high steroid levels that are characteristic of late pregnancy. The developing placenta itself augments its production of progesterone and estrogens, so by 8 weeks of gestation the placenta has become the major source of these steroids—the luteal-placental shift.

Estriol, which is not important in nonpregnant women, is a major estrogen during pregnancy.

After 8 weeks of gestation, the maternal-placental-fetal unit maintains high levels of progesterone and estrogens

Although it emerges as the major source of progesterone and estrogens, the human placenta cannot synthesize these hormones by itself; it requires the assistance of both mother and fetus. This joint effort in steroid biosynthesis has led to the concept of the **maternal-placental-fetal unit.** Fig. 56.7 illustrates the pathways that the maternal-placental-fetal unit uses to synthesize progesterone and the estrogens. Fig. 56.8 summarizes the exchange of synthetic intermediates among the three members of the maternal-placental-fetal unit.

Unlike the corpus luteum, which manufactures progesterone, estrone, and estradiol early in pregnancy (see Fig. 55.5), the placenta is an imperfect endocrine organ. First, the placenta cannot manufacture adequate cholesterol, the precursor for steroid synthesis. Second, the placenta lacks two crucial enzymes that are needed for synthesizing estrone and estradiol. Third, the placenta lacks a third enzyme that is needed to synthesize estriol.

The maternal-placental-fetal unit overcomes these placental shortcomings in two ways. First, the mother supplies most of the cholesterol as LDL particles (see ⊙ 46-8). Second, the fetal adrenal gland and liver supply the three enzymes that the placenta lacks.

RESPONSE OF THE MOTHER TO PREGNANCY

The **mean duration of human pregnancy** is ~266 days (38 weeks) from the time of ovulation or 280 days (40 weeks) from the first day of the last menstrual period. During this time, the mother experiences numerous and profound adaptive changes in her cardiovascular system, fluid volume, respiration, fuel metabolism, and nutrition. These orderly changes reflect the effects of various placental hormones as well as the increase in the size of the pregnant uterus. Key adaptations of maternal physiology in response to pregnancy include:

1. The maternal **blood volume** and **cardiac output** increase during the first trimester, expand rapidly during the second trimester, rise at a much lower rate during the third trimester, and finally achieve a plateau during the last several weeks of pregnancy. The increase in blood volume is needed to meet the demands of the enlarged pregnant uterus with its greatly hypertrophied vascular system.
2. Mild insulin resistance provides the fetus more time to extract nutrients from the maternal compartment after each meal.

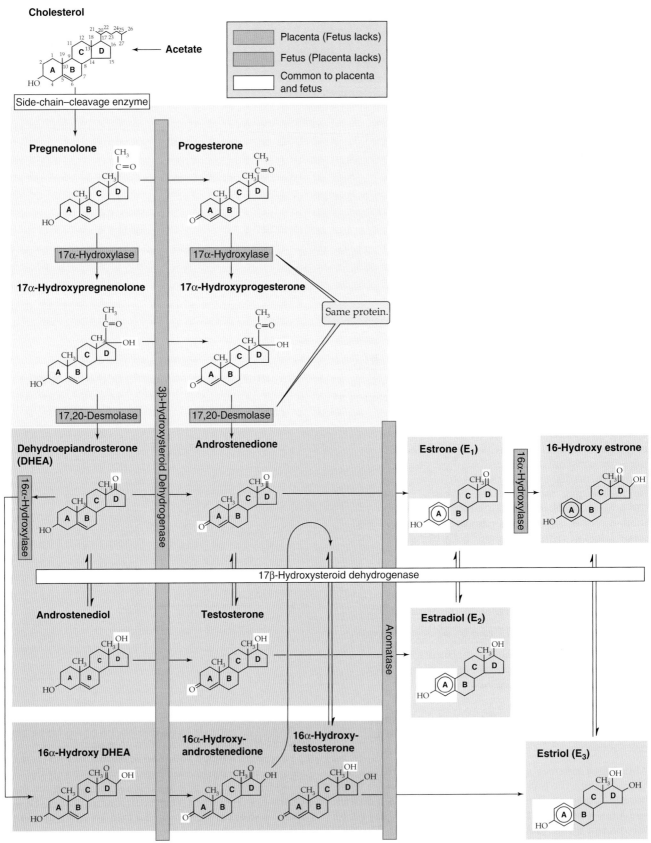

Fig. 56.7 Synthesis of progesterone and the estrogens by the maternal-placental-fetal unit. Individual enzymes are shown in *horizontal* and *vertical bars.* The *blue, brown,* and *white colors* of the bars code the location of enzymes.

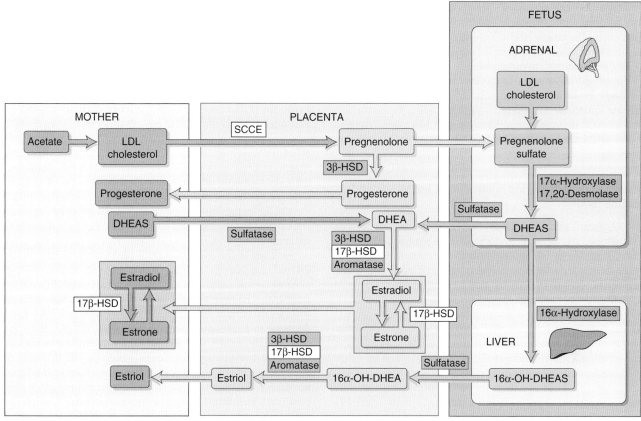

Fig. 56.8 Interactions of the maternal-placental-fetal unit. The details of the enzymatic reactions are provided in Fig. 56.7. *DHEAS,* Dehydroepiandrosterone, sulfated; *HSD,* hydroxysteroid dehydrogenase; *SCCE,* the side-chain-cleavage enzyme.

3. Increased levels of progesterone during pregnancy lead to an increase in alveolar ventilation.
4. Altered maternal appetite increases intake of dietary protein and iron.
5. Weight gain establishes energy stores needed for lactation.

PARTURITION

Human birth usually occurs at around the 40th week of gestation

Human birth usually occurs at around the 40th week of gestation. After birth, the fetus—now a neonate—must maintain physiological homeostasis even though it has lost its placenta and has been thrust into a markedly altered environment. Therefore, birth should occur only after organ systems have matured sufficiently to allow the neonate to survive outside the uterus. At the ~40th week of gestation, critical organ systems, especially those that interface with the environment (e.g., lungs, gut, and immune system) and those that maintain homeostasis (e.g., the hypothalamic-pituitary-adrenal axis, kidneys, liver, and pancreas), are functionally competent, and with maternal nurturing, the neonate has a high probability of survival. However, birth prior to 40 weeks is associated with neonatal morbidity and mortality, the severity of which increases the earlier birth occurs.

Parturition—the process of birth—involves (1) transformation of the myometrium (smooth-muscle component of the uterine wall) from a quiescent to a highly contractile state to become the engine for birth, (2) remodeling of the uterine cervix such that it softens (effacement) and dilates to open the gateway for birth, (3) rupture of the fetal membranes, (4) expulsion of the uterine contents, and (5) return of the uterus to its prepregnant state.

Parturition occurs in distinct stages, numbered 0 to 3

Stage 0—Quiescence ⊙ 56-3 Throughout most of pregnancy the uterus is relaxed, quiescent, and relatively insensitive to uterotonins—hormones that stimulate contractions, such as prostaglandins (PGs) and **oxytocin (OT)**—and the uterine cervix remains closed and rigid. Weak and irregular contractions, known as **Braxton Hicks contractions,** occur toward the end of pregnancy and may increase in frequency and intensity near term.

Stage 1—Transformation/Activation Before labor, the myometrium transforms to a more contractile state. This awakening of myometrial cells involves increased expression of genes that encode factors collectively referred to as **contraction-associated proteins (CAPs).** The cervix also begins to express genes encoding enzymes that break down the collagen matrix to facilitate effacement and dilation.

Stage 2—Active Labor Three major factors induce the forceful and rhythmic contractions that, in association with effacement and dilation of the cervix, constitute the obstetrical definition of labor: (1) increased levels of PGs, (2) increased myometrial cell interconnectivity, and (3) increased myometrial responsiveness to PGs and OT.

Stage 3—Involution Immediately after expulsion of the uterine contents, it is mainly OT that causes the sustained and forceful myometrial contraction that helps constrict the spiral arterioles and thereby facilitates postpartum uterine hemostasis.

After initiation of uterine contractions, both PGs and OT sustain labor

Although not all of the factors controlling the initiation of parturition are known, endocrine and paracrine interactions, signals elicited in response to inflammation (e.g., in response to intrauterine infection), and mechanical stretching of the uterus appear to play key roles. Once labor is initiated, it is sustained by a series of positive-feedback mechanisms involving inflammation within the gestational tissues—myometrium, cervix, decidua, placenta, nonplacental chorion, and amnion—until the uterine contents are expelled. Once labor is initiated, it is sustained by other positive-feedback loops involving PGs and the pituitary hormone, OT, both of which are potent stimulators of uterine contractions. Uterine contractions stimulate local PG release, which itself increases the intensity of uterine contractions. Uterine activity also stretches the cervix, which stimulates OT release via the Ferguson reflex. Because OT stimulates further uterine contractions, these contractions become self-perpetuating.

LACTATION

The fundamental secretory unit of the breast (Fig. 56.9A) is the alveolus (Fig. 56.9B and C), which is surrounded by contractile myoepithelial cells and adipose cells. These alveoli are organized into secretory lobules, each of which drains into a ductule. A group of 15 to 20 ductules drain into a lactiferous duct, which widens at the ampulla—a small reservoir. The lactiferous ducts carry the secretions to the outside.

Breast development at puberty depends primarily on the estrogens and progesterone. During pregnancy, gradual increases in levels of estrogens and progesterone in conjunction with prolactin lead to full development of the breasts.

The epithelial alveolar cells of the mammary gland secrete the complex mixture of sugars, proteins, lipids, and other substances that constitute milk

Breast milk is an emulsion of fats in an aqueous solution containing sugar (lactose), proteins (lactalbumin and casein), and several cations (K^+, Ca^{2+}, and Na^+) and anions (Cl^- and phosphate). The composition of human milk differs from that of human **colostrum** (the thin, yellowish, milk-like substance secreted during the first several days after parturition).

The epithelial cells in the alveoli of the mammary gland secrete the complex mixture of constituents that make up milk by the five major routes summarized in Fig. 56.9D.

PRL is essential for milk production, and suckling is a powerful stimulus for PRL secretion

Prolactin (PRL) released in the anterior pituitary acts on the mammary glands and is the principal hormonal regulator of lactation by promoting mammary growth, the **mammogenic effect**; initiation of milk secretion, the **lactogenic effect**; and maintenance of milk production once it has been established, the **galactopoietic effect**. Although the initiation of lactation requires the coordinated action of several hormones, PRL is the classic lactogenic hormone and is the primary hormone responsible for maintaining milk production once it has been initiated.

Suckling is the most powerful physiological stimulus for PRL release. Nipple stimulation triggers PRL secretion via an afferent neural pathway through the spinal cord (Fig. 56.10).

During the first 3 weeks of the neonatal period, maternal PRL levels remain tonically elevated. Thereafter, PRL levels decrease to a constant baseline level that is higher than that observed in women who are not pregnant. If the mother does *not* nurse her young, PRL levels generally fall to nonpregnancy levels after 1 to 2 weeks. If the mother *does* breast-feed, increased PRL secretion is maintained for as long as suckling continues. Suckling causes episodic increases in PRL secretion with each feeding, thus producing peaks in PRL levels superimposed on the elevated baseline PRL levels. After the infant completes a session of nursing, PRL levels return to their elevated baseline and remain there until the infant nurses again.

⊙ 56-4 OT and psychic stimuli initiate milk ejection ("let-down")

OT, which can promote uterine contraction, also enhances milk ejection by stimulating the contraction of the network of myoepithelial cells surrounding the alveoli and ducts of the breast, the **galactokinetic effect**. Nursing can sometimes cause uterine cramps. During nursing, suckling stimulates nerve endings in the nipple and triggers rapid bursts of OT release (Fig. 56.10). This neurogenic reflex is transmitted through the spinal cord, the midbrain, and the hypothalamus, where it stimulates neurons in the paraventricular and supraoptic nuclei that release OT from their nerve endings in the *posterior pituitary*. From the posterior pituitary, OT enters the systemic circulation and eventually reaches the myoepithelial cells that are arranged longitudinally on the lactiferous ducts and around the alveoli in the breast (Fig. 56.9C and D). The result is to promote the release of pre-existing milk after 40 to 60 seconds, a process known as the **let-down reflex.**

In addition to the suckling stimulus, many different psychic stimuli emanating from the infant, as well as neuroendocrine factors, promote OT release. The site or sound of an infant may trigger milk let-down, a phenomenon observed in many mammals. Thus, the posterior pituitary releases OT episodically even in anticipation of suckling. Fear, anger, or other stresses suppress this psychogenic reflex, thus inhibiting OT release and suppressing milk outflow.

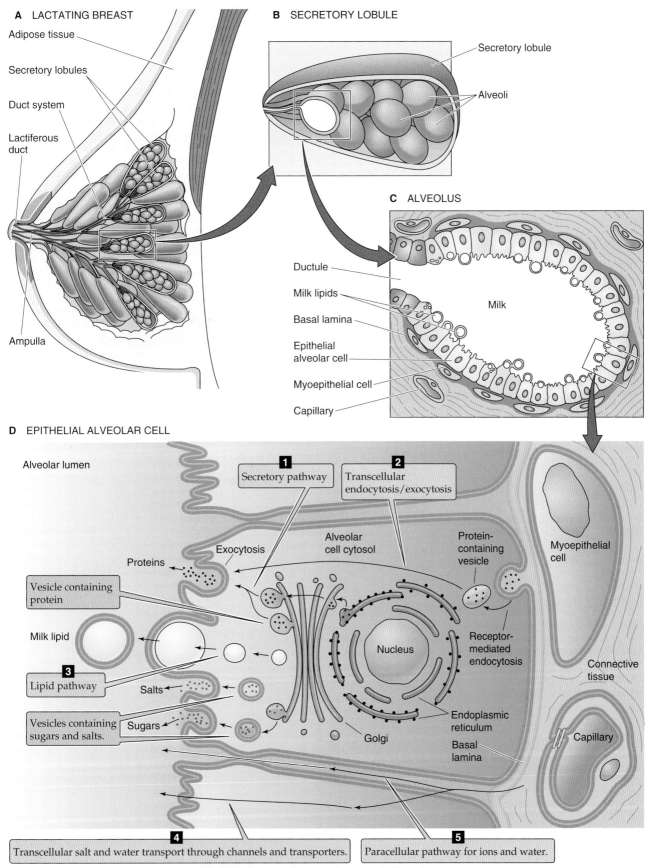

A LACTATING BREAST

Adipose tissue

Secretory lobules

Duct system

Lactiferous duct

Ampulla

B SECRETORY LOBULE

Secretory lobule

Alveoli

C ALVEOLUS

Ductule

Milk lipids

Basal lamina

Epithelial alveolar cell

Myoepithelial cell

Capillary

Milk

D EPITHELIAL ALVEOLAR CELL

Alveolar lumen

1 Secretory pathway

2 Transcellular endocytosis/exocytosis

Exocytosis

Alveolar cell cytosol

Protein-containing vesicle

Myoepithelial cell

Proteins

Vesicle containing protein

Milk lipid

3 Lipid pathway

Salts

Vesicles containing sugars and salts.

Sugars

Nucleus

Golgi

Receptor-mediated endocytosis

Endoplasmic reticulum

Basal lamina

Connective tissue

Capillary

4 Transcellular salt and water transport through channels and transporters.

5 Paracellular pathway for ions and water.

Fig. 56.9 Cross section of the breast and milk production.

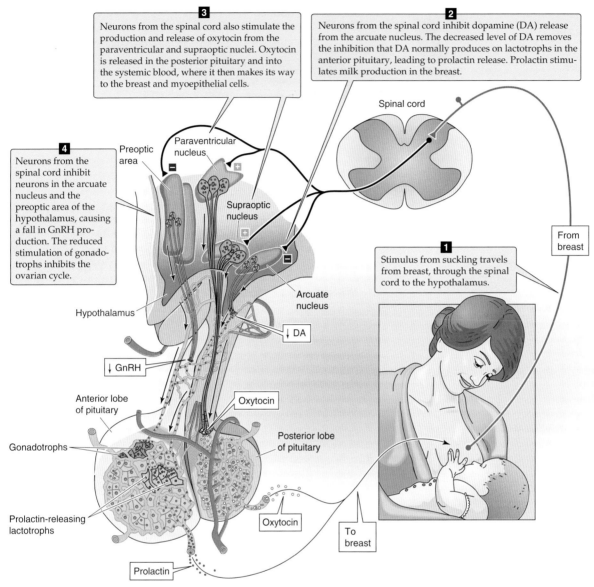

3 Neurons from the spinal cord also stimulate the production and release of oxytocin from the paraventricular and supraoptic nuclei. Oxytocin is released in the posterior pituitary and into the systemic blood, where it then makes its way to the breast and myoepithelial cells.

2 Neurons from the spinal cord inhibit dopamine (DA) release from the arcuate nucleus. The decreased level of DA removes the inhibition that DA normally produces on lactotrophs in the anterior pituitary, leading to prolactin release. Prolactin stimulates milk production in the breast.

4 Neurons from the spinal cord inhibit neurons in the arcuate nucleus and the preoptic area of the hypothalamus, causing a fall in GnRH production. The reduced stimulation of gonadotrophs inhibits the ovarian cycle.

1 Stimulus from suckling travels from breast, through the spinal cord to the hypothalamus.

Spinal cord

From breast

Preoptic area

Paraventricular nucleus

Supraoptic nucleus

Arcuate nucleus

Hypothalamus

↓ DA

↓ GnRH

Anterior lobe of pituitary

Gonadotrophs

Prolactin-releasing lactotrophs

Prolactin

Oxytocin

Posterior lobe of pituitary

Oxytocin

To breast

Fig. 56.10   Effect of suckling on the release of PRL, OT, and GnRH. Suckling has four effects, indicated by the four *numbered boxes.*

Suckling inhibits the ovarian cycle

Lactation generally inhibits cyclic ovulatory function by reducing GnRH release from the hypothalamus (Fig. 56.10, *box 4*). As a result, breast-feeding delays ovulation and normal menstrual cycles. However, if the mother continues to nurse her infant for a prolonged period, ovulatory cycles will eventually resume.

CHAPTER 57

FETAL AND NEONATAL PHYSIOLOGY

George Lister

Fetal development is a highly organized process. The transition to the extrauterine environment occurs abruptly and is likewise extraordinarily well orchestrated. After birth, the newborn must acclimate to its new milieu, where numerous homeostatic challenges confront the newly autonomous organs.

BIOLOGY OF FETAL GROWTH

Growth of the fetus begins soon after fertilization, when the first cell division occurs. Cell division, hypertrophy, and differentiation are well-coordinated events that result in the growth and development of specialized organ systems. The fetus, fetal membranes, and placenta develop and function as a unit throughout pregnancy, and their development is interdependent. The growth trajectory of fetal mass is relatively flat during the first trimester, increases linearly at the beginning of the second trimester, and rises rapidly during the third trimester.

Growth occurs by hyperplasia and hypertrophy

The growth of an organ occurs as a result of an increase in cell number (**hyperplasia**), an increase in cell size (**hypertrophy**), or both. Growth follows three sequential phases that are organ specific: (1) pure hyperplasia, (2) hyperplasia and concomitant hypertrophy, and (3) hypertrophy alone. For example, the **placenta** goes through all three phases of growth, but these phases are compressed because the placental life span is relatively short. In fact, simple hypertrophy is the primary form of placental growth. In contrast to placental growth and development, growth of the **fetus** occurs almost entirely by hyperplasia.

Growth depends primarily on genetic factors during the first half of gestation and on epigenetic factors thereafter

The fertilized egg contains the genetic material that directs cell multiplication and differentiation, and guides development of the human phenotype. For specific developmental events to occur at precise times, a programmed sequence of gene activation and suppression is necessary. Ignoring apoptosis, the fertilized egg (<1 ng) must undergo an average of ~42 divisions before newborn size is reached (~3 kg, an increase of >10^{12} fold). After birth, only approximately five additional divisions are necessary for the net increase in mass that is necessary to achieve adult size. Of course, many tissues (e.g., gastrointestinal tract, skin, blood cells) must continually undergo cell division to replenish cells lost by apoptosis.

During the first half of pregnancy, the fetus's own genetic program is the primary determinant of growth, and thus constrains patterns of growth. During the second half of pregnancy, the patterns of growth and development are more variable. The four primary epigenetic factors at work during the second half of pregnancy are placental, hormonal, environmental (e.g., maternal nutrition), and metabolic (e.g., diabetes). We discuss the first two factors (placental and hormonal) in the next two sections.

Increases in placental mass parallel periods of rapid fetal growth

The placenta plays several important roles in fetal growth and development. In addition to serving transport and storage functions, the placenta is involved in numerous biosynthetic activities. These include the synthesis of steroids, such as estrogen and progesterone, and of protein hormones, such as human chorionic gonadotropin (hCG) and the human chorionic somatomammotropins (hCSs; see ⊙ 56-2).

Fetal growth closely correlates with placental weight and trophoblast surface area. During periods of rapid fetal growth, placental weight increases. As the placental mass increases, the total surface area of the placental villi increases to sustain gas transport and fetal nutrition. Moreover, maternal blood flow to the uterus and fetal blood flow to the placenta also increase in parallel with the increase in placental mass. Placental growth increases linearly until ~4 weeks before birth, and adequate placental reserve is particularly important during the third trimester, when fetal growth is very rapid. **Fetal growth restriction** can occur as a result of decreased *placental reserve* caused by any insult. For example, mothers who smoke during pregnancy tend to have small placentas and are at high risk of delivering a low-birth-weight baby.

Insulin, the insulin-like growth factors, and thyroxine stimulate fetal growth

Glucocorticoids and Insulin Glucocorticoids in the fetus promote the storage of glucose as glycogen in the fetal liver, a process that increases greatly during the final month of gestation in preparation for the increased glycolytic activity required during and immediately after delivery. Near term, when fetal glucose metabolism becomes sensitive to **insulin,** this hormone contributes to the storage of glucose as glycogen, as well as to the uptake and utilization of amino acids and lipogenesis (see ⊙ 51-2).

Insulin-Like Growth Factors In the fetus, both IGF-1 and IGF-2, which are mitogenic peptides, are extremely important for growth. Birth weight correlates positively with IGF levels.

Thyroid Hormones The thyroid hormones are obligatory for normal growth and development (see ⊙ 49-5). Before the second trimester, most of the thyroxine (T_4) in the fetus is maternal. Fetal production of thyrotropin (or thyroid-stimulating hormone [TSH]) and T_4 begin to increase in the second trimester, concurrent with development of the hypothalamic-pituitary portal system.

DEVELOPMENT AND MATURATION OF THE CARDIOPULMONARY SYSTEM

Two distinct circulations—fetoplacental and uteroplacental—underlie the transfer of gases and nutrients

The fundamental difference between the circulatory system of the fetus and that of the infant/adult is the presence of the placenta, which produces essential hormones (e.g., progestins, estrogens, chorionic gonadotropins) and performs a number of vital functions (e.g., gas exchange, nutrient transport, fluid balance, and waste removal) that other systems provide in extrauterine life. The fetus accomplishes these tasks by directing a large fraction of fetal blood flow from the aorta via the two umbilical arteries to the **fetoplacental circulation** within chorionic villi. There the umbilical arteries branch into small tufts of vessels (villus capillaries) that come into apposition with the maternal **uteroplacental circulation,** which has a high blood flow. The placental membranes (the syncytiotrophoblast) that separate these two distinct circulations permit the efficient exchange of respiratory gases, fluid, and larger molecules that are critical to sustain growth and maintain homeostasis. Accordingly, disturbances in the placental circulation or delivery of nutritive substrates can have serious consequences for the growth and development of the fetus.

The transfer of respiratory gases occurs by diffusion, driven by the partial pressure differences of these gases in various compartments, as is the case in the lungs after birth (see ⊙ 30-1). The uterine arterial blood enters the placenta with a P_{O_2} of 80 to 100 mm Hg, whereas umbilical arterial blood enters with a P_{O_2} of ~20 mm Hg, so that O_2 diffuses from the uterine to the umbilical circulation. The result is that the effluent umbilical venous blood has a P_{O_2} of about 35 to 50 mm Hg, whereas the uterine venous P_{O_2} is consistently higher by 4 to 15 mm Hg. However, with some substances,

such as creatinine, the concentration is the same in fetal and maternal blood. Amino acids are transported across the syncytiotrophoblast and then diffuse into the fetal circulation.

An increase in cortisol, with other hormones, triggers pulmonary surfactant production in the third trimester

Two factors are required for gas exchange in the neonatal lung: (1) appropriate development of the lungs involving the structural growth and coincident branching of lung segments and blood vessels that creates an extensive alveolar-capillary interface for efficient diffusion of gases, and (2) the production of surfactant (see ⊙ 27-4), which permits lung expansion without excessive inspiratory effort.

⊙ **57-1** Hormones play a major role in controlling fetal lung growth and development in preparation for ex utero function. Numerous hormones stimulate surfactant biosynthesis, including glucocorticoids, thyroid hormones, thyrotropin-releasing hormone, and prolactin, as well as growth factors such as EGF. Glucocorticoids, in particular, play an essential role in stimulating fetal lung maturation by increasing the number of both type II pneumocytes and lamellar bodies within these cells. Fetal cortisol levels rise steadily during the third trimester and surge just before birth. Two thirds of this cortisol is of fetal origin; the rest crosses the placenta from the mother.

At ~32 weeks' gestation, cortisol stimulates in pneumocytes the expression of genes encoding several regulatory enzymes, leading to increased production of pulmonary surfactant late in gestation. Coincident with increased surfactant synthesis is a large increase in lung distensibility and stability on inflation. However, in infants born prematurely with insufficient surfactant and lungs that are not structurally mature, severe respiratory distress can result. Because of the surfactant deficiency, the infant must invest excessive work to create an adequate tidal volume with each breath and to maintain a normal functional residual capacity following expiration.

The fetal circulation has four unique pathways— placenta, ductus venosus, foramen ovale, and ductus arteriosus—to facilitate gas and nutrient exchange

One of the most crucial adaptations to extrauterine life is changes in the circulation from the fetal to the postnatal type. The fundamental difference between the fetal and postnatal circulations is that the placenta performs for the fetus functions that—at least in part—are performed by four organ systems in extrauterine life: (1) the lungs (gas exchange), (2) the gastrointestinal tract (nutrition), (3) the liver (nutrition, waste removal), and (4) the kidneys (fluid and electrolyte balance, waste removal).

Just as in the mature circulation, the fetal right ventricle pumps most of its output to the gas-exchange organ (i.e., the placenta). The fetal left ventricle pumps most of its output to systemic tissues. The key principle governing the unique pattern of fetal blood flow is the presence of three **shunts** that allow blood to bypass future postnatal routes and instead direct a large fraction of deoxygenated blood to the placenta. These are (1) the **ductus venosus** that directs blood from the left umbilical vein directly to the inferior vena cava, which allows oxygenated blood from the placenta to bypass the liver; (2) the **foramen ovale**, an oval hole in the wall between the atria of the heart that shunts oxygenated blood from the right atrium to the left atrium for distribution to the body; and (3) the **ductus arteriosus** that directs blood from the pulmonary artery to the aorta, thus bypassing the inactive fetal lungs.

CARDIOPULMONARY ADJUSTMENTS AT BIRTH

As the newborn exits the birth canal, it takes its first breath, which not only expands the lungs but also triggers a series of changes in the circulatory system. At the same time, the newborn loses its nutritional connection to the mother and confronts a cold new world. Three major challenges to metabolism accompany birth: *hypoxia, hypothermia,* and *hypoglycemia.* We discuss the adaptations of the respiratory and cardiovascular systems in this subchapter and adjustments of other organ systems in the next.

Loss of the placental circulation requires the newborn to breathe on its own

Although separation of the placenta does not occur until several minutes after birth, vasoconstriction in the umbilical *arteries* terminates the ability of the placenta to deliver oxygenated blood to the newborn immediately upon birth. Thus, even though the newborn may remain attached to its placenta during the first few moments of life, it is essential that the baby begins to breathe immediately. Because the umbilical *veins* do not constrict as do the umbilical arteries, blood flows from placenta to newborn if the infant is held below the level of the placenta, and if the umbilical cord is not clamped. This autotransfusion may constitute 75 to 100 mL, which is a substantial fraction of the newborn's total blood volume of ~300 mL (90 mL/kg).

At birth, the newborn must transform its circulatory system from one that supports gas exchange in the placenta to one that supports O_2 and CO_2 exchange in the lungs. In addition, other circulatory adjustments must occur as the gastrointestinal tract, liver, and kidneys assume their normal roles. As the lungs become functional at birth, the pulmonary and systemic circulations shift from interconnected and *parallel* systems to separate entities that function in *series.*

Mild hypoxia and hypercapnia, as well as tactile stimuli and cold skin, trigger the first breath

The first breath is the defining event for the newborn. Not only does it inflate the lungs, it also triggers circulatory changes that convert the fetal pattern of blood flow to the adult pattern.

The rapid onset of breathing immediately after delivery appears to be induced by a temporary state of **hypoxia** and **hypercapnia.** In most normal deliveries, these changes in P_{O_2} and P_{CO_2} result from the partial occlusion of the umbilical cord. Tactile stimulation and decreased skin temperature also promote the onset of breathing. When newborns do not begin to breathe immediately, hypercapnia and hypoxia increase and provide further simulation for the infant to breathe.

At birth, removal of the placenta increases systemic vascular resistance, whereas lung expansion decreases pulmonary vascular resistance

The fetal circulation has four unique pathways for blood flow absent in the adult: the placental circulation, ductus venosus, foramen ovale, and ductus arteriosus. Conversion to the postnatal blood flow pattern in which the lungs are the site for gas exchange requires that these pathways close soon after birth.

At birth, blood flow to the placenta ceases when the umbilical vessels are ligated, and the shunts progressively disappear over the ensuing hours to days. In addition, the pulmonary circulation, which received only ~7% of the cardiac output in the fetus, now accepts the entire cardiac output.

Removal of the Placental Circulation The placental circulation represents a major parallel path in the systemic circulation and accounts for the low vascular resistance of the fetal systemic circulation. When the placental circulation disappears at birth, the total peripheral resistance doubles. Because blood flow through the descending aorta is essentially unchanged, aortic and left ventricular systolic pressure must increase.

Increase in Pulmonary Blood Flow ⊙ 57-2 During fetal life pulmonary blood flow is markedly constricted and thereby blood diverts through the ductus arteriosus, which connects the pulmonary artery to the descending aorta causing oxygenated blood to bypass the fetal lungs. At birth, pulmonary vascular resistance abruptly decreases >5-fold with breathing (Fig. 57.1), owing to lung expansion and its sequelae—an increase in alveolar P_{O_2}, a decrease in alveolar P_{CO_2}—lifting the hypoxic vasoconstriction that prevailed during fetal life. As a result, blood flow through the pulmonary vasculature increases by ~4-fold at birth.

Closure of the ductus venosus within the first days of life forces portal blood to perfuse the liver

Although blood flow through the umbilical vein ceases soon after birth, the majority of the portal blood continues to flow through the ductus venosus. Thus, immediately after birth, portal flow through the liver remains low. However, within a few days after term birth (longer after preterm birth), constriction of the vascular smooth muscle within the ductus venosus causes functional closure of this shunt pathway. As a result, pressure in the portal vein increases markedly, thereby diverting blood into the liver.

Closure of the foramen ovale occurs as left atrial pressure begins to exceed right atrial pressure

After birth, the decrease in the pulmonary vascular resistance permits increased blood flow through the lungs, which increases venous return to the left atrium and elevates **left atrial pressure.** At the same time, the increase in pulmonary blood flow, the closing of the ductus arteriosus, and the increase in systemic resistance (due to removal of the

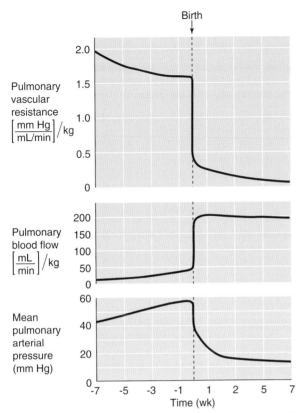

Figure 57.1 Effect of birth on pulmonary vascular resistance, blood flow, and mean arterial pressure. (Data from Rudolph AM: Congenital Diseases of the Heart: Clinical-Physiological Considerations. Armonk NY, Futura, 2001).

placenta) conspire to decrease blood flow down the descending aorta and thus the venous return to the right atrium. As a result, **right atrial pressure** falls. The net effect of the rise in left atrial pressure and the fall in right atrial pressure is a reversal of the pressure gradient across the atrial septum that pushes a flap of tissue—which previously protruded into the left atrium—back against the septum, functionally closing the foramen ovale (Fig. 57.2A). Closing the foramen usually prevents flow of blood from the left to the right atrium of the newborn.

Closure of the ductus arteriosus completes the separation between the pulmonary and systemic circulations

Immediately after birth, the ductus arteriosus remains open, but blood flow, which follows the path of least resistance, now begins to shunt (left to right) from the descending aorta to the pulmonary circulation because of the two events that change the relationship between pulmonary and systemic vascular resistance: (1) increased systemic resistance because of the removal of the placenta, and (2) decreased pulmonary resistance because of the expansion of the lungs.

Within a few hours after term birth, the ductus arteriosus closes *functionally* because its muscular wall constricts (Fig. 57.2A). Usually, all blood flow through the ductus arteriosus ceases within 1 week after birth. Within

a month or so, the lumen becomes obliterated *anatomically* because of thrombosis (i.e., blood clot within the lumen), intimal thickening, and loss of smooth-muscle cells.

NEONATAL PHYSIOLOGY

In humans, the **neonatal period** is defined as the first 4 weeks after birth. The newborn's ability to survive during this period depends on the adequate development and maturation of various fetal organ systems, adaptations of these organ systems to extrauterine life, and nurturing by a mother or other caretaker because of the neonate's extreme dependence. As the newborn loses its nutritional link with the placenta, the infant must now rely on its own gastrointestinal tract. Moreover, other functions normally carried out by the placenta are now entrusted to the liver and kidneys. Finally, on exiting its uterine "incubator," the newborn must stabilize body temperature.

Although the newborn is prone to hypothermia, nonshivering thermogenesis in brown fat helps to keep the neonate warm

The body loses heat to the environment by radiation, conduction, convection, and evaporation (see ⊙ 59-3). The newborn is particularly susceptible to thermal stress, owing to some important predisposing factors: (1) large skin surface area relative to small body mass (or volume); (2) limited ability to generate heat via shivering thermogenesis; (3) poor thermal insulation from the environment by adipose tissue; and (4) lack of behavioral adjustments, such as changing clothing or moving to a more favorable environment.

⊙ **57-3** Despite these factors, the newborn has important mechanisms for resisting hypothermia, including vasomotor responses, which divert warmed blood to or from the skin surface, and **nonshivering thermogenesis,** a process that occurs primarily in liver, brain, and brown fat.

Brown fat differs from white fat in having a high density of mitochondria; the cytochromes in these mitochondria give the brown fat cells their color. Newborns have particularly high levels of brown fat in the neck and midline of the upper back. Upregulation of a protein called **uncoupling protein 1** (**UCP1**) dissipates the H^+ gradient across the inner mitochondrial membrane. Thus, the mitochondria in brown fat can produce heat without producing useful energy in the form of ATP.

The neonate mobilizes glucose and fatty acids soon after delivery

Carbohydrate Metabolism The newborn depletes hepatic glycogen stores in the first 12 hours of life and is susceptible to hypoglycemia if feeding is delayed.

Low levels of blood glucose in the immediately postnatal period lead to a decrease in blood levels of **insulin** (see ⊙ 51-2) and a reciprocal increase of **glucagon** (see ⊙ 51-11). This hormonal milieu promotes the net release of glucose by the liver.

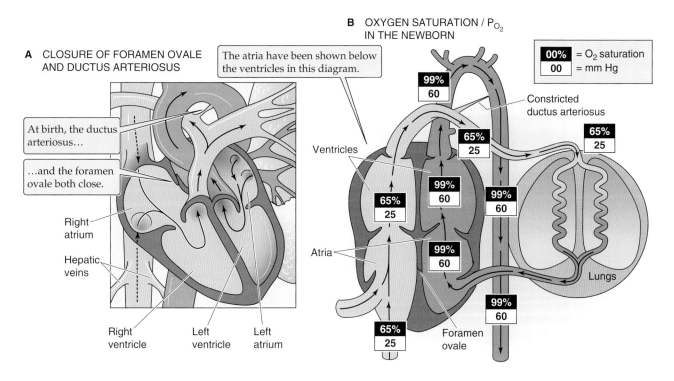

A CLOSURE OF FORAMEN OVALE AND DUCTUS ARTERIOSUS

The atria have been shown below the ventricles in this diagram.

B OXYGEN SATURATION / P$_{O_2}$ IN THE NEWBORN

At birth, the ductus arteriosus...

...and the foramen ovale both close.

Right atrium

Hepatic veins

Right ventricle

Left ventricle

Left atrium

00% = O$_2$ saturation
00 = mm Hg

Constricted ductus arteriosus

Ventricles

Atria

99% / 60

65% / 25

99% / 60

65% / 25

99% / 60

99% / 60

99% / 60

65% / 25

65% / 25

99% / 60

Foramen ovale

Lungs

Figure 57.2 Changes in the circulation at and around birth.

Fat Metabolism During the final 2 months of gestation, the fetus stores ~500 g of fat (i.e., ~15% of body weight), an important source of energy for the neonate. Decreased blood glucose just after birth raises levels of glucagon and epinephrine, which stimulate hormone-sensitive lipase in adipose tissue via cAMP (see ⊙ 58-9). This lipase breaks down triacylglycerols into glycerol and fatty acids (FAs), which enter the bloodstream. The liver can take up glycerol and ultimately synthesize glucose (i.e., gluconeogenesis).

Breast milk from a mother with a balanced diet satisfies all of the infant's nutritional requirements during the first several months of life

Provided the mother's diet is adequate during pregnancy, the newborn is in complete nutritional balance at birth. The newborn's natural nutrition for the first few days of life is **colostrum** (a milk-like substance secreted by the mammary glands), and thereafter it is **breast milk,** both of which the newborn's gastrointestinal tract can readily digest. The American Academy of Pediatrics recommends exclusive breast-feeding for the first 6 months, and then breast-feeding complemented with consumption of other foods until at least 1 year of age. If the infant is breast-fed, and if the mother's nutritional status is good, colostrum and breast milk meet all of the newborn's nutritional needs. Moreover, colostrum and breast milk make important contributions to the newborn's immune status. Both contain high concentrations of immunoglobulin A (or secretory) antibodies directed against bacteria and viruses, and they also contain macrophages. Breast milk contains factors that promote the growth of lactobacilli, which colonize the colon and may protect the infant from some virulent strains of *Escherichia coli.*

If the mother's dietary intake of iron is adequate during pregnancy, the infant's hepatic stores of **iron** will be adequate for hematopoiesis for 6 to 9 months following delivery.

The **calcium** in breast milk can meet the infant's needs for the rapid calcification of bones and teeth. Although the supply of calcium per se is unlikely to be a problem, **vitamin D** is necessary for the proper absorption of calcium by the intestines (see ⊙ 52-9). Vitamin D supplementation may be necessary if the newborn or the mother is not exposed to sufficient sunlight to generate vitamin D in the skin. Supplementation may also be required in formula-fed infants and in infants born prematurely. **Rickets** can develop rapidly in a vitamin D–deficient infant.

In premature newborns, immaturity of organ systems and fragility of homeostatic mechanisms exacerbate postnatal risks

The World Health Organization defines a **premature infant** as one born sooner than 37 weeks after the mother's last menstrual period, compared with the normal 40 weeks. Virtually all the challenges to the health of the neonate are made more severe by prematurity or intrauterine growth restriction, conditions that are therefore associated with reduced chances of survival. These problems generally reflect immaturity either of certain organ systems (e.g., lungs, intestines, liver, kidneys) or of homeostatic mechanisms (e.g., thermoregulation).

PHYSIOLOGY OF CELLS AND MOLECULES

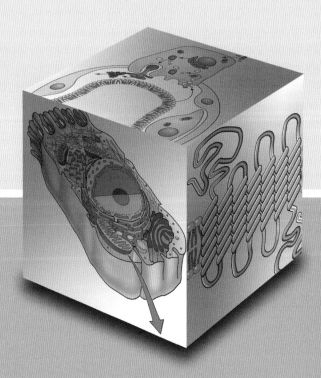

CHAPTER 58

METABOLISM

Gerald I. Shulman and Kitt Falk Petersen

58-1 Metabolism encompasses all chemical reactions necessary to sustain life in the body's cells. These chemical processes allow the body to grow, reproduce, maintain structure, and respond to changes in its environment. These processes can be **anabolic,** in which energy is used in the formation of substances such as proteins or nucleic acids, or **catabolic,** in which organic substances are broken down during cellular respiration to harvest energy to support cellular processes such as biosynthesis, transport of molecules or ions across cell membranes, or locomotion. A healthy, sedentary young man weighing 70 kg requires 2100 kcal (~30 kcal/kg body weight) to sustain resting metabolism for 1 day, an amount known as the **resting metabolic rate (RMR).** The number of calories increases with increased activity, illness, or other stress. The **basal metabolic rate (BMR)** is a clinical term for metabolism that is measured under standardized conditions in which the subject (1) has had a full night of restful sleep, (2) has been fasting for 12 hours, (3) is in a neutral thermal environment (see **59-5**), (4) has been resting physically for 1 hour, and (5) is free of psychic and physical stimuli. In adults the BMR (*units:* kilocalories per hour and per square meter of body surface area) is ~5% higher for males than for females and falls with age. The BMR is less than the RMR.

Regulation of energy metabolism in humans involves ingested nutrients, hormones, and interorgan exchanges of substrates to maintain a constant and adequate supply of fuel for all organs of the body. Because energy acquisition by the body is intermittent, whereas energy expenditure is continuous, the body needs to store and then parcel out energy in a carefully coordinated fashion. Insulin is the key hormone that orchestrates this exchange and distribution of substrates between tissues under fed and fasting conditions. Glucagon catecholamines, cortisol, and growth hormone play major roles in energy regulation at times of acute energy needs, which occur during exercise, under conditions of stress, or in response to hypoglycemia. The major organs involved in fuel homeostasis are (1) the liver, which is normally the major producer of glucose; (2) the brain, which in the fasted state is the major utilizer of glucose; and (3) the muscle and adipose tissue, which respond to insulin and store energy in the form of glycogen and fat, respectively.

FORMS OF ENERGY

Humans obtain their energy from food in three forms: (1) carbohydrates, (2) proteins, and (3) lipids. Moreover, each form consists of building blocks: monosaccharides (glucose, fructose, and galactose) for carbohydrates, amino acids for proteins, and fatty acids for lipids.

Carbohydrates, mainly in the form of glucose, contain 4.1 kcal/g of energy. The major storage form is **glycogen,** a polymer of glucose (10^6 to 10^8 Da) that consists of glucose molecules linked together by α-1,4 linkages in the straight portions of the polymer and by α-1,6 linkages at the frequent branch points (see Fig. 45.3). Virtually all cells of the body store glycogen; the highest concentrations occur in liver and muscle. Cells store glycogen in cytoplasmic granules that also contain the enzymes needed for glycogen synthesis and degradation. Glycogen is highly hydrophilic, containing 1 to 2 g of water per gram of glycogen, and thus provides a handy storage depot for glucose without affecting the osmotic pressure of the intracellular space. In contrast to the other potential stored forms of energy (lipid and protein), the liver can quickly break down glycogen by glycogenolysis to provide glucose for the brain during hypoglycemia.

58-2 The liver normally contains 75 to 100 g of glycogen but can store up to 135 g (9% of its weight) as glycogen. Muscle stores glycogen at much lower concentrations (1% to 1.5% of its weight). However, because of its larger mass, skeletal muscle has the largest store of glycogen in the body (nearly 300 g). A typical 70-kg human has up to ~400 g of glycogen (~0.6% of body weight). Thus, the total energy stored in the body in the form of glycogen can be about 1600 kcal (Table 58.1); this is enough to supply resting metabolism for less than a day, assuming 100% efficiency. Carbohydrate stores are essential because particularly the brain relies heavily on carbohydrates for fuel.

Proteins are linear polymers of L-amino acids, which have the general molecular structure $^+H_3N–HC(R)–COO^-$. Different functional R groups distinguish the 20 amino acids incorporated into nascent proteins during mRNA translation (Table 58.2). In α-amino acids, the amino group ($–NH_3^+$), the carboxyl group ($–COO^-$), and R all attach to the central or α-carbon atom. In proteins, the amino acids are linked together by peptide bonds that join the α-amino group of one amino acid with the α-carboxyl group of another. Nine of the amino acids are termed **essential amino acids** (Table 58.2) because the body cannot synthesize them at rates sufficient to sustain growth and normal functions. Thus, we must obtain these amino acids from our diet.

TABLE 58.1 Energy of Body Stores

CHEMICAL	WEIGHT (kg)	ENERGY DENSITY (kcal/g)	ENERGY (kcal)
Glycogen	0.7	1.5[a]	1,050
Protein	9.8/2 = 4.9[b]	4.3	21,000
Lipid	14	9.4	131,600

[a]Energy density of hydrated glycogen.
[b]Because only half of this protein can be mobilized as a fuel source, the total yield is only 21,000 kcal.

TABLE 58.2 Essential and Nonessential α-Amino Acids

ESSENTIAL	NONESSENTIAL
Histidine	Alanine
Isoleucine	Arginine
Leucine	Asparagine
Lysine	Aspartate
Methionine	Cysteine
Phenylalanine	Glutamate
Threonine	Glutamine
Tryptophan	Glycine
Valine	Proline
	Serine
	Tyrosine

Proteins contain 4.3 kcal/g, about the same as carbohydrates. A typical 70-kg human with 14% protein (9.8 kg)—only about half of which is available as a fuel source—can thus store ~21,000 kcal (Table 58.1) in the form of available protein. Unlike carbohydrate, protein is not a primary energy reserve in humans. Instead, proteins serve other important structural and functional roles. Structural proteins make up skin, collagen, ligaments, and tendons. Functional proteins include enzymes that catalyze reactions, muscle filaments such as myosin and actin, and various hormones. The body constantly breaks down proteins to amino acids, and vice versa, protein catabolism makes only a small contribution—much less than 5%—to normal resting energy requirements. During starvation, when carbohydrate reserves are exhausted, protein catabolism can contribute as much as 15% of the energy necessary to sustain the resting metabolic requirements by acting as major substrates for gluconeogenesis (see ◉ 58-4).

In the healthy human adult who is eating a weight-maintaining diet, amino acids derived from ingested protein replenish those proteins that have been oxidized in normal daily protein turnover. Once these protein requirements have been met, the body first oxidizes excess protein to CO_2 and then converts the remainder to glycogen or **triacylglycerols (TAGs).**

Lipids are the most concentrated form of energy storage because they represent, on average, 9.4 kcal/g. Lipids are dietary substances that typically occur in the form of TAGs. The gastrointestinal (GI) tract breaks down ingested TAGs (see ◉ 45-5) into **fatty acids (FAs)** and sn2-monoacylglycerols. FAs are composed of long carbon chains (14 to 24 carbon atoms) with a carboxyl terminus, and can be either *saturated* with hydrogen atoms or *unsaturated* (i.e., double bonds may connect one or more pairs of carbon atoms).

Fat is stored in a nonaqueous environment and therefore yields energy very close to its theoretical 9.4 kcal/g of TAGs. This greater efficiency of energy storage provided by fat is crucial for human existence to promote survival during famine. Therefore, fat serves as the major expendable fuel source. Most of the body's fat depots exist in the subcutaneous adipose tissue layers. A typical 70-k human with 20% fat (14 kg) thus carries 131,600 kcal of energy stored in adipose tissue (Table 58.1).

ENERGY BALANCE

Energy input to the body is the sum of energy output and storage

The **first law of thermodynamics** states that energy can be neither created nor destroyed; in a closed system, total energy is constant. This concept is illustrated in Fig. 58.1. Humans acquire all of their energy from ingested food, store it in different forms, and expend it in different ways. In the steady state, energy intake must equal energy output.

The GI tract breaks down ingested carbohydrates, proteins, and lipids into smaller components and then absorbs them into the bloodstream for transport to sites of metabolism.

◉ **58-3** The body's energy *inputs* must balance the sum of its energy *outputs* and the energy *stored*. When the body takes in more energy than it expends, the person is in **positive energy balance** and gains weight. Conversely, when energy intake is less than expenditure, this **negative energy balance** leads to weight loss, mostly from fat and, to a lesser extent, from protein in muscle.

A person can gain or lose weight by manipulating energy intake or output. An optimal strategy to encourage weight loss involves both increasing energy output and reducing energy intake.

Nitrogen balance—the algebraic sum of whole-body protein *degradation* and protein *synthesis*—is an indication of the *change* in whole-body protein stores. It is estimated from dietary protein intake and urinary nitrogen (i.e., urea) excretion.

The inefficiency of chemical reactions leads to loss of the energy available for metabolic processes

The **second law of thermodynamics** states that chemical transformations always result in a loss of the energy available to drive metabolic processes—the **Gibbs free energy (G).** The total internal energy (E) of the human body is the sum of the disposable or free energy (G) plus the unavailable or wasted energy, which ends up as heat (i.e., the product of absolute temperature, T, and entropy, S).

Some of the increased total energy will be stored as glycogen. However, because of the inefficiencies of the chemical reactions that convert glucose to glycogen, some of the total energy is wasted as heat.

Free energy, conserved as high-energy bonds in ATP, provides the energy for cellular functions

ATP consists of a nitrogenous ring (adenine), a 5-carbon sugar (ribose), and three phosphate groups. The last two phosphates are connected to the rest of the molecule by

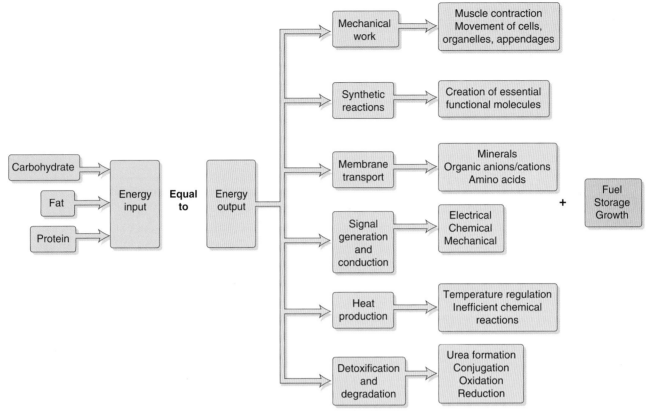

Figure 58.1 Energy balance.

high-energy bonds. The same is true for a related nucleotide, GTP. If we compare the free energies of phosphate bonds of various molecules, we see that the high-energy phosphate bonds of ATP lie toward the middle of the free-energy scale. Thus, in the presence of P_i, ADP can accept energy from compounds that are higher on the free-energy scale (e.g., phosphocreatine), whereas ATP can release energy in the formation of compounds that are lower on the free-energy scale (e.g., G6P). ATP can therefore *store* energy derived from energy-releasing reactions and *release* energy needed to drive other chemical reactions.

ENERGY INTERCONVERSION FROM CYCLING BETWEEN 6-CARBON AND 3-CARBON MOLECULES

Glycolysis converts the 6-carbon glucose molecule to two 3-carbon pyruvate molecules

The breakdown of glucose to pyruvate can occur in the presence of O_2 (aerobic glycolysis) or the absence of O_2 (anaerobic glycolysis). This process yields 47 kcal of free energy per mole of glucose. Of this energy, the cell can trap enough to yield directly 2 moles of ATP per mole of glucose, even under the relatively inefficient anaerobic conditions. Under *aerobic* conditions, the mitochondria can generate an additional three or five ATP molecules per glucose molecule from two **reduced nicotinamide adenine dinucleotide (NADH)** molecules.

Glycolysis occurs faster in anaerobic conditions than in aerobic conditions. This so-called **Pasteur effect** reflects the cell's attempt to maintain a constant $[ATP]_i$ by increasing the rate at which glycolysis breaks down glucose to generate ATP.

Under anaerobic conditions, cells convert pyruvate to lactate, which is accompanied by the accumulation of H+— **lactic acidosis.** This acidosis, in turn, can impede muscle contraction by decreasing muscle cell pH, which can result in muscle cramps and inhibition of key glycolytic enzymes needed for ATP synthesis.

⊙ 58-4 Gluconeogenesis converts nonhexose precursors to the 6-carbon glucose molecule

Gluconeogenesis is essential for life because the brain and **anaerobic tissues** (i.e., erythrocytes, leukocytes, bone marrow, and the renal medulla) normally depend on glucose as the primary fuel source. The daily glucose requirement of the brain in an adult is ~120 g, which accounts for most of the 180 g of glucose produced by the liver. The major site for gluconeogenesis is the liver, with the renal cortex making a much smaller contribution.

Although glycolysis converts glucose to pyruvate and gluconeogenesis converts pyruvate to glucose, gluconeogenesis is not simply glycolysis in reverse. The thermodynamic equilibrium of glycolysis lies strongly on the side of pyruvate formation. In contrast, gluconeogenesis requires energy, consuming four ATP, two GTP, and two NADH molecules for every glucose molecule formed. Gluconeogenesis bypasses three irreversible glycolytic reactions by using four different enzymes to reverse the overall direction to produce rather than to consume glucose.

The liver accomplishes gluconeogenesis by taking up, and converting to glucose, several nonhexose precursors, including lactate, pyruvate, and the major gluconeogenic amino acids **alanine** and **glutamine.**

The major gluconeogenic precursors are (1) lactate, which is derived from glycolysis in muscle and anaerobic tissues; (2) alanine, which is mostly derived from glycolysis and transamination of pyruvate in skeletal muscle; and (3) glycerol, which is derived from lipolysis in adipocytes.

Reciprocal regulation of glycolysis and gluconeogenesis minimizes futile cycling

The liver reciprocally and coordinately *regulates* the key glycolytic and gluconeogenic enzymes so that when one pathway (e.g., glycolysis) is active, the other pathway (gluconeogenesis in this case) is relatively inactive. Because glycolysis creates two ATP molecules and gluconeogenesis consumes four ATP and two GTP molecules, a full cycle from one glucose to two pyruvates and back again would have a net cost of two ATP and two GTP molecules. The liver regulates flux through these pathways in the short term mostly by allosteric regulation of enzyme activity, and in the long term by transcriptional regulation of gene expression.

Cells can convert glucose or amino acids into fatty acids

The liver can convert glucose to FAs. Glycolysis converts glucose to pyruvate, which can enter the mitochondrion via the **mitochondrial pyruvate carrier,** or **MPC.** When ATP demand is low, high levels of ATP, acetyl CoA, and NADH inside the mitochondria inhibit the enzyme that converts pyruvate to acetyl CoA—the normal entry point into the citric acid cycle (see Ⓞ 58-14). At the same time, high levels of ATP and acetyl CoA stimulate another enzyme that converts pyruvate to oxaloacetate, the last element in the citric acid cycle. The end result—in a process that requires the cytosolic enzyme **citrate lyase**—is to make acetyl CoA disappear from the mitochondrion and appear in the cytosol for FA synthesis.

Ⓞ **58-5** The rate-limiting step in FA synthesis is the conversion of acetyl CoA (2 carbons) to **malonyl CoA** (3 carbons). The next step is the sequential addition of 2-carbon units to a growing acyl chain, to produce an FA, catalyzed by **FA synthase.**

The cell esterifies the resulting FAs to glycerol to make **TAGs,** which the liver can package as **very-low-density lipoproteins** (VLDLs; see Ⓞ 46-7) for export to the blood.

The body permits only certain energy interconversions

The body has a hierarchy for energy interconversion. It can convert amino acids to glucose (gluconeogenesis) and fat, and it can convert glucose to fat and to certain amino acids. However, the body cannot convert fat to either glucose or amino acids. Fats can only be stored or oxidized. Thus, almost all carbon atoms in FAs end up as acetyl CoA, which enters the citric acid cycle.

ENERGY CAPTURE (ANABOLISM)

During feeding, the body stores excess calories as glycogen or fat. The process of digesting a mixed meal in the GI tract elevates the whole-body metabolic rate 20% to 25% higher than the RMR for ~90 minutes following a meal. In addition to this cost of digesting and absorbing, the energy cost of *storing* dietary carbohydrate as glycogen or dietary lipid as TAGs is 3% to 7% of the energy taken in. The cost of storing amino acids as protein is nearly 25% of the energy taken in. The cost of storing dietary carbohydrate as TAGs, or of storing amino acids as glycogen, is nearly 25% of the intake energy.

Ⓞ 58-6 After a carbohydrate meal, the body burns some ingested glucose and incorporates the rest into glycogen or TAGs

Three mechanisms maintain normoglycemia following carbohydrate ingestion: (1) suppression of hepatic glucose production; (2) stimulation of hepatic glucose uptake; and (3) stimulation of glucose uptake by peripheral tissues, predominantly muscle. Insulin (see Ⓞ 51-2) is the primary signal, which orchestrates the storage and metabolism of glucose via the insulin receptor. Glucose is the dominant signal for insulin secretion. With meals, other signals converge on the β cells of the pancreatic islets to coordinate insulin secretion. The incretins and neural signals prime the β cells, magnifying insulin release following meal-induced increases in blood glucose. This priming is absent when blood glucose increases as a result of hepatic glycogenolysis in response to stress.

Liver Following a carbohydrate meal, levels of insulin and glucose rise in the portal vein (similar to Fig. 51.1A), whereas glucagon levels fall. These changes suppress hepatic glucose production and promote net hepatic glucose uptake. Thus, the liver buffers the entry of glucose from the portal vein into the systemic circulation, thereby minimizing fluctuations in plasma [glucose] while promoting glucose storage. Once plasma [glucose] returns to baseline, the liver resumes net glucose production to maintain normoglycemia.

Ⓞ **58-7** Glucose taken up by the liver during the meal is predominantly stored as **glycogen.** The liver synthesizes glycogen by both a **direct pathway** from exogenous glucose and an **indirect pathway** from gluconeogenesis (Fig. 58.2A). When we ingest a meal following an overnight fast, these pathways contribute roughly equally to hepatic glycogen synthesis. A high-carbohydrate diet, hyperglycemia, and insulin promote the direct pathway, whereas reduced carbohydrate intake, lower plasma [glucose], and elevations in circulating [glucagon] stimulate the indirect pathway.

Because the liver has citrate lyase, it can also convert glucose that it takes up following a meal to FAs (Fig. 58.2A). The hepatocyte esterifies these FAs to glycerol to make **TAGs,** which it packages as **VLDLs** for export to the blood.

Muscle Glucose escaping the liver is cleared predominantly by striated muscle, which stores most of this glucose as glycogen (Fig. 58.2A). Muscle metabolizes the remaining glucose via the glycolytic pathway and then either oxidizes the products or recycles them to the liver, mostly as lactate and alanine.

A—CARBOHYDRATE MEAL

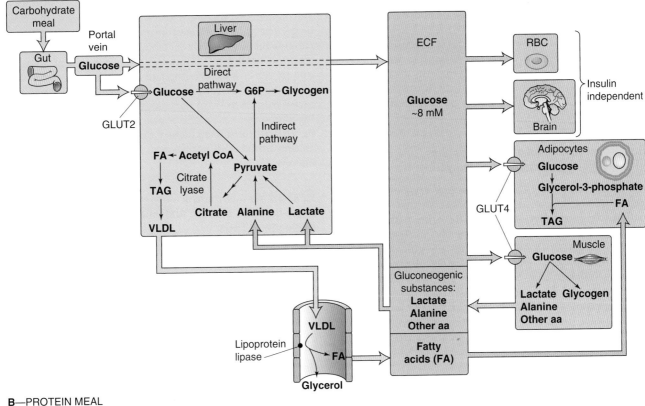

B—PROTEIN MEAL

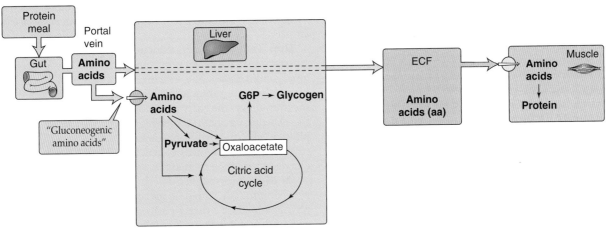

C—FATTY MEAL

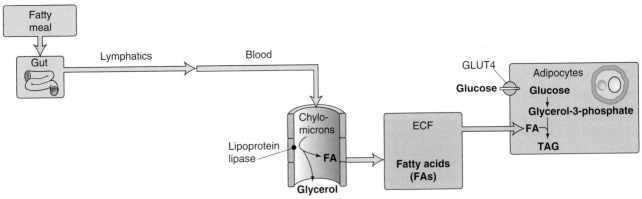

Figure 58.2   Energy storage following meals.

The uptake of glucose into muscle—as well as adipose tissue—is regulated predominantly by a rise in [insulin] and, to a lesser extent, by the hyperglycemia per se. Insulin, via the **phosphatidylinositol 3-kinase (PI3K)** pathway (see ⊙ **51-7**), promotes translocation of the **GLUT4** glucose transporter (see ⊙ **51-8**) to the plasma membrane, and stimulates glucose uptake by muscle and fat.

Adipose Tissue ⊙ **58-8** Although adipose tissue typically represents a large component of the peripheral mass (10% to 15% of body weight in men, 25% to 30% in women), adipocytes metabolize only a minor fraction of ingested glucose (Fig. 58.2C). The reason is that human adipocytes have a relatively low metabolic rate and contain relatively little citrate lyase, and thus have a low capability of converting glucose into FAs. However, adipocytes use glucose as the starting material for generating **glycerol-3-phosphate**, which serves as the backbone for TAG synthesis (Fig. 58.2A). In times of caloric and carbohydrate excess, the liver synthesizes FAs de novo from glucose and esterifies the FAs to generate TAGs, which it then exports in the form of VLDL particles (see Fig. 46.11). Lipoprotein lipase (LPL; see ⊙ **51-10**) hydrolyzes the TAGs in VLDLs and chylomicrons to FAs, which enter adipocytes for storage as TAGs.

After a protein meal, the body burns some ingested amino acids and incorporates the rest into proteins

Following a protein meal, the amino acids absorbed by the GI tract (see ⊙ **45-3**) have two major fates: they can either be oxidized to yield energy or be incorporated into protein. The liver removes a large fraction of amino acids that enter portal blood following a meal, particularly the gluconeogenic amino acids (Fig. 58.2B). In contrast, the liver less avidly removes the branched-chain amino acids (leucine, isoleucine, and valine), which muscle predominantly captures. Indeed, branched-chain amino acids are critical for the immediate repletion of muscle protein because they have a unique capacity to promote net protein accumulation, predominantly by inhibiting protein breakdown and to some extent by stimulating protein synthesis.

Insulin plays a major role in orchestrating protein anabolism, mostly by suppressing protein degradation. Therefore, the combination of the hyperinsulinemia and hyperaminoacidemia that follows a protein meal not only blocks proteolysis but also stimulates protein synthesis, resulting in net protein accumulation. Under such conditions, glucagon plays a critical role in preventing potential hypoglycemia by maintaining hepatic glucose production in the face of hyperinsulinemia.

After a fatty meal, the body burns some ingested FAs and incorporates the rest into TAGs

Following a fat-containing meal (Fig. 58.2C), lipases in the duodenum hydrolyze the TAGs to FAs and glycerol, which enterocytes in the small intestine take up, re-esterify into TAGs, and secrete as chylomicrons. The chylomicrons enter the lymphatics and then the systemic circulation.

Insulin, secreted in response to the carbohydrate or protein components of the meal, has three major effects on lipid metabolism. First, insulin induces synthesis of **LPL** (see ⊙ **51-10**), which promotes hydrolysis of TAGs to FAs and glycerol. The FAs enter the adipocytes for re-esterification into TAGs. Insulin promotes storage in muscle and adipose tissue of both *exogenous* TAGs (derived from a meal and carried in chylomicrons; Fig. 58.2C), and *endogenous* TAGs (produced by the liver and carried in VLDLs; Fig. 58.2A).

Second, insulin stimulates glucose uptake into adipocytes by stimulating **GLUT4.** The adipocytes transform the glucose to glycerol-3-phosphate (see ⊙ **58-8**), which is the backbone required for the re-esterification of FAs into TAGs.

⊙ **58-9** Third, in fat cells, insulin inhibits two enzymes that catalyze the hydrolysis of *stored* TAGs in adipocytes: **adipose triacylglycerol lipase (ATGL;** see ⊙ **51-9**), which releases an FA from a TAG to form a diacylglycerol, and **hormone-sensitive lipase (HSL),** which releases an FA from a DAG to form a monoacylglycerol.

ENERGY LIBERATION (CATABOLISM)

The general principle in energy catabolism is that the body first breaks down a complex storage polymer (e.g., glycogen or TAGs) to simpler compounds (e.g., glucose, FAs, lactate) that the cells can then metabolize to provide energy, mostly in the form of ATP, for cellular function.

The first step in energy catabolism is to break down glycogen or TAGs to simpler compounds

Skeletal Muscle ⊙ **58-10 Glycogenolysis** in skeletal muscle is catalyzed by glycogen phosphorylase (GP; Fig. 58.3A). In three ways, muscle contraction activates GP. First, **epinephrine** (see ⊙ **14-7**) binds to a β-adrenergic receptor and thereby promotes the formation of cAMP (see ⊙ **3-4**). The cAMP activates PKA, which in turn phosphorylates glycogen phosphorylase kinase (PK). In parallel, PKA inactivates phosphoprotein phosphatase 1 (see Fig. 3.5), thereby stabilizing the phosphorylated state of PK. The now active form of PK converts the inactive glycogen phosphorylase *b* (GPb) to the active **GPa.** Second, muscle activity increases the turnover of ATP, thereby raising $[AMP]_i$; the binding of AMP allosterically activates GPb. Third, intense activity of skeletal muscle causes $[Ca^{2+}]_i$ to rise; the binding of Ca^{2+} to PK allosterically activates this enzyme, and converts GPb to the active GPa. Skeletal muscle converts the product of glycogenolysis, glucose-1-phosphate (G1P), to G6P, which enters the glycolytic pathway within the muscle cell.

Liver ⊙ **58-11** GPa in hepatocytes converts glycogen to G1P. The signaling pathways that establish the GPa/GPb ratio are the same as in muscle, except that in the liver, it is mainly **glucagon** (see ⊙ **51-11**) in the portal blood—and, to a lesser extent, epinephrine—that triggers the increase in $[cAMP]_i$ (Fig. 58.3B). The liver then converts G1P to G6P, as in muscle. The liver contains the enzyme **G6Pase,** which cleaves the phosphate from G6P to yield glucose. Whereas glycogenolysis in skeletal muscle serves to meet *local* energy demands by releasing G6P, glycogenolysis in the liver serves

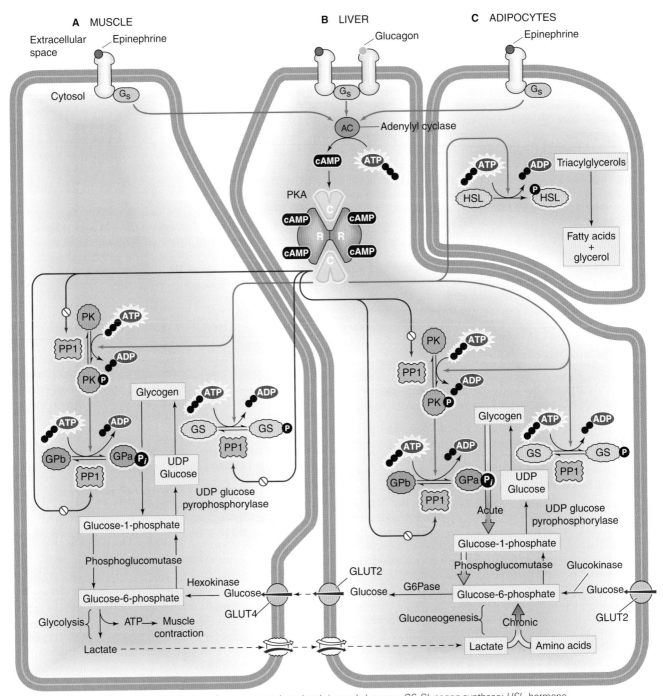

Figure 58.3 Mobilization of energy stores by epinephrine and glucagon. *GS,* Glycogen synthase; *HSL,* hormone-sensitive triacylglycerol lipase; *UDP,* uridine diphosphate. *Yellow halos* surround the active forms of enzymes.

to meet whole-body energy demands—mainly those of the central nervous system (CNS)—by releasing glucose to the *blood.*

Adipocytes ⊙ **58-12** In adipocytes, HSL catalyzes **lipolysis,** the hydrolysis of the ester linkages of TAGs to release FAs and glycerol. Nearly all (95%) of the available energy of TAGs resides in the FA moieties. Two hormones can stimulate lipolysis: **epinephrine,** which the adrenal medulla secretes under conditions of low blood glucose or stress, and **growth hormone** (see ⊙ **48-2**). Epinephrine acts through cAMP (Fig. 58.3C) to activate HSL and release FAs.

⊙ 58-13 The second step in TAG catabolism is β-oxidation of FAs

In carbohydrate catabolism, after the breakdown of glycogen, the second step is glycolysis. In TAG metabolism, after the breakdown to FAs, the second step is the β-oxidation of FAs, which takes place in the mitochondrial matrix. Before β-oxidation, the hepatocyte uses **FA transport protein 5** (**FATP5** or SLC27A5) to transport the FA from the extracellular fluid into the cytosol (Fig. 58.4), where **acyl CoA synthase** activates the FA to **acyl CoA** (i.e., the FA chain coupled to CoA). In a complex series of events (Fig. 58.4), this acyl CoA disappears

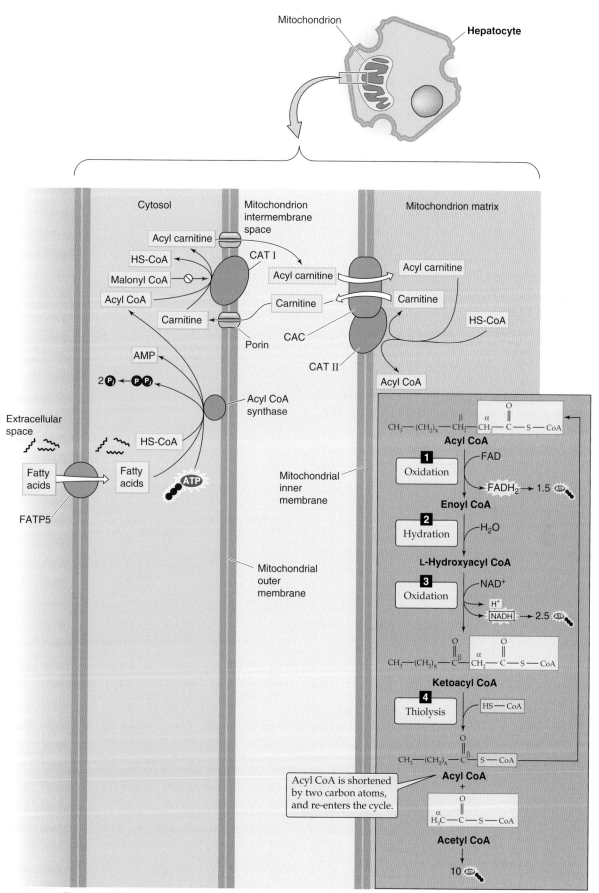

Figure 58.4 FA transport into mitochondrion and β-oxidation. *FAD/FADH₂*, Oxidized and reduced forms of flavin adenine dinucleotide, respectively; *NAD⁺/NADH*, oxidized and reduced forms of nicotinamide adenine dinucleotide, respectively.

from the cytosol and the acyl group reappears in the mitochondrial matrix (though linked to a different CoA) To deliver acyl CoA to the mitochondrial matrix, the cell uses **carnitine acyltransferase I (CAT I)** on the cytosolic side of the mitochondrial outer membrane to transfer the acyl group to carnitine. The resulting acylcarnitine moves through a porin in the mitochondrial outer membrane to enter the intermembrane space. The **carnitine/acylcarnitine transporter (CAC)** on the mitochondrial inner membrane moves acylcarnitine into the mitochondrial matrix. There, CAT II transfers the acyl group back to CoA to form acyl CoA and carnitine. The carnitine recycles to the cytosol via CAC and the porin, whereas the acyl CoA undergoes β-oxidation.

β-oxidation is a multistep process that removes a 2-carbon fragment from the end of an acyl CoA and releases the fragment as an acetyl CoA (Fig. 58.4). β-oxidation continues until it consumes the entire FA chain. The final cycle generates two acetyl CoA molecules. Unlike the breakdown of glucose, which can yield ATP even in the absence of O_2 (via glycolysis), the catabolism of FAs to yield energy in the form of ATP can occur only in the presence of O_2.

When energy levels are high, the cell generates malonyl CoA (see ⊚ 58-5) in the first committed step for FA *synthesis*. In contrast, malonyl inhibits CAT I and thereby inhibits β-*oxidation* (Fig. 58.4).

The final common steps in oxidizing carbohydrates, TAGs, and proteins to CO_2 are the citric acid cycle and oxidative phosphorylation

Under aerobic conditions, cells containing mitochondria typically convert most of the pyruvate they generate from carbohydrate metabolism to acetyl CoA, rather than to lactate. Pyruvate moves from the cytoplasm into the mitochondrial matrix for conversion to acetyl CoA. Acetyl CoA also forms in the mitochondria as the end product of the β-oxidation of FAs as well as amino-acid breakdown. The metabolism of the acetate moiety of acetyl CoA is the final common pathway of **aerobic catabolism,** which releases CO_2, H_2O, ATP, and heat.

Citric Acid Cycle ⊚ 58-14 A 2-carbon fragment—acetyl CoA—derived from glucose, FA, or amino-acid metabolism enters the citric acid cycle. The citric acid cycle conserves the liberated energy as GTP and the reduced electron carriers NADH and $FADH_2$. Cells tightly control the citric acid cycle by three *mechanisms*: substrate availability, product accumulation, and feedback inhibition of key enzymes.

Oxidative Phosphorylation ⊚ 58-15 The process by which mitochondria retrieve energy from $FADH_2$ and NADH is oxidative phosphorylation. These reduced nucleotides are products of glycolysis, β-oxidation (Fig. 58.4) conversion of pyruvate to acetyl CoA, and the citric acid cycle. Oxidative phosphorylation involves the transfer of electrons along a chain of molecules, and it ultimately traps the releasing energy in the formation of 1.5 ATP molecules per $FADH_2$ and 2.5 ATP molecules per NADH.

Ketogenesis ⊚ 58-16 Conditions such as prolonged fasting, consumption of a low-carbohydrate diet, or untreated diabetes mellitus lead to the production of three water-soluble byproducts of incomplete FA oxidation, substances collectively known as **ketone bodies:** acetoacetate, β-hydroxybutyrate, and acetone. The accelerated β-oxidation of FAs produces acetyl CoA faster than the citric acid cycle can consume it. As a result, excess

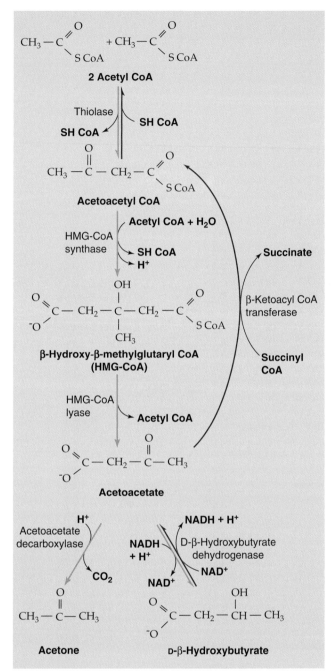

Figure 58.5 Ketogenesis and metabolism of ketone bodies. NAD^+/ NADH oxidized and reduced forms of nicotinamide adenine dinucleotide, respectively.

acetyl CoA spills over into the production of the three ketone bodies, primarily by liver mitochondria (Fig. 58.5, *downward orange arrows*). The first three reactions in ketogenesis have the net effect of condensing two molecules of acetyl CoA and one H_2O into one molecule of **acetoacetate,** two molecules of HS CoA, and one H^+. Thus, uncontrolled ketogenesis, which occurs in the absence of insulin (e.g., diabetic ketoacidosis), causes a metabolic acidosis (see ⊚ 28-6). The second and third reactions are essentially irreversible. Next, the liver can either reduce acetoacetate to **D-β-hydroxybutyrate** or decarboxylate the acetoacetate to **acetone.**

Extrahepatic tissues can consume either one D-β-hydroxybutyrate or one acetoacetate molecule (Fig. 58.5,

TABLE 58.3 Respiratory Quotients of the Major Foodstuffs

	ENERGY DENSITY (kcal/g)	RQ
Carbohydrate	4.1	1.00
Protein	4.3	0.80–0.85
Lipid	9.4	0.70

upward red arrows) to produce two acetyl CoA molecules that can then enter the citric acid cycle. Catalyzing the key step is β-**ketoacyl CoA transferase,** which is not present in hepatocytes.

Oxidizing different fuels yields similar amounts of energy per unit O_2 consumed

The **energy yield per unit of O_2** is only slightly greater for carbohydrate (5.0 kcal/L of O_2) than for lipid (4.7 kcal/L O_2). Carbohydrate, with its greater energy yield per O_2, is the body's preferred fuel for combustion during maximal exercise when O_2 availability is limited. However, fat is the preferred fuel during prolonged activity, when O_2 is available and fuel sources are abundant.

The metabolism of glucose by *aerobic* glycolysis and the citric acid cycle is far more efficient in providing energy in the form of ATP than *anaerobic* glycolysis in that complete oxidation of 1 molecule of glucose to CO_2 and H_2O via oxidative metabolism provides 30 to 32 molecules of ATP, whereas metabolism of 1 molecule of glucose to lactate by anaerobic glycolysis yields only ~2 molecules of ATP. However, anaerobic glycolysis has the major advantage of being able to supply much more ATP *per unit time* than oxidative metabolism of glucose or fat.

In the case of FA metabolism (Fig. 58.4), each cycle of β-oxidation yields a total of 14 ATP molecules. The total number of ATP molecules generated from the FA depends on the number of carbon atoms in the FA chain. For example, palmitic acid, a 16-carbon FA, needs seven β-oxidation cycles to form eight acetyl CoA molecules. The seven cycles generate 7 × 14 = 98 ATPs. The leftover acetyl CoA represents an additional 10 ATPs, for a total of 108 ATPs.

For each primary fuel source, Table 58.3 provides the **respiratory quotient (RQ;** see Equation 31.10) or ratio of moles of CO_2 produced per mole of O_2 consumed at the tissue level. The RQ reflects the density of oxygen atoms in the fuel source.

INTEGRATIVE METABOLISM DURING FASTING

The human body has two main priorities for energy liberation during fasting.

The first priority is to maintain a stable supply of energy for CNS function. The brain has little stored energy in the form of glycogen or TAGs and therefore depends on the liver (and under some circumstances the kidney) for a constant supply of energy in the form of glucose or ketone bodies (see ⊙ 58-16). In the fed state and early in the fasting state, the brain derives essentially all its energy from oxidation of glucose because ketone bodies are not present and the blood-brain barrier is mostly impermeable to FAs. Because a continuous supply of glucose is required to meet the energy demands of the CNS, humans have evolved elaborate, redundant mechanisms to maintain plasma [glucose] within a very narrow range, between 60 and 140 mg/dL (3.3 to 7.8 mM), between fasting and fed states.

Most other major organs of the body (liver, skeletal muscle, heart, kidney) fill their energy needs at this time by oxidizing FAs. In contrast to the well-regulated plasma [glucose], the concentrations of FAs and ketone bodies can vary by 10- and 100-fold, respectively, depending on the fed and fasted conditions. During prolonged fasting (>2 days), the liver metabolizes FAs to raise plasma levels of ketone bodies sufficiently to supply much of the brain's oxidative fuel needs and diminish the need for gluconeogenic substrate supply by proteolysis.

The second priority for the body is to maintain its protein reserves (i.e., contractile proteins, enzymes, nervous tissue, etc.) in times of fasting.

The body also has two main priorities for energy repletion after fasting. First, following a meal, liver and muscle replenish their limited glycogen reserves. Once these stores are full, liver and muscle convert any excess energy in the form of carbohydrate and protein to fat. The second priority during feeding is to replenish protein reserves.

During an overnight fast, glycogenolysis and gluconeogenesis maintain plasma glucose levels

The period after an overnight fast serves as a useful reference point because it represents the period before the transition from the fasted to the fed state. At this time, the concentrations of insulin, glucagon, and metabolic substrates that were altered by meal ingestion during the preceding day have returned to their basal levels.

Requirement for Glucose After an overnight fast, the decline in circulating insulin leads to a marked decrease in glucose uptake by insulin-sensitive tissues (e.g., muscle) and a shift toward the use by these tissues of FAs mobilized from fat stores. Maintaining plasma [glucose] in the presence of this ongoing glucose use, particularly by the brain, requires that the body produce glucose at rates sufficient to match its ongoing consumption.

Gluconeogenesis Versus Glycogenolysis Four to 5 hours after a meal (perhaps longer for a very large meal), a fall in plasma [insulin] (see ⊙ 51-2) and a rise in [glucagon] (see ⊙ 51-11) cause the liver to begin breaking down its stores of glycogen and releasing it as glucose. Moreover, both the liver and, to a lesser extent, the kidney generate glucose by gluconeogenesis. Net hepatic glycogenolysis and gluconeogenesis each contribute ~50% of whole-body glucose production during the first several hours of a fast.

Gluconeogenesis: The Cori Cycle ⊙ 58-17 In the first several hours of a fast, the brain consumes glucose at the rate of 4 to 5 g/hr, which is two thirds the rate of hepatic glucose production (~180 g/day). Obligate anaerobic tissues also metabolize glucose but convert it primarily to lactate and pyruvate. The liver takes up these products and uses gluconeogenesis to regenerate glucose at the expense of energy.

Gluconeogenesis: The Glucose-Alanine Cycle ⊙ 58-18 After an overnight fast, the body as a whole is in negative nitrogen balance, with muscle and splanchnic tissues being the principal sites of protein degradation and release of amino acids into the blood. During fasting, breakdown

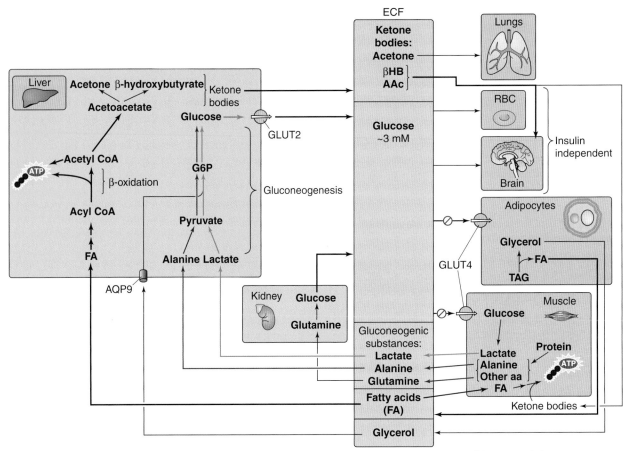

Figure 58.6 Metabolism during prolonged starvation. *aa,* Amino acids; *AAc,* acetoacetate; *AQP9,* aquaporin 9; *ECF,* extracellular fluid; *βHB,* β-hydroxybutyrate; *RBC,* red blood cell.

of muscle protein yields amino acids, which subsequently transfer their amino groups to α-ketoglutarate (supplied by the citric acid cycle) to form glutamate. Glutamine synthase can then add a second amino group to glutamate, thereby producing glutamine. Alternatively, alanine aminotransferase can transfer the amino group of glutamate to pyruvate (the product of glucose breakdown), generating alanine and α-ketoglutarate.

The amino acids taken up by the liver provide carbon for gluconeogenesis. On a molar basis, alanine is the principal amino acid taken up by the liver. Because the carbon backbone of alanine came from glucose metabolism in muscle, and the liver regenerates glucose from this alanine, the net effect is a **glucose-alanine cycle** between muscle and liver, analogous to the Cori cycle.

In addition to playing a role in gluconeogenesis, the glucose-alanine cycle is critical for **nitrogen metabolism** and thus provides a nontoxic alternative to ammonia for transferring amino groups—derived from muscle amino-acid catabolism—to the liver. The hepatocytes now detoxify the amino groups on alanine and other amino acids by generating urea (see Fig. 46.10), which the kidney then excretes. Another key amino acid in nitrogen metabolism is glutamine, which muscle releases into the blood for uptake by the gut and liver as well as the kidney. The kidney uses the carbon skeleton of glutamine for renal gluconeogenesis and converts the amino group to ammonia, which it excretes.

This ammonia excretion is particularly important in maintaining body acid-base balance during fasting. Combined, alanine and glutamine account for >40% of the amino-acid carbon used by liver and kidneys in gluconeogenesis.

Lipolysis Finally, the fall in plasma [insulin] after an overnight fast permits the release of FAs and glycerol from fat stores (see Fig. 51.6). This response appears to be more pronounced in visceral than peripheral fat depots. The decline in [insulin] and the ensuing lipolysis are sufficient to supply FAs to extracerebral tissues (e.g., muscle, heart, liver) for fuel and glycerol to the liver for gluconeogenesis. However, these changes are not sufficient to stimulate the hepatic conversion of FA to ketone bodies (see ◉ 58-16).

The body never completely suppresses gluconeogenesis. When an individual ingests a meal, gluconeogenic flux provides glucose for hepatic glycogen stores (*indirect pathway;* see ◉ 58-7). During fasting, the liver redirects the gluconeogenic flux to provide glucose for delivery to the circulation.

Starvation beyond an overnight fast enhances both gluconeogenesis and lipolysis.

Prolonged starvation moderates proteolysis but accelerates lipolysis, thereby releasing ketone bodies

As the duration of fasting increases, the body shifts from using its limited protein stores for gluconeogenesis to using its relatively large energy depots in fat for ketogenesis (Fig. 58.6).

Moreover, the brain shifts from oxidizing glucose to oxidizing two ketone bodies (see ⊙ **58-16**), β-hydroxybutyrate and acetoacetate, to meet most of its energy requirements.

Decreased Proteolysis Prolonged survival during starvation requires a major reduction in proteolysis. Indeed, urea excretion decreases from 10 to 15 g/day during the initial days of a fast to <1 g/day after 6 weeks of fasting. Because urea is the major obligatory osmolyte in the urine (see Fig. 38.3), this reduced urea production lessens obligatory water excretion and the daily water requirement.

Decreased Hepatic Gluconeogenesis The transition from protein to lipid degradation permits humans to extend their survival time during a prolonged fast from weeks to months, as long as fat stores are available and water intake is adequate. During this transition, hepatic gluconeogenesis decreases (Fig. 58.6), mostly because of diminished substrate delivery.

Increased Renal Gluconeogenesis Whereas hepatic gluconeogenesis falls, renal gluconeogenesis rises (Fig. 58.6) to reach as much as 40% of whole-body glucose production. Renal gluconeogenesis, which consumes H^+, most likely is an adaptation to the acidosis that accompanies ketogenesis (see ⊙ **58-16**). Indeed, acidosis stimulates renal ammoniagenesis in parallel with renal gluconeogenesis.

Increased Lipolysis and Ketogenesis During the first 3 to 7 days of fasting, hypoinsulinemia accelerates the mobilization of FAs from adipose tissue. As a result, plasma FA levels double and remain stable thereafter. The combination of low insulin and high glucagon (see ⊙ **51-12**) levels also increases hepatic oxidation of FAs, leading to a marked increase of hepatic ketogenesis (Fig. 58.6) or *ketogenic capacity*. The liver achieves peak rates of ketone body production (~100 g/day) by the third day and maintains them thereafter. Low insulin levels also progressively reduce the extraction of ketone bodies by peripheral tissues. The CNS receives an increasing supply of these water-soluble substrates, which eventually account for more than one half of the brain's energy requirements. Ketone bodies ultimately supplant the brain's dependency on glucose and, by limiting the brain's gluconeogenic demands, the body preserves protein stores.

As the fast progresses and fat stores are depleted, levels of leptin (see ⊙ **48-11**) decrease. This decrease is a protective signal that affects the hypothalamic-pituitary-gonadal axis, reducing the oscillations of luteinizing hormone and follicle-stimulating hormone and causing anovulation. In times of famine, this mechanism protects fertile women from the additional nutritional demands associated with pregnancy.

CHAPTER 59

REGULATION OF BODY TEMPERATURE

Shaun F. Morrison

HEAT AND TEMPERATURE: ADVANTAGES OF HOMEOTHERMY

Homeotherms maintain their activities over a wide range of environmental temperatures

The stable body temperature of homeotherms (species that regulate internal body temperature) is the consequence of neural networks that incorporate both anticipatory and negative-feedback controls. This arrangement creates an internal environment in which chemical reaction rates are relatively high and optimal and avoids the pathological consequences of wide fluctuations in body temperature (Table 59.1). The fundamental thermoregulatory system includes (1) thermal sensors; (2) thermosensory afferent pathways; (3) an integration system in the central nervous system (CNS); (4) efferent pathways; and (5) thermal effectors capable of heat generation (i.e., thermogenesis), such as brown adipose tissue and skeletal muscle (shivering), or effectors that modulate heat transfer, such as the circulation to the skin (which dissipates heat) and the sweat glands (which augment heat loss).

Body core temperature depends on time of day, physical activity, time in the menstrual cycle, and age

Temperature is a measure of heat content. The "normal" body temperature of an adult human is ~37°C (98.6°F), but it may be as low as 36°C or as high as 37.5°C in active, healthy people. *Body temperature* usually refers to the temperature of the internal body *core,* measured under the tongue (sublingually), in the ear canal, or in the rectum. For clinical purposes, the most reliable (although the least practical) among these three is the last, because it is least influenced by ambient (air) temperature. Measurement devices range from traditional mercury-in-glass thermometers to electronic digital-read-out thermistors. Nearly all such instruments are accurate to 0.1°C. The least invasive approach uses an infrared thermometer to measure the radiant temperature (see ⊙ 59-4) over the temporal artery.

Body core temperature (T_{core}) depends on many factors that alter either the activity of the CNS thermoregulatory network or the level of metabolism and heat content of the body, including the time of day, the stage of the menstrual cycle in women, and the individual's age.

All homeotherms maintain a circadian rhythm (~24-hour cycle) of body temperature, with variations of ~1°C. In humans, body temperature is usually lowest between 3:00 and 6:00 AM and peaks at 3:00 to 6:00 PM. The circadian rhythmicity in physiological variables is governed by groups of neurons in the suprachiasmatic nucleus in the anterior hypothalamus, whose activity is entrained by light-dark cues to a ~24-hour cycle but is independent of the sleep-wake cycle.

Reproductive hormones, and the CNS circuits that govern their production, influence the CNS thermoregulatory network. Indeed, in many women, body temperature increases ~0.5°C during the postovulatory phase of the menstrual cycle (see ⊙ 55-1). An abrupt increase in body temperature of 0.3°C to 0.5°C accompanies ovulation and may be useful as a fertility guide.

Infants and older people are less able than other age groups to maintain a stable normal body temperature, particularly in the face of external challenges. Newborns do not readily shiver or sweat and have a high surface-to-mass ratio, which renders them more susceptible to fluctuations in core temperature when exposed to hot or cold environments. However, they have large deposits of brown adipose tissue, which the sympathetic nervous system can stimulate to generate heat for cold defense.

Older people are also subject to greater fluctuations in core temperature. Aging is associated with a progressive deficit in the ability to sense heat and cold (see ⊙ 62-7), as well as reduced ability to generate heat (reduced metabolic rate and metabolic potential because of lower muscle mass) and to dissipate heat (reduced cardiovascular reserve and sweat gland atrophy from disuse).

The body's rate of heat production can vary from ~70 kcal/hr at rest to 600 kcal/hr during exercise

The body's metabolic rate, and thus its rate of heat production, is not constant. The **resting metabolic rate (RMR;** see ⊙ 58-1) is the energy consumption necessary to maintain the basal functions of resting cells, such as active solute transport across membranes as well as the activity of cardiac and respiratory muscles necessary for organismal survival. RMR is influenced by age, sex, circadian phase, season, digestive state, phylogeny, body size, and habitat. At an RQ of 0.8 (see Equation 31.10 and Table 58.3), the average person under sedentary (i.e., RMR) conditions has a resting V_{O_2} of 250 mL/min, which corresponds to an energy production of 72 kcal/hr (~85 watts)—dissipated as heat, as if the body were a zero-efficiency, 85-watt incandescent light bulb.

During physical exercise, an average adult can comfortably sustain an energy-consumption rate of 400 to 600 kcal/hr (e.g., a fast walk or a modest jog) for extended periods. A thermal load of this magnitude would raise core temperature by 1.0°C every 8 to 10 minutes if the extra heat could not escape the body. Physical activity would be limited to 25 to 30 minutes, at which time the effects of excessive hyperthermia (>40°C) would begin to impair body function. This impairment, of course, does not usually occur, primarily because of the effectiveness of the thermoregulatory heat-defense system.

⊙ 59-1 MODES OF HEAT TRANSFER

Maintaining a relatively constant body temperature requires a fine balance between heat production and heat losses

If body temperature is to remain unchanged, increases or decreases in heat production must be balanced by increases or decreases in heat loss, resulting in negligible heat storage within the body. If the body is at constant mass, the whole-body **heat-balance equation** expresses this concept as follows:

$$\underbrace{(M - W)}_{\text{Heat production (H)}} - \underbrace{(R + C + E)}_{\text{Heat losses}} = S$$

where Metabolism − Work done on environment − (Radiative heat loss + Convective heat loss + Evaporative heat loss) = Storage of heat

(59.1)

All terms in the foregoing equation have the units kcal/hr. **Metabolism (M)** is the consumption of energy from the cellular oxidation of carbohydrates, fats, and proteins. For an athlete, the **useful work on the environment (W)** might be the energy imparted to a soccer ball. However, because of a long list of inefficiencies, most metabolic energy consumption ends up as **heat production** (H = M − W).

Under conditions of maximal exercise (see Fig. 60.4), the rate of heat production could be 800 kcal/hr (~960 watts) for a brief period of time. Unless the body can dissipate this heat, death from hyperthermia and heat stroke (Table 59.1) would ensue rapidly.

Virtually all heat leaving the body must exit through the skin surface. In the following three sections, we consider the three major routes of heat elimination: **radiation (R), convection (C),** and **evaporation (E)**. As the heat-balance equation shows, the difference between heat production (M − W) and heat losses (R + C + E) is the **rate of heat storage (S)** within the body. The value of S may be positive or negative, depending on whether (M − W) > (R + C + E) or vice versa. A positive value of S results in a rise of T_{core}, such as during exercise, whereas a negative value of S results in a fall in T_{core}, as would occur shortly after entering very cold water.

Heat moves from the body core to the skin, primarily by convection

⊙ **59-2** Generally, all heat production occurs within the body's tissues, and all heat elimination occurs at the body surface. Fig. 59.1 illustrates a **passive system** in which heat flows depend on the size, shape, and composition of the body, as well as on the laws of physics. The circulating blood carries heat away from active tissues, such as muscle, to the body core—represented by the heart, lungs, and their central

TABLE 59.1 Consequences of Deviations in Body Temperature

TEMPERATURE (°C)	CONSEQUENCE
40–44	Heat stroke with multiple organ failure and brain lesions
38–40	Hyperthermia (as a result of fever or exercise)
36–38	Normal range
34–36	Mild hypothermia
30–34	Impairment of temperature regulation
27–29	Cardiac fibrillation

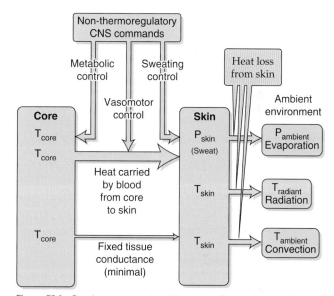

Figure 59.1 Passive or unregulated heat transfer. In the steady state, the rate of heat production by the body core must match the flow of heat from the core to the skin, and from the skin to the environment.

circulating blood volume. How does the body prevent its core from overheating? The answer is that the core transfers this heat to a dissipating heat sink. The organ serving as the body's greatest potential heat sink is the relatively cool **skin,** which is the largest organ in the body. Only a minor amount of the body's generated heat flows *directly* from the underlying body core to the skin by **conduction** across the body tissues. Most of the generated body heat flows in the blood—by **convection**—to the skin, and blood flow to the skin can increase markedly during heat defense. There, nearly all heat transferred to the skin will flow to the environment, as discussed in the next section.

The transfer of heat from core to skin occurs by passive conduction and by convection via blood.

Both conduction and convection are proportional to the temperature gradient from core to skin ($T_{core} - T_{skin}$), where T_{skin} is the average skin temperature. On very hot days, when skin temperature may be very high and close to T_{core}, even high skin blood flow may not be adequate to transfer sufficient heat to allow T_{core} to stabilize because the temperature gradient ($T_{core} - T_{skin}$) is too small.

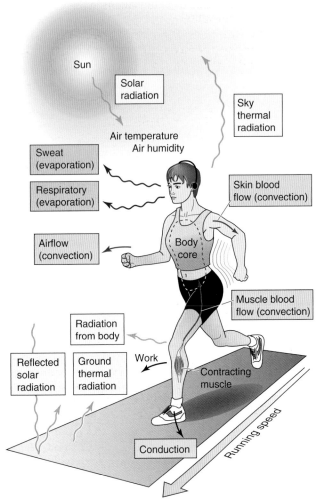

Figure 59.2 Model of energy transfer between the body and the environment.

59-3 Heat moves from the skin to the environment by radiation, conduction, convection, and evaporation

Fig. 59.2 is a graphic summary of the heat-balance equation (see Equation 59.1) for an athlete exercising in an outdoor environment. This illustration depicts the movement of heat within the body, its delivery to the skin surface, and its subsequent elimination to the environment by radiation, convection, and evaporation.

Radiation ⊙ **59-4** Heat transfer by radiation occurs between the skin and solid bodies in the environment. The exchange (gain or loss) of body heat with another object by radiation occurs at a rate that is proportional to the temperature difference between the skin and the object:

Rate of radiative heat loss		Radiative heat-transfer coefficient	Mean skin temp	Radiant temp of another object	Body surface area available for radiative heat exchange	**(59.2)**

$$\underbrace{R}_{\frac{kcal}{hr}} = \underbrace{h_{\text{radiative}}}_{\frac{kcal}{hr \times °C \times m^2}} \cdot \underbrace{(\overline{T}_{\text{skin}} - T_{\text{radiant}})}_{°C} \cdot \underbrace{A_{\text{radiative}}}_{m^2}$$

R is positive when the body loses heat and negative when it gains heat.

⊙ **59-5** The **radiant heat load** from the sun to the body on a cloudless summer day may exceed the RMR by a considerable amount. Conversely, on a winter evening, the **radiant heat loss** from the body to a cloudless, dark sky—which has a low radiant temperature—may exceed RMR. Thus, when walking past an uncurtained window, one may feel a sudden chill, caused by the sudden fall in skin temperature owing to increased radiant heat loss. Radiation of heat from the body accounts for ~60% of heat lost when the body is at rest in a neutral thermal indoor environment. A **neutral thermal environment** is a set of conditions (air temperature, airflow and humidity, and temperatures of surrounding radiating surfaces) in which the temperature of the body does not change when the subject is at rest (i.e., RMR) and is not shivering.

Conduction Heat transfer by conduction occurs when the body touches a solid material of different temperature. For example, lying on the hot sand causes one to gain heat by conduction. Conversely, placing an ice pack on a sore muscle causes heat loss by conduction.

Convection Heat transfer by convection occurs when a medium such as air or water carries the heat between the body and the environment. The convective heat loss is proportional to the difference between skin and ambient temperature:

Rate of convective heat loss		Convective heat-transfer coefficient	Mean skin temp	Ambient temp	Body surface area available for convective heat exchange	**(59.3)**

$$\underbrace{C}_{\frac{kcal}{hr}} = \underbrace{h_{\text{convective}}}_{\frac{kcal}{hr \times °C \times m^2}} \cdot \underbrace{(\overline{T}_{\text{skin}} - T_{\text{ambient}})}_{°C} \cdot \underbrace{A_{\text{convective}}}_{m^2}$$

C is positive when the body loses heat, and negative when it gains heat.

Whereas the radiative heat-transfer coefficient ($h_{\text{radiative}}$) is constant, the convective coefficient ($h_{\text{convective}}$) is variable and can increase up to 5-fold when air velocity is high. In the absence of air movement, the air immediately overlying the skin warms as heat leaves the skin. As this warmer and lighter air rises off the skin, cooler ambient air replaces it and, in turn, is warmed by the skin. This is the process of **natural convection**. However, with forced air movement, such as by wind or a fan, the cooler "ambient" air replaces the warmer air overlying the skin more rapidly. This change increases the effective convective heat transfer from the skin, even though the temperature of the ambient air is unchanged. This is a process of **forced convection**, which underlies the **wind chill factor**.

Evaporation ⊙ **59-6** Humans can dissipate nearly all the heat produced during exercise by evaporating sweat (see ⊙ **60-3**) from the skin surface. The evaporative rate is independent of the temperature gradient between skin and environment. Instead, it is proportional to the water vapor-pressure gradient between skin and environment:

Rate of evaporative heat loss		Evaporative heat-transfer coefficient	H_2O vapor pressure of skin	H_2O vapor pressure of environment	Body surface area available for evaporative heat exchange	

$$\underbrace{E}_{\frac{kcal}{hr}} = \underbrace{h_{\text{evaporative}}}_{\frac{kcal}{hr \times mm\, Hg \times m^2}} \cdot \underbrace{(P_{\text{skin}} - P_{\text{ambient}})}_{mm\, Hg} \cdot \underbrace{A_{\text{evaporative}}}_{m^2}$$

(59.4)

E is positive when the body loses heat by evaporation and negative when it gains heat by condensation.

As with convection, increased air velocity over the skin increases the effective vapor-pressure gradient between skin and the overlying air because of the faster movement of water vapor away from the skin.

The efficiency of heat transfer from the skin to the environment depends on both physiological and environmental factors. If ambient humidity is high, the gradient of water vapor pressure between skin and air will be low, thereby slowing evaporation and increasing the body's tendency to accumulate excess heat during exercise. This phenomenon underlies the temperature-humidity index—or **heat index.**

When the body is immersed in water, nearly all heat exchange occurs by convection, because essentially no exchanges can occur by radiation or evaporation. Because of the high conductivity and thermal capacity of water, the heat-transfer coefficient ($h_{convective}$) is ~100 times greater than that of air, so that the rate of body heat exchange is much greater in water than it is in air.

When heat gain exceeds heat loss, body core temperature rises

From the preceding three equations, we can calculate the body heat fluxes (R, C, and E). Knowing M (computed from V_{O_2} by indirect calorimetry; see ⊙ **49-3**) and W (if any), we can use the heat-balance equation (see Equation 59.1) to calculate the **rate of heat storage.** From this value, we can predict the rate of change in mean body temperature:

$$\underbrace{\frac{\Delta \overline{T}_{body}}{\Delta t}}_{\substack{\text{Rate of} \\ \text{temperature} \\ \text{increase} \\ \frac{°C}{hr}}} = \frac{\overbrace{Rate\ of\ heat\ storage}^{}}{\underbrace{0.83}_{\substack{\text{Specific} \\ \text{heat of} \\ \text{body} \\ \text{tissues}}} \cdot \underbrace{BW}_{\substack{\text{Body} \\ \text{weight}}}}_{\frac{kcal/hr}{[kcal/(kg°C)] \times kg}} \qquad \textbf{(59.5)}$$

The body has to deal with two types of heat load that tend to make its temperature rise. In the heat-balance equation (see Equation 59.1), the term (M − W) constitutes an **internal heat load.** Although the term (R + C + E) normally reflects a net heat *loss* from the body, it can also be a net heat *gain* by the body—an **external heat load,** which can occur if either the radiation (R) or convection (C) terms are heat *gains* rather than heat *losses.*

The clinician must understand *all* the terms of the heat-balance equation to treat thermally related illnesses. For example, excessive heat exposure can lead to **heat exhaustion,** in which T_{core} rises to as high as 39°C if the body cannot dissipate the heat load. Failure of the body's heat-defense mechanisms arises principally from dehydration (which reduces sweating) and hypovolemia (which reduces blood flow from muscle to core to skin). Heat exhaustion is the most common temperature-related abnormality in athletes. In more severe cases, excessive heat can lead to **heat stroke,** in which T_{core} rises to 41°C or more, due to impaired thermoregulatory mechanisms.

Clothing insulates the body from the environment and limits heat transfer from the body to the environment

Placing one or more layers of clothing between the skin and the environment insulates the body and retards heat transfer

between the core and the environment. In the presence of clothing, heat transfer from a warmer body to a cooler environment occurs by the same means as without clothing (i.e., radiation, conduction, convection, and evaporation), but from the clothing surface rather than from the skin surface.

⊙ 59-7 ACTIVE REGULATION OF BODY TEMPERATURE BY THE CENTRAL NERVOUS SYSTEM

Dedicated neural circuits in the CNS actively regulate body temperature. The central thermoregulatory network includes the following:

1. Afferent neurons that are the skin and visceral thermoreceptors
2. Thermal afferent pathways within the CNS
3. The thermoregulatory integration center in the preoptic anterior hypothalamus
4. Efferent pathways providing autonomic and somatomotor inputs to effectors
5. Thermal effectors that control heat transfer between the body and environment, and that control heat production by the body

This central thermoregulatory network is an **active system** that is superimposed on, and regulates, the *passive poikilothermic system* described earlier (see ⊙ **59-1**), in which the circulatory system and the laws of physics determine heat transfer between the body core and the environment.

⊙ 59-8 Thermoreceptors in the skin and temperature-sensitive neurons in the hypothalamus respond to changes in their local temperature

Skin Thermoreceptors The body has specialized sensory neurons (thermoreceptors) that provide the CNS with information about the thermal condition of the skin. The thermosensitive elements of thermoreceptors are free nerve endings that are distributed over the entire skin surface and contain cation channels that alter their conductance as the environmental temperature rises or falls. Peripheral thermoreceptors fall into two categories—**warmth** receptors and **cold** receptors.

Hypothalamic Temperature-Sensitive Neurons ⊙ **59-9** The principal mechanism through which the central thermoregulatory network senses changes in T_{core} is via temperature-sensitive neurons in the preoptic area of the anterior hypothalamus (see Fig. 47.2), where ~10% of neurons are warmth sensitive (i.e., their discharge rate increases as local temperature rises). Sensing of T_{core} by preoptic temperature-sensitive neurons is especially important during exercise, intake of hot fluids, or the resolution of a fever. In these conditions, heat storage increases more rapidly than heat dissipation, a situation calling for a prompt increase in heat loss to avoid a significant increase in T_{core}.

The CNS thermoregulatory network integrates thermal information and directs changes in efferent activity to modify rates of heat transfer and production

⊙ **59-10** Warming or cooling of the skin—via skin thermoreceptors—alters afferent neuronal activity (Fig. 59.3). Cutaneous warmth thermoreceptors—upon exposure to a

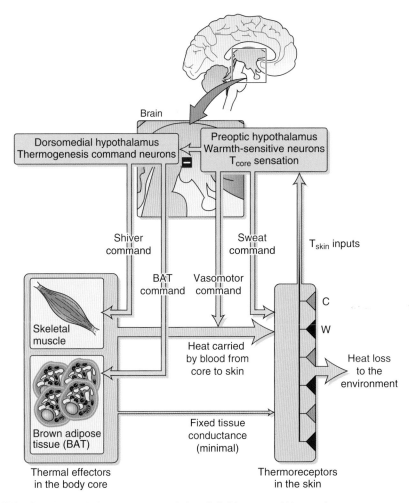

Figure 59.3 Overall model of temperature regulation. *C,* Cold receptor; *W,* warmth receptor.

warm environment—increase the activity of warmth sensory neurons in the thermal afferent pathway and thereby *stimulate* the discharge of the preoptic warmth-sensitive neurons. Conversely, cutaneous cold sensory signals *inhibit* the discharge of the preoptic warmth-sensitive neurons.

The preoptic warmth-sensitive neurons provide a variable level of *inhibition* to descending efferent pathways that otherwise would excite two types of spinal neurons: (1) sympathetic preganglionic neurons that promote cutaneous vasoconstriction (limiting heat transfer within and from the body) and brown adipose tissue thermogenesis, and (2) α motor neurons that cause shivering in skeletal muscle (generating heat).

⊙ 59-11 Thermal effectors include behavior, cutaneous circulation, sweat glands, and skeletal muscles responsible for shivering

As a thermal effector, **behavior** (from simply moving out of the hot sun to building a fire) is usually the central thermoregulatory system's first response to a change in environmental temperature, as sensed by skin thermoreceptors.

⊙ **59-12** The thermal effectors that modulate heat transfer are under the control of the sympathetic nervous system. Adjusting the smooth-muscle tone of cutaneous arterioles and of arteriovenous anastomoses (shunts) controls **cutaneous blood flow** (see ⊙ 24-4)—and therefore heat flow—from

the core to the skin surface, the primary site of heat dissipation to the environment.

Piloerection reduces the rate of heat loss by retaining a layer of warm air next to the skin and occurs by activation of the sympathetic input to smooth muscles in the hair follicles.

With a moderate heat load, the autonomic response primarily increases heat transfer from core to skin by elevating cutaneous blood flow. However, when the heat load is sufficiently great, the preoptic warmth-sensitive neurons also drive activation of the **eccrine sweat glands** (see ⊙ 60-3), which secrete sweat onto the skin surface. Sweating elevates the partial pressure of water vapor at the skin surface and promotes increased evaporation, which takes heat from the skin.

As cold stress increases, cutaneous vasoconstriction is supplemented with heat production—**thermogenesis**—initially in brown adipose tissue and subsequently through shivering. The sympathetic nervous system heavily innervates **brown adipocytes** (see ⊙ 57-3), releasing norepinephrine onto β_3-adrenergic receptors. The subsequent oxidation of fatty acids leads to the production not of ATP but of heat by virtue of the **uncoupling protein UCP1** (see ⊙ 49-4) and the abundant mitochondria.

Shivering begins with an often-unrecognized increase in basal skeletal muscle tone, followed by the familiar involuntary, clonic, rhythmic contractions and relaxations of skeletal muscles. Shivering can triple or quadruple the metabolic rate for brief intervals and double the metabolic rate for extended periods (hours) before fatigue occurs.

HYPOTHERMIA, HYPERTHERMIA, AND FEVER

Hypothermia or hyperthermia occurs when heat transfer to or from the environment overwhelms the body's thermoregulatory capacity

The most common environmental condition causing excessive **hypothermia** is prolonged immersion in cold water. Water has a specific heat per unit volume that is ~4000 times that of air and a thermal conductivity that is ~25 times that of air. Both properties contribute to a convective heat-transfer coefficient ($h_{convective}$ in Equation 59.3) that is ~100-fold greater in water than it is in air. The body's physiological defenses against hypothermia include peripheral vasoconstriction (which increases insulation) and shivering (which increases heat production), but even these measures do not prevent hypothermia during prolonged exposure because of water's high thermal conductivity.

Clothing adds insulation between skin and environment and thus reduces heat loss during exposure to the cold. The more skin one covers, the more one reduces the surface area for direct heat loss from skin to environment by convection and radiation. Adding *layers* of clothing increases the resistance of heat flow by trapping air, which is an excellent insulator. During heat exposure, the major avenue for heat loss is evaporation of sweat. Because evaporation also depends on the surface area available, the amount of clothing should be minimized. Wetting the clothing increases the rate of heat loss from the skin because water is a better conductor than air.

The most common environmental condition that results in excessive **hyperthermia** is prolonged simultaneous exposure to heat and high ambient humidity, particularly when accompanied by physical activity. The ability to dissipate heat by *radiation* falls as the radiant temperature of nearby objects increases (see Equation 59.2), and the ability to dissipate heat by *convection* falls as ambient temperature increases (see Equation 59.3). When ambient temperature reaches the mid-30s (°C), evaporation becomes the only effective avenue for heat dissipation. However, high ambient humidity reduces the skin-to-environment gradient for water vapor pressure, which reduces *evaporation* (see Equation 59.4). The combined reduction of heat loss by these three pathways can markedly increase the rate of heat storage (see Equation 59.5), causing progressive hyperthermia.

It is uncommon for radiative or convective heat gain to cause hyperthermia under conditions of low ambient humidity, because the body has a high capacity for dissipating the absorbed heat by evaporation.

⊙ 59-13 Exercise raises heat production, which is followed by a matching rise in heat loss, but at the cost of a steady-state hyperthermia of exercise

At the onset of muscular exercise, the rate of heat production increases in proportion to exercise intensity and exceeds the current rate of heat dissipation; thus, heat storage occurs and core temperature rises (Fig. 59.4). This rise in the temperature

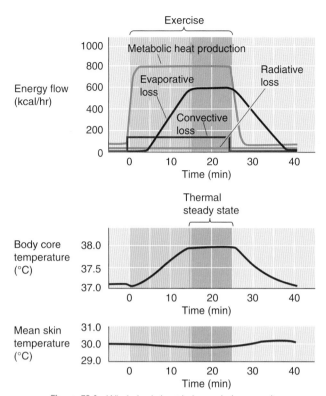

Figure. 59.4 Whole-body heat balance during exercise.

of the local environment of the preoptic warmth-sensitive neurons increases their discharge rate, which increases the neural output that activates heat dissipation (Fig. 59.3). As a result, skin blood flow and sweating increase as T_{core} rises, promoting an increase in the rate of heat transfer from core to environment and slowing the rate at which T_{core} rises. However, heat dissipation during exercise does not increase enough both to eliminate the already-acquired heat storage and to balance the ongoing heat production. Thus, the mildly elevated steady-state T_{core} persists as long as exercise continues.

In the example illustrated in Fig. 59.4, metabolic heat production rises rapidly to its maximal level for the particular level of exercise underway. However, evaporative heat loss increases only after a delay and then rises slowly to its maximal level, driven by increasing body temperature. In this example, the result is net storage during the first 15 minutes. The slight initial drop in T_{core} at the onset of exercise is caused by flushing out of blood from the cooler peripheral circulation when the muscle and skin beds vasodilate in response to the onset of exercise. Note also that mean skin temperature *decreases* during exercise because of the increased evaporative cooling of the skin caused by sweating.

Fever is a regulated hyperthermia

Whereas hyperthermia such as that resulting from exercise in a hot environment arise from incomplete compensation by the thermoregulatory system for an imposed heat load, fever is a *regulated* elevation of core temperature induced by the central thermoregulatory system itself.

In response to a variety of infectious and inflammatory stimuli, macrophages and, to a lesser extent, lymphocytes

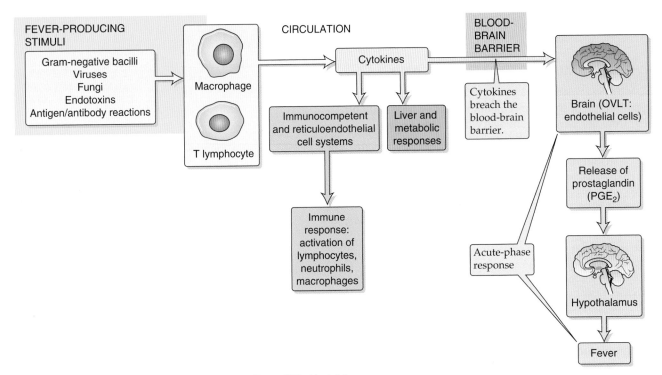

Figure. 59.5 Host defense response.

release cytokines into the circulation (Fig. 59.5). Cytokines are a diverse group of peptides and proteins involved in numerous tasks, among which are serving as the messenger molecules of the immune system. The first step in the host defense response is the **immune response** to foreign substances, including stimulation of T-lymphocyte proliferation, of natural killer cells, and of antibody production. The second is the **acute-phase response,** a diffuse collection of host reactions, including fever production, lethargy, and hyperalgesia, which apparently support the immunological response to, and the body's recovery from, infection or trauma. Finally, cytokines such as interleukin-1β (IL-1β) act as endogenous pyrogens in a signaling cascade that induces peripheral (e.g., in liver) and CNS production of **prostaglandin E$_2$ (PGE$_2$;** see Fig. 3.9). IL-1β, for example, could interact with the endothelial cells in a leaky portion of the blood-brain barrier (see ◉ 11-3) located in the capillary bed of the *organum vasculosum laminae terminalis* (OVLT). The OVLT is highly vascular tissue that lies in the wall of the third ventricle (above the optic chiasm) in the brain (see Fig. 11.3). IL-1β triggers endothelial cells within the OVLT to release PGE$_2$, which then diffuses into the adjacent preoptic hypothalamus to drive the febrile response.

PGE$_2$ inhibits warmth-sensitive neurons in the preoptic area—akin to the action of stimulated skin cold thermoreceptors—and activates the thermal effectors (see ◉ 59-12) for heat retention (cutaneous vasoconstriction) and heat production (brown adipose tissue thermogenesis, and shivering or "chills"), which results in an increase in T$_{core}$.

Once the PGE$_2$ production falls—perhaps due to administration of an anti-inflammatory drug that inhibits PGE$_2$ synthesis—the elevated T$_{core}$ can now produce a marked stimulation of the preoptic warmth-sensitive neurons, resulting in an inhibition of the thermal effectors for heat production and a strong stimulation of those for heat loss, and the fever "breaks."

During exercise, one *feels warm,* and this deviation from thermal comfort drives behaviors such as removing clothing or splashing cold water on the body to cool it. In contrast, during the onset of a fever, one *feels cold* and may choose to put on additional clothing or blankets to warm the body.

The value of fever in fighting infection is still debated. A popular hypothesis is that the elevated temperature enhances the host's response to infection. This view is supported by the observation that, in vitro, the rate of T-lymphocyte proliferation in response to interleukins is many-fold higher at 39°C than it is at 37°C.

CHAPTER 60

EXERCISE PHYSIOLOGY AND SPORTS SCIENCE

Steven S. Segal

Physical exercise is often the greatest stress that the body encounters in the course of daily life. Skeletal muscle typically accounts for 30% to 50% of the total body mass. Thus, with each bout of muscular activity, the body must make rapid, integrated adjustments at the level of cells and organ systems—and must tune these adjustments over time. The subdiscipline of exercise physiology and sports science focuses on the integrated responses that enable the body to convert chemical energy into mechanical work. To understand these interdependent processes, one must appreciate where regulation occurs, the factors that determine physical performance, and the adaptations that take place with repetitive use.

The cross-bridge cycle that underlies contraction of skeletal muscle requires energy in the form of ATP (see ◉ 9-8). Skeletal muscle converts only ~25% of the energy stored in carbon-carbon bonds into mechanical work. The rest appears as heat due to the inefficiencies of the biochemical reactions. Thus, the dissipation of this heat is central to cardiovascular function, fluid balance, and the ability to sustain physical effort—an example of an integrated organ-system response. Moreover, because muscle stores of ATP, phosphocreatine, and glycogen are limited, the ability to sustain physical activity requires another set of integrated cellular and organ-system responses to supply O_2 and energy sources to active muscles.

MOTOR UNITS AND MUSCLE FUNCTION

The motor unit is the functional element of muscle contraction

The **motor unit** (see ◉ 9-1) is the functional unit of skeletal muscle and consists of a single motor neuron and all the muscle fibers that it activates. A typical skeletal muscle such as the biceps brachii receives innervation from ~750 somatic motor neurons.

When the motor neuron generates an action potential, all fibers in the motor unit fire simultaneously. Thus, the fineness of control for movement varies with the **innervation ratio**—the number of muscle fibers per motor neuron. The small motor units that are recruited during sustained activity contain a high proportion of **type I** muscle fibers, which are highly oxidative and resistant to fatigue (see Table 9.1). The **type IIa** motor units have larger innervation ratios, contract faster, and have less oxidative capacity and fatigue resistance than type I

units. Still larger motor units—recruited for brief periods for rapid, powerful activity—typically consist of **type IIx** muscle fibers; these have less oxidative capacity (i.e., are more glycolytic) and are much more susceptible to fatigue than type IIa muscle. In practice, it may be best to view muscle fiber types and motor units as a continuum rather than distinct entities.

Within a whole muscle, muscle fibers of each motor unit intermingle with those of other motor units so extensively that a volume of muscle containing 100 muscle fibers is innervated by terminals from perhaps 50 different motor neurons. However, each muscle fiber is innervated by only one motor neuron.

Muscle force rises with the recruitment of motor units and an increase in their firing frequency

During contraction, the force exerted by a muscle depends on (1) how many motor units are recruited, and (2) how frequently each of the active motor neurons fires action potentials. Motor units are recruited in a progressive order, from the smallest motor neurons that innervate the fewest number of muscle fibers (and therefore the weakest motor units) to the largest neurons that innervate the greatest number of fibers (strongest)—the **size principle.**

At levels of force production lower than the upper limit of recruitment, gradations in force are accomplished via concurrent changes in the number of active motor units and the firing rate of those that have been recruited—**rate coding.** Once all the motor units in a muscle have been recruited, any further increase in force results from an increase in firing rate. The relative contribution of motor-unit recruitment and rate coding varies among muscles.

Compared with type I motor units, type II units are faster and stronger but more fatigable

Within a given motor unit, each muscle fiber is of the same **muscle fiber type.** The three human muscle fiber types—type I, type IIa, and type IIx (see Table 9.1)—differ in contractile and regulatory proteins, the content of myoglobin (and thus color) and of mitochondria and glycogen, and the metabolic pathways used to generate ATP (i.e., oxidative versus glycolytic metabolism). Physical training can modify these biochemical properties, which determine a range of functional parameters, including (1) speeds of contraction

A—TYPE I (SLOW)   **B**—TYPE IIa (FAST, FATIGUE-RESISTANT)   **C**—TYPE IIx (FAST, FATIGABLE)

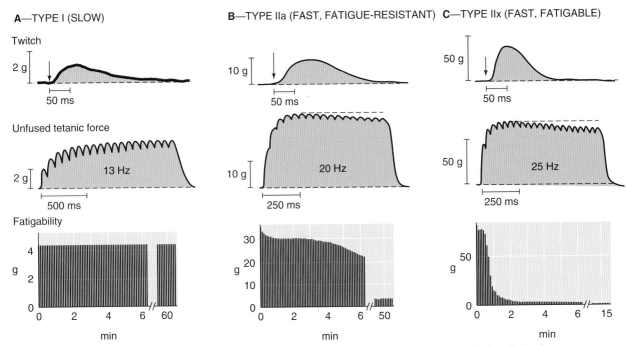

Figure 60.1 Properties of fiber types. The top row shows the tension developed during single twitches for each of the muscle types; the *arrows* indicate the time of the electrical stimulus. The middle row shows the tension developed during an unfused tetanus. The bottom row shows the degree to which each fiber type can sustain force during continuous stimulation. Note that the time scales become progressively larger from the top to bottom rows, with a break in the bottom row. Data from Burke RE, Levine DN, Tsairis P, et al: J Physiol 234:723–748, 1977.

and relaxation, (2) maximal force, and (3) susceptibility to fatigue (Fig. 60.1).

Fluid and energetically efficient movements require learning

To perform a desired movement—whether playing the piano or serving a tennis ball—the nervous system must activate a combination of muscles with the appropriate contractile properties, recruit motor units in defined patterns, and thereby create suitable mechanical interactions among body segments. When we perform movements with uncertainty—as in learning a new skill—actions tend to be stiff because of concurrent recruitment of motor units in antagonistic muscles that produce force in opposite directions. Such superfluous muscle fiber activity also increases the energy requirements for the activity. With learning, recruitment patterns become refined, and muscle fibers adapt to the task. Thus, movements become fluid and more energetically efficient.

Strength versus endurance training differentially alters the properties of motor units

The effects of physical activity on motor-unit physiology depend on the intensity and duration of the exercise. In general, sustained periods of activity of low to moderate intensity performed several times per week—**endurance (aerobic) training**—result in a greater oxidative capacity of muscle fibers and are manifested by increases in O_2 delivery, capillary supply, and mitochondrial content (see ⦿ **60-5**).

These adaptations reduce the susceptibility of the affected muscle fibers to fatigue (see ⦿ **60-2**). The lean and slender build of long-distance (i.e., endurance) runners reflects the abundance of highly oxidative type I and IIa muscle fibers of relatively small diameter, promoting O_2 and CO_2 diffusion between capillaries and mitochondria for high levels of aerobic energy production. Further, the high ratio of surface area to volume of the slender body also facilitates cooling of the body during prolonged activity and in hot environments.

In contrast, brief sets of high-intensity contractions performed several times per week—**strength (anaerobic) training**—result in type IIx motor units that can produce more force and can shorten against a given load at greater velocity by increasing the amount of contractile protein. The hypertrophied muscles of sprinters and weightlifters exemplify this type of adaptation, which relies more on rapid, *anaerobic* sources of energy production (see ⦿ **60-1**).

CONVERSION OF CHEMICAL ENERGY TO MECHANICAL WORK

At rest, skeletal muscle has a low metabolic rate. In response to contractile activity, the energy consumption of skeletal muscle can easily rise >100-fold. The body meets this increased energy demand by mobilizing energy stores both locally from muscle glycogen and triacylglycerols, and systemically from liver glycogen and adipose tissue triacylglycerols. The integrated physiological response to exercise involves the delivery of sufficient O_2 and fuel to ensure that the rate of **ATP** synthesis rises in parallel with the rate of ATP breakdown. Indeed, skeletal muscle precisely regulates the ratio of ATP to ADP even with these large increases in ATP turnover.

Physical performance can be defined in terms of power (work/time), speed, or endurance. Skeletal muscle has three energy systems, each designed to support a particular type of performance (Fig. 60.2). For power events, which typically last a few seconds or less (e.g., hitting a ball with a bat), the immediate energy sources include ATP and **phosphocreatine (PCr).** For spurts of activity that last several seconds to a minute (e.g., sprinting 100 m), muscles rely primarily on the rapid nonoxidative breakdown of carbohydrate stored as muscle glycogen to form ATP. For activities that last 2 minutes or longer but have low power requirements (e.g., jogging several kilometers), the generation of ATP through the oxidation of fat and glucose derived from the circulation becomes increasingly important.

ATP and PCr provide immediate but limited energy

At the onset of exercise, or during the transition to a higher intensity of contractile activity, the immediate energy sources are ATP and PCr. As for any other cell, muscle cells break down ATP to ADP and inorganic phosphate (P_i), releasing free energy (ΔG):

$$ATP \rightarrow ADP + P_i + \Delta G \qquad \textbf{(60.1)}$$

Muscle cells rapidly regenerate ATP from PCr in a reaction that is catalyzed by **creatine kinase:**

$$ADP + PCr \xrightarrow{\text{creatine kinase}} ATP + Creatine \qquad \textbf{(60.2)}$$

These two energy stores are sufficient to support intense contractile activity for only a few seconds (Fig. 60.2, *red curve*). When rates of ATP breakdown (see Equation 60.1) are high, ADP levels (normally very low) increase and can actually interfere with muscle contraction. Under such conditions, **adenylate kinase** (also known as **myokinase**) transfers the second phosphate group from one ADP to another, thereby regenerating ATP:

$$ADP + ADP \xrightarrow{\text{adenylate kinase}} ATP + AMP \qquad \textbf{(60.3)}$$

⊚ 60-1 Anaerobic glycolysis provides a rapid but self-limited source of ATP

When high-intensity exercise continues for more than several seconds, the breakdown of ATP and PCr is followed almost instantly by the accelerated breakdown of intramuscular glycogen to glucose—**glycogenolysis** (see ⊚ 58-10)—and then to pyruvate—**glycolysis**—and finally to lactate. This anaerobic metabolism of glucose has the major advantage of providing energy quickly to meet the increased metabolic demands of an intense workload, even before O_2, glucose, or fatty-acid delivery from blood increases. However, because of the low ATP yield of this pathway, muscle rapidly depletes its glycogen stores, which so that intense activity is limited to durations of ~1 minute (Fig. 60.2, *purple curve*).

The overall process generates two ATP molecules per glucose molecule:

$$\underset{\text{Glucose}}{C_6H_{12}O_6} + 2\,ADP + 2\,P_i \rightarrow 2\,\underset{\text{Lactate}}{C_3H_5O_3^-} + 2\,ATP + 2\,H^+ + heat$$

$$\textbf{(60.4)}$$

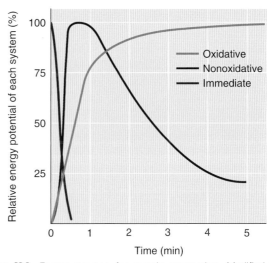

Figure 60.2 Energy sources for muscle contraction. Modified from Edington DW, Edgerton VR: The Biology of Physical Activity. Boston, Houghton Mifflin, 1976.

Oxidation of glucose, lactate, and fatty acids provides a slower but long-term source of ATP

Oxidation of Nonmuscle Glucose The aerobic metabolism of glucose, although slower than anaerobic glycolysis (see Equation 60.4), provides nearly 15-fold more ATP molecules per glucose molecule:

$$\overset{\text{Glucose}}{\overbrace{C_6H_{12}O_6}} + 6\,O_2 + 30\,ADP + 30\,P_i \rightarrow$$
$$6\,CO_2 + 6\,H_2O + 30\,ATP + heat \qquad \textbf{(60.5)}$$

The majority of glucose that contracting skeletal muscle oxidizes during aerobic energy production comes from circulating glucose, which in turn originates primarily from the breakdown of the hepatic glycogen stores of 75 to 100 g (see ⊚ 58-2).

Contracting skeletal muscle is an important sink for blood-borne glucose (Fig. 60.3). Moreover, contractile activity *per se* triggers the translocation of additional GLUT4 transporters (see ⊚ 5-5) from the cytosol to the plasma membrane.

Oxidation of Lactate During the first minutes of exercise, active muscle fibers use glycogenolysis to liberate glucose and then use glycolysis to form either pyruvate or lactate, depending on the relative activities of glycolysis and mitochondrial respiration. As blood flow and O_2 delivery increase during the initial minutes of the cardiovascular and respiratory adjustments to exercise, types I and IIa oxidative muscle fibers convert lactate back to pyruvate for uptake and subsequent oxidation by the mitochondria. In addition, glycolytic (type IIx) muscle fibers release lactate that can diffuse to nearby oxidative muscle fibers for aerobic production of ATP (Fig. 60.3).

Gluconeogenesis Hepatic gluconeogenesis (see ⊚ 58-4) becomes increasingly important as exercise is prolonged beyond an hour and hepatic glycogen stores become depleted. The most important substrates for hepatic gluconeogenesis are lactate and alanine. During prolonged exercise, the key substrate is lactate released into the circulation by contracting skeletal muscle (see below) for uptake by the liver, which resynthesizes glucose for uptake by the muscle—the **Cori cycle** (see ⊚ 58-17).

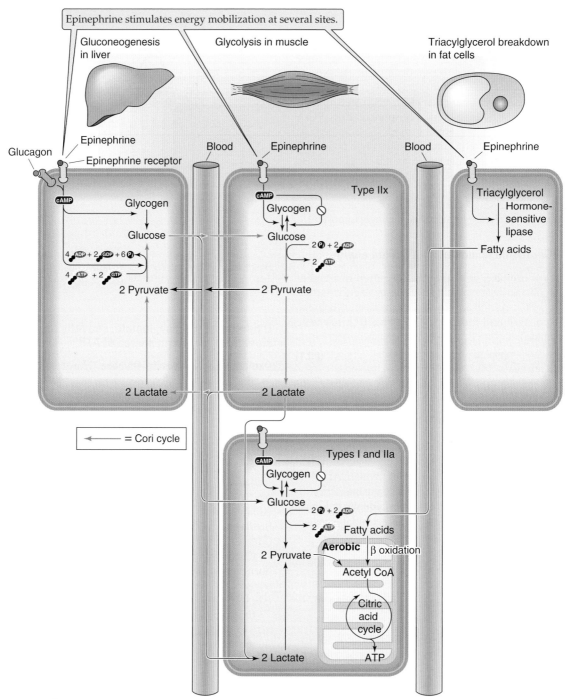

Figure 60.3   Steady-state energy supply to muscle from energy stores in muscle, liver, and adipose tissue. *CoA,* Coenzyme A.

Also during prolonged exercise, the oxidation of branched-chain amino acids by skeletal muscle leads to the release of alanine into the circulation for uptake by the liver, followed by hepatic gluconeogenesis and the release of glucose into the blood for uptake by muscle—the **glucose-alanine cycle** (see ◉ 58-18).

Oxidation of Nonmuscle Lipid   Most stored energy is in the form of triacylglycerols. The mobilization of lipid from adipocytes (see ◉ 58-12) during exercise is largely under the control of the sympathetic nervous system, complemented by the release of growth hormone during exercise lasting >30

to 40 minutes. The result of this mobilization is an increase in circulating levels of fatty acids, which can enter skeletal muscle—especially type I and IIa fibers (Fig. 60.3).

In the presence of adequate O_2, fatty acids provide up to 60% of the oxidized fuel supply of muscle during prolonged exercise. The oxidation of fatty acids (see ◉ 58-13), such as palmitate in the following example, has a very high yield of ATP:

$$\overbrace{C_{15}H_{31}COOH}^{\text{Palmitic acid}} + 23\,O_2 + 106\,ADP + 106\,P_i \rightarrow$$
$$16\,CO_2 + 16\,H_2O + 106\,ATP + heat \qquad \textbf{(60.6)}$$

⊙ 60-2 MUSCLE FATIGUE

Fatigued muscle produces less force and has a reduced velocity of shortening

Muscle fatigue is defined as the inability to maintain a desired power output—resulting from muscle contraction against a load—with a decline in both force and velocity of shortening. A decline in maximal force production with fatigue results from a reduction in the number of active cross-bridges as well as in the force produced per cross-bridge. Other characteristics of fatigued skeletal muscle are lower rates of both force production and relaxation, owing to impaired release and reuptake of Ca^{2+} by the sarcoplasmic reticulum (SR). As a result, fast movements become difficult or impossible, and athletic performance suffers accordingly.

Changes in the CNS produce central fatigue

Central fatigue reflects changes in the CNS and may involve altered input from muscle sensory nerve fibers, reduced excitatory input to motor control centers of the brain and spinal cord, and altered excitability of α and γ motor neurons (see Fig. 15.23). Central fatigue is likely to play only a minor role in limiting performance of highly trained athletes who have learned to pace themselves according to the task and are mentally conditioned to discomfort and stress. External sensory input, such as shouting and cheering, can often increase muscle force production and physical performance, which indicates that pathways proximal to corticospinal outputs can oppose central fatigue.

Impaired excitability and impaired Ca^{2+} release can produce peripheral fatigue

Under normal conditions, transmission block at the neuromuscular junction does not cause muscle fatigue, even though the release of neurotransmitter can decline. Thus, **peripheral fatigue** reflects a spectrum of events at the level of the muscle fiber, including impairments in the initiation and propagation of muscle action potentials, the release and handling of intracellular Ca^{2+} for cross-bridge activation, depletion of substrates for energy metabolism, and the accumulation of metabolic byproducts.

High-Frequency Fatigue With continuous firing of action potentials during intense exercise, Na^+ entry and K^+ exit exceed the ability of the Na-K pump to restore and maintain normal resting ion concentration gradients. A result is inactivation of voltage-gated Na^+ channels, which makes it more difficult to initiate and propagate action potentials. Within the T tubule, such depolarization impairs the ability of L-type Ca^{2+} channels to activate Ca^{2+}-release channels in the SR (see Fig. 9.3). Fatigue resulting from *impaired membrane excitability* is particularly apparent at high frequencies of stimulation during recruitment of *type II* motor units—**high-frequency fatigue.**

Low-Frequency Fatigue In prolonged moderate-intensity exercise, the release of Ca^{2+} from the SR falls, which apparently reflects changes in the Ca^{2+}-release channel or its associated proteins along with inhibition of the SERCA pump (see ⊙ 5-11) and thus diminished SR Ca^{2+} stores; this decrease in Ca^{2+} release leads to a depression in the amplitude of the $[Ca^{2+}]_i$ transient that accompanies the muscle twitch. Fatigue resulting from *impaired Ca^{2+} release* is thus particularly apparent at low frequencies of stimulation during recruitment of *type I* motor units—**low-frequency fatigue.** Recovery requires several hours.

Fatigue can result from ATP depletion, lactic acid accumulation, and glycogen depletion

ATP Depletion Intense stimulation of muscle fibers (particularly type IIx) requires high rates of ATP utilization, with PCr initially buffering $[ATP]_i$. As fatigue develops and $[PCr]_i$ diminishes, $[ATP]_i$ can fall from 5 mM to <2 mM, particularly at sites of cross-bridge interaction and in the vicinity of membrane pumps, so that respective ATPase activities are impaired.

Lactic Acid Accumulation Intense activity also activates glycolysis—again, particularly in type IIx fibers—which results in a high rate of lactic acid production and thus reduces pH_i to as low as 6.2. This fall in pH_i inhibits myosin ATPase activity, cross-bridge interactions, the binding of Ca^{2+} to troponin, the Na-K pump, as well as phosphofructokinase (the rate-limiting step of muscle glycolysis).

Glycogen Depletion During prolonged exercise of moderate intensity (~50% of maximal aerobic power), and with well-maintained O_2 delivery, the eventual decrease in glycogen stores in oxidative (type I and IIa) muscle fibers decreases power output. Long-distance runners describe this phenomenon as "hitting the wall." In long-distance running, endurance depends on the absolute amount of glycogen stored in the leg muscles before exercise. To postpone hitting the wall, the athlete must either begin the event with an elevated level of muscle glycogen or race more slowly. Because glycogen storage is primarily a function of diet, carbohydrate loading can increase resting muscle glycogen stores and postpone the onset of fatigue. Aerobic training can spare muscle glycogen by adaptations such as mitochondrial proliferation (see ⊙ 60-8) that shift the mix of oxidized fuels toward fatty acids.

DETERMINANTS OF MAXIMAL O_2 UPTAKE AND CONSUMPTION

The O_2 required for oxidative metabolism by exercising muscle travels from the atmosphere to the muscle mitochondria in discrete steps, discussed in the next three sections.

Maximal O_2 uptake by the lungs can exceed resting O_2 uptake by more than 20-fold

The respiratory and cardiovascular systems can readily deliver O_2 to active skeletal muscle at mild and moderate exercise intensities. As power output increases, the body eventually reaches a point at which the capacity of O_2 transport systems can no longer keep pace with demand, so the rate of O_2 uptake by the lungs ($\dot{V}_{O_2}$) plateaus (Fig. 60.4). At rest, $\dot{V}_{O_2}$ is typically 250 mL/min for a 70-kg person. **Maximal oxygen uptake measured at the lungs ($\dot{V}_{O_{2max}}$)** is an objective index of the functional capacity of the body's ability to generate aerobic power. In people who have a deficiency in any part of the O_2-transport system (e.g., chronic obstructive pulmonary disease or advanced heart disease), $\dot{V}_{O_{2max}}$ can be as low as 10 to 20 mL

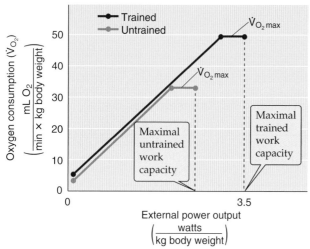

Figure 60.4 Dependence of O_2 consumption on mechanical power output in untrained and trained individuals.

$O_2/(min \times kg)$. The range for mildly active middle-aged adults is 30 to 40 mL $O_2/(min \times kg)$. In elite endurance athletes, $\dot{V}_{O_{2max}}$ may be as high as 80 to 90 mL $O_2/(min \times kg)$, more than a 20-fold elevation above the resting $\dot{V}_{O_2}$.

O_2 uptake by muscle is the product of muscle blood flow and O_2 extraction

During prolonged activity, the body must continually transport O_2 from the ambient air to the muscle mitochondria at a rate that is equivalent to the O_2 utilization by the muscle. This increased O_2 transport is accomplished by increasing alveolar ventilation to maintain alveolar P_{O_2} levels that are sufficient to saturate arterial blood fully with O_2 (see ⊙ 31-2) and by increasing cardiac output to ensure a sufficiently high flow of oxygenated blood to the active muscles (see ⊙ 20-5). The integrated organ-system response to the new, elevated metabolic load includes sophisticated reflexes to ensure matching of O_2 delivery and O_2 uptake.

The O_2-delivery rate is the product of cardiac output (i.e., heart rate × stroke volume) and arterial O_2 content:

$$\underset{\substack{\text{Arterial } O_2 \\ \text{delivery rate} \\ \text{to whole body} \\ \dot{V}a_{O_2} \\ \frac{mL\ O_2}{min}}}{} = \underset{\substack{\text{Heart} \\ \text{rate} \\ HR \\ \frac{beats}{min}}}{} \cdot \underset{\substack{\text{Cardiac} \\ \text{stroke} \\ \text{volume} \\ SV \\ \frac{mL\ blood}{beat}}}{} \cdot \underset{\substack{\text{Arterial} \\ O_2 \\ \text{content} \\ Ca_{O_2} \\ \frac{mL\ O_2}{mL\ blood}}}{} \quad (60.7)$$

The rate of O_2 uptake by skeletal muscle depends on both the O_2 delivery to skeletal muscle and the **extraction** of O_2 by the muscle, according to the Fick principle (see ⊙ 20-7):

$$\underset{\substack{\text{Rate of } O_2 \\ \text{uptake by} \\ \text{skeletal muscle} \\ \dot{V}_{O_2} \\ \frac{mL\ O_2}{min}}}{} = \underset{\substack{\text{Blood flow} \\ \text{to} \\ \text{skeletal muscle} \\ F \\ \frac{mL\ blood}{min}}}{} \cdot \underset{\substack{\text{a} - \text{v} \\ \text{difference of} \\ O_2 \text{ content} \\ (Ca_{O_2} - Cv_{O_2}) \\ \frac{mL\ O_2}{mL\ blood}}}{} \quad (60.8)$$

O_2 delivery by the cardiovascular system is the limiting step for maximal O_2 utilization

The transport of O_2 from atmosphere to muscle mitochondria occurs in three steps: uptake, delivery, and extraction. A limitation in any step could be rate limiting for maximal O_2 utilization by muscle.

Limited O_2 Uptake by the Lungs One view is that the lungs limit $\dot{V}_{O_{2max}}$. An inability of alveolar O_2 diffusion to saturate arterial blood fully (see Fig. 30.5C) occurs in a subset of elite athletes (including race horses).

Limited O_2 Delivery by the Cardiovascular System According to the prevalent view, a limitation in O_2 transport by the cardiovascular system determines $\dot{V}_{O_{2max}}$. That is, **maximal cardiac output,** and hence O_2 delivery, is the limiting step according to the **convective flow model.** Support for this view comes from the observation that training can considerably augment maximal cardiac output and muscle blood flow (see the following section).

Limited O_2 Extraction by Muscle A third view is that, with increasing demand, O_2 extraction by muscle from blood becomes inadequate despite adequate O_2 delivery. According to this **diffusive flow model,** a major limitation in O_2 transport is the kinetics of O_2 diffusion from hemoglobin in the red blood cell to the muscle mitochondrial matrix.

Effective circulating volume takes priority over cutaneous blood flow for thermoregulation

When we exercise in the heat, our circulatory systems must simultaneously support a large blood flow to both the skin (see ⊙ 59-2) and contracting muscles, which taxes the cardiac output and effective circulating volume (see ⊙ 23-26). Effective circulating volume depends on total blood volume, which in turn relies on extracellular fluid (ECF) volume and overall vasomotor (primarily venomotor) tone, which is important for distributing blood between central and peripheral blood vessels.

Effective circulating volume tends to fall during prolonged exercise, especially exercise in the heat, for three reasons (Fig. 60.5).

First, exercise causes a **shift in plasma water** from the intravascular to the interstitial space (Fig. 60.5, *numeral 2a*). This transcapillary movement of fluid during exercise primarily reflects increased capillary hydrostatic pressure as arterioles dilate (see ⊙ 20-13). In addition, increased osmolality within muscle cells removes water from the extracellular space.

Second, exercise causes a loss of total-body water through **sweating** (Fig. 60.5, *numeral 2b*). If exercise is prolonged without concomitant water intake, sweat loss will cost the body an important fraction of its total water. Early signs of heat-related illness include lightheadedness and disorientation, and represent **clinical dehydration.**

Third, exercise causes a **redistribution of blood volume** to the skin because of the increase in cutaneous blood flow in response to body heating (Fig. 60.5, *numeral 2c*). Venous volume *in the skin* increases as a result of the increased pressure in the compliant veins as blood flow to the skin rises. No compensatory venoconstriction occurs in the skin because of the overriding action of the temperature-control system.

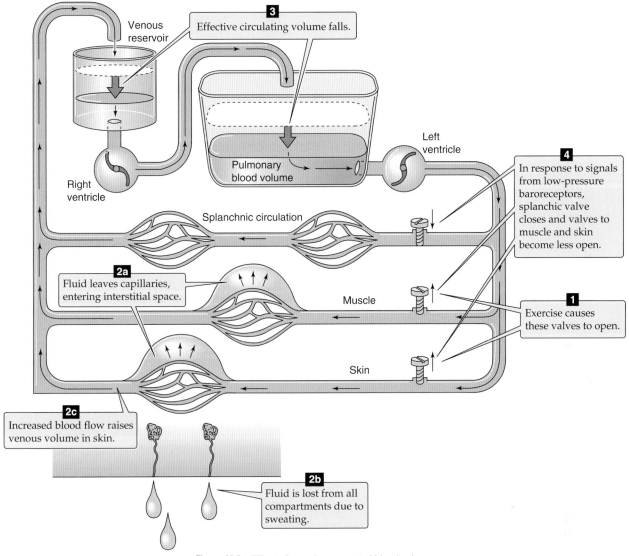

Figure 60.5   Effect of exercise on central blood volume.

In response to this decrease in effective circulating volume that occurs during exercise (Fig. 60.5, *numeral 3*), the cardiopulmonary low-pressure baroreceptors (see ⊙ **23-17**) initiate compensatory responses to increase total vascular resistance (Fig. 60.5, *numeral 4*). The sympathetic nervous system increases this resistance by (a) increasing the splanchnic vascular resistance, which directs cardiac output away from the gut; (b) offsetting some of the thermoregulatory system's vasodilatory drive to the skin; and (c) offsetting some of the vasodilatory drive to the active skeletal muscles.

SWEATING

⊙ 60-3 Eccrine, but not apocrine, sweat glands contribute to temperature regulation

Sweat glands are exocrine glands of the skin, formed by specialized infoldings of the epidermis into the underlying dermis. Sweat glands are of two types, apocrine and eccrine (Fig. 60.6A). The **apocrine** sweat glands, located in the axillary and anogenital regions of the body, are relatively few in number (~100,000) and large in diameter (2 to 3 mm). Their ducts empty into hair follicles.

Eccrine sweat glands are distributed over the majority of the body surface, are numerous (several million), and are small in diameter (50 to 100 μm). The palms of the hands and soles of the feet tend to have both larger and more densely distributed eccrine glands than elsewhere. The essential role of eccrine sweating is temperature regulation (see ⊙ **59-6**).

Eccrine sweat glands are tubules comprising a secretory coiled gland and a reabsorptive duct

⊙ **60-4** An eccrine sweat gland is a simple tubular epithelium composed of a coiled gland and a duct (Fig. 60.6B). A rich microvascular network surrounds the entire sweat gland. The **coiled gland,** located deep in the dermis, begins at a single blind acinus innervated by postganglionic sympathetic fibers that are cholinergic. The acinar cells secrete into the lumen a clear, odorless solution, similar in composition to protein-free plasma. This primary secretion flows through a long, wavy **duct** that passes outward through the dermis and

A—APOCRINE AND ECCRINE SWEAT GLANDS

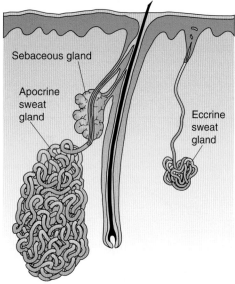

Sebaceous gland

Apocrine sweat gland

Eccrine sweat gland

B—COMPONENTS OF AN ECCRINE SWEAT GLAND

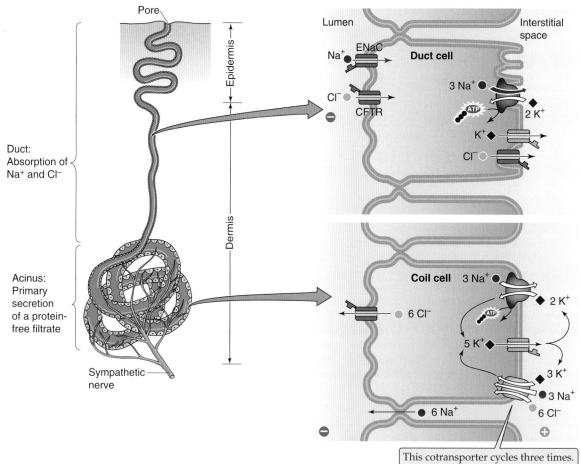

Pore

Epidermis

Dermis

Duct:
Absorption of
Na^+ and Cl^-

Acinus:
Primary
secretion
of a protein-
free filtrate

Sympathetic
nerve

Lumen   Interstitial space

Na^+ ENaC   **Duct cell**

Cl^- $3\,Na^+$

CFTR   ATP $2\,K^+$

K^+

Cl^-

Coil cell $3\,Na^+$

$2\,K^+$

$6\,Cl^-$ ATP

$5\,K^+$

$3\,K^+$

$3\,Na^+$

$6\,Na^+$ $6\,Cl^-$

This cotransporter cycles three times.

Figure 60.6   Sweat glands. The sebaceous gland—the duct of which empties into the hair follicle independently of the duct of the apocrine sweat gland—secretes sebum, a mixture of fat and the remnants of the cells that secrete the fat.

epidermis. Along the way, duct cells reabsorb salt and water until the fluid reaches the skin surface through an opening, the **sweat pore.**

Secretion by Coil Cells The primary secretion by coil cells (Fig. 60.6B, *lower inset*) occurs via the general mechanism for Cl^- secretion. An Na/K/Cl cotransporter mediates the uptake of Cl^- across the basolateral membrane, and the Cl^- exits across the apical membrane via a Cl^- channel (Fig. 60.6B, *lower inset*). As Cl^- diffuses into the lumen, the resulting lumen-negative voltage drives Na^+ secretion through the paracellular pathway.

The secretion of NaCl, as well as of urea and lactate, into the lumen sets up an osmotic gradient that drives the secretion of water, so the secreted fluid is nearly isotonic with plasma.

Reabsorption by Duct Cells As the secreted solution flows along the sweat gland duct, the duct cells reabsorb Na^+ and Cl^- (Fig. 60.6B, *upper inset*). Na^+ enters the duct cells across the apical membrane via epithelial Na^+ channels (ENaC), and Cl^- enters through the cystic fibrosis transmembrane conductance regulator (CFTR). The Na-K pump is responsible for the extrusion of Na^+ across the basolateral membrane, and Cl^- exits via a Cl^- channel. Because the water permeability of the epithelium lining the sweat duct is low, water reabsorption is limited, so that the final secretory fluid is always hypotonic to plasma.

Because sweat is hypotonic, sweating leads to the loss of **solute-free water,** that is, the loss of more water than salt.

The hyperthermia of exercise stimulates eccrine sweat glands

The rate of perspiration increases with body T_{core}, which in turn increases during exercise (see ◉ **59-13**). The major drive for increased perspiration is the sensing by the hypothalamic centers of increased T_{core}. Physical training increases the sensitivity of the hypothalamic drive to higher T_{core}. Indeed, the hyperthermia of exercise causes sweating to begin at a lower skin temperature than does sweating elicited by external heating. Postganglionic sympathetic cholinergic fibers (see Fig. 23.5) mediate the efferent limb of the sweating reflex.

ENDURANCE (AEROBIC) TRAINING

Aerobic training requires regular periods of stress and recovery

◉ **60-5** The body improves its capacity to perform work by responding to physical exertion. However, one must meet four conditions to achieve a **training effect,** or *adaptation* to exercise. First, the intensity of the activity must be higher than a critical threshold. For aerobic training (e.g., running, cycling, and swimming), the level of stress increases with the intensity of the activity. Second, each period of activity must be of sufficient duration. Third, one must repeat the activity over time on a regular basis (e.g., several times per week). Finally, sufficient rest must occur between each training session, because it is during the recovery period that the adaptations to exercise actually occur.

◉ 60-6 Aerobic training increases maximal O_2 delivery by increasing plasma volume and maximal cardiac output

$\dot{V}_{O_2 max}$ could increase as the result of either optimizing O_2 delivery to active muscle or optimizing O_2 extraction by active muscle. In fact, aerobic training improves both O_2 delivery and O_2 extraction.

$$\underbrace{\dot{V}_{aO_2 max}}_{\substack{mL\ O_2 \\ \overline{min}}} = \underbrace{\underbrace{HR_{opt}}_{\substack{\text{Maximal} \\ \text{cardiac output}}} \cdot \underbrace{SV_{opt}}_{\substack{mL\ blood \\ \overline{min}}}}_{} \cdot \underbrace{(Ca_{O_2} - Cv_{O_2 2})_{max}}_{\substack{mL\ O_2 \\ \overline{mL\ blood}}}$$

$$\text{(60.9)}$$

Maximal rate of O_2 uptake; Optimal heart rate; Optimal stroke volume; Maximal a−v difference of O_2 content

Maximizing Arterial O_2 Content Several factors could theoretically contribute to maximizing Ca_{O_2}:

1. Increasing the maximal alveolar ventilation enhances the driving force for O_2 uptake by the lungs (see Fig. 31.2).
2. Increasing the pulmonary diffusing capacity (see Fig. 30.5C) could enhance O_2 uptake at very high cardiac output, particularly at high altitude.
3. Improving the matching of pulmonary ventilation to perfusion should increase arterial P_{O_2} and the saturation of hemoglobin (see ◉ 31-9).
4. Increasing the concentration of hemoglobin enables a given volume of arterial blood to carry a greater amount of O_2 (see ◉ 29-4).

Maximizing Cardiac Output Factors that contribute to increasing maximal cardiac output include optimizing the increases in heart rate and cardiac stroke volume so that their product (i.e., cardiac output) is maximal (see Equation 60.9 and ◉ 25-3). Nearly all the increase in $\dot{V}_{O_2 max}$ that occurs with training is the result of an increase in maximal cardiac output, the product of optimal heart rate and optimal stroke volume (see Equation 60.9). The athlete achieves this increased cardiac output by increasing maximal cardiac stroke volume. Increased extraction, $(Ca_{O_2} - Cv_{O_2})_{max}$, in endurance training is a consequence of capillary proliferation and increased mitochondrial content of muscle fibers, which creates a greater O_2 sink under maximal aerobic conditions.

Maximal cardiac stroke volume increases during aerobic training because expansion of the plasma—and thus blood volume—increases the heart's preload, thereby increasing ventricular filling and proportionally increasing stroke volume (Starling's law of the heart; see ◉ 22-4).

◉ **60-7** The expansion of plasma volume probably reflects an increase in **albumin content.** This increase appears to be caused both by translocation from the interstitial compartment and by increased synthesis by the liver. The result of more colloid in the capillaries is a shift of fluid from the interstitium to the blood. Although the total volume of red blood cells also increases with aerobic training, the plasma volume expansion is greater than the red blood cell expansion, so that the hemoglobin concentration falls. This **sports anemia** occurs in highly trained endurance athletes, particularly those acclimatized to hot environments.

Aerobic training enhances O$_2$ diffusion into muscle

Whereas an increase in maximal cardiac output accounts for a major fraction of the increased O$_2$ uptake by muscle with training, a lesser fraction reflects increased O$_2$ extraction from blood. Fick's law describes the diffusion of O$_2$ between the alveolar air and pulmonary capillary blood (see Equation 30.2). A similar relationship describes the diffusion of O$_2$ from the systemic capillary blood to the mitochondria.

Finally, trained muscle can accommodate a greater maximal blood flow because of the growth of new microvessels, particularly capillaries. This increased capillary density increases D$_{O_2}$ because it provides a greater surface area for diffusion and also reduces the diffusion distance for O$_2$ between the capillary and muscle fibers (see Fig. 20.3).

⊙ 60-8 Aerobic training increases mitochondrial content

In untrained (but otherwise healthy) individuals, the maximum ability of mitochondria to consume O$_2$ is considerably greater than that of the cardiovascular system to supply O$_2$. Thus, mitochondrial content does not limit $\dot{V}_{O_{2max}}$ under non-training conditions. However, endurance training can increase the mitochondrial content of skeletal muscle fibers nearly 2-fold by stimulating the synthesis of mitochondrial enzymes and other proteins.

CHAPTER 61

ENVIRONMENTAL PHYSIOLOGY

Arthur DuBois[†]

The earth and its atmosphere provide environments that are compatible with an extraordinary number of diverse life forms, each adapted to its particular ecological niche. However, not all the earth's surface is equally friendly for *human* survival. Mountain climbers and deep-sea divers know the profound effects of **barometric pressure (P_B)** on human physiology, and astronauts quickly learn how the physically equivalent forces of **gravity** and **acceleration** affect the body. Humans can adapt to changes in P_B and gravity up to a point, but survival under extreme conditions requires special equipment.

THE ENVIRONMENT

Voluntary feedback control mechanisms can modulate the many layers of our external environment

Physiological control mechanisms—involuntary or voluntary—do not always work well. Physicians are acutely aware that factors such as medication, disease, or the extremes of age can interfere with involuntary feedback systems. These same factors can also interfere with voluntary feedback systems. For example, turning on the air conditioning is a difficult or even impossible task for an unconscious person, a bedridden patient, or a perfectly healthy baby. In these situations, a caregiver substitutes for the voluntary physiological control mechanisms. However, to perform this role effectively, the caregiver must understand how the environment would normally affect the care recipient and must anticipate how the involuntary and voluntary physiological control mechanisms would respond.

Environmental temperature provides conscious clues for triggering voluntary feedback mechanisms

Involuntary control mechanisms (see ◉ 59-7) can only go so far in stabilizing body core temperature in the face of extreme environmental temperatures. Thus, voluntary control mechanisms can become extremely important.

The usual range of body core temperature is 36°C to 38°C (see Table 59.1). At an environmental temperature of 26°C to 27°C and a relative humidity of 50%, a naked person is in a **neutral thermal environment** (see ◉ 59-5)—feeling comfortable and being within the zone of vasomotor regulation of body temperature. As ambient temperature rises, the person feels warm (28°C–29°C), slightly uncomfortable

(30C–32°C), hot and uncomfortable (35°C–37°C), and very hot and uncomfortable, and perhaps may unable to regulate core temperature (39°C–43°C). Finally, at 46°C, the heat is unbearable and heat stroke is imminent—the body heats rapidly, and the loss of extracellular fluid to sweat (see ◉ 60-3) may lead to circulatory collapse and death.

At the other extreme, we regard environmental temperatures of 24°C to 25°C as cool, 21°C to 22°C as slightly uncomfortable, and 19°C to 20°C as cold.

Room ventilation should maintain P_{O_2}, P_{CO_2}, and levels of toxic substances within acceptable limits

Ventilation of a room must be sufficient to supply enough O_2 and to remove enough CO_2 to keep the partial pressures of these gases within acceptable limits.

Acceptable Limits for P_{O_2} and P_{CO_2} In the United States, the Occupational Safety and Health Administration (OSHA) has adopted an **acceptable lower limit** for O_2 of 19.5% of dry air at sea level (i.e., 148 mm Hg).

According to OSHA, the **acceptable upper limit for P_{CO_2}** in working environments at sea level is 3.8 mm Hg, or 0.5% of dry air.

Carbon Monoxide More insidious than hypoxia, and less noticeable, is the symptomless encroachment of carbon monoxide (CO) gas on the oxyhemoglobin dissociation curve (see Fig. 29.2). CO can come from incomplete combustion of fuel, and suffocates people without their being aware of its presence. Detectors for this gas are thus essential for providing an early warning. CO can be lethal when it occupies approximately half of the binding sites on hemoglobin (Hb), which occurs at a P_{CO} of ~0.13 mm Hg or $0.13/760 \cong 170$ parts per million (ppm). The symptoms at ~12.5% CO saturation of Hb would be mild and nonspecific and would include headache, nausea, vomiting, and drowsiness. At 25% CO saturation, the symptoms would be more severe and would include impaired mental function and perhaps unconsciousness.

Tissues must resist the G force produced by gravity and other mechanisms of acceleration

Standing motionless on the earth's surface at sea level, we experience a gravitational force ($\mathcal{F}$)—our weight—that is the product of our mass and the acceleration due to gravity.

[†]Deceased.

A DIVING HELMET

B SCUBA SYSTEM

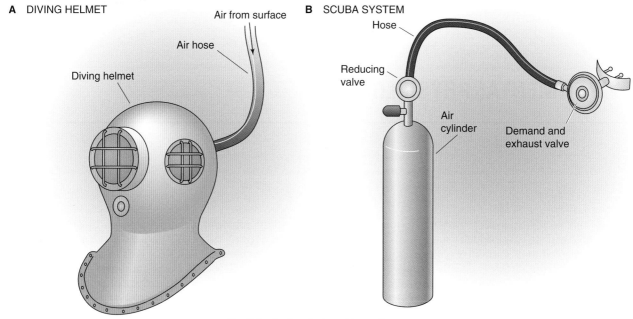

Fig. 61.1 Devices for breathing underwater.

Under a particular condition, we may experience a different acceleration from that due to gravity. The **G force** is a dimensionless number that describes force that we experience under a particular condition relative to the gravitational force. Thus, we normally experience a force of +1G that would cause us to fall with an acceleration of 9.8 m · s^{-2} if we were not supported in some way.

Accelerations besides that due to gravity also affect physiology. We can jump upward with an acceleration of ~3G and, upon landing, we strike the ground with a force of +3G.

With increasing age, bones tend to demineralize (see ⊙ 62-5) and weaken. Stepping off a curb, an elderly person with demineralized bones may fracture the neck of the femur or crush a vertebra.

The partial pressures of gases—other than water—inside the body depend on P$_B$

As discussed in the next two subchapters, extremely high or extremely low values of P$_B$ create special challenges for the physiology of the body. P$_B$ is the sum of the **partial pressures** of the individual gases in the air mixture (see Box 26.2). As P$_B$ increases during diving beneath the water, or as P$_B$ decreases during ascent to high altitude, the partial pressure of each constituent gas in dry ambient air (see Table 26.1)—aside from P$_{H_2O}$—changes in proportion to the change in P$_B$.

DIVING PHYSIOLOGY

Immersion raises P$_B$, thereby compressing gases in the lungs

The average P$_B$ at sea level is 760 mm Hg. When diving underwater, humans can experience extreme increases in P$_B$. A column of fresh water extending from the earth's surface upward 10.3 m exerts an additional pressure of 760 mm Hg. Because liquid water is virtually incompressible, P$_B$ increases linearly with the height (weight) of the column of water. Ten meters below the surface of the sea, P$_B$ is 2 atm, 1 atm for the atmospheric pressure plus 1 atm for the column of water. As the depth increases to 20 m and then to 30 m, P$_B$ increases to 3 atm, then 4 atm, and so on.

External pressure compresses each of the body's *air* compartments to an extent that depends on the compliance of the compartment. In compliant cavities such as the intestines, external pressure readily compresses internal gases. In relatively stiff cavities, or those that cannot equilibrate readily with external pressure, increases of external pressure can distort the cavity wall and result in pain or damage. For example, if the eustachian tube is blocked, the middle-ear pressure cannot equilibrate with external pressure, and blood fills the space in the middle ear or the tympanic membrane ruptures.

SCUBA divers breathe compressed air to maintain normal lung expansion

Divers first wore diving suits with spherical helmets over their heads (Fig. 61.1A). The air inside these helmets was pressurized to match exactly the pressure of the water in which they were diving. Jacques Cousteau perfected the *self-contained underwater breathing apparatus*, or **SCUBA,** that replaced cumbersome gear and increased the mobility and convenience of an underwater dive (Fig. 61.1B).

Increased alveolar P$_{N_2}$ can cause narcosis

Descending beneath the water causes the inspired P$_{N_2}$—nearly 600 mm Hg at sea level (see Table 26.1)—to increase as P$_B$ increases. According to **Henry's law** (see Box 26.2), the increased P$_{N_2}$ will cause more N$_2$ to dissolve in pulmonary-capillary blood and, eventually, the body's tissues. Because of its high lipid solubility, N$_2$ dissolves readily in adipocytes and in membrane lipids. A high P$_{N_2}$ reduces the ion conductance of membranes, and therefore neuronal excitability,

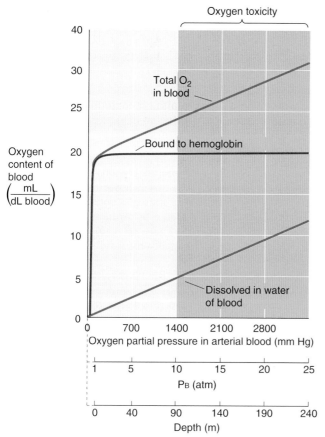

Fig. 61.2 O_2 content of blood at high pressures.

by mechanisms that are similar to those of gas anesthetics. Diving to increased depths (e.g., 4 to 5 atm) while breathing compressed air causes **nitrogen narcosis.**

Increased alveolar P_{O_2} can lead to O_2 toxicity

At sea level, dry inspired air has a P_{O_2} of 159 mm Hg. However, the *alveolar* P_{O_2} (PA_{O_2}) of a healthy person at sea-level air is ~101 mm Hg, reduced from 159 mm Hg by humidification in the airways and removal of O_2 by gas exchange with the blood. Arterial P_{O_2} (Pa_{O_2}) at sea level is very close to alveolar PA_{O_2} (within ~10 mm Hg) and nearly saturates Hb, to yield an arterial O_2 content of ~20 mL/dL blood (Fig. 61.2, *red curve*). As P_B—and therefore Pa_{O_2}—increases at greater depths, the O_2 bound to Hb increases very little. However, the O_2 that is physically dissolved in the water of blood increases linearly (Fig. 61.2, *black line*). Thus, the increment of total O_2 content at depth reflects dissolved O_2 (Fig. 61.2, *blue curve*).

During a breath-hold dive to 5 atm, or in a hyperbaric chamber pressurized to 5 atm, arterial P_{O_2} increases to ~700 mm Hg, slightly higher than when breathing 100% O_2 at sea level. Exposure to such a high P_{O_2} has no ill effects for up to several hours. However, prolonged exposure damages the airway epithelium and smooth muscle, causing bronchiolar and alveolar membrane inflammation and, ultimately, pulmonary edema, atelectasis, fibrin formation, and lung consolidation.

A prolonged elevation of P_{O_2} also has detrimental effects on nonpulmonary tissues, including the central nervous system (CNS). Exposure to an ambient P_{O_2} of ~1500 mm Hg

(e.g., breathing room air at ~10 atm) for as little as 30 to 45 minutes can cause seizures and coma. Preliminary symptoms of **O_2 toxicity** include muscle twitching, nausea, disorientation, and irritability.

After an extended dive, one must decompress slowly to avoid decompression illness

Although the preceding two sections have focused on problems divers face *while* at great depths, serious difficulties also arise if—*after* a prolonged, deep dive—the diver *returns* to the surface too quickly. At the end of such a dive, P_{N_2} is at the same high value in the alveoli and most tissues. As P_B falls during ascent, alveolar P_{N_2} will fall as well, which creates a P_{N_2} gradient from the mixed-venous blood to the alveolar air. Washout of N_2 from the blood creates a P_{N_2} gradient from tissues to blood. To allow enough time for the dissolved N_2 to move from tissues to blood to alveoli, a diver must rise to the surface slowly.

Too rapid an ascent causes the N_2 in the tissues—previously dissolved under high pressure—to leave solution and form bubbles as P_B falls.

During a too-rapid decompression, bubble formation can occur in any tissue in which N_2 has previously been dissolved. **Decompression illness (DCI)** is the general term for two major types of clinical disorder:
1. **Decompression sickness (DCS)** is caused by local bubble formation, either in tissues or in venous blood. In tissues, the distortion produced by these bubbles can affect function and cause itching or pain. In veins, the bubbles can cause obstruction, leading to capillary leaks.
2. **Arterial gas embolization (AGE)** is caused by bubbles that enter the systemic arterial blood via either tears in the alveoli or right-to-left shunts (e.g., a patent foramen ovale) and then become wedged in the brain or other organs.

The rate at which a diver should ascend to avoid DCI depends on both the depth and the duration of the dive. Divers use detailed tables to plan their rate of ascent from a deep dive.

The best treatment for DCI is to *recompress* the diver in a hyperbaric chamber. Recompression places the gases back under high pressure, forcing them to redissolve in the tissues, a process that instantly relieves many symptoms. Once the diver is placed under high pressure, decompression can be carried out at a deliberate and supervised pace.

HIGH-ALTITUDE PHYSIOLOGY

⊙ 61-1 P_B and ambient P_{O_2} on top of Mount Everest are approximately one third of their values at sea level

With increasing altitude, the number of gas molecules pressing down on a mountain climber falls exponentially; P_B falls by half for each ~5500 m of ascent.

Everest Base Camp At an altitude of 5500 m—which also happens to be the altitude of the first base camp used in most ascents of Mount Everest—P_B is half the value at sea level ($P_B \cong 380$ mm Hg), as is the ambient ($\cong 80$ mm Hg). At this altitude, arterial O_2 delivery (arterial blood O_2 content × cardiac output) can still meet O_2 demands in most healthy, active persons, even during mild physical activity.

Peak of Mount Everest   The peak of Mount Everest—8848 m above sea level—is the highest point on earth. P_B at the peak is ~255 mm Hg, approximately one third that at sea level, and the ambient P_{O_2} is only ~53 mm Hg. Hypoxia is thus a major problem at the summit of Mount Everest.

Air Travel   Pressurized cabins in passenger planes maintain an ambient pressure equivalent to ~1800 m of altitude (~79% of sea-level pressure) in cross-continental flights, or ~2400 m of altitude (~74% of sea-level pressure) in transoceanic flights. Most airline passengers are not bothered by the slight reduction in arterial O_2 saturation (89% saturation at 3000 m) associated with these airline cabin pressures. However, passengers with pulmonary disease may need to carry supplemental O_2 onto the plane even if they do not require it at sea level.

Up to modest altitudes, arterial O_2 content falls relatively less than P_B due to the shape of the Hb-O_2 dissociation curve

Although P_B and ambient P_{O_2} decrease by the same fraction with increasing altitude, the O_2 saturation of Hb in arterial blood decreases relatively little at altitudes up to ~3000 m. The reason is that at this altitude, arterial P_{O_2} is 60 to 70 mm Hg, which corresponds to the relatively flat portion of the O_2-Hb dissociation curve (see Fig. 29.2), so that arterial O_2 *content* is little affected. Thus, the characteristics of Hb protect the arterial O_2 content, despite modest reductions of P_{O_2}. At higher altitudes, where arterial O_2 content falls more steeply, aviators are advised to breathe supplemental O_2.

During the first few days at altitude, compensatory adjustments to hypoxemia include tachycardia and hyperventilation

A reduction in arterial P_{O_2} stimulates the peripheral chemoreceptors (see ⊙ 32-3) and causes an immediate increase in ventilation, which has two effects. First, it brings alveolar P_{O_2} (and thus arterial P_{O_2}) closer to the ambient P_{O_2}. Second, hyperventilation blows off CO_2, producing a respiratory alkalosis (see ⊙ 31-1) that inhibits the peripheral but especially the central chemoreceptors and thereby decreases ventilatory drive (see ⊙ 32-2). Thus, ventilation during an acute exposure to an altitude of 4500 m is only about twice that at sea level, whereas the hypoxia by itself would have produced a much larger stimulation. Accompanying the increased ventilatory drive during acute altitude exposure is an increase in heart rate, probably owing to the heightened sympathetic drive that accompanies acute hypoxemia (see ⊙ 23-16). The resultant increase in cardiac output enhances O_2 delivery.

During the next few days to weeks at an elevation of 4500 m, **acclimatization** causes ventilation to increase progressively by about the same amount as the acute response. As a result, P_{O_2} continues to rise, and P_{CO_2}, to fall. Two mechanisms appear to cause this slower phase of increased ventilation. First, the pH of the cerebrospinal fluid (CSF) decreases, which counteracts the respiratory alkalosis induced by the increase in ventilation and thus offsets the inhibition of central chemoreceptors. Second, the kidneys respond over a period of several days to the respiratory

alkalosis by decreasing their rate of acid secretion (see ⊙ 39-3) so that blood pH decreases toward normal (i.e., metabolic compensation for respiratory alkalosis). Another result of this compensation is that the unreabsorbed HCO_3^- produces an osmotic diuresis and an alkaline urine.

Long-term adaptations to altitude include increases in hematocrit, pulmonary diffusing capacity, capillarity, and oxidative enzymes

During prolonged residence at a high altitude, the reduced arterial P_{O_2} triggers profound adaptations that enhance O_2 delivery to tissues at a cost that is lower than that exacted by short-term compensatory strategies noted above. Many of these adaptations are mediated by an increase in **hypoxia-inducible factor 1 (HIF-1)** (see ⊙ 18-5), a transcription factor that activates genes involved in erythropoiesis, angiogenesis, and other processes.

Hematocrit   Red blood cell (RBC) mass slowly increases with prolonged hypoxemia. The Hb concentration of blood increases from a sea-level value of 14 to 15 g/dL to >18 g/dL, and hematocrit increases from 40% to 45% to >55%. Renal hypoxia and norepinephrine stimulate the production and release of **erythropoietin (EPO)** (see ⊙ 18-5), which stimulates production of proerythroblasts in bone marrow and also promotes accelerated development of RBCs from their progenitor cells.

Pulmonary Diffusing Capacity   Acclimatization to high altitude also causes a 2- to 3-fold increase in pulmonary diffusing capacity (see Equation 30.9) by at least four mechanisms: (1) a rise in the blood volume of pulmonary capillaries, (2) the associated increase in capillary surface area, (3) an increase in the depth of inspiration that increases surface area even further, and (4) right ventricular hypertrophy, which raises pulmonary arterial pressure, and raises perfusion to the upper regions of the lungs (see Fig. 31.5).

Capillary Density ⊙ 61-2   Hypoxia causes a dramatic increase in tissue vascularity. Tissue **angiogenesis** (see ⊙ 20-23) occurs within days of exposure to hypoxia, triggered by growth factors released by hypoxic tissues.

Oxidative Enzymes   Hypoxia promotes expression of oxidative enzymes in the mitochondria, thereby enhancing the tissues' ability to extract O_2 from the blood (see ⊙ 60-8).

High altitude causes mild symptoms in most people and acute or chronic mountain sickness in susceptible individuals

Symptoms of Hypoxia   A rapid ascent to high altitude may precipitate a constellation of relatively *mild symptoms*: drowsiness, fatigue, headache, nausea, and a gradual decline in cognition. These uncomfortable effects of acute hypoxia are progressive with increasing altitude. They occur in some people at altitudes as low as 2100 m and occur in most people at altitudes higher than 3500 m. Initially, these symptoms reflect an inadequate response (i.e., compensatory hyperventilation) to hypoxemia, which results in insufficient O_2 delivery to the brain. In the longer term, symptoms may stem from mild *cerebral edema*, which probably results from dilation of the cerebral arterioles leading to increased capillary filtration pressure and enhanced transudation (see ⊙ 20-12).

Acute Mountain Sickness Some people who ascend rapidly to altitudes as seemingly moderate as 3000 to 3500 m develop acute mountain sickness (AMS). The constellation of symptoms is more severe than those described in the previous paragraph and includes headache, fatigue, dizziness, dyspnea, sleep disturbance, peripheral edema, nausea, and vomiting. The symptoms usually develop within the first day and last for 3 to 5 days. The primary problem in AMS is hypoxia, and the symptoms probably have two causes. The first is thought to be a progressive, more severe case of **cerebral edema.** The second cause of the symptoms is **pulmonary edema,** which occurs as hypoxia leads to hypoxic pulmonary vasoconstriction (see ◉ 31-6), which in turn increases total pulmonary vascular resistance, pulmonary-capillary pressure, and transudation. Certain people have an exaggerated pulmonary vascular response to hypoxia, and they are especially susceptible to AMS. Cerebral or pulmonary edema can be fatal if the exposure to hypoxia is not rapidly reversed, first by providing supplemental O_2 to breathe and then by removing the individual from the high altitude.

Chronic Mountain Sickness After prolonged residence at high altitude, chronic mountain sickness may develop, due to an exaggerated production of RBCs. In such conditions, the hematocrit can exceed 60%—**polycythemia**—which dramatically increases blood viscosity and vascular resistance, and increases the risk of intravascular thrombosis. The combination of pulmonary hypoxic vasoconstriction and increased blood viscosity may eventually lead to *congestive heart failure* of the right ventricle.

FLIGHT AND SPACE PHYSIOLOGY

Acceleration in one direction shifts the blood volume in the opposite direction

Before liftoff, an astronaut experiences only the force of gravity, +1G. As a rocket blasts off from earth, the astronaut experiences higher G forces. Maximal G forces in the space shuttle were approximately +4G. Similarly, pilots of high-performance aircraft experience *positive* G forces as they pull out of a dive, and we all experience *negative* G forces when an aircraft hits turbulence, suddenly loses altitude, and lifts us out of our seats.

G forces propel the body's tissues in the direction opposite that of acceleration; these forces compress soft tissues against underlying structural elements (e.g., bone) or pull these tissues away from overlying structural elements. In addition, G forces tend to shift the blood volume away from the direction of acceleration, thereby adding to the other component forces that determine blood pressure (see ◉ 17-3).

In high-performance aircraft, the rapid motions associated with changes in flight direction or altitude produce G forces that can be considerable for several minutes, exceeding 8G. Even in relatively primitive aircraft, aerobatic maneuvers can shift blood volume away from the head, resulting in transient reductions in cerebral blood flow and O_2 delivery. If these reductions are sufficiently large, they can result in loss of consciousness. The early warnings of such an event are narrowing of the visual field (i.e., loss of peripheral vision) and loss of color perception as the retina is deprived of O_2, a phenomenon called **gray-out.** The term **blackout** describes a total loss of consciousness that occurs during acceleration that lasts for tens of seconds or minutes. Pilots of high-performance aircraft use G suits to provide counterpressure to the lower extremities. The counterpressure opposes the pooling of blood in the extremities and maintains sufficient cardiac filling, cardiac output, and blood flow to the brain, thereby reducing the tendency toward gray-out.

"Weightlessness" causes a cephalad shift of the blood volume and an increase in urine output

An astronaut in an orbiting spacecraft experiences "weightlessness," a state of near-zero G force, also called a **microgravity** environment because the centrifugal force of the spacecraft's orbital trajectory balances the earth's gravitational force. Thus, the astronaut has the sensation of weightlessness.

We are adapted to life at +1G, and arteriolar tone in the lower extremities prevents pooling of blood in the capacitance vessels, thereby ensuring adequate venous return to the right heart (see ◉ 25-1). The acute effects of microgravity on the circulatory system are exactly what one would expect for a system designed to oppose the effect of gravity in a standing person: blood volume redistributes toward the head. This cephalad shift of blood volume—away from the capacitance vessels of the legs—expands the **central blood volume,** increasing the cardiac preload and increasing the filtration of plasma water into the interstitium of the facial region. The resulting edema explains the dramatically bloated facial appearance of astronauts in microgravity within 24 hours of the launch.

Space flight leads to motion sickness and to decreases in muscle and bone mass

More than half of all astronauts experience motion sickness during the initial days of microgravity. **Motion sickness** (i.e., nausea and vomiting) results from conflicting sensory input to the brain regarding the position of the body. Nearly all cases of motion sickness resolve within the first 96 hours of microgravity exposure as the vestibular system or the CNS accommodates to the novel input.

Numerous other changes occur during prolonged residence in microgravity, many of which are related to the markedly diminished aerobic power output in space, where the force of gravity does not oppose muscle contraction. The major physiological alterations include reductions in body water content, plasma and RBC volume, muscle mass, and total-body calcium and phosphate (associated with a loss in bone mass). The bone loss appears to be continuous during time in a weightless environment, whereas the other changes occur only during the first weeks in space.

Exercise partially overcomes the deconditioning of muscles during space flight

The intermittent loading of muscles, bone, and the cardiovascular system prevents—to some extent—the *deconditioning* effects of space flight on muscle mass and performance. Aerobic activity in space, the impact of the feet on a treadmill, and the generation of physiological transmural pressure gradients appear to be sufficient to simulate exercise at +1G. This regimen can reduce or even eliminate the deconditioning effects of space flight.

Return to earth requires special measures to maintain arterial blood pressure

The problems associated with re-entry reflect a return to full gravity on earth's surface. The most dramatic effects result from reduced blood volume and decreased tone of the leg vessels. Both factors contribute to reductions in cardiac preload, orthostatic tolerance, and exercise capacity.

Astronauts employ various strategies just before re-entry to counter the adaptations to microgravity. The countermeasure to orthostatic intolerance is restoration of blood volume before re-entry. One means of attenuating the reduction of blood volume in space flight is an exercise program. Even a brief period (e.g., 30 minutes) of intense exercise expands plasma albumin content (see ◉ 60-7), increasing plasma oncotic pressure and plasma volume by 10% within 24 hours. Astronauts are maintained under continuous observation after re-entry until they have regained a normal orthostatic response. This usually occurs within hours, and certainly within 1 day, of re-entry.

CHAPTER 62

THE PHYSIOLOGY OF AGING

Edward J. Masoro[†]

Biomedical science paid surprisingly little attention to a remarkable change in human biology during the 20th century—the marked increase of human **life expectancy** in developed nations. Life expectancy is the projected mean length of life of those born in a given calendar year (e.g., 1990)—or those of a particular age (e.g., 30 years)—computed from the mortality characteristics of the entire population in a particular year (e.g., 2020). In the United States, life expectancy for men progressively increased from 47.9 years in 1900 to 76.4 years in 2012, and for women, from 50.7 years in 1900 to 81.2 years in 2012.

CONCEPTS IN AGING

During the 20th century, the age structure of populations in developed nations shifted toward older individuals

The fraction of the U.S. population ≥65 years of age was only 4% in 1900 but 12.4% in 2000. This trend in age structure is projected to continue. Moreover, because women have a greater life expectancy, they comprised 70.5% of the population >80 years of age in 1990 in developed nations.

The definition, occurrence, and measurement of aging are fundamental but controversial issues

The **age** of an organism usually refers to the length of time the individual has existed. Biogerontologists and members of the general public alike usually use aging to mean the process of **senescence.** For example, we may say that a person is young for her age, an expression meaning that the processes of senescence appear to be occurring slowly in that person. **Aging**—the synonym for senescence that we use throughout this chapter— *is the progressive deteriorative changes during the adult period of life that underlie an increasing vulnerability to challenges and thereby decrease the ability of the organism to survive.*

Biogerontologists distinguish **biological age** from **chronological age.** Although we easily recognize the biological aging of family members, friends, and pets, it would be helpful to have a quantitative measure of the rate of aging of an *individual.* **Biomarkers of aging**—morphological and functional changes that occur with time in the adult organism—could in principle serve as a measure of senescent deterioration. Alas, a generally agreed-on panel of biomarkers of aging has yet to emerge, so it is currently impossible to quantitate the aging of individuals.

Although measuring the aging of *individuals* is difficult, it has long been possible to measure the rate of aging of *populations.* The human **age-specific death rate** is the fraction of the population entering an age interval (e.g., 60 to 61 years of age) that dies during the age interval. After early adulthood, the age-specific death rate increases exponentially with increasing adult age.

Aging is an evolved trait

The current view is that aging evolved by default as the result of the absence of **forces of natural selection** that might otherwise eliminate mutations that promote senescence. For example, consider a cohort of a species that reaches reproductive maturity at age X. At that age, all members of the cohort will be involved in generating progeny. Furthermore, assume that this species is evolving in a hostile environment—the case for most species. As the age of this cohort increases past X, fewer and fewer members survive so that all members of the cohort die before exhibiting senescence. In this cohort, genes with detrimental actions expressed only at advanced ages would not be subjected to natural selection. If we now move the progeny of our cohort to a highly protective environment, many may well live to ages at which the deleterious genes can express their effects, thereby giving rise to the **aging phenotype.**

Human aging studies can be cross-sectional or longitudinal

Measuring the effects of aging on the human physiology presents investigators with a difficulty—the subjects' life span is longer than the investigator's scientific life span.

Cross-Sectional Design The usual approach to the foregoing difficulty is a cross-sectional design in which investigators study cohorts with several different age ranges (e.g., 20- to 29-year-olds, 30- to 39-year-olds) over a brief period (e.g., a calendar year). However, this design suffers from two serious potential confounders. One is the **cohort effect;** that is, different cohorts have had different environmental experiences. For example, in studies of the effects of aging on cognition, a confounding factor could be that younger cohorts have had the benefit of a relatively higher level of education. If aware of a potential confounder, the investigator may be able to modify the study's design to avoid the confounder.

[†]Deceased.

The second potential confounder is **selective mortality**—individuals with risk factors for diseases that cause death at a relatively young age are underrepresented in older age groups. For example, in a study on the effect of age on plasma lipoproteins, mortality at a young age from cardiovascular disease would preferentially eliminate individuals with the highest low-density lipoprotein levels.

Longitudinal Design To circumvent the confounders encountered in cross-sectional designs, investigators can repeatedly study a subject over a significant portion of his or her lifetime. However, this longitudinal design has other problems. Long-term longitudinal studies require a special organizational structure that can outlive an individual investigator and ensure completion of the study. Even shorter longitudinal studies are very costly. Some problems are inherent in the time course of longitudinal studies, including the effect of repeated measurements on the function being assessed, changes in subjects' lifestyle (e.g., diet), dropout of subjects from the study, and changes in professional personnel and technology.

Whether age-associated diseases are an integral part of aging remains controversial

Age-associated diseases are those that do not cause morbidity or mortality until advanced ages. Examples are coronary artery disease, stroke, many cancers, type 2 diabetes, osteoarthritis, osteoporosis, cataracts, Alzheimer disease, and Parkinson disease. These are either chronic diseases or acute diseases that result from long-term processes (e.g., atherogenesis).

Most gerontologists have held the view that age-associated diseases are *not* an integral part of aging. These gerontologists developed the concept of primary and secondary aging to explain why age-associated diseases occur in almost all elderly people. **Primary aging** refers to *intrinsic* changes occurring with age, unrelated to disease or environmental influences. **Secondary aging** refers to changes caused by the interaction of primary aging with environmental influences or disease processes.

CELLULAR AND MOLECULAR MECHANISMS OF AGING

In this subchapter, we consider three major classes of cellular and molecular processes that may be proximate causes of organismic aging: (1) damage caused by oxidative stress and other factors, (2) inadequate repair of damage, and (3) dysregulation of cell number. No one of these is *the* underlying mechanism of aging. Following development is a brief adult period when damage and repair are in balance, and then begins a long-term imbalance in favor of damage.

Oxidative stress and related processes that damage macromolecules may have a causal role in aging

Reactive Oxygen Species ⊙ **62-1** As illustrated in Fig. 62.1A, **reactive oxygen species (ROS)** include molecules such as **hydrogen peroxide (H_2O_2),** neutral free radicals such as the **hydroxyl radical (•OH),** and anionic radicals such as the

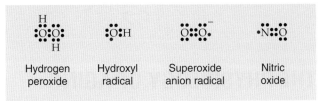

A   STRUCTURES

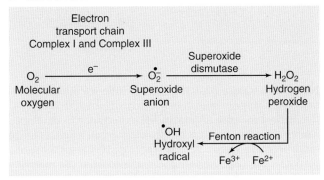

B   MITOCHONDRIAL GENERATION OF ROS

Fig. 62.1   Reactive oxygen species.

superoxide anion radical (O_2^-). Free radicals have an unpaired electron in the outer orbital, shown in *red* in Fig. 62.1A. These free radicals are extremely unstable because they react with target molecules. The target molecule left behind becomes a free radical, which initiates a chain reaction that continues until two free radicals meet to create a product with a covalent bond. ROS—particularly •OH, which is the most reactive of them all—have the potential to damage important biological molecules, such as proteins, lipids, and DNA.

⊙ **62-2** Quantitatively, the most important source of ROS is the mitochondrial electron transport chain. The enzyme **superoxide dismutase (SOD)** converts O_2^- to hydrogen peroxide, which in turn can yield the highly reactive •OH.

Only a small fraction of the oxygen used in aerobic metabolism (<1%) generates ROS. However, even that amount would be lethal in the absence of protective mechanisms. Fortunately, organisms have two potent antioxidant defenses. The major defense is enzymatic, specifically SODs, catalase, and glutathione peroxidase (Fig. 62.2). In addition, low-molecular-weight antioxidants, such as vitamins C and E, play a minor role in the defense against the metabolically produced radicals.

Because these antioxidant defense mechanisms are not fully protective, the dominant concept of the **oxidative stress theory of aging** is that an imbalance between the production and removal of ROS by antioxidant defenses is the major cause of aging.

Glycation and Glycoxidation ⊙ **62-3 Glycation** refers to nonenzymatic reactions between the carbonyl groups of reducing sugars (e.g., glucose) and the amino groups of macromolecules (e.g., proteins, DNA) to form **advanced glycation end products (AGEs).**

⊙ **62-4** The formation of AGEs is especially important for long-lived proteins and appears to play a role in the long-term complications of diabetes. The similarity between the aging phenotype and that of the patient with diabetes led to

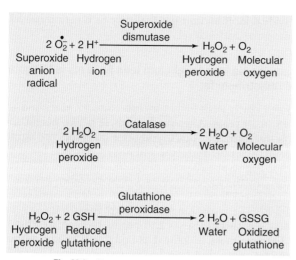

Fig. 62.2 Enzymatic defenses against ROS.

the **glycation hypothesis of aging.** The level of **glycemia** is a major factor in glycation, and periods of hyperglycemia contribute to enhanced glycation of proteins—including hemoglobin—in patients with diabetes. Proteins containing AGEs exhibit altered structural and functional properties. For example, AGE formation in lens proteins of the eye probably contributes to age-associated opacification.

Mitochondrial Damage Because mitochondria are the major *source* of ROS, they are also likely to be a major *target* of oxidative damage. Damage to mitochondrial DNA (mtDNA) increases greatly with age because, unlike genomic DNA, mtDNA is not protected by histones. According to the **mitochondrial theory of aging,** the damage to mtDNA results in the loss of cell function and hence aging.

Somatic Mutations Damage to genomic and mitochondrial DNA can occur as the result of radiation and other environmental agents, such as toxic chemicals. In recent years, oxidative stress has been recognized as a major source of DNA damage. Cells can repair much of the damage to DNA, and the level of damage is in a steady state between damaging and repair processes. According to the **DNA damage theory of aging,** accumulated DNA damage interferes with DNA replication and transcription, thereby impairing the ability of cells to function and causing aging.

Inadequacy of repair processes may contribute to the aging phenotype

Many biogerontologists believe that even more important than damage per se is the progressive age-associated loss in the ability to repair such damage.

DNA Repair The **DNA repair theory of aging** proposes that DNA repair declines with advancing age, which causes a rise in the steady-state level of damaged DNA and thereby compromises the integrity of the genome.

Protein Homeostasis Besides oxidative stress and nonenzymatic glycation, deamidation, racemization, and isomerization may lead to deterioration of proteins. Protecting the organism from an excessive accumulation of altered proteins are proteolytic degradation and replacement—**protein turnover.**

The rate of total-body protein turnover in humans decreases with age. Thus, the average lifetime of most but not all protein species increases with age. Long-lived proteins in the extracellular matrix, particularly collagen and elastin, undergo age-associated changes such as oxidation, glycation, and cross-linking.

Autophagy Degradation of cellular components by the lysosomes is referred to as autophagy, of which there are three types.

Macroautophagy involves the sequestering of proteins and other cytosolic components inside double-membrane vesicles called autophagosomes, the outer membrane of which fuses with a lysosome. The lysosomal enzymes degrade the cytosolic cargo.

In **microautophagy,** the lysosome membrane engulfs single damaged cytosolic molecules, exposing them to the lysosomal enzymes.

In **chaperone-mediated autophagy,** a complex of a damaged cytosolic protein and a chaperone traffics and then binds to a receptor on the lysosomal membrane. Lysosomal machinery then unfolds the protein and translocates it into the lysosome.

With increasing age, lysosomes in most tissues undergo marked changes, including an expansion of the lysosomal compartment, changes in lysosomal enzyme activities, and the accumulation of undegraded lysosomal products in the form of lipofuscin. A loss of lysosomal function adversely affects all three types of autophagy.

Dysfunction of the homeostasis of cell number may be a major factor in aging

For most cell types, the total number of cells remains nearly constant over much of adult life. An imbalance in favor of *cell division* results in hyperplasia, such as occurs in the prostates of elderly men, or in neoplasia (i.e., formation of new, abnormal cells), a disease process that also increases in frequency with age. An imbalance in favor of *cell removal* results in a reduction of cell number, such as occurs with age in some skeletal muscles. Of course, in cell types that are truly postmitotic in adult life, any age-associated loss of cells results in a decrease in number.

Limitations in Cell Division Human fibroblasts in culture divide only a limited number of times, a phenomenon known as the **Hayflick limit** that also applies to many other somatic cell types in culture. The intensive study of the Hayflick limit led to consideration of the role of telomeres in aging.

Telomeres are elements at the ends of linear chromosomes and are composed of repeated specific DNA sequences and associated proteins. The telomeres of human cells in culture shorten with each mitotic division. When the telomeres shorten to a critical length, the cell can no longer divide—a probable basis of the Hayflick limit.

Are the telomere findings in culture systems relevant to organismic senescence? A reduction in telomere length could play a role in cell types that exhibit an age-associated decrease in cell number. Clearly, a reduction in telomere length cannot be a factor in the aging of cells that are truly postmitotic during adult life. Telomeres do not shorten in the germline, which, unlike somatic cells, contains significant levels of **telomerase,** an enzyme that catalyzes the extension of telomere length. Cancer cells are also rich in telomerase.

Cell Removal Necrosis, apoptosis, and necroptosis are major processes by which the body loses cells. **Necrosis,** a cellular response to severe trauma, is manifested by uncontrolled breakdown of cellular structure, cell lysis, and an inflammatory response. The morphological characteristics of necrosis are cell swelling and loss of membrane integrity.

Apoptosis is a form of programmed cell death. It plays a key role in organogenesis and tissue renewal, and it also occurs in response to relatively mild damage. Apoptosis requires ATP, is gene driven, and is characterized by preservation of organelles, maintenance of membrane integrity, absence of inflammation, cell shrinkage, and fragmentation of the cell into multiple membrane-enclosed apoptotic bodies. Macrophages or neighboring cells remove the apoptotic bodies by phagocytosis.

Dysregulation of apoptosis promotes aging. For example, failure of apoptosis to remove damaged cells could result in abnormal function or increase the risk of cancer.

Necroptosis is a second important mode of regulated cell death. Like apoptosis, necroptosis involves a highly orchestrated sequence of intracellular signaling reactions. Notably, necroptosis is activated in response to many of the same microbial or environmental stresses that trigger apoptosis. In cells in which the stress or infectious stimuli suppress initiator caspases or executioner caspases, the cells activate the necroptotic cascade as an alternative to apoptosis. Indeed, some microbial pathogens express potent inhibitors of host cell caspases, which allows the pathogens to establish protected replicative niches within infected host cells. Engagement of the necroptosis pathway facilitates death of the infected host cells with consequent release of the internalized pathogens into extracellular compartments, where multiple innate immune mechanisms more readily destroy the pathogens. These mechanisms include complement-mediated cytolysis and neutrophil-mediated production of reactive oxygen and nitrogen species. Ischemia-reperfusion injury of organs such as the brain, kidney, and liver may trigger necroptosis and thus cell death.

AGING OF HUMAN PHYSIOLOGICAL SYSTEMS

The age-related changes just described at the cellular and molecular levels can also manifest themselves as deterioration of physiological systems. Although here we discuss *typical* age-related changes in physiological systems, the extent of change among individuals may range from barely perceptible to very marked. Indeed, a subset of individuals shows minimal physiological deterioration—these people have undergone "successful" aging. Many individuals show marked deterioration with age in all physiological systems, whereas other individuals exhibit little or no deterioration in one or more systems. Although the nature of the aging process is similar in the two sexes—except, of course, for the reproductive system—important quantitative differences exist. Because of the great reserve capacity or redundancy of some physiological systems, the effect of aging on a physiological process is often not apparent until either the individual faces an unusual challenge or function has fallen below some critical level.

Aging people lose height and lean body mass but gain and redistribute fat

Women reach peak height by age 16 to 17 years and men by 18 to 19 years. After reaching these peaks, height starts to decline, primarily due to compression of the cartilaginous disks between the vertebrae and loss of vertebral bone. This decline begins at ~20 years of age in women and at 25 years in men. By the age of 70 years, height has fallen 2.5% to 5% from the peak level.

⊙ **62-5** In most Americans, **body mass** increases until middle age in both sexes and begins to decrease after age 70. **Fat-free mass** is defined as body mass minus **adipose-tissue fat mass,** and **lean body mass** is defined as fat-free mass minus both bone mass and non–adipose-tissue fat mass. Both fat-free mass and lean body mass progressively decrease over most of adult life in both sexes.

Adipose-tissue fat mass increases with adult age, with the extent differing markedly among individuals. Although a sedentary lifestyle may be a factor, even physically fit individuals who do not exhibit an age-associated increase in body mass show a small but progressive increase in adipose-tissue fat mass (in parallel with the aforementioned decrease in fat-free body mass). In addition, the distribution of body fat changes with increasing age, with an accumulation of fat around abdominal viscera and in abdominal subcutaneous tissue. At the same time, a decrease in fat occurs in the extremities and the face; facial fat loss can give rise to a gaunt look. Visceral adipose tissue is an important source of cytokines (often referred to as adipokines) that promote inflammation, which in turn may play a role in the occurrence and progression of senescence.

Aging thins the skin and causes the musculoskeletal system to become weak, brittle, and stiff

Skin Intrinsic aging is manifest in skin areas protected from the sun, such as the buttocks. The additional damage caused by long-term exposure to the sun's ultraviolet radiation is called *photoaging*.

In intrinsic aging, the thickness of the **epidermis** decreases slightly, with no change in the outermost epidermal layer, the stratum corneum. The rate of generation of keratinocytes slows with age. The decreasing number of melanocytes reduces photoprotection, and the decreasing number of Langerhans cells reduces immune surveillance.

Intrinsic aging of the **dermis** affects mainly the extracellular matrix. The amount of elastin and collagen decreases, and their structures change. Glycosaminoglycan composition also changes. As a result, the dermis thins by ~20% and becomes stiffer, less malleable, and thus more vulnerable to injury.

Photoaging increases the extent of most intrinsic age changes in both the epidermis and dermis, and has additional effects, such as coarse wrinkles.

Aging also reduces the number and function of sweat glands as well as the production of sebum by sebaceous glands. The number of active melanocytes in hair follicles decreases, resulting in graying of hair. Nail growth also slows with increasing age.

Skeletal Muscle A steady loss in skeletal muscle mass—**sarcopenia**—occurs with aging, particularly beyond 50 years, and it primarily reflects a loss of number and, to a lesser extent, size of muscle fibers. The sarcopenia is due in part to inactivity, but also to a progressive loss of the motor neurons innervating type II motor units, which are recruited less frequently. The reduction in muscle strength and power is often a major cause of disability in the elderly. However, strength training in elderly persons can increase the *size* of the fibers and can thereby increase muscle mass.

Bone ⊙ **62-6** Remodeling of bone (see ⊙ **52-3**) occurs throughout adult life. During early adulthood, bone resorption and formation are in balance. However, starting late in the third decade of life, resorption exceeds formation, which leads to a slow progressive loss in bone mass. This loss is likely due to the action on **osteoblasts** of ROS, decreased insulin-like growth factor 1 (IGF-1), and increased parathyroid hormone. In women, bone loss accelerates for 5 to 10 years following menopause because of decreased levels of estrogen and increased levels of follicle-stimulating hormone (FSH). After this postmenopausal period, the rate of bone loss with increasing age in women returns to that of men. Bone loss can progress to **osteoporosis**, which is a major problem in geriatric medicine because of a heightened risk of bone fractures.

Synovial Joints With increasing adult age, joint flexibility falls, due mainly to the aging of **articular cartilage,** which thins and exhibits decreased tensile stiffness, fatigue resistance, and strength. These changes are partly due to decreases in water content. Aging impairs the function of **chondrocytes,** increases the cross-linking of collagen, and causes a loss of proteoglycans. The age-related changes in joint cartilage undoubtedly play a major role in the development of **osteoarthritis.**

The healthy elderly experience deficits in sensory transduction and speed of central processing

It is a common misconception that advancing age causes marked deterioration in the nervous system. However, in the absence of neurodegenerative disorders such as Alzheimer disease and Parkinson disease, impairment of the nervous system with age is much less severe than often believed.

Sensory Functions ⊙ **62-7** Most sensory systems exhibit some deterioration with age. Sensitivity to **touch** decreases, as do the abilities to sense vibration and to distinguish two spatially distinct points of contact. Proprioception, including the vestibular system of the inner ear, also deteriorates somewhat. The decrease of thermoregulatory ability, a serious problem for many elderly, occurs in part because of an impaired ability to sense heat and cold.

Hearing loss, particularly of high-frequency sound, is an almost invariable consequence of advancing age. This impairment is usually caused by loss of hair cells of the organ of Corti (see Fig. 15.16), but it can also stem from loss of nerve cells of the auditory nerve or from a reduced blood supply to the cochlea. A deficit in central processing can make it difficult for some elderly to distinguish spoken words from background noise.

Vision also deteriorates with increasing age. A progressive loss in the power of accommodation—**presbyopia**—occurs during adult life (see ⊙ **15-4**). Almost all elderly have a reduced number of retinal cones, lessened ability to alter pupil size in response to light intensity, and decreased ability of retinal rods to adapt to low intensity light (see ⊙ **15-7**). In addition, age-associated diseases—cataracts, glaucoma, and macular degeneration—can markedly decrease vision in many of the elderly.

The ability to detect and discriminate among sweet, sour, salty, and bitter **taste** qualities (see ⊙ **15-3**) deteriorates somewhat at advanced ages, along with a marked reduction in **olfaction** (see ⊙ **15-2**). Because "taste" involves both gustation and olfaction, many elderly live in a world of "pastel" food flavors.

Motor Functions A major effect of aging is the slowing of **reaction time:** the time elapsed between the occurrence of a stimulus and the motor response to it. This delay is observable in simple responses and becomes more pronounced as the complexity of the response increases (e.g., the need to make a choice among responses). Thus, a hallmark of nervous system aging is the slowing of **central processing.** One result is that the elderly tend to execute movements more slowly than the young.

The ability to maintain posture and balance deteriorates with increasing age. Slowing of central processing is a factor, but decreased muscle strength and deterioration of vision and proprioception also play important roles. Not surprisingly, the elderly have a high incidence of falls. Even when *capable* of walking at normal speeds, the healthy elderly *tend* to walk more slowly than the young and take shorter and more frequent steps. This walking pattern is less taxing for a person with knee and ankle joints that are less flexible, aids in maintaining balance, and enables a deteriorating sensory system to monitor hazards more effectively.

Cognitive Functions Although lay people generally believe that cognitive functions (e.g., intelligence, memory, learning) decline with advancing age, the cognitive decline is not marked in the absence of dementia. The decline that does occur in the healthy elderly may reflect the slowing of central processing. The capacity to use knowledge is not decreased in the healthy aged, but the ability to solve novel problems does decline. Certain types of memory deteriorate with advancing age, such as remembering where the car keys were left, but other types are not lost, such as retrieving conceptual information. Older people learn less quickly than younger people.

Aging causes decreased arterial compliance and increased ventilation-perfusion mismatching

In the absence of chronic cardiovascular or pulmonary disease, age-associated changes in these physiological systems are modest.

Cardiovascular Function Aging decreases the distensibility of arteries (see ⊙ **19-10**). The decreased compliance elevates systolic pressure, slightly decreases diastolic pressure, and thus widens pulse pressure. Afterload (see ⊙ **22-5**), the resistance to ejection of blood from the left ventricle, increases with advancing age, primarily because of reduced arterial compliance. The increased afterload causes thickening of the left ventricular wall, which involves an increase in size but not number of myocytes.

Many elderly experience postural hypotension (see ⊙ 25-2) because of age-associated blunting of the arterial baroreceptor reflex.

Pulmonary Function The strength and endurance of the respiratory muscles decrease with age. Lung volumes—both static volumes and forced expiratory volumes (e.g., FEV_1; see ⊙ 26-6) gradually decrease with age. In addition, small airways have an increased tendency to collapse (atelectasis) because of degeneration of the collagen and elastin support structure. The result is impaired ventilation of dependent lung regions, ventilation-perfusion mismatch, and reduced resting arterial P_{O_2}. In spite of these functional deteriorations, healthy elderly people do not experience a failure of either ventilation or gas exchange.

Exercise Maximal O_2 uptake ($\dot{V}_{O_2\,max}$; see Fig. 60.4) declines progressively with aging in physically trained individuals and even more so in untrained individuals of the same chronological age. Decreasing muscle mass as well as reduced cardiovascular and pulmonary function are probably all contributing factors.

The cardiovascular system responds to exercise differently in the elderly than in the young. For a given increase in cardiac output, heart rate rises less and stroke volume rises more in the elderly. Because the aging heart is less responsive to adrenergic stimulation, the increase in stroke volume is due primarily to the Frank-Starling mechanism (see ⊙ 22-4). Thus, during exercise, the left ventricular end-diastolic and end-systolic volumes increase, and maximal left ventricular ejection fraction falls.

The elderly exhibit a decrease in the pulmonary diffusing capacity (D_L)—due in part to decreased alveolar capillary volume—and an increase in the ventilation-perfusion mismatch. These alterations in pulmonary function have been implicated in the decrease in $\dot{V}_{O_2\,max}$.

Glomerular filtration rate falls with age in many but not all people

On average, renal blood flow decreases progressively with increasing age. Basal levels of renin and angiotensin II are lower in older adults. *Cross-sectional* studies show that glomerular filtration rate (GFR) starts to decline at 30 years of age and thereafter falls linearly with age. However, analysis of *longitudinal* data reveals that one third of the participants exhibited the GFR decline predicted from cross-sectional analysis, one third had a steeper decline, and one third had no decline at all. Thus, an age-associated decline in GFR is not inevitable.

Cross-sectional studies indicate that renal-tubule transport functions decrease with age. The kidneys do not respond as effectively to changes in sodium load, do not dilute or concentrate urine as effectively, and also have a somewhat impaired ability to excrete potassium, phosphate, and acid.

Many elderly men and women experience bladder symptoms. The capacity and compliance of the urinary bladder decrease with advancing age, and the number of uninhibited or inappropriate detrusor contractions increases. These changes make it more difficult to postpone voiding, a symptom known as **urgency.** A decrease in detrusor activity can contribute to a decreased rate of bladder emptying as well as an increase in residual bladder volume after voiding—poor emptying performance, which contributes to **nocturia** and **urinary frequency.**

Aging has only minor effects on gastrointestinal function

The gastrointestinal (GI) system functions in the healthy elderly about as well as in the young. A decreased ability to secrete gastric acid is limited to those infected with *Helicobacter pylori*. The loss of skeletal muscle at both ends of the GI tract can lead to minor age-related decreases in function (i.e., chewing, swallowing, fecal continence).

Aging causes modest declines in most endocrine functions

Total energy expenditure decreases with age, primarily due to decreases in physical activity. An age-associated decrease in the **resting metabolic rate** (**RMR;** see ⊙ 58-1) reflects a decrease in fat-free mass (see ⊙ 62-5); that is, the RMR per kilogram of fat-free mass does not decrease.

Insulin The impaired **glucose tolerance** (see Fig. 51.1) that usually occurs with aging is due primarily to increased **insulin resistance,** which in turn results mainly from increased adiposity and decreased physical activity. In addition, the elderly exhibit an age-associated decrease in insulin secretion that does not appear to be due to the lifestyle factors underlying insulin resistance.

Growth Hormone and Insulin-Like Growth Factor 1 Aging diminishes levels of growth hormone (GH) and, as a consequence, greatly reduces plasma IGF-1 levels (see ⊙ 48-7).

Adrenal Steroids The basal, circadian, and stimulated secretion of **cortisol** exhibits little age-related change. **Aldosterone** secretion is also well preserved. In contrast, the plasma concentration of the adrenal cortical hormone **dehydroepiandrosterone** (see Fig. 54.4) decreases markedly with increasing age.

Thyroid Hormones Thyroid function appears to be unaffected by age into the ninth decade of life.

Parathyroid Hormone Plasma **parathyroid** hormone levels increase with advancing age due to an increase in the rate of secretion by the parathyroid glands.

Gonadal Hormones Reproductive ability in women abruptly ceases at ~50 years of age with the occurrence of the **menopause** (see ⊙ 55-8). Men do not undergo an abrupt change in reproductive function during middle age. However, a progressive decrease in male reproductive and related functions does occur, often referred to as the **andropause.**

AGING SLOWLY

Slowing the aging process, and thereby extending life, has been a human goal throughout recorded history and probably in preliterate times as well. The marked increase in human life expectancy in the 20th century could be viewed as achieving this goal. However, much of that increase results from prevention of premature deaths related to infections and other environmental hazards. Over the centuries, the life span of the oldest of the old in human populations has

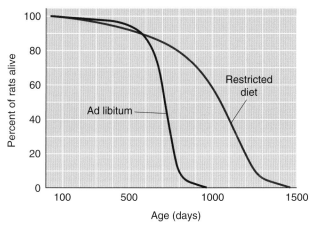

Fig. 62.3 Survival curves for a population of 115 male F344 rats fed ad libitum and 115 male F344 rats with restricted food intake (i.e., 60% of the ad libitum intake) starting at 6 weeks of age. Data from Yu BP, Masoro EJ, Murata I, et al: Life span of SPF Fischer 344 male rats fed ad libitum or restricted diets: Longevity, growth, lean body mass, and disease. J Gerontol 37:130–141, 1982. Copyright The Gerontological Society of America. Reproduced by permission of the publisher.

changed little, although the fraction of the population reaching these advanced ages has increased significantly.

Caloric restriction slows aging and extends life in several species, including some mammals

Restricting the food intake of rats, starting soon after weaning, increases both mean and maximum life span of both genders of several strains of rats (Fig. 62.3). The effect results from caloric restriction rather from than a specific dietary component.

For two reasons, most biogerontologists believe that food restriction retards aging processes. First, compared to rodents of the same age fed ad libitum, those on life-extending food-restriction regimens maintain physiological processes more like those of young animals. Second, life-extending food restriction delays the onset or progression of most age-associated diseases, including neoplastic, degenerative, and immune diseases.

The most popular view is that food restriction extends life by decreasing oxidative stress (see ◉ 62-1). Indeed, life-extending food restriction does decrease the accumulation of age-associated oxidative damage. It also causes a sustained reduction in plasma glucose levels, which could reduce glycation and glycoxidation (see ◉ 62-3), as well as a marked and sustained reduction in plasma levels of insulin and IGF-1. Genetic studies strongly indicate that decreasing insulin-like signaling (see ◉ 48-8 and ◉ 51-6) extends life. Thus, the decrease in the levels of insulin and IGF-1 may well play an important role in food restriction–induced life extension.

Inhibiting the mTOR pathway (see Fig. 51.3) by administering rapamycin extends the life of 600-day-old mice. Because the mTOR pathway senses nutrient status, it is possible that inhibiting the TOR pathway has a role in caloric restriction–induced life extension.

Another theory of the antiaging action of caloric restriction is **hormesis**—the beneficial effects resulting from cellular responses to mild repeated stress—would stimulate maintenance and repair processes and thereby retard aging. Food restriction at the level that extends life is a mild stress repeated daily.

Genetic alterations can extend life in several species

Caloric restriction is an example of environmental factors that determine longevity. It is also clear that genetics has a major role. For example, the large differences in life span among species (from <100 days in *Drosophila melanogaster* to <5 years in mice to >100 years in humans) are primarily, if not exclusively, due to genetic differences. Moreover, selective breeding within a species can produce populations that differ significantly in longevity.

Longevity probably depends on multiple genes. Among single-gene manipulations found to extend the life of *Caenorhabditis elegans*, *D. melanogaster*, *Saccharomyces cerevisiae*, and mice, many but not all involve a partial loss of function of the insulin-like signaling pathway.

Ames dwarf mice have a recessive point mutation in the *Prop-1* gene. Mice homozygous for the mutation have low levels of thyroid hormone, IGF-1 (see ◉ 48-8), and insulin and have an increased life span.

Further support for a role of reduced insulin-like signaling in life extension comes from studies of mice with a knockout of the *GHR/BP* gene, which encodes the GH receptor and its proteolytic cleavage product, GH-binding protein. This knockout mouse exhibits growth retardation, high plasma GH levels, low plasma IGF-1 levels, and significant life extension. Finally, overexpression of the KL gene in mice increases plasma levels of **Klotho** protein, which suppresses insulin and IGF-1 signaling and extends the life of mice.

Proposed interventions to slow aging and extend human life are controversial

The practice of **antiaging medicine** is becoming popular and plays an important role in preventing the occurrence and progression of certain age-associated diseases. For example, exercise and diet can reduce the incidence of coronary heart disease, stroke, and type 2 diabetes. However, some practitioners of antiaging medicine, as well as suppliers of pharmaceuticals and nutraceuticals, claim to have "magic bullets" that slow or even reverse aging. These purported magic bullets include antioxidants (e.g., vitamins E and C), amino acids (e.g., methionine), drugs (e.g., deprenyl), and hormones (e.g., melatonin, dehydroepiandrosterone, GH, estrogen, and testosterone). No credible evidence indicates that any of these agents reverses or even slows human aging. Aside from the question of efficacy is the possibility of long-term adverse effects of these supposed magic bullets. Combined estrogen and progestin therapy is a case in point. Although hailed for relieving the symptoms of menopause, this hormone replacement therapy was long in use before a well-designed study uncovered its harmful effects on the cardiovascular system.

INDEX

A

A bands, 103–104
Abdominal muscles, 325
Absolute refractory period, 78, 80
Absorptagogues, 482–483
Absorption, 450, 476
Acclimatization, 4, 646
Accommodation, 171
ACE. *See* Angiotensin-converting enzyme
Acetyl coenzyme A (CoA) carboxylase 2 (ACC2), 552–553
Acetylcholine (ACh), 146, 162, 251–252, 453, 459, 459f, 467–468
  M_3 muscarinic receptors for, 462
Acetylcholinesterase (AChE), 91
  inhibitors of, 99
Acid challenge, 435
Acid loader, 344
Acid secretion, 458–462, 459f
  three phases of, 460–462
Acid-base balance, 435–438, 436f
  maintenance of, 435–436
Acid-base disorders, 339t
Acid-base physiology, 336–345
  Davenport diagram, 338–343, 339t–340t, 340f–341f, 343f–344f
  pH and buffers, 336–338, 337t, 338f
Acid-base transport, 435–441
  at cellular and molecular levels, 438–440
  by different segments of nephron, 438
Acidemia, 421
Acidosis, 426
Acids, 336
  Hb-O_2 dissociation curve and, 349, 350f
  renal handling of, 435–438
  transport of, 435–441
Acinar cells, 466, 471
Acrosomal reaction, 596, 597f
ACTH. *See* Adrenocorticotropic hormone
Actin, 102–103
Actin cytoskeleton, 19
Action potentials, 62, 75–89, 101, 101f, 140, 140f, 453
  mechanisms of nerve and muscle, 75–80, 76f–80f
  propagation of, 86–89, 87f–88f
  of smooth muscles, 110, 111f
Activate protein kinase C, DAGs and, 27
Activation
  of egg cell, 596
  of platelets, 219
Active absorption, of bile acids, 506
Active labor stage, in parturition, 604
Active length-tension diagrams, 271

Active tension, 106
  elastic tension of vessels and, 232–233, 232f
Active transport, 6, 54
Active zones, of synaptic vesicles, 92, 97–98, 143
Activins, 587–588
Activity-related energy expenditure, 527
Acute acid load, 344
Acute mountain sickness, 647
Acute-phase response, fever and, 632
Adaptability, 4
Adenosine, 294
Adenosine triphosphate (ATP), 164
  depletion of, fatigue and, 637
  synthesis, 634–635, 635f
Adenylate kinase, 635
Adenylyl cyclase, 21, 24
  G proteins coupled to, 516–517
ADH. *See* Antidiuretic hormone
Adhering junctions, 16, 19
Adhesion, of platelets, 219
Adhesion molecules, 12
Adipocytes
  energy liberation and, 620
  insulin and, 554, 556f
Adipose tissue, energy capture, 619
Adipose triacylglycerol lipase (ATGL), 554
Adrenal androgens, 537
Adrenal cortex, 518, 537–541, 580
Adrenal gland, 537–546, 538f
Adrenal medulla, 305, 517, 537, 544–546
  in control of arterial pressure, 278–281, 280f
Adrenal steroids
  aging and, 654
  biosynthesis of, 539f
Adrenal zona fasciculata, 537–538
Adrenarche, 573–574
β adrenergic receptor kinase (β APK), 24
ß$_2$ adrenergic receptors, 462
α-adrenergic stimulation, 549
β-adrenergic stimulation, 549
Adrenoceptors, 518
Adrenocorticotropic hormone (ACTH), 538–539, 542–543
Adrenocorticotropic hormone receptor, 539–541
Adsorptive endocytosis, 503
Adult stem cells, 212
Affective states, modification by, 383
Afferent baroreceptor nerves
  increased arterial pressure and, 276, 277f
  medulla and, 276–277

Afferent nerves, 116
Afferent neural pathways, in neural reflex system, 275
Afferent neurons, 452–453
Afterhyperpolarization, 75
Afterload, 272
  end-systolic volume and, 284
ω-Agatoxin IVA, 84
Age, definition of, 649
Age-associated disease, 650
Age-specific death rate, 649
Aggregate resistance, 227
Aggregation, of platelets, 219
Aging
  biomarkers of, 649
  cellular and molecular mechanisms of, 650–652
  concepts of, 649–650
  disease and, 650
  distensibility of arteries and, 232, 232f
  glycation hypothesis of, 650–651
  of human physiological systems, 652–654
  oxidative stress theory of, 650
  phenotype, 649
  physiology of, 649–655
  slowly, 654–655
  studies for, 649–650
Agonists, 73
  of nicotinic AChR, 99
Air, composition of, 315t
Air pump, 317
Airflow, 330
  dilation and collapse of airways with, 335f
  redirection of, 372
Airway resistance, 331t, 332f
Akinase anchoring protein (AKAP), 24
Albumin, 212
Aldosterone, 410, 425, 474, 537, 541–544
  in disease, 543–544
  in K^+ secretion, 482
  role in normal physiology, 543
Aldosterone release, stimulation of, 445
Alkali, 336
All-trans retinal, 175
α cells, 547
Alternative 3' ends, 45
Alternative 3' splice sites, 44
Alternative 5' ends, 44
Alternative 5' splice sites, 44
Alternative splicing, 43–45, 45f
Alveolar air spaces, 319–320, 319f–321f
Alveolar dead space, 362–363

Note: Page numbers followed by *f* indicate figures, *t* indicate tables, and *b* indicate boxes.